CONTENTS

I WORKING IN LONG-TERM CARE SETTINGS
1 Working in Long-Term Care, 1
2 Resident Rights, 11
3 The Nursing Assistant in Long-Term Care, 19
4 Ethics and Laws, 32
5 Work Ethics, 44
6 Communicating With the Health Team, 59
7 Assisting With the Nursing Process, 74

II FOCUSING ON THE PERSON
8 Understanding the Resident, 82
9 Body Structure and Function, 97
10 The Older Person, 114
11 Sexuality, 128

III PROTECTING THE PERSON
12 Safety, 133
13 Preventing Falls, 156
14 Restraint Alternatives and Safe Restraint Use, 166
15 Preventing Infection, 182
16 Body Mechanics, 210
17 Safe Resident Handling, Moving, and Transfers, 219

IV ASSISTING WITH ACTIVITIES OF DAILY LIVING
18 The Resident's Unit, 252
19 Bedmaking, 265
20 Hygiene, 280
21 Grooming, 311
22 Urinary Elimination, 333
23 Bowel Elimination, 355
24 Nutrition and Fluids, 371
25 Nutritional Support and IV Therapy, 401
26 Exercise and Activity, 414
27 Comfort, Rest, and Sleep, 431
28 Oxygen Needs, 442
29 Respiratory Support and Therapies, 457
30 Assisted Living, 464

V ASSISTING WITH ASSESSMENT
31 Measuring Vital Signs, 473
32 Assisting With the Physical Examination, 496
33 Collecting and Testing Specimens, 502

VI ASSISTING WITH CARE NEEDS
34 Admissions, Transfers, and Discharges, 521
35 Wound Care, 535
36 Pressure Ulcers, 564
37 Hearing, Speech, and Vision Problems, 578
38 Cancer, Immune System, and Skin Disorders, 594
39 Nervous System and Musculo-Skeletal Disorders, 601
40 Cardiovascular and Respiratory Disorders, 617
41 Digestive and Endocrine Disorders, 625
42 Urinary and Reproductive Disorders, 634
43 Mental Health Problems, 642
44 Confusion and Dementia, 655
45 Developmental Disabilities, 673
46 Rehabilitation and Restorative Nursing Care, 682
47 Basic Emergency Care, 691
48 End-of-Life Care, 709

REVIEW QUESTION ANSWERS, 719

APPENDICES
A National Nurse Aide Assessment Program (NNAAP™) Written Examination Content Outline and Skills Evaluation, 722
B Minimum Data Set, 723
C Useful Spanish Vocabulary and Phrases, 756

GLOSSARY, 768

KEY ABBREVIATIONS, 777

INDEX, 779

evolve
learning system

To access your Student Resources, visit the web address below:

http://evolve.elsevier.com/Sorrentino/longterm/

Register today and gain access to:

- **Video Clips**
  Demonstrate important steps in procedures included in this textbook

- **Audio Glossary**
  Provides definitions of important terms in addition to audio pronunciations
  for selected key terms

- **Useful Spanish Vocabulary and Phrases**
  Includes helpful translations of common health care terms and phrases

- **Skills Evaluation Review**
  Reviews procedures that may be covered on certification reviews

- **Procedure Checklists**
  Step-by-step review of each procedure that allows for instructor use
  or student self-evaluation

ELSEVIER

Mosby's Textbook

for Long-Term Care Nursing Assistants

Sixth Edition

Sheila A. Sorrentino, PhD, RN
Curriculum and Health Care Consultant
Anthem, Arizona

• • •

Retired Author
Bernie Gorek, BS, MA
Gerontology Consultant
New England, North Dakota

ELSEVIER
MOSBY

ELSEVIER
MOSBY

3251 Riverport Lane
St. Louis, Missouri 63043

MOSBY'S TEXTBOOK FOR LONG-TERM CARE NURSING ASSISTANTS   ISBN: 978-0-323-07583-1

NOTICES

The content and procedures in this book are based on information currently available. They were reviewed by instructors and practicing professionals in various regions of the United States. However, center policies and procedures may vary from the information and procedures in this book. In addition, research and new information may require changes in standards and practices.

Standards and guidelines from the Centers for Disease Control and Prevention (CDC), Centers for Medicare & Medicaid Services (CMS), and the Occupational Safety and Health Administration (OSHA) may change as new information becomes available. Other federal and state agencies also may issue new standards and guidelines. So may accrediting agencies and national organizations. You are responsible for following the policies and procedures of your employer and the most current standards, practices, and guidelines as they relate to the safety of your work.

To the fullest extent of the law, neither the Publisher nor the authors or editors assume any liability for any injury and/or damage to persons or property as a matter of products liability, negligence or otherwise, or from any use or operation of any methods, products, instructions, or ideas contained in the material herein.

Previous editions copyrighted 2007, 2003, 1999, 1994, 1988

Library of Congress Cataloging-in-Publication Data
Sorrentino, Sheila A.
    Mosby's textbook for long-term care nursing assistants / Sheila A. Sorrentino, Bernie Gorek. -- 6th ed.
        p. cm.
    Includes index.
    ISBN 978-0-323-07583-1 (pbk. : alk. paper)
    1. Nurses' aides 2. Long-term care of the sick.   I. Gorek, Bernie.
II. Title: III. Title: Textbook for long-term care nursing assistants.
IV. Title: Long-term care nursing assistants.
    RT84.S67 2011
    610.7306'98--dc22

                                                                        2010031339

Senior Editor: Tamara Myers
Senior Developmental Editor: Maria Broeker
Publishing Services Manager: Jeff Patterson
Project Manager: Bill Drone
Designer: Paula Catalano

Printed in the United States of America

Last digit is the print number: 9 8 7 6 5 4 3

To my nephew,
Second Lieutenant Kyle Bookhout, United States Marine Corps
and his bride,
Second Lieutenant Katherine Bookhout, United States Marine Corps
2010 graduates of the United States Naval Academy.
For their honor, courage, and commitment
and wishing them a lifetime of love, health, and happiness.
God speed to them.

With much love,
Aunt Sheila

Sheila A. Sorrentino is currently a curriculum and health care consultant focusing on effective delegation and partnering with assistive personnel in hospitals, long-term care centers, and home care agencies.

Dr. Sorrentino was instrumental in the development and approval of CNA-PN-ADN programs in the Illinois Community College System and has taught in nursing assistant, practical nursing, associate degree, and baccalaureate and higher degree programs. Her career includes experiences as a nursing assistant, staff nurse, charge nurse, head nurse, nursing educator, assistant dean, dean, and consultant.

A Mosby author since 1982, Dr. Sorrentino is the author of *Mosby's Textbook for Nursing Assistants*, seventh edition, and several other textbooks for nursing assistive personnel. She was also involved in the development of *Mosby's Nursing Assistant Skills Videos* and *Mosby's Nursing Skills Videos*, winner of the 2003 *AJN* Book of the Year Award (electronic media). An earlier version of nursing assistant skills videos won the 1992 International Medical Films Award on caregiving.

Dr. Sorrentino has a bachelor of science degree in nursing, a master of arts in education, a master of science degree in community nursing, and a PhD in higher education administration. She is a member of Sigma Theta Tau International, the Honor Society of Nursing, and the Rotary Club of Anthem (Anthem, Arizona). She is a former member of the Provena Life Connections Board of Directors (Mokena, Illinois) and former member and chair of the Central Illinois Higher Education Health Care Task Force. She also served on the Iowa-Illinois Safety Council Board of Directors and the Board of Directors of Our Lady of Victory Nursing Center in Bourbonnais, Illinois.

In 1998 she received an alumni achievement award from Lewis University for outstanding leadership and dedication in nursing education. In 2005 she was inducted into the Illinois State University College of Education Hall of Fame. Her presentations at national and state conferences focus on delegation and other issues relating to nursing assistive personnel.

Dr. Sorrentino sponsors two nursing scholarships: one for a senior high school student from her high school alma mater intending to major in nursing and another for a nursing assistant working at one of the three agencies in which she worked during and after college (Heritage Manor, Peru, Illinois; Illinois Valley Community Hospital, Peru, Illinois; and St. Margaret's Hospital, Spring Valley, Illinois).

Mike Spinelli Photography, Phoenix, Arizona

Retired author Bernie Gorek is a gerontology consultant. She received her nursing diploma from St. Mary's School of Nursing in Rochester, Minnesota, and her bachelor's degree in Health Arts from the College of St. Francis in Joliet, Illinois. Bernie also received certification as a gerontological nurse practitioner from the University of Colorado in Denver and a master's degree in gerontology from the University of Northern Colorado in Greeley, Colorado, where she received the Dean's Citation for Excellence.

Bernie has had 26 years of experience in gerontological nursing: in a clinical role as a nurse practitioner and in administrative roles as Director of Community Health Services, Director of Nursing, and Director of Resident Care and Services at Bonell Good Samaritan Center in Greeley, Colorado. She has also had experience as a licensed nursing home administrator in Colorado and Wyoming.

Bernie has been a leader in developing and implementing innovative programs for residents in independent living and long-term health care settings. She was instrumental in the development and implementation of a community nursing assistant training program. She received a credential for Career and Technical Education from the Colorado State Board of Community Colleges and Occupational Education. She has consulted for the School of Nursing at the University of Northern Colorado in various grant-writing projects. Bernie served two terms as president of the National Conference of Gerontological Nurse Practitioners. She served on the editorial board for *Geriatric Nursing* for 3 years.

Photos by Jonathan, Dickinson, ND

CONSULTANT
Leighann N. Remmert, BSN, RN
Clinical Instructor
Capital Area School of Practical Nursing
Springfield, Illinois

REVIEWERS
Lynda Freeman, RN, BSN, MBA, PhD
Registered Nurse

Kimberly Gibbs, RN
Skills Lab Instructor
Spencerian College
Louisville, Kentucky

Arizinnia Hood, RN, BSN, MSN
Allied Health Coordinator
Cleveland Job Corps
Cleveland, Ohio

Alice Stone-Winkelblech, RN, BSN SD-CLTC
Nurse Practice Educator, CNA Instructor/Evaluator
Genesis Health Care
Phillipsburg, New Jersey

ACKNOWLEDGMENTS

Many individuals and agencies have contributed to this new, sixth edition of *Mosby's Textbook for Long-Term Care Nursing Assistants* by providing information, insights, and resources. We are especially grateful and appreciative of the efforts by:

- Lori Walsh (Administrator) and Deb Boyd (Director of Nursing) of LaSalle Healthcare (LaSalle, Illinois) for being valuable sources of information and insights and for coordinating and hosting our photo shoot. Their efforts allowed us to move through the session with ease.
- Rose Mary Carrico (Director of Medical/Surgical and ICU), Illinois Valley Community Hospital (Peru, Illinois), for her outstanding efforts in coordinating our photo shoot. We were in awe of her creativity and problem-solving abilities.
- Illinois Valley Community Hospital (Peru, Illinois) for once again hosting a photo shoot.
- Leighann N. Remmert, co-author of *Mosby's Essentials for Nursing Assistants*, fourth edition, and *Mosby's Textbook for Medication Assistants*, for serving as a consultant and helping with the production processes, including the tedious task of proofreading.
- Valerie Cooper of Abraham Lincoln Memorial Hospital (Lincoln, Illinois) for her assistance in obtaining a computerized documentation image.
- All the family, friends, and volunteers who participated in the photo shoot:
  - Anthony and Frances Sorrentino
  - Jerry and JoAnn Orlandini
  - Larry Huffman
  - Roger Tidaback
  - Pat Wlodarchak
  - John Apitado
  - Sue Fiesel
  - Michelle Lucas
  - Macee Lentz
  - Chuck Kellett
  - Kenneth Greening
  - Brianna Rebholz
  - Kayla Funtsinn
  - Tamara Cobb
  - Bekki Prokup
  - Miles McFadin
  - Maureen Rebholz

- Mary Beth Sorrentino Herron for providing clerical and technical support.
- The artists at Graphic World in St. Louis, Missouri, for their talented work.
- Photographer Mike DeFilipo of St. Louis, Missouri, for his great photos. He is very patient, cooperative, and flexible during photo shoots.
- Lynda Freeman, Kimberly Gibbs, Arizinnia Hood, and Alice Stone-Winkelblech for reviewing the manuscript and for their candor and suggestions. They have contributed to the thoroughness and accuracy of this book.
- Beth Welch (Columbus, Ohio) for serving as copy editor. It was a pleasure talking to her.
- And finally, to the talented and dedicated Elsevier/Mosby staff, especially:
  - Suzi Epstein (Executive Editor, retired) and Tamara Myers (Senior Editor)—they gave guidance and support and kept the project on track.
  - Maria Broeker (Senior Developmental Editor)—Maria handled numerous details, manuscript needs, tasks, and issues. She always has an empathetic ear and time to listen to author wants, needs, and frustrations. She is beyond terrific.
  - Sarah Graddy (Editorial Assistant)—Sarah provided prompt clerical and secretarial assistance. She is simply pleasant and a delight to work with.
  - Jeff Patterson (Publishing Services Manager), Bill Drone (Project Manager), and Kathy Teal (Production Assistant) for their production efforts. With all the design elements and layout considerations inherent in this book, they produced a user-friendly and attractive book.
  - Paula Catalano (Senior Book Designer)—Paula took all of our ideas, some rather abstract, and created a unique and colorful book and cover design. As always, the book is distinctive from the rest.

And to all those who contributed to this effort in any way, we are sincerely grateful.

Sheila A. Sorrentino

As with previous editions of *Mosby's Textbook for Long-Term Care Nursing Assistants,* the sixth edition serves to prepare students to function as nursing assistants in nursing centers. This textbook serves the needs of students and instructors in community colleges, technical schools, high schools, nursing centers, and other agencies. As students complete their education, the book is a valuable resource for the competency test review. As part of one's personal library, the book is a reference for the nursing assistant who seeks to review or learn additional information for safe care.

Residents are presented as *persons* with dignity and value who have a past, a present, and a future. Caring; understanding, protecting, and respecting the person's rights; and respecting residents as persons with dignity and value are attitudes conveyed throughout the book. Because of the importance of their protected rights, a new chapter—*Chapter 2: Resident Rights*—describes the rights provided for by the Omnibus Budget Reconciliation Act of 1987.

Nursing assistants of today and tomorrow must have a firm understanding of the legal principles affecting their role. Both federal and state laws directly and indirectly define their roles, range of functions, and limitations. Nursing assistant roles and functions also vary among states and nursing centers. Therefore emphasis is given to nursing assistant responsibilities, limitations, and professional boundaries which focus on the legal and ethical aspects of the role. This includes reporting abuse.

Nursing assistant functions and role limits also depend on effective delegation. Building on the delegation principles presented in Chapter 3, *Delegation Guidelines* boxes are presented as they relate to procedures. They empower the student to seek information from the nurse and the care plan about critical aspects of the procedure and the observations to report and record. Step 1 of most procedures refers the student to the appropriate *Delegation Guidelines* boxes.

Since the first edition, safety and comfort have been core values of *Mosby's Textbook for Long-Term Care Nursing Assistants.* Therefore *Promoting Safety and Comfort* boxes focus the student's attention on the need to be safe and cautious and to promote comfort when giving care. Step 1 of most procedures refers the student to the appropriate *Promoting Safety and Comfort* boxes.

Besides legal aspects, delegation, and safety and comfort, work ethics also affect how nursing assistants function. To foster a positive work ethic, Chapter 5 focuses on workplace behaviors and practices. The goal is for the nursing assistant to be a proud, professional member of the nursing and health teams.

Being a productive and efficient member of the nursing team requires teamwork, time management, and communication skills. Good communication skills are needed when interacting with residents. Two features address these issues:

- *Teamwork and Time Management* boxes suggest ways to efficiently work with and help other nursing team members.
- *Focus on Communication* boxes suggest what to say and questions to ask when interacting with residents, visitors, and the nursing team.

Persons with dementia present other challenges. *Residents With Dementia* boxes provide insights and care measures to promote the quality of life for persons with dementia.

A most exciting feature is the CD-ROM in this book. Using video clips and animations, key procedures are presented along with interactive exercises. The CD also includes an audio glossary and the *Body Spectrum* program.

Organizational Strategies

These concepts and principles—the resident as a person, ethical and legal aspects, delegation, safety and comfort, and work ethics—serve as the guiding framework for this book. Other organizational strategies and values include:

- Understanding the work setting and the individuals in that setting
- Respecting residents as physical, social, psychological, and spiritual beings with basic needs and protected rights
- Respecting personal choice and the person's dignity
- Appreciating the role of cultural heritage and religion in health and illness practices
- Understanding that knowledge about body structure and function is needed to give safe care and to safely perform nursing skills
- Following the principle that learning proceeds from the simple to the complex
- Recognizing that certain concepts and functions are foundational—safety, body mechanics, and preventing infection are central to other procedures
- Embracing the nursing process as the basis for planning and delivering nursing care and the role that nursing assistants play in assisting with the process

Content Issues

With every edition, revision and content decisions are made. When changes are made in laws or in guidelines and standards issued by government agencies, accrediting agencies, or associations, the decisions are easy Content and new figure decisions also are based on state curricula and competency testing services. Every attempt is made to make the book as up-to-date as possible with changes sometimes made right before publication.

Other content issues are more difficult. The learning needs and abilities of the student, instructor desires, work-related issues, course/program and book length, and production costs are among the factors considered. Also, because some chapters were long and were going to be longer because of new guidelines and content, they were divided into new ones to facilitate the teaching/learning process. With such issues in mind, new content includes:

New Chapters

- Chapter 2: Resident Rights
- Chapter 4: Ethics and Laws
- Chapter 29: Respiratory Support and Therapies
- Chapter 36: Pressure Ulcers
- Chapter 38: Cancer, Immune System, and Skin Disorders
- Chapter 39: Nervous System and Musculo-Skeletal Disorders
- Chapter 40: Cardiovascular and Respiratory Disorders
- Chapter 41: Digestive and Endocrine Disorders
- Chapter 42: Urinary and Reproductive Disorders

New Content

- Certification
- Working in Another State
- Nursing Assistant Standards
- Boundaries
- Color-Coded Wristbands
- Foodborne Illnesses
- Blood Glucose Testing
- Gallstones
- Cirrhosis
- Post-Traumatic Stress Disorder
- Suicide
- Paranoia
- Communication Problems (Chapter 44: Confusion and Dementia)
- Rummaging and Hiding Things
- Fragile X Syndrome
- Types of Care (Chapter 48: End-of-Life Care)

New Boxes

- Box 4-2 Rules for Maintaining Professional Boundaries
- Box 4-3 Boundary Signs

- Table 12-1 Water Temperature and Length of Exposure for a Third Degree Burn
- Box 12-2 Safety Measures to Prevent Poisoning
- Box 24-8 Common Causes of Dehydration
- Box 24-9 Signs and Symptoms of Foodborne Illnesses
- Box 37-3 Signs and Symptoms of Vision Problems
- Box 41-1 Signs and Symptoms of Gallstones
- Box 41-3 Persons at Risk for Hepatitis
- Box 41-4 Care of the Person With Cirrhosis
- Box 43-6 Risk Factors for Suicide
- Box 44-4 Signs and Symptoms of Delirium
- Box 44-6 Alzheimer's Disease and Normal Age-Related Changes
- Box 44-10 Family Caregivers—Taking Care of Yourself

New Focus on Communication Boxes

- The Interdisciplinary Health Care Team
- Refusing a Delegated Task
- Professional Boundaries
- Informed Consent
- Harassment
- Reporting and Recording
- Behavior Issues
- Effective Communication
- Applying Restraints
- Isolation Precautions
- Goggles and Face Shields
- Positioning the Person
- Noise
- Bathing
- Perineal Care
- Skin and Scalp Conditions
- Urinals
- Ambulation
- Coughing and Deep Breathing
- Taking Temperatures
- Using a Stethoscope
- The Midstream Specimen
- Tape
- Pressure Ulcer Stages
- Reporting and Recording (Chapter 36: Pressure Ulcers)
- Schizophrenia
- Suicide
- Care and Treatment
- Communication (Chapter 46: Rehabilitation and Restorative Nursing Care)
- Psychological and Social Aspects (Chapter 46: Rehabilitation and Restorative Nursing Care)
- Chain of Survival for Adults
- Culture and Spiritual Needs (Chapter 48: End-of-Life Care)

New Residents With Dementia Boxes

- Applying Restraints
- Safe Resident Handling, Moving, and Transfers
- The Person's Needs (Chapter 48: End-of-Life Care)

New Promoting Safety and Comfort Boxes

- Diarrhea
- *Clostridium difficile*
- Tracheostomies
- Suctioning
- Temperature Sites
- Behaviors and Problems
- Paranoia

New Procedure

- Measuring Blood Glucose

New Teamwork and Time Management box

- Wandering

Features and Design

Besides content issues, attention also is given to improving the book's features and designs. See "Student Preface."

May this book serve you and your students well. The intent is to provide you and your students with the current information needed to teach and learn safe and effective care during this time of dynamic change in health care.

Sheila A. Sorrentino, BSN, MA, MSN, PhD, RN

This book was designed for you. It was designed to help you learn. The book is a useful resource as you gain experience and expand your knowledge.

This preface gives some study guidelines and helps you use the book. When given a reading assignment, do you read from the first page to the last page without stopping? How much do you remember? You will learn more if you use a study system. A useful study system has these steps:

- Survey or preview
- Question
- Read and record
- Recite and review

Preview

Before you start a reading assignment, preview or survey the assignment. This gives you an idea of what the assignment covers. It also helps you recall what you already know about the subject. Carefully look over the assignment. Preview the chapter title, headings, subheadings, and terms or ideas in bold print or italics. Also survey the objectives, key terms, key abbreviations, boxes, and review questions at the end of the chapter. Previewing only takes a few minutes. Remember, previewing helps you become familiar with the material.

Question

After previewing, you need to form questions to answer while you read. Questions should relate to what might be asked on a test or how the information applies to giving care. Use the title, headings, and subheadings to form questions. Avoid questions that have one-word answers. Questions that begin with what, how, or why are helpful. While reading, you may find that a question does not help you study. If so, just change the question. Remember, questioning sets a purpose for reading. So changing a question only makes this step more useful.

Read and Record

Reading is the next step. Reading is more productive after determining what you already know and what you need to learn. Read to find answers to your questions. The purpose of reading is to:

- Gain new information
- Connect new information to what you already know

Break the assignment into smaller parts. Then answer your questions as you read each part. Also, mark important information—underline, highlight, or make notes. Underlining and highlighting remind you of what you need to learn. Go back and review the marked parts later. Making notes results in more immediate learning. To make notes, write down important information in the margins or in a notebook. Use words and statements to jog your memory about the material.

You need to remember what you read. To do so, work with the information. Organize information into a study guide. Study guides have many forms. Diagrams or charts show relationships or steps in a process. Note taking in outline format is also very useful. The following is a sample outline.

1. Main heading
   a. Second level
   b. Second level
      i. Third level
      ii. Third level
2. Main heading

Recite and Review

Finally, recite and review. Use your notes and study guides. Answer the questions you formed earlier. Also answer other questions that came up when reading and answering the Review Questions at the end of a chapter. Answer all questions out loud (recite).

Reviewing is more about when to study rather than what to study. You already determined what to study during the preview, question, and reading steps. The best times to review are right after the first study session, one week later, and before a quiz or test.

This book was also designed to help you study. Special design features are described on the next pages.

We hope you enjoy learning and your work. You and your work are important. You and the care you give make a difference in the person's life!

Sheila A. Sorrentino

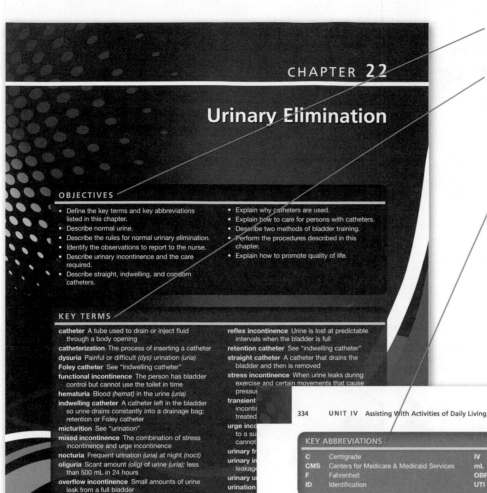

CHAPTER 22

Urinary Elimination

OBJECTIVES

- Define the key terms and key abbreviations listed in this chapter.
- Describe normal urine.
- Describe the rules for normal urinary elimination.
- Identify the observations to report to the nurse.
- Describe urinary incontinence and the care required.
- Describe straight, indwelling, and condom catheters.
- Explain why catheters are used.
- Explain how to care for persons with catheters.
- Describe two methods of bladder training.
- Perform the procedures described in this chapter.
- Explain how to promote quality of life.

KEY TERMS

catheter A tube used to drain or inject fluid through a body opening
catheterization The process of inserting a catheter
dysuria Painful or difficult *(dys)* urination *(uria)*
Foley catheter See "indwelling catheter"
functional incontinence The person has bladder control but cannot use the toilet in time
hematuria Blood *(hemat)* in the urine *(uria)*
indwelling catheter A catheter left in the bladder so urine drains constantly into a drainage bag; retention or Foley catheter
micturition See "urination"
mixed incontinence The combination of stress incontinence and urge incontinence
nocturia Frequent urination *(uria)* at night *(noct)*
oliguria Scant amount *(olig)* of urine *(uria);* less than 500 mL in 24 hours
overflow incontinence Small amounts of urine leak from a full bladder
polyuria Abnormally large amounts *(poly)* of urine *(uria)*

reflex incontinence Urine is lost at predictable intervals when the bladder is full
retention catheter See "indwelling catheter"
straight catheter A catheter that drains the bladder and then is removed
stress incontinence When urine leaks during exercise and certain movements that cause pressu...
transient incontin... treated...
urge inco... to a su... canno...
urinary fr...
urinary in... leakag...
urinary u...
urination ... bladde...
voiding S...

334   UNIT IV   Assisting With Activities of Daily Living

KEY ABBREVIATIONS

C	Centigrade	IV	Intravenous
CMS	Centers for Medicare & Medicaid Services	mL	Milliliter
F	Fahrenheit	OBRA	Omnibus Budget Reconciliation Act of 1987
ID	Identification	UTI	Urinary tract infection

Eliminating waste is a physical need. The respiratory, digestive, integumentary, and urinary systems remove body wastes. The digestive system rids the body of solid wastes. The lungs remove carbon dioxide. Sweat contains water and other substances. Blood contains waste products from body cells burning food for energy. The urinary system removes waste products from the blood. It also maintains the body's water balance.

NORMAL URINATION

The healthy adult produces about 1500 mL (milliliters) or 3 pints of urine a day. Many factors affect urine production. They include age, disease, the amount and kinds of fluid ingested, dietary salt, body temperature, perspiration, and drugs. Some substances increase urine production—coffee, tea, alcohol, and some drugs. A diet high in salt causes the body to retain water. When water is retained, less urine is produced.

Urination, micturition, and voiding mean the process of emptying urine from the bladder. The amount of fluid intake, habits, and available toilet facilities affect frequency. So do activity, work, and illness. People usually void at bedtime, after sleep, and before meals. Some people void every 2 to 3 hours. The need to void at night disturbs sleep.

Some persons need help getting to the bathroom. Others use bedpans, urinals, or commodes. Follow the rules in Box 22-1 and the person's care plan.

See *Focus on Communication: Normal Urination.*
See *Teamwork and Time Management: Normal Urination.*

Box 22-1   Rules for Normal Urination

- Practice medical asepsis.
- Follow Standard Precautions and the Bloodborne Pathogen Standard.
- Provide fluids as the nurse and care plan direct.
- Follow the person's voiding routines and habits. Check with the nurse and the care plan.
- Help the person to the bathroom when the request is made. Or provide the commode, bedpan, or urinal. The need to void may be urgent.
- Help the person assume a normal position for voiding if possible. Women sit or squat. Men stand.
- Warm the bedpan or urinal.
- Cover the person for warmth and privacy.
- Provide for privacy. Pull the curtain around the bed, close room and bathroom doors, and close window coverings. Leave the room if the person can be alone.
- Tell the person that running water, flushing the toilet, or playing music can mask voiding sounds. Voiding with others close by embarrasses some people.
- Stay nearby if the person is weak or unsteady.
- Place the signal light and toilet tissue within reach.
- Allow enough time. Do not rush the person.
- Promote relaxation. Some people like to read.
- Run water in a sink if the person cannot start the stream. Or place the person's fingers in warm water.
- Provide perineal care as needed (Chapter 20).
- Assist with hand washing after voiding. Provide a wash basin, soap, washcloth, and towel.
- Assist the person to the bathroom or offer the bedpan, urinal, or commode at regular times. Some people are embarrassed or are too weak to ask for help.

FOCUS ON COMMUNICATION
Normal Urination

Residents may not use "voiding" or "urinating" terms. The person may not understand what you are saying. Instead you can ask these questions:
- "Do you need to use the bathroom?"
- "Do you need to use the bedpan?"
- "Do you need to pass urine?"
- "Do you need to pee?"

TEAMWORK AND TIME MANAGEMENT
Normal Urination

The need to void may be urgent. Answer signal lights promptly. Also answer signal lights for co-workers. Otherwise incontinence may result. The person is wet and embarrassed. He or she is at risk for skin breakdown and infection. Your co-worker has extra work—changing linens and garments. You like help when you are busy. So do your co-workers.

**Annotations (right and left margins):**

Objectives tell what is presented in the chapter.

Key Terms are the important words and phrases in the chapter. Definitions are given for each term. The key terms introduce you to the chapter content. They are also a useful study guide.

Key Abbreviations are a quick reference of the abbreviations used in the chapter. They are listed after the "Key Terms."

Boxes and tables contain important rules, principles, guidelines, signs and symptoms, nursing measures, and other information in a list format. They identify important information and are useful study guides.

Blue, bolded type is used to highlight the key terms in the text. You again see the key term and read its definition. This helps reinforce your learning.

Teamwork and Time Management boxes suggest ways to efficiently work with and help nursing team members.

396   UNIT IV   Assisting With Activities of Daily Living

RESIDENTS WITH DEMENTIA
Feeding the Person

Residents with dementia may become distracted during meals. Some persons cannot sit long enough for a meal. Others forget how to use eating utensils. Some persons resist your efforts to assist them with eating. A confused person may throw or spit food.

The Alzheimer's Disease Education and Referral Center (ADEAR) recommends the following. The measures may be part of the person's care plan.
* Provide a calm, quiet setting for eating. Limit noise and other distractions. This helps the person focus on the meal.
* Limit the number of food choices.
* Offer several small meals throughout the day instead of larger ones.
* Use straws or cups with lids. These make drinking easier.
* Provide finger foods if the person has problems with utensils. A bowl may be easier to use than a plate.
* Provide healthy snacks. Keep snacks where the person can see them.

You must be patient. Talk to the nurse if you feel upset or impatient. Remember, the person has the right to be treated with dignity and respect.

DELEGATION GUIDELINES
Feeding the Person

Before feeding a person, you need this information from the nurse and the care plan:
* Why the person needs help
* How much help the person needs
* If the person can manage finger foods
* What the person's activity limits are
* What the person's dietary restrictions are
* What size portion to feed the person—⅓ teaspoonful or less
* What safety measures are needed if the person has dysphagia
* If the person can use a straw
* What observations to report and record:
  * The amount and kind of food eaten
  * Complaints of nausea or dysphagia
  * Signs and symptoms of dysphagia
  * Signs and symptoms of aspiration
* When to report observations
* What specific resident concerns to report at once

PROMOTING SAFETY AND COMFORT
Feeding the Person

Safety
Check food temperature. Very hot foods can burn the person.

Prevent aspiration. Check the person's mouth before offering more food or fluids. The person's mouth must be empty between bites and swallows.

Comfort
The person will eat better if not rushed. Sit to show the person that you have time for him or her. Standing communicates that you are in a hurry.

Wipe the person's hands, face, and mouth as needed during the meal. Use the napkin. If necessary, use a wet washcloth. Then dry the person with a towel.

Between-Meal Snacks

Many special diets involve between-meal snacks. Common snacks are crackers, milk, juice, a milkshake, cake, wafers, a sandwich, gelatin, and custard.

Snacks are served upon arrival on the nursing unit. Provide needed utensils, a straw, and a napkin. Follow the same considerations and procedures for serving meals and feeding persons.

Calorie Counts

Calorie records are kept for some people. On a flow sheet, note what the person ate and how much. For example, a chicken breast, rice, beans, a roll, pudding, and two pats of butter were served. The person ate all the chicken, half the rice, and the roll. One pat of butter was used. The beans and pudding were not eaten. Note these on the flow sheet. A nurse or dietitian converts these portions into calories. The nurse tells you which persons need calorie counts.

Fig. 24-13 A spoon is used to feed the person. The spoon is one-third full.

CHAPTER 20   Hygiene   281

...th. The skin ...ease. Intact ...e body and ...mbranes of ...e clean and ...vents body ...ses circula-

...giene. See ...people take ...at bedtime. ...quency also ...before work ...o not have ..., deodorant, ...ucts.

Many factors affect hygiene needs—perspiration, elimination, vomiting, drainage from wounds or body openings, bedrest, and activity. Illness and aging changes can affect self-care abilities. Some people need help with hygiene. The nurse uses the nursing process to meet the person's hygiene needs. Follow the nurse's directions and the care plan.

Some older persons resist your efforts to assist with hygiene. Illness, disability, dementia, and personal choice are common reasons. Follow the care plan to meet the person's needs.

See *Residents with Dementia: Hygiene.*
See *Focus on Communication: Hygiene.*
See *Focus on Rehabilitation: Hygiene.*

CARING ABOUT CULTURE
Personal Hygiene

Personal hygiene is very important to *East Indian Hindus.* Their religion requires at least one bath a day. Some believe bathing after a meal is harmful. Another belief is that a cold bath prevents a blood disease. Some believe that eye injuries can occur if a bath is too hot. Hot water can be added to cold water. However, cold water is not added to hot water. After bathing, the body is carefully dried with a towel.

From Giger JN, Davidhizar RE: Transcultural nursing: assessment and intervention, ed 5, St Louis, 2008, Mosby.

RESIDENTS WITH DEMENTIA
Hygiene

Persons with dementia may resist your efforts to assist with hygiene. Follow the care plan to meet the person's needs. Also see Chapter 44.

FOCUS ON COMMUNICATION
Hygiene

During hygiene procedures, make sure that the person is warm enough. You can ask:
* "Is the water warm enough?" "Is it too hot?" "Is it too cold?"
* "Are you warm enough?"
* "Do you need another bath blanket?"
* "Is the water starting to cool?"
* "Is the room warm enough?"

FOCUS ON REHABILITATION
Hygiene

Bending and reaching may be hard for older and disabled persons. Some have weak hand grips. They cannot hold soap or a washcloth. For independence, the person may use an adaptive device for hygiene (Fig. 20-1). Remember, let the person do as much for himself or herself as safely possible.

Fig. 20-1 Adaptive devices for hygiene. **A,** Tube squeezer for toothpaste. **B,** The wash mitt holds a bar of soap. **C,** A tap turner makes round knobs easy to turn. **D,** A long-handled sponge is used for hard-to-reach body parts. *(Courtesy ElderStore, Alpharetta, Ga.)*

Promoting Safety and Comfort boxes focus your attention on the need to be safe and cautious and promote comfort when giving care. "Safety" and "Comfort" subtitles are used.

Delegation Guidelines describe what information you need from the nurse and care plan before performing a procedure. They also tell you what information to report and record.

Color illustrations and photographs visually present key ideas, concepts, or procedure steps. They help you apply and remember the written material.

Caring About Culture boxes contain information about the various practices of other cultures.

Focus on Communication boxes suggest what to say and questions to ask when interacting with residents, visitors, and the nursing team.

Residents With Dementia boxes focus on information and care measures needed for persons with dementia.

Focus on Rehabilitation boxes alert you to considerations and insights about rehabilitation and restorative care.

Procedure icons in the title bar alert you to associated content areas. Heading icons and procedure icons are the same.

Procedures boxes are written in a step-by-step format. They are divided into *Quality of Life, Pre-Procedure, Procedure,* and *Post-Procedure* sections for easy studying. The Quality of Life section lists six simple courtesies that show respect for the resident as a person.

Video clip icons in the procedure title bar alert you to related video clips available online on *Evolve Student Learning Resources.*

NNAAP™ in the procedure title bar alerts you to those skills that are part of the National Nurse Aide Assessment Program (NNAAP™). Note: All states do not participate in NNAAP. Ask your instructor for a list of the skills tested in your state.

CD icons appear in the procedure box title bar for the skills included on the CD-ROM in the book.

Video icons in the procedure title bar alert you to procedures included on *Mosby's Nursing Assistant Video Skills 3.0.*

Heading icons alert you to associated procedures. Procedure boxes contain the same icon.

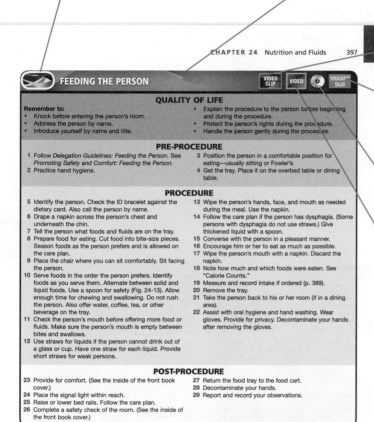

CHAPTER 24 Nutrition and Fluids 397

FEEDING THE PERSON

VIDEO CLIP · VIDEO · NNAAP™ Skill

QUALITY OF LIFE

Remember to:
- Knock before entering the person's room.
- Address the person by name.
- Introduce yourself by name and title.
- Explain the procedure to the person before beginning and during the procedure.
- Protect the person's rights during the procedure.
- Handle the person gently during the procedure.

PRE-PROCEDURE

1 Follow *Delegation Guidelines: Feeding the Person.* See *Promoting Safety and Comfort: Feeding the Person.*
2 Practice hand hygiene.
3 Position the person in a comfortable position for eating—usually sitting or Fowler's.
4 Get the tray. Place it on the overbed table or dining table.

PROCEDURE

5 Identify the person. Check the ID bracelet against the dietary card. Also call the person by name.
6 Drape a napkin across the person's chest and underneath the chin.
7 Tell the person what foods and fluids are on the tray.
8 Prepare food for eating. Cut food into bite-size pieces. Season foods as the person prefers and is allowed on the care plan.
9 Place the chair where you can sit comfortably. Sit facing the person.
10 Serve foods in the order the person prefers. Identify foods as you serve them. Alternate between solid and liquid foods. Use a spoon for safety (Fig. 24-13). Allow enough time for chewing and swallowing. Do not rush the person. Also offer water, coffee, tea, or other beverage on the tray.
11 Check the person's mouth before offering more food or fluids. Make sure the person's mouth is empty between bites and swallows.
12 Use straws for liquids if the person cannot drink out of a glass or cup. Have one straw for each liquid. Provide short straws for weak persons.
13 Wipe the person's hands, face, and mouth as needed during the meal. Use the napkin.
14 Follow the care plan if the person has dysphagia. (Some persons with dysphagia do not use straws.) Give thickened liquid with a spoon.
15 Converse with the person in a pleasant manner.
16 Encourage him or her to eat as much as possible.
17 Wipe the person's mouth with a napkin. Discard the napkin.
18 Note how much and which foods were eaten. See "Calorie Counts."
19 Measure and record intake if ordered (p. 389).
20 Remove the tray.
21 Take the person back to his or her room (if in a dining area).
22 Assist with oral hygiene and hand washing. Wear gloves. Provide for privacy. Decontaminate your hands after removing the gloves.

POST-PROCEDURE

23 Provide for comfort. (See the inside of the front book cover.)
24 Place the signal light within reach.
25 Raise or lower bed rails. Follow the care plan.
26 Complete a safety check of the room. (See the inside of the front book cover.)
27 Return the food tray to the food cart.
28 Decontaminate your hands.
29 Report and record your observations.

Providing Drinking Water

Residents need fresh drinking water each shift. They also need water whenever the pitcher is empty.

Some centers do not use the procedure that follows. Each person's pitcher is filled as needed. The pitcher is taken to an ice and water dispenser. If so, fill the pitcher with ice first. Then add water to the pitcher. Follow the center's procedure for providing fresh drinking water.

See *Delegation Guidelines: Providing Drinking Water.*
See *Promoting Safety and Comfort: Providing Drinking Water,* p. 398.

DELEGATION GUIDELINES
Providing Drinking Water

Before providing water, you need this information from the nurse and the care plan:
- The person's fluid orders
- If the person can have ice
- If the person uses a straw

- Describes education and licensing requirements for RNs and LPNs/LVNs.
- Protects the public from persons practicing nursing without a license. Persons who do not meet the state's requirements cannot perform nursing functions.

The law allows for denying, revoking, or suspending a nursing license. The purpose is to protect the public from unsafe nurses. Reasons include:
- Being convicted of a crime in any state
- Selling or distributing drugs
- Using the person's drugs for oneself
- Placing a person in danger from the over-use of alcohol or drugs
- Demonstrating grossly negligent nursing practice
- Being convicted of abusing or neglecting children or older persons
- Violating a nurse practice act and its rules and regulations
- Demonstrating incompetent behaviors
- Aiding or assisting another person to violate a nurse practice act and its rules and regulations
- Making medical diagnoses
- Prescribing drugs and treatments

Nursing Assistants A state's nurse practice act is used to decide what nursing assistants can do. Some nurse practice acts also regulate nursing assistant roles, functions, education, and certification requirements. Other states have separate laws for nursing assistants.

Legal and advisory opinions about nursing assistants are based on the state's nurse practice act. So are any state laws about their roles and functions. If you do something beyond the legal limits of your role, you could be practicing nursing without a license. This creates serious legal problems for you and the nurse supervising your work.

Nursing assistants must be able to function with skill and safety. Like nurses, nursing assistants can have their certification (p. 22) denied, revoked, or suspended. The National Council of State Boards of Nursing (NCSBN) lists these reasons for doing so:
- Substance abuse or dependency.
- Abandoning, abusing, or neglecting a resident.
- Fraud or deceit. Examples include:
  - Filing false personal information
  - Providing false information when applying for initial certification or to have it re-instated
- Violating professional boundaries (Chapter 4).
- Giving unsafe care.
- Performing acts beyond the nursing assistant role.
- Misappropriation (stealing, theft) or mis-using property.
- Obtaining money or property from a resident. Fraud, falsely representing oneself, and through force are examples.

- Having been convicted of a crime. Examples include murder, assault, kidnapping, rape or sexual assault, robbery, sexual crimes involving children, criminal mistreatment of children or a vulnerable adult (Chapter 4), drug trafficking, embezzlement (to take a person's property for one's own use), theft, and arson (starting fires).
- Failing to conform to the standards of nursing assistants (p. 25).
- Putting residents at risk for harm.
- Violating a resident's privacy.
- Failing to maintain the confidentiality of resident information.

The Omnibus Budget Reconciliation Act of 1987

The Omnibus Budget Reconciliation Act of 1987 (OBRA) is a federal law. Its purpose is to improve the quality of life of nursing center residents.

OBRA sets minimum training and competency evaluation requirements for nursing assistants. Each state must have a nursing assistant training and competency evaluation program (NATCEP). A nursing assistant must successfully complete a NATCEP to work in a nursing center, hospital long-term care unit, or home care agency receiving Medicare funds.

The Training Program OBRA requires at least 75 hours of instruction. Some states have more hours. At least 16 hours of supervised practical training are required. Such training occurs in a laboratory or clinical setting (Fig. 3-1, p. 22). Students perform nursing care and tasks on another person. A nurse supervises this practical training (clinical practicum or clinical experience).

The training program includes the knowledge and skills needed to give basic nursing care. Areas of study include:
- Communication
- Infection control
- Safety and emergency procedures
- Residents' rights
- Basic n...
- Persona...
- Feeding...
- Elimina...
- Skin ca...
- Transfe...
- Dressin...
- Helping...
- Range-...
- Signs a...
- How to...
  who ha...
  Compet...
has a writ...
The writt...

*(margin label:* OBRA-CMS) **

OBRA and CMS highlights inform you of requirements by the Omnibus Budget Reconciliation Act of 1987 (OBRA) and the Centers for Medicare & Medicaid Services (CMS).

QUALITY OF LIFE

The bed is the largest item in the resident's unit. The person, family, and visitors question the quality of care if the bed is unmade, messy, or dirty. They also question the person's quality of life. The bed must be neat, clean, and well made. It helps provide an orderly and pleasant setting. If the person stays in bed, straighten and tighten sheets and other linen as needed.

Some persons bring bedspreads, pillows, blankets, afghans, and quilts from home. Use these when making the bed. Such items are the person's property. Handle them with care and respect. Make sure they are labeled with the person's name. This protects them from loss. It also prevents them from becoming confused with the property of others.

Allow personal choice when possible. The center may use colored or printed linens. If so, let the person choose which linen to use. Also, let the person decide how many pillows or blankets to use. If possible, the person chooses when the bed is made. The more choices allowed, the greater the person's sense of control and quality of life.

REVIEW QUESTIONS

Circle T if the statement is TRUE. Circle F if the statement is FALSE.

1 T F   In nursing centers, complete linen changes are required for closed beds and surgical beds.
2 T F   Hem-stitching of the bottom sheet is placed away from the person.
3 T F   To remove crumbs from the bed, you shake linens in the air.
4 T F   The upper hem of the bedspread is even with the top of the mattress.
5 T F   Top linens are fan-folded to the foot of the bed for an open bed.
6 T F   A cotton drawsheet is used only with a waterproof drawsheet.
7 T F   Residents can bring bed coverings from home.

Circle the BEST answer.

8 Which requires a linen change?
   a The person will have visitors
   b Wet linen
   c Wrinkled linen
   d Crumbs in the bed
9 You will transfer a person from a stretcher to the bed. Which bed should you make?
   a A closed bed
   b An open bed
   c An occupied bed
   d A surgical bed
10 When handling linens
   a Put dirty linens on the floor
   b Hold linens away from your body and uniform
   c Shake linens to unfold them
   d Take extra linen to another person's room
11 A resident is out of the bed most of the day. Which bed should you make?
   a A closed bed
   b An open bed
   c An occupied bed
   d A surgical bed
12 A complete linen change is done when
   a The bottom linens are wet or soiled
   b The bed is made for a new person
   c The person will transfer from a stretcher to a bed
   d Linens are loose or wrinkled
13 You are using a waterproof drawsheet. Which is *true*?
   a A cotton drawsheet must completely cover the waterproof drawsheet.
   b Waterproof pads are needed.
   c The person's consent is needed.
   d The plastic or rubber is in contact with the person's skin.
14 To make an occupied bed, you do the following *except*
   a Cover the person with a bath blanket
   b Screen the person
   c Raise the far bed rail
   d Fan-fold top linens to the foot of the bed
15 A surgical bed is kept
   a In Fowler's position
   b In the lowest position
   c In the highest position
   d In the supine position

Answers to these questions are on p. 720.

Quality of Life boxes at the end of each chapter bridge the chapter's focus with how to promote the resident's rights and enhance quality of life when giving care.

Review Questions are useful study guides. They help you to review what you have learned. They can also be used when studying for a test or the competency evaluation. Answers are given at the back of the book beginning on p. 719.

CONTENTS

I WORKING IN LONG-TERM CARE SETTINGS

1 Working in Long-Term Care, 1

Long-Term Care Centers, 2
The Nursing Team, 5
Nursing Care Patterns, 5
The Interdisciplinary Health Care Team, 6
Paying For Health Care, 8
Meeting Standards, 9

2 Resident Rights, 11

Resident Rights, 12
Ombudsman Program, 17

3 The Nursing Assistant in Long-Term Care, 19

History and Current Trends, 20
Federal and State Laws, 20
Roles and Responsibilities, 23
Delegation, 25

4 Ethics and Laws, 32

Ethical Aspects, 33
Legal Aspects, 34
Reporting Abuse, 38

5 Work Ethics, 44

Health, Hygiene, and Appearance, 45
Getting a Job, 45
Preparing for Work, 52
Teamwork, 53
Managing Stress, 55
Harassment, 56
Resigning from a Job, 57
Losing a Job, 57
Drug Testing, 57

6 Communicating With the Health Team, 59

Communication, 60
The Medical Record, 60
The Kardex, 62
Resident Care Conferences, 62
Reporting and Recording, 62
Medical Terms and Abbreviations, 67
Computers and Other Electronic Devices, 70
Phone Communications, 70
Dealing With Conflict, 72

7 Assisting With the Nursing Process, 74

Assessment, 75
Nursing Diagnosis, 77
Planning, 77
Implementation, 80
Evaluation, 81
Your Role, 81

II FOCUSING ON THE PERSON

8 Understanding the Resident, 82

Caring for the Person, 83
Basic Needs, 83
Culture and Religion, 84
Effects of Illness and Disability, 85
Nursing Center Residents, 86
Behavior Issues, 87
Communicating With the Person, 88
Residents With Disabilities, 94
Family and Friends, 94

9 Body Structure and Function, 97

Cells, Tissues, and Organs, 98
The Integumentary System, 99
The Musculo-Skeletal System, 100
The Nervous System, 102
The Circulatory System, 105
The Respiratory System, 107
The Digestive System, 107
The Urinary System, 108
The Reproductive System, 109
The Endocrine System, 111
The Immune System, 112

10 The Older Person, 114

Growth and Development, 115
Psychological and Social Changes, 117
Physical Changes, 118
Housing Options, 122

11 Sexuality, 128

Sex and Sexuality, 129
Sexual Relationships, 129
Injury, Illness, and Surgery, 129
Sexuality and Older Persons, 130
Meeting Sexual Needs, 130
The Sexually Aggressive Person, 131
Sexually Transmitted Diseases, 132

III PROTECTING THE PERSON

12 Safety, 133

A Safe Setting, 134
Accident Risk Factors, 135
Identifying the Person, 135
Preventing Burns, 136
Preventing Poisoning, 137
Preventing Suffocation, 138
Preventing Infection, 141
Preventing Equipment Accidents, 141
Wheelchair and Stretcher Safety, 142
Handling Hazardous Substances, 143
Fire Safety, 145
Disasters, 149
Workplace Violence, 149
Risk Management, 152

13 Preventing Falls, 156

Causes and Risk Factors for Falls, 157
Fall Prevention Programs, 158
Transfer/Gait Belts, 162
The Falling Person, 163

14 Restraint Alternatives and Safe Restraint Use, 166

History of Restraint Use, 167
Restraint Alternatives, 168
Safe Restraint Use, 169

15 Preventing Infection, 182

Microorganisms, 183
Infection, 184
Medical Asepsis, 186
Isolation Precautions, 191
Bloodborne Pathogen Standard, 203
Surgical Asepsis, 205

16 Body Mechanics, 210

Principles of Body Mechanics, 211
Ergonomics, 213
Positioning the Person, 214

17 Safe Resident Handling, Moving, and Transfers, 219

Preventing Work-Related Injuries, 221
Moving Persons in Bed, 225
Turning Persons, 233
Sitting on the Side of the Bed (Dangling), 236
Transferring Persons, 238
Re-Positioning in a Chair or Wheelchair, 250

IV ASSISTING WITH ACTIVITIES OF DAILY LIVING

18 The Resident's Unit, 252

Comfort, 253
Room Furniture and Equipment, 254
General Rules, 262

19 Bedmaking, 265

Types of Beds, 266
Linens, 267
Making Beds, 268

20 Hygiene, 280

Daily Care, 282
Oral Hygiene, 282
Bathing, 290
The Back Massage, 302
Perineal Care, 305
Reporting and Recording, 309

21 Grooming, 311

Hair Care, 312
Shampooing, 317
Shaving, 319
Nail and Foot Care, 322
Changing Clothing and Hospital Gowns, 325

22 Urinary Elimination, 333

Normal Urination, 334
Urinary Incontinence, 342
Catheters, 344
Bladder Training, 353

23 Bowel Elimination, 355

Normal Bowel Elimination, 356
Factors Affecting Bowel Elimination, 356
Common Problems, 357
Bowel Training, 359
Enemas, 360
The Person With an Ostomy, 366

24 Nutrition and Fluids, 371

Basic Nutrition, 372
Factors Affecting Eating and Nutrition, 381
OBRA Dietary Requirements, 382
Special Diets, 383
Fluid Balance, 388
Meeting Food and Fluid Needs, 391
Foodborne Illnesses, 399

25 Nutritional Support and IV Therapy, 401

Enteral Nutrition, 402
Parenteral Nutrition, 407
IV Therapy, 408

26 Exercise and Activity, 414

Bedrest, 415
Range-of-Motion Exercises, 419
Ambulation, 424
Recreational Activities, 429

27 Comfort, Rest, and Sleep, 431

Comfort, 432
Pain, 432
Rest, 437
Sleep, 437

28 Oxygen Needs, 442

Factors Affecting Oxygen Needs, 443
Altered Respiratory Function, 444
Assisting With Assessment and Diagnostic
    Tests, 445
Promoting Oxygenation, 448
Assisting With Oxygen Therapy, 451

29 Respiratory Support and Therapies, 457

Artificial Airways, 458
Suctioning the Airway, 459
Mechanical Ventilation, 461
Chest Tubes, 462

30 Assisted Living, 464

Purpose, 466
ALR Residents, 466
Resident Rights, 466
Staff Requirements, 468
Service Plan, 468
Transfer, Discharge, and Eviction, 471

V ASSISTING WITH ASSESSMENT

31 Measuring Vital Signs, 473

Measuring and Reporting Vital Signs, 474
Body Temperature, 475
Pulse, 483
Respirations, 489
Blood Pressure, 490

32 Assisting With the Physical Examination, 496

Your Role, 497
Equipment, 497
Preparing the Person, 497
Positioning and Draping, 499
Assisting With the Exam, 500

33 Collecting and Testing Specimens, 502

Urine Specimens, 503
Stool Specimens, 511
Sputum Specimens, 515
Blood Glucose Testing, 516

VI ASSISTING WITH CARE NEEDS

34 Admissions, Transfers, and Discharges, 521

Admissions, 522
Moving the Person to a New Room, 531
Transfers and Discharges, 532

35 Wound Care, 535

Types of Wounds, 537
Skin Tears, 538
Circulatory Ulcers, 539
Wound Healing, 546
Dressings, 550
Binders, 554
Heat and Cold Applications, 555
Meeting Basic Needs, 561

36 Pressure Ulcers, 564

Risk Factors, 566
Persons at Risk, 567
Pressure Ulcer Stages, 567
Sites, 570
Prevention and Treatment, 570
Complications, 575
Reporting and Recording, 575

37 Hearing, Speech, and Vision Problems, 578

Ear Disorders, 579
Speech Disorders, 583
Eye Disorders, 584

38 Cancer, Immune System, and Skin Disorders, 594

Cancer, 595
Immune System Disorders, 597
Skin Disorders, 599

39 Nervous System and Musculo-Skeletal Disorders, 601

Nervous System Disorders, 602
Musculo-Skeletal Disorders, 607

40 Cardiovascular and Respiratory Disorders, 617

Cardiovascular Disorders, 618
Respiratory Disorders, 621

41 Digestive and Endocrine Disorders, 625

Digestive Disorders, 626
Endocrine Disorders, 631

42 Urinary and Reproductive Disorders, 634

Urinary System Disorders, 635
Reproductive Disorders, 639

43 Mental Health Problems, 642

Basic Concepts, 643
Anxiety Disorders, 643
Schizophrenia, 645
Mood Disorders, 646
Personality Disorders, 647
Substance Abuse and Addiction, 648
Suicide, 652
Care and Treatment, 653

44 Confusion and Dementia, 655

Confusion, 656
Dementia, 657
Alzheimer's Disease, 658
Care of Persons With AD and Other
   Dementias, 666

45 Developmental Disabilities, 673

Intellectual Disabilities, 674
Down Syndrome, 676
Fragile X Syndrome, 677
Cerebral Palsy, 677
Autism, 678
Spina Bifida, 679
Hydrocephalus, 680

46 Rehabilitation and Restorative Nursing
Care, 682

Restorative Nursing, 683
Rehabilitation and the Whole Person, 683
The Rehabilitation Team, 688
Rehabilitation Programs and Services, 689

47 Basic Emergency Care, 691

Emergency Care, 692
Basic Life Support for Adults, 693
Hemorrhage, 703
Fainting, 704
Shock, 704
Stroke, 705
Seizures, 705
Burns, 706

48 End-of-Life Care, 709

Terminal Illness, 710
Attitudes About Death, 710
The Stages of Dying, 712
Comfort Needs, 712
The Family, 714
Legal Issues, 714
Signs of Death, 715
Care of the Body After Death, 715

REVIEW QUESTION ANSWERS, 719

APPENDICES

A   National Nurse Aide Assessment Program
    (NNAAP™) Written Examination Content
    Outline and Skills Evaluation, 722
B   Minimum Data Set, 723
C   Useful Spanish Vocabulary and Phrases, 756

GLOSSARY, 768

KEY ABBREVIATIONS, 777

INDEX, 779

PROCEDURES

Procedures with this icon ⊙ are also on the CD-ROM in this book.

Procedures with this icon [VIDEO CLIP] have related video clips in the *Evolve Student Resources* for this book.

Procedures with this icon [VIDEO] are available in *Mosby's Nursing Assistant Video Skills 3.0*

Procedures with this icon [NNAAP Skill] are NNAAP™ skills.

Relieving Choking—Adult or Child (Over 1 Year of Age), 139

Using a Fire Extinguisher, 147

Applying a Transfer/Gait Belt, 163

Helping the Falling Person, 164

Applying Restraints, 179

Hand Washing, 189 [NNAAP Skill] ⊙ [VIDEO CLIP] [VIDEO]

Removing Gloves, 198 [NNAAP Skill] [VIDEO]

Donning and Removing a Gown, 199 [NNAAP Skill] [VIDEO]

Donning and Removing a Mask, 200 [VIDEO]

Sterile Gloving, 207

Raising the Person's Head and Shoulders, 226

Moving the Person Up in Bed, 228 [VIDEO]

Moving the Person Up in Bed With an Assist Device, 230

Moving the Person to the Side of the Bed, 232

Turning and Re-positioning the Person, 233 [NNAAP Skill] ⊙ [VIDEO CLIP] [VIDEO]

Logrolling the Person, 235

Sitting on the Side of the Bed (Dangling), 237

Transferring the Person to a Chair or Wheelchair, 240 [NNAAP Skill] ⊙ [VIDEO CLIP] [VIDEO]

Transferring the Person From a Chair or Wheelchair to Bed, 243

Transferring the Person Using a Mechanical Lift, 245 [VIDEO]

Transferring the Person to and From the Toilet, 247

Moving the Person to a Stretcher, 249

Making a Closed Bed, 270 [VIDEO CLIP] [VIDEO]

Making an Open Bed, 274

Making an Occupied Bed, 275 [NNAAP Skill] ⊙ [VIDEO]

Making a Surgical Bed, 278 [VIDEO]

Assisting the Person to Brush and Floss the Teeth, 284

Brushing and Flossing the Person's Teeth, 285 [NNAAP Skill] ⊙ [VIDEO CLIP] [VIDEO]

Providing Mouth Care for the Unconscious Person, 287 ⊙ [VIDEO CLIP] [VIDEO]

Providing Denture Care, 289 [NNAAP Skill] ⊙ [VIDEO CLIP] [VIDEO]

Giving a Complete Bed Bath, 294 [NNAAP Skill] ⊙ [VIDEO CLIP] [VIDEO]

Assisting With the Partial Bath, 297 [VIDEO CLIP] [VIDEO]

Assisting With a Tub Bath or Shower, 301 [VIDEO CLIP] [VIDEO]

Giving a Back Massage, 303 ⊙

Giving Female Perineal Care, 307 [NNAAP Skill] ⊙ [VIDEO CLIP] [VIDEO]

Giving Male Perineal Care, 308 [NNAAP Skill] ⊙ [VIDEO CLIP] [VIDEO]

Brushing and Combing the Person's Hair, 315 ⊙

Shampooing the Person's Hair, 318 ⊙ [VIDEO CLIP] [VIDEO]

Shaving the Person's Face With a Safety Razor, 321 [VIDEO]

Giving Nail and Foot Care, 323 [NNAAP Skill] ⊙ [VIDEO CLIP] [VIDEO]

Undressing the Person, 326 ⊙ [VIDEO]

Dressing the Person, 328 [NNAAP Skill] ⊙ [VIDEO CLIP] [VIDEO]

Changing the Gown of the Person With an IV, 331 [VIDEO]

Giving the Bedpan, 337 [NNAAP Skill] ⊙ [VIDEO CLIP] [VIDEO]

Giving the Urinal, 339 [VIDEO]

Helping the Person to the Commode, 341 [VIDEO]

Giving Catheter Care, 346 [NNAAP Skill] ⊙ [VIDEO CLIP] [VIDEO]

Changing a Leg Bag to a Drainage Bag, 349

Emptying a Urinary Drainage Bag, 350 [VIDEO]

Applying a Condom Catheter, 352 [VIDEO]

Giving a Cleansing Enema, 362 [VIDEO]

Giving a Small-Volume Enema, 364 [VIDEO]

Giving an Oil-Retention Enema, 366

Changing an Ostomy Pouch, 369 [VIDEO]

Measuring Intake and Output, 390

Preparing the Person for a Meal, 393

Serving Meal Trays, 394

Feeding the Person, 397

Providing Drinking Water, 398

Performing Range-of-Motion
   Exercises, 421

Helping the Person Walk, 425

Using a Pulse Oximeter, 447

Assisting With Deep-Breathing and Coughing
   Exercises, 449

Setting Up for Oxygen Administration, 455

Taking a Temperature With a Glass
   Thermometer, 478

Taking a Temperature With an Electronic
   Thermometer, 481

Taking a Radial Pulse, 486

Taking an Apical Pulse, 487

Taking an Apical-Radial Pulse, 488

Counting Respirations, 489

Measuring Blood Pressure, 493

Preparing the Person for an Examination, 498

Collecting a Random Urine Specimen, 504

Collecting a Midstream Specimen, 505

Collecting a 24-Hour Urine Specimen, 507

Testing Urine With Reagent Strips, 509

Straining Urine, 510

Collecting a Stool Specimen, 512

Testing a Stool Specimen for Blood, 514

Collecting a Sputum Specimen, 516

Measuring Blood Glucose, 518

Preparing the Person's Room, 523

Admitting the Person, 526

Measuring Weight and Height, 529

Measuring Height—The Person Is in Bed, 531

Moving the Person to a New Room, 532

Transferring or Discharging the Person, 533

Applying Elastic Stockings, 542

Applying Elastic Bandages, 544

Applying a Dry, Non-Sterile Dressing, 553

Applying Heat and Cold Applications, 559

Caring for Eyeglasses, 591

Adult CPR—One Rescuer, 700

Adult CPR—Two Rescuers, 701

Adult CPR With AED—Two Rescuers, 702

Assisting With Post-Mortem Care, 716

Working in Long-Term Care

OBJECTIVES

- Define the key terms and key abbreviations listed in this chapter.
- Describe the types, purposes, and organization of long-term care centers.
- Describe members of the nursing team.
- Describe the interdisciplinary health care team.

- Describe four nursing care patterns.
- Describe the programs that pay for health care.
- Explain why standards are met.
- Explain how to promote quality of life.

KEY TERMS

acute illness A sudden illness from which a person is expected to recover

Alzheimer's disease (AD) A disease that affects brain tissue; memory loss and confusion increase until the person cannot tend to simple personal needs

assisted living residence Provides housing, personal care, support services, health care, and activities in a home-like setting

board and care home Provides rooms, meals, laundry, and supervision to independent residents in a home-like setting; group home

case management A nursing care pattern; a case manager (an RN) coordinates a person's care from admission through discharge and into the home setting

chronic illness An ongoing illness, slow or gradual in onset; it has no cure; the illness can be controlled and complications prevented with proper treatment

functional nursing A nursing care pattern focusing on tasks and jobs; each nursing team member has certain tasks and jobs to do

group home See "board and care home"

hospice A health care agency or program for persons who are dying

independence Not relying on or requiring care from others

interdisciplinary health care team The many health care workers whose skills and knowledge focus on the person's total care; health team

licensed practical nurse (LPN) A nurse who has completed a 1-year nursing program and has passed a licensing test; called *licensed vocational nurse (LVN)* in some states

licensed vocational nurse (LVN) See "licensed practical nurse"

Medicaid A health care payment program sponsored by the federal government and operated by the states

Medicare A federal health insurance program for persons 65 years of age or older and younger people with certain disabilities

nursing assistant A person who gives basic nursing care under the supervision of a licensed nurse; nurse aide, nursing attendant, and health care assistant are some other titles

Continued

KEY TERMS—cont'd

nursing center Provides health care and nursing care to persons who need regular or continuous care; licensed nurses are required; nursing facility or nursing home

nursing facility (NF) See "nursing center"

nursing home See "nursing center"

nursing team Those who provide nursing care—RNs, LPNs/LVNs, and nursing assistants

primary nursing A nursing care pattern; an RN is responsible for the person's total care

registered nurse (RN) A nurse who has completed a 2-, 3-, or 4-year nursing program and has passed a licensing test

skilled nursing facility (SNF) Provides health care and nursing care for residents who have many or severe health problems or who need rehabilitation; may be part of a nursing center or a hospital

team nursing A nursing care pattern; a team of nursing staff is led by an RN who delegates care to other nurses; some nursing tasks and procedures are delegated to nursing assistants

KEY ABBREVIATIONS

AD	Alzheimer's disease	**LVN**	Licensed vocational nurse
ALR	Assisted living residence	**PPO**	Preferred provider organization
DON	Director of nursing	**RN**	Registered nurse
HMO	Health maintenance organization	**SNF**	Skilled nursing facility
LPN	Licensed practical nurse		

Working in long-term care offers many new and rewarding experiences. Your focus is the resident—the person needing care. You must provide quality care and promote the person's quality of life. This includes promoting his or her independence. Independence means not relying on or requiring care from others.

LONG-TERM CARE CENTERS

Long-term care centers provide health care to persons who cannot care for themselves at home. They do not need hospital care. Care needs range from simple to complex. Medical, nursing, dietary, recreational, rehabilitative, and social services are provided. So are housekeeping and laundry services.

Persons in long-term care centers are called *residents*. They are not *patients*. This is because the center is their temporary or permanent home.

Residents are older or disabled. Some are recovering from illness, injury, or surgery. Long-term care centers are designed to meet their needs. Some people return home when well enough. Others need nursing care until death.

Board and Care Homes

Board and care homes (group homes) provide rooms, meals, laundry and supervision to independent residents in a home-like setting. Care is given that meets the person's basic needs. A safe setting and supervision are provided. So are housekeeping and transportation services. There is an emergency call system and a 24-hour caregiver. This person may be a nursing assistant.

Residents can usually dress themselves. They usually tend to grooming and bathroom needs with little help. They receive help with personal care and drug reminders as needed.

Assisted Living Residences

Assisted living residences (ALRs) provide housing, personal care, support services, health care, and activities in a home-like setting (Chapter 30). Many look like apartment buildings. Some are part of retirement communities or nursing centers.

The person has a room or an apartment. Help is given as needed with personal care, meals, or taking drugs. Three meals a day are provided. So are housekeeping, laundry, and transportation services. Social and recreational activities are provided. There is access to health and medical care.

Nursing Centers

A nursing center provides health care and nursing care to persons who need regular or continuous care. Nursing facility (NF) and nursing home are other names. Licensed nurses are required.

Residents have more severe health problems than do board and care or ALR residents. These services are provided:

- Medical care
- Nursing care (Fig. 1-1)
- Dietary services
- Rehabilitation
- Recreation
- Social services
- Laundry
- Housekeeping
- Maintenance

Skilled nursing facilities (SNFs) provide health care and nursing care for residents who have many or severe health problems or who need rehabilitation. The SNF may be part of a nursing center or a hospital.

SNFs provide more complex care than nursing centers do. Many persons are admitted from hospitals. They need to recover or have rehabilitation after an illness, injury, or surgery. Some return home. Others do not.

Purposes and Goals Long-term care serves to *promote physical and mental health*. Most residents have one or more health problems. They are helped and encouraged to:

- Understand and accept the limits of their health problems
- Understand and accept physical and mental changes
- Function within those limits
- Focus on abilities, not disabilities
- Do as much for themselves as possible
- Change habits that make health problems worse
- Eat properly and exercise

The family needs to accept and understand what is happening to the loved one. The family is taught how to help the person maintain the highest possible level of function.

Long-term care also serves to *treat chronic illness*. A chronic illness is an on-going illness, slow or gradual in onset. It has no cure. The illness can be controlled and complications prevented with proper treatment. An acute illness is a sudden illness from which the person is expected to recover. An acute illness may require hospital care.

Fig. 1-1 A nursing assistant is helping a nurse with a resident's care.

Communicable diseases are prevented. A communicable disease can be spread from one person to another (Chapter 15). The common cold and influenza (flu) are examples. They can cause major health problems for older and disabled persons. Often you are the first person to detect signs and symptoms of a communicable disease.

Rehabilitation or restorative care helps persons return to their highest possible level of physical and mental function (Chapter 46). They are helped to become or remain as independent as possible. This includes persons who need nursing center care until death.

Rehabilitation starts when a person is admitted to the center. Weakness after an acute illness is common. *Deconditioning* is the process of becoming weak from illness or lack of exercise (Chapter 26). Strokes, fractures, and surgery are common causes. All staff members follow the rehabilitation plan.

Other Services Some nursing centers offer learning experiences for students. They study to become nurses, nursing assistants, doctors, or other health team members. All students focus on the center's purposes and goals.

Many nursing centers have special care units. Hospice and Alzheimer's disease units are common.

- *Hospices.* A hospice is a health care agency or program for persons who are dying. Such persons no longer respond to treatments aimed at cures. Usually they have less than 6 months to live. The physical, emotional, social, and spiritual needs of the person and family are met. The focus is on comfort, not cure. Children and pets can visit. Family and friends can assist with care. Hospice care is provided by hospitals, nursing centers, and home care agencies.

- *Alzheimer's Units (Dementia Care Units).* These units are for persons with Alzheimer's disease and other dementias (Chapter 44). Alzheimer's disease (AD) affects brain tissue (Chapter 44). Memory loss and confusion increase until the person cannot tend to simple personal needs. Over time, the person forgets names of self and others. The person may wander and become agitated and combative. The unit is usually closed off from the rest of the center. This provides a safe setting for residents to wander freely. AD worsens over time. When wandering is no longer a problem, a closed unit is no longer needed. The person is transferred to another unit in the center.
- *Rehabilitation and Subacute Care.* Some nursing centers and hospitals provide rehabilitation or subacute care. Often the stay is for a few weeks or months. Persons on these units are called *patients* or *clients*. If problems occur, the person may need long-term care.

Nursing Center Organization

Nursing centers are usually owned by an individual or a corporation. Some are owned by government agencies. The owners control policies to make sure that safe care is provided. Local, state, and federal rules must be followed.

Each center has an administrator. The administrator plans, directs, and oversees the delivery of health care. Department directors report to the administrator (Fig. 1-2). Most nursing centers have nursing, therapy, and food service departments. They also have housekeeping, maintenance, and laundry departments. A human resources director handles personnel matters such as hiring staff. A finance director handles resident billing. A social services director meets the social needs of residents and families. An activity director plans resident activities.

By law, nursing centers must have a medical director. This person is a doctor. This doctor consults with the staff about medical problems not handled by a resident's doctor. Guidance is given about resident care policies and programs.

Nursing Service

Nursing service is a large department. The director of nursing (DON) is an RN. The DON is responsible for the entire nursing staff. This includes giving safe care.

Nurse managers (usually RNs) assist the DON. They manage and carry out nursing department functions. Shift managers coordinate resident care for a certain shift. Other managers are responsible for a nursing area or a certain function. Staff development, restorative nursing, infection control, or continuous quality improvement are examples.

Each nursing unit usually has a charge nurse. Charge nurses are usually RNs. In some states, LPNs/LVNs

Fig. 1-2 Organization of a nursing center.

are charge nurses. The charge nurse is responsible for all resident care and for the actions of nursing staff on a unit. Staff RNs report to the charge nurse. LPNs/LVNs report to staff RNs or to the charge nurse. You report to the nurse supervising your work.

Nursing education (staff development) is part of nursing service. Nursing education staff:

- Plan and present educational programs (in-service programs)
- Provide the nursing team with new and changing information
- Teach the nursing team how to use new equipment and supplies
- Review key policies and procedures on a regular basis
- Educate and train nursing assistants
- Conduct new employee orientation programs
- Provide programs that meet federal and state educational requirements

THE NURSING TEAM

The nursing team involves those who provide nursing care—RNs, LPNs/LVNs, and nursing assistants. Their roles and responsibilities differ. All focus on the needs of residents and families.

Registered Nurses

A registered nurse (RN) has completed a 2-, 3-, or 4-year nursing program and has passed a licensing test:

- Community college programs—2 years
- Hospital-based diploma programs—2 or 3 years
- College or university programs—4 years

Nursing and the biological, social, and physical sciences are studied. The graduate nurse takes a licensing test offered by a state board of nursing. The nurse receives a license and becomes *registered* when the test is passed. RNs must have a license recognized by the state in which they work.

RNs assess, make nursing diagnoses, plan, implement, and evaluate nursing care (Chapter 7). They develop care plans for each person and provide care. They also delegate nursing care and tasks to the nursing team. They evaluate how the care plans and nursing care affect each person. RNs teach persons how to improve health and independence. They also teach the family.

RNs carry out the doctor's orders. They may delegate them to LPNs/LVNs or nursing assistants. RNs do not prescribe treatments or drugs. However, RNs can study to become *clinical nurse specialists* or *nurse practitioners*. These RNs have limited diagnosing and prescribing functions.

Licensed Practical Nurses and Licensed Vocational Nurses

A licensed practical nurse (LPN) has completed a 1-year nursing program and has passed a licensing test. Hospitals, community colleges, vocational schools, and technical schools offer programs. Some programs are 10 months long; others take 18 months. Some high schools offer 2-year programs.

Graduates take a licensing test for practical nursing. After passing the test, the person receives a license to practice and the title of *licensed practical nurse*. Licensed vocational nurse (LVN) is used in some states. LPNs/LVNs must have a license required by the state in which they work.

LPNs/LVNs are supervised by RNs, licensed doctors, and licensed dentists. They have fewer responsibilities and functions than RNs do. They need little supervision when the person's condition is stable and care is simple. They assist RNs in caring for acutely ill persons and with complex procedures.

Nursing Assistants

Nursing assistants give basic nursing care under the supervision of a licensed nurse. *Nurse aide, nursing attendant,* and *health care assistant* are some other titles.

Nursing assistants give much of the care provided in nursing centers. To work in a nursing center, they must have formal training and pass a competency test (Chapter 3).

NURSING CARE PATTERNS

Nursing care is given in many ways. The pattern used depends on how many persons need care, the staff, and the cost.

- Functional nursing focuses on tasks and jobs. Each nursing team member has certain tasks and jobs to do. For example, one nurse gives all drugs. Another gives all treatments. Nursing assistants give baths, make beds, and serve meals.
- Team nursing involves a team of nursing staff led by an RN ("team leader") who delegates care to other nurses. Some nursing tasks and procedures are delegated to nursing assistants. Delegation (Chapter 3) is based on the person's needs and team member abilities. Team members report to the team leader about observations made and the care given.
- Primary nursing involves total care. An RN is responsible for the person's total care. The nursing team assists as needed. The RN ("primary nurse") gives nursing care and makes discharge plans. The RN teaches and counsels the person and family.

See *Focus on Rehabilitation: Nursing Care Patterns,* p. 6.

Case management is often used in rehabilitation and sub-acute care. In **case management**, a case manager (an RN) coordinates a person's care from admission through discharge and into the home setting. He or she communicates with the person's doctor and the health team. There also is communication with the insurance company and community agencies as needed. The case manager also helps the health team work together.

THE INTERDISCIPLINARY HEALTH CARE TEAM

The **interdisciplinary health care team** (*health team*) involves the many health care workers whose skills and knowledge focus on the person's total care (Table 1-1). The team provides supportive services for the overall goal of quality resident care (Fig. 1-3, p. 8). They work together to meet each person's needs. Many health care workers are involved in the care of each person. Coordinated care is needed. An RN leads this team.

See *Focus on Communication: The Interdisciplinary Health Care Team*, p. 8.

Table 1-1 Health Team Members

Title	Description	Credentials
Activities director	Assesses, plans, and implements recreational needs	Varies with state and/or employer; ranges from no training to bachelor's degree
Audiologist	Tests hearing; prescribes hearing aids; works with persons who are hard-of-hearing	Master's degree or higher; state license
Cleric (clergyman; clergywoman)	Assists with spiritual needs	Priest, minister, rabbi, sister (nun), deacon, or other pastoral training
Clinical laboratory technologist	Performs complicated laboratory tests on blood, urine, and other body fluids, secretions, and excretions; organizes, supervises, and performs diagnostic analyses	Bachelor's degree; national certification test; license in some states
Clinical nurse specialist	Provides nursing care and consults in a nursing specialty—geriatrics, critical care, diabetes, rehabilitation, and wound care are examples	RN with master's degree or doctorate as a clinical nurse specialist
Dental hygienist	Focuses on preventing dental disorders; supervised by a licensed dentist	Completion of a dental hygiene program; state license
Dentist	Prevents and treats disorders and diseases of the teeth, gums, and oral structures	Doctor of dental science (DDS) or doctor of dental medicine (DMD); state license
Dietitian and nutritionist	Assesses and plans for nutritional needs; teaches good nutrition, food selection, and preparation	Bachelor's degree; registered dietitian (RD) must pass a national registration test; license or certification in some states
Licensed practical/ vocational nurse (LPN/LVN)	Provides direct nursing care, including giving drugs, under the direction of an RN	State-approved program (usually 1 year in length); state license
Medical or clinical laboratory technician	Collects samples and performs laboratory tests on blood, urine, and other body fluids, secretions, and excretions	Associate's degree; national certifying test; license in some states
Medical records and health information technician	Maintains medical records; transcribes medical reports; files records; completes required reports	Associate's degree; credentialing test

Table 1-1 Health Team Members—cont'd

Title	Description	Credentials
Medication assistant-certified (MA-C)	Gives drugs as allowed by state law under the supervision of an RN or LPN/LVN	Certified nursing assistant with additional education and training as required by state law; state certification
Nurse practitioner	Plans and provides care with the health team; does physical exams, health assessments, and health education	RN with master's degree or higher and clinical experience in an area of nursing; certification test may be required
Nursing assistant	Assists nurses and gives nursing care; supervised by an RN or LPN/LVN	Completion of a state-approved training and competency evaluation program to work in long-term care or in home care agencies receiving Medicare funds; state registry; state certification or license
Occupational therapist registered (OTR)	Assists persons to learn or retain skills needed to perform daily activities; designs adaptive equipment for daily living	Master's degree or higher; national certification; state license
Occupational therapy assistant	Performs tasks and services supervised by an OT	Associate's degree; national certification; license in some states
Pharmacist	Fills drug orders written by doctors; monitors and evaluates drug interactions; consults with doctors and nurses about drug actions and interactions	Pharm. D. degree; state license
Physical therapist (PT)	Assists persons with musculo-skeletal problems to restore function and prevent disability	Master's degree or higher; state license
Physical therapy assistant	Performs tasks and services supervised by a PT	Associate's degree; national certification or license in some states
Physician (doctor)	Diagnoses and treats diseases and injuries	Medical school graduation (MD), residency, and national board certification; state license
Physician's assistant (PA)	Assists in diagnosis and treatment; performs medical tasks supervised by a doctor	Associate's degree or higher; national certification exam; license in some states
Podiatrist	Prevents, diagnoses, and treats foot disorders	Doctor of podiatric medicine (DPM); state license
Radiographer/radiologic technologist	Takes x-rays and processes film for viewing	Associate's degree or higher; license in some states
Registered nurse (RN)	Assesses, makes nursing diagnoses, plans, implements, and evaluates nursing care; supervises LPNs/LVNs and nursing assistants	Associate's degree, diploma, or bachelor's degree; state license
Respiratory therapist (RT)	Assists in treating lung and heart disorders; gives respiratory treatments and therapies	Associate's degree; national certification test; license in most states
Social worker	Deals with social, emotional, and environmental issues affecting illness and recovery; coordinates community agencies to assist patients, residents, and families	Bachelor's degree or higher; 2 years supervised work experience for clinical social workers; license, certification, or registration
Speech-language pathologist	Evaluates speech and language and treats persons with speech, voice, hearing, communication, and swallowing disorders	Master's degree; supervised work experience and national test for licensure in most states

Modified from Bureau of Labor Statistics, U.S. Department of Labor, Occupational Handbook, 2010-2011 edition.

Fig. 1-3 Members of the health team. The person is the focus of care.

PAYING FOR HEALTH CARE

Health care is a major focus in society. The goals are to provide health care to everyone and to reduce the high cost of care. Hospital and nursing center care is costly. So are doctor visits, drugs, medical supplies, and home care. Most people cannot afford these costs. Some avoid medical care because they cannot pay. Others pay doctor bills but go without food or drugs. Health care bills cause worry, fear, and emotional upset. If the person has insurance, some care costs are covered. Rarely is the total cost of care covered.

These programs help pay for health care:
- *Private insurance* is bought by individuals and families. The insurance company pays for some or all health care costs.
- *Group insurance* is bought by groups or organizations for individuals. This is often an employee benefit.

- **Medicare** is a federal health insurance program for persons 65 years of age or older. Some younger people with certain disabilities are covered. Part A pays for some hospital, SNF, hospice, and home care costs. Part B helps pay for doctors' services, outpatient hospital care, physical and occupational therapists, some home care, and many other services. Part B is voluntary. The person pays a monthly premium.
- **Medicaid** is a health care payment program. Sponsored by the federal government, it is operated by the states. People with low incomes usually qualify. So do some older, blind, and disabled persons. There is no insurance premium. The amount paid for covered services is limited.

See *Promoting Safety and Comfort: Paying for Health Care.*

Prospective Payment Systems

Prospective payment systems limit the amount paid by insurers, Medicare, and Medicaid. Prospective means *before* care.

- *Medicare Severity-adjusted diagnosis-related groups (MS-DRGs)* are for hospital costs.
- *Resource utilization groups (RUGs)* are for SNF payments.
- *Case mix groups (CMGs)* are used for rehabilitation centers.

Length of stay and treatment costs are determined for each group. If the treatment costs are less than the amount paid, the agency keeps the extra money. If costs are greater, the agency takes the loss.

Managed Care

Managed care deals with health care delivery and payment (Box 1-1). Insurers contract with doctors and hospitals for reduced rates or discounts. The insured person uses doctors and agencies providing the lower rates. If others are used, care is covered in part or not at all. The person pays for costs not covered by insurance.

Managed care limits the choice of where to go for health care. It also limits the care that doctors provide. Managed care is common for Medicaid and Medicare coverage.

Managed Care as Pre-Approval for Services Many insurers must approve the need for health care services. If the need is approved, the insurer pays for the services. If the need is not approved, the person pays for the costs. The pre-approval process depends on the insurer.

This pre-approval process is also called *managed care.* It includes monitoring care. The purpose is to reduce unneeded services and procedures. The insurer decides what to pay. With HMOs and PPOs, the insurer may decide where the person goes for services.

MEETING STANDARDS

Nursing centers must meet certain standards. Standards are set by the federal and state governments. They also are set by accrediting agencies. Standards relate to center policies and procedures, budget and finances, and quality of care. A center must meet standards for:

- *Licensure.* A license is issued by the state. A center must have a license to operate and provide care.
- *Certification.* This is required to receive Medicare and Medicaid funds.
- *Accreditation.* This is voluntary. It signals quality and excellence.

The Survey Process

Surveys are done to see if the center meets set standards. A survey team will:

- Review policies and procedures
- Review medical records
- Interview staff, residents, and families
- Observe how care is given
- Observe if dignity and privacy are promoted
- Check for cleanliness and safety
- Review budgets and finances
- Make sure the staff meets state requirements (Are doctors and nurses licensed? Are nursing assistants on the state registry?)

The survey team decides if the center meets the standards. If standards are met, the center receives a license, certification, or accreditation.

Sometimes problems are found. A problem is called a *deficiency* (Box 1-2, p. 10). The center is given time to correct it. Usually 60 days are given. Sometimes less time is given. The agency can be fined for uncorrected or serious deficiencies. Or it can lose its license, certification, or accreditation.

Your Role

You have an important role in meeting standards and in the survey process. You must:

- Provide quality care.
- Protect the person's rights.
- Provide for the person's and your own safety.
- Help keep the center clean and safe.
- Conduct yourself in a professional manner.
- Have good work ethics.
- Follow center policies and procedures.
- Answer questions honestly and completely.

Box 1-1 Types of Managed Care

Health Maintenance Organization (HMO)—provides health care services for a pre-paid fee. For the fee, persons receive needed services offered by the HMO. Some have an annual physical exam. Others need hospital care. Whatever services are used, the cost is covered by the pre-paid fee. HMOs focus on preventing disease and maintaining health. Keeping someone healthy costs far less than treating illness.

Preferred Provider Organization (PPO)—is a group of doctors and hospitals. They provide health care at reduced rates. Usually the agreement is between the PPO and an employer or an insurance company. Employees or those insured receive reduced rates for the services used. The person can choose any doctor or hospital in the PPO.

Box 1-2   Common Nursing Center Deficiencies

Surveyors cited nursing homes because they failed to:

- Watch each resident carefully and provide assistive devices to prevent accidents
- Provide the care and services needed to attain or maintain the highest quality of life possible
- Protect residents from abuse, mistreatment, neglect, and/or theft of personal property
- Keep each resident free from unneeded physical restraints
- Provide activities to meet each person's needs
- Listen to resident or family groups or act on their complaints or suggestions
- Hire only people with no legal history of abusing, neglecting, or mistreating residents
- Report or investigate any acts of abuse, neglect, or mistreatment
- Keep the nursing home area free of dangers that cause accidents

From www.medicare.gov.

QUALITY OF LIFE

Nursing center care is always focused on the resident. The interdisciplinary health care team helps all residents to become or remain as independent as possible. This promotes their quality of life. Always remember to let residents do as much for themselves as safely possible. This helps their feelings of independence. Do not do or take over tasks that residents can do themselves.

REVIEW QUESTIONS

Circle the BEST answer.

1 Helping persons return to their highest physical and mental function is called
   a Maintaining independence
   b Promoting health
   c Preventing disease
   d Rehabilitation

2 Which provides 24-hour nursing care?
   a Board and care homes
   b Assisted living residences
   c Nursing centers
   d Residential care facilities

3 Rehabilitation starts when the
   a Person is ready to leave the center
   b Person is admitted to the center
   c Doctor writes the order
   d Health team thinks the person is ready

4 Who controls policy in a nursing center?
   a The director of nursing
   b The owner
   c The health team
   d Medicare and Medicaid

5 A health care program for dying persons is a
   a Hospice
   b Board and care home
   c Skilled nursing facility
   d Home care agency

6 The nursing team does *not* include
   a Doctors
   b LPNs/LVNs
   c Nursing assistants
   d RNs

7 Who is responsible for the entire nursing staff?
   a The case manager
   b The RN
   c The director of nursing
   d The medical director

8 Nursing assistants are supervised by
   a RNs and LPN/LVNs
   b Other nursing assistants
   c The health team
   d The medical director

9 The nursing assistant's role is to
   a Meet Medicare and Medicaid standards
   b Assist nurses in giving care
   c Carry out the doctor's orders
   d Manage care

10 Nursing tasks are delegated according to a person's needs and staff member abilities. This nursing care pattern is called
   a Team nursing
   b Functional nursing
   c Case management
   d Primary nursing

11 Medicare is for persons who
   a Are 65 years of age and older
   b Are part of a PPO
   c Have group insurance
   d Have low incomes

12 A survey team is at your center. A team member asks you some questions. You should
   a Refer all questions to the nurse
   b Answer as the DON tells you to
   c Give as little information as possible
   d Give honest and complete answers

Answers to these questions are on p. 719.

Resident Rights

OBJECTIVES

- Define the key terms and key abbreviation listed in this chapter.
- Describe the purpose and requirements of the Omnibus Budget Reconciliation Act of 1987 (OBRA).

- Identify the person's rights under OBRA.
- Explain how to protect the person's rights.
- Explain the ombudsman role.
- Explain how to promote quality of life.

KEY TERMS

involuntary seclusion Separating a person from others against his or her will, keeping the person to a certain area, or keeping the person away from his or her room without consent

ombudsman Someone who supports or promotes the needs and interests of another person

representative Any person who has the legal right to act on the resident's behalf when he or she cannot do so for himself or herself

treatment The care provided to maintain or restore health, improve function, or relieve symptoms

KEY ABBREVIATIONS

CMS   Centers for Medicare & Medicaid Services

OBRA   Omnibus Budget Reconciliation Act of 1987

In 1987 the U.S. Congress passed the *Omnibus Budget Reconciliation Act (OBRA)*. This federal law applies to all 50 states. OBRA requires that nursing centers provide care in a manner and in a setting that maintains or improves each person's quality of life, health, and safety. It also requires nursing assistant training and competency evaluation (Chapter 3). Resident rights are a major part of OBRA.

RESIDENT RIGHTS

Residents have rights as United States citizens. For example, they have the right to vote. They also have rights relating to their everyday lives and care in a nursing center. These rights are protected by federal and state laws. Nursing centers must protect and promote such rights. The center cannot interfere with a resident's rights.

Some residents are incompetent (not able). They cannot exercise their rights. A representative (partner, adult child, court-appointed guardian) does so for them. A representative is any person who has the legal right to act on the resident's behalf when he or she cannot do so for himself or herself.

Nursing centers must inform residents of their rights. Centers must also inform residents of all rules about resident conduct and responsibilities in the center. This is done orally and in writing. Such information is given before or during admission to the center, as needed during the person's stay, and when laws (state or federal) or center rules change. It is given in the language the person uses and understands.

- Medical terms are avoided to the extent possible.
- An interpreter is used if the person speaks and understands a foreign language or communicates by sign language.
- Written translations are provided in the foreign languages common in the center's geographic area.
- Sign language and other communication aids are used as necessary.
- Large-print texts are available for persons with impaired vision.

Resident rights (Box 2-1) are posted throughout the center (Fig. 2-1). Those that affect your role are described in this chapter.

Information

The *right to information* means access to all records about the person. They include the medical record, contracts, incident reports, and financial records. The request can be oral or written.

The person has the right to be fully informed of his or her health condition. Information is given in a language and in words the person can understand. Interpreters are used as needed. Sign language or other aids are used for those with hearing losses.

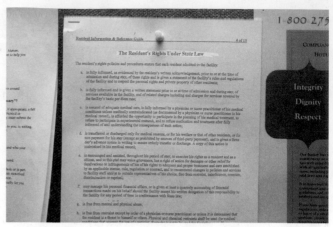

Fig. 2-1 Resident rights are posted in the nursing center.

The person must also have information about his or her doctor. This includes the doctor's name, specialty, and how to contact the doctor.

Report any request for information to the nurse. *You do not give the information described above to the person or family (Chapter 3).*

Refusing Treatment

The person has *the right to refuse treatment.* Treatment means the care provided to maintain or restore health, improve function, or relieve symptoms. A person who does not give consent (Chapter 4) or refuses treatment cannot be treated against his or her wishes. The center must find out what the person is refusing and why. For example, a person learned to walk after a hip fracture. However, the person refuses to walk. The center must:

- Find out the reason for the refusal.
- Educate the person about the problems that can result from not walking.
- Offer other treatment options.
- Continue to provide all other services.

Advance directives are part of the right to refuse treatment (Chapter 48). They include living wills and instructions about life support. *Advance directives* are written instructions about health care when the person is not able to make such decisions.

Report any treatment refusal to the nurse. The nurse may change the person's care plan.

Privacy and Confidentiality

Residents have the *right to personal privacy.* Staff must provide care in a manner that maintains privacy of the person's body. The person's body is exposed only as necessary. Only staff directly involved in care and treatments are present. The person must give consent for others to be present. For example, a student wants to observe a treatment. The person's consent is needed for the student to observe.

Box 2-1 Resident Rights

- To be treated with dignity and respect. And to receive quality care.
- To exercise one's rights as a center resident and as a citizen of the United States.
- To be informed orally and in writing of one's rights and center rules. This is done in a language the person understands.
- To access all records about himself or herself including current clinical records.
- To obtain copies of one's records. This is at the resident's expense.
- To refuse treatment.
- To refuse to take part in experimental research. This is the development and testing of new treatments and drugs.
- To make advance directives (Chapter 48).
- To be informed of Medicare benefits and services. This includes costs and charges covered and not covered.
- To file complaints with the appropriate state agency about abuse, neglect, and the mis-use of one's property.
- To be informed of center services and of the charges for those services.
- To choose one's doctor.
- To know the name, specialty, and how to contact the doctor responsible for his or her care.
- To be fully informed of his or her total health status, including his or her medical condition.
- To be informed of:
  - Any accident or injury that may need medical attention
  - A change in one's physical, mental, or psycho-social status
  - The need to stop, change, or add a treatment
  - A decision to transfer or discharge the person
  - A change in the person's room or roommate
  - A change in the person's rights under federal or state law
- To manage one's personal and financial affairs.
- To be fully informed in advance about one's care and treatment. This includes changes in care and treatment.
- To privacy and confidentiality:
  - Of personal and medical records
  - Of treatment and personal care
  - Of written and phone communications
  - During visits with family and friends
  - When meeting with resident groups

- To voice grievances and have them solved promptly.
- To see the results of federal and state surveys. The person also has the right to see the plans to correct problems or areas of weakness.
- To perform services for the center or to refuse to perform services.
- To send and receive mail that is not open. To buy supplies to send mail.
- To receive information from one's doctor and community and state agencies responsible for protecting developmentally disabled and mentally ill persons.
- To have and use personal items and clothing.
- To share a room with one's spouse (husband, wife) when married residents live in the same center (Chapter 11).
- To take one's drugs without help if able.
- To receive notice before one's room or roommate is changed.
- To refuse to change to a different room.
- To have reasonable notice about a transfer or discharge (Chapter 34).
- To be free from physical and chemical restraints (Chapter 14).
- To be free from abuse (verbal, sexual, physical), bodily punishment, and involuntary seclusion (Chapter 4).
- To be cared for in a manner and in a setting that maintains or enhances quality of life.
- To choose activities, schedules, and health care that meets one's interest.
- To interact with community members inside and outside of the center.
- To make choices about one's life in the center.
- To organize and take part in resident groups.
- To take part in social, religious, and community activities.
- To a setting and services that consider one's needs and choices.
- To be informed of his or her health and medical condition in a language that he or she understands. That language is used when he or she takes part in care planning.
- To a clean, comfortable, and home-like setting. This includes temperature, lighting, and sound levels.
- To attain or maintain one's highest level of function.
- To closet space.
- To visit with one's spouse, family, and friends at any reasonable hour.

OBRA-CMS

A person has the right to use the bathroom in private. Privacy is maintained for all personal care measures. Bathing and dressing are examples. Protect privacy by:
- Closing privacy curtains, doors, and window coverings
- Removing residents from public view
- Providing clothes or draping the person to prevent unnecessary exposure of body parts
- Practicing the measures listed in Chapter 4

Leaving the person without a gown or bed covers violates the person's right to privacy. So does leaving the room door open when the person uses the bathroom or bedpan.

Residents have the right to visit with others in private—in areas where others cannot see or hear them. If requested, the center must provide private space. Offices, chapels, dining rooms, and meeting rooms are used as needed.

Fig. 2-2 A resident is talking privately on the phone.

Fig. 2-3 A resident is choosing what clothing to wear.

Residents have the right to make phone calls in private (Fig. 2-2). The calls must not be where they can be overheard. Therefore phones are not used in offices or at the nurses' station. Centers provide cordless phones or phone jacks in resident rooms. Phones are at the correct height for use by persons in wheelchairs. Phones for hearing-impaired persons are also available. Some residents have their own wireless phones.

The right to privacy also involves mail. The person has the right to send and receive mail without others interfering. No one can open mail the person sends or receives without his or her consent. Unopened mail is given to the person within 24 hours of delivery to the center. Mail the person sends is delivered to the postal service within 24 hours when there is regular delivery or pick-up service.

Information about the person's care, treatment, and condition is kept confidential. So are medical and financial records. Consent is needed to release them to other agencies or persons.

You must provide privacy and protect confidentiality. Doing so shows respect for the person. It also protects the person's dignity. Privacy and confidentiality are discussed in Chapters 3 and 4.

Personal Choice

Residents have the *right to make their own choices*. They can choose their own doctors. They also have the right to take part in planning and deciding about their care and treatment. They can choose activities, schedules, and care based on their preferences. They can choose when to get up and go to bed, what to wear, how to spend time, and what to eat (Fig. 2-3). They can choose friends and visitors inside and outside the center.

Personal choice promotes quality of life, dignity, and self-respect. You must allow personal choice whenever safely possible.

Grievances

Residents have the *right to voice concerns, questions, and complaints about treatment or care*. The problem may involve another person. It may be about care that was given or not given. The center must promptly try to correct the matter. No one can punish the person in any way for voicing the grievance.

Work

The person does not work for care, care items, or other things or privileges. The person is not required to perform services for the center.

However, the person has *the right to work or perform services if he or she wants to*. Some people like to garden, repair or build things, clean, sew, mend, or cook. Other persons need work for rehabilitation or activity reasons. The desire or need for work is part of the person's care plan. Residents volunteer or are paid for their services.

Taking Part in Resident Groups

The person has the *right to form and take part in resident groups*. Families have the right to meet with other families. These groups can discuss concerns and suggest center improvements. They also can support each other, plan activities, and take part in educational activities.

Residents have the *right to take part in social, cultural, religious, and community events*. They have the *right to help in getting to and from events of their choice*.

Personal Items

Residents have the *right to keep and use personal items*. This includes clothing and some furnishings. The type

OBRA-CMS

and amount of personal items allowed depend on space needs and the health and safety of others.

Treat the person's property with care and respect. The items may not have value to you. However, they having meaning to the person. They also relate to personal choice, dignity, a home-like setting, and quality of life.

The person's property is protected. Items are labeled with the person's name. The center must investigate reports of lost, stolen, or damaged items. Police help is sometimes needed. The person and family are advised not to keep jewelry and other costly items in the center.

Protect yourself and the center from being accused of stealing a person's property. Do not go through a person's closet, drawers, purse, or other space without the person's knowledge and consent. A nurse may ask you to inspect closets and drawers. Center policy should require that a co-worker and the person or legal representative be present. The co-worker is a witness to your activities. Follow center policy for reporting and recording the inspection.

Freedom From Abuse, Mistreatment, and Neglect

Residents have the *right to be free from verbal, sexual, physical, and mental abuse* (Chapter 4). *Abuse* means:
- The willful infliction of injury, unreasonable confinement, intimidation (to threaten to hurt or punish), or punishment that results in physical harm, pain, or mental anguish
- Depriving the person of the goods or services needed to attain or maintain well-being

They also have the right to be free from involuntary seclusion:
- Separating a person from others against his or her will
- Keeping the person confined to a certain area
- Keeping the person away from his or her room without consent

No one can abuse, neglect, or mistreat a resident. This includes center staff, volunteers, and staff from other agencies or groups. It also includes other residents, family members, friends, visitors, and legal representatives. Nursing centers must investigate suspected or reported cases of abuse. They cannot employ persons who:
- Were found guilty of abusing, neglecting, or mistreating others by a court of law.
- Have a finding entered into the state's nursing assistant registry (Chapter 3) about abuse, neglect, mistreatment, or wrongful acts involving the person's money or property. A *finding* means that a state has determined that the employee abused, neglected, mistreated, or wrongfully used the person's money or property.

Freedom From Restraint

Residents have the *right not to have body movements restricted*. Restraints and certain drugs can restrict body movements. Some drugs can restrain the person because they affect mood, behavior, and mental function. Sometimes residents are restrained to protect them from harming themselves or others. A doctor's order is needed for restraint use. Restraints are not used for staff convenience or to discipline a person. They are used only if required to treat the person's medical symptoms. Restraints are discussed in Chapter 14.

Quality of Life

Residents have the *right to quality of life*. Nursing centers must care for residents in a manner and in a setting that promotes dignity and respect for self. This means that staff provide care in a manner that maintains or enhances the person's self-esteem and feelings of self-worth. Staff must promote physical, mental, and psychosocial well-being. Protecting resident rights promotes quality of life. It shows respect for the person.

The person is spoken to in a polite and courteous manner. Good, honest, and thoughtful care enhances the person's quality of life. Box 2-2, p. 16 lists OBRA-required actions that promote dignity and privacy.

Activities

Residents have the *right to activities that enhance each person's physical, mental, and psycho-social well-being*. The intent is to promote self-esteem, pleasure, comfort, education, creativity, success, and independence. They must have a purpose and relate to the person's needs, interests, culture, and background. Centers also provide religious services for spiritual health. Activities must have meaning for the person. They are meaningful when they:
- Reflect the person's interests and life-style
- Are enjoyed by the person
- Help the person feel useful or produce something useful
- Provide a sense of belonging

Activities may involve large or small groups. A concert is a large group activity. A card game is a small group activity. Other activities involve two people. Or the person does something alone. Writing a letter and playing a computer game are examples.

You assist residents to and from activity programs. You may need to help them with activities.

See *Teamwork and Time Management: Activities* p. 16.
See *Focus on Communication: Activities* p. 16.

OBRA-CMS

Box 2-2   OBRA-Required Actions to Promote Dignity and Privacy

Courteous and Dignified Interactions
- Use the right tone of voice.
- Use good eye contact.
- Stand or sit close enough as needed.
- Use the person's proper name and title. For example: "Mrs. Crane."
- Gain the person's attention before interacting with him or her.
- Use touch if the person approves.
- Respect the person's social status.
- Listen with interest to what the person is saying.
- Do not yell at, scold, or embarrass the person.

Privacy and Self-Determination
- Drape properly during care and procedures to avoid exposure and embarrassment.
- Drape properly in chair.
- Use privacy curtains or screens during care and procedures.
- Close the room door during care and procedures as the person desires. Also close window coverings.
- Knock on the door before entering. Wait to be asked in.
- Close the bathroom door when the person uses the bathroom.

Maintain Personal Choice and Independence
- Person smokes in allowed areas.
- Person takes part in activities according to his or her interests.
- Person takes part in scheduling activities and care.

Maintain Personal Choice and Independence—cont'd
- Person gives input into the care plan about preferences and independence.
- Person is involved in room or roommate change.
- The person's items are moved or inspected only with the person's consent.

Courteous and Dignified Care
- Groom hair, beards, and nails as the person wishes.
- Assist with dressing in the right clothing for time of day and personal choice.
- Promote independence and dignity in dining.
- Respect private space and property. For example, change radio or TV stations only with the person's consent.
- Assist with walking and transfers. Do not interfere with independence.
- Assist with bathing and hygiene preferences. Do not interfere with independence.
  - Appearance is neat and clean.
  - The person is clean shaven or has a groomed beard and mustache.
  - Nails are trimmed and clean.
  - Dentures, hearing aids, eyeglasses, and other devices are used correctly.
  - Clothing is clean.
  - Clothing is properly fitted and fastened.
  - Shoes, hose, and socks are properly applied and fastened.
  - Extra clothing is worn for warmth as needed. Sweaters and lap blankets are examples.

TEAMWORK AND TIME MANAGEMENT
Activities

Residents may need help getting to and from activity programs. Know when an activity begins and ends. Do the following before assisting residents to activity areas:
- Assist with elimination needs and hand washing.
- Assist with grooming measures such as brushing and combing hair. A person may want to apply some perfume or make-up.
- Make sure the person wears the correct clothing and footwear for the activity.
- Make sure the person has needed assistive devices. Eyeglasses, hearing aids, canes, and walkers are examples.

Allow 15 to 20 minutes to assist residents to and from the activity area. Help your co-workers as needed.

You may have to help residents with activities (Fig. 2-4). If not, use the activity time wisely. Provide needed care and visit residents who cannot leave their rooms. You can also clean and straighten rooms, bathrooms, shower rooms, and utility rooms.

FOCUS ON COMMUNICATION
Activities

You may need help assisting residents to and from activity programs. Politely ask a co-worker to help you. Share this information with your co-worker:
- What time you need the help.
- How much of the co-worker's time you need.
- The residents you need help with.
- If the person walks or uses a wheelchair.
- What assistive devices are used. Eyeglasses, hearing aids, canes, and walkers are examples.

Be sure to say "please" when asking for help. And thank the person for helping you. For example:

"Jane, can you please help me assist two residents to the concert? It starts at 1:00 so I'll need your help at 12:45. Mr. Harris needs his glasses and hearing aid. He'll use a walker. Mrs. Janz uses a wheelchair. She needs her glasses and a blanket for her lap. The blanket is in her wheelchair. The concert is over at 2:00. Please help me then, too. Thank you so much for helping me."

Fig. 2-4 A nursing assistant is helping residents in an activity program.

Environment

Residents have the *right to a safe, clean, comfortable, and home-like setting*. The person is allowed to have and use personal items to the extent possible.

The center must provide a setting and services that meet the person's needs and preferences. The setting and staff must promote the person's independence, dignity, and well-being. The center must try to change schedules, call systems, and room arrangements to meet the person's desires and needs.

For example, the center must make changes when a person:

- Refuses a bath because he or she prefers a shower.
- Prefers to have a shower at a different time or day.
- Refuses a shower because of the fear of falling.
- Is uneasy about the staff assigned to help him or her.
- Is worried about falling.
- Cannot reach or use the signal light.
- Cannot reach personal items.
- Does not like the food served.

OMBUDSMAN PROGRAM

The Older Americans Act is a federal law. It requires a long-term care ombudsman program in every state. An ombudsman is someone who supports or promotes the needs and interests of another person. Long-term care ombudsmen are employed by a state agency. Some are volunteers. They are not nursing center employees. They act on behalf of nursing center and assisted-living residents.

Ombudsmen protect the health, safety, welfare, and rights of residents. They:

- Investigate and resolve complaints.
- Provide services to assist residents.
- Provide information about long-term care services.
- Monitor nursing center care.
- Monitor nursing center conditions.
- Provide support to resident and family groups.
- Help the resident and family resolve conflicts within the family.
- Help the center manage difficult problems.
- Educate residents, families, and the public about long-term care issues and concerns.
- Represent residents' interests before local, state, and federal governments.

Residents have the right to voice grievances and disputes. They also have the right to communicate privately with anyone of their choice. They can share concerns with anyone outside the center.

OBRA requires that nursing centers post the names, addresses, and phone numbers of local and state ombudsmen. This information must be posted where residents can easily see it.

A resident or family may share a concern with you. You must know state and center policies and procedures for contacting an ombudsman. Ombudsman services are useful when:

- There is concern about a person's care or treatment.
- Someone interferes with a person's rights, health, safety, or welfare.

QUALITY OF LIFE

OBRA is concerned with the quality of life, health, and safety of residents. All care must maintain or improve each person's quality of life. The information and procedures in this book help you provide the best quality care. Everything you do must maintain or improve each person's quality of life, health, and safety. If you remember this, your job will be rewarding and enjoyable.

REVIEW QUESTIONS

Circle the BEST answer.

1 OBRA is a
  a State law
  b Federal law
  c State agency
  d Federal agency

2 A son has the legal right to act on his mother's behalf. The son is his mother's legal
  a Ombudsman
  b Representative
  c Caregiver
  d Health care provider

3 A daughter wants to read her father's medical record. What should you do?
  a Give her the medical record.
  b Ask the resident if you can give the daughter the record.
  c Tell the nurse.
  d Tell her that she cannot do so.

4 A resident refuses to have a shower. What should you do?
  a Tell her that she cannot refuse a shower.
  b Tell her daughter.
  c Give her a bath instead.
  d Tell the nurse.

5 Which violates the person's right to privacy?
  a Closing the bathroom door when the person uses the bathroom
  b Opening the window blinds when assisting with bathing
  c Covering the person when giving personal care
  d Asking the person's permission to observe a treatment

6 A resident has a phone in his room. He wants to make a phone call. What should you do?
  a Leave the room.
  b Tell the nurse.
  c Ask him to use the phone at the nurses' station.
  d Close the privacy curtain so you can stay in the room to finish your tasks.

7 Who decides how to style a person's hair?
  a The person
  b The nurse
  c You
  d The ombudsman

8 Residents do *not* have a right to
  a A private room
  b Refuse treatment
  c Contact an ombudsman
  d Make personal choices

9 A person brought furniture and other items from home. They are
  a Sent home with the family
  b Labeled with the person's name
  c Arranged as you prefer
  d Shared with other residents

10 Residents have the right to be free from the following *except*
  a Disease
  b Abuse
  c Involuntary seclusion
  d Neglect

11 Who selects activities for a resident?
  a The nurse
  b You
  c The person's representative
  d The person

12 The center must provide the following *except*
  a A safe and clean setting
  b A comfortable setting
  c A home-like setting
  d A noise-free setting

13 A long-term care ombudsman
  a Is employed by the nursing center
  b Investigates resident complaints
  c Grants a nursing center a license or certification
  d Can prevent a resident from leaving the center

14 Which action does *not* promote a person's dignity?
  a Restraining the person
  b Providing privacy during personal care
  c Making sure the person has needed assistive devices
  d Listening to the person

15 Which is the correct way to address a person?
  a "Hello, sweetie."
  b "Hello, Mrs. Smith."
  c "Hello, Jim."
  d "Hello, Grandpa."

16 Which does *not* promote dignity or privacy?
  a Knocking before entering the person's room
  b Closing the bathroom door when the person uses the bathroom.
  c Assisting with bathing and hygiene preferences
  d Moving the person's items as you prefer

Circle T if the statement is TRUE. Circle F if the statement is FALSE.

17 T F   OBRA applies to all 50 states.
18 T F   Nursing center residents have rights as U.S. citizens.
19 T F   Residents are informed of their rights only in writing.
20 T F   You should open the person's mail within 24 hours of it being delivered to the center.
21 T F   A resident complains about the food. The center must try to provide desired foods.
22 T F   Residents must provide some type of work for the center.
23 T F   Resident groups can discuss ideas for activity programs.
24 T F   An employee was found guilty of abusing a resident. The center can continue to employ the person.
25 T F   You can restrain a resident to provide care.

Answers to these questions are on p. 719.

The Nursing Assistant in Long-Term Care

OBJECTIVES

- Define the key terms and key abbreviations listed in this chapter.
- Explain the history and current trends affecting nursing assistants.
- Explain the laws that affect nursing assistants.
- List the reasons for denying, suspending, or revoking a nursing assistant's certification, license, or registration.
- Describe the training and competency evaluation requirements for nursing assistants.
- Identify the information in the nursing assistant registry.
- Explain how to obtain certification, a license, or registration in another state.

- Describe what nursing assistants can do and their role limits.
- Describe the standards for nursing assistants developed by the National Council of State Boards of Nursing.
- Explain why a job description is important.
- Describe the delegation process.
- Explain your role in the delegation process.
- Explain how to accept or refuse a delegated task.
- Explain how to promote quality of life.

KEY TERMS

accountable Being responsible for one's actions and the actions of others who performed delegated tasks; answering questions about and explaining one's actions and the actions of others

delegate To authorize another person to perform a nursing task in a certain situation

job description A document that describes what the center expects you to do

nursing task Nursing care or a nursing function, procedure, activity, or work that can be delegated to nursing assistants when it does not require an RN's professional knowledge or judgment

responsibility The duty or obligation to perform some act or function

Federal and state laws and nursing center policies combine to define the roles and functions of each health team member. Everyone must protect residents from harm. To do so, you need to know:

- What you can and cannot do
- Your legal limits

Laws, job descriptions, and the person's condition shape your work. So does the amount of supervision you need.

HISTORY AND CURRENT TRENDS

For decades, nursing assistants have helped nurses with basic nursing care. Often called *nurse's aides*, they gave baths and made beds. They helped with grooming, elimination, and other needs. Their work was similar in hospitals and nursing centers. Until the 1980s, training was not required by law. Nurses gave on-the-job training. Some hospitals, nursing centers, and schools offered nursing assistant courses.

Before the 1980s, team nursing was common. A registered nurse (RN) was the team leader. The RN assigned care to nurses and nursing assistants. Care was assigned according to each person's needs and condition. It also depended on the staff member's education and experiences.

Primary nursing was common in the 1980s. RNs planned and gave care. Many hospitals only hired RNs. Meanwhile, nursing centers relied on nursing assistants for resident care.

Home care increased during the 1980s. Prospective payment systems limit health care payments (Chapter 1). To reduce care costs, hospital stays also are limited. Therefore patients are discharged earlier than in the past. Often they are still quite ill and need home care.

Efforts to reduce health care costs include:

- *Hospital closings.* Many do not make enough money to stay open.
- *Hospital mergers.* Hospitals merge to share resources and to avoid the same costly services. For example, one hospital offers heart surgery. The other serves women and children.
- *Health care systems.* Agencies join together as one provider of care. A system often has hospitals, nursing centers, and home care agencies. It also has hospice settings, ambulance services, and doctors. For example, a hospital patient needs long-term care. The person transfers from the hospital to a system nursing center. The person is transported by the system-owned ambulance service. After rehabilitation, the person returns home. The system-owned home care agency provides needed services in the home setting. The person's care stays within the system from the hospital to the home setting.
- *Managed care.* Insurers have contracts with doctors, hospitals, and health care systems for reduced rates. See Chapter 1.
- *Staffing mix.* Hospitals hire RNs, licensed practical nurses/licensed vocational nurses (LPNs/LVNs), and nursing assistants. Most hospitals require a state-approved nursing assistant training and competency evaluation for employment. More training is given for tasks not in the training program.

FEDERAL AND STATE LAWS

The U.S. Congress makes federal laws that all 50 states must follow. State legislatures make state laws. For example, the New York legislature makes state laws for New York. The Texas legislature makes state laws for Texas. You must know the federal and state laws that affect your work. They provide direction for what you can do.

See Chapter 4 for other laws affecting your work.

Nurse Practice Acts

Each state has a nurse practice act. It protects the public's welfare and safety by regulating nursing practice in that state. A nurse practice act:

- Defines RN and LPN/LVN.
- Describes the scope of practice for RNs and LPNs/LVNs.

- Describes education and licensing requirements for RNs and LPNs/LVNs.
- Protects the public from persons practicing nursing without a license. Persons who do not meet the state's requirements cannot perform nursing functions.

The law allows for denying, revoking, or suspending a nursing license. The purpose is to protect the public from unsafe nurses. Reasons include:

- Being convicted of a crime in any state
- Selling or distributing drugs
- Using the person's drugs for oneself
- Placing a person in danger from the over-use of alcohol or drugs
- Demonstrating grossly negligent nursing practice
- Being convicted of abusing or neglecting children or older persons
- Violating a nurse practice act and its rules and regulations
- Demonstrating incompetent behaviors
- Aiding or assisting another person to violate a nurse practice act and its rules and regulations
- Making medical diagnoses
- Prescribing drugs and treatments

Nursing Assistants A state's nurse practice act is used to decide what nursing assistants can do. Some nurse practice acts also regulate nursing assistant roles, functions, education, and certification requirements. Other states have separate laws for nursing assistants.

Legal and advisory opinions about nursing assistants are based on the state's nurse practice act. So are any state laws about their roles and functions. If you do something beyond the legal limits of your role, you could be practicing nursing without a license. This creates serious legal problems for you and the nurse supervising your work.

Nursing assistants must be able to function with skill and safety. Like nurses, nursing assistants can have their certification (p. 22) denied, revoked, or suspended. The National Council of State Boards of Nursing (NCSBN) lists these reasons for doing so:

- Substance abuse or dependency.
- Abandoning, abusing, or neglecting a resident.
- Fraud or deceit. Examples include:
  - Filing false personal information
  - Providing false information when applying for initial certification or to have it re-instated
- Violating professional boundaries (Chapter 4).
- Giving unsafe care.
- Performing acts beyond the nursing assistant role.
- Misappropriation (stealing, theft) or mis-using property.
- Obtaining money or property from a resident. Fraud, falsely representing oneself, and through force are examples.

- Having been convicted of a crime. Examples include murder, assault, kidnapping, rape or sexual assault, robbery, sexual crimes involving children, criminal mistreatment of children or a vulnerable adult (Chapter 4), drug trafficking, embezzlement (to take a person's property for one's own use), theft, and arson (starting fires).
- Failing to conform to the standards of nursing assistants (p. 25).
- Putting residents at risk for harm.
- Violating a resident's privacy.
- Failing to maintain the confidentiality of resident information.

OBRA-CMS

The Omnibus Budget Reconciliation Act of 1987

The Omnibus Budget Reconciliation Act of 1987 (OBRA) is a federal law. Its purpose is to improve the quality of life of nursing center residents.

OBRA sets minimum training and competency evaluation requirements for nursing assistants. Each state must have a nursing assistant training and competency evaluation program (NATCEP). A nursing assistant must successfully complete a NATCEP to work in a nursing center, hospital long-term care unit, or home care agency receiving Medicare funds.

The Training Program OBRA requires at least 75 hours of instruction. Some states have more hours. At least 16 hours of supervised practical training are required. Such training occurs in a laboratory or clinical setting (Fig. 3-1, p. 22). Students perform nursing care and tasks on another person. A nurse supervises this practical training (clinical practicum or clinical experience).

The training program includes the knowledge and skills needed to give basic nursing care. Areas of study include:

- Communication
- Infection control
- Safety and emergency procedures
- Residents' rights
- Basic nursing skills
- Personal care skills
- Feeding methods
- Elimination procedures
- Skin care
- Transferring, positioning, and turning methods
- Dressing
- Helping the person walk
- Range-of-motion exercises
- Signs and symptoms of common diseases
- How to care for cognitively impaired persons (those who have problems with thinking and memory)

Competency Evaluation The competency evaluation has a written test and a skills test (Appendix A, p. 722). The written test has multiple-choice questions. Each

Fig. 3-1 Nursing assistant training program. **A,** Students study in a classroom setting. **B,** An instructor demonstrates a skill in a laboratory setting.

has 4 choices. Only 1 answer is correct. The number of questions varies from state to state.

The skills test involves performing nursing skills. You will perform certain skills learned in your training program.

You take the competency evaluation after your training program. Your instructor tells you when and where the tests are given. He or she helps you complete the application. There is a fee for the evaluation. If working in a nursing center, the employer pays this fee. You are told the place and time of the tests after your application is processed. Some states give a choice of test dates and sites.

Your training prepares you for the competency evaluation. If you listen, study hard, and practice safe care, you should do well. If the first attempt was not successful, you can retest. OBRA allows at least 3 attempts to successfully complete the evaluation.

Nursing Assistant Registry OBRA requires a nursing assistant registry in each state. It is an official record or listing of persons who have successfully completed that state's approved NATCEP. The registry has information about each nursing assistant:

- Full name, including maiden name and any married names.
- Last known home address.
- Registry number and the date it expires.
- Date of birth.
- Last known employer, date hired, and date employment ended.
- Date the competency evaluation was passed.
- Information about findings of abuse, neglect, or dishonest use of property. It includes the nature of the offense and supporting evidence. If a hearing was held, the date and its outcome are included. The person has the right to include a statement disputing the finding. All information stays in the registry for at least 5 years.

Any agency (hospital, nursing center, home care agency) can access registry information. You also receive a copy of your registry information. The copy is provided when the first entry is made and when information is changed or added. You can correct wrong information.

Other OBRA Requirements Retraining and a new competency evaluation program are required for nursing assistants who have not worked for 24 months. It does not matter how long you worked as a nursing assistant. What matters is how long you did *not* work. States can require:

- A new competency evaluation
- Both retraining and a new competency evaluation

Nursing centers must provide 12 hours of educational programs to nursing assistants every year. Performance reviews also are required. That is, your work is evaluated. These requirements help ensure that you have the current knowledge and skills to give safe, effective care.

See *Teamwork and Time Management: Other OBRA Requirements.*

Certification

Each state's NATCEP must meet OBRA requirements. Some states require more training hours. And each state has its own competency evaluation program. After successfully completing your state's NATCEP, you have the title used in your state:

- Certified nursing assistant (CNA) or certified nurse aide (CNA). CNA is used in most states.
- Licensed nursing assistant (LNA).
- Registered nurse aide (RNA).

OBRA-CMS

OBRA-CMS

Educational programs in nursing centers are commonly called *in-service programs* or *in-service training.* Some are required; others are optional. Program announcements and schedules are posted on bulletin boards on nursing units, in staff locker rooms and lounges, and by the time clock. Some are included with your paycheck. Know where your agency posts in-service information. Check those areas often.

Such training is scheduled before your shift begins, during your shift, or after your shift. If scheduled before work, plan to arrive early. If scheduled after work, plan to stay late. Arrange for transportation and childcare as needed (Chapter 5).

If the program is during your shift, plan with your co-workers. Some staff stay on the unit while others attend the program. Staff on the unit tend to all residents. A person may have special care needs while you are off the unit. Share this information with the staff who will provide such care. When you return to the unit, thank your co-workers for helping you. Help your co-workers when they leave the unit to attend in-service programs.

Working in Another State To work in another state, you must meet that state's registry requirements. First, contact the state agency responsible for NATCEPs and the nursing assistant registry. To find that agency, do one of the following:

- Contact your current nursing assistant registry.
- Go to the National Council of State Boards of Nursing website. Find the link to the state agency.

Then apply to the state agency to be a CNA (LNA, RNA). The state uses one of these terms: *endorsement, reciprocity,* or *equivalency.* The terms mean that:

- Your application for CNA (LNA, RNA) is reviewed to see if you meet the state's requirements:
  - Your certification (license, registration) is current and in good standing
  - You meet that state's education, work, and legal requirements
- Certification (a license, registration) is granted if the requirements are met.

Follow the application instructions. Expect to:

- Complete the required forms.
- Provide proof of successfully completing a NATCEP. You may need to send a copy of the certificate of completion from your NATCEP. Do not send the original.
- Request written registry verification from the state in which you are currently certified (licensed, registered). Pay the required fee.
- Provide fingerprints.
- Pay the required application fee.

A criminal background check is done. Registry information is checked. Expect an investigation if the check shows a criminal history or if the check shows findings of abuse, neglect, dishonest use of property, or other action against you.

You must be truthful. False or misleading information may result in:

- Denial of certification (a license, registration)
- Disciplinary action
- A fine

The review results in one or more of the following:

- Being granted or denied certification (a license, registration).
- Having to take a competency test. This may be the written test, the skills test, or both.
- Having to take a NATCEP in that state.

ROLES AND RESPONSIBILITIES

Nurse practice acts, OBRA, state laws, and legal and advisory opinions direct what you can do. To protect persons from harm, you must understand what you can do, what you cannot do, and the legal limits of your role. In some states, this is called *scope of practice.* The NCSBN calls it *range of functions.*

Licensed nurses supervise your work. You assist them in giving care. You also perform nursing tasks related to the person's care. A **nursing task** is the nursing care or a nursing function, procedure, activity, or work that can be delegated to nursing assistants when it does not require an RN's professional knowledge or judgment. Often you function without a nurse in the room. At other times you help nurses give care. In some centers, you assist doctors with procedures. The rules in Box 3-1 will help you understand your role.

The range of functions for nursing assistants varies among states and centers. Before you perform a nursing task make sure that:

- Your state allows nursing assistants to do so
- It is in your job description
- You have the necessary education and training
- A nurse is available to answer questions and to supervise you

You perform nursing tasks to meet the person's hygiene, safety, comfort, nutrition, exercise, and elimination needs. You also handle and move persons, make observations, and collect specimens. You help admit and discharge residents. You also measure temperatures, pulses, respirations, and blood pressures. And you help promote the person's mental comfort.

Box 3-2 describes the limits of your role—the nursing tasks that you should never do. State laws differ. You must know what you can do in the state in which you are working. For example, you move from Vermont to Maine. You must learn the laws and rules in Maine. Or you might work in two states. For example, you work in centers in Illinois and Iowa. You must know the laws and rules of both states.

State laws and rules limit nursing assistant functions. Your job description reflects those laws and rules. A center can further limit what you can do. So can a nurse based on the person's needs. However, no center or nurse can expand your range of functions beyond what your state's laws and rules allow.

Box 3-1   Rules for Nursing Assistants

- You are an assistant to the nurse.
- A nurse assigns and supervises your work.
- You report observations about the person's physical and mental status to the nurse (Chapter 7). Report changes in the person's condition or behavior at once.
- The nurse decides what should be done for a person. The nurse decides what should not be done for a person. You do not make these decisions.
- Review directions and the care plan with the nurse before going to the person.
- Perform only those tasks for which you are trained.
- Ask a nurse to supervise you if you are not comfortable performing a nursing task.
- Perform only the nursing tasks that your state and job description allow.

Box 3-2   Role Limits for Nursing Assistants

- ***Never give drugs (medications, medicines).*** This includes drugs given orally, rectally, vaginally, and by injection. It also includes drugs given by application to the skin, eyes, ears, and nose. Nor do you give drugs directly into the bloodstream or through an intravenous (IV) line. Nurses give drugs. Many states allow nursing assistants to give drugs after completing a state-approved medication assistant training program. The function must be in your job description. And you must have the necessary supervision.
- ***Never insert tubes or objects into body openings. Do not remove them from the body.*** You must not insert tubes into a person's bladder, esophagus, trachea, nose, ears, bloodstream, or surgically created body openings. Exceptions to this rule are the procedures you will study during your training. Giving enemas is an example. To perform them, they must be in your job description. And you must have the necessary supervision.
- ***Never take oral or phone orders from doctors.*** Politely give your name and title, and ask the doctor to wait for a nurse. Promptly find a nurse to speak with the doctor.
- ***Never perform procedures that require sterile technique.*** With sterile technique, all objects in contact with the person are free of microorganisms (Chapter 15). Sterile technique and procedures require skills, knowledge, and judgment beyond your training. You can assist a nurse with a sterile procedure. However, you will not perform the procedure yourself.
- ***Never tell the person or family the person's diagnosis or medical or surgical treatment plans.*** This is the doctor's responsibility. Nurses may clarify what the doctor has said.
- ***Never diagnose or prescribe treatments or drugs for anyone.*** Doctors diagnose and prescribe.
- ***Never supervise others including other nursing assistants.*** This is a nurse's legal responsibility. You will not be trained to supervise others. Supervising others can have serious legal problems.
- ***Never ignore an order or request to do something. This includes nursing tasks that you can do, those you cannot do, and those that are beyond your legal limits.*** Promptly and politely explain to the nurse why you cannot carry out the order or request. The nurse assumes you are doing what you were told to do unless you explain otherwise. You cannot neglect the person's care.

Box 3-3   Nursing Assistant Standards

The nursing assistant:

- Performs nursing tasks within the range of functions allowed by the state's nurse practice act and its rules.
- Is honest and shows integrity in performing nursing tasks. (*Integrity* involves following a code of ethics. See Chapter 4.)
- Bases nursing tasks on his or her education and training. Also bases them on the nurse's directions.
- Is accountable (p. 28) for his or her behavior and actions while assisting the nurse and helping residents.
- Performs delegated aspects of the person's nursing care.
- Assists the nurse in observing residents. Also assists in identifying their needs.
- Communicates:
  - Progress toward completing delegated nursing tasks
  - Problems in completing delegated nursing tasks
  - Changes in the person's status
- Asks the nurse to clarify what is expected when unsure.
- Uses educational and training opportunities as available.
- Practices safety measures to protect the person, others, and self.
- Respects the person's rights, concerns, decisions, and dignity.
- Functions as a member of the health team. Helps implement the care plan (Chapter 7).
- Respects the person's property and the property of others.
- Protects confidential information unless required by law to share the information.

Modified from National Council of State Boards of Nursing, Inc.: Model nursing practice act and model nursing administrative rules, Chicago, Ill, 2009, Author.

Nursing Assistant Standards

OBRA defines the basic range of functions for nursing assistants. All NATCEPs include those functions (p. 21). Some states allow other functions. NATCEPs also prepare nursing assistants to meet the standards listed in Box 3-3.

Job Description

The **job description** is a document that describes what the center expects you to do (Fig. 3-2, pp. 26–27). It also states educational requirements.

Always obtain a written job description when you apply for a job. Ask questions about it during your job interview. Before accepting a job, tell the employer about:
- Functions you did not learn.
- Functions you cannot do for moral or religious reasons.

FOCUS ON COMMUNICATION
Job Description

Your training prepares you to perform certain nursing tasks. The center may not let you do everything you learned. Other centers may want you to do things that you did not learn. Use your job description if you need to discuss these issues with the nurse.

For example, Mr. Wey is in the bathroom when the nurse brings a drug to him. The nurse tells you to give him the drug when he comes out of the bathroom. If you give the drug, you are performing a task and responsibility beyond the limits of your role. With respect, you must firmly refuse to follow the nurse's direction. You can say:

"I'm sorry, but I cannot give Mr. Wey that drug. I was not trained to give drugs, and that task is not in my job description. I'll let you know when Mr. Wey comes out of the bathroom."

Clearly understand what is expected before taking a job. Do not take a job that requires you to:
- Act beyond the legal limits of your role
- Function beyond your training limits
- Perform acts that are against your morals or religion

No one can force you to do something beyond the legal limits of your role. Sometimes jobs are threatened for refusing to follow a nurse's orders. Often staff obey out of fear. That is why you must understand:
- Your roles and responsibilities
- What you can safely do
- The things you should never do
- Your job description
- The ethical and legal aspects of your role (Chapter 4)
See *Focus on Communication: Job Description.*

DELEGATION

Nurse practice acts give nurses certain responsibilities. They also give them the legal authority to perform nursing actions. A **responsibility** is the duty or obligation to perform some act or function. For example, RNs are responsible for supervising LPNs/LVNs and nursing assistants. Only RNs can carry out this responsibility.

Delegate means to authorize another person to perform a nursing task in a certain situation. The person must be competent to perform a task in a given situation. For example, you know how to give a bed bath. However, Mr. Jones is a new resident. The RN wants to spend time with him and assess his nursing needs. You do not assess. Therefore the RN gives the bath.

Text continued on p. 28

POSITION DESCRIPTION/PERFORMANCE EVALUATION

Job Title: Certified Nursing Assistant (CNA), Skilled Nursing Facility   Supervised by: Licensed Nurse

Prepared by: _____   Date: _____   Approved by: _____   Date: _____

Job Summary: Provides direct and indirect resident care activities under the direction of an RN or LPN. Assists residents with activities of daily living, provides for personal care and comfort, and assists in the maintenance of a safe and clean environment for an assigned group of residents.

DUTIES AND RESPONSIBILITIES:

E=Exceeds the Standard   M=Meets the Standard   NI=Needs Improvement

Demonstrates Competency in the Following Areas:	E	M	NI
Assists in the preparation for admission of residents.	2	1	0
Assists in and accompanies residents in the admission, transfer, and discharge procedures.	2	1	0
Provides morning care, which may include bed bath, shower or whirlpool, oral hygiene, combing hair, back massage, dressing resident, changing bed linen, cleaning overbed table and bedside stand, straightening room, and other general care as necessary throughout the day.	2	1	0
Provides evening care, which includes hand/face washing as needed, oral hygiene, back massage, pericare, freshening linen, cleaning overbed table, straightening room, and other general care as needed.	2	1	0
Notifies RN/LPN when resident complains of pain.	2	1	0
Assists with post-mortem care.	2	1	2
Assists nurses in treatment procedures.	2	1	0
Provides general nursing care such as positioning residents, lifting and turning residents, applying/utilizing special equipment, assisting in use of bedpan or commode, and ambulating the residents.	2	1	0
Performs all aspects of resident care in an environment that optimizes resident safety and reduces the likelihood of medical/health care errors.	2	1	0
Measures and records temperature, pulse, respiration, weight, blood pressure, and intake-output.	2	1	0
Makes rounds with outgoing shift. Knows whereabouts of assigned residents.	2	1	0
Makes rounds with oncoming shift to ensure the unit is left in good condition.	2	1	0
Adheres to policies and procedures of the center and the Department of Nursing.	2	1	0
Participates in socialization activities on the unit.	2	1	0
Turns and positions residents as ordered and/or as needed, making sure no rough surfaces are in direct contact with the body. Moves and turns with proper and safe body mechanics and with available resources.	2	1	0
Checks for reddened areas or skin breakdown and reports to RN or LPN.	2	1	0
Ensures residents are dressed properly and assists, as necessary. Ensures that clothing is properly stored in bedside stand or on hangers in closet. Ensures that all residents are clean and dry at all times.	2	1	0
Checks unit for adequate linen. Cleans linen cart. Provides clean linen and clothing. Makes beds.	2	1	0
Treats residents and their families with respect and dignity.	2	1	0
Follows center policies and procedures when caring for persons who are restrained.	2	1	0
Prepares residents for meals. Serves and removes food trays. Assists with meals or feeds residents, if necessary.	2	1	0
Distributes drinking water and other nourishments to residents.	2	1	0
Performs general care activities for residents on Isolation Precautions.	2	1	0
Answers residents' signal lights promptly. Anticipates residents' needs and makes rounds to assigned residents.	2	1	0
Assists residents with handling and care of clothing and other personal property (including dentures, eyeglasses, contact lenses, hearing aids, and prosthetic devices).	2	1	0
Transports residents to and from various departments, as requested.	2	1	0
Reports and, when appropriate, records any changes observed in condition or behavior of residents and unusual incidents.	2	1	0
Participates in and contributes to Resident Care Conferences.	2	1	0
Follows directions, both oral and written, and works cooperatively with other staff members.	2	1	0

Fig. 3-2 Nursing assistant job description. Note that the job description is also a performance evaluation tool. *(Modified from Medical Consultants Network, Inc., Englewood, Colo.)*

POSITION DESCRIPTION/PERFORMANCE EVALUATION—cont'd

	E	M	NI
Establishes and maintains interpersonal relationships with residents, family members, and other center personnel while assuring confidentiality of resident information.	2	1	0
Has the ability to acquire knowledge of and develop skills in basic nursing procedures and simple charting.	2	1	0
Attends in-service education programs, as assigned, to learn new treatments, procedures, skills, etc.	2	1	0
Maintains personal health in order to prevent absence from work due to health problems.	2	1	0

Professional Requirements:	E	M	NI
Meets dress code standards. Appearance is neat and clean.	2	1	0
Completes annual education requirements.	2	1	0
Maintains regulatory requirements.	2	1	0
Meets center's standards for attendance.	2	1	0
Consistently completes and maintains assigned duties.	2	1	0
Wears identification while on duty.	2	1	0
Practices careful, efficient, and non-wasteful use of supplies and linen. Follows established charge procedure for resident charge items.	2	1	0
Attends annual review and department in-services, as scheduled.	2	1	0
Attends at least 75% of staff meetings. Reads and returns all monthly staff meeting minutes.	2	1	0
Represents the center in a positive and professional manner.	2	1	0
Actively participates in the Continuous Quality Improvement (CQI) activities.	2	1	0
Complies with all center policies regarding ethical business practices.	2	1	0
Communicates the mission, ethics, and goals of the center, as well as the focus statement of the department.	2	1	0
Possesses a genuine interest and concern for older and disabled persons.	2	1	0

TOTAL POINTS _____ _____ _____

Regulatory Requirements:

- High school graduate or equivalent
- Current Certified Nursing Assistant (CNA) certification
- Current Basic Life Support for Healthcare Providers certification within three (3) months of hire date

Language Skills:

- Ability to read and communicate effectively in English
- Additional languages preferred

Skills:

- Basic computer knowledge

Physical Demands:

- See "Physical Demands" policy.

I have received, read, and understand the Position Description/Performance Evaluation above.

_____   _____
Name/Signature   Date Signed

Fig. 3-2, cont'd For legend, see facing page.

Who Can Delegate

RNs can delegate nursing tasks to LPNs/LVNs and nursing assistants. In some states, LPNs/LVNs can delegate tasks to nursing assistants. RNs and LPNs/LVNs can only delegate tasks within their scope of practice. And they can only delegate the tasks in your job description.

Delegation decisions must protect the person's health and safety. The delegating nurse is legally accountable for the nursing task. Accountable means to be responsible for one's actions and the actions of others who performed the delegated tasks. It also involves answering questions about and explaining one's actions and the actions of others.

The delegating nurse must make sure that the task was completed safely and correctly. If the RN delegates, the RN is responsible for the delegated task. If the LPN/LVN delegates, he or she is responsible for the delegated task. The RN also supervises LPNs/LVNs. Therefore the RN is legally accountable for the tasks that LPNs/LVNs delegate to nursing assistants. The RN is accountable for all nursing care.

Nursing assistants cannot delegate. You cannot delegate any task to other nursing assistants or to any other worker. You can ask someone to help you. But you cannot ask or tell someone to do your work.

Delegation Process

To make delegation decisions, the nurse follows a process. The person's needs, the nursing task, and the staff member doing the task must fit. The nurse decides whether or not to delegate the task to you. The person's needs and the task may require a nurse's knowledge, judgment, and skill. You may be asked to assist.

Do not get offended or angry if you cannot perform a task usually delegated to you. The nurse decides what is best for the person at the time. That decision is also best for you at that time. You must not do something that requires a nurse's judgment. For example, you always care for Mrs. Mills. Now she is weak and not eating well. The nurse wants to observe and evaluate the changes in her condition. The nurse gives needed care. At this time Mrs. Mills needs the nurse's judgment and knowledge.

The person's circumstances are central factors in delegation decisions. Delegation decisions must result in the best care for the person. Otherwise the person's health and safety are at risk. Also, the nurse may face serious legal problems. If you perform a task that places the person at risk, you may face serious legal problems.

The NCSBN describes the delegation process in four steps.

Step 1—Assess and Plan Step 1 is done by the nurse. To safely delegate, the nurse needs to understand the person's needs. And the nurse needs to know your knowledge, skills, and job description.

When assessing the person's needs, the nurse answers these questions:
- What is the nature of the person's needs? How complex are the needs? How can they vary? How urgent are the care needs?
- What are the most important long-term needs? What are the most important short-term needs?
- How much judgment is needed to meet the person's needs and give care?
- How predictable is the person's health status? How does the person respond to health care?
- What problems might arise from the nursing task? How severe might they be?
- What actions are needed if a problem arises? How complex are those actions?
- What emergencies or incidents might arise? How likely might they occur?
- How involved is the person in health care decisions? How involved is the family?
- How will delegating the nursing task help the person? What are the risks to the person?

To assess your knowledge and skills, the nurse answers these questions.
- What knowledge and skills are needed to safely perform the nursing task?
- What is your role in the center? What is in your job description?
- What are the conditions under which the nursing task will be performed?
- What is expected after the nursing task is performed?
- What problems can arise from the nursing task? What problems might the person develop during the nursing task?

The nurse then decides if it is safe to delegate the nursing task. It must be safe for the person and safe for you. If unsafe, the nurse stops the delegation process. If it is safe for the person and you, the nurse moves to step 2.

Step 2—Communication This step involves the nurse and you. The nurse must provide clear and complete directions about:
- How to perform and complete the task
- What observations to report and record
- When to report observations
- What specific resident concerns to report at once
- Priorities for nursing tasks
- What to do if the person's needs change or condition changes

The nurse must make sure that you understand the directions. The nurse asks you questions to make sure you understand. He or she may ask you to explain what you are going to do. Do not be insulted by such questions. The nurse must make sure that you give safe care. This protects the person and you.

Before performing a delegated nursing task, you must have the opportunity to discuss the task with the nurse. Make sure that you:

- Ask questions about the delegated task.
- Ask questions about what you are expected to do.
- Tell the nurse if you have not done the task before. Also tell the nurse if you have not done it often.
- Ask for needed training or supervision.
- Restate what is expected of you.
- Restate what specific resident concerns to report to the nurse.
- Explain how and when you will report your progress in completing the task.
- Know how to contact the nurse for an emergency.
- Know what the nurse wants you to do during an emergency.

After completing a delegated task, you report and record the care given. You also report and record your observations. See "Reporting and Recording" in Chapter 6.

Step 3—Surveillance and Supervision *Surveillance* means to keep a close watch over someone or something. *Supervise* means to oversee, direct, or manage. In this step, the nurse observes the care you give. The nurse makes sure that you complete the task correctly. The nurse also observes the person's condition and response to your care. How often the nurse makes observations depends on:

- The person's health status and needs
- If the person's condition is stable or unstable
- If the nurse can predict the person's responses and risks to care
- The setting where the nursing task occurs
- The resources and support available
- If the nursing task is simple or complex

The nurse must follow up on any problems or concerns. For example, the nurse takes action if:

- You did not complete the nursing task in a timely manner.
- The task did not meet expectations.
- There is an unexpected change in the person's condition.

The nurse is alert for signs and symptoms that signal a possible change in the person's condition. This way the nurse, with your help, can take action before the person's condition changes in a major way.

Sometimes problems arise in completing a nursing task. By supervising you, the nurse can detect and solve problems early. This helps you complete the task safely and on time.

After you complete the task, the nurse may review and discuss what happened with you. This helps you learn. If a similar situation happens in the future, you have ideas about how to adjust.

Step 4—Evaluation and Feedback This step is done by the nurse. *Evaluate* means to judge. The nurse decides if the delegation was successful. The nurse answers these questions:

- Was the nursing task done correctly?
- Did the person respond to the task as expected?
- Was the outcome (the result) as desired? Was it a good or bad result?
- Was communication between you and the nurse timely and effective?
- What went well? What were the problems?
- Does the care plan need to change (Chapter 7)? Or can the plan stay the same?
- Did the nursing task present ways for the nurse or you to learn?
- Did the nurse give you the right feedback? *Feedback* means to respond. The nurse tells you what you did correctly. If you did something wrong, the nurse tells you that too. Feedback is another way for you to learn and improve the care you give.
- Did the nurse thank you for completing the nursing task?

The Five Rights of Delegation

The NCSBN's *Five Rights of Delegation* is another way to view the delegation process. To use the "five rights," the nurse answers the questions listed in the four steps described above. The *Five Rights of Delegation* are:

- *The right task.* Can the task be delegated? Is the nurse allowed to delegate the task? Is the task in your job description?
- *The right circumstances.* What are the person's physical, mental, emotional, and spiritual needs at this time?
- *The right person.* Do you have the training and experience to safely perform the task for this person?
- *The right directions and communication.* The nurse must give clear directions. The nurse tells you what to do and when to do it. The nurse tells you what observations to make and when to report back. The nurse allows questions and helps you set priorities.
- *The right supervision.* In this step, the nurse:
  - Guides, directs, and evaluates the care you give.
  - Demonstrates tasks as necessary and is available to answer questions. The less experience you have with a task, the more supervision you need. Complex tasks require more supervision than do basic tasks. Also, the person's circumstances affect how much supervision you need.
  - Assesses how the task affected the person and how well you performed the task.
  - Tells you what you did well and how to improve your work. This helps you learn and give better care.

Your Role in Delegation

You perform delegated nursing tasks for or on *a person*. You must protect the person from harm. You have two

| Box 3-4 | The *Five Rights of Delegation* for Nursing Assistants |

The Right Task
- Does your state allow you to perform the task?
- Were you trained to do the task?
- Do you have experience performing the task?
- Is the task in your job description?

The Right Circumstances
- Do you have experience performing the task given the person's condition and needs?
- Do you understand the purposes of the task for the person?
- Can you perform the task safely under the current circumstances?
- Do you have the equipment and supplies to safely complete the task?
- Do you know how to use the equipment and supplies?

The Right Person
- Are you comfortable performing the task?
- Do you have concerns about performing the task?

The Right Directions and Communication
- Did the nurse give clear directions and instructions?
- Did you review the task with the nurse?
- Do you understand what the nurse expects?

The Right Supervision
- Is a nurse available to answer questions?
- Is a nurse available if the person's condition changes or if problems occur?

Modified from National Council of State Boards of Nursing, Inc.: The Five Rights of Delegation, Chicago, Ill, 2006, Author.

choices when a task is delegated to you. You either *agree* or *refuse* to do the task. Use the *Five Rights of Delegation* in Box 3-4.

Accepting a Task   When you agree to perform a task, you are responsible for your own actions. What you do or fail to do can harm the person. *You must complete the task safely.* Ask for help when you are unsure or have questions about a task. Report to the nurse what you did and the observations you made.

Refusing a Task   You have the right to say "no." Sometimes refusing to follow the nurse's directions is your right and duty. You should refuse to perform a task when:
- The task is beyond the legal limits of your role.
- The task is not in your job description.
- You were not prepared to perform the task.
- The task could harm the person.
- The person's condition has changed.
- You do not know how to use the supplies or equipment.
- Directions are not ethical or legal.
- Directions are against center policies.
- Directions are not clear or not complete.
- A nurse is not available for supervision.

Use common sense. This protects you and the person. Ask yourself if what you are doing is safe for the person.

Never ignore an order or a request to do something. Tell the nurse about your concerns. If the task is within the legal limits of your role and in your job description, the nurse can help increase your comfort with the task. The nurse can:
- Answer your questions
- Demonstrate the task
- Show you how to use supplies and equipment
- Help you as needed
- Observe you performing the task
- Check on you often
- Arrange for needed training

Do not refuse a task because you do not like it or do not want to do it. You must have sound reasons. Otherwise, you place the person at risk for harm. You also could lose your job.

See *Focus on Communication: Refusing a Task.*

FOCUS ON COMMUNICATION
Refusing a Task

A nurse may delegate a task that you did not learn in your training program. The task is in your job description. You can say:

"I know this task is in my job description, but I did not learn it in school. Can you show me what to do and then observe me doing it? That would really help me."

A nurse may ask you to do something that is not in your job description. With respect, you must firmly refuse the nurse's request. You can say:

"I'm sorry. I am not trained to do that. That task is not in my job description. Can I help you with something else?"

QUALITY OF LIFE

The work you do is important for the person's quality of life. The work you do has value. By continuing to learn, you increase your skills and knowledge. It adds to your value. It offers you more opportunities. Your current training is just the start of a life-time of learning and possibilities.

Some states have higher levels of nursing assistants. Medication assistant-certified (MA-C) is an example. MA-Cs are nursing assistants with extra training. Supervised by a licensed nurse, they give drugs as allowed by state law.

You can continue to learn in many ways. Find out the options available in your state and center. Take advantage of them. Be proud of your training. And never stop learning!

REVIEW QUESTIONS

Circle the BEST answer.

1 Nursing practice is regulated by
   a The National Council of State Boards of Nursing
   b Nurse practice acts
   c Medicare
   d Medicaid

2 What state law affects what nursing assistants can do?
   a Standards for nursing assistants
   b OBRA
   c Nurse practice act
   d Medicaid

3 Your nursing assistant certification can be revoked for
   a Refusing a nursing task
   b Asking the nurse questions
   c Performing acts beyond your role
   d Keeping the person's information confidential

4 Which requires a training and competency evaluation program for nursing assistants?
   a Medicare
   b Medicaid
   c NCSBN
   d OBRA

5 As a nursing assistant, you
   a Must perform all nursing tasks as directed by the nurse
   b Make decisions about a person's care
   c Need a written job description before employment
   d Give a drug when a nurse tells you to

6 As a nursing assistant, you
   a Can take verbal or phone orders from doctors
   b Are responsible for your own actions
   c Can remove tubes from the person's body
   d Can ignore a nursing task if it is not in your job description

7 Which statement is *false*?
   a You are accountable for your actions.
   b You must be honest when performing nursing tasks.
   c You can use the person's property for your own needs.
   d A law can require you to share the person's confidential information.

8 Who assigns and supervises your work?
   a Other nursing assistants
   b The health team
   c Nurses
   d Doctors

9 You are responsible for
   a Supervising other nursing assistants
   b Delegation decisions
   c Completing delegated tasks safely
   d Deciding what treatments are needed

10 You perform a task not allowed by your state. Which is *true*?
   a If a nurse delegated the task, there is no legal problem.
   b You could be practicing nursing without a license.
   c You can perform the task if it is in your job description.
   d If you complete the task safely, there is no legal problem.

11 These statements are about delegation. Which is *false*?
   a Nurses can delegate their responsibilities to you.
   b A delegated task must be safe for the person.
   c The delegated task must be in your job description.
   d The delegating nurse is responsible for the safe completion of the task.

12 A task is in your job description. Which is *false*?
   a The nurse must delegate the task to you.
   b The nurse can delegate the task if the person's circumstances are right.
   c You must have the necessary education and training to complete the task.
   d You must have clear directions before you perform the task.

13 A nurse delegates a task to you. You must
   a Complete the task
   b Decide to accept or refuse the task
   c Delegate the task if you are busy
   d Ignore the request if you do not know what to do

14 You can refuse to perform a task for these reasons *except*
   a The task is beyond the legal limits of your role
   b The task is not in your job description
   c You do not like the task
   d A nurse is not available to supervise you

15 You decide to refuse a task. What should you do?
   a Delegate the task to a nursing assistant.
   b Communicate your concerns to the nurse.
   c Ignore the request.
   d Talk to the director of nursing.

Answers to these questions are on p. 719.

Ethics and Laws

OBJECTIVES

- Define the key terms and key abbreviations listed in this chapter.
- Describe ethical conduct.
- Describe the rules of conduct for nursing assistants.
- Explain how to maintain professional boundaries.
- Explain how to prevent negligent acts.

- Give examples of false imprisonment, defamation, assault, battery, and fraud.
- Describe how to protect the right to privacy.
- Explain the purpose of informed consent.
- Explain your role in relation to wills.
- Describe elder, child, and domestic abuse.
- Explain how to promote quality of life.

KEY TERMS

abuse The willful infliction of injury, unreasonable confinement, intimidation, or punishment that results in physical harm, pain, or mental anguish; depriving the person (or the person's caretaker) of the goods or services needed to attain or maintain well-being

assault Intentionally attempting or threatening to touch a person's body without the person's consent

battery Touching a person's body without his or her consent

boundary crossing A brief act or behavior outside the helpful zone

boundary sign An act, behavior, or thought that warns of a boundary crossing or violation

boundary violation An act or behavior that meets your needs, not the person's

civil law Laws concerned with relationships between people

crime An act that violates a criminal law

criminal law Laws concerned with offenses against the public and society in general

defamation Injuring a person's name and reputation by making false statements to a third person

ethics Knowledge of what is right conduct and wrong conduct

false imprisonment Unlawful restraint or restriction of a person's freedom of movement

fraud Saying or doing something to trick, fool, or deceive a person

invasion of privacy Violating a person's right not to have his or her name, photo, or private affairs exposed or made public without giving consent

law A rule of conduct made by a government body

libel Making false statements in print, writing, or through pictures or drawings

malpractice Negligence by a professional person

neglect Failure to provide the person with the goods or services needed to avoid physical harm, mental anguish, or mental illness

negligence An unintentional wrong in which a person did not act in a reasonable and careful manner and a person or the person's property was harmed

KEY TERMS—cont'd

professional boundary That which separates helpful behaviors from behaviors that are not helpful

professional sexual misconduct An act, behavior, or comment that is sexual in nature

protected health information Identifying information and information about the person's health care that is maintained or sent in any form (paper, electronic, oral)

self-neglect A person's behaviors that threaten his or her health and safety

slander Making false statements orally

standard of care The skills, care, and judgments required by a health team member under similar conditions

tort A wrong committed against a person or the person's property

vulnerable adult A person 18 years old or older who has a disability or condition that makes him or her at risk to be wounded, attacked, or damaged

will A legal document of how a person wants property distributed after death

KEY ABBREVIATIONS

HIPAA Health Insurance Portability and Accountability Act of 1996

OBRA Omnibus Budget Reconciliation Act of 1987

Nurse practice acts, your training and job description, and safe delegation serve to protect residents from harm (Chapter 3). Protecting them from harm also involves a complex set of rules and standards of conduct. They form the ethical and legal aspects of care.

ETHICAL ASPECTS

Ethics is knowledge of what is right conduct and wrong conduct. Morals are involved. It also deals with choices or judgments about what should or should not be done. An ethical person behaves and acts in the right way. He or she does not cause a person harm.

Ethical behavior also involves not being *prejudiced* or *biased.* To be prejudiced or biased means to make judgments and have views before knowing the facts. Judgments and views usually are based on one's values and standards. They are based in the person's culture, religion, education, and experiences. The person's situation may be very different from your own. For example:

- Children want their mother to have nursing home care. In your culture, children care for older parents at home.
- A person has many tattoos and body piercings. You do not like tattoos or body piercings.
- An 83-year-old man does not want life-saving measures. You believe that everything must be done to save a life.

Do not judge the person by your values and standards. Do not avoid persons whose standards and values differ from your own.

Ethical problems involve making choices. You must decide what is the right thing to do. For example:

- You find a co-worker in an empty room drinking from a cup. You smell alcohol on her breath. She asks you not to tell anyone.
- A resident has bruises all over her body. She told the nurse that she fell. She tells you that her son is very mean to her. She asks you not to tell the nurse.

Professional groups have codes of ethics. The code has rules, or standards of conduct, for group members to follow. The American Nurses Association (ANA) has a code of ethics for registered nurses (RNs). The National Federation of Licensed Practical Nurses (NFLPN) has one for licensed practical nurses/licensed vocational nurses (LPNs/LVNs). The rules of conduct in Box 4-1, p. 34 can guide your thinking and behavior. See Chapter 5 for ethics in the workplace.

Boundaries

A *boundary* limits or separates something. For example, a fence forms a boundary. You stay inside or outside of the fenced area. As a nursing assistant, you help residents and families. Therefore you enter into a helping relationship with them. The helping relationship has professional boundaries.

Box 4-1   Code of Conduct for Nursing Assistants

- Respect each person as an individual.
- Know the limits of your role and knowledge.
- Perform only those tasks that are within the legal limits of your role.
- Perform only those tasks that you have been prepared to do.
- Perform no act that will cause the person harm.
- Take drugs only if prescribed and supervised by a doctor.
- Carry out the directions and instructions of the nurse to your best possible ability.
- Follow the center's policies and procedures.
- Complete each task safely.
- Be loyal to your employer and co-workers.
- Act as a responsible citizen at all times.
- Keep the person's information confidential.
- Protect the person's privacy.
- Protect the person's property.
- Consider the person's needs to be more important than your own.
- Report errors and incidents at once.
- Be accountable for your actions.

PROFESSIONAL BOUNDARIES

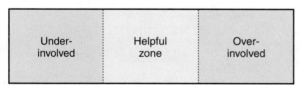

Fig. 4-1 Professional boundaries. *(Modified from National Council of State Boards of Nursing, Inc.: Professional boundaries: a nurse's guide to the importance of appropriate professional boundaries, Chicago, Ill, 2010, Author.)*

Professional boundaries separate helpful behaviors from behaviors that are not helpful (Fig. 4-1). The boundaries create a helpful zone. If your behaviors are outside the helpful zone, you are over-involved with the person or under-involved. The following can occur:

- **Boundary crossing.** This is a brief act or behavior outside the helpful zone. The act or behavior may be thoughtless or something you did not mean to do. Or it could be on purpose if it meets the person's needs. For example, you give a crying patient a hug. The hug meets the person's needs at that time. If giving a hug meets your needs, the act is wrong. Also, it is wrong to hug the person every time you see him or her.

- **Boundary violation.** This is an act or behavior that meets your needs, not the person's. The act or behavior is not ethical. It violates the code of conduct in Box 4-1. The person could be harmed. Boundary violations include:
  - Abuse (p. 38).
  - Giving a lot of information about yourself. You tell a person about your personal relationships or problems.
  - Keeping secrets with the person.

- **Professional sexual misconduct.** This is an act, behavior, or comment that is sexual in nature. It is sexual misconduct even if the person consents or makes the first move.

Some boundary violations and some types of professional sexual misconduct also are crimes. To maintain professional boundaries, follow the rules in Box 4-2. Be alert to boundary signs. **Boundary signs** are acts, behaviors, or thoughts that warn of a boundary crossing or violation (Box 4-3).

See *Focus on Communication: Professional Boundaries.*

LEGAL ASPECTS

Ethics is about what you *should or should not do.* Laws tell you what you *can and cannot do.* A **law** is a rule of conduct made by a government body. The U.S. Congress and state legislatures make laws. Enforced by the government, laws protect the public welfare.

Criminal laws are concerned with offenses against the public and society in general. An act that violates a criminal law is called a **crime.** If found guilty of a crime, the person is fined or sent to prison. Murder, robbery, rape, kidnapping, and abuse (p. 38) are crimes.

Civil laws are concerned with relationships between people. Examples of civil laws are those that involve contracts and nursing practice. A person found guilty of breaking a civil law usually has to pay a sum of money to the injured person.

Torts

Tort comes from the French word meaning wrong. Torts are part of civil law. A **tort** is a wrong committed against a person or the person's property. Some torts are *unintentional.* Harm was not intended. Some torts are *intentional.* Harm was intended.

Unintentional Torts **Negligence** is an unintentional wrong. The negligent person did not act in a reasonable and careful manner. As a result, a person or the person's property was harmed. The person causing the harm did not intend or mean to cause harm. The person failed to do what a reasonable and careful person *would have done.* Or he or she did what a reasonable and careful person *would not have done.* The negligent person may have to pay damages (a sum of money) to the one injured.

Box 4-2 Rules for Maintaining Professional Boundaries

- Follow the code of conduct listed in Box 4-1.
- Talk to the nurse if you sense a boundary sign, crossing, or violation.
- Avoid caring for family, friends, and people with whom you do business. This may be hard to do in a small community. Always tell the nurse if you know the person. The nurse may change your assignment.
- Do not date, flirt with, kiss, or have a sexual relationship with current residents. The same applies to family members of current residents.
- Do not make sexual comments or jokes.
- Do not use offensive language.
- Do not discuss your sexual relationships with residents or their families.
- Do not say or write things that could suggest a romantic or sexual relationship with a resident or family member.
- Use touch correctly (Chapter 8). Only touch or handle sexual and genital areas when necessary to give care. Such areas include the breasts, nipples, perineum, buttocks, and anus of both males and females.
- Do not accept gifts, loans, money, credit cards, or other valuables from a resident or family member.
- Do not give gifts, loans, money, credit cards, or other valuables to a resident or family member.
- Do not borrow from a resident or family member. This includes money, personal items, and transportation.
- Maintain a professional relationship at all times. Do not develop any personal relationship or friendship with the resident or family member.
- Do not visit or spend extra time with a resident who is not part of your assignment.
- Do not share personal or financial information with a resident or family member.
- Do not help a resident or family member with his or her finances.
- Do not take a resident home with you. This includes for holidays or other events.
- Ask these questions before you date or marry a person whom you cared for. Be aware of the risk for sexual misconduct.
  - How long ago did you assist with the person's care?
  - Was the person's care short-term or long-term?
  - What kind and how much information do you have about the person? How will that information affect your relationship with the person?
  - Will the person need more care in the future?
  - Does dating or marrying the person place the person at risk for harm?

Box 4-3 Boundary Signs

- You think about the person when you are not at work.
- You organize your work and provide other care around the person's needs.
- You spend free time with the person. You visit with the person during breaks, meal times, when off duty, and so on.
- You trade assignments with other staff so you can provide the person's care.
- You give more care or attention to the person at the expense of other residents.
- You believe that you are the only person who understands the person and his or her needs.
- The person gives you gifts or money.
- You give the person gifts or money.
- You share information about yourself with the person.
- You talk about your work situation with the person.
- You flirt with the person.
- You make comments that have a sexual message.
- You tell the person "off-color" jokes.
- You notice more touch between you and the person.
- You use foul, vulgar, or offensive language when talking to the person.
- You and the person have secrets.
- You choose the person's side when he or she disagrees with other staff or the family.
- You select what you report and record. You do not give complete information.
- You do not like questions about the care you give or your relationship with the person.
- You change how you dress or your appearance when you will work with the person.
- You receive gifts from the person after he or she leaves the center.
- You have contact with the person after he or she leaves the center.

FOCUS ON COMMUNICATION
Professional Boundaries

Some residents and families want to thank the staff for the care given. Some send thank-you cards and letters. Some offer gifts—candy, cookies, money, gift certificates, flowers, and so on. Accepting gifts is a boundary violation. When offered a gift, you can say:
- "Thank you so much for thinking of me. It's very kind of you. However, it is against center policy to accept gifts of any kind. I do appreciate your offer."
- "Thank you for wanting me to have the flowers your friend sent. They are lovely. However, it is against center policy to receive gifts. Let me help you find a way to take them home."

Malpractice is negligence by a professional person. A person has professional status because of training and the service provided. Nurses, doctors, dentists, and pharmacists are examples.

What you do or do not do can lead to a lawsuit if harm results to the person or property of another. Standard of care refers to skills, care, and judgments required by a health team member under similar conditions. Standards of care come from:

- Laws, including nurse practice acts.
- Textbooks.
- Center policy and procedure manuals (Fig. 4-2). These explain how to perform certain procedures.
- Manufacturer instructions for equipment and supplies.
- Job descriptions.
- Approval and accrediting agency standards.
- Standards and guidelines issued by government agencies.

The following actions could lead to charges of negligence:

- A nurse asks you to apply a hot soak. You fail to test water temperature. The water is too hot. The person is burned.
- Mrs. Parks needs help getting to the bathroom. You do not answer her signal light promptly. She gets up without help. She falls and breaks an arm.
- You use a mechanical lift to transfer Mr. Brown from bed to a chair. You do not follow the manufacturer's instructions for using the lift. Mr. Brown slips out of the lift and falls to the floor. He fractures a hip.
- Mrs. Clark complains of chest pain. You do not tell the nurse. Mrs. Clark has a heart attack and dies.
- Two residents have the same last name. You do not identify the person before a procedure. You perform the procedure on the wrong person. Both residents are harmed. One had a procedure that was not ordered. The other did not have a needed procedure.

Fig. 4-2 A nurse and nursing assistant review the policy and procedure manual. It is kept at the nurses' station.

You are legally responsible (liable) for your own actions. The nurse is liable as your supervisor. However, you still have personal liability. Remember, sometimes refusing to follow the nurse's directions is your right and duty (Chapter 3).

Intentional Torts Intentional torts are acts meant to be harmful. The act is done on purpose.

Defamation is injuring a person's name and reputation by making false statements to a third person. Libel is making false statements in print, writing, or through pictures or drawings. Slander is making false statements orally. Never make false statements about a resident, co-worker, or any other person. Examples of defamation include:

- Implying or suggesting that a person uses drugs
- Saying that a person is insane or mentally ill
- Implying or suggesting that a person steals money from the staff

False imprisonment is the unlawful restraint or restriction of a person's freedom of movement. It involves:

- Threatening to restrain a person
- Restraining a person
- Preventing a person from leaving the agency

Invasion of privacy is violating a person's right not to have his or her name, photo, or private affairs exposed or made public without giving consent. You must treat the person with respect and ensure privacy. Only staff involved in the person's care should see, handle, or examine his or her body. See Box 4-4 for measures to protect privacy.

Box 4-4   Protecting the Right to Privacy

- Keep all information about the person confidential.
- Cover the person when he or she is being moved in hallways.
- Screen the person. Close the privacy curtain as in Figure 4-3. Close the door when giving care. Also close window coverings.
- Expose only the body part involved in care or a procedure.
- Do not discuss the person or the person's treatment with anyone except the nurse supervising your work. "Shop talk" is a common cause of invasion of privacy.
- Ask visitors to leave the room when care is given.
- Do not open the person's mail.
- Allow the person to visit with others in private.
- Allow the person to use the phone in private.
- Follow center policies and procedures required to protect privacy.

Fig. 4-3 Pulling the privacy curtain around the bed helps protect the person's privacy.

The Health Insurance Portability and Accountability Act of 1996 (HIPAA) protects the privacy and security of a person's health information. **Protected health information** refers to identifying information and information about the person's health care that is maintained or sent in any form (paper, electronic, oral). Failure to follow HIPAA rules can result in fines, penalties, and criminal action including jail time. Always follow center policies and procedures. Direct any questions about the person or the person's care to the nurse. Also follow the rules for using computers and other electronic devices (Chapter 6).

Fraud is saying or doing something to trick, fool, or deceive a person. The act is fraud if it does or could harm a person or the person's property. Telling a person or family that you are a nurse is fraud. So is giving wrong or incomplete information on a job application.

Assault and battery may result in both civil and criminal charges. **Assault** is intentionally attempting or threatening to touch a person's body without the person's consent. The person fears bodily harm. Threatening to "tie down" a person is an example of assault. **Battery** is touching a person's body without his or her consent. Consent is the important factor in assault and battery. The person must consent to any procedure, treatment, or other act that involves touching the body. The person has the right to withdraw consent at any time.

Protect yourself from being accused of assault and battery. Explain to the person what you are going to do and get the person's consent. Consent may be verbal—"yes" or "okay." Or it can be a gesture—a nod, turning over for a back rub, or holding out an arm for you to take a pulse.

Informed Consent

A person has the right to decide what will be done to his or her body and who can touch his or her body. The doctor is responsible for informing the person about all aspects of treatment. Consent is informed when the person clearly understands:

- The reason for a treatment, procedure, or care measure
- What will be done
- How it will be done
- Who will do it
- The expected outcomes
- Other treatment, procedure, or care options
- The effects of not having the treatment, procedure, or care measure

Persons under legal age (usually 18 years) cannot give consent, nor can mentally incompetent persons. Such persons are unconscious, sedated, or confused. Or they have certain mental health problems. Informed consent is given by a responsible party—a wife, husband, daughter, son, or a legal representative.

Consent is given when the person enters the center. A form is signed giving general consent to treatment. Special consent forms are required before admission to a secured Alzheimer's unit (Chapter 44). Certain procedures performed by the doctor require special consents. The doctor informs the person about all aspects of the procedure. The nurse may be given this responsibility.

You are never responsible for obtaining written consent. In some centers, you can witness the signing of a consent. When a witness, you are present when the person signs the consent.

See *Focus on Communication: Informed Consent.*

FOCUS ON COMMUNICATION
Informed Consent

There are different ways to give consent:
- *Written consent.* The person signs a form agreeing to a treatment or procedure. You are not responsible for obtaining written consent.
- *Verbal consent.* The person says aloud that he or she consents. "Yes" and "okay" are examples.
- *Implied consent.* For example, you ask Mr. Jones if you can check his blood pressure. He extends his arm. His movement implies consent.

Before any procedure, explain the steps to the person. This is how you obtain verbal or implied consent. Also explain each step during a procedure. This allows the person the chance to refuse at any time.

Wills

A will is a legal document of how a person wants property distributed after death. You can ethically and legally witness a will signing. Or you can refuse to do so without fear of legal action.

A person may ask you to prepare a will. You must politely refuse. Explain that you do not have the legal knowledge or ability to prepare a will. Report the request to the nurse. The nurse will speak to the person or family member about contacting a lawyer.

Do not witness a will signing if you are named in the will. To do so prevents you from getting what was left to you. As a witness, be prepared to testify that:

- The person was of sound mind when the will was signed
- The person stated that the document was his or her last will

Many centers do not let staff witness wills. Know your center's policy before you agree to witness a will. If you have questions, ask the nurse. If you witness a will, tell the nurse.

REPORTING ABUSE

Some persons are mistreated or harmed on purpose. This is abuse. Abuse is:

- The willful infliction of injury, unreasonable confinement, intimidation, or punishment that results in physical harm, pain, or mental anguish. *Intimidation* means to make afraid with threats of force or violence.
- Depriving the person (or the person's caregiver) of the goods or services needed to attain or maintain well-being.

Abuse also includes involuntary seclusion (Chapter 2). Abuse is a crime. All persons must be protected from abuse. This includes persons in a coma.

The abuser is usually a family member or caregiver—spouse, partner, adult child, and others. The abuser can be a friend, neighbor, landlord, or other person. Both men and women are abusers. Both men and women are abused.

State laws, accrediting agencies, and the Omnibus Budget Reconciliation Act of 1987 (OBRA) do not allow centers to employ persons who were convicted of abuse, neglect, or mistreatment. Before hiring, the center must thoroughly check the applicant's work history. All references are checked. Efforts must be made to find out about any criminal records.

The center also checks the nursing assistant registry for findings of abuse, neglect, or mistreatment. It also is checked for mis-using or stealing a person's property.

OBRA-CMS

RESIDENTS WITH DEMENTIA
Vulnerable Adults

Some persons have behaviors that threaten his or her health and safety. This is called self-neglect. Causes include declining health and chronic disease. Other causes are disorders that impair judgment or memory. Alzheimer's disease and dementia are examples. The warning signs of self-neglect are:

- Hoarding. The person saves, hides, or stores things. Newspapers, magazines, food containers, and shopping bags are examples.
- Not having food, water, heat, and other necessities.
- Not taking needed drugs.
- Refusing medical treatment for serious illnesses.
- Dehydration—poor urinary output, dry skin, dry mouth, confusion.
- Poor hygiene.
- Wearing the wrong clothing for the weather.
- Confusion.

Vulnerable Adults

Vulnerable comes from the Latin word *vulnerare,* which means *to wound.* Vulnerable adults are persons 18 years old or older who have disabilities or conditions that make them at risk to be wounded, attacked, or damaged. They have problems caring for or protecting themselves due to:

- A mental, emotional, physical, or developmental disability. See Chapter 45 for "Developmental Disabilities."
- Brain damage.
- Changes from aging.

All residents, regardless of age, are vulnerable. Older persons and children are at risk for abuse.

See *Residents With Dementia: Vulnerable Adults.*

Elder Abuse

Elder abuse is any knowing, intentional, or negligent act by a caregiver or any other person to an older adult. The act causes harm or serious risk of harm. Elder abuse can take these forms:

- *Physical abuse.* This involves inflicting, or threatening to inflict, physical pain or injury. Grabbing, hitting, slapping, kicking, pinching, hair-pulling, or beating are examples. It also includes *corporal punishment*—punishment inflicted directly on the body. Beatings, lashings, and whippings are examples. Depriving the person of a basic need also is physical abuse.

- *Neglect.* Failure to provide the person with the goods or services needed to avoid physical harm, mental anguish, or mental illness is called **neglect.** This includes failure to provide health care or treatment, food, clothing, hygiene, shelter, or other needs. In health care, neglect includes but is not limited to:
  - Leaving persons lying or sitting in urine or feces
  - Keeping persons alone in their rooms or other areas
  - Failing to answer signal lights
- *Verbal abuse.* Using oral or written words or statements that speak badly of, sneer at, criticize, or condemn the person. It includes unkind gestures, threats of harm, or saying things to frighten the person. For example, a person is told that he or she will never see family members again.
- *Involuntary seclusion.* Confining the person to a certain area. People have been locked in closets, basements, attics, bathrooms, and other spaces.
- *Financial exploitation or misappropriation.* To *exploit* means to use unjustly. *Misappropriate* means to dishonestly, unfairly, or wrongly take for one's own use. The older person's resources (money, property, assets) are mis-used by another person. Or the resources are used for the other person's profit or benefit. The person's money is stolen or used by another person. It is also mis-using a person's property. For example, a son sells his mother's house without her consent.
- *Emotional or mental abuse.* This involves inflicting mental pain, anguish, or distress through verbal or nonverbal acts. Humiliation, harassment, ridicule, and threats of punishment are examples. It includes being deprived of needs such as food, clothing, care, a home, or a place to sleep.
- *Sexual abuse.* The person is harassed about sex or is attacked sexually. The person may be forced to perform sexual acts out of fear of punishment or physical harm.
- *Abandonment.* *Abandon* means to leave or desert someone. The person is deserted by someone who is supposed to give his or her care.

There are many signs of elder abuse. The abused person may show only some of the signs in Box 4-5.

Federal and state laws require the reporting of elder abuse. If abuse is suspected, it must be reported. Where and how to report abuse vary among states. You may suspect abuse. If so, discuss the matter and your observations with the nurse. Give as many details as possible. The nurse contacts health team members as needed.

The nurse also contacts community agencies that investigate elder abuse. They act at once if the problem is life-threatening. Sometimes the police or courts are involved.

Box 4-5   Signs of Elder Abuse

- Living conditions are unsafe, unclean, or inadequate.
- Personal hygiene is lacking. The person is not clean. Clothes are dirty.
- Weight loss—there are signs of poor nutrition and poor fluid intake.
- Assistive devices are missing or broken—eyeglasses, hearing aids, dentures, cane, walker, and so on.
- Medical needs are not met.
- Frequent injuries—conditions behind the injuries are strange or seem impossible.
- Old and new injuries—bruises, pressure marks, welts, scars, fractures, punctures, and so on.
- Complaints of pain or itching in the genital area.
- Bleeding and bruising around the breasts or in the genital area.
- Burns on the feet, hands, buttocks, or other parts of the body. Cigarettes and cigars cause small circle-like burns.
- Pressure ulcers (Chapter 36) or contractures (Chapter 26).
- The person seems very quiet or withdrawn.
- Unexplained withdrawal from normal activities.
- The person seems fearful, anxious, or agitated.
- Sudden change in alertness.
- Depression.
- Sudden changes in finances.
- The person does not seem to want to talk or answer questions.
- The person is restrained. Or the person is locked in a certain area for long periods.
- The person cannot reach toilet facilities, food, water, and other needed items.
- Private conversations are not allowed. The caregiver is present during all conversations.
- Strained or tense relationships with a caregiver.
- Frequent arguments with a caregiver.
- The person seems anxious to please the caregiver.
- Drugs are not taken properly. Drugs are not bought. Or too much or too little of the drug is taken.
- Emergency room visits may be frequent.
- The person may change doctors often. Some people do not have a doctor.

Helping abused older persons is not always easy or possible. Some abuse is not reported or recognized. Or the investigating agency cannot gain access to the person. Sometimes older persons are abused by a spouse or adult child. A victim may want to protect the spouse or child. Some victims are embarrassed or believe abuse is deserved. A victim may fear what will happen. He or she may think that the present situation is better than no care at all. Some people fear not being believed if they report the abuse themselves.

OBRA-CMS

Abuse in Nursing Centers OBRA requires these actions if abuse is suspected within the center:

- The incident is reported at once to the administrator. It also is reported at once to other officials as required by federal and state laws.
- All claims of abuse are thoroughly investigated.
- The center must prevent further potential for abuse while the investigation is in progress.
- Investigation results are reported to the center administrator within 5 days of the incident. They also are reported to other officials as required by federal and state laws.
- Corrective actions are taken if the claim is found to be true.

Box 4-6 lists some severe cases of elder abuse. The abusers were convicted of crimes.

The examples of abuse that follow are more common. However, such abuse is still wrong. It will be investigated. You can lose your job. Your state nursing assistant registry will be notified. Nursing assistants have lost their certification (license, registration) because of elder abuse.

- A person constantly crying out for help is taken to his room. He is left alone with the door closed.
- A person is told to be nice, otherwise care will not be given.
- A person cannot control her bowels. She is called "dirty" and "disgusting."
- A person is turned in a rough and hurried manner.
- The nurse uses the person's phone to call a friend.
- A person lies in a wet and soiled bed all night.
- Money is taken from a person's wallet.
- A person uses the signal light a lot. It is taken away from the person.
- A person's mouth is forced open. Food is forced into the person's mouth.
- A person is told that her son does not visit because she is so mean.

Child Abuse and Neglect

Child abuse and neglect involve the following:

- A child 18 years old or younger
- Any recent act or failure to act on the part of a parent or caregiver
- The act or failure to act results in death, serious physical or emotional harm, sexual abuse, or exploitation
- The act or failure to act presents a likely or immediate risk for harm

Child abuse and neglect occur at every social level. They occur in low-, middle-, and high-income families. The abuser may have little education or be highly educated. The abuser usually is a household member—parent, a parent's partner, brother or sister, nanny. Usually an abuser is someone the family knows. Risk factors for child abuse include:

- Stress
- Family crisis (divorce, unemployment, moving, poverty, crowded living conditions)
- Drug or alcohol abuse
- Abuser history of being abused as a child
- Discipline beliefs that include physical punishment
- Lack of emotional attachment to the child
- A child with birth defects or chronic illness
- A child with personality or behaviors that the abuser considers "different" or not acceptable
- Unrealistic expectations for the child's behavior or performance
- Families that move often and do not have family or friends nearby

---

Box 4-6 Prosecuted Cases of Elder Abuse

- A resident was complaining of pain while being cleaned. To stop him from complaining, a nursing assistant stuck a rag down his throat.
- A patient was screaming. To stop the patient from screaming, a nurse poured water down her throat.
- A nursing assistant beat and kicked a 92-year-old man who was lying on the floor.
- A nursing assistant stepped on a resident's face.
- A person was visiting his grandmother. While there, he sexually abused a patient with head injuries.
- A female patient in a wheelchair was dragged into a room by a nursing assistant. The nursing assistant forced the patient to have sex with him.
- A nursing assistant teased and taunted a resident with dementia.
- A health care worker repeatedly insulted an older woman because her son was gay.
- A nursing assistant forced a person to urinate in bed. Then the nursing assistant made fun of the person.
- Two older women lived in a board and care home. Both had Alzheimer's disease. They were left in a room with blood splattered on the walls. The carpet was caked with feces, vomitus, and urine. The women were partially dressed. One woman was tied to the bed with a sheet.
- A nursing assistant failed to feed a resident who could not feed herself. A video camera caught the nursing assistant dumping the person's food into trash cans.
- A resident could not talk. She totally depended on the staff for care. She did not have a bowel movement for 26 days. She was given a laxative every 3 days. No other treatment was given for her constipation.
- Caregivers willfully neglected to give drugs to residents.

From American Society on Aging: Elder abuse and neglect: prosecution and prevention, *San Francisco, Calif, Author.*

Types of Child Abuse and Neglect Child abuse and neglect can take different forms. Often more than one type is present.

- *Physical abuse* is injuring the child on purpose. It can cause death. Forms of physical abuse include striking, kicking, burning, or biting the child. It is any action that causes physical impairment of the child.
- *Neglect* can be physical or emotional. *Physical neglect* means to deprive the child of food, clothing, shelter, and medical care. *Emotional neglect* is not meeting the child's need for affection and attention.
- *Sexual abuse* is using, persuading, or forcing a child to engage in sexual conduct. It can take many forms:
  - *Rape or sexual assault*—forced sexual acts with a person against his or her will.
  - *Molestation*—sexual advances toward a child. It includes kissing, touching, or fondling sexual areas. The abuser may kiss, touch, or fondle the child. Or the child is forced to kiss, touch, or fondle the abuser.
  - *Incest*—sexual activity between family members. The abuser may be a parent, brother or sister, step-brother or step-sister, aunt or uncle, cousin, or grandparent.
  - *Child pornography*—taking pictures or videotaping a child involved in sexual acts or poses.
  - *Child prostitution*—forcing a child to engage in sexual activity for money. Usually the child is forced to have many sexual partners.
- *Emotional abuse* is injuring the child mentally. The child has changes in behavior, emotional responses, thinking, reasoning, learning, and so on. The child may show anxiety, depression, withdrawal, or aggressive behaviors.
- *Substance abuse* is part of child abuse and neglect in some states. A *controlled substance* is a drug or chemical substance whose possession and use are controlled by law. Substance abuse involves:
  - Making a controlled substance in the presence of a child or on the premises occupied by a child
  - Allowing a child to be present where there are chemicals or equipment used to make or store a controlled substance
  - Selling, distributing, or giving drugs or alcohol to a child
  - Using a controlled substance that impairs the caregiver's ability to adequately care for the child
  - Exposing the child to equipment and supplies for using, selling, or distributing drugs
  - Exposing the child to other drug-related activities
- *Abandonment* is when a parent's identity or whereabouts are unknown. The child was left in circumstances where the child suffers serious harm. Or the parent fails to maintain contact with the child or provide support for the child.

Box 4-7 (p. 42) lists the signs of child abuse and neglect. Report any changes in the child's body or behavior. Child and parent behaviors may signal that something is wrong. The child may be quiet and withdrawn. He or she may fear adults. Sometimes children are afraid to go home. Sudden behavior changes are common in sexual abuse. Bed-wetting, thumb-sucking, loss of appetite, poor grades, and running away from home are examples. Some children attempt suicide.

Parents give different stories about what happened. Injuries are blamed on play accidents or other children. Frequent emergency room visits are common.

Child abuse is complex. Many more behaviors, signs, and symptoms are present than discussed here. The health team must be alert for signs and symptoms of child abuse. All states require the reporting of suspected child abuse. However, someone should not be falsely accused.

If you suspect child abuse, share your concerns with the nurse. Give as much detail as you can. The nurse contacts health team members and child protection agencies as needed.

Domestic Abuse

Domestic abuse—also called domestic violence, intimate partner abuse, partner abuse, and spousal abuse—occurs in relationships. One partner has power and control over the other through abuse. Fear and harm occur. Usually more than one of the following is present:

- *Physical abuse*—unwanted punching, slapping, grabbing, choking, poking, biting, pulling hair, twisting arms, or kicking. It may involve burns and weapons. Physical injuries occur. Death is a constant threat.
- *Sexual abuse*—unwanted sexual contact.
- *Verbal abuse*—unkind and hurtful remarks. They make the person feel unwhole, unattractive, and without value.
- *Economic abuse*—controlling money. Having or not having a job is controlled by the abuser. So are paychecks, money gifts from family and friends, and money for household expenses (food, clothing).
- *Social abuse*—controlling friendships and other relationships. The abuser controls phone calls, car use, leaving the home, and visits with family and friends.

Residents can suffer from domestic abuse. For example, a husband slaps his wife during a visit. Or a wife uses her husband's money for herself rather than buying her husband's drugs.

Box 4-7   Signs and Symptoms of Child Abuse and Neglect

Physical Abuse
- Bruises on the face (eyes, lips, mouth, cheeks), back, buttocks, abdomen, chest, and inner thighs.
- Welts on the face (lips, mouth, cheeks), back, buttocks, abdomen, chest, and inner thighs.
  - The shape of the object causing the welt may be seen. The shape may be of a belt, belt buckle, wooden spoon, chain, clothes hanger, rope, or other object.
- Burns and scalds on the feet, hands, back, buttocks, or other body parts.
  - Intentional burns leave a pattern from the item causing the burn: cigarettes, irons, curling irons, ropes, stove burners, and radiators are examples.
  - In scalds, the area put in hot liquid is clearly marked. For example, a scald to the hand looks like a glove. A scald to the foot looks like a sock.
- Fractures of the nose, skull, arms, or legs.
- Bite marks.

Neglect
- Fails to gain weight.
- Shows great affection to others.
- Wants to eat large amounts of food.
- Steals food.
- Is dirty or has a severe body odor.
- Lacks the correct clothing for the weather.
- Abuses alcohol or drugs.
- States that no one is home.

Sexual Abuse
- Bleeding, cuts, and bruises of the genitalia, anus, breasts, or mouth.
- Stains or blood on underclothing.
- Painful urination.
- Signs and symptoms of urinary tract infection (Chapter 42).
- Vaginal discharge.
- Genital odor.
- Genital pain.
- Difficulty walking or sitting.
- Pregnancy.
- Fearful behaviors—nightmares, depression, unusual fears, attempts to run away.
- Sexual behavior that does not fit with one's age.

Emotional Abuse
- Sudden changes in self-confidence.
- Headaches.
- Stomach aches.
- Abnormal fears.
- Nightmares.
- Attempts to run away.

Domestic abuse is a safety issue. Like child and elder abuse, domestic abuse is complex. The victim often hides the abuse. He or she may protect the abusive partner. State laws vary about reporting domestic abuse. However, the health team has an ethical duty to give information about safety and community resources. If you suspect domestic abuse, share your concerns with the nurse. The nurse gathers information to help the person.

OBRA-CMS

Under OBRA, the resident has the right to be free from abuse, mistreatment, or neglect. If a resident is abused by anyone, the abuse must be reported. This includes abuse by a partner.

QUALITY OF LIFE

Residents have the right to a comfortable and safe setting. To protect them from harm, you must understand your roles and responsibilities. What you do and how you do it affects their quality of life.

OBRA's purpose is to improve the quality of life of nursing center residents. The law requires training and competency evaluation programs for nursing assistants working in long-term care. These programs provide nursing assistants with the knowledge and skills needed to give basic nursing care. You must always practice within the legal limits of your role.

Residents have the right to be free from abuse, mistreatment, and neglect. Nursing centers have procedures for investigating all cases of suspected abuse. Be alert for signs and symptoms of abuse. If you suspect that a person is being abused, report the matter to the nurse. Share your observations with the nurse.

REVIEW QUESTIONS

Circle the BEST answer.

1 Ethics is
   a Making judgments before you have the facts
   b Knowledge of what is right and wrong conduct
   c A behavior that meets your needs, not the person's
   d Skills, care, and judgments required of a health team member

2 Which is ethical behavior?
   a Sharing information about a resident with your family
   b Accepting gifts from a resident's family
   c Reporting errors
   d Calling your family before answering a signal light

3 On your days off, you call the center to check on a resident. This is a
   a Professional boundary
   b Boundary crossing
   c Boundary violation
   d Boundary sign

4 To maintain professional boundaries, your behaviors must
   a Help the person
   b Meet your needs
   c Be biased
   d Show that you care

5 A friend is admitted to the center. You helped with the person's care. This is a
   a Professional boundary
   b Boundary crossing
   c Boundary violation
   d Boundary sign

6 Which is *not* a crime?
   a Abuse
   b Murder
   c Negligence
   d Robbery

7 These statements are about negligence. Which is *false*?
   a It is an unintentional tort.
   b The negligent person did not act in a reasonable manner.
   c Harm was caused to a person or a person's property.
   d A prison term is likely.

8 Threatening to touch the person's body without the person's consent is
   a Assault
   b Battery
   c Defamation
   d False imprisonment

9 Restraining a person's freedom of movement is
   a Assault
   b Battery
   c Defamation
   d False imprisonment

10 Photos of Mr. Blue are shown to others without his consent. This is
   a Battery
   b Fraud
   c Invasion of privacy
   d Malpractice

11 A person asks if you are a nurse. You answer "yes." This is
   a Negligence
   b Fraud
   c Libel
   d Slander

12 Informed consent is when the person
   a Fully understands all aspects of his or her treatment
   b Signs a consent form
   c Is admitted to the center
   d Decides how to distribute property after his or her death

13 Who is at risk for being wounded, attacked, or damaged?
   a Children
   b Older adults
   c Persons with disabilities
   d All residents

14 You scold an older person for not eating lunch. This is
   a Physical abuse
   b Neglect
   c Emotional abuse
   d Verbal abuse

15 Which is *not* a sign of elder abuse?
   a Stiff joints and joint pain
   b Old and new bruises
   c Poor personal hygiene
   d Frequent injuries

16 A child is deprived of food, clothing, and shelter. This is
   a Physical abuse
   b Neglect
   c Abandonment
   d Emotional abuse

17 A child has a black eye, bruises on her face, and bite marks on her arms. These are signs of
   a Physical abuse
   b Sexual abuse
   c Neglect
   d Substance abuse

18 You find blood stains on a child's underpants. This is a sign of
   a Physical abuse
   b Sexual abuse
   c Neglect
   d Substance abuse

19 These statements are about domestic abuse. Which is *true*?
   a It always involves physical harm.
   b It always involves violence.
   c One partner has control over the other partner.
   d Only one type of abuse is usually present.

20 You suspect a person was abused. What should you do?
   a Tell the family.
   b Call the police.
   c Tell the nurse.
   d Ask the person about the abuse.

Answers to these questions are on p. 719.

Work Ethics

OBJECTIVES

- Define the key terms and key abbreviations listed in this chapter.
- Identify good health and hygiene practices.
- Describe how to look professional.
- Describe the qualities and traits of a successful nursing assistant.
- Explain how to get a job.
- Explain how to plan for childcare and transportation.
- Describe ethical behavior on the job.
- Explain how to manage stress.
- Explain the aspects of harassment.
- Explain how to resign from a job.
- Identify the common reasons for losing a job.
- Explain the reasons for drug testing.
- Explain how to promote quality of life.

KEY TERMS

confidentiality Trusting others with personal and private information

courtesy A polite, considerate, or helpful comment or act

gossip To spread rumors or talk about the private matters of others

harassment To trouble, torment, offend, or worry a person by one's behavior or comments

preceptor A staff member who guides another staff member; mentor

priority The most important thing at the time

professionalism Following laws, being ethical, having good work ethics, and having the skills to do your work

stress The response or change in the body caused by any emotional, physical, social, or economic factor

stressor The event or factor that causes stress

work ethics Behavior in the workplace

KEY ABBREVIATIONS

NATCEP Nursing assistant training and competency evaluation program

OBRA Omnibus Budget Reconciliation Act of 1987

As a nursing assistant, you must act and function in a professional manner. **Professionalism** involves following laws, being ethical, having good work ethics, and having the skills to do your work. Laws and ethics are discussed in Chapter 4. Laws are rules of conduct made by government bodies. Ethics deals with right and wrong conduct. It involves choices and judgments about what to do or what not to do. An ethical person does the right thing. In the workplace, certain behaviors (conduct), choices, and judgments are expected. **Work ethics** deals with behavior in the workplace. Your conduct reflects your choices and judgments. Work ethics involves:

* How you look
* What you say
* How you behave
* How you treat others
* How you work with others

To get and keep a job, you must conduct yourself in the right way.

HEALTH, HYGIENE, AND APPEARANCE

Residents, families, and visitors expect the health team to look and act healthy. For example, a person is told to stop smoking, yet he or she sees health team members smoking. If you are not clean, people wonder if you give good care. You are part of the health team. Your health, appearance, and hygiene need careful attention.

Your Health

You must give safe and effective care. To do so, you must be physically and mentally healthy. Otherwise you cannot function at your best.

* *Diet.* You need a balanced diet (Chapter 24). Start your day with a good breakfast. To maintain your weight, balance the calories you take in with your energy needs. To lose weight, take in fewer calories than your energy needs. Avoid foods high in fat, oil, and sugar. Also avoid salty foods and crash diets.
* *Sleep and rest.* Sleep and rest are needed for health and to do your job well. Most adults need about 7 hours of sleep daily. Fatigue, lack of energy, and irritability mean you need more rest and sleep.
* *Body mechanics.* You will bend, carry heavy objects, and handle, move, and turn persons. These tasks place stress and strain on your body. You need to use your muscles correctly (Chapter 16).
* *Exercise.* Exercise is needed for muscle tone, circulation, and weight loss. Walking, running, swimming, and biking are good forms of exercise. Regular exercise helps you feel better physically and mentally. Consult your doctor before starting a vigorous exercise program.

* *Your eyes.* You will read instructions and take measurements. Wrong readings can cause the person harm. Have your eyes checked. Wear needed eyeglasses or contact lenses. Provide enough light for reading and fine work.
* *Smoking.* Smoking causes lung, heart, and circulatory disorders. Smoke odors stay on your breath, hands, clothing, and hair. Hand washing and good personal hygiene are needed.
* *Drugs.* Some drugs affect thinking, feeling, behavior, and function. Working under the influence of drugs affects the person's safety. Only take drugs ordered by a doctor. Take them in the prescribed way.
* *Alcohol.* Alcohol is a drug that depresses the brain. It affects thinking, balance, coordination, and mental alertness. Never report to work under the influence of alcohol. Do not drink alcohol while working. Like other drugs, alcohol affects the person's safety.

Your Hygiene

Personal hygiene needs careful attention. Bathe daily. Use a deodorant or antiperspirant to prevent body odors. Brush your teeth often—upon awakening, before and after meals, and at bedtime. Use a mouthwash to prevent breath odors. Shampoo often. Style hair in a simple, attractive way. Keep fingernails clean, short, and neatly shaped.

Menstrual hygiene is important. Change tampons or sanitary pads often, especially if flow is heavy. Wash your genital area with soap and water at least twice a day. Also practice good hand washing.

Foot care prevents odors and infection. Wash your feet daily. Dry thoroughly between the toes. Cut toenails straight across after bathing or soaking them.

Your Appearance

Good health and hygiene practices help you look and feel well. Follow the practices in Box 5-1, p. 46. They help you look clean, neat, and professional (Fig. 5-1, p. 46).

GETTING A JOB

There are easy ways to find out about jobs and places to work:

* Newspaper ads
* Local state employment services
* Centers you would like to work at
* Phone book yellow pages
* People you know—your instructor, family, and friends
* The Internet
* Your school's or college's job placement counselors
* Your clinical experience site

Box 5-1   Practices for a Professional Appearance

- Practice good hygiene.
- Wear uniforms that fit well. They are modest in length and style. Follow the center's dress code.
- Keep uniforms clean, pressed, and mended. Sew on buttons. Repair zippers, tears, and hems.
- Wear a clean uniform daily.
- Wear your name badge or photo ID at all times when on duty. Make sure it can be seen. Wear it according to center policy.
- Wear undergarments that are clean and fit properly. Change them daily.
- Wear undergarments in the correct color for your skin tone. Do not wear colored (red, pink, blue, and so on) ones. They can be seen through white and light-colored uniforms.
- Cover tattoos (body art). They may offend others.
- Follow the center's dress code for jewelry. Wedding and engagement rings may be allowed. Rings and bracelets can scratch a person. Confused or combative persons can easily pull on jewelry (necklaces, dangling earrings). So can young children.
- Do not wear jewelry in pierced eyebrows, nose, lips, or tongue while on duty.
- Follow the center's dress code for earrings. Usually small, simple earrings are allowed. For multiple ear piercings, usually only one set of earrings is allowed.
- Wear a wristwatch with a second (sweep) hand.
- Wear clean stockings and socks that fit well. Change them daily.
- Wear shoes that fit properly, are comfortable, give needed support, and have non-skid soles. Do not wear sandals or open-toed shoes.
- Clean and polish shoes often. Wash and replace laces as needed.
- Keep fingernails clean, short, and neatly shaped. Long nails can scratch a person. Nails must be natural.
- Do not wear nail polish. Chipped nail polish may provide a place for microbes to grow.
- Have a simple, attractive hairstyle. Hair is off your collar and away from your face. Use simple pins, combs, barrettes, and bands to keep long hair up and in place.
- Keep beards and mustaches clean and trimmed.
- Use makeup that is modest in amount and moderate in color. Avoid a painted and severe look.
- Do not wear perfume, cologne, or after-shave lotion. The scents may offend, nauseate, or cause breathing problems in residents.

Your clinical experience site is an important source. The staff always looks at students as future employees. They look for good work ethics. They watch how students treat residents and co-workers. They look for the qualities and traits described in Box 5-2. If that center is not hiring, the staff may suggest other places to apply.

Fig. 5-1 This nursing assistant is well-groomed. Her uniform and shoes are clean. Her hair has a simple style. It is away from her face and off of her collar. She does not wear jewelry.

What Employers Look For

If you owned a business, who would you want to hire? Your answer helps you better understand the employer's point of view. Employers want people who:
- Are dependable
- Are well-groomed
- Have needed job skills and training
- Have values and attitudes that fit with the center

Good work ethics involves the qualities and traits described in Box 5-2. They are necessary for you to function well (Fig. 5-2).

Applicants who look good communicate many things to the employer. You have one chance to make a good first impression. A well-groomed person will likely get the job. A sloppy person with wrinkled or dirty clothes may not get the job, nor will someone with body or breath odors. See p. 48 for how to dress for an interview.

Being dependable is important. You must be at work on time and when scheduled. Undependable people cause everyone problems. Other staff take on extra work. Fewer people give care. Quality of care suffers. You want co-workers to work when scheduled. Otherwise, you have extra work. You have less time to spend with residents. Likewise, co-workers also expect you to work when scheduled.

Box 5-2 Qualities and Traits for Good Work Ethics

- **Caring.** Have concern for the person. Help make the person's life happier, easier, or less painful.
- **Dependable.** Report to work on time and when scheduled. Perform delegated tasks. Keep obligations and promises.
- **Considerate.** Respect the person's physical and emotional feelings. Be gentle and kind toward residents, families, and co-workers.
- **Cheerful.** Greet and talk to people in a pleasant manner. Do not be moody, bad-tempered, or unhappy while at work.
- **Empathetic.** Empathy is seeing things from the person's point of view—putting yourself in the person's place. How would you feel if you had the person's problems?
- **Trustworthy.** Residents and staff have confidence in you. They believe you will keep information confidential. They trust you not to gossip about residents or the health team.
- **Respectful.** Residents have rights, values, beliefs, and feelings. They may differ from yours. Do not judge or condemn the person. Treat the person with respect and dignity at all times. Also show respect for the health team.
- **Courteous.** Be polite and courteous to residents, families, visitors, and co-workers. See p. 54 for common courtesies in the workplace.
- **Conscientious.** Be careful, alert, and exact in following instructions. Give thorough care. Do not lose or damage the person's property.
- **Honest.** Accurately report the care given, your observations, and any errors.
- **Cooperative.** Willingly help and work with others. Also take that "extra step" during busy and stressful times.
- **Enthusiastic.** Be eager, interested, and excited about your work. Your work is important.
- **Self-aware.** Know your feelings, strengths, and weaknesses. You need to understand yourself before you can understand the residents.

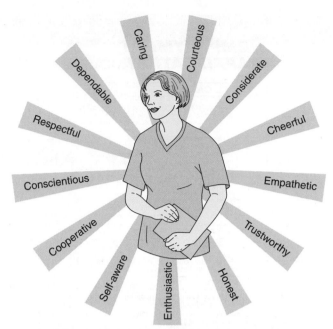

Fig. 5-2 Good work ethics involves these qualities and traits.

Job Skills and Training Employers need to know that you have the required job skills. To work in long-term care, you must complete a state-approved nursing assistant training and competency evaluation program (NATCEP). This is a requirement of the Omnibus Budget Reconciliation Act of 1987 (OBRA). The employer checks the nursing assistant registry and requests proof of training:

- A certificate of course completion
- A high school, college, or technical school transcript
- An official grade report (report card)

Give the employer only a *copy* of your certificate, transcript, or grade report. Never give the original to the employer. Keep it for future use. The employer may want a transcript sent directly from the school or college.

Job Applications

You get a job application from the *personnel office* or *human resources office* (Fig. 5-3, pp. 48-49). You can complete the application there. Or you can take it home and return it by mail or in person. You must be well-groomed and behave pleasantly when seeking or returning a job application. It may be your first chance to make a good impression.

To complete a job application, follow the guidelines in Box 5-3, p. 50. How you fill out the application may mean getting or not getting the job. Often the application is your first chance to impress the employer. A neat, readable, and complete application gives a good image. A sloppy or incomplete one does not.

Some centers provide job applications on-line. Follow the center's instructions for completing and sending an on-line application.

The Job Interview

A job interview is the employer's chance to get to know and evaluate you. You also find out more about the center.

The interview may be when you complete the job application. Some centers schedule interviews after reviewing applications. Write down the interviewer's name and the interview date and time. If you need directions to the center, ask for them at this time.

OBRA-CMS

EMPLOYMENT APPLICATION

APPLICANT INSTRUCTIONS

If you need help filling out this application form or for any phase of the employment process, please notify the person that gave you this form and every effort will be made to accommodate your needs in a reasonable amount of time.

1. Please read "APPLICANT NOTE" below.
2. Complete both sides of this page.
3. If more space is needed to complete any question, use comments section at the bottom of this page.
4. Print clearly: incomplete or illegible applications will not be processed. PLEASE NOTE "NOT APPLICABLE" IF NOT ANSWERING A QUESTION.
5. Provide only requested information. Failure to do so may result in disqualification of your application.
6. Some packets may include an AFFIRMATIVE ACTION QUESTIONNAIRE. This information is being gathered for affirmative action under Section 503 of the Rehabilitation Act of 1973. The information requested is voluntary and will be kept confidential. An applicant will not be subject to any adverse treatment for refusing to complete the questionnaire.
7. DO NOT FILL OUT ANY OTHER ATTACHED FORMS OR PAGES UNTIL INSTRUCTED.

TODAY'S DATE: _____

NAME: _____
          LAST   FIRST   MI

SOCIAL SECURITY NUMBER: _____

HOME PHONE: _____ WORK PHONE: _____

CURRENT ADDRESS: _____
                              STREET

_____
          CITY   STATE   ZIP

PRIOR ADDRESS: _____
                            STREET

_____
          CITY   STATE   ZIP

APPLICANT NOTE

This application form is intended for use in evaluating your qualifications for employment. This is not an employment contract. Please answer all appropriate questions completely and accurately. False or misleading statements during the interview and on this form are grounds for terminating the application process or, if discovered after employment, terminating employment. All qualified applicants will receive consideration without discrimination based on sex, marital status, race, color, age, creed, national origin, sexual orientation, military reserve membership, ancestry, religion, height, weight, use of a guide or support animal because of blindness, deafness or physical handicap, or the presence of disabilities. A conviction will not necessarily bar an applicant from employment. Additional testing of job-related skills and for the presence of drugs in your body may be required prior to employment. After an offer of employment, and prior to reporting to work, you may be required to submit to a medical review. Depending on company policy and the needs of the job, you will be required to complete a medical history form and may be required to be examined by a medical professional designated by the company.

AVAILABILITY

For which position are you applying? _____

What date can you start? _____ What category would you prefer? ❑ Full time   ❑ Part time   ❑ Temporary   ❑ Labor pool

For which schedules are you available?* ❑ Weekdays   ❑ Weekends   ❑ Evenings   ❑ Nights   ❑ Overtime   ❑ Shift   ❑ Other_____
*reasonable efforts will be made to accommodate sincerely held moral and ethical beliefs, (WI) religious beliefs and practices (All other States)

JOB-RELATED SKILLS

NOTE: Do not fill out any part of this section you believe to be non-job related.

❑ Yes   ❑ No   If the job requires, do you have the appropriate valid drivers license?
                                Name on license _____ DL# _____ Type _____ State of Issue _____

❑ Yes   ❑ No   Have you had any moving violations within the last seven years? Please describe. _____
                                Please list any other skills, licenses or certificates that may be job-related or that you feel would be of value to this job or company. _____

❑ Yes   ❑ No   Have you been given a job description or had the essential functions of the job explained to you?

❑ Yes   ❑ No   Do you understand these essential functions?

❑ Yes   ❑ No   Can you perform the essential functions of this job with or without reasonable accommodation?

SECURITY

List states and counties of residence for the past seven years: _____
_____

❑ Yes   ❑ No   Have you used any names or Social Security Numbers other than given above? If so, please list in comments, below.

❑ Yes   ❑ No   Have you been convicted of a crime in the past seven years? If so, please describe in the boxes below. (Conviction will not necessarily be a bar to employment. In accordance with company policy and applicable state and federal laws, factors such as age at time of the offense, remoteness of the offense, time since last conviction, nature of the job sought and rehabilitation effort will be reviewed.)

INCIDENT	CITY/STATE	CHARGE
1.		
2.		

COMMENTS   (ASK FOR AN ADDITIONAL PAGE IF NECESSARY)
_____
_____
_____
_____

© ADP SCREENING & SELECTION SERVICES 2002

Fig. 5-3 A sample job application. *(Courtesy ADP Screening and Selection Services, Ft. Collins, Colorado.)*

Box 5-4, p. 50 lists common interview questions. Prepare your answers before the interview. Also prepare a list of your skills. Give the list to the interviewer.

Preparing for the Interview You must present a good image. You need to be neat, clean, and well-groomed. How you dress is important. Follow the guidelines in Box 5-5, p. 51.

Be on time. It shows you are dependable. Go to the center some day before your interview. Note how long it takes to get there and where to park. Also find the personnel office. A *dry run* (practice run) gives an idea of how long it takes to get from your home to the personnel office.

PREVIOUS EMPLOYERS

PLEASE NOTE: Your application will not be considered unless every question in this section is answered. Since we will make every effort to contact previous employers, the **correct telephone numbers of past employers are critical.** Ask for a phone book or call information if necessary. FOR EMPLOYERS OUTSIDE THE U.S., A CURRENT FAX NUMBER IS MANDATORY.

MOST RECENT EMPLOYER   ❑ Yes ❑ No   Are you currently working for this employer?
❑ Yes ❑ No   If yes, may we contact?

PHONE ( )
FAX ( )

COMPANY NAME _____ CITY _____ STATE _____
FROM _____ TO _____
DATES EMPLOYED   JOB TITLE _____ SUPERVISOR NAME _____
DUTIES _____
SALARY _____ PER (HOUR, WEEK, MONTH)   REASON FOR LEAVING _____

SECOND MOST RECENT EMPLOYER

PHONE ( )
FAX ( )

COMPANY NAME _____ CITY _____ STATE _____
FROM _____ TO _____
DATES EMPLOYED   JOB TITLE _____ SUPERVISOR NAME _____
DUTIES _____
SALARY _____ PER (HOUR, WEEK, MONTH)   REASON FOR LEAVING _____

THIRD MOST RECENT EMPLOYER

PHONE ( )
FAX ( )

COMPANY NAME _____ CITY _____ STATE _____
FROM _____ TO _____
DATES EMPLOYED   JOB TITLE _____ SUPERVISOR NAME _____
DUTIES _____
SALARY _____ PER (HOUR, WEEK, MONTH)   REASON FOR LEAVING _____

REFERENCES   Include only individuals familiar with your work ability. Do not include relatives.

NAME	ADDRESS/PHONE	YEARS KNOWN/RELATIONSHIP
1.		
2.		

EDUCATION   NOTE: Do not fill out any part of this section you believe to be non-job related.
Please circle highest grade completed.   7   8   9   10   11   12   13   14   15   16   16+

If your school records are under a different name than listed on page 1, please enter that name _____

NAME	CITY/STATE	GRADUATED	DEGREE?
HIGH SCHOOL			
COLLEGE			
OTHER			

CERTIFICATION AND RELEASE   I certify that I have read and understand the applicant note on page one of this form and that the answers given by me to the foregoing questions and the statements made by me are complete and true to the best of my knowledge and belief. I understand that any false information, omissions or misrepresentations of facts called for in this application, whether on this document or not, may result in rejection of my application or discharge at any time during my employment. I authorize the company and/or its agents, including consumer reporting bureaus, to verify any of this information. I authorize all former employers, persons, schools, companies and law enforcement authorities from any liability for any damage whatsoever for issuing this information. I also understand that the use of illegal drugs is prohibited during employment. If company policy requires, I am willing to submit to drug testing to detect the use of illegal drugs prior to and during employment.

SIGNATURE _____ DATE _____

© ADP SCREENING & SELECTION SERVICES 2002

Fig. 5-3, cont'd For legend, see facing page.

When you arrive for the interview, turn off your wireless phone or pager. Tell the receptionist your name and why you are there. Also give the interviewer's name. Then sit quietly in the waiting area. Do not smoke, chew gum, or use your phone. While you wait, review your answers to the common interview questions. Waiting may be part of the interview. The interviewer may ask the receptionist about how you acted while waiting. Smile, and be polite and friendly.

Box 5-3 Guidelines for Completing a Job Application

- Read and follow the directions. They may ask you to print using black ink. You need to follow directions on the job. Employers look at job applications to see if you can follow directions.
- Write neatly. Your writing must be readable. A messy application gives a bad image. Readable writing gives the correct information. The center cannot contact you if unable to read your phone number. You may miss getting the job.
- Complete the entire form. Something may not apply to you. If so, write "non-applicable" or "N/A" for non-applicable. Or draw a line through the space. This tells the employer that you read the section. It also shows that you did not skip the item on purpose.
- Report any felony arrests or convictions as directed. Write "no" or "none" as appropriate. Criminal background and fingerprint checks are common requirements.
- Give information about employment gaps. If you did not work for a time, the employer wonders why. Provide this information to give a good impression about your honesty. Some reasons are an illness, going to school, raising your children, or caring for an ill or older family member.

- Tell why you left a job, if asked. Be brief, but honest. People leave jobs for one that pays better. Some leave for career advancement. Other reasons include those given for employment gaps. If you were fired from a job, give an honest but positive response. Do not talk badly about a former employer.
- Provide references. Be prepared to give names, titles, addresses, and phone numbers of at least four references who are not relatives. You should have this information written down before completing an application. (Always ask references if an employer can contact them.) You may get the job faster or over another applicant if the employer can quickly check references. If they are missing or not complete, the employer waits for all of the information. This wastes your time and the employer's time. Also, the employer wonders if you are hiding something with incomplete reference information.
- Be prepared to provide the following:
  - Social Security number
  - Proof of citizenship or legal residency
  - Proof of required training and competency evaluation
  - Identification—driver's license or government-issued ID card
- Give honest responses. Lying on an application is fraud. It is grounds for being fired.
- Keep a file of your education and work history.

Box 5-4 Common Interview Questions

What the Interviewer May Ask You:
- Tell me about yourself.
- Tell me about your career goals.
- What are you doing to reach these goals?
- Describe your idea of *professional* behavior.
- Tell me about your last job. Why did you leave?
- What did you like the most about your last job? What did you like the least?
- What would your supervisor and co-workers tell me about you? Your dependability? Your skills? Your flexibility?
- Which functions are the hardest for you? How do you handle this difficulty?
- How do you set your priorities?
- How have your experiences prepared you for this job?
- What would you like to change about your last job?
- How do you handle problems with residents and co-workers?
- Why do you want to work here?
- Why should this center hire you?

Questions to Ask the Interviewer:
- Which job functions do you think are the most important?
- What employee qualities and traits are the most important to you?
- What nursing care pattern is used here (Chapter 1)?
- Who will I work with?
- When are performance evaluations done? Who does them? How are they done?

Questions to Ask the Interviewer—cont'd
- What performance factors are evaluated?
- How does the supervisor handle problems?
- What are the most common reasons that nursing assistants lose their jobs here?
- What are the most common reasons that nursing assistants resign from their jobs here?
- How do you see this job in the next year? In the next 5 years?
- What is the greatest reward from this job?
- What is the greatest challenge from this job?
- What do you like the most about nursing assistants who work here? What do you like the least?
- Why should I work here rather than in another center?
- Why are you interested in hiring me?
- How much will I make an hour?
- What hours will I work?
- What uniforms are required?
- What benefits do you offer?
  - Health and disability insurance?
  - Continuing education?
  - Vacation time?
- Does the center have a new employee orientation program?
- May I have a tour of the center and the unit I will work on? Will you introduce me to the nurse manager and unit staff?
- Can I have a few minutes to talk to the nurse manager?

Fig. 5-4 A, A simple suit is worn for a job interview. **B,** This man wears slacks and a shirt and tie for his interview.

Box 5-5 Grooming and Dressing for an Interview

- Bathe and brush your teeth. Wash your hair.
- Use deodorant or antiperspirant.
- Make sure your hands and fingernails are clean.
- Apply makeup in a simple, attractive manner.
- Style your hair in a neat and attractive way. Wear it as you would for work.
- Do not wear jeans, shorts, tank tops, halter tops, or other casual clothing.
- Iron clothing. Sew on loose buttons and mend garments as needed.
- Wear clothing that covers tattoos (body art).
- Wear a simple dress, skirt and blouse, or suit (women). Men wear a suit or dark slacks and a shirt and tie. A jacket is optional. A long-sleeved white or light blue shirt is best (Fig. 5-4).
- Wear socks (men and women) or hose (women). Hose should be free of runs and snags.
- Make sure shoes are clean and in good repair.
- Avoid heavy perfumes, colognes, and after-shave lotions. A lightly scented fragrance is okay.
- Wear only simple jewelry that complements your clothes. Avoid adornments in body piercings. If you have multiple ear piercings, wear only one set of earrings.
- Stop in the restroom when you arrive for the interview. Check your hair, makeup, and clothes.

During the Interview Politely greet the interviewer. A firm handshake is correct for men and women. Address the interviewer as Miss, Mrs., Ms., Mr., or Doctor. Stand until asked to take a seat. When sitting, use good posture. Sit in a professional manner. If offered a beverage, you may accept. Be sure to thank the person.

Good eye contact is needed. Look directly at the interviewer when you answer or ask questions. Poor eye contact sends negative information—being shy, insecure, dishonest, or lacking interest.

Watch your body language (Chapter 8). Body language involves facial expressions, gestures, posture, and body movements. What you say is important. However, how you use and move your body also tells a great deal. Avoid distracting habits—biting nails; playing with jewelry, clothing, or your hair; crossing your arms; and swinging legs back and forth. Keep your mind on the interview. Do not touch or read things on the person's desk.

The interview lasts 15 to 45 minutes. Give complete and honest answers. Speak clearly and with confidence. Avoid short and long answers. "Yes" and "no" answers give little information. Briefly explain "yes" and "no" responses (Chapter 8).

The interviewer will ask about your skills. Share your skills list. He or she may ask about a skill not on your list. Explain that you are willing to learn the skill if your state allows nursing assistants to perform the task.

Find the right job for you. An employer wants to hire someone who will be happy in the job and the center. Box 5-4 lists some questions for you to ask at the end of the interview. The person's answers will help you decide if the job is right for you.

Review the job description with the interviewer. If you have questions about it, ask them at this time. Advise the interviewer of functions you cannot perform because of training, legal, ethical, or religious reasons. Honesty now prevents problems later.

The interviewer signals when the interview is over. You may be offered a job at this time. Or you are told when to expect a call or letter. Follow-up is acceptable. Ask when you can check on your application. Before leaving, thank the interviewer. Say that you look forward to hearing from him or her. Shake the person's hand before you leave.

```
December 12

Dear Ms. O'Neal,

Thank you for the interview yesterday. I enjoyed meeting you
and learning more about the nursing center. I was impressed
by the friendliness of the staff and would enjoy working in that
environment.

Again, thank you. I look forward to hearing from you soon.

Sincerely,
Alison M.Teal
```

Fig. 5-5 Sample thank-you note written after a job interview.

After the Interview A thank-you letter or note is advised (Fig. 5-5). Write this within 24 hours after the interview. Write neatly and clearly. Use a computer or typewriter if your writing is hard to read. The thank-you note should include:

- The date
- The interviewer's formal name using Miss, Mrs., Ms., Mr., or Dr.
- A statement thanking the person for the interview
- Comments about the interview, the center, and your eagerness to hear about the job
- Your signature using your first and last names

Accepting a Job

Accept the job that is best for you. You can apply many places and have many interviews. Think about all offers before accepting one. You might have more questions about a center. Ask them before accepting the job. To help decide what to do, discuss the offer with a family member, friend, co-worker, or your instructor.

When you accept a job, agree on a starting date, pay rate, and work hours. Find out where to report on your first day. Ask for such information in writing. That way you and the center have the same understanding of the job offer. Use the written offer later if questions arise. Also ask for the employee handbook and other center information. Read everything before you start working.

New Employee Orientation

Centers have orientation programs for new employees. The center's policy and procedure manual is reviewed. Your skills are checked. That is, the center has you perform the procedures in your job description. This is to make sure that you do them safely and correctly. Also, you are shown how to use the center's supplies and equipment.

Many centers have preceptor programs. A preceptor (mentor) is a staff member who guides another staff member. A nurse or nursing assistant:

- Helps you learn the center's layout so you can find what you need
- Introduces you to residents and staff
- Helps you organize your work
- Helps you feel comfortable as a part of the nursing team
- Answers questions about the policy and procedure manual

A nursing assistant preceptor is not your supervisor. Only nurses can supervise. A preceptor program usually lasts 2 to 4 weeks. Its purpose is to help you succeed in your role. It also helps ensure quality care. After the preceptor program, you should feel comfortable with the setting and your role. If not, ask for more orientation time.

PREPARING FOR WORK

You successfully completed a NATCEP. You had a successful job interview. To keep your job, you must function well and work well with others. You must:

- Work when scheduled
- Get to work on time
- Stay the entire shift

Absences and tardiness (being late) are common reasons for losing a job. Childcare and transportation issues often interfere with getting to work. Plan for them in advance.

Childcare

Someone needs to care for your children when you leave for work, while you are at work, and before you get home from work. Also plan for emergencies:

- Your childcare provider is ill or cannot care for your children that day.
- A child becomes ill while you are at work.
- You will be late getting home from work.

Transportation

Plan for how you get to and from work. If you drive, keep your car in good working order. Keep enough gas in the car. Or leave early to get gas.

Carpooling is an option. Carpool members depend on each other. If the driver is late leaving, everyone is late for work. If one person is not ready when the driver arrives, everyone is late for work. Carpool with persons you trust to be ready and on time. When you drive, leave and pick up others on time. As a passenger, be ready to be picked up on time.

Know your bus or train schedule. Know what other bus or train to take if delays occur. Always carry enough money for fares to and from work.

Always have a back-up plan for getting to work. Your car may not start, the carpool driver may not go to work, or public transportation may not operate.

TEAMWORK

How you look, how you behave, and what you say affect everyone in the center. Practice good work ethics:
- Work when scheduled.
- Be cheerful and friendly.
- Perform delegated tasks.
- Be available to help others. Help willingly.
- Be kind to others.

The *Employee Handbook* of OSF Saint Francis Medical Center (Peoria, Ill) says it best:

You are what people see when they arrive here; yours are the eyes they look into when they're frightened and lonely. Yours are the voices people hear when they ride the elevators, when they try to sleep, and when they try to forget their problems. You are what they hear on their way to appointments which could affect their destinies, and what they hear after they leave those appointments. Yours are the comments people hear when you think they can't.

Yours is the intelligence and caring that people hope they'll find here. If you're noisy, so is the medical center. If you're rude, so is the medical center. And if you're wonderful, so is the medical center.

You are an important member of the health team. Quality of care is affected by how you work with others and how you feel about your job.

Attendance

Report to work when scheduled and on time. The entire unit is affected when just one person is late. Call the center if you will be late or cannot go to work. Follow the center's attendance policy in your employee handbook. Poor attendance can cause you to lose your job.

Be *ready to work* when your shift starts. Store your coat, purse, backpack, and other items before your shift starts. Use the restroom when you arrive at the center. Arrive on your nursing unit a few minutes early. This gives you time to greet others and settle yourself.

Attendance also means staying the entire shift. Prepare for childcare emergencies. Watching the clock for when your shift ends gives a bad image. You may need to work over-time. Prepare to stay longer if necessary. When it is time to leave, report off duty to the nurse.

See *Teamwork and Time Management: Attendance.*

Your Attitude

You need a good attitude (see Box 5-2). Show that you enjoy your work. Listen to others. Be willing to learn. Stay busy, and use your time well.

TEAMWORK AND TIME MANAGEMENT
Attendance

Sometimes a staff member is late for work or does not show up for work. Until a replacement arrives, you and other staff members have extra work. Resident care cannot suffer.

To promote teamwork and manage your time:
- Ask the nurse how you can help.
- Do not complain about not having enough staff.
- Ask the nurse to list the most important tasks and care measures.

Your work is very important. Nurses, residents, and families rely on you to give good care. They expect you to be pleasant and respectful. You must believe that you and your work have value.

Always think before you speak. These statements signal a bad attitude:
- "That's not my resident."
- "I can't. I'm too busy."
- "I didn't do it."
- "I don't feel like it."
- "It's not my fault."
- "Don't blame me."
- "It's not my turn. I did it yesterday."
- "Nobody told me."
- "That's not my job."
- "You didn't say that you needed it right away."
- "I work harder than anyone else."
- "No one appreciates what I do."
- "I'm tired of this place."
- "Is it time to leave yet?"
- "Good luck. I had a horrible day."

Gossip

To **gossip** means to spread rumors or talk about the private matters of others. Gossiping is unprofessional and hurtful. To avoid being a part of gossip:
- Remove yourself from a group or setting where people are gossiping.
- Do not make or repeat any comment that can hurt a person, family member, visitor, co-worker, or the center.
- Do not make or repeat any comment that you do not know is true. Making or writing false statements about another person is defamation (Chapter 4).
- Do not talk about residents, family members, visitors, co-workers, or the center at home or in social settings.

Confidentiality

The person's information is private and personal. **Confidentiality** means trusting others with personal and private information. The person's information is shared only among health team members involved in

OBRA-CMS

his or her care. Privacy and confidentiality are rights protected by OBRA. Center, family, and co-worker information also is confidential.

Avoid talking about residents, families, the center, or co-workers when others are present. Share information only with the nurse. Do not talk about residents, families, the center, or co-workers in hallways, elevators, dining areas, or outside the center. Others may overhear you. Residents and visitors are very alert to comments. They think you are talking about them or their loved ones. This leads to wrong information and wrong impressions about the person's condition. You can easily upset the person or family. Be very careful about what, how, when, and where you say things.

Do not eavesdrop. To eavesdrop means to listen in or overhear what others are saying. It invades a person's privacy.

Many centers have intercom systems. They allow for communication between the bedside and the nurses' station (Chapter 18). The person uses the intercom to signal when help is needed. Someone at the nurses' station answers the intercom. The nursing team also uses the intercom to communicate with each other. Be careful what you say over the intercom. It is like a loud speaker. Others nearby can hear what you are saying.

See *Focus on Communication: Confidentiality.*

Hygiene and Appearance

How you look affects the way people think about you and the center. If the staff are clean and neat, people think the center is clean and neat. They think the center is unclean if the staff are messy and not tidy. People also wonder about the quality of care given.

Home and social attire is often improper at work. You cannot wear jeans, halter tops, tank tops, or short skirts. Clothing must not be tight, revealing, or sexual. Females cannot show cleavage, the tops of breasts, or upper thighs. Males must avoid tight pants and exposing their chests. Only the top shirt button is open. Follow the practices in Box 5-1.

FOCUS ON COMMUNICATION
Confidentiality

Your family members and friends may ask you about people they know in the center. They may ask about residents, their families, or employees. For example, your mother says: "Mrs. Drew goes to our church. I heard that she's in your nursing home. What's wrong with her?"

Do not share any information with your family and friends. Doing so violates the person's right to privacy and confidentiality (Chapters 2 and 4). You can say:

"I'm sorry, but I can't tell you about anyone in the center. It is unprofessional and against center policies. And it violates the person's right to privacy and confidentiality. Please don't ask me about anyone in the center."

Speech and Language

Your speech and language must be professional. Speech and language used in home and social settings may be improper at work. Words used with family and friends may offend residents, families, visitors, and co-workers. Remember the following:

- Do not swear or use foul, vulgar, or abusive language.
- Do not use slang.
- Control the volume and tone of your voice. Speak softly and gently.
- Speak clearly. The person may have a hearing problem (Chapter 37).
- Do not shout or yell.
- Do not fight or argue with a person, family member, visitor, or co-worker.

Courtesies

A courtesy is a polite, considerate, or helpful comment or act. Courtesies are easy. They take little time or energy. And they mean so much to people. Even the smallest kind act can brighten someone's day:

- Address others by Miss, Mrs., Ms., Mr., or Doctor. Use a first name only if the person asks you to do so.
- Say "please." Begin or end each request with "please."
- Say "thank you" whenever someone does something for you.
- Apologize. Say "I'm sorry" when you make a mistake or hurt someone. Even little things—like bumping someone in the hallway—need an apology.
- Be thoughtful. Compliment others. Wish others a happy birthday, a happy day or weekend off, or a happy holiday.
- Wish the person and family well when they leave the center. "Stay well" or "stay healthy" are good phrases to use.
- Hold doors open for others. If you are at the door first, open the door and let others pass through.
- Hold elevator doors open for others coming down the hallway.
- Let residents, families, and visitors enter elevators first.
- Stand to greet visitors and families.
- Help others willingly when asked.
- Give praise. If you see a co-worker do or say something that impresses you, tell that person. Also tell your co-workers.
- Do not take credit for another person's deeds. Give the person credit for the action.

Personal Matters

You were hired to do a job. Personal matters cannot interfere with the job, otherwise care is neglected. You could lose your job for tending to personal matters while at work. To keep personal matters out of the workplace:

- Make personal phone calls during meals and breaks. Use a pay phone or your wireless phone.
- Do not let family and friends visit you on the unit. If they must see you, have them meet you during a meal or break.
- Make appointments (doctor, dentist, lawyer, and others) for your days off.
- Do not use the center's computers, printers, fax machines, copiers, or other equipment for your personal use.
- Do not take center supplies (pens, paper, and others) for your personal use.
- Do not discuss personal problems.
- Control your emotions. If you need to cry or express anger, do so in a private place. Get yourself together quickly and return to your work.
- Do not borrow money from or lend it to co-workers. This includes meal money and bus or train fares. Borrowing and lending can lead to problems with co-workers.
- Do not sell things or engage in fund-raising. For example, do not sell your child's candy or raffle tickets to co-workers.
- Turn off personal pagers and wireless phones.
- Do not send or check text messages.

Meals and Breaks

Meal breaks are usually 30 minutes. Other breaks are usually 15 minutes. Meals and breaks are scheduled so that some staff are always on the unit. Staff remaining on the unit cover for the staff on break.

Staff members depend on each other. Leave for and return from breaks on time. That way other staff can have their turn. Do not take longer than allowed. Tell the nurse when you leave and return to the unit.

Job Safety

You must protect residents, families, visitors, co-workers, and yourself from harm. Everyone is responsible for safety. Negligent behavior affects the safety of others (Chapter 4). Safety practices are presented throughout this book. These guidelines apply to everything you do:

- Understand the roles, functions, and responsibilities in your job description.
- Know the contents and policies in the employee handbook and policy and procedure manuals.
- Know what is right and wrong.
- Know what you can and cannot do.
- Develop the desired qualities and traits of nursing assistants.
- Follow the nurse's directions and instructions.
- Question unclear directions and things you do not understand.
- Help others willingly when asked.
- Follow center rules.
- Ask for any training that you might need.
- Report measurements, observations, the care given, the person's complaints, and any errors accurately (Chapter 6).
- Accept responsibility for your actions. Admit when you are wrong or make mistakes. Do not blame others. Do not make excuses for your actions. Learn what you did wrong and why. Always try to learn from your mistakes.
- Handle the person's property carefully and prevent damage.

Planning Your Work

You will give care and perform routine tasks on the nursing unit. Some tasks are done at certain times. Others are done by the end of the shift.

The nurse, the Kardex, the care plan, and your assignment sheet help you decide what to do and when (Chapters 6 and 7). This is called *priority setting*. A priority is the most important thing at the time. Setting priorities involves deciding:

- Which person has the greatest or most life-threatening needs
- What tasks the nurse or person needs done first
- What tasks need to be done at a set time
- What tasks need to be done when your shift starts
- What tasks need to be done at the end of your shift
- How much time it takes to complete a task
- How much help you need to complete a task
- Who can help you and when

Priorities change as the person's needs change. A person's condition can improve or worsen. New residents are admitted. Others are transferred to other nursing units or discharged. These and many other factors can cause priorities to change.

Setting priorities is hard at first. It becomes easier as you gain experience. You can ask the nurse to help you set priorities. Plan your work to give safe, thorough care and to make good use of your time (Box 5-6, p. 56).

MANAGING STRESS

Stress is the response or change in the body caused by any emotional, physical, social, or economic factor. Stress is normal. It occurs every minute of every day. It occurs in everything you do.

A stressor is the event or factor that causes stress. Many stressors are pleasant—watching a child play, planning a party, laughing with family and friends, enjoying a nice day. Some are not pleasant—illness, injury, family problems, death of loved ones, divorce, money concerns. Many parts of your job are stressful.

Box 5-6   Planning Your Work

- Discuss priorities with the nurse.
- Know the routine of your shift and nursing unit.
- Follow unit policies for shift reports.
- List tasks that are on a schedule. For example, some persons are turned or offered the bedpan every 2 hours.
- Judge how much time you need for each person and task.
- Identify the tasks to do while residents are eating, visiting, or involved with activities or therapies.
- Plan care around meal times, visiting hours, and therapies. Also consider recreation and social activities.
- Identify when you will need help from a co-worker. Ask a co-worker to help you. Give the time when you will need help and for how long.
- Schedule equipment or rooms for the person's use. The shower room is an example.
- Review delegated tasks. Gather needed supplies beforehand.
- Do not waste time. Stay focused on your work.
- Leave a clean work area. Make sure rooms are neat and orderly. Also clean utility areas.
- Be a self-starter. Have initiative. Ask others if they need help. Follow unit routines, stock supply areas, and clean utility rooms. Stay busy.

No matter the cause, stress affects the whole person:

- *Physically*—sweating, increased heart rate, faster and deeper breathing, increased blood pressure, dry mouth, and so on
- *Mentally*—anxiety, fear, anger, dread, depression, and using defense mechanisms (Chapter 43)
- *Socially*—changes in relationships, avoiding others, needing others, blaming others, and so on
- *Spiritually*—changes in beliefs and values and strengthening or questioning one's belief in God or a higher power

Prolonged or frequent stress can threaten your health. Physical and mental health problems can occur. Some problems are minor—headaches, stomach upset, sleep problems, muscle tension, and so on. Others are life-threatening—high blood pressure, heart attack, stroke, ulcers, and so on.

Dealing with stress is important. If your job causes stress, it affects your family and friends. If you have stress in your personal life, it affects your work. Stress affects you, the care you give, the person's quality of life, and how you relate to co-workers. These guidelines can help you reduce or cope with stress:

- Exercise regularly. It has physical and mental benefits—cardiovascular health, weight control, tension release, emotional well-being, and relaxation.
- Get enough rest and sleep.
- Eat healthy.

- Plan personal and quiet time for you. Read, take a hot bath, go for a walk, meditate, or listen to music. Do what makes you feel good.
- Use common sense about what you can do. Do not try to do everything that family and friends ask you to do. Consider the amount of time and energy that you have.
- Do one thing at a time. The demands on you may seem overwhelming. List each thing that you have to do. Set priorities.
- Do not judge yourself harshly. Do not try to be perfect or expect too much from yourself.
- Give yourself praise. You do good and wonderful things every day.
- Have a sense of humor. Laugh at yourself. Laugh with others. Spend time with those who make you laugh.
- Talk to the nurse if your work or a person is causing too much stress. The nurse can help you deal with the matter.

HARASSMENT

Harassment means to trouble, torment, offend, or worry a person by one's behavior or comments. Harassment can be sexual. Or it can involve age, race, ethnic background, religion, or disability. You must respect others. Do not offend others by your gestures, remarks, or use of touch. Do not offend others with jokes, photos, or other pictures (drawings, cartoons, and so on). Harassment is not legal in the workplace.

See *Focus on Communication: Harassment.*

Sexual Harassment

Sexual harassment involves unwanted sexual behaviors by another. The behavior may be a sexual advance, or it may be a request for a sexual favor. Some remarks, comments, and touching are sexual. The behavior affects the person's work and comfort. In extreme cases, the person's job is threatened if sexual favors are not granted.

Victims of sexual harassment may be men or women. Men harass women or men. Women harass men or women. You might feel that you are being harassed. If so, report the matter to the nurse and the human resource officer.

FOCUS ON COMMUNICATION
Harassment

You have the right to feel safe and unthreatened. If someone's comments make you uncomfortable, you can say: "Please don't say things like that. It's unprofessional." If someone's actions make you uneasy, you can say: "Please don't do that. It's unprofessional." Leave the area. Report the person's statements or actions to the nurse.

Box 5-7 Common Reasons for Losing a Job

- Poor attendance—not going to work or excessive tardiness (being late).
- Abandonment—leaving the job during your shift.
- Falsifying a record—job application or a person's medical record.
- Violent behavior in the workplace.
- Having weapons in the work setting—guns, knives, explosives, or other dangerous items.
- Having, using, or distributing alcohol in the work setting.
- Having, using, or distributing drugs in the work setting. This excludes taking drugs ordered by a doctor.
- Taking a person's drugs for your own use or giving it to others.
- Harassment.
- Using offensive speech and language.
- Stealing the center's or a person's property.
- Destroying the center's or a person's property.
- Showing disrespect to residents, families, visitors, co-workers, or supervisors.
- Abusing or neglecting a person.
- Invading a person's privacy.
- Failing to maintain resident, family, center, or co-worker confidentiality. This includes access to computer and other electronic information.
- Using the center's supplies and equipment for your own use.
- Defamation—see Chapter 4 and "Gossip," p. 53.
- Abusing meal breaks and break periods.
- Sleeping on the job.
- Violating the center's dress code.
- Violating any center policy.
- Failing to follow center care procedures.
- Tending to personal matters while on duty.

Be careful about what you say or do. Even innocent remarks and behaviors can be viewed as harassment. Employee orientation programs address harassment. You might not be sure about your own or another person's remarks or behaviors. If so, discuss the matter with the nurse. You cannot be too careful.

RESIGNING FROM A JOB

A job closer to home, better pay, or new opportunities may prompt you to leave your job. School, childcare, and illness are other reasons. Whatever the reason, tell your employer. Do one of the following:

- Give a written notice.
- Write a resignation letter.
- Complete a form in the human resource office.

Giving 2-weeks' notice is a good practice. Do not leave a job without notice. Doing so can affect resident care. Include the following in your notice:

- Reason for leaving
- The last date you will work
- Comments thanking the employer for the opportunity to work in the center

An exit interview is common practice. You and the employer talk before you leave the center. The employer asks what you liked about the center and your job. Often employees are asked how the center can improve.

LOSING A JOB

A job is a privilege. You must perform your job well and protect residents from harm. No pay raise or losing your job results from poor performance. Failure to follow center policy is often grounds for termination. So is failure to get along with others. Box 5-7 lists the many reasons why you can lose your job. To protect your job, function at your best. Always practice good work ethics.

DRUG TESTING

Drug and alcohol use affects resident and staff safety. Quality of care suffers. Those who use drugs or alcohol are late to work or absent more often than staff who do not use such substances. Therefore drug testing policies are common. Review your center's policy for when and how you might be tested.

QUALITY OF LIFE

Your job as a nursing assistant is important. Residents, families, and visitors believe that you will give safe and effective care. They trust that you will:

- Work when scheduled
- Arrive at work on time
- Stay the entire shift
- Complete your assignments
- Be well-groomed
- Be pleasant and courteous

Your work ethics impact quality of life. Good work ethics help persons feel safe, secure, loved, and cared for. If you want to make their lives happier, easier, and less painful, you will practice good work ethics.

REVIEW QUESTIONS

Circle T if the statement is TRUE. Circle F if the statement is FALSE.

1. T F You wear needed eyeglasses. This helps protect the person's safety.
2. T F Childcare requires planning before you go to work.
3. T F Being on time for work means arriving at the center when your shift begins.

Continued

4 T F You share information about a person with a friend. This is grounds for losing your job.

5 T F You must be careful what you say over the intercom system.

6 T F You do not follow the center's dress code. You could lose your job.

7 T F You can use the center's computer for your homework.

8 T F You can keep your wireless phone turned on while at work.

9 T F You must know your center's attendance policy.

10 T F Harassment is legal in the workplace.

Circle the BEST answer.

11 Which will *not* help you do your job well?
a Enough rest and sleep
b Regular exercise
c Using drugs and alcohol
d Good nutrition

12 Which is *not* a good hygiene practice?
a Bathing daily
b Using a deodorant
c Brushing teeth after meals
d Having long and polished fingernails

13 You are getting ready for work. Which is *not* a good practice?
a Wearing jewelry
b Ironing your uniform
c Wearing your name badge
d Styling hair up and off your collar

14 When should you ask questions about your job description?
a After completing the job application
b Before completing the job application
c When your interview is scheduled
d During the interview

15 Lying on a job application is
a Negligence
b Fraud
c Libel
d Defamation

16 You are completing a job application. You should do the following *except*
a Write neatly and clearly
b Provide references
c Give information about employment gaps
d Leave spaces blank that do not apply to you

17 Which of the following do employers look for the *most*?
a Cooperation
b Courtesy
c Dependability
d Empathy

18 Empathy is
a Feeling sorry for a person
b Seeing things from the other person's point of view
c Being polite to others
d Saying kind things

19 What should you wear to a job interview?
a A uniform
b Party clothes
c A simple dress or suit
d What is most comfortable

20 Which is a poor behavior during a job interview?
a Good eye contact with the interviewer
b Shaking hands with the interviewer
c Asking the interviewer questions
d Crossing your arms and legs

21 Which is the best response to an interview question?
a "Yes" or "no"
b Long answers
c Brief explanations
d A written response

22 Which statement reflects a good work attitude?
a "It's not my fault."
b "I'm sorry. I didn't know."
c "That's not my job."
d "I did it yesterday. It's your turn."

23 A co-worker says that a doctor and nurse are dating. This is
a Gossip
b Eavesdropping
c Confidential information
d Sexual harassment

24 Which is professional speech and language?
a Speaking clearly
b Using vulgar words
c Shouting
d Arguing

25 Which is *not* a courteous act?
a Saying "please" and "thank you"
b Wanting others to open doors for you
c Saying "I'm sorry"
d Complimenting others

26 You are on a meal break. Which is *false*?
a You can make personal phone calls.
b Family members can meet you.
c You can take a few extra minutes if needed.
d The nurse needs to know that you are off the unit.

27 You are planning your work. You should do the following *except*
a Discuss priorities with the nurse
b Ask others if they need help
c Stay busy
d Plan care so that you can watch the person's TV

28 These statements are about stress. Which is *false*?
a Stress affects the whole person.
b A stressor is an event that causes stress.
c All stress is unpleasant.
d Stress is normal.

29 Which does *not* help reduce stress?
a Exercise, rest, and sleep
b Blaming yourself for things you did not do
c Planning quiet time
d Having a sense of humor

30 Which is *not* harassment?
a Using touch to comfort a person
b Joking about a person's religion
c Asking for a sexual favor
d Acting like a disabled person

31 A resignation letter should *not* include
a Your reasons for leaving
b The last day you will work
c A thank-you to the employer
d Problems you had during your work

32 Which is *not* a reason for losing your job?
a Leaving the job during your shift
b Using alcohol in the work setting
c Sleeping on the job
d Taking a meal break

Answers to these questions are on p. 719.

Communicating With the Health Team

OBJECTIVES

- Define the key terms and key abbreviations listed in this chapter.
- Explain why health team members need to communicate.
- Describe the rules for good communication.
- Explain the purpose, parts, and information found in the medical record.
- Describe the legal and ethical aspects of medical records.
- Describe the purpose of the Kardex.
- List the information you need to report to the nurse.

- List the rules for recording.
- Use the 24-hour clock, medical terminology, and abbreviations.
- Explain how computers and other electronic devices are used in health care.
- Explain how to protect the right to privacy when using computers and other electronic devices.
- Describe the rules for answering phones.
- Explain how to problem solve and deal with conflict.
- Explain how to promote quality of life.

KEY TERMS

abbreviation A shortened form of a word or phrase

chart See "medical record"

communication The exchange of information—a message sent is received and correctly interpreted by the intended person

conflict A clash between opposing interests or ideas

Kardex A type of card file that summarizes information found in the medical record—drugs, treatments, diagnoses, routine care measures, equipment, and special needs

medical record A written account of a person's condition and response to treatment and care; chart or clinical record

prefix A word element placed before a root; it changes the meaning of the word

progress note A written description of the care given and the person's response and progress

recording The written account of care and observations; charting

reporting The oral account of care and observations

root A word element containing the basic meaning of the word

suffix A word element placed after a root; it changes the meaning of the word

word element A part of a word

Health team members communicate with each other to give coordinated and effective care. They share information about:

- What was done for the person
- What needs to be done for the person
- The person's response to treatment

For example, the doctor ordered a blood test for Mrs. Carter. Food and fluids affect the test results. Mrs. Carter must fast for 10 hours before the blood is drawn. A nurse tells the dietary department that Mrs. Carter will have breakfast later. She explains the breakfast delay to you and Mrs. Carter. A technician tells the nurse the blood sample was drawn. The nurse orders the meal. A dietary worker brings the tray to the nursing unit. You serve Mrs. Carter's tray. After she is done eating, you remove the tray and observe what she ate. You report your observations to the nurse. The nurse records your observations in Mrs. Carter's medical record.

Team members communicated with each other and Mrs. Carter. Her care was coordinated and effective. She knew that she was not neglected or forgotten.

You need to understand the basic aspects and rules of communication. Then you can learn how to communicate information to the nursing and health teams.

COMMUNICATION

Communication is the exchange of information—a message sent is received and correctly interpreted by the intended person. For good communication:

- Use words that mean the same thing to you and the receiver of the message. Avoid words with more than one meaning. What does "far" mean—10 feet, 50 feet, or 100 feet?
- Use familiar words. You will learn medical terms. If someone uses a strange term, ask what it means. You must understand the message. Otherwise communication does not occur. Likewise, avoid terms that the person and family do not understand.
- Be brief and concise. Do not add unrelated or unnecessary information. Stay on the subject. Do not wander in thought or get wordy.

- Give information in a logical and orderly manner. Organize your thoughts. Present them step-by-step.
- Give facts and be specific. Give the receiver a clear picture of what you are saying. You report a pulse rate of 110. It is more specific and factual than saying the "pulse is fast."

THE MEDICAL RECORD

The medical record (chart) is a written account of a person's condition and response to treatment and care. (OBRA calls it the clinical record.) The health team uses it to share information about the person. The record is permanent. Sometimes it is used months or years later if the person's health history is needed. The record is a legal document. It can be used in court as legal evidence of the person's problems, treatment, and care.

The record has many forms. Each page has the person's name, room and bed number, and other identifying information. This helps prevent errors and improper placement of records. The record includes the person's:

- Admission sheet
- Health history
- Physical examination results
- Doctor's orders
- Doctor's progress note
- Progress notes (nursing team and health team)
- Graphic sheet
- Flow sheets
- Laboratory results
- X-ray reports
- IV (intravenous) therapy record
- Respiratory therapy record
- Consultation reports
- Assessments from nursing, social services, dietary services, and recreational therapy
- Special consents

Health team members record on the forms for their departments. Other team members read the information. It tells the care provided and the person's response (Fig. 6-1).

Nursing centers have policies about medical records and who can see them. Policies address:

- Who records
- When to record
- Abbreviations
- Correcting errors
- Ink color
- Signing entries

Some centers allow nursing assistants to record observations and care. Others do not. You must know your center's policies.

Professional staff involved in a person's care can review charts. Cooks and laundry, housekeeping, and office staff do not need to read charts. Some centers let nursing assistants read charts. If not, the nurse shares needed information.

You have an ethical and legal duty to keep the person's information confidential. You may know someone in the center. If you are not involved in the person's care, you have no right to review the person's chart. To do so is an invasion of privacy.

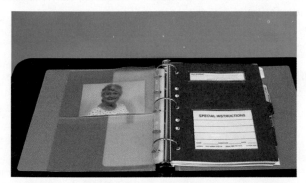

Fig. 6-1 A medical record.

OBRA-CMS

Under OBRA, residents have the right to the information in their medical records. A resident or a legal representative may ask you for the chart. Report the request to the nurse. The nurse deals with the request.

The following parts of the medical record relate to your work.

The Admission Sheet

The admission sheet is completed when the person is admitted to the center. It has the person's identifying information—legal name, birth date, age, gender (male or female), address, and marital status. It also has the person's Medicare or Social Security number. The name of the person's legal representative is included. Other information includes known allergies, diagnoses, date and time of admission, doctor's name, religion, and church or place of worship.

Each person receives an identification (ID) number. It is on the admission sheet. So is information about advance directives. An advance directive is a document stating a person's wishes about life support measures (Chapter 48).

Use the admission sheet to fill out other forms that require the same information. That way the person does not have to answer the same question many times.

Progress Notes

The progress note is a written description of the care given and the person's response and progress (Fig. 6-2). The nurse records:

- Signs and symptoms
- Information about treatments and drugs
- Information about teaching and counseling
- Procedures performed by the doctor
- Visits by other health team members

Date	Time	Nursing Margin	Other Depts Margin
3-19	1700	Out with family for dinner. Jane Doe, LPN	
	1930	Returned from outing accompanied by her son. States she had a pleasant time Mary Smith, CNA	
3-20	0900	In bed. Complains of headache. T 98.4 orally, radial pulse 72 and regular, respirations 18 and unlabored. BP 134/84 left arm lying down. Alice Jones, RN notified of resident complaint and vital signs. Ann Adams, CNA	
	0910	In bed resting. States she has had a headache for about 1/2 hour. Denies nausea and dizziness. No other complaints. PRN Tylenol given. Instructed resident to use signal light if headache worsens or other symptoms occur. Alice Jones, RN	
	0945	Resting quietly. Denies headache at this time. T 98.4 orally, radial pulse 70 and regular, respirations 18 and unlabored. BP 132/84 left arm lying down. Alice Jones, RN	

Fig. 6-2 Progress notes. Note that other members of the health team also can record on this form.

Activities of Daily Living Flow Sheet

ORDER/INSTRUCTION	TIME	1	2	3	4	5	6	7	8	9
		JAN		FEB		(MAR)		APR		
Bowel Movements L = Large M = Medium S = Small IC = Incontinent	11-7	M								
	7-3			L						
	3-11									
Bladder Elimination I = Independent IC = Incontinent FC = Foley catheter	11-7	/	/	/	/					
	7-3	/	/	/	/					
	3-11	/	IC	/	/					
Weight Bearing Status TT = Toe touch AT = As tol. P = Partial F = Full NWB = No weight bearing	11-7	AT	AT	AT	AT					
	7-3	AT	AT	AT	AT					
	3-11	AT	AT	AT	AT					
Transfer Status ML = Mech lift SBA = Stand by assist; Assist of 1 or 2	11-7	SBA	SBA	SBA	SBA					
	7-3	SBA	SBA	SBA	SBA					
	3-11	SBA	SBA	SBA	A-1					
Activity A = Ambulate GC = Gerichair T = Turn every 2 hrs. W/C = Wheelchair	11-7	T	T	T	T					
	7-3	A	A	A	A					
	3-11	A	A	A	A					
Safety LT = Lap tray BR = Bed rails BA = Bed alarm SB = Seat belt	11-7									
	7-3									
	3-11									
Feeding Status I = Independent S = Set up F = Staff feed SP = Swallow precautions TL = Thickened liquids	Breakfast	8	8	8	8					
	Lunch	8	8	8	8					
	Supper	8	8	8	8					
Amount of food taken in %	Breakfast	75	100	100	75					
	Lunch	75	75	100	75					
	Supper	50	50	50	75					
Bath and Shampoo every _Monday_ & _Thursday_ on _7-3_ shift T = Tub S = Shower B = Bed bath	11-7									
	7-3	T								
	3-11									
Oral Care Own/Dentures/No teeth I = Independent S = Set up A = Assist	11-7	8	8	8	8					
	7-3	8	8	8	8					
	3-11	8	8	8	8					
Dressing I = Independent S = Set up A = Assist T = Total care	11-7	A	A	S	S					
	7-3									
	3-11	A	A	A	A					
Grooming: Washing Face and Hands Combing Hair I = Independent S = Set up A = Assist T = Total care	11-7	A	A	A	A					
	7-3	A	A	A	A					
	3-11	A	A	A	A					
Trim Fingernails weekly _Thursday_	11-7									
	7-3		✓							
	3-11									
Lotion Arms and Legs twice daily	11-7									
	7-3	✓	✓	✓	✓					
	3-11	✓	✓	✓	✓					
Shave Men daily Shave Women every _Monday_ & _Thursday_ on _7-3_ shift	11-7									
	7-3		✓							
	3-11									
Amount Between-Meal Nourishment taken in %	AM	100	75	100	50					
	PM	100	100	75	75					
	HS	50	75	75	75					
Intake and Output	11-7									
	7-3									
	3-11									
Vital Signs Every _Thursday_	11-7									
	7-3		✓							
	3-11									
Weight Every _Thursday_	11-7		✓							
	7-3									
	3-11									

Fig. 6-3 Some items on an activities of daily living flow sheet.

Progress notes are written when there is an unusual event, a problem, or a change in the person's condition. OBRA requires that summaries of care be written at least every 3 months. They reflect the person's progress toward the goals set in the care plan (Chapter 7). They also reflect the person's response to care. Some centers require summaries more often.

Flow Sheets

The activities of daily living (ADL) flow sheet is used to record a person's ability to perform ADL (Fig. 6-3). This flow sheet addresses hygiene, food and fluids, elimination, rest and sleep, activities, and social interactions.

Other flow sheets are used to record frequent measurements and observations. Measuring fluid intake and output is an example (Chapter 24).

THE KARDEX

The Kardex is a type of card file. It summarizes information found in the medical record—drugs, treatments, diagnoses, routine care measures, equipment, and special needs. The Kardex is a quick, easy source of information about the person (Fig. 6-4).

RESIDENT CARE CONFERENCES

OBRA requires two types of resident care conferences:
- *Interdisciplinary care planning (IDCP) conference.* This is held regularly to review and update care plans. It also is held to develop care plans for new residents. The nurse, doctor, and other health team members attend.
- *Problem-focused conference.* This is held when one problem affects a person's care. Only staff directly involved with the problem attend.

The person has the right to take part in these planning conferences. Often the family is involved. The person may refuse actions suggested by the health team.

You may be asked to attend these conferences. Always share your ideas and observations.

REPORTING AND RECORDING

The health team communicates by reporting and recording. Reporting is the oral account of care and observations. Recording (*charting*) is the written account of care and observations.

See *Focus on Communication: Reporting and Recording, p. 64.*

DIET	NOURISHMENT/SPECIAL FEEDING	INTAKE/OUTPUT

DIET _Regular_

Hold:

NOURISHMENT/SPECIAL FEEDING _Health shake at Bedtime._

INTAKE/OUTPUT
Encourage/(Restrict) Fluids __2000__ mL/24 Hr.
7-3 __1000__   3-11 __800__   11-7 __200__

FUNCTIONAL STATUS

	SELF	ASSIST	TOTAL	OTHER	SPECIFY
Feeding	□	☒	□	□	
Bathing	□	☒	□	□	
Toileting	□	☒	□	□	
Oral Care	□	☒	□	□	
Positioning	☒	□	□	□	
Transferring	☒	□	□	□	
Wheeling	□	□	□	□	
Walking	☒	□	□	□	
	□	□	□	□	

ACTIVITIES
Bedrest & BRP _____
Bedside Commode _____
Up ad Lib __X__
Chair _____
Ambulatory __X__
Ambulate & Assist _____
Turn _____
Dangle _____
Mode of Travel _____

ELIMINATION
Bladder - Cont. (Incont)
Catheter _____
Date Changed _____
Irrigations _____
Bowel - (Cont.)/ Incont.
Ostomy _____
Irrigations _____

VITALS
Temp. _daily_
Pulse _daily_
Resp. _daily_
BP _daily_
Weight _daily_
Other:
Pulse OX
daily

COMMUNICATION DEFICITS   □ None
Hearing _Hard-of-hearing_
Vision _Impaired_
Speech _____
Language _Impaired_

SPECIAL CONDITIONS (Paralysis, Pressure Ulcers, Etc.)

SAFETY/SUPPORTIVE MEASURES
Bed rails: □ Nights Only □ Constant □ No Need
Restraints: _____
Support Devices: □ PRN   □ Constant

PROSTHESIS   □ None
Glasses __X__   Dentures __X__
Contacts _____   Limb _____
Hearing Aid _L ear_

RESPIRATORY THERAPY
Aerosol
IPPB
Ultrasonic
Rx Med _____

OXYGEN
__2__ Liter/Minute
☒ PRN   □ Constant
___ Tent   ___ Catheter
___ Mask   __X__ Cannula

SPECIAL EQUIPMENT/PROCEDURES/ANCILLARY SERVICES/ETC.

Speech therapy 3 times/wk.

DATE	TREATMENTS/MISCELLANEOUS

ORDERED	SCHEDULED	COMPLETED	X-RAY AND SPECIAL DIAGNOSTIC EXAMS
10-20	10-20	10-20	Chest x-ray

START DATE	SCHEDULED MEDICATIONS	STOP DATE	RENEW	START DATE	STOP OR RENEW	SITE	IV FLUID & RATE	DATE & TIME CHANGED TUBING	DRESS.	SITE
10-19	Lasix 40 mg PO daily									
10-19	Lanoxin 0.25 mg PO daily									

DATE	ONE TIME ORDERS

DATE	DAILY/REPEATING ORDERS
10-20	Serum potassium daily

DATE	TIME	PRN MEDICATIONS
10-19	2100	Ativan 0.25 mg PO q4h PRN anxiety

MISCELLANEOUS

ALLERGIES:
☒ None Known

NURSING ALERTS:

EMERGENCY CONTACT:
Name: _Parker, Marie_   Telephone No.   Home: _555-1212_
Relationship: _Wife_   Bus: _____

ROOM	NAME	PHYSICIAN	ADMITTING DIAGNOSIS/PROBLEM	HOSP. NO.
310	Parker, Edwin	Dr. S Epstein	1. CHF 2. Dementia	1035B

Fig. 6-4 A sample Kardex. (Modified from Briggs Corporation, Des Moines, Iowa.)

FOCUS ON COMMUNICATION
Reporting and Recording

"Small," "moderate," and "large" mean different things to different people. Is small the size of a dime? Or is it the size of a quarter? In health care, different meanings can cause serious problems. Give accurate descriptions and measurements. If you have a question, ask the nurse to look at what you are trying to describe.

Reporting

You report care and observations to the nurse. Report to the nurse at these times:

- Whenever there is a change from normal or a change in the person's condition. Report these changes at once.
- When the nurse asks you to do so.
- When you leave the unit for meals, breaks, or for other reasons.
- Before the end-of-shift report.
  When reporting, follow the rules in Box 6-1, p. 65.

End-of-Shift Report The nurse gives a report at the end of the shift. This is called the *end-of-shift report*. It is given to the nursing team of the on-coming shift. The nurse reports about:

- The care given
- The care to give during other shifts
- The person's current condition
- Likely changes in the person's condition

In some centers, the entire nursing team hears the end-of-shift report as they come on duty. In other centers, only nurses hear the report. After the report, information is shared with nursing assistants.

See *Teamwork and Time Management: End-of-Shift Report.*

See *Promoting Safety and Comfort: End-of-Shift Report.*

TEAMWORK AND TIME MANAGEMENT
End-of-Shift Report

Two staffs are present at the end of a shift—the staff going off duty and the staff coming on duty. The entire on-coming shift may attend the end-of-shift report. If so, staff members going off duty answer all signal lights, provide care, and tend to routine tasks. If only nurses attend the end-of-shift report, nursing assistants of the on-coming shift also answer signal lights, provide care, and tend to routine tasks.

The end-of-shift is a time for good teamwork. Continue to do your job. Your attitude is important. If going off duty, avoid saying or thinking the following:

- "I'm ready to go home. Let them do it."
- "It's their turn. I've been here all day (evening or night)."
- "No one helped us when we came on duty."

Some centers have clear duties for the two shifts. For example, those going off duty continue to answer signal lights. They know about changes in the person's condition and care plan and about new orders. They also know about the care needs of new residents. The on-coming shift has yet to learn this information. The on-coming shift uses this time to perform routine tasks for the shift and to collect needed supplies and equipment.

PROMOTING SAFETY AND COMFORT
End-of-Shift Report

Safety

You may not hear the end-of-shift report as you come on duty. Yet you need to answer signal lights and give care before the nurse shares new information with you. To give safe care:

- Check the care plan before granting a request. The person's condition or care plan may have changed. There may be new orders from the doctor.
- Ask a nurse about the care needs of new residents. If necessary, politely interrupt the end-of-shift report to ask your questions.
- Do not take directions or orders from another nursing assistant. Remember, nursing assistants cannot supervise or delegate to other nursing assistants.

Box 6-1 Rules for Reporting and Recording

Reporting

- Be prompt, thorough, and accurate.
- Give the person's name and room and bed number.
- Give the time your observations were made or the care was given.
- Report only what you observed or did yourself.
- Report care measures that you expect the person to need. For example, you expect that the person will need the bedpan during your meal break.
- Report expected changes in the person's condition. For example, you expect that the person may be tired after physical therapy.
- Give reports as often as the person's condition requires. Or give them when the nurse asks you to.
- Report any changes from normal or changes in the person's condition. Report these changes at once. See Chapter 7.
- Use your written notes to give a specific, concise, and clear report (Fig. 6-5).

Recording

General Rules

- Follow center policies and procedures for recording. Ask for needed training.
- Include the date and time for every recording. Use conventional time (AM or PM) or 24-hour clock time according to center policy (p. 66).
- Use only center-approved abbreviations (p. 69).
- Use correct spelling, grammar, and punctuation.
- Do not use ditto marks.
- Sign all entries with your name and title as required by center policy.
- Make sure each form has the person's name and other identifying information.
- Record only what you observed and did yourself. Do not record for another person.
- Never chart a procedure, treatment, or care measure until after it is completed.
- Be accurate, concise, and factual. Do not record judgments or interpretations.
- Record in a logical and sequential manner.

Recording—cont'd

General Rules—cont'd

- Be descriptive. Avoid terms with more than one meaning.
- Use the person's exact words whenever possible. Use quotation marks to show that the statement is a direct quote.
- Chart any changes from normal or changes in the person's condition. Also chart that you informed the nurse (include the nurse's name), what you told the nurse, and the time you made the report.
- Do not omit information.
- Record safety measures. Examples include placing the signal light within reach, assisting a person when up, or reminding a person not to get out of bed.

Paper Charting

- Always use ink. Use the ink color required by the center.
- Make sure writing is readable and neat.
- Never erase or use correction fluid. Draw a line through the incorrect part. Date and initial the line. Write "mistaken entry" over it if this is center policy. Then re-write the part. Follow center policy for correcting errors.
- Do not skip lines. Draw a line through the blank space of a partially completed line or to the end of the page. This prevents others from recording in a space with your signature.

Electronic Charting

- Log in using your username and password. Do not chart using another person's username.
- Check the time your entry is made. Make sure it is the intended time.
- Check for accuracy. Review your entry before saving.
- Save your entries. Unsaved data will be lost.
- Follow the manufacturer's instructions for changing or un-charting a mistaken entry. Most electronic charting systems keep a record of what was entered before a change was made. This works in the same manner as drawing a line through a mistaken entry in paper charting. The first entry is still visible.
- Log off after you are done charting. This prevents others from charting under your username.

Fig. 6-5 The nursing assistant uses notes to report to the nurse.

Recording

When recording on the person's chart, you must communicate clearly and thoroughly. Follow the rules in Box 6-1. The charting sample in Figure 6-6, p. 66 shows how the rules apply.

Anyone who reads your charting should know:

- What you observed
- What you did
- The person's response

Date	Time	Nursing Margin	Other Depts Margin
4/10	1045	Requested assistance to lie down. States, "I don't feel well. I have a little upset stomach."	
		Denies pain. VS taken. T-99(O). P-76 regular rate and rhythm. R-18 unlabored.	
		BP 134/84 L arm lying down. Signal light within reach. Paula Jones, RN notified at 1040	
		of resident's complaint and VS. Mary Jensen, CNA	
	1100	Asleep in bed. Appears to be resting comfortably. Color good. No signs of	
		discomfort or distress noted at this time. Paula Jones, RN	
	1145	Refused to go to the dining room for lunch. Complains of nausea. Denies	
		abdominal pain. Has not had an emesis. Abdomen soft to palpation. Good bowel	
		sounds. VS taken. T-~~98.2~~ 99.2. P-76 regular rate and rhythm. R-18 unlabored.	
		(Mistaken entry 4-10, PJ)	
		BP-134/84. States she will try to eat something. Full liquid room tray ordered.	
		Paula Jones, RN	

Fig. 6-6 Charting sample.

Reporting and Recording Time The 24-hour clock (military time or international time) has four digits (Fig. 6-7). The first two digits are for the hours: 0100 = 1:00 AM; 1300 = 1:00 PM. The last two digits are for minutes: 0110 = 1:10 AM. The AM and PM abbreviations are not used.

As Box 6-2 shows, the hour is the same for morning times, but AM is not used. For PM times add 12 to the clock time. If it is 2:00 PM, add 12 and 2 for 1400. For 8:35 PM, add 12 and 835 for 2035.

Some centers use 0000 for midnight. Others use 2400. Follow center policy.

Box 6-2   24-Hour Clock

Conventional Time	24-Hour Clock
1:00 AM	0100
2:00 AM	0200
3:00 AM	0300
4:00 AM	0400
5:00 AM	0500
6:00 AM	0600
7:00 AM	0700
8:00 AM	0800
9:00 AM	0900
10:00 AM	1000
11:00 AM	1100
12:00 NOON	1200
1:00 PM	1300
2:00 PM	1400
3:00 PM	1500
4:00 PM	1600
5:00 PM	1700
6:00 PM	1800
7:00 PM	1900
8:00 PM	2000
9:00 PM	2100
10:00 PM	2200
11:00 PM	2300
12:00 MIDNIGHT	2400 or 0000

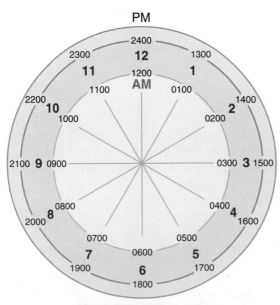

Fig. 6-7 The 24-hour clock.

MEDICAL TERMS AND ABBREVIATIONS

Medical terms and abbreviations are used in health care. Someone may use a word or phrase that you do not understand. If so, ask a nurse to explain its meaning. Otherwise, communication does not occur. A medical dictionary is useful for learning new words.

Like all words, medical terms are made up of parts or word elements—prefixes, roots, and suffixes (Box 6-3, pp. 68 and 69). Most are from Greek or Latin. They are combined to form medical terms. To translate a term, the word is separated into its elements.

Prefixes, Roots, and Suffixes

A prefix is a word element placed before a root. It changes the meaning of the word. The prefix *olig* (scant, small amount) is placed before the root *uria* (urine) to make *oliguria*. It means a scant amount of urine. Prefixes are always combined with other word elements. They are never used alone.

The root is the word element that contains the basic meaning of the word. It is combined with another root, with prefixes, and with suffixes. A vowel (an *o* or an *i*) is added when two roots are combined or when a suffix is added to a root. The vowel makes the word easier to pronounce.

A suffix is a word element placed after a root. It changes the meaning of the word. Suffixes are not used alone. When translating medical terms, begin with the suffix. For example, *nephritis* means inflammation of the kidney. It was formed by combining *nephro* (kidney) and *itis* (inflammation).

Medical terms are formed by combining word elements. Remember, prefixes always come before roots. Suffixes always come after roots. A root can be combined with prefixes, roots, and suffixes. The prefix *dys* (difficult) is combined with the root *pnea* (breathing). This forms *dyspnea*. It means difficulty breathing.

Roots can be combined with suffixes. The root *mast* (breast) combined with the suffix *ectomy* (excision or removal) forms *mastectomy*. It means the removal of a breast.

Combining a prefix, root, and suffix is another way to form medical terms. Endocarditis has the prefix *endo* (inner), the root *card* (heart), and the suffix *itis* (inflammation). *Endocarditis* means inflammation of the inner part of the heart.

Abdominal Regions

The abdomen is divided into regions (Fig. 6-8). They are used to describe the location of body structures, pain, or discomfort. The regions are:
- Right upper quadrant (RUQ)
- Left upper quadrant (LUQ)
- Right lower quadrant (RLQ)
- Left lower quadrant (LLQ)

Directional Terms

Certain terms describe the position of one body part in relation to another. These terms give the direction of the body part when a person is standing and facing forward (Fig. 6-9):
- *Anterior (ventral)*—at or toward the front of the body or body part
- *Distal*—the part farthest from the center or from the point of attachment
- *Lateral*—away from the midline; at the side of the body or body part
- *Medial*—at or near the middle or midline of the body or body part
- *Posterior (dorsal)*—at or toward the back of the body or body part
- *Proximal*—the part nearest to the center or to the point of origin

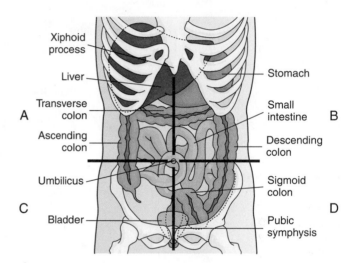

Fig. 6-8 The four abdominal regions. **A,** Right upper quadrant. **B,** Left upper quadrant. **C,** Right lower quadrant. **D,** Left lower quadrant.

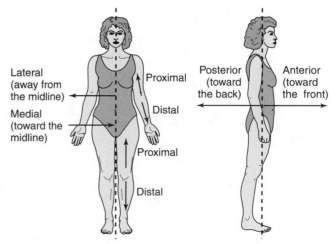

Fig. 6-9 Directional terms describe the position of one body part in relation to another.

Box 6-3   Medical Terminology

Prefix	Meaning
a-, an-	without, not, lack of
ab-	away from
ad-	to, toward, near
ante-	before, forward, in front of
anti-	against
auto-	self
bi-	double, two, twice
brady-	slow
circum-	around
contra-	against, opposite
de-	down, from
dia-	across, through, apart
dis-	apart, free from
dys-	bad, difficult, abnormal
ecto-	outer, outside
en-	in, into, within
endo-	inner, inside
epi-	over, on, upon
eryth-	red
eu-	normal, good, well, healthy
ex-	out, out of, from, away from
hemi-	half
hyper-	excessive, too much, high
hypo-	under, decreased, less than normal
in-	in, into, within, not
inter-	between
intra-	within
intro-	into, within
leuk-	white
macro-	large
mal-	bad, illness, disease
meg-	large
micro-	small
mono-	one, single
neo-	new
non-	not
olig-	small, scant
para-	beside, beyond, after
per-	by, through
peri-	around
poly-	many, much
post-	after, behind
pre-	before, in front of, prior to
pro-	before, in front of
re-	again, backward
retro-	backward, behind
semi-	half
sub-	under, beneath
super-	above, over, excess
supra-	above, over
tachy-	fast, rapid
trans-	across
uni-	one

Root (combining vowel)	Meaning
abdomin (o)	abdomen
aden (o)	gland
adren (o)	adrenal gland
angi (o)	vessel
arterio	artery
athr (o)	joint
broncho	bronchus, bronchi
card, cardi (o)	heart
cephal (o)	head
chole, chol (o)	bile
chondr (o)	cartilage
colo	colon, large intestine
cost (o)	rib
crani (o)	skull
cyan (o)	blue
cyst (o)	bladder, cyst
cyt (o)	cell
dent (o)	tooth
derma	skin
duoden (o)	duodenum
encephal (o)	brain
enter (o)	intestines
fibr (o)	fiber, fibrous
gastr (o)	stomach
gloss (o)	tongue
gluc (o)	sweetness, glucose
glyc (o)	sugar
gyn, gyne, gyneco	woman
hem, hema, hemo, hemat (o)	blood
hepat (o)	liver
hydr (o)	water
hyster (o)	uterus
ile (o), ili (o)	ileum
laparo	abdomen, loin, flank
laryng (o)	larynx
lith (o)	stone
mamm (o)	breast, mammary gland
mast (o)	mammary gland, breast
meno	menstruation
my (o)	muscle
myel (o)	spinal cord, bone marrow
necro	death
nephr (o)	kidney
neur (o)	nerve
ocul (o)	eye
oophor (o)	ovary
ophthalm (o)	eye
orth (o)	straight, normal, correct
oste (o)	bone
ot (o)	ear
ped (o)	child, foot

Box 6-3 Medical Terminology—cont'd

Root (combining vowel)—cont'd	Meaning
pharyng (o)	pharynx
phleb (o)	vein
pnea	breathing, respiration
pneum (o)	lung, air, gas
proct (o)	rectum
psych (o)	mind
pulmo	lung
py (o)	pus
rect (o)	rectum
rhin (o)	nose
salping (o)	eustachian tube, uterine tube
splen (o)	spleen
sten (o)	narrow, constriction
stern (o)	sternum
stomat (o)	mouth
therm (o)	heat
thoraco	chest
thromb (o)	clot, thrombus
thyr (o)	thyroid
toxic (o)	poison, poisonous
toxo	poison
trache (o)	trachea
urethr (o)	urethra
urin (o)	urine
uro	urine, urinary tract, urination
uter (o)	uterus
vas (o)	blood vessel, vas deferens
ven (o)	vein
vertebr (o)	spine, vertebrae

Suffix	Meaning
-algia	pain
-asis	condition, usually abnormal
-cele	hernia, herniation, pouching
-centesis	puncture and aspiration of
-cyte	cell
-ectasis	dilation, stretching
-ectomy	excision, removal of
-emia	blood condition
-genesis	development, production, creation
-genic	producing, causing
-gram	record
-graph	a diagram, a recording instrument
-graphy	making a recording
-iasis	condition of
-ism	a condition
-itis	inflammation
-logy	the study of
-lysis	destruction of, decomposition
-megaly	enlargement
-meter	measuring instrument
-oma	tumor
-osis	condition
-pathy	disease
-penia	lack, deficiency
-phagia	to eat or consume, swallowing
-phasia	speaking
-phobia	an exaggerated fear
-plasty	surgical repair or reshaping
-plegia	paralysis
-ptosis	falling, sagging, dropping down
-rrhage, -rrhagia	excessive flow
-rrhaphy	stitching, suturing
-rrhea	profuse flow, discharge
-scope	examination instrument
-scopy	examination using a scope
-stasis	maintenance, maintaining a constant level
-stomy, -ostomy	creation of an opening
-tomy, -otomy	incision, cutting into
-uria	condition of the urine

Abbreviations

Abbreviations are shortened forms of words or phrases. They save time and space when recording. Each center has a list of accepted abbreviations. Obtain the list when you are hired. Use only those accepted by the center. If not sure that an abbreviation is acceptable, write the term out in full. This promotes accurate communication.

Common abbreviations are on the inside of the back book cover for easy use.

Common Terms and Phrases

Some terms and phrases apply to basic care and safety. Because they are used throughout this book, they are presented in Box 6-4, p. 70. Some are presented as key terms in other chapters.

Box 6-4   Common Health Care Terms and Phrases

activities of daily living (ADL)	The activities usually done during a normal day in a person's life
assistive device	Any item used by the person or staff to promote the person's function or safety (hand rails, grab bars, transfer lifts, canes, walkers, wheelchairs, and so on)
atrophy	The decrease in size or the wasting away of tissue
care plan	A written guide about the person's care
cognitive function	Involves memory, thinking, reasoning, ability to understand, judgment, and behavior
contracture	The lack of joint mobility caused by abnormal shortening of a muscle
dementia	The loss of cognitive and social function caused by changes in the brain; the loss of cognitive function
dysphagia	Difficulty (dys) swallowing (phagia)
dyspnea	Difficult, labored, or painful (dys) breathing (pnea)
feces	The semi-solid mass of waste products in the colon that are expelled through the anus
fever	Elevated body temperature
Fowler's position	A semi-sitting position; the head of the bed is raised between 45 and 60 degrees
incontinence	Not being able to control urination (urinary incontinence) or defecation (fecal incontinence)
pressure ulcer	A localized injury to the skin and/or underlying tissue, usually over a bony prominence
prone	Lying on the abdomen with the head turned to one side
semi-Fowler's position	The head of the bed is raised 30 degrees; or the head of the bed is raised 30 degrees and the knee portion is raised 15 degrees
signal light	Part of the call system that allows the person to signal the nurses' station for help
supine	The back-lying or dorsal recumbent position
vital signs	Temperature, pulse, respirations, and blood pressure
voiding	Urinating

COMPUTERS AND OTHER ELECTRONIC DEVICES

Computer systems collect, send, record, and store information. Information is retrieved when needed. Many centers store charts and care plans (Chapter 7) on computers. Entering data on a computer is often easier and faster than paper charting.

The health team uses computers and faxes to send messages and reports to the nursing unit. This reduces clerical work and phone calls. And information is sent with greater speed and accuracy.

Computers are used for measurements such as blood pressures, temperatures, and heart rates. The computer senses normal and abnormal measurements. When the abnormal is sensed, an alarm alerts the nursing staff. Computer monitoring is common in hospitals and in skilled nursing units.

Computers and other electronic devices save time. Quality care and safety are increased. Fewer errors are made in recording. Records are more complete (Fig. 6-10). Staff is more efficient.

Computers store vast amounts of information. Therefore the right to privacy must be protected. Each staff member using computers and other electronic devices is issued a username and password. They are used to access, send, receive, or store protected health information (PHI).

You must follow the center's policies when using computers and other electronic devices. You must keep PHI and electronic protected health information (ePHI, EPHI) confidential. Follow the rules in Box 6-5 and the ethical and legal rules about privacy, confidentiality, and defamation (Chapter 4).

PHONE COMMUNICATIONS

You will answer phones at the nurses' station or in resident rooms. You need good communication skills. The caller cannot see you, but you give much information by your tone of voice, how clearly you speak, and your attitude. Behave as if you are speaking to someone face-to-face. Be professional and courteous. Also practice good work ethics. Follow the center's policy and the guidelines in Box 6-6, p. 72.

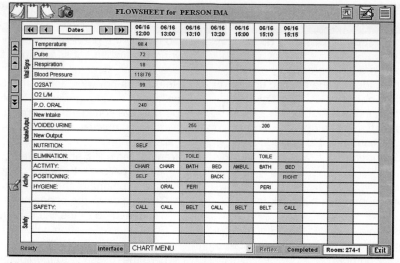

Fig. 6-10 Computer charting. *(Courtesy Abraham Lincoln Memorial Hospital, Lincoln, Ill.)*

FLOWSHEET for PERSON IMA	06/16 12:00	06/16 13:00	06/16 13:10	06/16 13:20	06/16 15:00	06/16 15:10	06/16 15:15			
Temperature	98.4									
Pulse	72									
Respiration	18									
Blood Pressure	118/76									
O2SAT	99									
O2 L/M										
P.O. ORAL	240									
New Intake										
VOIDED URINE			250			200				
New Output										
NUTRITION:	SELF									
ELIMINATION:			TOILE			TOILE				
ACTIVITY:	CHAIR	CHAIR	BATH	BED	AMBUL	BATH	BED			
POSITIONING:	SELF			BACK		RIGHT				
HYGIENE:		ORAL	PERI			PERI				
SAFETY:	CALL	CALL	BELT	CALL	BELT	BELT	CALL			

Ready   Interface CHART MENU   Reflex Completed Room: 274-1 Exit

Box 6-5 Using the Center's Computer and Other Electronic Devices

Computers

- Do not tell anyone your username or password. If someone has your information, he or she can access, record, send, receive, or store PHI under your name. It will be hard to prove that someone else did so and not you.
- Do not write down, post, or expose your username or password in a manner that is not secure. For example, do not write them on a notepad or post them at your work station.
- Change your password often. Follow center policy.
- Do not use another person's username or password.
- Follow the rules for recording (see Box 6-1).
- Enter data carefully. Double-check your entries.
- Prevent others from seeing what is on the screen:
  - Position the monitor so the screen cannot be seen in the hallway or by others.
  - Be aware of anyone standing behind you.
  - Stand or sit with your back to the wall if recording on a mobile computer unit.
  - Do not leave the computer unattended.
- Log off after making an entry.
- Do not leave printouts where others can read them or pick them up.
- Shred or destroy computer-printed documents or worksheets. Follow center policy.
- Send e-mail and messages only to those needing the information.
- Do not use e-mail for information or messages that require immediate reporting. Give the report in person. (The person may not read the e-mail in a timely manner.)
- Do not use e-mail or messages to report confidential information. This includes addresses, phone numbers, and Social Security numbers. The computer system may not be secure.

Computers—cont'd

- Do not use the center's computer to:
  - Send personal e-mail messages
  - Send or receive e-mail or messages that are offensive, not legal, or sexual
  - Send or receive e-mail or messages for illegal activities, jokes, politics, gambling (including football and other pools), chain letters, or other non-work activities
  - Post information, opinions, or comments on Internet message boards
  - Take part in Internet discussion groups
  - Upload, download, or send materials containing a copyright, trademark, or patent
- Remember that any communication can be read or heard by someone other than the intended person.
- Remember that deleted communications can be retrieved by authorized staff.
- Remember that the center has the right to monitor your use of computers or other electronic devices. This includes Internet use.
- Do not open another person's e-mail or messages.
- Follow center policy for mis-directed e-mails.

Faxes

- Use the center's approved "cover sheet." The sheet has instructions about:
  - The confidentiality of PHI
  - The receiver's responsibilities about PHI and if the fax is received in error (mis-directed fax)
- Complete the "cover sheet" according to center policy:
  - Name of the person to receive the PHI
  - Receiver's fax number
  - Date
  - Number of pages being faxed
  - Department name
  - Name and phone number of the person sending the fax
- Follow center policy for a mis-directed fax.
- Do not leave sent or received faxes unattended in the fax machine or lying around.

Box 6-6   Guidelines for Answering Phones

- Answer the call after the first ring if possible. Be sure to answer by the fourth ring.
- Do not answer the phone in a rushed or hasty manner.
- Give a courteous greeting. Identify the nursing unit, and give your name and title. For example: "Good morning. Three center. Mark Wills, nursing assistant."
- Write the following information when taking a message:
  - The caller's name and phone number (include area code and extension number)
  - The date and time
  - The message
- Repeat the message and phone number back to the caller.
- Ask the caller to "Please hold" if necessary. First find out who is calling. Then ask if the caller can hold. Do not put callers with an emergency on hold.
- Do not lay the phone down or cover the receiver with your hand when not speaking to the caller. The caller may overhear confidential conversations.
- Return to a caller on hold within 30 seconds. Ask if the caller can wait longer or if the call can be returned.
- Do not give confidential information to any caller. Resident and employee information is confidential. Refer such calls to a nurse.
- Transfer the call if appropriate:
  - Tell the caller that you are going to transfer the call.
  - Give the name of the department if appropriate.
  - Give the caller the phone number in case the call gets disconnected or the line is busy.
  - End the conversation politely. Thank the person for calling, and say good-bye.
  - Give the message to the appropriate person.

DEALING WITH CONFLICT

People bring their values, attitudes, opinions, experiences, and expectations to the work setting. Differences often lead to conflict. Conflict is a clash between opposing interests or ideas. People disagree and argue. There are misunderstandings and unrest.

Conflicts arise over issues or events. Work schedules, absences, and the amount and quality of work performed are examples. The problems must be worked out. Otherwise, unkind words or actions may occur. The work setting becomes unpleasant. Care is affected.

To resolve conflict, identify the real problem. This is part of *problem solving*. The problem solving process involves these steps:

- Step 1: Define the problem. *A nurse ignores me.*
- Step 2: Collect information about the problem. Do not include unrelated information. *The nurse does not look at me. The nurse does not talk to me. The nurse does not respond when I ask for help. The nurse does not ask me to help with tasks that require two people. The nurse talks to other staff members.*
- Step 3: Identify possible solutions. *Ignore the nurse. Talk to my supervisor. Talk to co-workers about the problem. Change jobs.*
- Step 4: Select the best solution. *Talk to my supervisor.*
- Step 5: Carry out the solution. *See below.*
- Step 6: Evaluate the results. *See below.*

Communication and good work ethics help prevent and resolve conflicts. Identify and solve problems before they become major issues. To deal with conflict:

- Ask your supervisor for some time to talk privately. Explain the problem. Give facts and specific examples. Ask for advice in solving the problem.
- Approach the person with whom you have the conflict. Ask to talk privately. Be polite and professional.
- Agree on a time and place to talk.
- Talk in a private setting. No one should hear you or the other person.
- Explain the problem and what is bothering you. Give facts and specific behaviors. Focus on the problem. Do not focus on the person.
- Listen to the person. Do not interrupt.
- Identify ways to solve the problem. Offer your thoughts. Ask for the co-worker's ideas.
- Set a date and time to review the matter.
- Thank the person for meeting with you.
- Carry out the solution.
- Review the matter as scheduled.
  See *Focus on Communication: Dealing With Conflict.*

FOCUS ON COMMUNICATION
Dealing With Conflict

You may find it hard to talk to someone with whom you have a conflict. This is hard for many people. However, letting the problem or issue continue only makes the matter worse. The following may help you to start talking to the person:

- "You say 'no' when I ask you to help me. I help you when you ask me to. This really bothers me. Can we talk privately for a few minutes?"
- "I heard you tell John that you saw me sitting in Mrs. Gordon's room. You seemed angry when you said it. Can we talk privately? I want to explain why I was sitting and find out why that bothers you."
- "The new schedule shows me working every weekend this month. Please tell me why. The employee handbook says that we work every other weekend."

QUALITY OF LIFE

Health team members must communicate with each other for effective and coordinated care. Communication must be factual, concise, and understandable. It must be presented in a logical way. This helps the health team provide high-quality resident care. False or incomplete information can harm the person.

Resident information is personal and confidential. Always protect the right to privacy. Share information only with the health team members involved in the person's care. Never share it with the person's family or friends without the person's consent.

REVIEW QUESTIONS

Circle T if the statement is TRUE. Circle F if the statement is FALSE.

1 T   F   You help with Mrs. Gordon's care. Reading her medical record violates her right to privacy.
2 T   F   You can access all medical records in the center.
3 T   F   You can attend the interdisciplinary care conference.
4 T   F   You can give information about the person over the phone.

Circle the BEST answer.

5 To communicate, you should do the following *except*
   a Use terms with many meanings
   b Be brief and concise
   c Present information logically and in sequence
   d Give facts and be specific
6 Mr. Drake is discharged from the center. His medical record is
   a Destroyed   c Permanent
   b Sent home with him   d Stored on a computer
7 These statements are about medical records. Which is *false?*
   a They are used to communicate information about residents.
   b They are a written or electronic account of illness and response to treatment.
   c They can be used as evidence of the care given.
   d Anyone working in the center can read them.
8 A person is weighed daily. The measurement is recorded on the
   a Admission sheet
   b Kardex
   c Flow sheet
   d Progress notes
9 Where does the nurse describe the nursing care given?
   a Admission sheet
   b Activities of daily living flow sheet
   c Progress notes
   d Kardex

10 When recording, you do the following *except*
    a Use ink
    b Include the date and time
    c Erase errors
    d Sign all entries with your name and title
11 These statements are about recording. Which is *false?*
    a Use the person's exact words when possible.
    b Record only what you did and observed.
    c Sign your initials to a mistaken entry.
    d Chart a procedure before completing it.
12 In the evening the clock shows 9:26. In 24-hour clock time this is
    a 9:26 PM
    b 1926
    c 0926
    d 2126
13 A suffix is
    a Placed at the beginning of a word
    b Placed after a root
    c A shortened form of a word or phrase
    d The main meaning of the word
14 Which term relates to the side of the body?
    a Anterior
    b Lateral
    c Posterior
    d Proximal
15 These statements are about computers in health care. Which is *false?*
    a Computers are used to collect, send, record, and store information.
    b The person's privacy must be protected.
    c All employees have the same password.
    d Computers link one department to another.
16 You have access to the center's computer. Which is *true?*
    a E-mail and messages are sent only to those needing the information.
    b E-mail is used for reports the nurse needs at once.
    c You can open another person's e-mail.
    d You can use the computer for your personal needs.
17 You answer a person's phone. How should you answer?
    a "Good morning. Mrs. Park's room."
    b "Good morning. Third floor."
    c "Hello."
    d "Good morning. Tammy Brown, nursing assistant, speaking."
18 A co-worker is often late for work. This means extra work for you. To resolve the conflict you should do the following *except*
    a Explain the problem to your supervisor
    b Discuss the matter during the end-of-shift report
    c Give facts and specific behaviors
    d Suggest ways to solve the problem

Answers to these questions on p. 719.

Assisting With the Nursing Process

KEY TERMS

assessment Collecting information about the person; a step in the nursing process

comprehensive care plan A written guide about the care a person should receive; developed by the health team; care plan

evaluation To measure if goals in the planning step were met; a step in the nursing process

goal That which is desired for or by a person as a result of nursing care

implementation To perform or carry out nursing measures in the care plan; a step in the nursing process

medical diagnosis The identification of a disease or condition by a doctor

nursing diagnosis Describes a health problem that can be treated by nursing measures; a step in the nursing process

nursing intervention An action or measure taken by the nursing team to help the person reach a goal

nursing process The method nurses use to plan and deliver nursing care; its five steps are assessment, nursing diagnosis, planning, implementation, and evaluation

objective data Information that is seen, heard, felt, or smelled by an observer; signs

observation Using the senses of sight, hearing, touch, and smell to collect information

planning Setting priorities and goals; a step in the nursing process

signs See "objective data"

subjective data Things a person tells you about that you cannot observe through your senses; symptoms

symptoms See "subjective data"

triggers Clues for the Care Area Assessments (CAAs)

Nurses communicate with each other about the person's strengths, problems, needs, and care. This information is shared through the nursing process. The nursing process is the method nurses use to plan and deliver nursing care. It has five steps:

- Assessment
- Nursing diagnosis
- Planning
- Implementation
- Evaluation

The nursing process focuses on the person's nursing needs. The person and nursing team need good communication.

Each step is important. If done in order with good communication, nursing care is organized and has purpose. All nursing team members do the same things for the person. They have the same goals. The person feels safe and secure with consistent care.

The nursing process is used for all age-groups. It is on-going. New information is gathered and the person's needs may change. However, the steps are the same. You will see the continuous nature of the nursing process as each step is explained.

ASSESSMENT

Assessment involves collecting information about the person. Nurses use many sources. A health history is taken. This tells about current and past health problems. The family's health history is important. Many diseases are genetic. That is, the risk for certain diseases is inherited from parents. For example, a mother had breast cancer. Her daughters are at risk. Information from the doctor is reviewed. So are test results and past medical records.

An RN (registered nurse) assesses the person's body systems and mental status. You play a key role in assessment. You make many observations as you give care and talk to the person.

Observation is using the senses of sight, hearing, touch, and smell to collect information:

- You *see* how the person lies, sits, or walks. You see flushed or pale skin. You see red and swollen body areas.

- You *listen* to the person breathe, talk, and cough. You use a stethoscope to listen to the heartbeat and to measure blood pressure.
- Through *touch*, you feel if the skin is hot or cold, or moist or dry. You use touch to take the person's pulse.
- *Smell* is used to detect body, wound, and breath odors. You also smell odors from urine and bowel movements.

Objective data (signs) are seen, heard, felt, or smelled by an observer. You can feel a pulse. You can see urine color. Subjective data (symptoms) are things a person tells you about that you cannot observe through your senses. You cannot feel or see the person's pain, fear, or nausea.

Box 7-1, p. 76 lists the basic observations you need to make and report to the nurse. Box 7-2, p. 77 lists the observations that you must report at once. Make notes of your observations. Use them to report and record observations. Carry a note pad and pen in your pocket. Note your observations as you make them. The center may provide electronic devices for this purpose (Fig. 7-1, p. 77).

The assessment step never ends. New information is collected with every resident contact. New observations are made. The person shares more information. Often the family adds more information.

The Omnibus Budget Reconciliation Act of 1987 (OBRA) requires the Minimum Data Set (MDS) for nursing center residents (Appendix B, p. 723). The MDS is an assessment and screening tool. It provides extensive information about the person. Examples include memory, communication, hearing and vision, physical function, and activities.

The nurse uses your observations to complete the MDS. The MDS is begun when the person is admitted to the center. The RN responsible for the person's care makes sure the MDS is complete. The MDS is updated before each care conference. It is completed once a year and whenever a significant change occurs in the person's health status. An RN signs the MDS. A signed MDS means that it is complete and accurate.

OBRA-CMS

Box 7-1 Basic Observations

Ability to Respond

- Is the person easy or hard to wake up?
- Can the person give his or her name, the time, and location when asked?
- Does the person identify others correctly?
- Does the person answer questions correctly?
- Does the person speak clearly?
- Are instructions followed correctly?
- Is the person calm, restless, or excited?
- Is the person conversing, quiet, or talking a lot?

Movement

- Can the person squeeze your fingers with each hand?
- Can the person move arms and legs?
- Are the person's movements shaky or jerky?
- Does the person complain of stiff or painful joints?

Pain or Discomfort

- Where is the pain located? (Ask the person to point to the pain.)
- Does the pain go anywhere else?
- How does the person rate the severity of the pain—mild, moderate, severe?
- How does the person rate the pain on a scale of 0 to 10 (Chapter 27)?
- When did the pain begin?
- What was the person doing when the pain began?
- How long does the pain last?
- How does the person describe the pain?
  - Sharp
  - Severe
  - Knife-like
  - Dull
  - Burning
  - Aching
  - Comes and goes
  - Depends on position
- Was a pain-relief drug given?
- Did the pain-relief drug relieve the pain? Is the pain still present?
- Is the person able to sleep and rest?
- What is the position of comfort?

Skin

- Is the skin pale or flushed?
- Is the skin cool, warm, or hot?
- Is the skin moist or dry?
- What color are the lips and nail beds?
- Is the skin intact? Are there broken areas? If so, where?
- Are sores or reddened areas present?
- Are bruises present? Where are they located?
- Does the person complain of itching? If yes, where?

Eyes, Ears, Nose, and Mouth

- Is there drainage from the eyes? What color is the drainage?
- Are the eyelids closed? Do they stay open?
- Are the eyes reddened?
- Does the person complain of spots, flashes, or blurring?
- Is the person sensitive to bright lights?
- Is there drainage from the ears? What color is the drainage?
- Can the person hear? Is repeating necessary? Are questions answered appropriately?

Eyes, Ears, Nose, and Mouth—cont'd

- Is there drainage from the nose? What color is the drainage?
- Can the person breathe through the nose?
- Is there breath odor?
- Does the person complain of a bad taste in the mouth?
- Does the person complain of painful gums or teeth?

Respirations

- Do both sides of the person's chest rise and fall with respirations?
- Is breathing noisy?
- Does the person complain of pain or difficulty breathing?
- What is the amount and color of sputum?
- What is the frequency of the person's cough? Is it dry or productive?

Bowels and Bladder

- Is the abdomen firm or soft?
- Does the person complain of gas?
- What are the amount, color, and consistency of bowel movements?
- What is the frequency of bowel movements?
- Can the person control bowel movements?
- Does the person have pain or difficulty urinating?
- What is the amount of urine?
- What is the color of urine?
- Is the urine clear? Are there particles in the urine?
- Does the urine have a foul smell?
- Can the person control the passage of urine?
- What is the frequency of urination?

Appetite

- Does the person like the food served?
- How much of the meal is eaten?
- What foods does the person like?
- Can the person chew food?
- What is the amount of fluid taken?
- What fluids does the person like?
- How often does the person drink fluids?
- Can the person swallow food and fluids?
- Does the person complain of nausea?
- What is the amount and color of material vomited?
- Does the person have hiccups?
- Is the person belching?
- Does the person cough when swallowing?

Activities of Daily Living

- Can the person perform personal care without help?
  - Bathing?
  - Brushing teeth?
  - Combing and brushing hair?
  - Shaving?
- Which does the person use: toilet, commode, bedpan, or urinal?
- Does the person feed himself or herself?
- Can the person walk?
- What amount and kind of help is needed?

Other

- Is the person bleeding from any body part? If yes, where and how much?

Box 7-2 Observations to Report at Once

- A change in the person's ability to respond
  - A responsive person is no longer responding.
  - A non-responsive person is now responding.
- A change in the person's mobility
  - The person cannot move a body part.
  - The person is now able to move a body part.
- Complaints of sudden, severe pain
- A sore or reddened area on the person's skin
- Complaints of a sudden change in vision
- Complaints of pain or difficulty breathing
- Abnormal respirations
- Complaints of or signs of difficulty swallowing
- Vomiting
- Bleeding
- Vital signs outside their normal ranges

Fig. 7-1 The nursing assistant uses a computer to note observations.

NURSING DIAGNOSIS

The RN uses assessment information to make a nursing diagnosis. A **nursing diagnosis** describes a health problem that can be treated by nursing measures (Box 7-3, pp. 78 and 79). The problem may exist or develop.

Nursing diagnoses and medical diagnoses are not the same. A **medical diagnosis** is the identification of a disease or condition by a doctor. Cancer, stroke, heart attack, infection, and diabetes are examples. Doctors order drugs, therapies, and surgery to cure or heal.

A person can have many nursing diagnoses. They deal with the total person—physical, emotional, social, and spiritual needs. They may change as assessment information changes. Or new nursing diagnoses are added. For example, "Acute pain" is added after surgery.

PLANNING

Planning involves setting priorities and goals. Nursing measures or actions are chosen to help the person meet the goals. The person, family, and health team help the RN plan care.

Priorities relate to what is most important for the person. Maslow's theory of basic needs is useful for setting priorities (Chapter 8). The needs are arranged in order of importance. Some needs are required for life and survival (oxygen, water, and food). They must be met before all other needs. They have priority and must be done first.

Goals are then set. A **goal** is that which is desired for or by a person as a result of nursing care. Goals are aimed at the person's highest level of well-being and function—physical, emotional, social, spiritual. Goals promote health and prevent health problems. They also promote rehabilitation.

Nursing interventions are chosen after goals are set. An *intervention* is an action or measure. A **nursing intervention** is an action or measure taken by the nursing team to help the person reach a goal. *Nursing intervention, nursing action,* and *nursing measure* mean the same thing. A nursing intervention does not need a doctor's order. However, some nursing measures come from a doctor's order. For example, a doctor orders that Mrs. Lange walk 50 yards 2 times a day. The nurse includes this order in the care plan.

OBRA-CMS

Interdisciplinary Care Planning Conference

OBRA requires regular interdisciplinary care planning (IDCP) conferences for each person (Chapter 6). The **comprehensive care plan** (care plan) is a written guide about the care a person should receive. The health team develops it. The resident and family give input. The care plan includes nursing diagnoses and goals. It has the person's problems, goals for care, and actions to take to help the person solve health problems.

The problems identified on the MDS give **triggers** (clues) for the Care Area Assessments (CAAs). (See Appendix B, p. 754). For example, Mr. Smith is weak from illness and lack of exercise. The MDS shows that he cannot do activities of daily living (ADL). This triggers the CAAs. A care plan is developed to solve the problem. The goal is for Mr. Smith to perform his own ADL. Staff from occupational therapy, physical therapy, and

Box 7-3   Nursing Diagnoses Approved by the North American Nursing Diagnosis Association International (NANDA-I)

- Activity Intolerance
- Activity Intolerance, Risk for
- Activity Planning, Ineffective
- Airway Clearance, Ineffective
- Anxiety
- Aspiration, Risk for
- Autonomic Dysreflexia
- Autonomic Dysreflexia, Risk for
- Bathing Self-Care Deficit
- Bleeding, Risk for
- Body Image, Disturbed
- Body Temperature, Risk for Imbalanced
- Breathing Pattern, Ineffective
- Cardiac Output, Decreased
- Caregiver Role Strain
- Caregiver Role Strain, Risk for
- Comfort, Impaired
- Comfort, Readiness for Enhanced
- Communication, Impaired Verbal
- Communication, Readiness for Enhanced
- Community Coping, Ineffective
- Community Coping, Readiness for Enhanced
- Confusion, Acute
- Confusion, Chronic
- Confusion, Risk for Acute
- Constipation
- Constipation, Perceived
- Constipation, Risk for
- Contamination
- Contamination, Risk for
- Coping, Defensive
- Coping, Ineffective
- Coping, Readiness for Enhanced
- Death Anxiety
- Decisional Conflict
- Decision Making, Readiness for Enhanced
- Denial, Ineffective
- Dentition, Impaired
- Development, Risk for Delayed
- Diarrhea
- Dignity, Risk for Compromised Human
- Disuse Syndrome, Risk for
- Diversional Activity, Deficient
- Dressing Self-Care Deficit
- Electrolyte Imbalance, Risk for
- Energy Field, Disturbed
- Environmental Interpretation Syndrome, Impaired
- Failure to Thrive, Adult
- Falls, Risk for
- Family Coping, Compromised
- Family Coping, Disabled
- Family Coping, Readiness for Enhanced
- Family Processes, Dysfunctional
- Family Processes, Interrupted
- Family Processes, Readiness for Enhanced

- Fatigue
- Fear
- Feeding Self-Care Deficit
- Fluid Balance, Readiness for Enhanced
- Fluid Volume, Deficient
- Fluid Volume, Excess
- Fluid Volume, Risk for Deficient
- Fluid Volume, Risk for Imbalanced
- Gas Exchange, Impaired
- Gastro-Intestinal Motility, Dysfunctional
- Gastro-Intestinal Motility, Risk for Dysfunctional
- Gastro-Intestinal Perfusion, Risk for Ineffective
- Glucose Level, Blood, Risk for Unstable
- Grieving
- Grieving, Complicated
- Grieving, Risk for Complicated
- Growth and Development, Delayed
- Health Behavior, Risk-Prone
- Health Maintenance, Ineffective
- Hope, Readiness for Enhanced
- Hopelessness
- Hyperthermia
- Hypothermia
- Immunization Status, Readiness for Enhanced
- Incontinence, Bowel
- Incontinence, Urinary, Functional
- Incontinence, Urinary, Overflow
- Incontinence, Urinary, Reflex
- Incontinence, Urinary, Stress
- Incontinence, Urinary, Urge
- Incontinence, Urinary, Urge, Risk for
- Infection, Risk for
- Injury, Risk for
- Insomnia
- Intracranial Adaptive Capacity, Decreased
- Knowledge, Deficient
- Knowledge, Readiness for Enhanced
- Latex Allergy Response
- Latex Allergy Response, Risk for
- Lifestyle, Sedentary
- Liver Function, Risk for Impaired
- Loneliness, Risk for
- Memory, Impaired
- Mobility, Impaired Bed
- Mobility, Impaired Physical
- Mobility, Impaired Wheelchair
- Moral Distress
- Nausea
- Neglect, Self
- Neglect, Unilateral
- Noncompliance
- Nutrition, Imbalanced: Less Than Body Requirements
- Nutrition, Imbalanced: More Than Body Requirements
- Nutrition, Imbalanced: More Than Body Requirements, Risk for

Nursing diagnoses common in long-term care. Nursing Diagnosis—Definitions and Classification 2009-2011, ©2009, 2007, 2005, 2003, 2001, 1998, 1996, 1994, NANDA International. Used by arrangement with Wiley-Blackwell Publishing; a company of John Wiley & Sons, Inc. In order to make safe and effective judgments using NANDA-I diagnoses it is essential that nurses refer to the definitions and defining characteristics of the diagnoses listed in this work.

Box 7-3	Nursing Diagnoses Approved by the North American Nursing Diagnosis Association International (NANDA-I)—cont'd

- Nutrition, Readiness for Enhanced
- Oral Mucous Membrane, Impaired
- Pain, Acute
- Pain, Chronic
- Peripheral Neurovascular Dysfunction, Risk for
- Personal Identity, Disturbed
- Poisoning, Risk for
- Post-Trauma Syndrome
- Post-Trauma Syndrome, Risk for
- Power, Readiness for Enhanced
- Powerlessness
- Powerlessness, Risk for
- Protection, Ineffective
- Rape-Trauma Syndrome
- Relationship, Readiness for Enhanced
- Religiosity, Impaired
- Religiosity, Readiness for Enhanced
- Religiosity, Risk for Impaired
- Relocation Stress Syndrome
- Relocation Stress Syndrome, Risk for
- Renal Perfusion, Risk for Ineffective
- Resilience, Impaired Individual
- Resilience, Readiness for Enhanced
- Resilience, Risk for Compromised
- Role Performance, Ineffective
- Self-Care, Readiness for Enhanced
- Self-Concept, Readiness for Enhanced
- Self-Esteem, Chronic Low
- Self-Esteem, Situational Low
- Self-Esteem, Situational Low, Risk for
- Self-Health Management, Ineffective
- Self-Health Management, Readiness for Enhanced
- Self-Mutilation
- Self-Mutilation, Risk for
- Sensory Perception, Disturbed (Specify type: Visual, Auditory, Kinesthetic, Gustatory, Tactile, Olfactory)
- Sexual Dysfunction

- Sexuality, Ineffective Pattern
- Shock, Risk for
- Skin Integrity, Impaired
- Skin Integrity, Risk for Impaired
- Sleep Deprivation
- Sleep Pattern, Disturbed
- Sleep, Readiness for Enhanced
- Social Interaction, Impaired
- Social Isolation
- Sorrow, Chronic
- Spiritual Distress
- Spiritual Distress, Risk for
- Spiritual Well-Being, Readiness for Enhanced
- Stress, Overload
- Suffocation, Risk for
- Suicide, Risk for
- Surgical Recovery, Delayed
- Swallowing, Impaired
- Therapeutic Regimen Management, Ineffective Family
- Thermoregulation, Ineffective
- Tissue Integrity, Impaired
- Tissue Perfusion, Cardiac, Risk for Decreased
- Tissue Perfusion, Cerebral, Risk for Ineffective
- Tissue Perfusion, Peripheral, Ineffective
- Toileting Self-Care Deficit
- Transfer Ability, Impaired
- Trauma, Risk for
- Trauma, Vascular, Risk for
- Urinary Elimination, Impaired
- Urinary Elimination, Readiness for Enhanced
- Urinary Retention
- Ventilation, Impaired Spontaneous
- Ventilatory Weaning Response, Dysfunctional
- Violence, Risk for Other-Directed
- Violence, Risk for Self-Directed
- Walking, Impaired
- Wandering

nursing work to solve the problem. The actions to help Mr. Smith reach the goal are:

- Occupational therapy to work with Mr. Smith on ADL daily
- Physical therapy to work with Mr. Smith on exercises daily
- Nursing staff member to walk Mr. Smith 20 yards twice daily

The care plan states the person's strengths. For example, Mrs. Jones can walk without help. This strength increases her independence. The health team helps Mrs. Jones continue to walk on her own.

A comprehensive care plan is developed for each person. Care plan suggestions are welcomed from all health team members, including nursing assistants. You use the care plan to give care. It is a communication tool. It tells what care to give and when.

Care plan forms vary in each center. It may be in the person's chart, in a notebook, in a Kardex, or on a computer. The plan must be carried out. The care plan is revised as the person's needs change.

See *Focus on Communication: Interdisciplinary Care Planning Conference,* p. 80.

FOCUS ON COMMUNICATION
Interdisciplinary Care Planning Conference

You spend a lot of time with the residents. You see what they like and do not like. You see what they can do and what they cannot do. Residents talk to you. They tell you about their families and interests. You make observations every time you are with them. Share this information during care conferences. Also share your ideas about the person's care. Your sharing can improve the person's quality of life. For example, you can say:

- "Mr. Antonio never eats his squash. He says that he misses the fresh green beans and broccoli from his garden. Can he have those more often?"
- "Mrs. Clark can use her feet to propel her wheelchair. Why do we have to push her wheelchair?"
- "Miss Walsh never talks when her family visits. She just sits there. Yet she talks to her roommate all the time."

IMPLEMENTATION

To *implement* means to perform or carry out. The **implementation** step is performing or carrying out nursing measures in the care plan. Care is given in this step.

Nursing care ranges from simple to complex. The nurse delegates nursing tasks that are within your legal limits and job description. The nurse may ask you to assist with complex measures.

You report the care given to the nurse. In some centers, you record the care given. Report and record *after* giving care, not before. Also report and record your observations. Observing is part of assessment. New observations may change the nursing diagnoses. If so, care plan changes are made. To give correct care, you need to know about any changes in the care plan.

Assignment Sheets

The nurse communicates delegated tasks to you. An assignment sheet is used for this purpose (Fig. 7-2). The assignment sheet tells you about:

- Each person's care.
- What measures and tasks need to be done.
- Which nursing unit tasks to do. Cleaning kitchenettes and utility rooms and stocking shower rooms are examples.

Talk to the nurse about any unclear assignment. You can also check the care plan and Kardex if you need more information.

See *Teamwork and Time Management: Assignment Sheets.*

Assignment Sheet

Date: _9–10_
Shift: _Day_
Nursing assistant: _John Reed_
Supervisor: _Mary Adams, RN_

Breaks: _1000_   _1400_
Lunch: _1230_
Unit Tasks: _Pass ice water at 0900_
Clean utility room at 1430

***Check the care plan for other care measures and information**

Room # _501A_ Name: _Mrs. Ann Lopez_	**Functional status/other care measures and procedures**
ID Number: _S1514491530_ Date of birth: _11/04/1925_ VS: _Daily at 0700_ T _____ P _____ R _____ BP _____ Wt: _Weekly (Monday at 0700)_ _____ Intake _____ BM _____ Bath: Portable tub Shampoo Bed rails	Total assist with ADL Stand-pivot transfers Uses w/c Incontinent of bowel and bladder – uses briefs Bilateral passive ROM exercises to extremities twice daily Turn and reposition q2h when in bed Wears eyeglasses and dentures Diet: High fiber (Total Assist)
Room # _510B_ Name: _Mr. Mark Monroe_	**Functional status/other care measures and procedures**
ID Number: _D4468947762_ Date of birth: _12/29/1926_ VS: _2 times daily, at 0700 and 1500_ 0700: T _____ P _____ R _____ BP _____ 1500: T _____ P _____ R _____ BP _____ Wt: _Daily at 0700_ _____ Intake _____ Output _____ BM _____ Bath: Shower	Independent with ADL Independent with ambulation Attends exercise group every morning Continent of bowel and bladder – q4h bathroom schedule to maintain continence Wears eyeglasses Coughing and deep breathing exercises q4h Diet: Sodium-controlled (Independent)

Fig. 7-2 Sample assignment sheet. NOTE: This assignment sheet is a computer printout.

TEAMWORK AND TIME MANAGEMENT
Assignment Sheets

Use your assignment sheet to organize your work and to set priorities:

- What do you need to do first?
- What can be done while the person is having breakfast, lunch, or dinner?
- What can you do while the person is at therapy (physical, occupational, and so on) or an activity?
- Do you need to reserve a room (shower room, tub room) or equipment (portable tub, shower chair)?
- What do you need help with?
- How many co-workers are needed to complete tasks such as turning and transferring a person?
- Ask a co-worker to help you. Tell the person what you need help with, when you need the help, and how long the task will take.
- Check off tasks as you complete them.

EVALUATION

Evaluation means to measure. The **evaluation** step involves measuring if the goals in the planning step were met. Progress is evaluated. Goals may be met totally, in part, or not at all. Assessment information is used for this step. Changes in nursing diagnoses, goals, and the care plan may result.

The nursing process never ends. Nurses constantly collect information about the person. Nursing diagnoses, goals, and the care plan may change as the person's needs change.

YOUR ROLE

You have a key role in the nursing process. The nurse uses your observations for nursing diagnoses and planning. You may help develop the care plan. In the implementation step, you perform tasks in the care plan. Your assignment sheet tells you what to do. Your observations are used for the evaluation step.

QUALITY OF LIFE

The resident has the right to take part in his or her care planning. OBRA requires that the person be included in the process. The person may refuse actions suggested by the health team. Involving the person in the care planning process helps the team better meet the person's needs. You are a key member of the team. Share your observations and ideas. They can help the team provide better care.

REVIEW QUESTIONS

Circle the BEST answer.

1. Which is *not* a step in the nursing process?
   - a Observation
   - b Assessment
   - c Planning
   - d Implementation

2. The nursing process
   - a Involves guidelines for care plans
   - b Is a care conference
   - c Involves triggers
   - d Is the method nurses use to plan and deliver nursing care

3. What happens during assessment?
   - a Goals are set.
   - b Information is collected.
   - c Nursing measures are carried out.
   - d Progress is evaluated.

4. Which is a symptom?
   - a Redness
   - b Vomiting
   - c Pain
   - d Pulse rate of 78

5. Which is a sign?
   - a Nausea
   - b Headache
   - c Dizziness
   - d Dry skin

6. Which should you report at once?
   - a The person had a bowel movement.
   - b The person complains of sudden, severe pain.
   - c The person does not like the food served for lunch.
   - d The person complains of stiff, painful joints.

7. Which should you report at once?
   - a The person can no longer move a body part.
   - b The person answers questions correctly.
   - c The person has a breath odor.
   - d The person walked to the dining room.

8. Measures in the nursing care plan are carried out. This is
   - a A nursing diagnosis
   - b Planning
   - c Implementation
   - d Evaluation

9. Which statement about the nursing process is *true*?
   - a It is done without the person's input.
   - b You are responsible for it.
   - c It is used to communicate the person's care.
   - d Steps can be done in any order.

10. The comprehensive care plan is
    - a Written by the doctor
    - b The measures to help the person
    - c The same for all persons
    - d Also called the Kardex

11. What is used to communicate the nursing tasks delegated to you?
    - a The care plan
    - b The Kardex
    - c An assignment sheet
    - d Care conferences

12. Which is a nursing diagnosis?
    - a Cancer
    - b Heart attack
    - c Kidney failure
    - d Pain

Answers to these questions are on p. 719.

CHAPTER 8

Understanding the Resident

OBJECTIVES

- Define the key terms listed in this chapter.
- Identify the parts that make up the whole person.
- Explain Abraham Maslow's theory of basic needs.
- Explain how culture and religion influence health and illness.
- Identify the emotional and social effects of illness.
- Describe persons cared for in nursing centers.
- Identify the elements needed for good communication.

- Describe how to use verbal and nonverbal communication.
- Explain the methods and barriers to good communication.
- Explain how to communicate with persons who have behavior problems.
- Explain how to communicate with persons who have disabilities or who are comatose.
- Explain why family and visitors are important to the person.
- Identify the courtesies given to the person, family, and friends.
- Explain how to promote quality of life.

KEY TERMS

body language Messages sent through facial expressions, gestures, posture, hand and body movements, gait, eye contact, and appearance

comatose Being unable to respond to stimuli

culture The characteristics of a group of people—language, values, beliefs, habits, likes, dislikes, customs—passed from one generation to the next

disability Any lost, absent, or impaired physical or mental function

esteem The worth, value, or opinion one has of a person

holism A concept that considers the whole person; the whole person has physical, social, psychological, and spiritual parts that are woven together and cannot be separated

need Something necessary or desired for maintaining life and mental well-being

nonverbal communication Communication that does not use words

optimal level of function A person's highest potential for mental and physical performance

paraphrasing Restating the person's message in your own words

religion Spiritual beliefs, needs, and practices

self-actualization Experiencing one's potential

self-esteem Thinking well of oneself and seeing oneself as useful and having value

verbal communication Communication that uses written or spoken words

The resident is the most important person in the center. Age, religion, and nationality make each person unique. So do culture, education, occupation, and life-style. Each person is important and special. Each has value. The person is treated as someone who thinks, acts, feels, and makes decisions.

You will care for many residents. Most are old. Each person has fears, needs, and rights. Each has suffered losses—loss of home, family, friends, and body functions. Family and community roles have been lost, too.

CARING FOR THE PERSON

For effective care, you must consider the whole person. Holism means *whole*. **Holism** is a concept that considers the whole person. The whole person has physical, social, psychological, and spiritual parts. These parts are woven together and cannot be separated (Fig. 8-1).

Each part relates to and depends on the others. As a social being, a person speaks and communicates with others. Physically, the brain, mouth, tongue, lips, and throat structures must function for speech. Communication is also psychological. It involves thinking and reasoning.

To consider only the physical part is to ignore the person's ability to think, make decisions, and interact with others. It also ignores the person's experiences, life-style, culture, religion, joys, sorrows, and needs.

Disability and illness affect the whole person. For example, Mrs. Butler had a stroke. She needs help with her physical needs. She had to leave her home. Relationships with her husband and children are changed. She is angry with God for letting this happen to her. The health team plans care to help her deal with her problems.

Addressing the Person

You must know and respect the whole person to provide effective, quality care. Too often a person is referred to as a room number. For example: "12A needs the bedpan," rather than "Mrs. Brown in 12A needs the bedpan." This strips the person of his or her identity. It reduces the person to a thing.

Residents are not things. They are not your relatives or children. They are complex, adult human beings. Follow these rules to address them with dignity and respect:

- Call residents by their titles—Mrs. Jones, Mr. Smith, Miss Turner, or Dr. Gonzalez.
- Do not call residents by their first names unless they ask you to.
- Do not call residents by any other name unless they ask you to.
- Do not call residents Grandma, Papa, Sweetheart, Honey, or other names.

BASIC NEEDS

A **need** is something necessary or desired for maintaining life and mental well-being. According to Abraham Maslow, a famous psychologist, basic needs must be met for a person to survive and function. According to this theory, the needs are arranged in order of importance (Fig. 8-2). Lower-level needs must be met before the higher-level needs. Basic needs, from the lowest level to the highest level, are:

- Physical needs
- Safety and security needs
- Love and belonging needs
- Self-esteem needs
- The need for self-actualization

People normally meet their own needs. When they cannot, it is usually because of disease, illness, injury, or advanced age. Those who are ill or injured usually seek health care.

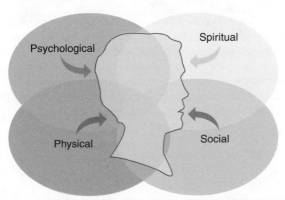

Fig. 8-1 A person is a physical, psychological, social, and spiritual being. The parts overlap and cannot be separated.

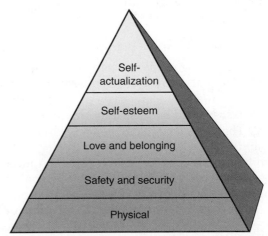

Fig. 8-2 Basic needs for life as described by Maslow. *(From Maslow AH: Frager RD (Editor), Fadiman J (Editor): Motivation and personality, ed 3, ©1987. Reprinted by permission of Pearson Education, Inc., Upper Saddle River, NJ.)*

Physical Needs

Oxygen, food, water, elimination, rest, and shelter are needed for life. They are needed to survive. A person dies within minutes without oxygen. Without food or water, a person feels weak and ill within a few hours. The kidneys and intestines must function. Otherwise, poisonous wastes build up in the blood. This can cause death. Without enough rest and sleep, a person becomes very tired. Without shelter, the person is exposed to extremes of heat and cold.

You help the person meet physical needs. You need to truly understand their importance. When choking, how do you feel? How do you feel when you are thirsty or hungry? How do you react without enough sleep? What are your fears when you need to use the bathroom right away?

Safety and Security Needs

Safety and security needs relate to feeling safe from harm, danger, and fear. Many people are afraid of nursing centers. Some care involves strange equipment. Some care causes pain or discomfort. People feel safer and more secure if they know what will happen. For every task, even a simple bath, the person should know:

* Why it is needed
* Who will do it
* How it will be done
* What sensations or feelings to expect

Many persons do not feel safe and secure when admitted to a nursing center. They are not in their usual, secure home settings. They are in a strange place with strange routines. Strangers care for them. Some become scared and confused.

Be kind and understanding. Show them the new setting. Listen to their concerns. Explain all routines and procedures. You may have to repeat information many times. Sometimes the information may need repeating for many days or weeks until the person feels safe and secure. Be patient.

Love and Belonging Needs

Love and belonging needs relate to love, closeness, and affection. They also involve meaningful relationships with others. There are many cases in which people became weaker or died because they lacked love and belonging. This is seen in older persons who have outlived family and friends.

Family, friends, and the health team can meet love and belonging needs. The center is the person's home. You must help the person feel loved and accepted. Remind the person that you are there to help him or her.

Self-Esteem Needs

Esteem is the worth, value, or opinion one has of a person. Self-esteem means to think well of oneself and to see oneself as useful and having value. People often lack self-esteem when ill, injured, older, or disabled. For example:

* An older man once built his own home and worked a farm. He supported and raised a family. Now he cannot dress or feed himself.
* Cancer treatments caused a woman to lose her hair. She does not feel attractive or whole.
* A person has a slow, crippling disease.
* A person had a leg amputated.

You must treat all persons with respect. Although it takes more time, encourage them to do as much for themselves as possible. This helps increase self-esteem.

The Need for Self-Actualization

Self-actualization means experiencing one's potential. It involves learning, understanding, and creating to the limit of a person's capacity. This is the highest need. Rarely, if ever, is it totally met. Most people constantly try to learn and understand more. This need can be postponed, and life will continue.

CULTURE AND RELIGION

Culture is the characteristics of a group of people—language, values, beliefs, habits, likes, dislikes, and customs. They are passed from one generation to the next. The person's culture influences health beliefs and practices. Culture also affects thinking and behavior during illness and when in a nursing center.

People come from many cultures, races, and nationalities. Their family practices and food choices may differ from yours. So might their hygiene habits and clothing styles. Some speak a foreign language. Some cultures have beliefs about what causes and cures illness. (See *Caring About Culture: Health Care Beliefs.*) They may perform rituals to rid the body of disease. (See *Caring About Culture: Sick Care Practices.*) Many have beliefs and rituals about dying and death (Chapter 48). Culture also is a factor in communication.

CARING ABOUT CULTURE
Health Care Beliefs

Some *Mexican Americans* believe that illness is caused by prolonged exposure to hot or cold. If hot causes illness, cold is used for the cure. Likewise, hot is used to cure illnesses caused by cold. Hot and cold are found in body organs, medicines (drugs), the air, and food. For example, an earache may occur from cold air entering the body. Hot remedies are used to cure the earache.

The hot-cold balance is also a belief of some *Vietnamese Americans*. Illnesses, food, drugs, and herbs are hot or cold. Hot is given to balance cold illnesses. Cold is given for hot illnesses.

Modified from Giger JN, Davidhizar RE: Transcultural nursing: assessment and intervention, *ed 5, St Louis, 2008, Mosby.*

CARING ABOUT CULTURE
Sick Care Practices

Folk practices are common among some *Vietnamese Americans.* They include *cao gio* ("rub wind")—rubbing the skin with a coin to treat the common cold. Skin pinching *(bat gio—"catch wind")* is used for headaches and sore throats. Herbs, oils, and soups are used for many signs and symptoms.

Some *Russian Americans* practice folk medicine. Herbs are taken through drinks or enemas. For headaches, an ointment is placed behind the ears and temples and at the back of the neck. A backache treatment involves placing a dough of dark rye flour and honey on the spine.

Folk healers are used by some *Mexican Americans.* Folk healers may be family members or from outside the family. A *yerbero* uses herbs and spices to prevent or cure disease. A *curandero* (*curandera* if female) deals with serious physical and mental illnesses. Witches use magic. A *brujos* is a male witch. A *brujas* is a female witch.

Modified from Giger JN, Davidhizar RE: Transcultural nursing: assessment and intervention, *ed 5, St Louis, 2008, Mosby.*

Fig. 8-3 Residents attend a religious service at a nursing center.

Religion relates to spiritual beliefs, needs, and practices. A person's religion influences health and illness practices. Religions may have beliefs and practices about daily living, behaviors, relationships with others, diet, healing, days of worship, birth and birth control, drugs, and death.

Many people find comfort and strength from religion during illness. They may want to pray and observe religious practices. Nursing centers offer religious services. Many have chapels or meditation areas for prayer. Assist residents to attend services as needed (Fig. 8-3). Some leave the center to worship.

A person may want to see a spiritual leader or advisor. Report this to the nurse. Make sure the room is neat and orderly. Have a chair ready for the cleric. Provide privacy during the visit.

The nursing process reflects the person's culture and religion. The care plan includes the person's cultural and religious practices.

You must respect and accept the person's culture and religion. You will meet people from other cultures and religions. Learn about their beliefs and practices. This helps you understand the person and give better care.

A person may not follow all beliefs and practices of his or her culture or religion. Some people do not practice a religion. Each person is unique. Do not judge the person by your standards. And do not force your ideas on the person.

EFFECTS OF ILLNESS AND DISABILITY

People do not choose sickness or injury. When they occur, they have physical, psychological, and social effects. Some result in disabilities. A **disability** is any lost, absent, or impaired physical or mental function. It may be temporary or permanent.

Normal activities—work, driving, fixing meals, yard work, hobbies—may be hard or impossible. Daily activities bring pleasure, worth, and contact with others. People often feel angry, upset, and useless when unable to perform them. These feelings may increase if others must help with routine functions.

Some people feel alone and isolated after out-living family and friends. Those who are disabled or have chronic illnesses may have many fears and concerns about nursing centers. They may feel lonely and abandoned by family and friends. They may fear depending on strangers. Many fear increasing loss of function. Some express their fears. Others do not or cannot.

Anger is a common response to illness and disability. Persons who need nursing center care are often angry. The person may direct anger at you. However, the person is usually angry at the situation. You might have problems dealing with the person's anger. If so, ask the nurse for help.

You can help the person feel safe, secure, and loved. Take an extra minute to "visit," to hold a hand, or to give a hug. (Remember to maintain professional boundaries. See Chapter 4.) Show that you are willing to help with personal needs. Respond promptly. Treat each person with respect and dignity.

Optimal Level of Function

Sometimes the health team cannot prevent increasing loss of function. However, residents are helped to maintain their **optimal level of function.** This is the person's highest potential for mental and physical performance. Encourage the person to be as independent as possible. Always focus on the person's abilities. Do not focus on disabilities.

Hospital patients are often treated as sick, dependent people. Promoting this "sick role" in a nursing center reduces quality of life. The health team focuses on improving the person's quality of life. You must help each person regain or maintain as much physical and mental function as possible.

Fig. 8-4 This older man needs nursing center services.

NURSING CENTER RESIDENTS

Most residents are older. Some are alert and oriented. Often they have chronic health problems that prevent them from living alone or with family (Fig. 8-4). Others are very confused and disoriented. They cannot care for themselves. Still others are recovering from fractures, acute illnesses, or surgery. Some residents are terminally ill (dying). They need special care to maintain comfort and make their last days as peaceful as possible.

Alert, Oriented Residents

Alert and oriented residents know who they are and where they are. They know the year and the time of day. These people need nursing center care because of physical problems. Some are paralyzed from a stroke, injury, or birth defect. Others are disabled from arthritis or multiple sclerosis. Still others have chronic heart, liver, kidney, or respiratory diseases.

The amount of care required depends on the degree of disability. Because these persons are alert and oriented, they may have problems adjusting to a nursing center. The care plan includes measures to help the person accept the nursing center as home.

Confused and Disoriented Residents

Many persons are mildly to severely confused and disoriented. Some cannot find the dining room. Others do not know the month or year. Others have more severe problems. For example, a man thinks he is waiting for a train. Or an older woman wants to feed her baby. The most severely disoriented persons do not know who they are.

Sometimes confusion and disorientation are temporary. This is especially true for new residents. Some persons have Alzheimer's disease and other dementias. Confusion and disorientation are permanent and become worse (Chapter 44).

Complete Care Residents

Some people are very disabled. They also are confused and disoriented. They need total assistance with all activities. They cannot meet any of their own needs. Nor can they say what they need or want. The health team must keep them clean, safe, and comfortable. You must treat them with respect and compassion. Touch, massage, and music may provide comfort and decrease loneliness.

Short-Term Residents

Some people need nursing center care to recover from fractures, acute illness, or surgery. Often they are younger than most residents. They may need tube feedings, wound care, rehabilitation, or other treatments. Others may need therapy programs: physical, occupational, speech and language, or respiratory. Some need restorative nursing care (Chapter 46). The goal is to help them regain their optimal level of function so they can return home.

Some people are cared for at home. They are admitted to nursing centers for short stays. This is *respite care.* Respite means rest or relief. The caregiver can take a vacation, tend to business, or simply rest. Respite care may last from a few days to several weeks.

Life-Long Residents

Birth defects and childhood injuries and diseases can cause disabilities. Intellectual disabilities (mental retardation) and Down syndrome are common causes. A disability occurring before 22 years of age is called a *developmental disability* (Chapter 45). It may be a physical impairment, intellectual impairment, or both.

The person with a developmental disability has limited function in at least three of these areas:
- Self-care
- Understanding or expressing language
- Learning
- Mobility
- Self-direction
- Independent living
- Financial support for one's self

The person needs life-long assistance, support, and special devices. Some nursing centers admit developmentally disabled children and adults.

Residents with Mental Health Problems

Some people have problems coping or adjusting to stress (Chapter 43). Their behavior and function are affected. In severe cases, self-care and independent living are impaired. Some persons have physical and mental illnesses.

Terminally Ill Residents

Terminally ill persons are dying. They may have advanced cancer, liver, kidney, respiratory, or other diseases. Some are alert and oriented. Others are comatose. *Comatose* means being unable to respond to stimuli (p. 94). The person may still feel pain. Often pain is shown by grimacing or groaning.

Some persons have severe pain. They need frequent care to maintain comfort. Promptly report any sign of discomfort to the nurse. Drugs for pain relief are important. So is the care you give. Turning and re-positioning, gentle back rubs, and touch promote comfort and peace. So does holding a hand. Many centers work with hospice programs. The goal is to provide quality care to persons who are dying (Chapters 1 and 48).

BEHAVIOR ISSUES

Many people accept illness and disability as part of aging. Others do not adjust well. They have some of the following behaviors. These behaviors are new for some people. For others, they are life-long. They are part of one's personality.

- *Anger.* Anger is a common emotion. Causes include fear, pain, and dying and death. Loss of function and loss of control over health and life are causes. Anger is a symptom of some diseases that affect thinking and behavior. Some people are generally angry. Anger is communicated verbally and nonverbally (p. 89). Verbal outbursts, shouting, raised voices, and rapid speech are common. Some people are silent. Others are not cooperative. They may refuse to answer questions. Nonverbal signs include rapid movements, pacing, clenched fists, and a red face. Glaring and getting close to you when speaking are other signs. Violent behaviors can occur.
- *Demanding behavior.* Nothing seems to please the person. The person is critical of others. He or she wants care given at a certain time and in a certain way. Loss of independence, loss of health, and loss of control of life are causes. So are unmet needs.
- *Self-centered behavior.* The person cares only about his or her own needs. The needs of others are ignored. The person demands the time and attention of others. The person becomes impatient if needs are not met.

- *Aggressive behavior.* The person may swear, bite, hit, pinch, scratch, or kick. Fear, anger, pain, and dementia (Chapter 44) are causes. Protect the person, others, and yourself from harm (Chapter 12).
- *Withdrawal.* The person has little or no contact with family, friends, and staff. He or she spends time alone and does not take part in social or group events. This may signal physical illness or depression. Some people are generally not social. They prefer to be alone.
- *Inappropriate sexual behavior.* Some people make inappropriate sexual remarks. Or they touch others in the wrong way. Some disrobe or masturbate in public. These behaviors may be on purpose. Or they are caused by disease, confusion, dementia, or drug side effects.

Some behaviors are not pleasant. You cannot avoid the person or lose control. Good communication is needed. Behaviors are addressed in the care plan. The care plan may include some of the guidelines in Box 8-1.

See *Teamwork and Time Management: Behavior Issues*, p. 88.

See *Focus on Communication: Behavior Issues*, p. 88.

Box 8-1   Dealing With Behavior Issues

- Recognize frustrating and frightening situations. Put yourself in the person's situation. How would you feel? How would you want to be treated?
- Treat the person with dignity and respect.
- Answer questions clearly and thoroughly. Ask the nurse to answer questions you cannot answer.
- Keep the person informed. Tell the person what you are going to do and when.
- Do not keep the person waiting. Answer signal lights promptly. If you tell the person that you will do something for him or her, do it promptly.
- Explain the reason for long waits. Ask if you can get or do something to increase the person's comfort.
- Stay calm and professional, especially if the person is angry or hostile. Often the person is not angry at you. He or she is angry at another person or situation.
- Do not argue with the person.
- Listen and use silence (p. 93). The person may feel better if able to express his or her feelings.
- Protect yourself from violent behaviors (Chapter 12).
- Report the person's behavior to the nurse. Discuss how to deal with the person.

COMMUNICATING WITH THE PERSON

You communicate with residents every time you give care. You give information to the person. The person gives information to you. Your body sends messages all the time—at the bedside, in hallways, at the nurses' station, in the dining room, and elsewhere. The person and family are aware of what you say and what you do. Good work ethics and understanding the person are needed for good communication. What you say and do also are important.

Effective Communication

For effective communication between you and the person, you must:
- Follow the rules of communication (Chapter 6):
  - Use words that have the same meaning for you and the person.
  - Avoid medical terms and words not familiar to the person.
  - Communicate in a logical and orderly manner. Do not wander in thought.
  - Give facts and be specific.
  - Be brief and concise.
- Understand and respect the resident as a person.
- View the person as a physical, psychological, social, and spiritual human being.

- Appreciate the person's problems and frustrations.
- Respect the person's rights.
- Respect the person's religion and culture.
- Give the person time to understand the information that you give.
- Repeat information as often as needed. Repeat what you said. Use the exact same words. Do not give the person a new message to process. If the person does not seem to understand after repeating, try re-phrasing the message. This is very important for persons with hearing problems.
- Ask questions to see if the person understood you.
- Be patient. People with memory problems may ask the same question many times. Do not say that you are repeating information. Accept the memory loss as a disability.
- Include the person in conversations when others are present. This includes when a co-worker is assisting you with care.

  See *Residents With Dementia: Effective Communication.*

Verbal Communication

Words are used in verbal communication. Words are spoken or written. You talk to the person. You find out how the person is feeling and share information. Most verbal communication involves the spoken word. Follow these rules:
- Face the person. Look directly at the person.
- Position yourself at the person's eye level. You may have to sit or squat by the person.
- Control the loudness and tone of your voice.
- Speak clearly, slowly, and distinctly.
- Do not use slang or vulgar words.
- Repeat information as needed.
- Ask one question at a time. Wait for an answer.
- Do not shout, whisper, or mumble.
- Be kind, courteous, and friendly.

The written word is used when the person cannot speak or hear but can read. The nurse and care plan tell you how to communicate with the person. The devices shown in Figure 8-5 are often used. The person also may have poor vision. When writing messages:

- Keep them brief and concise.
- Use a black felt pen on white paper.
- Print in large letters.

Some persons cannot speak or read. Ask questions that have "yes" or "no" answers. The person can nod, blink, or use other gestures for "yes" and "no." Follow the care plan. A picture board may be helpful (Fig. 8-6, p. 90).

Persons who are deaf may use sign language (Fig. 8-7, p. 90). See Chapter 37.

Nonverbal Communication

Nonverbal communication does not use words. Messages are sent with gestures, facial expressions, posture, body movements, touch, and smell. Nonverbal messages more accurately reflect a person's feelings than words do. They are usually involuntary and hard to control. A person may say one thing but act another way. Watch the person's eyes, hand movements, gestures, posture, and other actions. Sometimes they tell you more than words.

Fig. 8-5 Communication aids. **A,** Picture board in English and Spanish. *Continued*

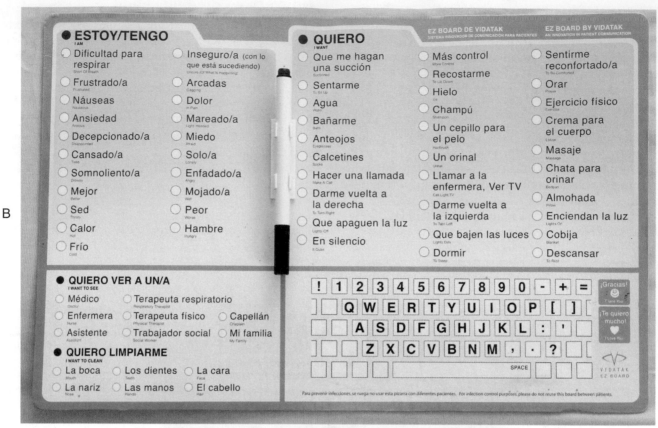

● ESTOY/TENGO
I AM

- Dificultad para respirar
  Short Of Breath
- Frustrado/a
  Frustrated
- Náuseas
  Nauseous
- Ansiedad
  Anxious
- Decepcionado/a
  Disappointed
- Cansado/a
  Tired
- Somnoliento/a
  Drowsy
- Mejor
  Better
- Sed
  Thirsty
- Calor
  Hot
- Frío
  Cold
- Inseguro/a (con lo que está sucediendo)
  Unsure (Of What Is Happening)
- Arcadas
  Gagging
- Dolor
  In Pain
- Mareado/a
  Light Headed
- Miedo
  Afraid
- Solo/a
  Lonely
- Enfadado/a
  Angry
- Mojado/a
  Wet
- Peor
  Worse
- Hambre
  Hungry

● QUIERO VER A UN/A
I WANT TO SEE

- Médico
  Doctor
- Enfermera
  Nurse
- Asistente
  Assistant
- Terapeuta respiratorio
  Respiratory Therapist
- Terapeuta físico
  Physical Therapist
- Trabajador social
  Social Worker
- Capellán
  Chaplain
- Mi familia
  My Family

● QUIERO LIMPIARME
I WANT TO CLEAN

- La boca
  Mouth
- La nariz
  Nose
- Los dientes
  Teeth
- Las manos
  Hands
- La cara
  Face
- El cabello
  Hair

● QUIERO
I WANT

EZ BOARD DE VIDATAK
SISTEMA INNOVADOR DE COMUNICACIÓN PARA PACIENTES
EZ BOARD BY VIDATAK
AN INNOVATION IN PATIENT COMMUNICATION

- Que me hagan una succión
  Be Suctioned
- Sentarme
  To Sit Up
- Agua
  Water
- Bañarme
  Bath
- Anteojos
  Eyeglasses
- Calcetines
  Socks
- Hacer una llamada
  Make A Call
- Darme vuelta a la derecha
  To Turn Right
- Que apaguen la luz
  Lights Off
- En silencio
  It Quiet
- Más control
  More Control
- Recostarme
  To Lie Down
- Hielo
  Ice
- Champú
  Shampoo
- Un cepillo para el pelo
  Hairbrush
- Un orinal
  Urinal
- Llamar a la enfermera, Ver TV
  Call Light, TV
- Darme vuelta a la izquierda
  To Turn Left
- Que bajen las luces
  Lights Dim
- Dormir
  To Sleep
- Sentirme reconfortado/a
  To Be Comforted
- Orar
  Prayer
- Ejercicio físico
  Exercise
- Crema para el cuerpo
  Lotion
- Masaje
  Massage
- Chata para orinar
  Bedpan
- Almohada
  Pillow
- Enciendan la luz
  Lights On
- Cobija
  Blanket
- Descansar
  To Rest

```
! 1 2 3 4 5 6 7 8 9 0 - + =   ¡Gracias!
  Q W E R T Y U I O P [ ]     Thank You
   A S D F G H J K L : '      ¡Te quiero mucho!
    Z X C V B N M , . ?       I Love You
              SPACE           VIDATAK EZ BOARD
```

Para prevenir infecciones, se ruega no usar esta pizarra con diferentes pacientes. For infection control purposes, please do not reuse this board between patients.

Fig. 8-5, cont'd Communication aids. **B,** Communication board in Spanish. **C,** Magic Slate.

Fig. 8-6 A resident uses a picture board and picture cards to communicate.

Fig. 8-7 Sign language is used to communicate.

CARING ABOUT CULTURE
Touch Practices

Touch practices vary among cultural groups. Touch is a friendly gesture in the *Philippine* culture. Touch is used often in *Mexico*. Some people believe that using touch while complimenting a person is important. It is thought to neutralize the power of the evil eye *(mal de ojo)*.

Persons from the *United Kingdom* tend to reserve touch for persons they know well. Within limits, touch is acceptable in *Poland.* Its use depends on age, gender, and the relationship.

In *India*, men shake hands with other men. Men do not shake hands with women. Instead, they place their palms together and bow slightly to women. As a sign of respect or to seek a blessing, people touch the feet of older adults.

In *Vietnam*, a person's head is not touched by others. It is considered the center of the soul. Men do not touch women whom they do not know. Men commonly shake hands with men.

People from *China* do not like touching by strangers. A nod or slight bow is given during introductions. Health care workers of the same gender are preferred.

In *Ireland*, a firm handshake is preferred. Only family and close friends are embraced.

Modified from D'Avanzo CE, Geissler EM: Pocket guide to cultural health assessment, ed 4, St Louis, 2008, Mosby.

CARING ABOUT CULTURE
Facial Expressions

Through facial expressions, *Americans* communicate:
- *Coldness*—there is a constant stare. Face muscles do not move.
- *Fear*—eyes are open wide. Eyebrows are raised. The mouth is tense with the lips drawn back.
- *Anger*—eyes are fixed in a hard stare. Upper lids are lowered. Eyebrows are drawn down. Lips are tightly compressed.
- *Tiredness*—eyes are rolled upward.
- *Disapproval*—eyes are rolled upward.
- *Disgust*—narrowed eyes. The upper lip is curled. There are nose movements.
- *Embarrassment*—eyes are turned away or down. The face is flushed. The person pretends to smile. He or she rubs the eyes, nose, or face. He or she twitches the hair, beard, or mustache.
- *Surprise*—direct gaze with raised eyebrows.

Italian, Jewish, African-American, and *Hispanic* persons smile readily. They use many facial expressions and gestures for happiness, pain, or displeasure. *Irish, English,* and *Northern European* persons tend to have less facial expression.

In some cultures, facial expressions mean the opposite of what the person is feeling. For example, *Asians* may conceal negative emotions with a smile.

Modified from Giger JN, Davidhizar RE: Transcultural nursing: assessment and intervention, ed 5, St Louis, 2008, Mosby.

Touch Touch is a very important form of nonverbal communication. It conveys comfort, caring, love, affection, interest, trust, concern, and reassurance. Touch means different things to different people. The meaning depends on age, gender (male or female), experiences, and culture.

Cultural groups have rules or practices about touch. They relate to who can touch, when it can occur, and where to touch the body. (See *Caring About Culture: Touch Practices.*)

Some people do not like to be touched. However, touch can show caring and warmth. Stroking or holding a hand can comfort a person. Touch should be gentle. It should not be hurried, rough, or sexual. To use touch, follow the person's care plan. Remember to maintain professional boundaries.

Body Language People send messages through their **body language**:
- Facial expressions (See *Caring About Culture: Facial Expressions.*)
- Gestures
- Posture
- Hand and body movements
- Gait
- Eye contact
- Appearance (dress, hygiene, jewelry, perfume, cosmetics, tattoos, body piercings, and so on)

Slumped posture may mean the person is not happy or not feeling well. A person may deny pain. However, he or she protects the affected body part by standing, lying, or sitting in a certain way. Many messages are sent through body language.

Your actions, movements, and facial expressions send messages. So do how you stand, sit, walk, and look at the person. Your body language should show interest and enthusiasm. It should show caring and respect for the person. Often you will need to control your body language. Control reactions to odors from body fluids, secretions, excretions, or the person's body. Many odors are beyond the person's control. Embarrassment and humiliation increase if you react to odors.

CARING ABOUT CULTURE
Eye Contact Practices

In the *American* culture, eye contact signals a good self-concept. It also shows openness, interest in others, attention, honesty, and warmth. Lack of eye contact can mean:

* Shyness
* Lack of interest
* Humility
* Guilt
* Embarrassment
* Low self-esteem
* Rudeness
* Dishonesty

For some *Asian* and *American Indian* cultures, eye contact is impolite. It is an invasion of privacy. In certain *Indian* cultures, eye contact is avoided with persons of higher or lower socio-economic class. It is also given a special sexual meaning.

In *Iraq*, men and women avoid direct eye contact. Long, direct eye contact is rude in *Mexico*. In rural parts of *Vietnam*, it is not respectful to look at another person while talking. Blinking means that a message is received. In the *United Kingdom*, looking directly at a speaker means the listener is paying attention.

Modified from Giger JN, Davidhizar RE: Transcultural nursing: assessment and intervention, ed 5, St Louis, 2008, Mosby. Modified from D'Avanzo CE, Geissler EM: Pocket guide to cultural health assessment, ed 4, St Louis, 2008, Mosby.

Communication Methods

Certain methods help you communicate with others. They result in better relationships. More information is gained for the nursing process.

Listening Listening means to focus on verbal and nonverbal communication. You use sight, hearing, touch, and smell. You focus on what the person is saying. You observe nonverbal clues. They can support what the person says. Or they can show other feelings. For example, Mr. Hart says, "I want to stay here. That way my daughter won't have to care for me." You see tears, and he looks away from you. His verbal says *happy*. His nonverbal shows *sadness*.

Listening requires that you care and have interest. Follow these guidelines:

* Face the person.
* Have good eye contact with the person. See *Caring About Culture: Eye Contact Practices.*
* Lean toward the person (Fig. 8-8). Do not sit back with your arms crossed.
* Respond to the person. Nod your head. Say "uh huh," "mmm," and "I see." Repeat what the person says. Ask questions.
* Avoid communication barriers.

Fig. 8-8 Listen by facing the person. Have good eye contact. Lean toward the person.

Paraphrasing Paraphrasing is restating the person's message in your own words. You use fewer words than the person did. Paraphrasing:

* Shows you are listening
* Lets the person see if you understand the message
* Promotes further communication

The person usually responds to your statement. For example:

Mr. Hart: My wife was crying after she spoke with the doctor. I don't know what they talked about.

You: You don't know why your wife was crying.

Mr. Hart: He must have told her that I have a tumor.

Direct Questions Direct questions focus on certain information. You ask the person something you need to know. Some direct questions have "yes" or "no" answers. Others require more information. For example:

You: Mr. Hart, do you want to shave this morning?

Mr. Hart: Yes.

You: Mr. Hart, when would you like to do that?

Mr. Hart: Could we start in 15 minutes? I'd like to call my son first.

You: Yes, we can start in 15 minutes. Did you have a bowel movement today?

Mr. Hart: No.

You: You said you didn't eat well this morning. Can you tell me what you ate?

Mr. Hart: I only had toast and coffee. I just don't feel like eating this morning.

Open-Ended Questions Open-ended questions lead or invite the person to share thoughts, feelings, or ideas. The person chooses what to talk about. He or she controls the topic and the information given. Answers require more than a "yes" or "no." For example:

* "What do you like about living with your daughter?"
* "Tell me about your grandson."
* "What was your wife like?"
* "What do you like about being retired?"

The person chooses how to answer. Responses to open-ended questions are longer. They give more information than do responses to direct questions.

CARING ABOUT CULTURE
The Meaning of Silence

In the *English* and *Arabic* cultures, silence is used for privacy. Among *Russian, French,* and *Spanish* cultures, silence means agreement between parties. In some *Asian* cultures, silence is a sign of respect, particularly to an older person.

Modified from Giger JN, Davidhizar RE: Transcultural nursing: assessment and intervention, *ed 5, St Louis, 2008, Mosby.*

Clarifying Clarifying lets you make sure that you understand the message. You can ask the person to repeat the message, say you do not understand, or restate the message. For example:

- "Could you say that again?"
- "I'm sorry, Mr. Hart. I don't understand what you mean."
- "Are you saying that you want to go home?"

Focusing Focusing is dealing with a certain topic. It is useful when a person rambles or wanders in thought. For example, Mr. Hart talks at length about food and places to eat. You need to know why he did not eat much breakfast. To focus on breakfast you say: "Let's talk about breakfast. You said you don't feel like eating."

Silence Silence is a very powerful way to communicate. Sometimes you do not need to say anything. This is true during sad times. Just being there shows you care. At other times, silence gives time to think, organize thoughts, or choose words. Silence is useful when making decisions. It also helps when the person is upset and needs to gain control. Silence on your part shows caring and respect for the person's situation and feelings.

Sometimes pauses or long silences are uncomfortable. You do not need to talk when the person is silent. The person may need silence. Dealing with silence gets easier as you gain experience in your role. See *Caring About Culture: The Meaning of Silence.*

Communication Barriers

Communication barriers prevent the sending and receiving of messages. Communication fails. You must avoid these barriers:

- *Using unfamiliar language.* You and the person must use and understand the same language. If not, messages are not accurately interpreted. See Appendix C, p. 756, for useful Spanish words and phrases.
- *Cultural differences.* The person may attach different meanings to verbal and nonverbal communication. See *Caring About Culture: Communicating With Persons From Other Cultures.*
- *Changing the subject.* Someone changes the subject when the topic is uncomfortable. Avoid changing the subject whenever possible.

CARING ABOUT CULTURE
Communicating With Persons From Other Cultures

To communicate with persons from other cultures:
- Ask the nurse about the beliefs and values of the person's culture. You can also ask the resident and family. Learn as much as you can about the person's culture.
- Do not judge the person by your own attitudes, values, beliefs, and ideas.
- Follow the person's care plan. It includes the person's cultural beliefs and customs.
- Do the following when communicating with foreign-speaking persons:
  - Convey comfort by your tone of voice and body language.
  - Do not speak loudly or shout. It will not help the person understand English.
  - Speak slowly and distinctly.
  - Keep messages short and simple.
  - Be alert for words the person seems to understand.
  - Use gestures and pictures.
  - Repeat the message in other ways.
  - Avoid using medical terms and abbreviations.
  - Be alert for signs the person is pretending to understand. Nodding and answering "yes" to all questions are signs that the person does not understand what you are saying.

Modified from Giger JN, Davidhizar RE: Transcultural nursing: assessment and intervention, *ed 5, St Louis, 2008, Mosby.*

- *Giving your opinion.* Opinions involve judging values, behaviors, or feelings. Let others express feelings and concerns without adding your opinion. Do not make judgments or jump to conclusions.
- *Talking a lot when others are silent.* Talking too much is usually because of nervousness and discomfort with silence. Silences have meaning. They show acceptance, rejection, and fear. They also show the need for quiet and time to think.
- *Failure to listen.* Do not pretend to listen. It shows lack of interest and caring. This causes poor responses. You miss complaints of pain, discomfort, or other symptoms that you must report to the nurse.
- *Pat answers.* "Don't worry." "Everything will be okay." "Your doctor knows best." These make the person feel that you do not care about his or her concerns, feelings, and fears.
- *Illness and disability.* Some illnesses, injuries, and birth defects affect speech, hearing, vision, cognitive function, and body movements. Verbal and nonverbal communication are affected.
- *Age.* Values and communication styles vary among age-groups.

RESIDENTS WITH DISABILITIES

A person may acquire a disability any time from birth through old age. Disease and injury are common causes. For example, children can develop hearing problems from ear infections. Head injuries from accidents can impair cognitive function. Spinal cord injuries can affect movements. And loud noise (music, machines) is linked to hearing loss. The cause of disability or the age of onset does not matter. The person does not choose to have a disability.

The person has to adjust to the disability. For many people, this can be long and hard (Chapter 46).

You will care for many people with disabilities. Your attitude is important for effective communication. People with disabilities have the same basic needs as you and everyone else. They feel joy, sorrow, happiness, sadness, and other emotions just like you and everyone else. They laugh, cry, have families, go to school, work, get married, and pay bills just like you and everyone else. And they have the right to dignity and respect just like you and everyone else.

To communicate with persons who have certain disabilities, see persons:

- Who have speech impairments—Chapter 37
- Who are hard-of-hearing—Chapter 37
- Who are blind—Chapter 37
- Who are confused—Chapter 44
- With Alzheimer's disease and other dementias—Chapter 44

Common courtesies and manners (etiquette) apply to any person with a disability. See Box 8-2 for disability etiquette. The guidelines are from Easter Seals, an organization that helps persons with disabilities and their families.

The Person Who Is Comatose

Comatose means being unable to respond to stimuli. The person who is comatose is unconscious. The person cannot respond to others. Often the person can hear and can feel touch and pain. Pain may be shown by grimacing or groaning. Assume that the person hears and understands you. Use touch and give care gently. Practice these measures:

- Knock before entering the person's room.
- Tell the person your name, the time, and the place every time you enter the room.
- Give care on the same schedule every day.
- Explain what you are going to do. Explain care measures step-by-step as you do them.
- Tell the person when you are finishing care.
- Use touch to communicate care, concern, and comfort.
- Tell the person what time you will be back to check on him or her.
- Tell the person when you are leaving the room.

Box 8-2   Disability Etiquette

- Extend the same courtesies to the person as you would to anyone else.
- Allow the person privacy.
- Do not hang on or lean on a person's wheelchair.
- Treat adults as adults. Do not use the person's first name unless he or she asks you to do so.
- Do not pat a person who is in a wheelchair on the head.
- Speak directly to the person. Do not address questions intended for the person to his or her companion.
- Do not be embarrassed if you use words that relate to a disability. For example, you say "Did you see that?" to a person with a vision problem.
- Sit or squat to talk to a person in a wheelchair or chair. This puts you and the person at eye level.
- Ask the person if he or she needs help before acting. If the person says "no," respect the person's wishes. If the person wants help, ask the person what to do and how to do it.
- Think before giving directions to a person in a wheelchair. Think about distance, weather conditions, stairs, curbs, steep hills, and other obstacles.
- Allow the person extra time to say or do things. Let the person set the pace in walking, talking, or other activities.

Modified from Disability Etiquette, *Easter Seals, 2010.*

FAMILY AND FRIENDS

Family and friends help meet safety and security, love and belonging, and self-esteem needs. They offer support and comfort. They lessen loneliness. Some also help with the person's care. This helps both the person and family. The family knows they are doing something to help the person. And the person's physical and emotional needs are met. The presence or absence of family or friends affects the person's quality of life.

The person has the right to visit with family and friends in private and without unnecessary interruptions (Fig. 8-9). You may need to give care when visitors are there. Protect the right to privacy. Do not expose the person's body in front of them. Politely ask them to leave the room. Show them where to wait. Promptly tell them when they can return. A partner or family member may want to help you. If the resident consents, you may allow the person to stay.

Treat family and friends with courtesy and respect. They have concerns about the person's condition and care. They need support and understanding. However, do not discuss the person's condition with them. Refer their questions to the nurse.

Fig. 8-9 A resident visits with his family.

CARING ABOUT CULTURE
Family Roles in Sick Care

In *Vietnam,* family members are involved in the person's hospital care. They stay at the bedside and sleep in the person's bed or on straw mats. In *Vietnam* and *China,* family members provide food, hygiene, and comfort.

In *Pakistani* hospitals, there are different sections for females and males. Adult family members of the opposite sex are not allowed to stay overnight.

Modified from D'Avanzo CE, Geissler EM: Pocket guide to cultural health assessment, *ed 4, St Louis, 2008, Mosby.*

QUALITY OF LIFE

The resident is the most important person in the nursing center. Each person has physical, psychological, social, and spiritual needs. You must know and respect the whole person to provide quality care. This includes promoting physical, mental, spiritual, and social well-being. Try to not focus on physical needs alone. Consider the person's thoughts and feelings. Small gestures make a difference. For example, give a person time to pray before eating if this is something he or she values. While giving care, ask about his or her friends and family. Or simply say: "How are you feeling today?" Respect all of the person's needs. All interact and affect the person's well-being. Provide care that focuses on the person as a whole.

You will care for people from different cultures and religions. Learn as much as you can about a person's religious and cultural beliefs and practices. This will help you understand the person and give better care.

Illness and disability affect quality of life. Normal tasks and activities that bring pleasure and contact with others may be hard or impossible. People often feel angry, frustrated, and useless. You can help by treating each person with dignity and respect. You also help each person reach or maintain his or her optimal level of function. Always focus on the person's abilities. Do not focus on disabilities.

Family and visitors are important to the person. They can offer support and comfort, and enhance the person's quality of life. Always treat them with respect.

Visiting rules depend on center policy and the person's condition. Dying persons usually can have family members present all the time. This is policy for hospice units. Know your center's visiting policies and what is allowed for the person.

A visitor may upset or tire a person. Report your observations to the nurse. The nurse will speak with the visitor about the person's needs.

See *Caring About Culture: Family Roles in Sick Care.*

REVIEW QUESTIONS

Circle the BEST answer.

1 You work in a nursing center. You focus on
   a The person's care plan
   b The person's physical, safety and security, and self-esteem needs
   c The person as a physical, psychological, social, and spiritual being
   d The person's cultural and spiritual needs
2 Which basic need is the *most* essential?
   a Self-actualization
   b Self-esteem
   c Love and belonging
   d Safety and security
3 Based on Maslow's theory of basic needs, which person's needs must be met *first*?
   a The person who wants another blanket
   b The person who wants mail opened
   c The person who asks for more water
   d The person who is crying

Continued

4 A person says "What are they doing to me?" Which basic needs are *not* being met?

   a Physical needs

   b Safety and security needs

   c Love and belonging needs

   d Self-esteem needs

5 A person has a garden behind the nursing center. This relates to

   a Self-actualization   **c** Love and belonging

   b Self-esteem   **d** Safety and security

6 Which is *false*?

   a Culture influences health and illness practices.

   b Culture and religion influence food practices.

   c Cultural and religious practices are allowed in nursing centers.

   d A person must follow all beliefs and practices of his or her culture or religion.

7 These are statements about illness and disability. Which is *false*?

   a They are matters of personal choice.

   b They affect normal activities.

   c Anger is a common response.

   d A goal is for the person to maintain optimal level of function.

8 Alert and oriented residents need nursing center care because they

   a Are very disabled and confused

   b Have trouble remembering things

   c Have physical problems

   d Are dying

9 A person wants care given at a certain time and in a certain way. Nothing seems to please the person. The person is most likely demonstrating

   a Angry behavior   **c** Withdrawn behavior

   b Demanding behavior   **d** Aggressive behavior

10 A person is demonstrating problem behavior. You should do the following *except*

   a Put yourself in the person's situation

   b Tell the person what you are going to do and when

   c Ask the person to be nicer

   d Listen and use silence

11 Which is *false*?

   a Verbal communication uses the written or spoken word.

   b Verbal communication is the truest reflection of a person's feelings.

   c Messages are sent by facial expressions, gestures, posture, and body movements.

   d Touch means different things to different people.

12 To communicate with a person you should

   a Use medical words and phrases

   b Change the subject often

   c Give your opinions

   d Be quiet when the person is silent

13 Which might mean that you are *not* listening?

   a You sit facing the person.

   b You have good eye contact with the person.

   c You sit with your arms crossed.

   d You ask questions.

14 Which is a direct question?

   a "Do you feel better now?"

   b "What are your plans for home?"

   c "What will you do at home?"

   d "Why can't you sleep?"

15 A person wants to take a shower. You say "You would like to take shower." This is

   a A communication barrier

   b A direct question

   c Paraphrasing

   d An open-ended question

16 Focusing is useful when

   a A person is rambling

   b You want to make sure you understand the message

   c You want the person to share thoughts and feelings

   d You need certain information

17 Which promotes communication?

   a "Don't worry."

   b "Everything will be just fine."

   c "This is a good nursing center."

   d "Why are you crying?"

18 Which is *not* a barrier to communication?

   a Using silence

   b Giving your opinions

   c Changing the subject

   d Illness

19 A person uses a wheelchair. For effective communication, you should

   a Lean on the wheelchair

   b Pat the person on the head

   c Direct questions to the companion

   d Sit or squat next to the person

20 A person is comatose. Which action is *not correct*?

   a Assume that the person can hear and can feel touch.

   b Explain what you are going to do.

   c Use listening and silence to communicate.

   d Tell the person when you are leaving the room.

21 A person has many visitors. Which is *false*?

   a They can help meet basic needs.

   b Privacy should be allowed.

   c The nurse answers their questions about the person's care.

   d Visitors can stay in the room when care is given.

22 A visitor seems to tire a person. What should you do?

   a Ask the person to leave.

   b Tell the nurse.

   c Stay in the room to observe the person and visitor.

   d Find out the visitor's relationship to the person.

Answers to these questions are on p. 719.

Body Structure and Function

OBJECTIVES

- Define the key terms and key abbreviations listed in this chapter.
- Identify the basic structures of the cell.
- Explain how cells divide.

- Describe four types of tissue.
- Identify the structures of each body system.
- Identify the functions of each body system.
- Explain how to promote quality of life.

KEY TERMS

artery A blood vessel that carries blood away from the heart

capillary A tiny blood vessel; food, oxygen, and other substances pass from the capillaries into the cells

cell The basic unit of body structure

digestion The process of physically and chemically breaking down food so that it can be absorbed for use by the cells

hemoglobin The substance in red blood cells that carries oxygen and gives blood its color

hormone A chemical substance secreted by the endocrine glands into the bloodstream

immunity Protection against a disease or condition; the person will not get or be affected by the disease

menstruation The process in which the lining of the uterus breaks up and is discharged from the body through the vagina

metabolism The burning of food for heat and energy by the cells

organ Groups of tissues with the same function

peristalsis Involuntary muscle contractions in the digestive system that move food down the esophagus through the alimentary canal

respiration The process of supplying the cells with oxygen and removing carbon dioxide from them

system Organs that work together to perform special functions

tissue A group of cells with similar functions

vein A blood vessel that returns blood to the heart

KEY ABBREVIATIONS

GI	Gastro-intestinal	**WBC**	White blood cell
RBC	Red blood cell		

You help residents meet basic needs. Their bodies do not work at peak levels because of illness, disease, or injury. Your care promotes comfort, healing, and recovery. You need to know the body's normal structure and function. It will help you understand signs, symptoms, and the reasons for care and procedures. You will give safe and more efficient care.

See Chapter 10 for changes in body structure and function that occur with aging.

CELLS, TISSUES, AND ORGANS

The basic unit of body structure is the **cell**. Cells have the same basic structure. Function, size, and shape may differ. Cells are very small. You need a microscope to see them. Cells need food, water, and oxygen to live and function.

Figure 9-1 shows the cell and its structures. The *cell membrane* is the outer covering. It encloses the cell and helps it hold its shape. The *nucleus* is the control center of the cell. It directs the cell's activities. The nucleus is in the center of the cell. The *cytoplasm* surrounds the nucleus. Cytoplasm contains smaller structures that perform cell functions. *Protoplasm* means "living substance." It refers to all structures, substances, and water within the cell. Protoplasm is a semi-liquid substance much like an egg white.

Chromosomes are thread-like structures in the nucleus. Each cell has 46 chromosomes. Chromosomes contain *genes*. Genes control the traits children inherit from their parents. Height, eye color, and skin color are examples.

The nucleus controls cell reproduction. Cells reproduce by dividing in half. The process of cell division is called *mitosis*. It is needed for tissue growth and repair. During mitosis, the 46 chromosomes arrange themselves in 23 pairs. As the cell divides, the 23 pairs are pulled in half. The two new cells are identical. Each has 46 chromosomes (Fig. 9-2).

Cells are the body's building blocks. Groups of cells with similar functions combine to form **tissues**:

- *Epithelial tissue* covers internal and external body surfaces. Tissue lining the nose, mouth, respiratory tract, stomach, and intestines is epithelial tissue. So are the skin, hair, nails, and glands.
- *Connective tissue* anchors, connects, and supports other tissues. It is in every part of the body. Bones, tendons, ligaments, and cartilage are connective tissue. Blood is a form of connective tissue.
- *Muscle tissue* stretches and contracts to let the body move.
- *Nerve tissue* receives and carries impulses to the brain and back to body parts.

Nucleus

Cell membrane

Cytoplasm

Fig. 9-1 Parts of a cell.

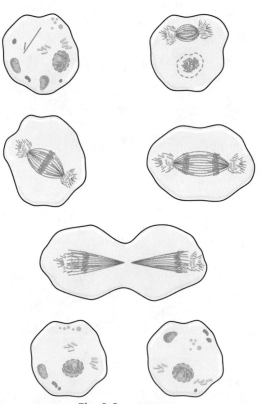

Fig. 9-2 Cell division.

Groups of tissue with the same function form **organs**. An organ has one or more functions. Examples of organs are the heart, brain, liver, lungs, and kidneys. **Systems** are formed by organs that work together to perform special functions (Fig. 9-3).

THE INTEGUMENTARY SYSTEM

The *integumentary system*, or *skin*, is the largest system. *Integument* means covering. The skin covers the body. It has epithelial, connective, and nerve tissue. It also has oil glands and sweat glands. There are two skin layers (Fig. 9-4):

* The *epidermis* is the outer layer. It has living cells and dead cells. The dead cells were once deeper in the epidermis. They were pushed upward as the cells divided. Dead cells constantly flake off. They are replaced by living cells. Living cells also die and flake off. Living cells of the epidermis contain *pigment*. Pigment gives skin its color. The epidermis has no blood vessels and few nerve endings.
* The *dermis* is the inner layer. It is made up of connective tissue. Blood vessels, nerves, sweat glands, and oil glands are found in the dermis. So are hair roots.

The epidermis and dermis are supported by *subcutaneous tissue*. The subcutaneous tissue is a thick layer of fat and connective tissue.

Oil glands and *sweat glands, hair,* and *nails* are skin appendages:
* *Hair*—covers the entire body, except the palms of the hands and the soles of the feet. Hair in the nose and ears and around the eyes protects these organs from dust, insects, and other foreign objects.
* *Nails*—protect the tips of the fingers and toes. Nails help fingers pick up and handle small objects.
* *Sweat glands*—help the body regulate temperature. Sweat consists of water, salt, and a small amount of wastes. Sweat is secreted through pores in the skin. The body is cooled as sweat evaporates.
* *Oil glands*—lie near the hair shafts. They secrete an oily substance into the space near the hair shaft. Oil travels to the skin surface. This helps keep the hair and skin soft and shiny.

The skin has many functions:
* It is the body's protective covering.
* It prevents microorganisms and other substances from entering the body.
* It prevents excess amounts of water from leaving the body.
* It protects organs from injury.
* Nerve endings in the skin sense both pleasant and unpleasant stimulation. Nerve endings are over the entire body. They sense cold, pain, touch, and pressure to protect the body from injury.
* It helps regulate body temperature. Blood vessels dilate (widen) when the temperature outside the body is high. More blood is brought to the body surface for cooling during evaporation. When blood vessels constrict (narrow), the body retains heat. This is because less blood reaches the skin.

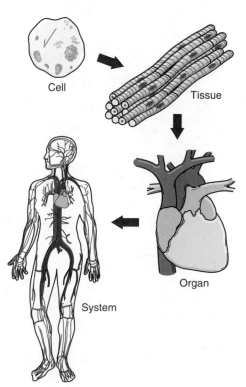

Fig. 9-3 Organization of the body.

Fig. 9-4 Layers of the skin.

THE MUSCULO-SKELETAL SYSTEM

The musculo-skeletal system provides the framework for the body. It lets the body move. This system also protects and gives the body shape.

Bones

The human body has 206 *bones* (Fig. 9-5). There are four types of bones:

- *Long bones* bear the body's weight. Leg bones are long bones.
- *Short bones* allow skill and ease in movement. Bones in the wrists, fingers, ankles, and toes are short bones.
- *Flat bones* protect the organs. They include the ribs, skull, pelvic bones, and shoulder blades.
- *Irregular bones* are the vertebrae in the spinal column. They allow various degrees of movement and flexibility.

Bones are hard, rigid structures. They are made up of living cells. They are covered by a membrane called *periosteum*. Periosteum contains blood vessels that supply bone cells with oxygen and food. Inside the hollow centers of the bones is a substance called *bone marrow*. Blood cells are formed in the bone marrow.

Joints

A *joint* is the point at which two or more bones meet. Joints allow movement (Chapter 26). *Cartilage* is the connective tissue at the end of the long bones. It cushions the joint so that the bone ends do not rub together. The *synovial membrane* lines the joints. It secretes *synovial fluid*. Synovial fluid acts as a lubricant so the joint can move smoothly. Bones are held together at the joint by strong bands of connective tissue called *ligaments*.

There are three major types of joints (Fig. 9-6):

- *Ball-and-socket joint* allows movement in all directions. It is made up of the rounded end of one bone and the hollow end of another bone. The rounded end of one fits into the hollow end of the other. The joints of the hips and shoulders are ball-and-socket joints.
- *Hinge joint* allows movement in one direction. The elbow is a hinge joint.
- *Pivot joint* allows turning from side to side. A pivot joint connects the skull to the spine.

Ball and socket

Hinge

Pivot

Fig. 9-6 Types of joints.

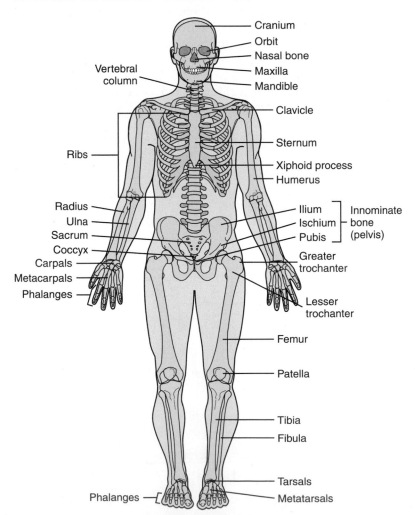

Fig. 9-5 Bones of the body.

Muscles

The human body has more than 500 *muscles* (Figs. 9-7 and 9-8). Some are voluntary. Others are involuntary.

* *Voluntary muscles* can be consciously controlled. Muscles attached to bones *(skeletal muscles)* are voluntary. Arm muscles do not work unless you move your arm; likewise for leg muscles. Skeletal muscles are *striated.* That is, they look striped or streaked.
* *Involuntary muscles* work automatically. You cannot control them. They control the action of the stomach, intestines, blood vessels, and other body organs. Involuntary muscles also are called *smooth muscles.* They look smooth, not streaked or striped.
* *Cardiac muscle* is in the heart. It is an involuntary muscle. However, it appears striated like skeletal muscle.

Muscles have three functions:

* Movement of body parts
* Maintenance of posture
* Production of body heat

Strong, tough connective tissues called *tendons* connect muscles to bones. When muscles contract (shorten), tendons at each end of the muscle cause the bone to move. The body has many tendons. See the Achilles tendon in Figure 9-8. Some muscles constantly contract to maintain the body's posture. When muscles contract, they burn food for energy. Heat is produced. The more muscle activity, the greater the amount of heat produced. Shivering is how the body produces heat when exposed to cold. Shivering is from rapid, general muscle contractions.

Fig. 9-7 Anterior view of the muscles of the body.

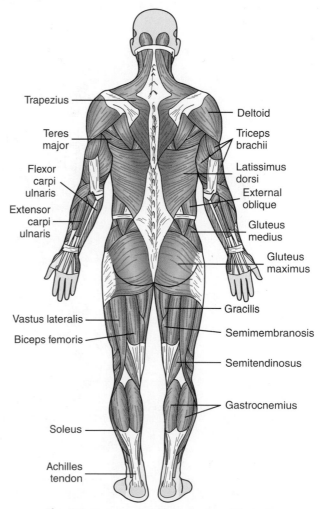

Fig. 9-8 Posterior view of the muscles of the body.

THE NERVOUS SYSTEM

The nervous system controls, directs, and coordinates body functions. Its two main divisions are:

- The *central nervous system* (CNS). It consists of the brain and spinal cord (Fig. 9-9).
- The *peripheral nervous system*. It involves the *nerves* throughout the body (Fig. 9-10).

Nerves carry messages or impulses to and from the brain. Nerves connect to the spinal cord. They are easily damaged and take a long time to heal. Some nerve fibers have a protective covering called a *myelin sheath*. The myelin sheath also insulates the nerve fiber. Nerve fibers covered with myelin conduct impulses faster than those fibers without it.

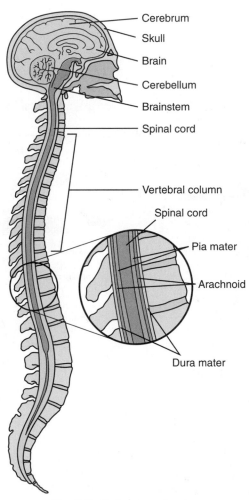

Fig. 9-9 Central nervous system.

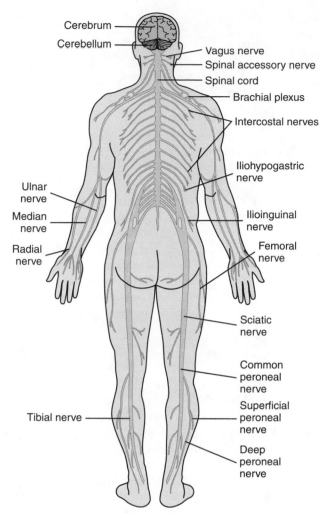

Fig. 9-10 Peripheral nervous system.

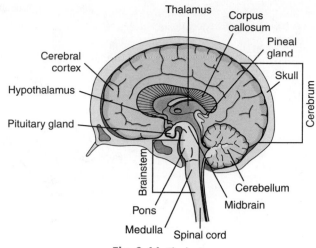

Fig. 9-11 The brain.

The Central Nervous System

The *brain* and *spinal cord* make up the central nervous system. The brain is covered by the skull. The three main parts of the brain are the *cerebrum,* the *cerebellum,* and the *brainstem* (Fig. 9-11).

The cerebrum is the largest part of the brain. It is the center of thought and intelligence. The cerebrum is divided into two halves called the *right* and *left hemispheres.* The right hemisphere controls movement and activities on the body's left side. The left hemisphere controls the right side.

The outside of the cerebrum is called the *cerebral cortex.* It controls the highest functions of the brain. These include reasoning, memory, consciousness, speech, voluntary muscle movement, vision, hearing, sensation, and other activities.

The cerebellum regulates and coordinates body movements. It controls balance and the smooth movements of voluntary muscles. Injury to the cerebellum results in jerky movements, loss of coordination, and muscle weakness.

The brainstem connects the cerebrum to the spinal cord. The brainstem contains the *midbrain, pons,* and *medulla.* The midbrain and pons relay messages between the medulla and the cerebrum. The medulla is below the pons. The medulla controls heart rate, breathing, blood vessel size, swallowing, coughing, and vomiting. The brain connects to the spinal cord at the lower end of the medulla.

The spinal cord lies within the spinal column. The cord is 17 to 18 inches long. It contains pathways that conduct messages to and from the brain.

The brain and spinal cord are covered and protected by three layers of connective tissue called meninges:

- The outer layer lies next to the skull. It is a tough covering call the *dura mater.*
- The middle layer is the *arachnoid.*
- The inner layer is the *pia mater.*

The space between the middle layer (arachnoid) and inner layer (pia mater) is the *arachnoid space.* The space is filled with *cerebrospinal fluid.* It circulates around the brain and spinal cord. Cerebrospinal fluid protects the central nervous system. It cushions shocks that could easily injure brain and spinal cord structures.

The Peripheral Nervous System

The peripheral nervous system has 12 pairs of *cranial nerves* and 31 pairs of *spinal nerves.* Cranial nerves conduct impulses between the brain and the head, neck, chest, and abdomen. They conduct impulses for smell, vision, hearing, pain, touch, temperature, and pressure. They also conduct impulses for voluntary and involuntary muscles. Spinal nerves carry impulses from the skin, extremities, and the internal structures not supplied by cranial nerves.

Some peripheral nerves form the *autonomic nervous system.* This system controls involuntary muscles and certain body functions. The functions include the heartbeat, blood pressure, intestinal contractions, and glandular secretions. These functions occur automatically.

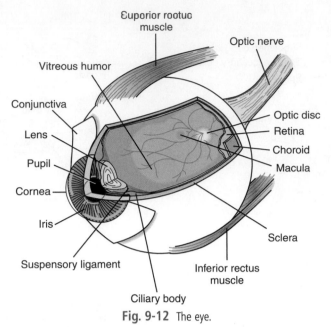

Fig. 9-12 The eye.

The autonomic nervous system is divided into the *sympathetic nervous system* and the *parasympathetic nervous system*. They balance each other. The sympathetic nervous system speeds up functions. The parasympathetic nervous system slows functions. When you are angry, scared, excited, or exercising, the sympathetic nervous system is stimulated. The parasympathetic system is activated when you relax or when the sympathetic system is stimulated for too long.

The Sense Organs

The five senses are *sight, hearing, taste, smell,* and *touch.* Receptors for taste are in the tongue. They are called *taste buds.* Receptors for smell are in the nose. Touch receptors are in the dermis, especially in the toes and fingertips.

The Eye Receptors for vision are in the *eyes* (Fig. 9-12). The eye is easily injured. Bones of the skull, eyelids and eyelashes, and tears protect the eyes from injury. The eye has three layers:

* The *sclera*, the white of the eye, is the outer layer. It is made of tough connective tissue.
* The *choroid* is the second layer. Blood vessels, the *ciliary muscle,* and the *iris* make up the choroid. The iris gives the eye its color. The opening in the middle of the iris is the *pupil.* Pupil size varies with the amount of light entering the eye. The pupil constricts (narrows) in bright light. It dilates (widens) in dim or dark places.
* The *retina* is the inner layer. It has receptors for vision and the nerve fibers of the *optic nerve.*

Light enters the eye through the *cornea.* It is the transparent part of the outer layer that lies over the eye. Light rays pass to the *lens,* which lies behind the pupil. The light is then reflected to the retina. Light is carried to the brain by the optic nerve.

The *aqueous chamber* separates the cornea from the lens. The chamber is filled with a fluid called *aqueous humor.* The fluid helps the cornea keep its shape and position. The *vitreous humor* is behind the lens. It is a gelatin-like substance that supports the retina and maintains the eye's shape.

The Ear The *ear* is a sense organ (Fig. 9-13). It functions in hearing and balance. It has three parts: the *external ear, middle ear,* and *inner ear.*

The external ear (outer part) is called the *pinna* or *auricle.* Sound waves are guided through the external ear into the *auditory canal.* Glands in the auditory canal secrete a waxy substance called *cerumen.* The auditory canal extends about 1 inch to the *eardrum.* The eardrum (*tympanic membrane*) separates the external and middle ear.

The middle ear is a small space. It contains the *eustachian tube* and three small bones called *ossicles.* The eustachian tube connects the middle ear and the throat. Air enters the eustachian tube so that there is equal pressure on both sides of the eardrum. The ossicles amplify sound received from the eardrum and transmit the sound to the inner ear. The three ossicles are:

* The *malleus.* It looks like a hammer.
* The *incus.* It looks like an anvil.
* The *stapes.* It is shaped like a stirrup.

The inner ear consists of *semicircular canals* and the *cochlea.* The cochlea looks like a snail shell. It contains fluid. The fluid carries sound waves from the middle

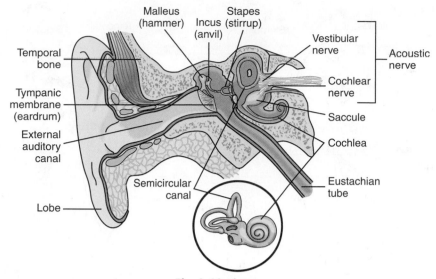

Fig. 9-13 The ear.

ear to the *acoustic nerve.* The acoustic nerve then carries the message to the brain.

The three semicircular canals are involved with balance. They sense the head's position and changes in position. They send messages to the brain.

THE CIRCULATORY SYSTEM

The circulatory system is made up of the *blood, heart,* and *blood vessels.* The heart pumps blood through the blood vessels. The circulatory system has many functions:

- Blood carries food, oxygen, and other substances to the cells.
- Blood removes waste products from cells.
- Blood and blood vessels help regulate body temperature. The blood carries heat from muscle activity to other body parts. Blood vessels in the skin dilate to cool the body. They constrict to retain heat.
- The system produces and carries cells that defend the body from microbes that cause disease.

The Blood

The blood consists of blood cells and *plasma.* Plasma is mostly water. It carries blood cells to other body cells. Plasma also carries substances that cells need to function. This includes food (proteins, fats, and carbohydrates), hormones (p. 111), and chemicals.

Red blood cells (RBCs) are called *erythrocytes.* They give blood its red color because of a substance in the RBC called **hemoglobin.** As RBCs circulate through the lungs, hemoglobin picks up oxygen. Hemoglobin carries oxygen to the cells. When blood is bright red, hemoglobin in the RBCs is saturated (filled) with oxygen. As blood circulates through the body, oxygen is given to the cells. Cells release carbon dioxide (a waste

product). It is picked up by the hemoglobin. RBCs saturated with carbon dioxide make the blood look dark red.

The body has about 25 trillion (25,000,000,000,000) RBCs. About 4½ to 5 million cells are in a cubic millimeter of blood (the size of a tiny drop). RBCs live for 3 or 4 months. They are destroyed by the liver and spleen as they wear out. New RBCs are formed in the bone marrow. About 1 million RBCs are produced every second.

White blood cells (WBCs) are called *leukocytes.* They have no color. They protect the body against infection. There are about 5,000 to 10,000 WBCs in a cubic millimeter of blood. At the first sign of infection, WBCs rush to the infection site. There they multiply rapidly. The number of WBCs increases when there is an infection. WBCs are formed by the bone marrow. They live about 9 days.

Platelets (thrombocytes) are needed for blood clotting. They are formed by the bone marrow. There are about 200,000 to 400,000 platelets in a cubic millimeter of blood. A platelet lives about 4 days.

The Heart

The heart is a muscle. It pumps blood through the blood vessels to the tissues and cells. The heart lies in the middle to lower part of the chest cavity toward the left side (Fig. 9-14, p. 106). The heart is hollow and has three layers (Fig. 9-15, p. 106):

- The *pericardium* is the outer layer. It is a thin sac covering the heart.
- The *myocardium* is the second layer. It is the thick, muscular part of the heart.
- The *endocardium* is the inner layer. A membrane, it lines the inner surface of the heart.

Fig. 9-14 Location of the heart in the chest cavity.

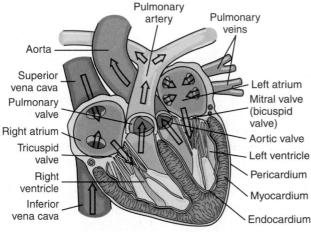

Fig. 9-15 Structures of the heart.

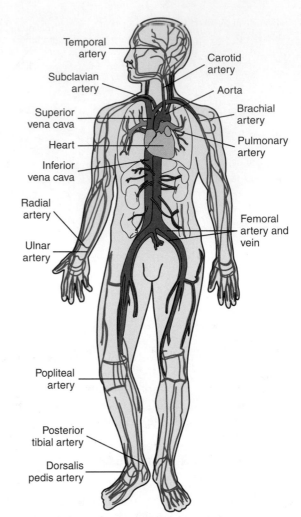

Fig. 9-16 Arterial and venous systems. Arterial system is red. Venous system is blue.

The heart has four chambers (see Fig. 9-15). Upper chambers receive blood and are called *atria*. The *right atrium* receives blood from body tissues. The *left atrium* receives blood from the lungs. Lower chambers are called *ventricles*. Ventricles pump blood. The *right ventricle* pumps blood to the lungs for oxygen. The *left ventricle* pumps blood to all parts of the body.

Valves are between the atria and ventricles. The valves allow blood flow in one direction. They prevent blood from flowing back into the atria from the ventricles. The *tricuspid valve* is between the right atrium and the right ventricle. The *mitral valve (bicuspid valve)* is between the left atrium and left ventricle.

Heart action has two phases:
- *Diastole.* It is the resting phase. Heart chambers fill with blood.
- *Systole.* It is the working phase. The heart contracts. Blood is pumped through the blood vessels when the heart contracts.

The Blood Vessels

Blood flows to body tissues and cells through the blood vessels. There are three groups of blood vessels: arteries, capillaries, and veins.

Arteries carry blood away from the heart. Arterial blood is rich in oxygen. The *aorta* is the largest artery. It receives blood directly from the left ventricle. The aorta branches into other arteries that carry blood to all parts of the body (Fig. 9-16). These arteries branch into smaller parts within the tissues. The smallest branch of an artery is an *arteriole*.

Arterioles connect to **capillaries.** Capillaries are very tiny blood vessels. Food, oxygen, and other substances pass from capillaries into the cells. The capillaries pick up waste products (including carbon dioxide) from the cells. Veins carry waste products back to the heart.

Veins return blood to the heart. They connect to the capillaries by *venules*. Venules are small veins. Venules branch together to form veins. The many veins also branch together as they near the heart to form two main veins (see Fig. 9-16). The two main veins are the *inferior vena cava* and the *superior vena cava*. Both empty into the right atrium. The inferior vena cava carries blood from the legs and trunk. The superior vena cava carries blood from the head and arms. Venous blood is dark red. It has little oxygen and a lot of carbon dioxide.

Blood flow through the circulatory system is shown in Figure 9-15. The path of blood flow is as follows:

- Venous blood, poor in oxygen, empties into the right atrium.
- Blood flows through the tricuspid valve into the right ventricle.
- The right ventricle pumps blood into the lungs to pick up oxygen.
- Oxygen-rich blood from the lungs enters the left atrium.
- Blood from the left atrium passes through the mitral valve into the left ventricle.
- The left ventricle pumps the blood to the aorta. It branches off to form other arteries.
- Arterial blood is carried to the tissues by arterioles and to the cells by capillaries.
- Cells and capillaries exchange oxygen and nutrients for carbon dioxide and waste products.
- Capillaries connect with venules.
- Venules carry blood that has carbon dioxide and waste products.
- Venules form veins.
- Veins return blood to the heart.

THE RESPIRATORY SYSTEM

Oxygen is needed to live. Every cell needs oxygen. Air contains about 21% oxygen. This meets the body's needs under normal conditions. The respiratory system (Fig. 9-17) brings oxygen into the lungs and removes carbon dioxide. **Respiration** is the process of supplying the cells with oxygen and removing carbon dioxide from them. Respiration involves *inhalation* (breathing in) and *exhalation* (breathing out). The terms *inspiration* (breathing in) and *expiration* (breathing out) also are used.

Air enters the body through the *nose*. The air then passes into the *pharynx* (throat). It is a tube-shaped passageway for air and food. Air passes from the pharynx into the *larynx* (voice box). A piece of cartilage, the *epiglottis*, acts like a lid over the larynx. The epiglottis prevents food from entering the airway during swallowing. During inhalation the epiglottis lifts up to let air pass over the larynx. Air passes from the larynx into the *trachea* (windpipe).

The trachea divides at its lower end into the *right bronchus* and the *left bronchus*. Each bronchus enters a lung. Upon entering the lungs, the bronchi divide many times into smaller branches. The smaller branches are called *bronchioles*. Eventually the bronchioles subdivide. They end up in tiny one-celled air sacs called *alveoli*.

Alveoli look like small clusters of grapes. They are supplied by capillaries. Oxygen and carbon dioxide are exchanged between the alveoli and capillaries. Blood in

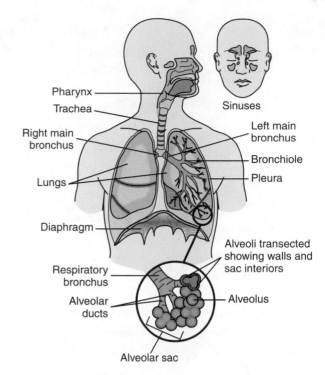

Fig. 9-17 Respiratory system.

the capillaries picks up oxygen from the alveoli. Then the blood is returned to the left side of the heart and pumped to the rest of the body. Alveoli pick up carbon dioxide from the capillaries for exhalation.

The lungs are spongy tissues. They are filled with alveoli, blood vessels, and nerves. Each lung is divided into lobes. The right lung has three lobes; the left lung has two. The lungs are separated from the abdominal cavity by a muscle called the *diaphragm.*

Each lung is covered by a two-layered sac called the *pleura.* One layer is attached to the lung and the other to the chest wall. The pleura secretes a very thin fluid that fills the space between the layers. The fluid prevents the layers from rubbing together during inhalation and exhalation. A bony framework made up of the ribs, sternum, and vertebrae protects the lungs.

THE DIGESTIVE SYSTEM

The digestive system breaks down food physically and chemically so it can be absorbed for use by the cells. This process is called **digestion.** The digestive system is also called the *gastro-intestinal (GI) system.* The system also removes solid wastes from the body.

The digestive system involves the *alimentary canal (GI tract)* and the accessory organs of digestion (Fig. 9-18, p. 108). The alimentary canal is a long tube. It extends from the mouth to the anus. Its major parts are the mouth, pharynx, esophagus, stomach, small intestine, and large intestine. Accessory organs are the teeth, tongue, salivary glands, liver, gallbladder, and pancreas.

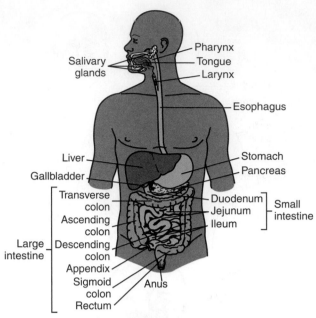

Fig. 9-18 Digestive system.

Digestion begins in the *mouth.* The mouth also is called the *oral cavity.* It receives food and prepares it for digestion. Using chewing motions, the *teeth* cut, chop, and grind food into small particles for digestion and swallowing. The *tongue* aids in chewing and swallowing. Taste buds on the tongue's surface contain nerve endings. Taste buds allow sweet, sour, bitter, and salty tastes to be sensed. *Salivary glands* in the mouth secrete *saliva.* Saliva moistens food particles to ease swallowing and begin digestion. During swallowing, the tongue pushes food into the *pharynx.*

The pharynx (throat) is a muscular tube. Swallowing continues as the pharynx contracts. Contraction of the pharynx pushes food into the *esophagus.* The esophagus is a muscular tube about 10 inches long. It extends from the pharynx to the *stomach.* Involuntary muscle contractions called **peristalsis** move food down the esophagus through the alimentary canal.

The stomach is a muscular, pouch-like sac. It is in the upper left part of the abdominal cavity. Strong stomach muscles stir and churn food to break it up into even smaller particles. A mucous membrane lines the stomach. It contains glands that secrete *gastric juices.* Food is mixed and churned with the gastric juices to form a semi-liquid substance called *chyme.* Through peristalsis, the chyme is pushed from the stomach into the small intestine.

The *small intestine* is about 20 feet long. It has three parts. The first part is the *duodenum.* There, more digestive juices are added to the chyme. One is called *bile.* Bile is a greenish liquid made in the *liver.* Bile is stored in the *gallbladder.* Juices from the *pancreas* and small intestine are added to the chyme. Digestive juices chemically break down food so it can be absorbed.

Peristalsis moves the chyme through the two other parts of the small intestine: the *jejunum* and the *ileum.* Tiny projections called *villi* line the small intestine. Villi absorb the digested food into the capillaries. Most food absorption takes place in the jejunum and the ileum.

Some chyme is not digested. Undigested chyme passes from the small intestine into the *large intestine (large bowel* or *colon).* The colon absorbs most of the water from the chyme. The remaining semi-solid material is called *feces.* Feces contain a small amount of water, solid wastes, and some mucus and germs. These are the waste products of digestion. Feces pass through the colon into the *rectum* by peristalsis. Feces pass out of the body through the *anus.*

THE URINARY SYSTEM

The digestive system rids the body of solid wastes. The lungs rid the body of carbon dioxide. Water and other substances leave the body through sweat. There are other waste products in the blood from cells burning food for energy. The urinary system (Fig. 9-19):
- Removes waste products from the blood
- Maintains water balance within the body

The *kidneys* are two bean-shaped organs in the upper abdomen. They lie against the back muscles on each side of the spine. They are protected by the lower edge of the rib cage.

Fig. 9-19 Urinary system.

Fig. 9-20 A nephron.

Fig. 9-21 Male reproductive system.

Each kidney has over a million tiny *nephrons* (Fig. 9-20). Each nephron is the basic working unit of the kidney. Each nephron has a *convoluted tubule*, which is a tiny coiled tubule. Each convoluted tubule has a *Bowman's capsule* at one end. The capsule partly surrounds a cluster of capillaries called a *glomerulus*. Blood passes through the glomerulus and is filtered by the capillaries. The fluid part of the blood is squeezed into the Bowman's capsule. The fluid then passes into the tubule. Most of the water and other needed substances are re-absorbed by the blood. The rest of the fluid and the waste products form *urine* in the tubule. Urine flows through the tubule to a *collecting tubule*. All collecting tubules drain into the *renal pelvis* in the kidney.

A tube, called the *ureter*, is attached to the renal pelvis of the kidney. Each ureter is about 10 to 12 inches long. The ureters carry urine from the kidneys to the *bladder*. The bladder is a hollow, muscular sac. It lies toward the front in the lower part of the abdominal cavity.

Urine is stored in the bladder until the need to urinate is felt. This usually occurs when there is about a half pint (250 milliliters [mL]) of urine in the bladder. Urine passes from the bladder through the *urethra*. The opening at the end of the urethra is the *meatus*. Urine passes from the body through the meatus. Urine is a clear, yellowish fluid.

THE REPRODUCTIVE SYSTEM

Human reproduction results from the union of a male sex cell and a female sex cell. The male and female reproductive systems are different. This allows for the process of reproduction.

The Male Reproductive System

The male reproductive system is shown in Figure 9-21. The *testes (testicles)* are the male sex glands. Sex glands also are called *gonads*. The two testes are oval or almond-shaped glands. Male sex cells are produced in the testes. Male sex cells are called *sperm* cells.

Testosterone, the male hormone, is produced in the testes. This hormone is needed for reproductive organ function. It also is needed for the development of the male secondary sex characteristics. There is facial hair; pubic and axillary (underarm) hair; and hair on the arms, chest, and legs. Neck and shoulder sizes increase.

The testes are suspended between the thighs in a sac called the *scrotum*. The scrotum is made of skin and muscle.

Sperm travel from a testis to the *epididymis*. The epididymis is a coiled tube on top and to the side of the testis. From the epididymis, sperm travel through a tube called the *vas deferens*. Each vas deferens joins a seminal vesicle. The two seminal vesicles store sperm and produce *semen*. Semen is a fluid that carries sperm from the male reproductive tract. The ducts of the seminal vesicles unite to form the *ejaculatory duct*. It passes through the *prostate gland*.

The prostate gland lies just below the bladder. It is shaped like a donut. The gland secretes fluid into the semen. As the ejaculatory ducts leave the prostate, they join the *urethra*. The urethra runs through the prostate gland. The urethra is the outlet for urine and semen. The urethra is contained within the *penis*.

The penis is outside of the body and has *erectile* tissue. When a man is sexually excited, blood fills the erectile tissue. The penis enlarges and becomes hard and erect. The erect penis can enter a female's vagina. The semen, which contains sperm, is released into the vagina.

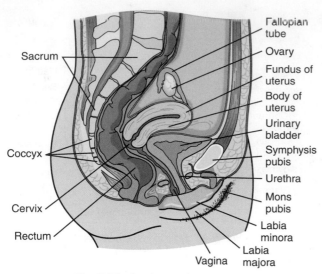

Fig. 9-22 Female reproductive system.

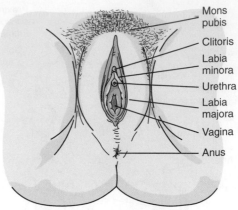

Fig. 9-23 External female genitalia.

The Female Reproductive System

Figure 9-22 shows the female reproductive system. The female gonads are two almond-shaped glands called *ovaries*. An ovary is on each side of the uterus in the abdominal cavity.

The ovaries contain *ova* or eggs. Ova are the female sex cells. One ovum (egg) is released monthly during the woman's reproductive years. Release of an ovum is called *ovulation*.

The ovaries secrete the female hormones *estrogen* and *progesterone*. These hormones are needed for reproductive system function. They also are needed for the development of secondary sex characteristics in the female. These include increased breast size, pubic and axillary (underarm) hair, slight deepening of the voice, and widening and rounding of the hips.

When an ovum is released from an ovary, it travels through a *fallopian tube*. There are two fallopian tubes, one on each side. The tubes are attached at one end to the uterus. The ovum travels through the fallopian tube to the *uterus*.

The *uterus* is a hollow, muscular organ shaped like a pear. It is in the center of the pelvic cavity behind the bladder and in front of the rectum. The main part of the uterus is the *fundus*. The neck or narrow section of the uterus is the *cervix*. Tissue lining the uterus is called the *endometrium*. The endometrium has many blood vessels. If sex cells from the male and female unite into one cell, that cell implants into the endometrium. There the cell grows into a baby. The uterus serves as a place for the *fetus* (unborn baby) to grow and receive nourishment.

The cervix of the uterus projects into a muscular canal called the *vagina*. The vagina opens to the outside of the body. It is just behind the urethra. The vagina receives the penis during intercourse. It also is part of the

birth canal. Glands in the vaginal wall keep it moistened with secretions. In young girls, the external vaginal opening is partially closed by a membrane called the *hymen*. The hymen ruptures when the female has intercourse for the first time.

The external female genitalia are called the *vulva* (Fig. 9-23):
- The *mons pubis* is a rounded, fatty pad over a bone called the *symphysis pubis*. The mons pubis is covered with hair in the adult female.
- The *labia majora* and *labia minora* are two folds of tissue on each side of the vaginal opening.
- The *clitoris* is a small organ composed of erectile tissue. It becomes hard when sexually stimulated.

The *mammary glands (breasts)* secrete milk after childbirth. The glands are on the outside of the chest. They are made up of glandular tissue and fat (Fig. 9-24). The milk drains into ducts that open onto the *nipple*.

Menstruation The endometrium is rich in blood to nourish the cell that grows into a fetus. If pregnancy does not occur, the endometrium breaks up. It is discharged from the body through the vagina. This process is called **menstruation.** Menstruation occurs about every 28 days. Therefore it is called the *menstrual cycle.*

The first day of the menstrual cycle begins with menstruation. Blood flows from the uterus through the vaginal opening. Menstrual flow usually lasts 3 to 7 days. Ovulation occurs during the next phase. An ovum matures in an ovary and is released. Ovulation usually occurs on or about day 14 of the cycle.

Meanwhile, estrogen and progesterone (the female hormones) are secreted by the ovaries. These hormones cause the endometrium to thicken for pregnancy. If pregnancy does not occur, the hormones decrease in amount. This causes the blood supply to the endometrium to decrease. The endometrium breaks up. It is discharged through the vagina. Another menstrual cycle begins.

Fig. 9-24 The female breast.

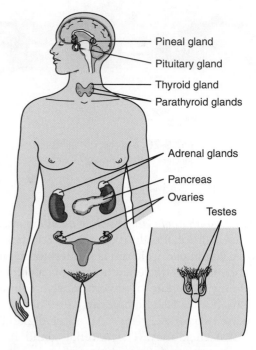

Fig. 9-25 Endocrine system.

Fertilization

To reproduce, a male sex cell (sperm) must unite with a female sex cell (ovum). The uniting of the sperm and ovum into one cell is called *fertilization.* A sperm has 23 chromosomes. An ovum has 23 chromosomes. When the two cells unite, the fertilized cell has 46 chromosomes.

During intercourse, millions of sperm are deposited into the vagina. Sperm travel up the cervix, through the uterus, and into the fallopian tubes. If a sperm and an ovum unite in a fallopian tube, fertilization results. Pregnancy occurs. The fertilized cell travels down the fallopian tube to the uterus. After a short time, the fertilized cell implants in the thick endometrium and grows during pregnancy.

THE ENDOCRINE SYSTEM

The endocrine system is made up of glands called the *endocrine glands* (Fig. 9-25). The endocrine glands secrete chemical substances called hormones into the bloodstream. Hormones regulate the activities of other organs and glands in the body.

The *pituitary gland* is called the *master gland.* About the size of a cherry, it is at the base of the brain behind the eyes. The pituitary gland is divided into the *anterior*

pituitary lobe and the *posterior pituitary lobe.* The anterior pituitary lobe secretes:

- *Growth hormone (GH)*—needed for growth of muscles, bones, and other organs. It is needed throughout life to maintain normal-size bones and muscles. Growth is stunted if a baby is born with deficient amounts of growth hormone. Too much of the hormone causes excessive growth.
- *Thyroid-stimulating hormone (TSH)*—needed for thyroid gland function.
- *Adrenocorticotropic hormone (ACTH)*—stimulates the adrenal gland.

The anterior lobe also secretes hormones that regulate growth, development, and function of the male and female reproductive systems.

The posterior pituitary lobe secretes *antidiuretic hormone (ADH)* and *oxytocin.* ADH prevents the kidneys from excreting excessive amounts of water. Oxytocin causes uterine muscles to contract during childbirth.

The *thyroid gland,* shaped like a butterfly, is in the neck in front of the larynx. *Thyroid hormone (TH, thyroxine)* is secreted by the thyroid gland. It regulates metabolism. Metabolism is the burning of food for heat and energy by the cells. Too little TH results in slowed body processes, slowed movements, and weight gain. Too much TH causes increased metabolism, excess energy, and weight loss. Some babies are born with deficient amounts of TH. Their physical growth and mental growth are stunted.

Fig. 9-26 A phagocyte digests and destroys a microorganism. *(From Thibodeau GA, Patton KT: Structure and function of the body, ed 11, St Louis, 2000, Mosby.)*

The four *parathyroid glands* secrete *parathormone*. Two lie on each side of the thyroid gland. Parathormone regulates calcium use. Calcium is needed for nerve and muscle function. Insufficient amounts of calcium cause *tetany*. Tetany is a state of severe muscle contraction and spasm. If untreated, tetany can cause death.

There are two *adrenal glands.* An adrenal gland is on the top of each kidney. The adrenal gland has two parts: the *adrenal medulla* and the *adrenal cortex*. The adrenal medulla secretes *epinephrine* and *norepinephrine*. These hormones stimulate the body to quickly produce energy during emergencies. Heart rate, blood pressure, muscle power, and energy all increase.

The adrenal cortex secretes three groups of hormones needed for life:

- *Glucocorticoids*—regulate the metabolism of carbohydrates. They also control the body's response to stress and inflammation.
- *Mineralocorticoids*—regulate the amount of salt and water that is absorbed and lost by the kidneys.
- Small amounts of *male and female sex hormones*—pp. 109-110.

The *pancreas* secretes *insulin*. Insulin regulates the amount of sugar in the blood available for use by the cells. Insulin is needed for sugar to enter the cells. If there is too little insulin, sugar cannot enter the cells. If sugar cannot enter the cells, excess amounts of sugar build up in the blood. This condition is called *diabetes*.

The *gonads* are the glands of human reproduction. Male sex glands (testes) secrete *testosterone*. Female sex glands (ovaries) secrete *estrogen* and *progesterone*.

THE IMMUNE SYSTEM

The immune system protects the body from disease and infection. Abnormal body cells can grow into tumors. Sometimes the body produces substances that cause the body to attack itself. Microorganisms (bacteria, viruses, and other germs) can cause an infection. The immune system defends against threats inside and outside the body.

The immune system gives the body **immunity**. Immunity means that a person has protection against a disease or condition. The person will not get or be affected by the disease:

- *Specific immunity* is the body's reaction to a certain threat.
- *Nonspecific immunity* is the body's reaction to anything it does not recognize as a normal body substance.

Special cells and substances function to produce immunity:

- *Antibodies*—normal body substances that recognize other substances. They are involved in destroying abnormal or unwanted substances.
- *Antigens*—substances that cause an immune response. Antibodies recognize and bind with unwanted antigens. This leads to the destruction of unwanted substances and the production of more antibodies.
- *Phagocytes*—white blood cells that digest and destroy microorganisms and other unwanted substances (Fig. 9-26).
- *Lymphocytes*—white blood cells that produce antibodies. Lymphocyte production increases as the body responds to an infection.
- *B lymphocytes (B cells)*—cause the production of antibodies that circulate in the plasma. The antibodies react to specific antigens.
- *T lymphocytes (T cells)*—cells that destroy invading cells. *Killer T cells* produce poisons near the invading cells. Some T cells attract other cells. The other cells destroy the invaders.

When the body senses an antigen from an unwanted substance, the immune system acts. Phagocyte and lymphocyte production increases. Phagocytes destroy the invaders through digestion. The lymphocytes produce antibodies that identify and destroy the unwanted substances.

QUALITY OF LIFE

The human body is made up of systems. Each has its own structures and functions. The systems are related to and depend on each other to properly function and survive. Injury or disease of one part of a system affects the entire system and the whole body.

Basic knowledge of the body's normal structure and function should result in safe, quality care. It will help you better understand the reasons for the care you give. Always treat the person and the person's body with dignity and respect.

REVIEW QUESTIONS

Circle the BEST answer.

1 The basic unit of body structure is the
   a Cell   c Nephron
   b Neuron   d Ovum

2 The outer layer of the skin is called the
   a Dermis   c Integument
   b Epidermis   d Myelin

3 Which is *not* a function of the skin?
   a Provides the protective covering for the body
   b Regulates body temperature
   c Senses cold, pain, touch, and pressure
   d Provides the shape and framework for the body

4 Which allows movement?
   a Bone marrow   c Joints
   b Synovial membrane   d Ligaments

5 Skeletal muscles
   a Are under involuntary control
   b Appear smooth
   c Are under voluntary control
   d Appear striped and smooth

6 The highest functions in the brain take place in the
   a Cerebral cortex   c Brainstem
   b Medulla   d Spinal nerves

7 The ear is involved with
   a Regulating body movements
   b Balance
   c Smoothness of body movements
   d Controlling involuntary muscles

8 The liquid part of the blood is the
   a Hemoglobin   c Plasma
   b Red blood cell   d White blood cell

9 Which part of the heart pumps blood to the body?
   a Right atrium   c Right ventricle
   b Left atrium   d Left ventricle

10 Which carry blood away from the heart?
   a Capillaries   c Venules
   b Veins   d Arteries

11 Oxygen and carbon dioxide are exchanged
   a In the bronchi
   b Between the alveoli and capillaries
   c Between the lungs and pleura
   d In the trachea

12 Digestion begins in the
   a Mouth   c Small intestine
   b Stomach   d Colon

13 Most food absorption takes place in the
   a Stomach
   b Small intestine
   c Colon
   d Large intestine

14 Urine is formed by the
   a Jejunum
   b Kidneys
   c Bladder
   d Liver

15 Urine passes from the body through the
   a Ureters
   b Urethra
   c Anus
   d Nephrons

16 The male sex gland is called the
   a Penis
   b Semen
   c Testis
   d Scrotum

17 The male sex cell is the
   a Semen
   b Ovum
   c Gonad
   d Sperm

18 The female sex gland is the
   a Ovary
   b Cervix
   c Uterus
   d Vagina

19 The discharge of the lining of the uterus is called
   a The endometrium
   b Ovulation
   c Fertilization
   d Menstruation

20 The endocrine glands secrete
   a Hormones
   b Mucus
   c Semen
   d Insulin

21 The immune system protects the body from
   a Low blood sugar
   b Disease and infection
   c Loss of fluid
   d Stunted growth

Answers to these questions are on p. 719.

The Older Person

- Define the key terms and key abbreviations listed in this chapter.
- Identify the developmental tasks for each age-group.
- Identify the psychological and social changes common in older adulthood.
- Describe the physical changes from aging and the care required.
- Describe housing options for older persons.
- Explain how to promote quality of life.

KEY TERMS

development Changes in mental, emotional, and social function

developmental task A skill that must be completed during a stage of development

dysphagia Difficulty (*dys*) swallowing (*phagia*)

dyspnea Difficult, labored, or painful (*dys*) breathing (*pnea*)

geriatrics The care of aging people

gerontology The study of the aging process

growth The physical changes that are measured and that occur in a steady, orderly manner

menopause When menstruation stops and there has been at least 1 year without a menstrual period

presbyopia Age-related (*presby*) farsightedness (*opia* means eye)

KEY ABBREVIATIONS

CCRC Continuing care retirement community

CMS Centers for Medicare & Medicaid Services

OBRA Omnibus Budget Reconciliation Act of 1987

People live longer than ever before. They are healthier and more active. U.S. government reports show the following for the United States:

- In 2009, there were nearly 39,600,000 people age 65 and older.
- In 2008, there were 16,500,000 men age 65 and older. There were 22,400,000 women age 65 and older.
- In 2008, there were more older men who were married than older women.
- In 2008, there were 5,700,000 people age 85 and older. In 2020, the number of people age 85 and older is expected to increase to 6,600,000.

Chronic illness is common in older persons. Disability often results. Most older persons have at least one disability. Disabilities increase and become more severe with aging. They can interfere with:

- Self-care—bathing, dressing, eating, elimination
- Mobility and getting around one's home setting
- Fixing meals, shopping, doing housework
- Managing money
- Using a phone
- Taking drugs
- Leisure and recreational activities

Still, most older people live in a family setting. They live with a partner, children, brothers or sisters, or other family. Some live alone or with friends. Still others live in nursing centers. The need for nursing center care increases with aging.

GROWTH AND DEVELOPMENT

Throughout life, people grow and develop. Growth is the physical changes that are measured and that occur in a steady, orderly manner. Growth is measured in height and weight. Changes in appearance and body functions also measure growth (Fig. 10-1).

Development relates to changes in mental, emotional, and social function. A person behaves and thinks in certain ways in each stage of development. A 2-year-old thinks in simple terms. A 40-year-old thinks in complex ways. The entire person is affected.

Growth and development occur in a sequence, order, and pattern. Certain skills must be completed during each stage. A developmental task is a skill that must be completed during a stage of development. A stage cannot be skipped. Each stage is the basis for the next stage. Each stage has its own characteristics and developmental tasks (Box 10-1, p. 116).

Late Adulthood (65 Years and Older)

Late adulthood ranges from 65 years of age and older. The *oldest-old* are 85 years of age and older.

Gerontology is the study of the aging process. Geriatrics is the care of aging people. Aging is normal. It is not a disease. Normal changes occur in body structure and function. They increase the risk for illness, injury, and disability. Psychological and social changes also occur. Often changes are slow. Most people adjust well to these changes. They lead happy, meaningful lives. The developmental tasks of late adulthood are listed in Box 10-1, p. 116.

There are many myths about aging and older persons. A *myth* is a widely believed story that is not true. To provide good care, you need to know the facts about older persons and aging. See Box 10-2, p. 116 for some common myths and facts.

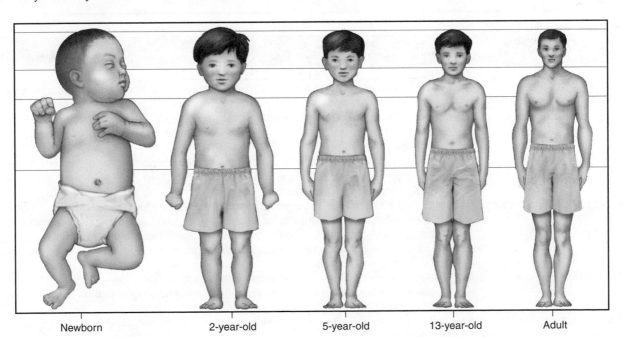

Newborn   2-year-old   5-year-old   13-year-old   Adult

Fig. 10-1 Body appearance changes during growth. *(From Thibodeau GA, Patton KT: The human body in health & disease, ed 5, St Louis, 2010, Mosby.)*

Box 10-1 Stages of Growth and Development

Infancy (Birth to 1 Year)
- Learning to walk
- Learning to eat solid foods
- Beginning to talk and communicate with others
- Learning to trust
- Beginning to have emotional relationships with parents, brothers, and sisters
- Developing stable sleep and feeding patterns

Toddlerhood (1 to 3 Years)
- Tolerating separation from parents or primary caregivers
- Gaining control of bowel and bladder function
- Using words to communicate
- Becoming less dependent on parents or primary caregivers

Preschool (3 to 6 Years)
- Increasing the ability to communicate and understand others
- Performing self-care
- Learning gender (male, female) differences and developing sexual modesty
- Learning right from wrong and good from bad
- Learning to play with others
- Developing family relationships

School Age (6 to 9 or 10 Years)
- Developing social and physical skills needed for playing games
- Learning to get along with children of the same age and background (peers)
- Learning gender-appropriate behaviors and attitudes
- Learning basic reading, writing, and arithmetic skills
- Developing a conscience and morals
- Developing a good feeling and attitude about oneself

Late Childhood (9 or 10 to 12 Years)
- Becoming independent of adults and learning to depend on oneself
- Developing and keeping friendships with peers

Late Childhood (9 or 10 to 12 Years)—cont'd
- Understanding the physical, psychological, and social roles of one's sex
- Developing moral and ethical behavior
- Developing greater muscular strength, coordination, and balance
- Learning how to study

Adolescence (12 to 18 Years)
- Accepting changes in the body and appearance
- Developing appropriate relationships with males and females of the same age
- Accepting the male or female role appropriate for one's age
- Becoming independent from parents and adults
- Preparing for marriage and family life
- Preparing for a career
- Developing the morals, attitudes, and values needed to function in society

Young Adulthood (18 to 40 Years)
- Choosing education and a career
- Selecting a partner
- Learning to live with a partner
- Becoming a parent and raising children
- Developing a satisfactory sex life

Middle Adulthood (40 to 65 Years)
- Adjusting to physical changes
- Having grown children
- Developing leisure-time activities
- Adjusting to aging parents

Late Adulthood (65 Years and Older)
- Adjusting to decreased strength and loss of health
- Adjusting to retirement and reduced income
- Coping with a partner's death
- Developing new friends and relationships
- Preparing for one's own death

Box 10-2 Myths and Facts About Aging

Myth	Fact
All old people are the same.	Each person is unique. People age in different ways. Culture, religion, education, income, and life experiences affect aging. People develop throughout life.
Aging means illness and disability.	Older persons are at risk for health problems and disabilities. However, most are healthy. Not smoking, good nutrition, and exercise can reverse or slow many changes blamed on aging.
Older persons lose interest in sex.	Aging does not mean that sexual activity and expression must end. Many older people enjoy a fulfilling sex life. Sexuality is important throughout life. Intimacy, love, and companionship are needed.
Older people are lonely and isolated.	Most older people have frequent contact with their children. Older parents commonly live within 10 miles of their children. Most see a child at least once a week and take part in family activities. Regular contact with sisters and brothers is common. They can provide support and companionship. Many older persons have jobs, do volunteer work, and enjoy hobbies.
Mental function declines with age.	Older persons may receive and process information more slowly than younger people. However, people learn until very late in life. Many 90-year-olds have high levels of mental function.
Most older persons live in nursing centers.	In 2008, only 1,600,000 (4.1%) of the people 65 years and older lived in long-term care settings.
Old people are crabby and rude.	Some old people are crabby and rude. So are people of all ages. Older persons who are crabby and rude were probably crabby and rude when younger.

PSYCHOLOGICAL AND SOCIAL CHANGES

Graying hair, wrinkles, and slow movements are physical reminders of growing old. These changes affect self-esteem. They threaten self-image and feelings of self-worth. They also threaten independence.

Social roles also change. A parent may depend on an adult child for care. Retirees need activities to replace the work role. Adjusting to the death of a partner, family members, and friends is common. The person faces his or her own death.

People cope with aging in their own way. How they cope depends on health status, life experiences, finances, education, and social support systems.

Retirement

Age 65 is the usual retirement age. Some retire earlier. Others work into their 70s. Retirement is a reward for a life-time of work. The person can relax and enjoy life (Fig. 10-2). Travel, leisure, and doing what one wants to are retirement "benefits." Many people enjoy retirement. Others are not so lucky. They are ill or disabled. Poor health and medical bills can make retirement very hard.

Work helps meet love, belonging, and self-esteem needs. The person feels fulfilled and useful. Friendships form. Co-workers share daily events. Leisure time, recreation, and companionship often involve co-workers. Some retired people want to work. They have part-time jobs or do volunteer work (Fig. 10-3).

Reduced Income Retirement usually means reduced income. Social Security may provide the only income.

The retired person still has expenses. Rent or house payments continue. Food, clothing, utility bills, and taxes are other expenses. Car expenses, home repairs, drugs, and health care are other costs. So are entertainment and gifts.

Reduced income may force life-style changes. Examples include:
- Limiting social and leisure events
- Buying cheaper food, clothes, and household items
- Moving to cheaper housing
- Living with children or other family
- Avoiding health care or needed drugs
- Relying on children or other family for money or needed items

Severe money problems can result. Some people plan for retirement. They have savings, investments, retirement plans, and insurance. They are financially comfortable during retirement.

Social Relationships

Social relationships change throughout life. (See *Caring About Culture: Foreign-Born Persons.*) Children grow up and leave home. They have their own families. Some live far away from parents. Older family members and friends die, move away, or are disabled. Yet most older people have regular contact with children, grandchildren, family, and friends. Others are lonely. Separation from children is a common cause. So is lack of companionship with people their own age (Fig. 10-4, p. 118).

Fig. 10-3 This retired woman is a nursing center volunteer.

Fig. 10-2 A retired couple enjoys golf as a leisure time activity.

> ### CARING ABOUT CULTURE
> #### Foreign-Born Persons
>
> Some older persons speak and understand a foreign language. Communication occurs with family and friends who speak the same language. They also share cultural values and practices. These relatives and friends may move away or die. The person may not have anyone to talk to. He or she may not be understood by others. The person feels greater loneliness and isolation.

Fig. 10-4 Older people enjoy being with others of their own age.

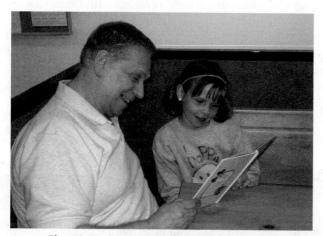

Fig. 10-5 An older man reads with his grandchild.

Fig. 10-6 An older couple takes part in family activities.

Many older people adjust to these changes. Hobbies, religious and community events, and new friends help prevent loneliness. Some community groups sponsor bus trips to ball games, shopping, plays, and concerts.

Grandchildren can bring great love and joy (Fig. 10-5). Family times help prevent loneliness. They help the older person feel useful and wanted (Fig. 10-6).

See *Focus on Communication: Social Changes.*

> **FOCUS ON COMMUNICATION**
> **Social Changes**
>
> The social changes of aging can cause loneliness. If nursing center care is needed, the loneliness can seem even greater. The person may be in the same building with other people. However, those people do not replace relationships with family and friends. To help the person feel less lonely, you can:
> - Suggest that the person call a family member or friend. Offer to assist with finding phone numbers and dialing.
> - Keep the phone within the person's reach. This helps him or her place or answer calls with ease.
> - Suggest that the person read cards and letters. Offer to assist.
> - Visit with the person a few times during your shift.
> - Introduce new residents to other residents and staff.

Children as Caregivers

Some children care for older parents. Parents and children change roles. The child cares for the parent. This helps some older persons feel more secure. Others feel unwanted, in the way, and useless. Some lose dignity and self-respect. Tensions may occur among the child, parent, and other household members. Lack of privacy is a cause. So are disagreements and criticisms about housekeeping, raising children, cooking, and friends.

Death of a Partner

As couples age, the chances increase that a partner will die. Women usually live longer than men. Therefore many women become widows.

A person may try to prepare for a partner's death. When death occurs, the loss is crushing. No amount of preparation is ever enough for the emptiness and changes that result. The person loses a lover, friend, companion, and confidant. Grief may be very great. The person's life will likely change. Serious physical and mental health problems may result. Some lose the will to live. Some attempt suicide.

PHYSICAL CHANGES

Physical changes occur with aging (Box 10-3). They happen to everyone. Body processes slow down. Energy level and body efficiency decline. The rate and degree of change vary with each person. They depend on such factors as diet, health, exercise, stress, environment, and heredity. Changes are slow over many years. Often they are not seen for a long time.

Normal aging does not mean loss of health. Quality of life does not have to decline. The person can adjust to many of the changes.

Box 10-3   Common Physical Changes During the Aging Process

Integumentary System
- Skin becomes less elastic
- Skin loses strength
- Brown spots ("age spots" or "liver spots") on the wrists and hands
- Fewer nerve endings
- Fewer blood vessels
- Fatty tissue layer is lost
- Skin thins and sags
- Skin is fragile and easily injured
- Folds, lines, and wrinkles appear
- Blood vessels in the dermis become more fragile
- Decreased secretion of oil and sweat glands
- Dry skin
- Itching
- Increased sensitivity to heat and cold
- Decreased sensitivity to pain
- Nails become thick and tough
- Whitening or graying hair
- Facial hair in some women
- Loss or thinning of hair
- Drier hair

Musculo-Skeletal System
- Muscles atrophy
- Strength, tone, and contractility decrease
- Bone mass decreases
- Bones become weaker
- Bones become brittle; can break easily
- Vertebrae shorten
- Joints become stiff and painful
- Hip and knee joints become flexed
- Gradual loss of height; trunk becomes shorter
- Decreased mobility

Nervous System
- Brain and spinal cord lose nerve cells
- Nerve cells send messages at a slower rate
- Reflexes slow
- Reduced blood flow to the brain
- Abnormal structures can form in the brain
- Brain tissue may shrink (atrophy)
- Changes in brain cells
- Shorter memory
- Forgetfulness
- Slower ability to respond
- Confusion
- Dizziness
- Sleep patterns change
- Reduced sensitivity to touch
- Reduced sensitivity to pain
- Smell and taste decrease
- Eyelids thin and wrinkle
- Less tear secretion
- Pupils less responsive to light
- Decreased vision at night or in dark rooms
- Problems seeing green and blue colors
- Poor vision
- Changes in auditory nerve
- Eardrums atrophy
- High-pitched sounds are not heard
- Decreased ear wax secretion
- Hearing loss

Circulatory System
- Heart pumps with less force
- Heart valves thicken and become stiff
- Heart rate may slow
- Abnormal heart rhythms may occur
- Heart may enlarge slightly
- Heart walls thicken
- Arteries narrow and become stiffer
- Less blood flows through narrowed arteries
- Weakened heart works harder to pump blood through narrowed vessels
- Number of red blood cells decreases

Respiratory System
- Respiratory muscles weaken
- Some lung tissue is lost
- Lung tissue becomes less elastic
- Chest is less able to stretch to breathe
- Difficulty breathing (dyspnea [p. 121])
- Decreased strength for coughing and clearing the airway

Digestive System
- Decreased saliva production
- Difficulty swallowing (dysphagia [p. 121])
- Decreased appetite
- Decreased secretion of digestive juices
- Difficulty digesting fried and fatty foods
- Indigestion
- Loss of teeth
- Decreased peristalsis causing flatulence and constipation

Urinary System
- Kidney function decreases
- Reduced blood supply to kidneys
- Kidneys atrophy
- Urine becomes concentrated
- Bladder tissue less able to stretch
- Bladder muscles weaken
- Bladder may not empty completely when urinating
- Urinary frequency
- Urinary urgency may occur
- Urinary incontinence may occur
- Night-time urination may occur

Reproductive System
- Men
  - Testosterone decreases slightly
  - Erections take longer
  - Longer phase between erection and orgasm
  - Less forceful orgasms
  - Erections lost quickly
  - Longer time between erections
- Women
  - Menopause (p. 122)
  - Estrogen and progesterone decrease
  - Uterus, vagina, and genitalia shrink (atrophy)
  - Thinning of vaginal walls
  - Vaginal dryness
  - Arousal takes longer
  - Less intense orgasms
  - Quicker return to pre-excitement state

The Integumentary System

The skin loses its elasticity, strength, and fatty tissue layer. The skin thins and sags. Wrinkles appear. Secretions from oil and sweat glands decrease. Dry skin and itching occur. The skin is fragile and easily injured. The skin's blood vessels are fragile. Skin breakdown, skin tears, and pressure ulcers are risks (Chapters 35 and 36). So are bruising and delayed healing. This is because the skin's blood vessels are fragile.

Brown spots appear on sun-exposed areas. They are called "age spots" or "liver spots." They are common on the wrists and hands.

Loss of the skin's fatty tissue layer affects body temperature. The person is more sensitive to cold. Protect the person from drafts and cold. Sweaters, lap blankets, socks, and extra blankets are helpful. So are higher thermostat settings.

Dry skin causes itching. It is easily damaged. A shower or bath twice a week is enough for hygiene. Partial baths are taken at other times. Mild soaps or soap substitutes are used to clean the underarms, genitals, and under the breasts. Often soap is not used on the arms, legs, back, chest, and abdomen. Lotions and creams prevent drying and itching. Deodorants may not be needed because sweat gland secretion is decreased. See Chapter 20 for hygiene.

Nails become thick and tough. Feet usually have poor circulation. A nick or cut can lead to a serious infection. See Chapter 21 for nail and foot care.

The skin has fewer nerve endings. This affects the sensing of heat, cold, pressure, and pain. Burns are great risks. Fragile skin, poor circulation, and decreased ability to sense heat and cold increase the risk of burns. Older persons often complain of cold feet. Socks provide warmth. Hot water bottles and heating pads are not used because of the risk for burns.

White or gray hair is common. Hair loss occurs in men. Hair thins on men and women. Thinning occurs on the head, in the pubic area, and under the arms. Women and men may choose to wear wigs. Some color hair to cover graying. Facial hair (lip and chin) may occur in women.

Hair is drier from decreases in scalp oils. Brushing promotes circulation and oil production. Shampoo frequency depends on personal choice. Usually it decreases with age. It is done as needed for hygiene and comfort.

Skin disorders increase with age. They rarely cause death if treated early. The risk of skin cancers increases with age. Prolonged sun exposure is a cause.

Skin changes can be seen. Gray hair, hair loss, brown spots, wrinkles, and sagging skin are some examples. These changes can affect self-esteem and body image.

The Musculo-Skeletal System

Muscle cells decrease in number. Muscles atrophy (shrink). They decrease in strength.

Bones lose minerals, especially calcium. Bones lose strength. They become brittle and break easily. Sometimes just turning in bed can cause fractures (broken bones).

Vertebrae shorten. Joints become stiff and painful. Hip and knee joints flex (bend) slightly. These changes cause gradual loss of height and strength. Mobility also decreases.

Older persons need to stay active. Activity, exercise, and diet help prevent bone loss and loss of muscle strength. Walking is good exercise. Exercise groups and range-of-motion exercises are helpful (Chapter 26). A diet high in protein, calcium, and vitamins is needed.

Bones can break easily. Protect the person from injury and prevent falls (Chapters 12 and 13). Turn and move the person gently and carefully (Chapter 17). Some persons need help and support getting out of bed. Some need help walking.

The Nervous System

Nerve cells are lost. Nerve conduction and reflexes slow. Responses are slower. For example, an older person slips. The message telling the brain of the slip travels slowly. The message from the brain to prevent the fall also travels slowly. The person falls.

Blood flow to the brain is reduced. Dizziness may occur. It increases the risk for falls. Practice measures to prevent falls (Chapter 13). Remind the person to get up slowly from bed or a chair. This helps prevent dizziness (Chapter 26).

Changes occur in brain cells. This affects personality and mental function. So does reduced blood flow to the brain. Memory is shorter. Forgetfulness increases. Responses slow. Confusion, dizziness, and fatigue may occur. Older persons often remember events from long ago better than recent ones. Many older people are mentally active and involved in current events. They show fewer personality and mental changes. (See Chapter 44 for confusion and dementia.)

Sleep patterns change. Falling asleep is harder for older persons. Sleep periods are shorter. They wake often at night and have less deep sleep. Less sleep is needed. Loss of energy and decreased blood flow may cause fatigue. They may rest or nap during the day. They may go to bed early and get up early.

The Senses Aging affects touch, smell, taste, sight, and hearing.

Touch. Touch and sensitivity to pain and pressure are reduced. So is sensing heat and cold. These changes increase the risk for injury. The person may not notice painful injuries or diseases. Or the person feels minor pain. You need to:

- Protect older persons from injury (Chapters 12 and 13).
- Follow safety measures for heat and cold (Chapter 35).
- Check for signs of skin breakdown (Chapters 20, 35, and 36).
- Give good skin care (Chapter 20).
- Prevent skin tears (Chapter 35) and pressure ulcers (Chapter 36).

Taste and Smell. Taste and smell dull. Appetite decreases. Taste buds decrease in number. The tongue senses sweet, salty, bitter, and sour tastes. Sweet and salty tastes are lost first. Older people often complain that food has no taste or tastes bitter. They like more salt and sugar on food.

The Eye. Eyelids thin and wrinkle. Tear secretion is less. Dust and pollutants can irritate the eyes.

The pupil becomes smaller and responds less to light. Vision is poor at night or in dark rooms. The eye takes longer to adjust to lighting changes. Vision problems occur when going from a dark to a bright room. They also occur when going from a bright to a dark room.

Clear vision is reduced. Eyeglasses are needed. The lens of the eye yellows. Therefore greens and blues are harder to see.

Older persons become more farsighted. This is called presbyopia. (*Presby* relates to aging. *Opia* means eye.) The lens becomes more rigid with age. It is harder for the eye to shift from far to near vision and from near to far vision. These changes increase the risk of falls and accidents. The risk is greater on stairs and where lighting is poor. Eyeglasses are worn as needed. Keep rooms well-lit. Night-lights help at night.

The Ear. Changes occur in the auditory nerve. Eardrums atrophy (shrink). High-pitched sounds are hard to hear. Severe hearing loss occurs if these changes progress. A hearing aid may be needed. It must be clean and correctly placed in the ear.

Wax secretion decreases. Wax becomes harder and thicker. It is easily impacted (wedged in the ear). This can cause hearing loss. A doctor or nurse removes the wax.

The Circulatory System

The heart muscle weakens. It pumps blood with less force. Problems may not occur at rest. Activity, exercise, excitement, and illness increase the body's need for oxygen and nutrients. A damaged or weak heart cannot meet these needs.

Arteries narrow and are less elastic. Less blood flows through them. Poor circulation occurs in many body parts. A weak heart must work harder to pump blood through narrowed vessels.

Exercise helps maintain health and well-being. Many older persons exercise daily. They walk, jog, golf, and bicycle. They also hike, ski, play tennis, swim, and play other sports. Older persons need to be as active as possible.

Sometimes circulatory changes are severe. Rest is needed during the day. Over-exertion is avoided. The person should not walk far, climb many stairs, or carry heavy things. Personal care items, TV, phone, and other needed items are kept nearby. Some exercise helps circulation. It also prevents blood clots in leg veins. Some persons need to stay in bed. They need range-of-motion exercises (Chapter 26). Doctors may order certain exercises and activity limits.

The Respiratory System

Respiratory muscles weaken. Lung tissue becomes less elastic. Often lung changes are not noted at rest. Difficult, labored, or painful breathing (dyspnea) may occur with activity. (*Dys* means difficult. *Pnea* means breathing.) The person may lack strength to cough and clear the airway of secretions. Respiratory infections and diseases may develop. These can threaten the older person's life.

Normal breathing is promoted. Avoid heavy bed linens over the chest. They prevent normal chest expansion. Turning, re-positioning, and deep breathing are important. They help prevent respiratory complications from bedrest. Breathing usually is easier in semi-Fowler's position (Chapter 16). The person should be as active as possible.

The Digestive System

Salivary glands produce less saliva. This can cause difficulty swallowing (dysphagia). (*Dys* means difficult. *Phagia* means swallowing.) Dry foods may be hard to swallow. Taste and smell dull. This decreases appetite.

Secretion of digestive juices decreases. As a result, fried and fatty foods are hard to digest. They may cause indigestion.

Loss of teeth and ill-fitting dentures cause chewing problems. This causes digestion problems. Hard-to-chew foods are avoided. Ground or chopped meat is easier to chew and swallow.

Peristalsis decreases. The stomach and colon empty slower. Flatulence and constipation can occur (Chapter 23).

Dry, fried, and fatty foods are avoided. This helps swallowing and digestion problems. Oral hygiene and denture care improve taste. Some people do not have teeth or dentures. Their food is pureed or ground.

High-fiber foods help prevent constipation. However, they are hard to chew and can irritate the intestines. They include apricots, celery, and fruits and vegetables with skins and seeds. Persons with chewing problems or constipation often need foods that provide soft bulk. They include whole-grain cereals and cooked fruits and vegetables.

Fewer calories are needed. Energy and activity levels decline. More fluids are needed for chewing, swallowing, digestion, and kidney function. Foods are needed to prevent constipation and bone changes. High-protein foods are needed for tissue growth and repair. However, some older persons lack protein in their diets. High-protein foods (meat and fish) are costly.

The Urinary System

Kidney function decreases. The kidneys shrink (atrophy). Blood flow to the kidneys is reduced. Waste removal is less efficient. Urine is more concentrated.

The ureters, bladder, and urethra lose tone and elasticity. Bladder muscles weaken. Bladder size decreases. Therefore the bladder stores less urine. Urinary frequency or urgency may occur. Many older persons have to urinate during the night. Urinary incontinence (inability to control the passage of urine from the bladder) may occur (Chapter 22).

In men, the prostate gland enlarges. This puts pressure on the urethra. Difficulty urinating or frequent urination occurs.

Urinary tract infections are risks. Adequate fluids are needed. The person needs water, juices, milk, and gelatin. Provide fluids according to the care plan. Remind the person to drink. Offer fluids often to those who need help. Most fluids should be taken before 1700 (5:00 PM). This reduces the need to urinate during the night.

Persons with incontinence may need bladder training programs. Sometimes catheters are needed. See Chapter 22.

The Reproductive System

Reproductive organs change with aging. For the effects of aging on sexuality, see Chapter 11.

- *Men.* The hormone *testosterone* decreases slightly. It affects strength, sperm production, and reproductive tissues. These changes affect sexual activity. An erection takes longer. The phase between erection and orgasm also is longer. Orgasm is less forceful than when younger. Erections are lost quickly. The time between erections also is longer. Older men may need the penis stimulated for arousal. Fatigue, over-eating, and drinking too much alcohol affect erections. Some men fear performance problems. They may avoid closeness.

- *Women.* Menopause is when menstruation stops and there has been at least 1 year without a menstrual period. The woman can no longer have children. This occurs around 50 years of age. Female hormones (*estrogen* and *progesterone*) decrease. The uterus, vagina, and genitalia shrink (atrophy). Vaginal walls thin. There is vaginal dryness. These changes make intercourse uncomfortable or painful. Arousal takes longer. Orgasm is less intense. The pre-excitement state returns more quickly.

HOUSING OPTIONS

A person's home is more than a place to live. A home has family memories. It is a link to neighbors and the community. It brings pride and self-esteem. Aging can lead to changes in a person's home setting.

Most older people live in their own homes. Some choose smaller homes when children are gone. Some retire to warmer climates. Others move closer to children and family. Still others have to give up their homes. Reduced income, taxes, home repairs, and yard work are factors. Some people cannot care for themselves.

Many housing options meet the needs of older people. A new home setting could maintain or improve the person's quality of life.

Living With Family

Sometimes older brothers, sisters, and cousins live together. They:
- Provide companionship
- Share living expenses
- Provide care during illness or disability

Living with children is an option. The older parent (or parents) moves in with the child. Or the child moves to the parent's home. The parent may be healthy, may need some help, or may be ill or disabled. Some adult children give care to avoid nursing center care. A nursing center is an option if they cannot give needed care.

Living with an adult child is a social change. Everyone in the home must adjust. Sleeping plans may change if there is no spare bedroom. The parent may need a hospital bed. It can go in a family or living room, dining room, den, or bedroom.

The adult child's family needs time alone. Other family members may help give care. Respite care (Chapter 8) is an option for weekends and vacations. Home care agencies can provide nurses or home health care aides. Many community and church groups have volunteers who help give care.

Fig. 10-7 An adult day-care center.

Fig. 10-8 This man enjoys gardening.

Adult Day-Care Centers Many children need to work even though the parent cannot stay alone. Adult day-care centers provide meals, supervision, and activities (Fig. 10-7). Some provide rides to and from the center. Some serve persons with dementia (Chapter 44).

Requirements vary. Some require that the person be able to walk. A cane or walker is used as needed. Others allow wheelchairs. Most require that the person perform some self-care.

Many activities are offered. Cards, board games, movies, crafts, dancing, walks, exercise groups, and lectures are common. Some provide bowling and swimming. All activities are supervised. Needed help is given.

Some areas have inter-generational day-care centers. Children and older persons are in the same center. They work together on some activities. They eat and play together. Young children bring much joy to older persons. They give older persons purpose, love, and affection. In turn, children learn about aging. They also receive love and affection from older persons.

Elder Cottage Housing Opportunity

Elder Cottage Housing Opportunity (ECHO) homes are small homes designed for older and disabled persons. The portable home is placed in the yard of a single-family home. The older person lives independently but near family or friends.

Apartments

Some older persons live in apartments. They pay rent and utility bills. The owner provides maintenance, yard work, snow removal, and appliance repair. Older persons remain independent. They can keep personal items. Many older persons like to garden or do yard work (Fig. 10-8). Apartment living usually does not provide such activities.

An *accessory dwelling unit (ADU)* is a separate living area in a home. It has a kitchen, bedroom, and bathroom. Some have a small living room. The older person lives independently near other people. Some children have these apartments for older parents. Or the older person's home may have an apartment. ADUs are also called an "in-law apartment," an "accessory apartment," and a "second unit."

Residential Hotels

Some cities have residential hotels. Private rooms or small apartments are rented. Food services may include a dining room, cafeteria, or room service. Some provide recreational activities and emergency medical services. Most hotels are close to shopping, places of worship, and other civic services.

Congregate Housing

Congregate means a group, gathering, or a cluster. In congregate housing, apartments are for older people. Buildings have wheelchair access, hand rails, elevators, and other safety features. Apartments are designed to meet the needs of older persons. Some are furnished.

Services are many. A doctor or nurse is on call. Someone checks on the person daily. A dining room is common. Rides are provided to places of worship, the doctor, or shopping areas. Tenants pay monthly rent.

Senior Citizen Housing In many areas, state and federal funds support apartment complexes for older and disabled persons. Such persons have low to moderate incomes. Monthly rents are lower. The rent depends on the person's monthly income.

Home-Sharing

Two or more people share a house or apartment. Each person has a bedroom. They share other living spaces—kitchen, bathroom, living room. They share household chores and expenses. Or cooking, cleaning, and yard work are exchanged for rent.

Shared housing is a way to avoid living alone. It provides companionship. Some people feel safer when living with another person.

Assisted Living Residences

Assisted living residences are for persons who need help with daily living (Chapters 1 and 30). The person has social contact with others in a home-like setting. Health care and 24-hour over-sight are provided. Nursing care is not provided.

Board and Care Homes

Board and care homes provide a room, meals, laundry, and supervision (Chapter 1). Some homes are for older persons. Others are for people with certain problems. Dementia, mental health problems, and developmental disabilities are examples.

Homes vary in size—from housing 4 to 30 people or more. The care provided and rules vary from state to state. The person pays monthly rent. Some board and care homes receive government funds.

Adult Foster Care

Adult foster care can take two forms:
* An older person lives with a family.
* A single family home serves 4 to 5 persons with special needs. They may be older, disabled, or mentally ill.

The person receives help with daily living. A room, meals, and laundry are provided. Help is given with shopping and transportation. The person receives needed health care.

Continuing Care Retirement Communities

Continuing care retirement communities (CCRCs) offer many services. They range from independent living units to 24-hour nursing care. A CCRC has housing, activity, and health care services. It meets the changing needs of older persons living alone or with a partner. CCRCs usually provide:
* Nursing care and other health care services
* Meals (including special diets)
* Housekeeping
* Transportation
* Personal assistance
* Recreational and educational activities

Independent living units are small apartments. Residents perform self-care and take their own drugs. Food service is provided. Help is nearby if needed. Many people have their own cars. They travel or drive about as desired. Rides are provided for those who need them.

Services are added as the person's needs change. Over time, some persons need nursing center care. They move into the nursing center within the CCRC. Many older couples find comfort in this plan. One partner needs nursing care. The other is close by and can visit often.

The person signs a contract with the CCRC. The contract is for a certain time or for the person's lifetime. The contract lists services provided and the required fees.

Nursing Centers

Some older persons cannot care for themselves. Nursing centers are options for them (Chapter 1). Some people stay in nursing centers until death. Others stay until they can return home. The nursing center is the person's temporary or permanent home. The setting is as home-like as possible (Fig. 10-9).

The person needing nursing center care may suffer some or all of these losses:
* Loss of identity as a productive member of a family and community
* Loss of possessions—home, household items, car, and so on
* Loss of independence
* Loss of real-world experiences—shopping, traveling, cooking, driving, hobbies, and so on
* Loss of health and mobility

The person may feel useless, powerless, and hopeless. The health team helps the person cope with loss and improve quality of life. Treat the person with dignity and respect. Also practice good communication skills. Follow the care plan.

Fig. 10-9 A, A nursing center is as home-like as possible. **B,** Some centers allow residents to bring their own bed and furniture from home.

Nursing centers serve to meet the needs of older and disabled persons. Physical changes of aging are considered in the center's design. So are safety needs. Programs and services meet the person's basic needs. Box 10-4 lists the features of a quality nursing center.

Some center designs, programs, and services follow the *Eden Alternative*™. Animals, plants, and children play a key role in giving residents dignity and purpose. The goal is to prevent residents from feeling lonely, helpless, and bored. "Household," "neighborhood," and "community" are other nursing center models and designs.

Box 10-4 Features of a Quality Nursing Center

Basic Information
- The center is Medicare-certified.
- The center is Medicaid-certified.
- The center provides the level of care needed. Rehabilitation, dementia, and ventilator services are examples.
- The center is located close enough for family and friends to visit.

Resident Appearance
- Residents are clean and well-groomed.
- Residents are dressed appropriately for the season or time of day.

Living Spaces
- The center is free from overwhelming, unpleasant odors.
- The center appears clean and well-kept.
- The temperature is comfortable for the residents.
- The center has good lighting.
- Noise levels in the dining room are comfortable.
- Noise levels in common areas are comfortable.
- Smoking is not allowed. If allowed, it is restricted to certain areas.
- Furnishings are sturdy, comfortable, and attractive.

Staff
- The relationship between the staff and residents appears to be warm, polite, and respectful.
- All staff wear name tags.
- Staff knock on the person's door before entering the room.
- Staff refer to residents by name.
- The center offers a training and continuing education program for all staff.
- The center does background checks on all staff.
- The center has licensed nurses on staff 24 hours a day. An RN is present at least 8 hours a day, 7 days a week.
- The same nursing team (including nursing assistants) works with the same resident 4 to 5 days a week.
- Nursing assistants work with a reasonable number of residents.
- Nursing assistants take part in care planning meetings.
- The center has a full-time social worker on staff.
- A licensed doctor is on staff. He or she is there daily and can be reached at all times.
- The center's management team has worked together for at least 1 year. This includes the administrator and director of nursing.

Residents' Rooms
- Residents may have personal belongings in their rooms.
- Residents may have personal furniture in their rooms.
- Each resident has storage space (closet and drawers) in his or her room.
- Each resident has a window in his or her room.
- Residents have access to a personal telephone.
- Residents have access to a personal TV.
- Residents have a choice of roommates.
- The resident can reach his or her water pitcher.
- The center has policies and procedures to protect residents' belongings.

Hallways, Stairs, Lounges, and Bathrooms
- Exits are clearly marked.
- The center has quiet areas where residents can visit with family and friends.
- The center has smoke detectors and sprinklers.
- All common areas, resident rooms, and doorways are designed for wheelchair use.
- The center has hand rails in the hallways.
- The center has grab bars in bathrooms.

Menus and Food
- Residents have a choice of food items at each meal.
- The person's favorite foods are served.
- Nutritious snacks are available upon request.
- Staff help residents eat and drink if help is needed.

Activities
- Residents may choose to take part in a variety of activities. This includes residents who cannot leave their rooms.
- The center has outdoor areas for resident use. Staff help residents to go outside.
- The center has an active volunteer program.

Safety and Care
- The center has an emergency evacuation plan.
- Regular fire drills are held. Residents, including bed-bound residents, are moved to safety.
- Residents receive preventive care to stay healthy. Yearly flu shots are an example.
- Residents may see their personal doctors.
- The center has an arrangement with a nearby hospital for emergencies.
- Care plan meetings are held with residents and family members.
- The center has corrected all problems on its last state inspection report.

Modified from Centers for Medicare & Medicaid Services: Guide to choosing a nursing home, Baltimore, Md, revised November 2009, U.S. Department of Health and Human Services.

Most nursing centers receive Medicare or Medicaid funds. They must meet requirements of the Omnibus Budget Reconciliation Act of 1987 (OBRA). OBRA protects the person's rights and promotes quality of life. The Centers for Medicare & Medicaid Services (CMS) has rules and regulations for OBRA. See Box 10-5. The CMS is a federal agency. It has the power to issue standards, rules, and regulations. These are called agency-made laws. Employers and employees must comply with them. Unannounced surveys are conducted to see if nursing centers are meeting OBRA and CMS requirements.

Box 10-5   Environment Requirements

- The person's care equipment is clean and properly stored. This includes toothbrushes, dentures, denture cups, glasses and water pitchers, emesis basins, hair brushes and combs, bedpans, urinals, feeding tubes, leg bags and catheter bags, pads, and positioning devices.
- Bed linens are clean and in good condition.
- There are clean towels and washcloths for each person.
- The person has closet space with shelves. The person can reach the shelves.
- Lighting levels are comfortable and adequate.
- Temperature levels are comfortable and safe. The temperate is between 71° and 81° F (Fahrenheit).
- Sound levels are comfortable. Sound levels allow for hearing, privacy, and social interaction.
- Safety precautions are followed for persons who smoke. See Chapter 12.
- Hand rails, assistive devices, and other surfaces are in good repair. They are free from sharp edges or other hazards.
- Furniture is appropriate for the residents.
- The person's setting is as free from accident hazards as possible.
  - Resident care equipment is used following the manufacturer's instructions.
  - Safety measures are practiced for hazardous substances (Chapter 12).
  - Safety measures are practiced to prevent burns from hot water temperatures (Chapter 12).
  - Safety measures are practiced to prevent equipment accidents (Chapter 12). This includes electrical safety.
  - Safety measures are practiced to prevent accidents from assistive devices and equipment. This includes canes, walkers, wheelchairs, mechanical lifts, restraints, bed rails, mattresses, and so on.

Modified from Centers for Medicare & Medicaid Services: State operations manual, Baltimore, Md, January 6, 2009, U.S. Department of Health and Human Services.

QUALITY OF LIFE

Moving to a nursing center can cause feelings of loneliness and isolation. Making new friends helps the person adjust. It also improves quality of life. Some residents cannot visit with friends or get to activities without help. Offer to take them to visit in a friend's room or to an activity.

Some people are trying to cope with many losses. They may have a hard time talking to others. Encourage them to talk about losses. They may find that other residents have similar losses.

Urinary problems may cause older persons to avoid social events. Help them to the bathroom before the event or visit. Follow the care plan if other measures are needed (Chapter 22).

Feeling good about one's appearance and setting is important to feel comfortable with others. These measures can help residents:

- Make sure their clothes and linens are clean and dry.
- Help them with grooming—shaving, makeup, hair care, and so on.
- Help them dress in clothes of their choice.
- Make sure dentures, eyeglasses, and hearing aids are in place.
- Keep their rooms clean and orderly.
- Help them display personal items if asked. Do not touch items without the person's permission.
- Treat each person as if you were in his or her home.
- Respect them and their settings.

Some quiet, private persons avoid social contacts. Respect their wishes for privacy.

REVIEW QUESTIONS

Circle the BEST answer.

1 People aged 85 and older are
   a The young-old
   b Old
   c The oldest-old
   d Elderly

2 The study of the aging process is called
   a Geriatrics
   b Dysphagia
   c Gerontology
   d Dyspnea

3 Retirement usually means
   a Lowered income
   b Changes from aging
   c Less free time
   d Financial security

4 Which does *not* cause loneliness in older persons?
   a Children moving away
   b The death of family and friends
   c Problems communicating with others
   d Contact with other older persons

5   Older persons living with their children often feel
    a   Independont
    b   Wanted and a part of things
    c   Useless
    d   Dignified
6   These statements are about a partner's death. Which is *false*?
    a   The person loses a lover, friend, companion, and confidant.
    b   Preparing for the event lessens grief.
    c   The survivor may develop health problems.
    d   The survivor's life will likely change.
7   Skin changes occur with aging. Care should include the following *except*
    a   Providing for warmth
    b   Applying lotion
    c   A daily bath with soap
    d   Providing good skin care
8   An older person complains of cold feet. You should
    a   Provide socks
    b   Apply a hot water bottle
    c   Soak the feet in hot water
    d   Apply a heating pad
9   Aging causes changes in the musculo-skeletal system. Which is *false*?
    a   Bones become brittle. They can break easily.
    b   Bedrest is needed for loss of strength.
    c   Joints become stiff and painful.
    d   Exercise slows musculo-skeletal changes.
10 Changes occur in the nervous system. Which is *true*?
    a   Less sleep is needed than when younger.
    b   The person forgets events from long ago.
    c   Sensitivity to pain increases.
    d   Confusion occurs in all older persons.
11 Changes occur in the eye. Which is *false*?
    a   Night vision decreases.
    b   Blue and green colors are easy to see.
    c   Eyelids thin and wrinkle.
    d   The eye is easily irritated by dust.
12 Which is *not* a common cause of hearing loss in older persons?
    a   Changes in the auditory nerve
    b   Atrophy of the eardrums
    c   Impacted ear wax
    d   Ear infections
13 Arteries narrow and lose their elasticity. These changes result in
    a   A slower heart rate
    b   Lower blood pressure
    c   Poor circulation to many body parts
    d   Less blood in the body
14 An older person has cardiovascular changes. Care includes the following *except*
    a   Placing needed items nearby
    b   A moderate amount of daily exercise
    c   Avoiding exertion
    d   Long walks

15 Respiratory changes occur with aging. Which is *false*?
    a   Heavy bed linens are avoided.
    b   The person is turned often if on bedrest.
    c   The side-lying position is best for breathing.
    d   The person should be as active as possible.
16 Older persons should avoid dry foods because of
    a   Decreases in saliva
    b   Loss of teeth or ill-fitting dentures
    c   Decreased amounts of digestive juices
    d   Decreased peristalsis
17 Changes occur in the digestive system. Older persons should eat
    a   Fruits and vegetables with skins and seeds
    b   Dry and fatty foods
    c   Raw apricots and celery
    d   Protein foods
18 Changes occur in the urinary system. Which is *true*?
    a   Kidneys increase in size.
    b   Fluids are needed for kidney function.
    c   The bladder becomes larger.
    d   Blood flow to the kidneys increases.
19 The doctor orders increased fluid intake for an older person. You should
    a   Give most of the fluid before 1700 (5:00 PM)
    b   Provide mostly water
    c   Start a bladder training program
    d   Insert a catheter
20 Most older people live
    a   In nursing centers
    b   In a family setting
    c   With children
    d   In senior citizen housing
21 These statements are about adult day-care centers. Which is *false*?
    a   They provide meals, supervision, and activities.
    b   Usually the person must do some self-care.
    c   All activities are supervised.
    d   Personal care is provided.
22 Which housing option provides lodging, meals, and some help with personal care?
    a   Apartments
    b   Senior citizen housing
    c   Board and care homes
    d   Residential hotels
23 A continuing care retirement community provides the following *except*
    a   Independent living units
    b   A nursing center
    c   Adult foster care
    d   Meals, transportation, and recreational activities
24 A quality nursing center
    a   Is Medicare-certified and Medicaid-certified
    b   Is owned by doctors and nurses
    c   Has independent living units
    d   Provides adult and child day care

Answers to these questions are on p. 719.

CHAPTER 11

Sexuality

OBJECTIVES

- Define the key terms and key abbreviations listed in this chapter.
- Describe sex, sexuality, and sexual relationships.
- Explain why sexuality is important throughout life.
- Explain how injury and illness can affect sexuality.
- Explain how aging can affect sexuality in older persons.
- Explain how the nursing team can promote sexuality.
- Explain why some persons become sexually aggressive.
- Describe how to deal with sexually aggressive persons.
- Explain how to promote quality of life.

KEY TERMS

bisexual A person who is attracted to both sexes

erectile dysfunction (ED) See "impotence"

heterosexual A person who is attracted to members of the other sex

homosexual A person who is attracted to members of the same sex

impotence The inability of the male to have an erection; erectile dysfunction

sex Physical activities involving the reproductive organs; done for pleasure or to have children

sexuality The physical, emotional, social, cultural, and spiritual factors that affect a person's feelings and attitudes about his or her sex

transgender A broad term used to describe people who express their sexuality or gender in other than the expected ways; persons who are undergoing hormone therapy or surgery for sexual reassignment (female to male; male to female)

transsexual A person who believes that he or she is a member of the other sex

transvestite A person who dresses and behaves like the other sex for emotional and sexual relief; cross-dresser

KEY ABBREVIATIONS

CMS	Centers for Medicare & Medicaid Services	**OBRA**	Omnibus Budget Reconciliation Act of 1987
ED	Erectile dysfunction		

Residents are viewed as whole persons. They have physical and safety needs. They also have love and belonging, self-esteem, and self-actualization needs. Their physical, emotional, social, and spiritual needs are considered.

Sexuality involves the whole person. Illness, injury, and aging can affect sexuality.

SEX AND SEXUALITY

Sex is the physical activities involving the reproductive organs (Chapter 9). It is done for pleasure or to have children. Sexuality is the physical, emotional, social, cultural, and spiritual factors that affect a person's feelings and attitudes about his or her sex. Sexuality involves the personality and the body. It affects how a person behaves, thinks, dresses, and responds to others.

Sexuality develops when a baby's sex is known. It is shown in names, colors, and toys. Blue is for boys and pink for girls. Dolls are for girls. Trains are for boys. By the age of 2, children know their own sex. Three-year-olds know the sex of other children. They learn male and female roles from adults (Fig. 11-1). Children learn that boys and girls each behave in certain ways.

As children grow older, interest increases about the body and how it works. Teens are more aware of sex and the body. Their bodies respond to stimulation. They engage in sexual behaviors. They kiss, embrace, pet, or have intercourse. Pregnancy and sexually transmitted diseases (Chapter 42) are great risks.

Sex has more meaning as young adults mature. Attitudes and feelings are important. Partners are selected. They decide about sex before marriage and birth control.

Sexuality is important throughout life. Attitudes and sex needs change with aging. They are affected by life events. These include divorce, death of a partner, injury, illness, and surgery.

Fig. 11-1 This little girl is learning female roles from her mother.

SEXUAL RELATIONSHIPS

A heterosexual is attracted to members of the other sex. Men are attracted to women. Women are attracted to men. Sexual behavior is male-female.

A homosexual is attracted to members of the same sex. Men are attracted to men. Women are attracted to women. *Gay* refers to homosexuality. Homosexual men are called *gay men*. *Lesbian* refers to a female homosexual. Before the 1960s and 1970s, many gay persons were secret about their sexual orientation. Now many gay persons openly express their sexual preferences and relationships.

Bisexuals are attracted to both sexes. Some have same-gender and male-female behaviors. They often marry and have children. They may seek a same-gender relationship or experience outside of marriage.

Transvestites dress and behave like the other sex for emotional and sexual relief. Commonly called *cross-dressers*, most are men. Often they marry and are heterosexual. They dress as men most of the time. They usually dress as women in private. Some dress completely as women. Others focus on bras and panties. The sex partner may not know about the practice. Some partners take part in cross-dressing activities. Some transvestites have same-gender friends with similar interests.

Transsexuals believe that they are members of the other sex. A male believes that he is a female in a man's body. A female believes that she is a male in a woman's body. They often feel "trapped" in the wrong body. Most have always had these feelings. As children they usually behave like the other sex. Many seek mental health treatment. Some have sex-change operations.

Transgender is a broad term used to describe people who express their sexuality or gender in other than the expected ways. The term also is used to describe persons who are undergoing hormone therapy or surgery for sexual reassignment (female to male; male to female).

INJURY, ILLNESS, AND SURGERY

Injury, illness, and surgery can affect sexual function. Sometimes the nervous, circulatory, and reproductive systems are involved. One or more systems may be affected. Sexual ability may change. Most chronic illnesses affect sexual function. Heart disease, stroke, diabetes, and chronic obstructive pulmonary disease are examples.

Reproductive system surgeries have physical and mental effects. Removal of the uterus, ovaries, or a breast affects women. Prostate or testes removal affects erections.

Impotence (erectile dysfunction; ED) is the inability of the male to have an erection. Diabetes, spinal cord injuries, and multiple sclerosis are causes. So are prostate problems and alcoholism. Heart and circulatory disorders, drugs, drug abuse, and psychological factors are other causes. Some drugs for high blood pressure cause ED. So do other drugs. Some drugs treat ED.

Emotional changes are common. The person may feel unclean, unwhole, unattractive, or mutilated. Attitudes may change. The person may feel unfit for closeness and love. Therefore some problems are emotional. Time and understanding are helpful. So is a caring partner. Some need counseling.

Changes in sexual function greatly impact the person. Fear, anger, worry, and depression are common. They are seen in the person's behavior and comments. The person's feelings are normal and expected. Follow the care plan. It has measures to help the person deal with his or her feelings.

SEXUALITY AND OLDER PERSONS

Love, affection, and intimacy are needed throughout life (Fig. 11-2). Older persons love, fall in love, hold hands, and embrace. Many have intercourse.

Older persons have many losses. Children leave home. Family and friends die. People retire. Health problems occur. Strength decreases. Appearance changes. It helps to feel close to another person.

Reproductive organs change with aging (Chapter 10). Frequency of sex decreases for many older persons.

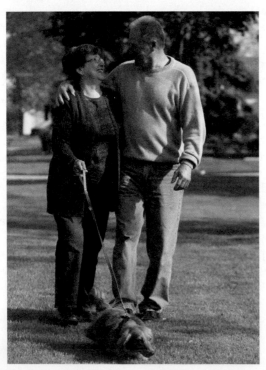

Fig. 11-2 Love and affection are important to persons of all ages.

Reasons relate to weakness, fatigue, and pain. Reduced mobility, aging, and chronic illness are factors.

Some older people do not have intercourse. This does not mean loss of sexual needs or desires. Often needs are expressed in other ways. They hold hands, touch, caress, and embrace. These bring closeness and intimacy.

Sexual partners are lost through death, divorce, and relationship break-ups. Or a partner needs hospital or nursing center care. These situations occur in adults of all ages.

MEETING SEXUAL NEEDS

The nursing team promotes the meeting of sexual needs. The measures in Box 11-1 may be part of the person's care plan.

Box 11-1   Promoting Sexuality

- Let the person practice grooming routines. Assist as needed. For women, this includes applying makeup, nail polish, and cologne. Many women shave their legs and underarms and pluck eyebrows. Men may use after-shave lotion and cologne. Hair care is important to men and women.
- Let the person choose clothing. Hospital gowns embarrass both men and women. Street clothes are worn if the person's condition permits.
- Protect the right to privacy. Do not expose the person. Drape and screen the person.
- Accept the person's sexual relationships. The person may not share your sexual attitudes, values, or practices. The person may have a homosexual, premarital, or extramarital relationship. Do not judge or gossip about relationships.
- Allow privacy. You can usually tell when people want to be alone. If the person has a private room, close the door for privacy. Some centers have *Do Not Disturb* signs for doors. Let the person and partner know how much time they have alone. For example, remind them about meal times, drugs, and treatments. Tell other staff members that the person wants time alone.
- Knock before you enter any room. This is a simple courtesy that shows respect for privacy.
- Consider the person's roommate. Privacy curtains provide little privacy. They do not block sound. Arrange for privacy when the roommate is out of the room. Sometimes roommates offer to leave for a while. If the roommate cannot leave, the nurse finds a private area.
- Allow privacy for masturbation. It is a normal form of sexual expression. Close the privacy curtain and the door. Knock before you enter any room. This saves you and the person embarrassment. Sometimes confused persons masturbate in public areas. Lead the person to a private area. Or distract him or her with an activity.

Fig. 11-3 Relationships develop in nursing centers.

Married couples in nursing centers can share the same room. This is a requirement of the Omnibus Budget Reconciliation Act of 1987 (OBRA). The couple has lived together a long time. Long-term care is no reason to keep them apart. They can share the same bed if their conditions permit. A double, queen-size, or king-size bed is provided by the couple or the center.

Single persons may develop relationships. They are allowed time together, not kept apart (Fig. 11-3).

THE SEXUALLY AGGRESSIVE PERSON

Some persons want the health team to meet their sexual needs. They flirt or make sexual advances or comments. Some expose themselves, masturbate, or touch the staff. This can anger and embarrass the staff member. These reactions are normal. Often there are reasons for the person's behavior. Understanding this helps you deal with the matter.

Sexually aggressive behaviors have many causes. They include:

- Nervous system disorders
- Confusion, disorientation, and dementia
- Drug side effects
- Fever
- Poor vision

The person may confuse someone with his or her partner. Or the person cannot control behavior. The cause is changes in mental function. The healthy person controls sexual urges. Changes in the brain make control difficult. Sexual behavior in these cases is usually innocent.

Sometimes touch serves to gain attention. For example, Mr. Green cannot speak. He cannot move his right side. Your buttocks are near him. To get your attention, he touches your buttocks. His behavior is not sexual.

Sometimes masturbation is a sexually aggressive behavior. Some persons touch and fondle the genitals for sexual pleasure. However, urinary or reproductive system disorders can cause genital soreness or itching. So can poor hygiene and being wet or soiled from urine or feces. Touching genitals could signal a health problem.

Sometimes the purpose of touch is sexual. For example, a person wants to prove that he or she is attractive and can perform sexually. You must be professional about the matter.

- Ask the person not to touch you. State the places where you were touched.
- Tell the person that you will not do what he or she wants.
- Tell the person what behaviors make you uncomfortable. Politely ask the person not to act that way.
- Allow privacy if the person is becoming aroused. Provide for safety. Complete a safety check of the room (see the inside of the front book cover). Tell the person when you will return.
- Discuss the matter with the nurse. The nurse can help you understand the behavior.
- Follow the care plan. It has measures to deal with sexually aggressive behaviors. They are based on the cause of the behavior. Many centers have classes to help staff deal with such behavior.

See *Focus on Communication: The Sexually Aggressive Person.*

FOCUS ON COMMUNICATION
The Sexually Aggressive Person

Confronting the sexually aggressive person is difficult. This is true for young and older staff and for new and experienced staff. Ask yourself these questions:

- Does the person have a health problem that affects impulse control? If yes, the behavior may not have a sexual purpose.
- Is the person's behavior on purpose? Is the intent sexual? If yes, you must confront the behavior. Be direct and matter-of-fact. For example, you can say:
  - "You brushed your hand across my breast (or other body part) two times this morning. Please don't do that again."
  - "No, I cannot kiss you. It would be unprofessional for me to do so."
  - "You exposed yourself to me again today. Please do not do that again."

The sexually aggressive person needs the nurse's attention. Discuss the matter with the nurse. Report what happened and when. Also report what you said and did. The nurse must deal with the problem. If other staff are reporting such behaviors, the nurse views the problem in a broader and different way.

Protecting the Person

The person must be protected from unwanted sexual comments and advances. This is sexual abuse (Chapter 4). Tell the nurse right away. No one should be allowed to sexually abuse another person. This includes staff members, residents, family members or other visitors, and volunteers.

SEXUALLY TRANSMITTED DISEASES

Some diseases are spread by sexual contact. They are discussed in Chapter 42.

QUALITY OF LIFE

Sexuality is part of the total person. Illness or injury does not make it of little concern. Nor does surgery or aging. How sexuality is expressed may change. To meet the person's sexual needs, follow the care plan. Always provide for privacy.

Do not judge or gossip about a person's sexuality. Healthy, pleasurable sexual relationships and intimacy enhance the quality of life for people of all ages.

REVIEW QUESTIONS

Circle the BEST answer.

1 Sex involves
   a The organs of reproduction
   b Attitudes and feelings
   c Cultural and spiritual factors
   d Masturbation
2 Sexuality is important to
   a Small children
   b Teenagers and young adults
   c Middle-age adults
   d Persons of all ages
3 Impotence is
   a When menstruation stops
   b A reaction to illness
   c Not being able to achieve an erection
   d No sexual activity
4 Reproductive organs change with aging.
   a True
   b False
5 Mr. and Mrs. Green live in a nursing center. Which will *not* promote their sexuality?
   a Allowing their normal grooming routines
   b Having them wear hospital gowns
   c Allowing them privacy
   d Accepting their relationship

6 Two residents are holding hands. Nursing staff should keep them apart.
   a True
   b False
7 Mr. and Mrs. Green want some time alone. The nursing team can do the following *except*
   a Close the room door
   b Put a *Do Not Disturb* sign on the door
   c Tell other staff that they want some time alone
   d Close the privacy curtain so no one can hear them
8 Mr. and Mrs. Green should each have a room. This is an OBRA requirement.
   a True
   b False
9 A person is masturbating in the dining room. You should do the following *except*
   a Cover the person and quietly take the person to his or her room
   b Scold the person
   c Provide privacy
   d Tell the nurse
10 A person touches you sexually and asks for a kiss. You should do the following *except*
   a Discuss the matter with the nurse
   b Do what the person asks
   c Explain that the behaviors make you uncomfortable
   d Ask the person not to touch you

Answers to these questions are on p. 719.

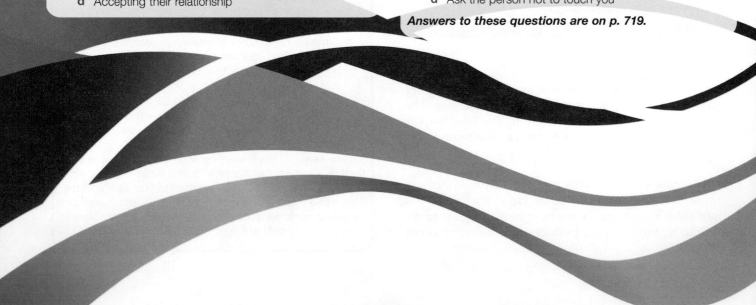

Safety

OBJECTIVES

- Define the key terms and key abbreviations listed in this chapter.
- Describe accident risk factors.
- Explain why you identify a person before giving care.
- Explain how to correctly identify a person.
- Describe the safety measures to prevent burns, poisoning, and suffocation.
- Identify the signs and causes of choking.
- Explain how to prevent equipment accidents.
- Explain how to handle hazardous substances.
- Describe safety measures for fire prevention and oxygen use.

- Explain what to do during a fire.
- Give examples of natural and human-made disasters.
- Explain how to report accidents and errors.
- Explain how to protect yourself from workplace violence.
- Describe your role in risk management.
- Perform the procedures described in this chapter.
- Explain how to promote quality of life.

KEY TERMS

coma A state of being unaware of one's surroundings and being unable to react or respond to people, places, or things

dementia The loss of cognitive and social function caused by changes in the brain

disaster A sudden catastrophic event in which people are injured and killed and property is destroyed

electrical shock When electrical current passes through the body

ground That which carries leaking electricity to the earth and away from an electrical item

hazard Any thing in the person's setting that may cause injury or illness

hazardous substance Any chemical in the workplace that can cause harm

hemiplegia Paralysis on one side of the body

incident Any event that has harmed or could harm a resident, visitor, or staff member

paralysis Loss of muscle function, loss of sensation, or loss of both muscle function and sensation

paraplegia Paralysis in the legs and lower trunk

quadriplegia Paralysis in the arms, legs, and trunk; tetraplegia

suffocation When breathing stops from the lack of oxygen

tetraplegia See "quadriplegia"

workplace violence Violent acts (including assault and threat of assault) directed toward persons at work or while on duty

Safety is a basic need. Residents are at great risk for accidents and falls. (See Chapter 13 for falls.) Some accidents and injuries cause death.

The health team must provide for safety. This includes you. Ordinary and sometimes extraordinary measures are needed to prevent accidents and keep residents safe. The goal is to decrease the person's risk of accidents and injuries without limiting mobility and independence.

The Omnibus Budget Reconciliation Act of 1987 (OBRA) requires that nursing centers follow safety policies and procedures. So do accrediting agency standards. The intent is to keep residents, visitors, and staff safe. Measures to protect residents must not interfere with their rights (Chapter 2).

Common sense and simple safety measures can prevent most accidents. You must protect residents, visitors, yourself, and co-workers. The safety measures in this chapter apply to nursing and everyday life. The care plan lists other safety measures for the person.

A SAFE SETTING

In a safe setting, a person has little risk of illness or injury. The person's setting is free of hazards to the extent possible. A hazard is any thing in the person's setting that may cause injury or illness.

The person feels safe and secure physically and mentally. The risk of infection, falls, burns, poisoning, and other injuries is low. Temperature and noise levels are comfortable. Smells are pleasant. There is enough room and light to move about safely. The person and the person's property are safe from fire and intruders. The person is not afraid. He or she has few worries and concerns.

The person must receive the right care and treatment. The person is protected from falls, burns, poisoning, suffocation, and infection. To protect the person from harm, follow the person's care plan. Also practice the safety measures in this chapter.

See *Teamwork and Time Management: A Safe Setting.*

TEAMWORK AND TIME MANAGEMENT
A Safe Setting

The entire health team must provide a safe setting. You may see something unsafe. Correct the matter right away if it is something you can do. For example:
- You see a water spill. Wipe up the spill right away. Do so even if you did not cause the spill.
- You see a person sliding out of a wheelchair. Position the person correctly in the chair. Do so even if a co-worker is responsible for the person's care.
- A person is having problems holding a cup of coffee. Offer to help the person.
- Food is left unattended in a microwave oven. Turn off the device. Then tell your co-worker the reason for your action.
- A grab bar is loose in the bathroom. Tell the nurse. Follow center policy for reporting the problem.

You cannot correct some safety issues. Follow center policy for reporting such problems. They include:
- Electrical outlets or switches coming out of the wall
- Electrical outlets that do not work
- Water leaks from windows, doors, ceilings, pipes, faucets, tubs, showers, toilets, hot water heaters, fountains, and other water sources
- Toilets that do not work properly
- Water from faucets that does not warm up or that is very hot
- Broken windows
- Windows and doors that do not work properly
- Knobs and handles that are broken or do not work properly
- Hand rails and grab bars that are loose or need repair
- Odd smells and odors
- Odd sounds
- Signs of rodents, flies, or other pests
- Broken or damaged furniture
- Lights and lamps that do not work or have burnt-out bulbs
- Flooring (carpeting, tiles) in need of repair

ACCIDENT RISK FACTORS

Some people cannot protect themselves. They present dangers to themselves and others. They rely on others for safety. Know the factors that increase a person's risk of accidents and injuries. Follow the person's care plan to provide for safety.

- *Age.* Changes from aging increase the risk for falls and other injuries. Older persons have decreased strength and move slowly. Some are unsteady. Often balance is affected. These changes prevent quick and sudden movements to avoid dangers and prevent falls. Older persons also are less sensitive to heat and cold. They have poor vision, hearing problems, and a dulled sense of smell. Confusion, poor judgment, memory problems, and disorientation may occur (Chapter 44).
- *Awareness of surroundings.* People need to know their surroundings to protect themselves from injury. Coma is a state of being unaware of one's surroundings and being unable to react or respond to people, places, or things. A coma can occur from illness or injury. The person in a coma relies on others for protection. Confused and disoriented persons may not understand what is happening to and around them. See *Residents With Dementia: Accident Risk Factors (Awareness of Surroundings).*
- *Agitated and aggressive behaviors.* Pain can cause these behaviors. So can confusion, decreased awareness of surroundings, and fear of what may happen.
- *Vision loss.* Persons with poor vision have problems seeing things. They can fall or trip over toys, rugs, equipment, furniture, and cords. Some have problems reading labels on cleaners and other containers. Poisoning can result. It also can result from taking the wrong drug or the wrong dose.

- *Hearing loss.* Persons with hearing loss have problems hearing explanations and instructions. They may not hear warning signals or fire alarms. Some cannot hear approaching meal carts, drug carts, stretchers, or people in wheelchairs. They do not know to move to safety.
- *Impaired smell and touch.* Illness and aging affect smell and touch. The person may not detect smoke or gas odors. When touch is reduced, burns are a risk. The person has problems sensing heat and cold. Some people have a decreased pain sense. They may be unaware of injury. For example, Mrs. Parks does not feel a blister from her shoes. She has poor circulation to her legs and feet. The blister can become a serious wound.
- *Impaired mobility.* Some diseases and injuries affect mobility. A person may know there is danger but cannot move to safety. Some persons cannot walk or propel wheelchairs. Some persons are paralyzed. Paralysis means loss of muscle function, loss of sensation, or loss of both muscle function and sensation. Paraplegia is paralysis in the legs and lower trunk. Quadriplegia (tetraplegia) is paralysis in the arms, legs, and trunk. Hemiplegia is paralysis on one side of the body.
- *Drugs.* Drugs have side effects. They include loss of balance, drowsiness, and lack of coordination. Reduced awareness, confusion, and disorientation can occur. The person may be fearful and uncooperative. Report behavior changes to the nurse. Also report the person's complaints.

IDENTIFYING THE PERSON

You will care for many people. Each has different treatments, therapies, and activity limits. You must give the right care to the right person. Life and health are threatened if the wrong care is given.

The person may receive an identification (ID) bracelet when admitted to the center (Fig. 12-1). The bracelet has the person's name, room and bed number, birth date, age, doctor, and center name. Other identifying information may include the person's ID number given by the center. Some centers include the person's religion.

RESIDENTS WITH DEMENTIA
Accident Risk Factors (Awareness of Surroundings)

Some persons suffer from dementia. Dementia is the loss of cognitive and social function caused by changes in the brain (Chapter 44). Memory and the ability to think and reason are lost. Dementia is caused by diseases and injuries.

Persons with dementia are confused and disoriented. Their awareness of surroundings is reduced. They may not understand what is happening to and around them. Judgment is poor. They no longer know what is safe and what are dangers. They may access closets, cupboards, or other unsafe and unlocked areas. They may eat or drink cleaning products, drugs, or poisons. Accidents and injuries are great risks. The health team must meet all safety needs.

Fig. 12-1 ID bracelet.

Fig. 12-2 The ID bracelet is checked against the assignment sheet to accurately identify the person.

Fig. 12-3 The person's photo is at the head-board. Her name is under the photo. The nursing assistant is using the photo to identify the person.

You use the bracelet to identify the person before giving care. The assignment sheet states what care to give. To identify the person:

- Compare identifying information on the assignment sheet with that on the ID bracelet (Fig. 12-2). Carefully check the information. Some people have the same first and last names. For example, John Smith is a very common name.
- Use at least two identifiers. An identifier cannot be the person's room or bed number. Some centers require that the person state his or her name and birth date. Others require using the person's ID number. Always follow center policy.
- Call the person by name when checking the ID bracelet. This is a courtesy given as you touch the person and before giving care. Just calling the person by name is not enough to identify him or her. Confused, disoriented, drowsy, hard-of-hearing, or distracted persons may answer to any name.

Alert and oriented residents may choose not to wear ID bracelets. This is noted on the person's care plan. Follow center policy and the care plan to identify the person.

Some nursing centers have photo ID systems (Fig. 12-3). The person's photo is taken on admission. Then it is placed in the person's medical record. If your center uses such a system, learn to use it safely.

See *Promoting Safety and Comfort: Identifying the Person.*

PREVENTING BURNS

Burns are a leading cause of death among children and older persons. Smoking, spilled hot liquids, electrical items, and very hot water (hand sinks, tubs, showers) are some causes in nursing centers. Risk factors for burns in older persons are decreased skin thickness, decreased sensitivity to heat, reduced reaction time, decreased mobility, communication problems, confusion, and dementia.

PROMOTING SAFETY AND COMFORT
Identifying the Person

Safety
Always identify the person before you begin a task or procedure. Do not identify the person and then leave the room to collect supplies and equipment. You could go to the wrong room and give care to the wrong person. And the person for whom the care was intended would not receive it. This too could cause harm.

Sometimes ID bracelets become damaged from water, spilled food and fluids, and everyday wear and tear. Make sure you can read the information on the ID bracelet. If you cannot, tell the nurse. The nurse can have a new bracelet made for the person.

Comfort
Make sure the person's ID bracelet is not too tight. You should be able to slide 1 or 2 fingers under the bracelet. If it is too tight, tell the nurse.

Burn severity depends on water temperature and length of exposure (Table 12-1). The person's condition also is a factor.

- *Superficial (first degree) burn*—involves the epidermis (top layer of skin). Sunburn is an example. The skin is red and painful to touch. There may be mild swelling.
- *Partial-thickness (second degree) burn*—involves the epidermis and dermis. The skin appears deep red. The person has pain and blisters. The skin may appear glossy from leaking fluid.
- *Full-thickness (third degree) burn*—the epidermis and dermis, fat, muscle, and bone may be injured or destroyed. These burns are not painful. Nerve endings are destroyed. The skin appears charred or has white, brown, or black patches.

The safety measures in Box 12-1 can prevent burns.

Table 12-1	Water Temperature and Length of Exposure for a Third Degree Burn	

Fahrenheit (F)	Centigrade (C)	Time Required for a Third Degree Burn to Occur
155° F	68° C	1 second
148° F	64° C	2 seconds
140° F	60° C	5 seconds
133° F	56° C	15 seconds
127° F	52° C	1 minute
124° F	51° C	3 minutes
120° F	48° C	5 minutes
100° F	37° C	Usually a safe temperature for bathing

Modified from Centers for Medicare & Medicaid Services: State operations manual, *Baltimore, Md, April 10, 2009, U.S. Department of Health and Human Services.*

Box 12-1   Safety Measures to Prevent Burns

Eating and Drinking
- Assist with eating and drinking as needed. Spilled hot food or fluids can cause burns.
- Be careful when carrying hot foods and fluids near older persons.

Water
- Turn on cold water first, then hot water. Turn off hot water first, then cold water.
- Measure bath or shower water temperature (Chapter 20). Check it before a person gets into the tub or shower.
- Check for "hot spots" in bath water. Move your hand back and forth.

Appliances
- See "Preventing Equipment Accidents" (p. 141).
- Do not allow the use of space heaters.
- Do not let the person sleep with a heating pad.
- Do not let the person use an electric blanket.
- Turn off curling irons, electric rollers, and hair dryers when not in use.

Smoking
- Be sure residents smoke only in smoking areas.
- Do not leave smoking materials at the bedside. They are only left at the bedside if the person is trusted to smoke alone in smoking areas. Follow the care plan.
- Supervise the smoking of persons who cannot protect themselves.
- Do not allow smoking in bed.
- Do not allow smoking where oxygen is used or stored (Chapter 28).
- Be alert to ashes that may fall onto an older person.

Other
- Follow safety guidelines when applying heat and cold (Chapter 35).

PREVENTING POISONING

Poisoning also is a health hazard and a major cause of death. Older persons are at risk. Drugs and household products are common poisons. Poisoning in adults may be from carelessness, confusion, or poor vision when reading labels. As a result, a person may take too much of a drug. Sometimes poisoning is a suicide attempt.

The measures in Box 12-2 can prevent poisoning.

Box 12-2   Safety Measures to Prevent Poisoning

- Keep harmful products in locked areas.
- Keep child-resistant caps on all harmful products.
- Store personal care items according to center policy. Soap, mouthwash, lotion, deodorant, and shampoo are examples. These items could cause harm when swallowed.
- Use and store harmful products according to the manufacturer's instructions (p. 143).
- Do not leave harmful products unattended when in use.
- Make sure all harmful products are labeled (p. 144).
- Do not mix cleaning products.
- Read all labels carefully. Have good lighting.
- Keep harmful products in their original containers. Do not store them in food containers.
- Do not store harmful products near food.
- Discard harmful products that are outdated.
- Keep emergency numbers by the telephone: poison control center (1-800-222-1222), police, ambulance, hospital, and doctor.

PREVENTING SUFFOCATION

Suffocation is when breathing stops from the lack of oxygen. Death occurs if the person does not start breathing. Common causes include choking, drowning, inhaling gas or smoke, strangulation, and electrical shock (p. 141).

Carbon monoxide poisoning is another cause. Carbon monoxide is a colorless, odorless, and tasteless gas. It is produced by burning fuel. For example, motor vehicles, furnaces, gas water heaters, gas stoves, and gas dryers use fuel. These devices must be in good working order and used correctly. Otherwise, dangerous levels of carbon monoxide may result. Instead of breathing in oxygen, the person breathes in air filled with carbon monoxide. Headache, nausea, and dizziness are common. So are confusion, breathing problems, sleepiness, and cherry-pink skin. Death can occur.

Measures to prevent suffocation are listed in Box 12-3. Clear the airway if the person is choking.

Choking

Foreign bodies can obstruct the airway. This is called *choking* or *foreign-body airway obstruction (FBAO)*. Air cannot pass through the air passages to the lungs. The body does not get enough oxygen. It can lead to cardiac arrest. *Cardiac arrest* is when the heart stops suddenly and without warning (Chapter 47).

Box 12-3   Safety Measures to Prevent Suffocation

- Cut food into small, bite-sized pieces for persons who cannot do so themselves.
- Make sure dentures fit properly and are in place.
- Make sure the person can chew and swallow the food served.
- Report loose teeth or dentures.
- Check the care plan for swallowing problems before providing food (including snacks) or fluids. The person may ask for something that he or she cannot swallow.
- Tell the nurse at once if the person has swallowing problems.
- Do not give oral food or fluids to persons with feeding tubes (Chapter 25).
- Follow aspiration precautions (Chapter 24).
- Do not leave a person unattended in a bathtub or shower.
- Move all persons from the area if you smell smoke.
- Position the person in bed properly (Chapter 16).
- Use bed rails correctly (Chapter 13).
- Use restraints correctly (Chapter 14).
- Prevent entrapment in the bed system (Chapter 18).
- See "Preventing Equipment Accidents" (p. 141).

Choking often occurs during eating. A large, poorly chewed piece of meat is the most common cause. Weakness, dentures that fit poorly, dysphagia (difficulty swallowing), and chronic illness are also causes. So are laughing and talking while eating and excessive alcohol intake.

Unconscious persons can choke. Common causes are aspiration of vomitus and the tongue falling back into the airway. These also occur during cardiac arrest.

Foreign bodies can cause mild or severe airway obstruction. With *mild airway obstruction*, some air moves in and out of the lungs. The person is conscious and usually can speak. Often forceful coughing can remove the object. Breathing may sound like wheezing between coughs. For mild airway obstruction:

- Stay with the person.
- Encourage the person to keep coughing to expel the object.
- Do not interrupt the person's efforts to clear the airway. If breathing and coughing, abdominal thrusts are not needed.
- If the obstruction persists, call for help.

Difficulty breathing occurs with *severe airway obstruction*. Air does not move in and out of the lungs. The person may not be able to breathe, speak, or cough. If able to cough, the cough is of poor quality. When the person tries to inhale, there is no noise or a high-pitched noise. The person may appear pale and cyanotic (bluish color).

The conscious person clutches at the throat (Fig. 12-4). Clutching at the throat is often called the "universal sign of choking." The conscious person is very frightened. If the obstruction is not removed, the person will die. Severe airway obstruction is an emergency.

Fig. 12-4 A choking person clutches at the throat.

Relieving Choking Abdominal thrusts are used to relieve severe airway obstruction. Abdominal thrusts are quick, upward thrusts to the abdomen. They force air out of the lungs and create an artificial cough. They are done to try to expel the foreign body from the airway.

Abdominal thrusts are not used for very obese persons or pregnant women. Chest thrusts are used (p. 140).

You may observe a person choking. And you may perform emergency measures to relieve choking. Report and record what happened, what you did, and the person's response (Fig. 12-5).

Relief of choking occurs when the foreign body is removed. Or it occurs when you feel air move and see the chest rise and fall when giving rescue breaths. The person may still be unresponsive.

Self-Administered Abdominal Thrusts. You may choke when by yourself. Perform abdominal thrusts to relieve the obstructed airway.

1 Make a fist with one hand.
2 Place the thumb side of the fist above your navel and below the lower end of the sternum.
3 Grasp your fist with your other hand.
4 Press inward and upward quickly.
5 Press the upper abdomen against a hard surface if the thrust did not relieve the obstruction. Use the back of a chair, a table, or railing.
6 Use as many thrusts as needed.

The Unresponsive Adult. You may find an adult who is unresponsive. You did not see the person lose consciousness, and you do not know the cause. Do not assume the cause is choking. Check to see if the person is responding. If not, start cardiopulmonary resuscitation (CPR). See Chapter 47.

	Date	Time	Nursing Margin	Other Depts Margin
9-10	1215	While eating lunch, Mrs. Rand began coughing and clutching at her throat. Her		
		tablemate shouted "she's choking". I went to Mrs. Rand's table. She mouthed the words		
		"I can't breathe". I performed abdominal thrusts with Mrs. Rand sitting in her		
		chair. After three abdominal thrusts, she coughed out a pecan-sized piece of meat. She		
		then began breathing. Mary Jones, RN arrived and took over the care of Mrs. Rand.		
		Ben Armes, CNA.		

Fig. 12-5 Charting sample for choking.

RELIEVING CHOKING—ADULT OR CHILD (OVER 1 YEAR OF AGE)

PROCEDURE

1 Ask the person if he or she is choking. Help the person if he or she nods "yes" and cannot talk.
2 Have someone call for help:
   a *In a public area,* have someone activate the Emergency Medical Services (EMS) system by calling 911. Send someone to get an automated external defibrillator (AED). See Chapter 47.
   b *In a center,* call the emergency response system. This team quickly responds to give care in life-threatening situations. Send someone to get the AED.
3 *If the person is sitting or standing,* give abdominal thrusts:
   a Stand or kneel behind the person.
   b Wrap your arms around the person's waist.

c Make a fist with one hand.
d Place the thumb side of the fist against the abdomen. The fist is slightly above the navel in the middle of the abdomen and well below the end of the sternum (breastbone). See Figure 12-6, *A,* p. 140.
e Grasp the fist with your other hand (Fig. 12-6, *B,* p. 140).
f Press your fist into the person's abdomen with a quick, upward thrust.
g Repeat thrusts until the object is expelled or the person becomes unresponsive.

Continued

PROCEDURE—cont'd

4 *If the person is lying down but responsive,* give abdominal thrusts (Fig. 12-7).

  a Straddle the person's thighs.

  b Place the heel of one hand against the abdomen. It is in the middle slightly above the navel and well below the end of the sternum (breastbone).

  c Place your second hand on top of your first hand.

  d Press both hands into the abdomen with a quick, upward thrust.

  e Repeat thrusts until the object is expelled or the person becomes unresponsive.

5 *If the person is obese or pregnant,* give chest thrusts:

  a Stand behind the person.

  b Place your arms under the person's underarms. Wrap your arms around the person's chest.

  c Make a fist. Place the thumb side of the fist on the middle of the sternum (breastbone).

  d Grasp the fist with your other hand.

  e Give thrusts to the chest until the object is expelled or the person becomes unresponsive.

6 *If the object is dislodged,* encourage the person to go to the hospital. Injuries can occur from abdominal or chest thrusts.

7 *If the person becomes unresponsive,* lower the person to the floor or ground. Position the person supine (lying flat on the back). Make sure EMS or the emergency response system was called (step 2). If alone, provide 5 cycles (2 minutes) of CPR first. Then call EMS or the emergency response system.

8 Start CPR. See Chapter 47.

  a Do not check for a pulse. Begin with compressions. Give 30 compressions. Chest compressions help dislodge an obstruction.

  b Use the head tilt-chin lift method to open the airway (Fig. 12-8). Open the person's mouth. The mouth should be wide open. Look for an object. Remove the object if you see it and can remove it easily. Use your fingers.

  c Give 2 breaths.

  d Continue cycles of 30 compressions and 2 breaths. Look for an object every time you open the airway for rescue breaths.

9 *If you relieve choking in an unresponsive person:*

  a Check for a response, breathing, and a pulse.

    (1) *If no response, normal breathing, or pulse*—continue CPR. Attach an AED (Chapter 47).

    (2) *If no response and no normal breathing but there is a pulse*—give rescue breaths. For an adult, give 1 breath every 5 to 6 seconds (10 to 12 breaths per minute). For a child, give 1 breath every 3 to 5 seconds (12 to 20 breaths per minute). Check for a pulse every 2 minutes. If no pulse, begin CPR.

    (3) *If the person has normal breathing and a pulse*—place the person in the recovery position if there is no response (Chapter 47). Continue to check the person until help arrives. Encourage the person to go to the hospital if the person responds.

Fig. 12-6 Hand positioning for abdominal thrusts. **A,** The fist is slightly above the navel in the midline of the abdomen. **B,** The other hand clasps the fist.

Fig. 12-7 Abdominal thrusts with the person lying down.

Airway closed

Airway open

Fig. 12-8 The head tilt-chin lift method opens the airway. One hand is on the person's forehead. Pressure is applied to lift the head back. The chin is lifted with the fingers of the other hand.

PREVENTING INFECTION

The spread of infection is a major hazard in nursing centers. Infections are caused by microorganisms that easily spread from one person to another. Infection is a risk for persons who are older, chronically ill, or disabled. Infections increase their health problems. They often cause death. Chapter 15 describes how to prevent infections.

PREVENTING EQUIPMENT ACCIDENTS

All equipment is unsafe if broken, not used correctly, or not working properly. This includes hospital beds. Inspect all equipment before use. Check glass and plastic items for cracks, chips, and sharp or rough edges. They can cause cuts, stabs, or scratches. Follow the Bloodborne Pathogen Standard (Chapter 15).

Electrical items must work properly and be in good repair. Frayed cords (Fig. 12-9) and over-loaded electrical outlets (Fig. 12-10) can cause fires, burns, and electrical shocks. Electrical shock is when electrical current passes through the body. It can burn the skin, muscles, nerves, and other tissues. It can affect the heart and cause death.

Three-pronged plugs (Fig. 12-11) are used on all electrical items. Two prongs carry electrical current. The third prong is the ground. A ground carries leaking electricity to the earth and away from an electrical item. If a ground is not used, leaking electricity can be conducted to the person. It can cause electrical shocks and possible death. If you receive a shock, report it at once. Do not use the item.

Warning signs of a faulty electrical item include:
- Shocks
- Loss of power or a power outage
- Dimming or flickering lights
- Sparks
- Sizzling or buzzing sounds
- Burning odor
- Loose plugs

Do not use or give damaged items to residents. Take the item to the nurse. The nurse will have you do one of the following:
- Discard the item following center policy.
- Tag the item and send it for repair following center policy.

Practice the safety measures in Box 12-4, p. 142 when using equipment. An incident report (p. 153) is completed if a resident, visitor, or staff member has an equipment-related accident. The Safe Medical Devices Act requires that centers report equipment-related illnesses, injuries, and deaths.

Fig. 12-9 A frayed electrical cord.

Fig. 12-11 A three-pronged plug.

Fig. 12-10 An over-loaded electrical outlet.

Box 12-4   Safety Measures to Prevent Equipment Accidents

General Safety

- Follow center policies and procedures.
- Follow the manufacturer's instructions. Use equipment correctly.
- Read all caution and warning labels.
- Do not use an unfamiliar item. Ask for needed training. Also ask a nurse to supervise you the first time you use an item.
- Use an item only for its intended purpose.
- Make sure the item works before you begin.
- Make sure you have all needed equipment. For example, you need to plug in an item. There must be an outlet.
- Show a broken or damaged item to the nurse. Follow the nurse's instructions and center policies for discarding items or sending them for repair.
- Do not try to repair broken or damaged items.
- Do not use broken or damaged items.

Electrical Safety

- Inspect electrical cords and appliances for damage. Make sure they are in good repair.
- Use three-pronged plugs on all electrical devices.
- Use extension cords for only one device. This prevents over-loading a circuit.
- Do not use power strips for care equipment.
- Do not cover power cords with rugs, carpets, linens, or other materials. Do not run power cords under rugs.
- Connect a bed power cord directly to a wall outlet. Do not connect a bed power cord to an extension cord or outlet strip.
- Do not use electrical items owned by the person until they are safety checked. The maintenance staff does this.
- Keep electrical items away from water.
- Keep work areas clean and dry. Wipe up spills right away.
- Do not touch electrical items if you are wet, if your hands are wet, or if you are standing in water.
- Do not put a finger or any item into an outlet.
- Turn off equipment before unplugging it. Sparks occur when electrical items are unplugged while turned on.
- Hold onto the plug (not the cord) when removing it from an outlet (Fig. 12-12).
- Do not give showers or tub baths during electrical storms. Lightning can travel through pipes.
- Do not use electrical items or phones during storms.
- Do not use water to put out an electrical fire. If possible, turn off or unplug the item.
- Do not touch a person who is experiencing an electrical shock. If possible, turn off or unplug the item. Call for help at once.
- Keep electrical cords away from heating vents and other heat sources.
- Turn off the electrical device when done using the item.
- Unplug all electrical devices when not in use.

WHEELCHAIR AND STRETCHER SAFETY

Some people cannot walk or they have severe problems walking. A wheelchair may be useful (Fig. 12-13). If able, the person propels the chair using the handrims. Some use their feet to move the chair. Other wheelchairs are propelled by motors. The person moves the chair with hand, chin, mouth, or other controls. If the person cannot propel the wheelchair, another person pushes it using the handgrips/push handles.

Stretchers are used to transport persons who cannot use wheelchairs. They cannot sit up or must lie down.

Follow the safety measures in Box 12-5 when using wheelchairs and stretchers. The person can fall from the wheelchair or stretcher. Or the person can fall during transfers to and from the wheelchair or stretcher.

Fig. 12-12 Hold onto the plug to remove it from an outlet.

1. Handgrip/push handle
2. Back upholstery
3. Armrest
4. Seat upholstery
5. Front rigging
6. Footplate
7. Caster
8. Crossbrace
9. Wheel lock/brake
10. Wheel and handrim
11. Tipping lever

Fig. 12-13 Parts of a wheelchair.

Box 12-5 Wheelchair and Stretcher Safety

Wheelchair Safety

- Check the wheel locks (brakes). Make sure you can lock and unlock them.
- Check for flat or loose tires. A wheel lock will not work on a flat or loose tire.
- Make sure the wheel spokes are intact. Damaged, broken, or loose spokes can interfere with moving the wheelchair or locking the wheels.
- Make sure the casters point forward. This keeps the wheelchair balanced and stable.
- Position the person's feet on the footplates.
- Make sure the person's feet are on the footplates before moving the chair. The person's feet must not touch or drag on the floor when the chair is moving.
- Push the chair forward when transporting the person. Do not pull the chair backward unless going through a doorway.
- Lock both wheels before you transfer a person to or from the wheelchair.
- Follow the care plan for keeping the wheels locked when not moving the wheelchair. Locking the wheels prevents the chair from moving if the person wants to move to or from the chair. (Locking the wheelchair may be viewed as a restraint. See Chapter 14.)
- Do not let the person stand on the footplates.
- Do not let the footplates fall back onto the person's legs.
- Make sure the person has needed wheelchair accessories—safety belt, pouch, tray, lap-board, cushion.

Wheelchair Safety—cont'd

- Remove the armrests (if removable) when the person transfers to the bed, toilet, commode, tub, or car (Chapter 17).
- Swing front rigging out of the way for transfers to and from the wheelchair. Some front riggings detach for transfers.
- Clean the wheelchair according to center policy.
- Ask a nurse or physical therapist to show you how to propel wheelchairs up steps and ramps and over curbs.
- Follow the safety measures to prevent equipment accidents (Box 12-4).

Stretcher Safety

- Ask two co-workers to help you transfer the person to or from the stretcher (Chapter 17).
- Lock the stretcher wheels before the transfer.
- Fasten the safety straps when the person is properly positioned on the stretcher.
- Ask a co-worker to help with the transport.
- Raise the side rails. Keep them up during the transport.
- Make sure the person's arms, hands, legs, and feet do not dangle through the side rail bars.
- Stand at the head of the stretcher. Your co-worker stands at the foot of the stretcher.
- Move the stretcher feet first (Fig. 12-14).
- Do not leave the person alone.
- Follow the safety measures to prevent equipment accidents (Box 12-4).

Fig. 12-14 A person is transported by stretcher. The stretcher is moved feet first.

HANDLING HAZARDOUS SUBSTANCES

A hazardous substance is any chemical in the workplace that can cause harm. The Occupational Safety and Health Administration (OSHA) requires that health care employees:

- Understand the risks of hazardous substances.
- Know how to safely handle them.

Physical hazards can cause fires or explosions. *Health hazards* are chemicals that can cause acute or chronic health problems. Acute problems occur rapidly and last a short time. They usually are from short-term exposure. Chronic problems usually result from long-term exposure. They occur over a long time.

Health hazards can:

- Cause cancer
- Affect blood cell formation and function
- Damage the kidneys, nervous system, lungs, skin, eyes, or mucous membranes
- Cause birth defects, miscarriages, and fertility problems from reproductive system damage

Exposure to hazardous substances can occur under normal working conditions. It also can happen during certain emergencies. Examples include equipment failures, container ruptures, or the uncontrolled release of a hazard into the workplace. Hazardous substances include:

- Drugs used in cancer therapy (chemotherapy, anti-cancer drugs)
- Anesthesia gases
- Gases used to sterilize equipment
- Oxygen
- Disinfectants and cleaning agents
- Radiation used for x-rays and cancer treatments
- Mercury (found in thermometers and blood pressure devices [Chapter 31])

OSHA requires a hazard communication program. The program includes container labeling, material safety data sheets (MSDSs), and employee training. The center also provides eyewash and total body wash stations in areas where hazardous substances are used.

Labeling

Hazardous substance containers include bags, barrels, bottles, boxes, cans, cylinders, drums, and storage tanks. All need warning labels (Fig. 12-15). The manufacturer supplies all labels. Warning labels identify:

- Physical and health hazards. Health hazards include the organs affected and potential health problems.
- Precaution measures. For example, "Do not use near open flame." Or "Avoid skin contact."
- What personal protective equipment to wear—gown, mask, gloves, goggles, and so on.
- How to use the substance safely.
- Storage and disposal information.

Words, pictures, and symbols communicate the warnings. A container must have a label. If a warning label is removed or damaged, do not use the substance. Take the container to the nurse, and explain the problem. Do not leave the container unattended.

Material Safety Data Sheets

Every hazardous substance has an MSDS. It provides detailed information about the substance:

- The chemical name and any common names
- The ingredients in the substance
- Physical and chemical characteristics (appearance, color, odor, boiling point, and others)
- Potential physical effects (fire, explosion)
- Conditions that could cause a chemical reaction
- How the chemical enters the body (inhalation, ingestion, skin contact, or absorption)
- Health hazards including signs and symptoms
- Protective measures (how to use, handle, and store the substance)
- Emergency and first aid procedures
- Explosion information and fire-fighting measures (including what type of fire extinguisher to use [p. 146])
- How to clean up a spill or leak
- Personal protective equipment needed during clean-up
- How to dispose of the hazardous substance
- Manufacturer information (name, address, and a telephone number for more information)

Employees must have ready access to MSDSs. They are in a binder at a certain place on each nursing unit. Some centers access the MSDS through the internet or an 800-hotline number (Fig. 12-16). Check the MSDS before using a hazardous substance, cleaning up a leak or spill, or disposing of the substance. Tell the nurse about a leak or spill right away. Do not leave a leak or spill unattended.

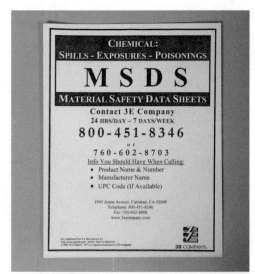

Fig. 12-16 The 800-hotline number for material safety data sheets (MSDSs) is posted.

Fig. 12-15 Warning labels on hazardous substances.

Box 12-6	Safety Measures for Hazardous Substances

- Read all warning labels.
- Follow the safety measures on the warning label and MSDS.
- Make sure each container has a warning label that is not damaged.
- Use a leak-proof container to carry or transport a hazardous substance.
- Wear personal protective equipment to clean spills and leaks. The warning label or MSDS tells you what to wear (mask, gown, gloves, eye protection, safety boots).
- Clean up spills at once. Work from clean areas to dirty areas using circular motions.
- Dispose of hazardous waste in sealed bags or containers.
- Stand behind a lead shield during x-ray or radiation therapy procedures.
- Do not enter a room while a person is having x-rays or radiation therapy.
- Wash your hands after handling hazardous substances.
- Work in well-ventilated areas to avoid inhaling gases.
- Store a hazardous substance according to the MSDS.

Employee Training

Your employer provides hazardous substance training. You are told about hazards, exposure risks, and protection measures. You learn to read and use warning labels and MSDSs.

Each hazardous substance requires certain protection measures. Box 12-6 lists general rules to safely handle hazardous substances.

FIRE SAFETY

Fire is a constant danger. Faulty electrical equipment and wiring, over-loaded electrical circuits, and smoking are major causes of fires. The entire health team must prevent fires. They must act quickly and responsibly during a fire.

Fire and the Use of Oxygen

Three things are needed for a fire:
- A spark or flame
- A material that will burn
- Oxygen

FOCUS ON COMMUNICATION
Fire and the Use of Oxygen

You may have to remind a resident or visitor not to smoke inside the center. You can simply say:
- "Mrs. Murphy, this is a smoke-free area. Here is an ashtray to put out your cigarette. If you want to smoke, I'll be happy to show you the smoking area outside."
- "Mr. Garcia, please don't smoke inside the center. We have a smoking area outside the back entrance on hallway 2. I'll be happy to show you the way."

Tell the nurse what happened, what you said, and what you did. The nurse may need to speak with the person about not smoking.

Air has some oxygen. However, some people need extra oxygen (Chapter 28). Safety measures are needed where oxygen is used and stored:
- "No Smoking" signs are placed on the door and near the bed.
- The person and visitors are reminded not to smoke in the room.
- Smoking materials (cigarettes, cigars, and pipes), matches, and lighters are removed from the room.
- Electrical items are turned off *before* being unplugged.
- Wool blankets and synthetic fabrics that cause static electricity are removed from the person's room.
- The person wears a cotton gown or pajamas.
- Electrical items are in good working order. This includes electric shavers, TVs, radios, computers, and other electronic devices.
- Lit candles, incense, and other open flames are not allowed.
- Materials that ignite easily are removed from the room. They include oil, grease, nail polish remover, and so on.

Centers have no-smoking policies and smoke-free areas. No smoking is allowed inside the buildings. Signs are posted on all entry doors. Some people ignore such rules. Remind them about the no-smoking rules.

See *Focus on Communication: Fire and the Use of Oxygen.*

Preventing Fires

Fire prevention measures were described in relation to burns, equipment accidents, and oxygen use. Other fire safety measures are listed in Box 12-7, p. 146.

Box 12-7   Fire Prevention Measures

- Follow the safety measures for oxygen use.
- Smoke only where allowed to do so. Do not smoke in residents' rooms.
- Be sure all ashes, cigars, cigarettes, and other smoking materials are out before emptying ashtrays.
- Empty ashtrays into a metal container partially filled with sand or water. Do not empty ashtrays into plastic containers or wastebaskets lined with paper or plastic bags.
- Provide ashtrays for persons who are allowed to smoke.
- Supervise persons who smoke. This is very important for persons who are confused, disoriented, or sedated.
- Follow safety practices when using electrical items.
- Keep matches, lighters, and flammable liquids and materials away from confused or disoriented persons.
- Do not leave cooking unattended on stoves, in ovens, or in microwave ovens.
- Store flammable liquids in their original containers. Keep the containers where residents cannot reach them.
- Do not smoke or light matches or lighters around flammable liquids or materials.
- Follow the safety measures to prevent equipment accidents (Box 12-4).

PROMOTING SAFETY AND COMFORT
What to Do During a Fire

Safety

Touch doors before opening them. Do not open a hot door. Use another way out of the room or building.

If your clothing is on fire, do not run. Drop to the floor or ground. Cover your face. Roll to smother flames. If another person's clothing is on fire, get the person to the floor or ground. Roll the person, or cover the person with a blanket, bedspread, or coat. This smothers the flames.

If smoke is present, cover your nose and mouth with a damp cloth. Do the same for residents, visitors, and other staff. Have everyone crawl to the nearest exit.

Do the following if you cannot get out of the building because of flames or smoke:

- Call 911 or the fire department. Tell the operator where you are. Give exact information: center name, address, phone number, and where you are in the building.
- Cover your nose and mouth with a damp cloth. Do the same for residents, visitors, and other staff.
- Move away from the fire. Go to a room with a window. Close the room door. Stuff wet towels, blankets, sheets, or bedspreads at the bottom of the door.
- Open the window.
- Hang something from the window (towel, sheet, blanket, clothing). This helps firefighters find you.

Rescue   Alarm   Confine   Extinguish

Fig. 12-17 During a fire, remember RACE: **R**escue, **A**larm, **C**onfine, and **E**xtinguish.

What to Do During a Fire

Know your center's policies and procedures for fire emergencies. Know where to find fire alarms, fire extinguishers, and emergency exits. Fire drills are held to practice emergency fire procedures. Remember the word *RACE* (Fig. 12-17):

- R—for *rescue.* Rescue persons in immediate danger. Move them to a safe place.
- A—for *alarm.* Sound the nearest fire alarm. Notify the operator.
- C—for *confine.* Close doors and windows to confine the fire. Turn off oxygen or electrical items used in the general area of the fire.
- E—for *extinguish.* Use a fire extinguisher on a small fire that has not spread to a larger area.

Clear equipment from all normal and emergency exits. *Do not use elevators if there is a fire.*

See *Promoting Safety and Comfort: What to Do During a Fire.*

Using a Fire Extinguisher

Centers require that all employees demonstrate use of a fire extinguisher. Different extinguishers are used for different kinds of fires:

- Oil and grease fires
- Electrical fires
- Paper and wood fires

A general procedure for using a fire extinguisher is presented. Remember the word *PASS* used by the National Fire Protection Association:

- *P*—for *pull the safety pin*. Doing so unlocks the handle on many types of fire extinguishers.
- *A*—for *aim low*. Direct the hose or nozzle at the base of the fire. Do not try to spray the tops of the flames.
- *S*—for *squeeze the lever*. Squeeze or push down on the lever, handle, or button to start the stream. Release the lever, handle, or button to stop the stream.
- *S*—for *sweep back and forth*. Sweep the stream back and forth (side to side) at the base of the fire.

 USING A FIRE EXTINGUISHER

PROCEDURE

1 Pull the fire alarm.
2 Get the nearest fire extinguisher.
3 Carry it upright.
4 Take it to the fire.
5 Follow the word *PASS*:
   a *P*—for *pull the safety pin* (Fig. 12-18, *A*). This unlocks the handle.
   b *A*—for *aim low* (Fig. 12-18, *B*). Direct the hose or nozzle at the base of the fire. Do not try to spray the tops of the flames.
   c *S*—for *squeeze the lever* (Fig. 12-18, *C*). Squeeze or push down on the lever, handle, or button to start the stream. Release the lever, handle, or button to stop the stream.
   d *S*—for *sweep back and forth* (Fig. 12-18, *D*). Sweep the stream back and forth (side to side) at the base of the fire.

Fig. 12-18 Using a fire extinguisher. **A,** *Pull* the safety pin. **B,** *Aim* the hose at the base of the fire. **C,** *Squeeze* the top handle down. **D,** *Sweep* back and forth.

Fig. 12-19 Swing-carry technique. **A,** Assist the person to a sitting position. A co-worker grasps the person's ankles as you both turn the person so that he sits on the side of the bed. **B,** Pull the person's arm over your shoulder. With one arm, reach across the person's back to your co-worker's shoulder. Reach under the person's knees and grasp your co-worker's arm. Your co-worker does the same.

Fig. 12-20 One-rescuer carry. **A,** Spread a blanket on the floor. Make sure the blanket will extend beyond the person's head. Assist the person to sit on the side of the bed. Grasp the person under the arms, and cross your hands over her chest. Lower the person to the floor by sliding her down one of your legs. **B,** Wrap the blanket around the person. Grasp the blanket over the head area. Pull the person to a safe area.

Evacuating Centers have evacuation policies and procedures. If evacuation is necessary, residents closest to the fire are taken out first. Those who can walk are given blankets to wrap around themselves. A staff member takes them to a safe place. Figures 12-19 and 12-20 show how to rescue persons who cannot walk. Once firefighters arrive, they direct rescue efforts.

DISASTERS

A disaster is a sudden catastrophic event. People are injured and killed. Property is destroyed. Natural disasters include tornadoes, hurricanes, blizzards, earthquakes, volcanic eruptions, floods, and some fires. Human-made disasters include auto, bus, train, and airplane accidents. They also include fires, bombings, nuclear power plant accidents, riots, gas or chemical leaks, explosions, and wars.

The center has procedures for disasters that could occur in your area. Follow them to keep residents, visitors, staff, and yourself safe.

Communities, fire and police departments, and health care agencies have disaster plans. They include procedures to deal with the people needing treatment. The plan generally provides for:

- Discharging residents who can go home
- Assigning staff and equipment to an emergency area
- Assigning staff to transport persons from treatment areas
- Calling off-duty staff to work

A disaster may damage the center. The disaster plan includes evacuation procedures.

Bomb Threats

Centers have procedures for bomb threats. You must follow them if a caller makes a bomb threat or if you find an item that looks or sounds strange. Often bomb threats are sent by phone, mail, e-mail, messenger, or other means. Or the person can leave a bomb in the center. If you see a stranger in the center, tell the nurse at once. You cannot be too safe.

WORKPLACE VIOLENCE

Workplace violence is violent acts (including assault or threat of assault) directed toward persons at work or while on duty. It includes:

- Murders
- Beatings, stabbings, and shootings
- Rapes and sexual assaults
- Use of weapons—firearms, bombs, or knives
- Kidnapping
- Robbery
- Threats—obscene phone calls; threatening oral, written, or body language; and harassment of any nature (being followed, sworn at, or shouted at)

Workplace violence can occur in any place where an employee performs a work-related duty. It can be a permanent or temporary place. This includes buildings, parking lots, field sites, homes, and travel to and from work assignments. Workplace violence can occur anywhere in the center.

According to OSHA, more assaults occur in health care settings than in other industries. Nurses and nursing assistants are at risk. They have the most contact with residents and visitors. Risk factors include:

- People with weapons.
- Police holds—persons arrested or convicted of crimes.
- Acutely disturbed and violent persons seeking health care.
- Alcohol and drug abuse.
- Mentally ill persons who do not take needed drugs, do not have follow-up care, and are not in hospitals unless they are an immediate threat to themselves or others.
- Pharmacies have drugs and are a target for robberies.
- Gang members and substance abusers are patients, residents, or visitors.
- Upset, agitated, and disturbed family and visitors.
- Long waits for emergency or other services.
- Being alone with the person during care or transport to other areas.
- Low staff levels during meals, emergencies, and at night.
- Poor lighting in hallways, rooms, parking lots, and other areas.
- Lack of training in recognizing and managing potentially violent situations.

OSHA has guidelines for violence prevention programs. The goal is to prevent or reduce employee exposure to situations that can cause death or injury. Worksite hazards are identified. Prevention measures are developed and followed. Also, employees receive safety and health training. You need to:

- Understand and follow your center's workplace violence prevention program.
- Understand and follow safety and security measures.
- Voice safety and security concerns.
- Report strange or suspicious persons right away.
- Report violent incidents promptly and accurately.
- Serve on health and safety committees that review workplace violence.
- Attend training programs that help you recognize and manage agitation, assaultive behavior, and criminal intent.

Box 12-8, p. 150 lists some measures to prevent or control workplace violence. Box 12-9, p. 151 lists personal safety practices. Follow them all the time. Complete an incident report (p. 153), as needed, for workplace violence.

The nurse assesses the behavior and the behavioral history of new and transferred residents. Restraints may be ordered if persons are a threat to themselves or others (Chapter 14). Persons with mental health problems are supervised as they move throughout the center. Aggressive and agitated persons are treated in open areas. Privacy and confidentiality are maintained. Security officers deal with agitated, aggressive, or disruptive persons.

Box 12-8 Measures to Prevent or Control Workplace Violence

Agitated or Aggressive Persons

- Stand away from the person. Judge the length of the person's arms and legs. Stand far enough away so that the person cannot hit or kick you.
- Stand close to the door. Do not become trapped in the room.
- Be aware of items in the room that can be used as weapons. Move away from such objects. Examples include vases, phones, radios, letter openers, paper weights, and belts.
- Know where to find panic buttons, signal lights, alarms, closed-circuit monitors, and other security devices.
- Keep your hands free.
- Stay calm. Talk to the person in a calm manner. Do not raise your voice or argue, scold, or interrupt the person.
- Be aware of your body language. Do not point a finger or glare at the person. Do not put your hands on your hips.
- Do not touch the person.
- Tell the person that you will get the nurse to speak to him or her.
- Leave the room as soon as you can. Make sure the person is safe.
- Tell the nurse or security officer about the matter. Report items in the room that can be used as weapons.

Safety Devices

- Alarm systems, closed-circuit video monitoring, panic buttons, hand-held alarms, wireless phones, two-way radios, and phone systems are installed (Fig. 12-21). These systems have a direct line to security staff or the police.
- Metal detectors are at entrances to identify guns, knives, or other weapons.
- Curved mirrors are at hallway intersections and hard-to-see areas.
- Bullet-resistant, shatter-proof glass is at nurses' stations.
- Staff do not turn off door alarms.
- Staff do not share security codes with anyone.

Weapons

- Jewelry and scarves that can serve as weapons are not worn. For example, a person can grab earrings and bracelets. Or a person can strangle someone with a necklace or scarf.
- Long hair is worn up and off the collar (Chapter 5). A person can pull long hair and cause head injuries.

Weapons—cont'd

- Keys, scissors, pens, or other items that can serve as weapons are not visible.
- Pictures, vases, and other items that can serve as weapons are few in number.
- Tools or items left by maintenance staff or visitors are removed if they can serve as weapons.

Family and Visitors

- Visitors sign in and receive a pass to access resident areas.
- Visiting hours and policies are enforced.
- A list of "restricted visitors" is made for residents with a history of violence or who are victims of violence.
- Waiting rooms and lounges are comfortable and reduce stress.
- Family and visitors are informed in a timely manner.

Building Safety and Security

- Unused doors are locked.
- Bright lights are inside and outside buildings.
- Broken lights, windows, and door locks are replaced or repaired.
- Staff restrooms lock and prevent access to visitors.
- Access to the pharmacy and drug storage areas is controlled.
- Furniture is placed to prevent entrapment. This includes furniture in resident rooms and in therapy areas, dining rooms, and lounges.
- Keys are not left unattended.

Staff Safety Measures

- Staff members are not alone when caring for persons with agitated or aggressive behaviors.
- Staff wear ID badges that prove employment.
- A "buddy system" is used when using elevators, stairways, restrooms, and low-traffic areas.
- Uniforms fit well. Tight uniforms limit running. An attacker can grab loose uniforms.
- Shoes have good soles. Shoes that cause slipping limit running.
- Vehicles are locked and in good repair.
- Security escort services are used for walking to vehicles, bus stops, or train stations.

Fig. 12-21 People entering and leaving the center are monitored on closed-circuit TV.

Box 12-9 Personal Safety Practices

General Measures

- Know the area where you are going. Ask questions about the area.
- Make a "dry run" of the area. Know the route in advance. The shortest route is not always the safest.
- Let someone know where you are at all times. Let someone know when you leave and when you arrive at your destination. If you do not call in when expected, the person knows something is wrong.
- Make it known that you do not carry drugs, needles, or syringes.
- Do not carry large amounts of money or valuables. Leave them at home or in the locked car trunk. If someone wants what you have, give it. The only thing of value is *you*.
- Carry wallets, purses, and backpacks safely. Men should carry wallets in an inside coat pocket or in a side pant pocket. Never carry a wallet in the rear pocket. Keep a firm grip on a purse. Keep it close to your body.
- Keep your wireless phone in your hand.
- Carry a whistle or shriek alarm.
- Avoid ATM machines at night.
- Be careful when getting on elevators and when entering stairways.
- Do not approach a stranger or someone acting in a suspicious manner. Report the matter right away.

Home Settings

- Keep doors and windows to the home locked at all times.
- Do not open doors to strangers. Ask for identification.
- Do not let a stranger into the home to use a phone or bathroom. Offer to call the police if the person needs help.
- Do not give personal information to callers or people at the door.

Car Safety

- Have plenty of gas in your car.
- Keep your car in good working order.
- Keep these in your car—local map, flashlight with working batteries, flares, a fire extinguisher, and a first aid kit.
- Raise the hood and use the flares if the car breaks down. Stay in the car. Call the police if you have a wireless phone. If someone stops by to help, ask that person to call the police.
- Lock your car. Sometimes you may want to leave it unlocked. If you need to get in the car fast, you do not want to fumble with keys. Use your judgment. Do not leave anything in the car if you leave it unlocked.
- Have your car key ready so you can get into the car quickly. Do not fumble for keys on the way to or at the car.
- Check under the car as you approach it. A person hiding under the car can grab your ankle or leg. Leave at once if someone is under the car. The person under the car may be working with a buddy who is waiting to attack you while you are being held or injured at the leg or ankle.
- Check the back seat before getting into the car. Make sure no one is in the car. Leave at once if someone is in the car.
- Lock car doors when you get in the car. Keep windows rolled up.

Car Safety—cont'd

- Do not open the car door or window to talk to a person approaching your car.
- Do not get out of the car to remove something from the windshield.
- Keep purses, backpacks, and other valuables under the seat or near your side. Do not leave them on the seat. They are easy targets for smash-and-grab robbers.
- Do not hitchhike or pick up hitchhikers.

Parking Your Car

- Check for places to park. Choose a well-lit area. If using a parking garage, park near entrances, exits, and on the lower level. Try to get close to the attendant if possible. The closest space to your destination is not always the safest for parking.
- Park your car so that you can leave quickly and easily. Park at street corners so no one can park in front of you. In parking lots, back in. You can see more from the front windshield than from the back window.

Walking

- Do not wear headphones or earbuds when walking. They keep you from hearing cars and people around you.
- Use well-lit and busy streets if you have to walk. Avoid vacant lots, alleys, wooded areas, and construction sites. The shortest way is not always the safest.
- Walk near the curb. Stay away from doorways, shrubs, and bushes.
- Note the location of phone booths. And carry a wireless phone. Know your location, and keep phone calls simple.
- Go to a police or fire station or a store if you think someone is following you.

Public Transportation

- Carry money for phone calls and for bus, train, or taxi fares. Have money in your pocket to avoid fumbling with a purse or wallet.
- Stand with others and near the ticket booth. Sit near the driver or conductor.
- Keep your wireless phone in your hand.

If You Are Threatened or Attacked

- Scream as loud and as long as you can. Keep screaming. Men and women should scream.
- Yell "FIRE," not "help." Most people will respond to "FIRE."
- Use your car keys as a weapon. Carry them in your strong hand. Have one key extended (Fig. 12-22, p. 152). Hold the key firmly. If you are attacked, go for the person's face. Slash the person's face with the key. Do not use poking motions. Do not try for a certain target because you might miss. Do not be shy—your attacker will not be.
- Remember, you have two arms, two hands, two feet, and two knees. You can attack from more than one direction at once. Do not be shy—your attacker will not be. Push, pull, yank, and so on. You can attack a man's or woman's genitals.
- Use your thumbs as weapons. Go for the eyes and push hard.
- Carry a travel size can of aerosol hair spray. Go for the face.

Fig. 12-22 A car key is used as a weapon.

Fig. 12-23 Color-coded wristbands. The alert is printed on the band.

RISK MANAGEMENT

Risk management involves identifying and controlling risks and safety hazards affecting the center. The intent is to:

- Protect everyone in the center—residents, visitors, and staff
- Protect center property from harm or danger
- Protect the person's valuables
- Prevent accidents and injuries

Risk management deals with these and other safety issues:

- Accident and fire prevention
- Negligence and malpractice
- Resident abuse
- Workplace violence
- Federal and state requirements

Risk managers work with all center departments. They look for patterns and trends in incident reports, resident complaints, staff complaints, and accident and injury investigations. Risk managers look for and correct unsafe situations. They also make procedure changes and training recommendations as needed.

Color-Coded Wristbands

Color-coded wristbands are used to promote the person's safety and prevent harm. They quickly communicate an alert or warning (Fig. 12-23). The type of alert is printed on the band. The printing is useful in dim lighting and for persons who are color blind. Many states use these three colors:

- Red—means an "allergy alert." Red is a warning to "stop." A red wristband is used to warn of allergies to food, drugs, treatment supplies such as tape or latex gloves, dust, plants, grass, and so on. Allergies are not listed on the wristband. Some persons have too many allergies to list on the wristband.
- Yellow—means a "fall risk." Yellow implies "caution." The person is at risk for falling. Yellow wristbands are used for persons with a history of falls. Or they are used for persons at risk for falls because of dizziness, balance problems, confusion, and so on. See Chapter 13.
- Purple—means the person has a "do not resuscitate" (DNR) order. See Chapter 48.

Some centers use other colors for other alerts. For example, pink is used for a "limb alert." This means that an arm or leg is not used for blood pressure measurements, blood draws, or intravenous infusions. To safely use color-coded wristbands:

- Know the wristband colors used in your center. Colors may vary among centers.
- Check the care plan and your assignment sheet when you see a color-coded wristband. You need to know the reason for the wristband and the care measures needed. Ask the nurse if you have questions.
- Do not confuse "social cause" bands with your center's color-coded wristbands. "Live Strong" is an example.
- Check for wristbands on persons transferred from another agency. That agency may use different colored wristbands. Or the colors' meanings may differ from those in your center. The nurse needs to remove wristbands from another agency.
- Tell the nurse if you think a person needs a color-coded wristband.

Personal Belongings

The person's belongings must be kept safe. Often they are sent home with the family. A personal belongings list is completed (Fig. 12-24). Each item is listed and described. The staff member and person sign the completed list.

A valuables envelope is used for jewelry and money. Each jewelry item is listed and described on the envelope. Describe what you see. For example, describe a ring as having a white stone with six prongs in a yellow setting. Do not assume the stone is a diamond in a gold setting. For valuables:

- Count money with the person.
- Put money and each jewelry item in the envelope with the person watching. Seal the envelope. Sign the envelope like a personal belongings list.
- Give the envelope to the nurse. The nurse takes it to the safe or sends it home with the family.

INVENTORY LIST

QTY.	ARTICLES	QTY.	APPLIANCES	QTY.	PROSTHETIC DEVICES	ACQUIRED AFTER ADMISSION
	Belts		T.V. - Ser. #:		Dentures: ☐ Upper	Date / Item
	Blouses		Radio - Ser. #:		☐ Lower ☐ Partial	
	Coats		Hair Dryer		Eye Wear	
	Dresses		Electric Razor		Cane	
	Gloves				Walker - Ser. #:	
	Hats				W/chair - Ser. #:	
	Housecoats - Robes		JEWELRY		Brace	
	Jackets		Ring (Describe)			
	Nightgowns - Pajamas					
	Purses		Watch (Describe)		OTHER	
	Shaving Kit					
	Shoes		Other			
	Shorts					
	Slacks					
	Slippers					
	Slips		FURNITURE			
	Socks/Hose					
	Suitcases					
	Suits				VALUABLES RELEASED FROM SAFE	
	Sweaters					
	Ties					
	Undershirts					
	Underwear					

(ON DISCHARGE)

I received on discharge in satisfactory condition the above articles and a copy of this list.
Disposition of belongings: _____

▶ _____   ▶ _____
Signature of Patient/Resp. Party   Date   Signature of Facility Representative   Date

NOTE ▶ Patient/Responsible Party is responsible for assuring that all personal belongings are properly marked. All items brought in after admission are added to this inventory at the request of Patient/Responsible Party.

QTY.	ARTICLES	QTY.	APPLIANCES	QTY.	PROSTHETIC DEVICES	ACQUIRED AFTER ADMISSION
	Belts		T.V. - Ser. #:		Dentures: ☐ Upper	Date / Item
	Blouses		Radio - Ser. #:		☐ Lower ☐ Partial	
	Coats		Hair Dryer		Eye Wear	
	Dresses		Electric Razor		Cane	
	Gloves				Walker - Ser. #:	
	Hats				W/chair - Ser. #:	
	Housecoats - Robes		JEWELRY		Brace	
	Jackets		Ring (Describe)			
	Nightgowns - Pajamas					
	Purses		Watch (Describe)		OTHER	
	Shaving Kit					
	Shoes		Other			
	Shorts					
	Slacks					
	Slippers					
	Slips		FURNITURE			
	Socks/Hose					
	Suitcases					
	Suits				VALUABLES LOCKED IN SAFE	
	Sweaters					
	Ties					
	Undershirts					
	Underwear					

(ON ADMISSION)

I certify that this is a correct list of my clothes and belongings which I wish to retain in my possession and for which I take ENTIRE RESPONSIBILITY. I have received a copy of this list.

▶ _____   ▶ _____
Signature of Patient/Resp. Party   Date   Signature of Facility Representative   Date

If the patient is unable to sign, state reason: _____
▶ Signature of Witness: _____

PATIENT NAME—LAST	FIRST	MIDDLE	HOSP. NO.	RO

INVENTORY LIST

Form 883/2   BRIGGS, Des Moines, Iowa 50306 PRINTED IN U.S.A.

Fig. 12-24 Personal belongings list. *(Courtesy Briggs Corp., Des Moines, Iowa.)*

Dentures, eyeglasses, hearing aids, watches, some jewelry, radios, computers, and other electronic devices are kept at the bedside. Items kept at the bedside are listed in the person's record. Some people keep money for newspapers and personal items. The amount kept is noted in the person's record.

Clothing and shoes are labeled with the person's name. So are other items brought from home.

Reporting Incidents

An **incident** is any event that has harmed or could harm a resident, visitor, or staff member. It includes accidents and errors in giving care. See Box 12-10, p. 154 for examples.

Report accidents and errors at once. This includes:
- Accidents involving residents, visitors, or staff.
- Errors in care. This includes giving the wrong care, giving care to the wrong person, or not giving care.
- Broken or lost items owned by the person. Dentures, hearing aids, and eyeglasses are examples.
- Lost money or clothing.
- Hazardous substance incidents.
- Workplace violence incidents.

An *incident report* is completed as soon as possible after the incident. The following information is required:

- Names of those involved
- Date and time of the accident or error
- Location of the accident or error
- A complete description of what happened
- Names of witnesses
- Any other requested information

Not part of the medical record, incident reports are reviewed by risk management and a committee of health care workers. They look for patterns and trends of accidents or errors. For example, are falls occurring on the same shift and on the same unit? Are lost or missing items being reported on the same shift or same unit? Are residents being injured on the same shift or same unit? There may be new policies and procedures to prevent future incidents.

Box 12-10   Common Incidents

- A resident's dentures are found broken in the laundry.
- A confused resident is found sleeping in bed with another resident.
- An agitated resident strikes another person.
- A resident is sitting on the porch of a house four blocks from the center.
- A resident is sleeping in a visitor's car.
- A visitor slips and falls on a wet floor.
- A housekeeper drops and breaks a resident's clock while dusting.
- A resident is found sitting on the floor by the bed.
- A nurse gives the wrong drug to a resident.
- A resident is burned while taking a bath.
- A resident drops a hearing aid into the toilet.
- A resident suffers a skin tear while resisting staff efforts to assist with dressing.
- A nursing assistant wears a ring with a large stone. A resident is scratched during care.
- A resident bites a staff member.
- A nurse leaves a needle on a resident's bed. A nursing assistant receives a needle-stick injury when making the bed.
- A resident is given the wrong meal tray. The error is found after the person is done eating.
- The maintenance staff left tools in a resident's room. The person is injured on the tools.
- A resident is bruised from a restraint.
- A resident falls in the hallway.
- A resident was not re-positioned for 6 hours. A pressure ulcer develops.
- A nursing assistant receives an electrical shock from a bed.
- A resident's dentures drop and break.
- Visitors are shouting in the hallway. Security is called.
- A resident reports missing money and jewelry.

QUALITY OF LIFE

Most accidents can be prevented. Remember, persons who are older and disabled are at great risk for accidents. To promote safety:

- Know the common safety hazards
- Know the causes of accidents
- Know who you need to protect
- Use common sense

The entire health team must provide a safe setting. You may see something unsafe. Do what you can to correct the matter.

Chronic illness, advanced age, disability, drugs, strange settings, and special equipment increase a person's risk for injury. Practice safety measures. Use safety devices as needed. Follow the person's care plan to give safe care.

Always identify the person before giving care. You can threaten a person's life and health if you give the wrong care or omit care. Use the ID bracelet to correctly identify the person. Two residents could have the same last name. Some may have the same first and last names.

To prevent fires, follow the safety measures for smoking and electrical items. Extra measures are needed when oxygen is used. Residents who smoke present fire safety concerns. Ask the nurse if the person can have smoking materials at the bedside. Know where to find fire alarms, fire extinguishers, and emergency exits. Also know your center's procedure for a fire.

Follow procedures for handling hazardous substances. Physical hazards can cause fires and explosions. Some chemicals can cause acute or chronic health problems.

Workplace violence is a danger in health care settings. Practice measures to prevent and control workplace violence. Everyone must keep the center safe for residents, visitors, and staff.

REVIEW QUESTIONS

Circle the BEST answer.

1 Who provides a safe setting for residents and visitors?
   a The health team   c The administrator
   b The nursing team   d The risk manager
2 Which is *not* a risk factor for accidents?
   a Needing eyeglasses
   b Hearing problems
   c Memory problems
   d Oriented to person, time, and place
3 A person in a coma
   a Has suffered an electrical shock
   b Has dementia
   c Is unaware of surroundings
   d Has stopped breathing
4 A person with dementia
   a Cannot think and reason
   b Is not aware of his or her surroundings
   c Is paralyzed
   d Has suffered an electrical shock

REVIEW QUESTIONS—cont'd

5 A person with dementia
 a Is at high risk for accidents and injuries
 b Knows what is safe
 c Knows when to move away from danger
 d Is agitated and aggressive

6 A person with quadriplegia is paralyzed
 a From the waist down
 b From the neck down
 c On the right side of the body
 d On the left side of the body

7 To identify a person, you
 a Call the person by name
 b Ask the person his or her name
 c Compare information on the ID bracelet against your assignment sheet
 d Ask both roommates their names

8 Burns are caused by the following *except*
 a Smoking   c Very hot bath water
 b Spilled hot liquids   d Oxygen

9 Safety measures to prevent poisoning include the following *except*
 a Keeping harmful products in low storage areas
 b Keeping child-resistant caps on harmful products
 c Making sure all harmful products have labels
 d Storing harmful products away from food

10 Which can cause suffocation?
 a Reporting loose teeth or dentures
 b Using electrical items that are in good repair
 c Cutting food into small, bite-size pieces
 d Restraints

11 The most common cause of choking in adults is
 a A loose denture   c Marbles
 b Meat   d Candy

12 If severe airway obstruction occurs, the person usually
 a Clutches at the throat
 b Can speak, cough, and breathe
 c Is calm
 d Has a seizure

13 These statements are about relieving FBAO. Which is *false*?
 a Abdominal thrusts can be self-administered.
 b A person is pregnant. Give abdominal thrusts.
 c Injuries can occur from abdominal or chest thrusts.
 d CPR is started if the responsive victim loses consciousness.

14 You need to shave a new resident. Before using the person's electric shaver
 a You need to inspect it
 b The maintenance staff must do a safety check
 c You need to check for a frayed cord
 d You need an electrical outlet

15 You are using equipment. Which measure is *not* safe?
 a Following the manufacturer's instructions
 b Keeping electrical items away from water and spills
 c Pulling on the cord to remove a plug from an outlet
 d Turning off electrical items after using them

16 A person uses a wheelchair. Which measure is *not* safe?
 a The wheels are locked for transfers.
 b The chair is pulled backward to transport the person.
 c The feet are positioned on the footplates.
 d The casters point forward.

17 Stretcher safety involves the following *except*
 a Locking the wheels for transfers
 b Fastening the safety straps
 c Raising the side rails
 d Moving the stretcher head first

18 You spilled a hazardous substance. You should do the following *except*
 a Read the material safety data sheet
 b Cover the spill and go tell the nurse
 c Wear personal protective equipment to clean up the spill
 d Complete an incident report

19 The fire alarm sounds. The following is done *except*
 a Turning off oxygen
 b Using elevators
 c Closing doors and windows
 d Moving residents to a safe place

20 Your clothing is on fire. You should do the following *except*
 a Run to get help   c Cover your face
 b Drop to the floor   d Roll to smother the
   or ground   flames

21 A severe weather alert was issued for your area. What should you do?
 a Take cover.
 b Follow the center's disaster plan.
 c Make sure your family is safe.
 d Pull the fire alarm.

22 A person is agitated and aggressive. You should do the following *except*
 a Stand away from the person
 b Stand close to the door
 c Use touch to show you care
 d Talk to the person without raising your voice

23 A person has a yellow wristband. This means that the person
 a Is at risk for bleeding   c Is at risk for falling
 b Has an allergy   d Has an acute illness

24 You work the night shift. Which is *unsafe*?
 a Parking in a well-lit area
 b Locking your car
 c Finding your keys after getting into the car
 d Checking under the car and in your back seat

25 A resident brought a radio from home. Which helps prevents property loss?
 a Completing a personal belongings list
 b Labeling the item with the person's name
 c Putting the item in a safe
 d Using a wheelchair pouch for the item

26 You gave a person the wrong treatment. Which is *true*?
 a Report the error at the end of the shift.
 b Take action only if the person was injured.
 c You are guilty of negligence.
 d You must complete an incident report.

Answers to these questions are on p. 719.

CHAPTER 13

Preventing Falls

OBJECTIVES

- Define the key terms listed in this chapter.
- Identify the causes and risk factors for falls.
- Describe the safety measures that help prevent falls.
- Explain how to use bed rails safely.
- Explain the purpose of hand rails and grab bars.
- Explain how to use wheel locks safely.
- Describe how to use transfer/gait belts.
- Explain how to help the person who is falling.
- Perform the procedures described in this chapter.
- Explain how to promote quality of life.

KEY TERMS

bed rail A device that serves as a guard or barrier along the side of the bed; side rail

gait belt See "transfer belt"

transfer belt A device used to support a person who is unsteady or disabled; gait belt

KEY ABBREVIATIONS

CMS Centers for Medicare & Medicaid Services

OBRA Omnibus Budget Reconciliation Act of 1987

The risk of falling increases with age. Often falling is a sign of other health problems. Persons older than 65 years are at risk. A history of falls increases the risk of falling again. Falls are the most common accidents in nursing centers.

According to the Centers for Disease Control and Prevention (CDC):

- About 1800 nursing center residents die each year from falls.
- Nursing center falls can cause serious injury including fractures. Fractures of the spine, hip, forearm, leg, ankle, pelvis, upper arm, and hand are the most common. Hip fractures and head trauma increase the risk of death.
- Falls result in disability, decline in function, and reduced quality of life.
- Fear of falling can cause further loss of function, depression, feelings of helplessness, and social isolation. This may increase the person's risk of falling again.

CAUSES AND RISK FACTORS FOR FALLS

Most falls occur in resident rooms and bathrooms. Poor lighting, cluttered floors, incorrect bed height, and out-of-place furniture are causes. So are wet and slippery floors, bathtubs, and showers. Wheelchairs can cause falls if they do not fit the person or are in poor repair. Needing to use the bathroom, usually to urinate, is a major cause of falls. For example, Mrs. Hines has an urgent need to urinate. She falls trying to get to the bathroom.

Most falls occur between 1600 (4:00 PM) and 2000 (8:00 PM). Falls also are more likely during shift changes. During shift changes, staff are busy going off and coming on duty. Confusion can occur about who gives care and answers signal lights. Shift changes vary among centers. They often occur between these hours:

- 0600 (6:00 AM) and 0800 (8:00 AM)
- 1400 (2:00 PM) and 1600 (4:00 PM)
- 2200 (10:00 PM) and 2400 (midnight)

The accident risk factors described in Chapter 12 can lead to falls. The problems listed in Box 13-1 also increase a person's risk of falling.

See *Teamwork and Time Management: Causes and Risk Factors for Falls.*

Box 13-1   Factors Increasing the Risk of Falls

Care Setting
- Bed: incorrect height
- Care equipment: IV (Intravenous) poles, drainage tubes and bags, and others
- Cluttered floors
- Furniture out of place
- Lighting: poor
- Setting: strange and unfamiliar
- Throw rugs
- Wet and slippery floors, bathtubs, and showers
- Wheelchairs, walkers, canes, and crutches: improper use or fit

The Person
- Alcohol: over-use
- Balance problems
- Blood pressure: low or high
- Confusion
- Depression
- Disorientation
- Dizziness; dizziness on standing
- Drug side effects
  - Low blood pressure when standing or sitting
  - Drowsiness
  - Fainting
  - Dizziness
  - Coordination: poor
  - Unsteadiness
  - Urination: frequent
  - Diarrhea
  - Confusion and disorientation
- Elimination needs
- Falls: history of
- Foot problems
- Incontinence: urinary and fecal
- Joint pain and stiffness
- Judgment: poor
- Light-headedness
- Memory problems
- Mobility: decreased
- Muscle weakness
- Reaction time: slow
- Shoes that fit poorly
- Vision problems
- Weakness

TEAMWORK AND TIME MANAGEMENT
Causes and Risk Factors for Falls

The entire health team must protect the person from harm. If you see something unsafe, tell the nurse at once. Do not assume the nurse knows or that someone is tending to the matter.

Answer all signal lights promptly. This includes the signal lights of residents assigned to co-workers.

Know your role during shift changes. Nursing staff going off duty and those of the on-coming shift must work together to prevent falls.

FALL PREVENTION PROGRAMS

Nursing centers have fall prevention programs. The measures listed in Box 13-2 are part of such programs and the person's care plan. The care plan also lists measures for the person's specific risk factors.

Common sense and simple safety measures can prevent many falls. The health team works with the person and family to reduce the risk of falls. The goal is to prevent falls without decreasing the person's quality of life.

See *Focus on Communication: Fall Prevention Programs*.

See *Promoting Safety and Comfort: Fall Prevention Programs*.

Box 13-2   Safety Measures to Prevent Falls

Basic Needs
- Fluid needs are met.
- Eyeglasses and hearing aids are worn as needed. Reading glasses are not worn when up and about.
- Tasks are explained before and while performing them.
- Help is given with elimination needs. It is given at regular times and whenever requested. Assist the person to the bathroom. Or provide the bedpan, urinal, or commode.
- The bedpan, urinal, or commode is kept within easy reach if the person can use the device without help.
- A warm drink, soft lights, or a back massage is used to calm the person who is agitated.
- Barriers are used to prevent wandering (Fig. 13-1).
- The person is properly positioned when in bed, a chair, or a wheelchair. Use pillows, wedge pads, or seats as the nurse and care plan direct (Chapter 16).
- Correct procedures are used for transfers (Chapter 17).
- The person is involved in meaningful activities.
- Exercise programs are followed. They help improve balance, strength, walking, and physical function.

Bathrooms and Shower/Tub Rooms
- Tubs and showers have non-slip surfaces or non-slip bath mats.
- Grab bars (safety bars) are in showers. They also are by tubs and toilets.
- Bathrooms have grab bars.
- Shower chairs are used (Chapter 20).
- Safety measures for tub baths and showers are followed (Chapter 20).

Floors
- Carpeting (if used) is wall-to-wall or tacked down.
- Scatter, area, and throw rugs are not used.
- Floor covers are one color. Bold designs can cause dizziness in older persons.
- Floors have non-glare, non-slip surfaces.
- Non-skid wax is used on hardwood, tiled, or linoleum floors.
- Loose floor boards and tiles are reported. So are frayed rugs and carpets.
- Floors and stairs are free of clutter, cords, and other items that can cause tripping.
- Floors are free of spills. Wipe up spills at once. Put a "Wet Floor" sign by the wet area.
- Floors are free of excess furniture and equipment.
- Electrical and extension cords are out of the way. This includes power strips.
- Equipment and supplies are kept on one side of the hallway.

Furniture
- Furniture is placed for easy movement.
- Furniture is kept in place. It is not re-arranged.
- Chairs have armrests. Armrests give support when standing or sitting.
- A phone, lamp, and personal belongings are within the person's reach.

Beds and Other Equipment
- The bed is at the correct height for the person.
- The bed is in the lowest horizontal position, except when giving bedside care. The distance from the bed to the floor is reduced if the person falls or gets out of bed.
- Bed rails are used according to the care plan (p. 160).
- A mattress, special mat, or floor cushion is placed on the floor beside the bed (Fig. 13-2, p. 160). This reduces the chance of injury if the person falls or gets out of bed.
- Wheelchairs, walkers, canes, and crutches fit properly. They are in good repair. Another person's equipment is not used.
- Crutches, canes, and walkers have non-skid tips.
- Correct equipment is used for transfers (Chapter 17). Follow the care plan.
- Positioning devices are used as directed (Chapter 16).
- Wheelchair and stretcher safety is followed (Chapter 12).
- Wheel locks on beds (p. 162), wheelchairs, and stretchers are in working order.
- Bed and wheelchair or stretcher wheels are locked for transfers.
- Linens are checked for sharp objects and for the person's property (dentures, eyeglasses, hearing aids, and so on).

Lighting
- Rooms, hallways, and stairways have good lighting. So do bathrooms and shower/tub rooms.
- Light switches (including those in bathrooms) are within reach and easy to find.
- Night-lights are in bedrooms, hallways, and bathrooms.

Shoes and Clothing
- Non-skid footwear is worn. Socks, bedroom slippers, and long shoelaces are avoided.
- Clothing fits properly. Clothing is not loose. It does not drag on the floor. Belts are tied or secured in place.

Box 13-2   Safety Measures to Prevent Falls—cont'd

Signal Lights and Alarms

- The person is taught how to use the signal light (Chapter 18).
- The signal light is always within the person's reach. This includes when sitting in the chair, on the commode, and when in the bathroom and tub/shower room.
- The person is asked to call for assistance when help is needed:
  - When getting out of bed or a chair
  - With walking
  - With getting to or from the bathroom or commode
  - With getting on or off the bedpan
- Signal lights are answered promptly. The person may need help right away. He or she may not wait for help.
- Bed, chair, door, floor mat, and belt alarms are used. They sense when the person tries to get up, get out of bed, or open a door (Fig. 13-3, p. 160).
- Alarms are responded to at once.

Other

- Color-coded alerts are used to warn of a fall risk. Yellow is the common color for a fall alert. Besides wristbands (Chapter 12), some centers also use color-coded blankets, non-skid footwear, socks, and magnets or stickers to place on room doors.
- The person is checked often. This may be every 15 minutes or as required by the care plan. Careful and frequent observation is important.

Other—cont'd

- Frequent checks are made on persons with poor judgment or memory. This may be every 15 minutes or as required by the care plan.
- Persons at risk for falling are close to the nurses' station.
- Hand rails are on both sides of stairs and hallways.
- The person uses hand rails when walking or using stairs.
- The person uses grab bars in bathrooms and shower/tub rooms.
- Family and friends are asked to visit during busy times. Mealtimes and shift changes are examples. They also are asked to visit during the evening and night shifts.
- Companions are provided. Sitters, companions, or volunteers are with the person.
- Non-slip strips are on the floor next to the bed and in the bathroom. They are intact.
- Caution is used when turning corners, entering corridor intersections, and going through doors. You could injure a person coming from the other direction.
- Pull (do not push) wheelchairs, stretchers, carts, and other wheeled equipment through doorways. This allows you to lead the way and to see where you are going.
- A safety check is made of the room after visitors leave. (See the inside of the front book cover.) They may have lowered a bed rail, removed a signal light, or moved a walker out of reach. Or they may have brought an item that could harm the person.

FOCUS ON COMMUNICATION
Fall Prevention Programs

Often falls occur when the person tries to get needed items. The person has to reach too far and falls out of bed or from a chair. Or the person tries to get up without help. Prevent falls by asking the person these questions:

- "What things would you like near you?"
- "Can I move this closer to you?"
- "Can you reach the signal light?"
- "Can you reach your cane?" (Walker and wheelchair are other examples.)
- "Do you need to use the bathroom now?"
- "Is there anything else you need before I leave the room?"

PROMOTING SAFETY AND COMFORT
Fall Prevention Programs

Safety

Some people are visually impaired or blind. Besides the measures in Box 13-2, other safety measures are needed to protect them from falling. See Chapter 37.

Fig. 13-1 Barriers are used to prevent wandering.

Fig. 13-2 Floor cushion. *(Image Courtesy Posey Company, Arcadia, Calif.)*

Fig. 13-4 Bed rails. The far bed rail is raised. The near bed rail is lowered.

Fig. 13-3 Chair alarm. *(Image courtesy Posey Company, Arcadia, Calif.)*

Bed Rails

A **bed rail** *(side rail)* is a device that serves as a guard or barrier along the side of the bed. Bed rails are raised and lowered (Fig. 13-4). They lock in place with levers, latches, or buttons. Bed rails are half, three quarters, or the full length of the bed. When half-length rails are used, each side may have two rails. One is for the upper part of the bed, the other for the lower part.

The nurse and care plan tell you when to raise bed rails. They are needed by persons who are unconscious or sedated with drugs. Some confused or disoriented people need them. If a person needs bed rails, keep them up at all times except when giving bedside nursing care.

Bed rails present hazards. The person can fall when trying to climb over them. Or the person cannot get out of bed or use the bathroom. *Entrapment* is a risk (Chapter 18). That is, the person can get caught, trapped, entangled, or strangled.

Bed rails prevent the person from getting out of bed. They are considered restraints by the Omnibus Budget Reconciliation Act of 1987 (OBRA) and the Centers for Medicare & Medicaid Services (CMS) if:

- The person cannot get out of bed
- The person cannot lower them without help

Bed rails cannot be used unless needed to treat a person's medical symptoms. Some people feel safer with bed rails up. Others use them to change positions in bed. The person or legal representative must give consent for raised bed rails. The need for bed rails is carefully noted in the person's medical record and the care plan.

Accrediting agency standards and federal and state laws affect bed rail use. They are allowed when the person's condition requires them. Bed rails must be in the person's best interests.

The procedures in this book include using bed rails. This helps you learn to use them correctly. The nurse, the care plan, and your assignment sheet tell you which people use bed rails. If a person does not use them, omit the "raise bed rails" or "lower bed rails" steps.

If a person uses bed rails, check the person often. Report to the nurse that you checked the person. If you are allowed to chart, record when you check the person and your observations (Fig. 13-5).

See *Promoting Safety and Comfort: Bed Rails.*

Date	Time	Nursing Margin	Other Depts Margin		
11/10	0900	I turned Mr. Adams from his back to his L side. One pillow placed under his head, one against his back, and one supporting his R leg. Full bed rails raised according to the care plan. Bed lowered to its lowest position. Water pitcher and filled water glass c̄ straw placed on the overbed table within Mr. Adam's reach. Phone and box of tissue on the bedside table within reach. Urinal hung on the bed rail per Mr. Adam's request. Signal light attached to the bed rail within reach. Mr. Adams states he is comfortable and that needed items are within his reach. I told him that I would be checking on him every 15 minutes and that he should use the signal light if he needed anything. Gwen Rider, CNA.			

Fig. 13-5 Charting sample.

PROMOTING SAFETY AND COMFORT
Bed Rails

Safety
You raise the bed to give care. Follow these safety measures to prevent the person from falling:
- *For a person who uses bed rails.* Always raise the far bed rail if you are working alone. Raise both bed rails if you need to leave the bedside for any reason.
- *For the person who does not use bed rails.* Ask a co-worker to help you. The co-worker stands on the far side of the bed. This protects the person from falling.
- Never leave the person alone when the bed is raised.
- Always lower the bed to its lowest position when you are done giving care.

Comfort
The person has to reach over raised bed rails for items on the bedside stand and overbed table. Such items include the water pitcher and cup, tissues, phone, and TV and light controls. Adjust the overbed table so it is within the person's reach. Ask if the person wants other items nearby. Place them on the overbed table too. Always make sure needed items, including the signal light, are within the person's reach.

Hand Rails and Grab Bars

Hand rails are in hallways and stairways (Fig. 13-6). They give support to persons who are weak or unsteady when walking.

Grab bars (safety bars) are in bathrooms and in shower/tub rooms (Fig. 13-7, p. 162). They provide support for sitting down or getting up from a toilet. They also are used for getting in and out of the shower or tub.

Fig. 13-6 Hand rails provide support when walking.

Fig. 13-7 Grab bars in a shower.

Fig. 13-8 Lock on a bed wheel.

Fig. 13-9 Transfer/gait belt. The belt buckle is positioned off center. Excess strap is tucked under the belt. The nursing assistant grasps the belt from underneath.

Wheel Locks

Bed legs have wheels. They let the bed move easily. Each wheel has a lock to prevent the bed from moving (Fig. 13-8). Wheels are locked at all times except when moving the bed. Make sure bed wheels are locked:

- When giving bedside care
- When you transfer a person to and from the bed

Wheelchair and stretcher wheels also are locked during transfers (Chapters 12 and 17). You or the person can be injured if the bed, wheelchair, or stretcher moves.

TRANSFER/GAIT BELTS

A **transfer belt (gait belt)** is a device used to support a person who is unsteady or disabled (Fig. 13-9). It helps prevent falls and injuries. When used to transfer a person (Chapter 17), it is called a *transfer belt*. When used to help a person walk, it is called a *gait belt*.

The belt goes around the person's waist. Grasp under the belt to support the person during the transfer or when assisting the person to walk.

See *Promoting Safety and Comfort: Transfer/Gait Belts.*

PROMOTING SAFETY AND COMFORT
Transfer/Gait Belts

Safety

Transfer/gait belts are routinely used in nursing centers. If the person needs help, a belt is required. To use one safely, always follow the manufacturer's instructions.

Some transfer/gait belts have a quick-release buckle. Position the quick-release buckle at the person's back where he or she cannot reach it. This prevents the person from releasing the buckle during the procedure. Injury could result if the buckle is released.

Do not leave excess strap dangling. Tuck the excess strap under the belt.

Remove the belt after the procedure. Do not leave the person alone while he or she is wearing a transfer/gait belt.

Using a transfer/gait belt is unsafe for some persons. The belt could cause pressure or rub against care equipment. Check with the nurse and the care plan before using a transfer/gait belt if the person has:

- An ostomy—colostomy, ileostomy, urostomy (Chapters 23 and 42).

Safety—cont'd

- A gastrostomy tube (Chapter 25).
- Chronic obstructive pulmonary disease (Chapter 40).
- An abdominal wound, incision, or drainage tube (Chapter 35).
- A chest wound, incision, or drainage tube (Chapter 29).
- Monitoring equipment.
- A hernia–part of an organ that protrudes or projects through an opening in a muscle wall. Hernias often involve a loop of bowel or the stomach.
- Other conditions or care equipment involving the chest or abdomen.

Comfort

A transfer belt is always applied over clothing. It is never applied over bare skin. Also, it is applied under the breasts. Breasts must not be caught under the belt. The belt buckle is never positioned over the person's spine.

 APPLYING A TRANSFER/GAIT BELT

QUALITY OF LIFE

Remember to:
- Knock before entering the person's room.
- Address the person by name.
- Introduce yourself by name and title.

- Explain the procedure to the person before beginning and during the procedure.
- Protect the person's rights during the procedure.
- Handle the person gently during the procedure.

PROCEDURE

1 See *Promoting Safety and Comfort: Transfer/Gait Belts.*
2 Practice hand hygiene.
3 Identify the person. Check the identification (ID) bracelet against the assignment sheet. Also call the person by name.
4 Provide for privacy.
5 Assist the person to a sitting position.
6 Apply the belt around the person's waist over clothing. Do not apply it over bare skin.
7 Secure the buckle. The buckle is in front.

8 Tighten the belt so it is snug. It should not cause discomfort or impair breathing. You should be able to slide your open, flat hand under the belt.
9 Make sure that a woman's breasts are not caught under the belt.
10 Turn the belt so the quick-release buckle is at the person's back. The buckle is not over the spine.
11 Tuck any excess strap under the belt.

THE FALLING PERSON

A person may start to fall when standing or walking. The person may be weak, light-headed, or dizzy. Fainting may occur. See p. 157 for the risk factors for falls.

Do not try to prevent the fall. You could injure yourself and the person while twisting and straining to prevent the fall. Balance is lost as the person falls. If you try to prevent the fall, you could lose your balance. Thus both you and the person could fall or cause the other person to fall. Head, wrist, arm, hip, knee, and other injuries could occur.

If a person starts to fall, ease him or her to the floor. This lets you control the direction of the fall. You can also protect the person's head. Do not let the person move or get up before the nurse checks for injuries. Calmly explain that the nurse will check for injuries such as broken bones.

If you find a person on the floor, do not move the person. Stay with the person, and call for the nurse.

An incident report is completed after all falls. The nurse may ask you to help with the report.

See *Residents With Dementia: The Falling Person*, p. 164.

HELPING THE FALLING PERSON

PROCEDURE

1   Stand behind the person with your feet apart. Keep your back straight.
2   Bring the person close to your body as fast as possible. Use the transfer/gait belt (Fig. 13-10, *A*). Or wrap your arms around the person's waist. If necessary (but not preferred), you can also hold the person under the arms.
3   Move your leg so the person's buttocks rest on it (Fig. 13-10, *B*). Move the leg near the person.
4   Lower the person to the floor. The person slides down your leg to the floor (Fig. 13-10, *C*). Bend at your hips and knees as you lower the person.
5   Call a nurse to check the person. Stay with the person.
6   Help the nurse return the person to bed. Ask other staff to help if needed.

POST-PROCEDURE

7   Provide for comfort. (See the inside of the front book cover.)
8   Place the signal light within reach.
9   Raise or lower bed rails. Follow the care plan.
10   Complete a safety check of the room. (See the inside of the front book cover.)
11   Report and record the following:
   • How the fall occurred
   • How far the person walked
   • How activity was tolerated before the fall
   • Complaints before the fall
   • How much help the person needed while walking
12   Complete an incident report.

Fig. 13-10 The falling person. **A,** The falling person is supported with the gait belt. **B,** The person's buttocks rest on the nursing assistant's leg. **C,** The person is eased to the floor on nursing assistant's leg.

RESIDENTS WITH DEMENTIA
The Falling Person

Some older persons are confused. A confused person may not understand why you do not want him or her to move or get up after a fall. Forcing a person not to move may injure the person and you. You may need to let the person move for his or her safety and your own. Never use force to hold a person down. Stay calm, and protect the person from injury. Talk to the person in a quiet, soothing voice. Call for help.

QUALITY OF LIFE

Older persons have fragile bones that break easily. The risk of a fracture is great. A fall can seriously affect a person's quality of life. For example: Ms. Polk has a broken wrist from a fall. She cannot fasten undergarments, button her blouse, pull up her pants, or tie her shoes. She cannot wipe herself after urinating or having a bowel movement. She depends on others to help her.

QUALITY OF LIFE—cont'd

You must help prevent falls. However, you must not interfere with the person's rights. Sometimes preventing falls and the right to personal choice are in conflict. For example, Ms. Polk wants to wear socks without non-skid footwear. The socks could cause her to slip and fall. You need to respect her choice, but explain why it is best to wear shoes too. Then have her choose what shoes to wear.

Sometimes safety measures to prevent falls are time consuming. Perhaps you cannot find a transfer belt. Or you need to get a walker. Or you must put on the person's shoes. Resist the urge to take short cuts. Take the time to:
- Find and use assistive devices.
- Put proper footwear on the person.
- Raise or lower the bed and side rails as appropriate.
- Lock wheels on beds, stretchers, and wheelchairs.
- Ask others to help if needed.

Residents have the right to feel safe. Fear of falling does not make a person feel safe. Before moving a person, explain what you are going to do and what he or she needs to do. Also give step-by-step instructions as you progress. Do not move the person without telling him or her first. These measures help increase the person's comfort. See Chapter 17 for how to safely handle, move, and transfer the person. Good communication promotes comfort. It supports the person's right to safety and security.

Some persons may feel restricted by the use of safety devices. They may feel it limits their independence. For example, Ms. Mills does not like having her bed rails up. She says: "I feel trapped. Do those have to be up?" Ms. Mills has fallen out of bed at night. The care plan includes having bed rails up while she is in bed.

Listen to the person's concerns. Kindly explain the reason for the safety device. If the person still refuses, tell the nurse. Do not let the person talk you out of performing a safety measure or using a safety device. Safety is always a priority.

REVIEW QUESTIONS

Circle the BEST answer.

1 Most falls occur in
  a Resident rooms and bathrooms
  b Dining rooms
  c Lounges
  d Hallways

2 Most falls occur
  a In the morning   c In the afternoon
  b At lunch time   d During the evening

3 A person's care plan includes fall prevention measures. Which should you question?
  a Assist with elimination needs.
  b Keep phone, lamp, and TV controls within reach.
  c Check the person every 2 hours.
  d Complete a safety check after visitors leave the room.

4 You observe the following in the person's room. Which is *not* safe?
  a The lamp cord is by the chair.
  b The chair has armrests.
  c The night-light works.
  d The bed is in the lowest horizontal position.

5 You note the following after a person got dressed. Which is safe?
  a The person is wearing non-skid shoes.
  b Pant cuffs are dragging on the floor.
  c The belt is not fastened.
  d The shirt is too big.

6 A co-worker is helping Mr. Polk today. His chair alarm goes off. What should you do?
  a Find your co-worker.
  b Tell the nurse.
  c Assist Mr. Polk.
  d Wait for someone to respond to the alarm.

7 To help prevent falls, you need to report
  a Equipment and supplies being on one side of the hallway
  b A mattress on the floor beside the bed
  c A co-worker pulling a wheelchair through a doorway
  d Clutter on stairways

8 Bed rails are used
  a When you think they are needed
  b When the bed is raised
  c According to the care plan
  d To support persons who are weak or unsteady

9 You are going to transfer a person from the bed to a chair. Bed wheels must be locked.
  a True
  b False

10 A transfer/gait belt is applied
  a To the skin   c Over the breasts
  b Over clothing   d Under the robe

11 To safely use a transfer/gait belt, you must
  a Follow the manufacturer's instructions
  b Raise the bed rails
  c Lock the bed wheels
  d Set the bed alarm

12 You apply a transfer/gait belt. What should you do with the excess strap?
  a Cut it off.
  b Wrap it around the person's waist.
  c Tuck it under the belt.
  d Let it dangle.

13 A person starts to fall. Your first action is to
  a Try to prevent the fall
  b Call for help
  c Bring the person close to your body as fast as possible
  d Lower the person to the floor

14 You found a person lying on the floor. What should you do?
  a Call for the nurse.
  b Help the person back to bed.
  c Apply a transfer belt.
  d Lock the bed wheels.

Answers to these questions are on p. 719.

CHAPTER 14

Restraint Alternatives and Safe Restraint Use

KEY TERMS

chemical restraint Any drug that is used for discipline or convenience and not required to treat medical symptoms

freedom of movement Any change in place or position of the body or any part of the body that the person is physically able to control

medical symptom An indication or characteristic of a physical or psychological condition

physical restraint Any manual method or physical or mechanical device, material, or equipment attached to or near the person's body that he or she cannot remove easily and that restricts freedom of movement or normal access to one's body

remove easily The manual method, device, material, or equipment used to restrain the person that can be removed intentionally by the person in the same manner it was applied by the staff

KEY ABBREVIATIONS

CMS Centers for Medicare & Medicaid Services
FDA Food and Drug Administration

OBRA Omnibus Budget Reconciliation Act of 1987
TJC The Joint Commission

Chapters 12 and 13 have many safety measures. However, some persons need extra protection. They may present dangers to themselves or others (including staff). For example:

- Mrs. Perez forgets to call for help when getting up and with walking. Falling is a risk.
- Mrs. Wilson tries to pull out her feeding tube. The tube is part of her treatment.
- Ms. Walsh scratches and picks at a wound. This can damage her skin or the wound.
- Mr. Ross wanders. He may wander into traffic or get lost in neighborhoods, parks, forests, or other areas. Exposure to hot or cold weather presents other dangers.
- Mr. Winters tries to hit, pinch, and bite the staff. They are at risk for harm.

The Centers for Medicare & Medicaid Services (CMS) have rules for using restraints. Like the Omnibus Budget Reconciliation Act of 1987 (OBRA), CMS rules protect the person's rights and safety. This includes the right to be free from restraint or seclusion. Restraints may only be used to treat a medical symptom or for the immediate physical safety of the person or others. Restraints may only be used when less restrictive measures fail to protect the person or others. They must be discontinued at the earliest possible time.

The CMS uses these terms:

- *Physical restraint*—is any manual method or physical or mechanical device, material, or equipment attached to or near the person's body that he or she cannot remove easily and that restricts freedom of movement or normal access to one's body.
- *Chemical restraint*—is any drug that is used for discipline or convenience and not required to treat medical symptoms. The drug or dosage is not a standard treatment for the person's condition.
- *Freedom of movement*—is any change in place or position of the body or any part of the body that the person is physically able to control.
- *Remove easily*—means that the manual method, device, material, or equipment used to restrain the person can be removed intentionally by the person in the same manner it was applied by the staff. For example, the person can put bed rails down, untie a knot, unclasp a buckle.

To meet the person's safety needs, a resident care conference is held. The health team reviews and updates the person's care plan. Every attempt is made to protect the person without using restraints. Sometimes they are needed. Restraints are used only as a *last resort* to protect persons from harming themselves or others.

HISTORY OF RESTRAINT USE

Restraints were once thought to *prevent* falls. Research shows that restraints *cause* falls. Falls occur when persons try to get free of the restraints. Injuries are more serious from falls in restrained persons than in those not restrained.

Restraints also were used to prevent wandering or interfering with treatment. They were often used for persons who showed confusion, poor judgment, or behavior problems. Older persons were restrained more often than younger persons were. Restraints were viewed as necessary devices to protect a person. However, they can cause serious harm (Box 14-1). They can even cause death.

Besides the CMS, the Food and Drug Administration (FDA), state agencies, and The Joint Commission (TJC—an accrediting agency) have guidelines for the use of restraints. They do not forbid the use of restraints. However, *they require considering or trying all other appropriate alternatives first.*

Every center has policies and procedures about restraints. They include identifying persons at risk for harm, harmful behaviors, restraint alternatives, and proper restraint use. Staff training is required.

Box 14-1 Risks of Restraint Use

- Agitation
- Anger
- Constipation
- Contractures
- Cuts and bruises
- Decline in physical function (ability to walk, muscle condition)
- Dehydration
- Delirium
- Depression
- Dignity: loss of
- Embarrassment and humiliation
- Falls
- Fractures
- Head trauma
- Incontinence
- Infections: pneumonia and urinary tract
- Mistrust
- Nerve injuries
- Pressure ulcers
- Self-respect: loss of
- Social contact: reduced
- Strangulation
- Withdrawal

OBRA-CMS

Box 14-2   Alternatives to Restraint Use

- Diversion is provided—TV, videos, music, games, relaxation tapes, and so on.
- Life-long habits and routines are in the care plan. For example, showers before breakfast; reads in the bathroom; walks outside before lunch; watches TV after lunch; and so on.
- Family and friends make videos of themselves for the person to watch.
- Videos are made of visits with family and friends for the person to watch.
- Time is spent in supervised areas (dining room, lounge, near the nurses' station).
- Pillows, wedge cushions, and posture and positioning aids are used.
- The signal light is within reach.
- Signal lights are answered promptly.
- Food, fluid, hygiene, and elimination needs are met.
- The bedpan, urinal, or commode is within the person's reach.
- Back massages are given.
- Family, friends, and volunteers visit.
- The person has companions or sitters.
- Time is spent with the person.
- Extra time is spent with a person who is restless.
- Reminiscing is done with the person.
- A calm, quiet setting is provided.
- The person wanders in safe areas.
- The entire staff is aware of persons who tend to wander. This includes staff in housekeeping, maintenance, the business office, dietary, and so on.

- Exercise programs are provided.
- Outdoor time is planned during nice weather.
- The person does jobs or tasks he or she consents to.
- Warning devices are used on beds, chairs, and doors.
- Knob guards are used on doors.
- Padded hip protectors are worn under clothing (Fig. 14-1).
- Floor cushions are placed next to beds (Chapter 13).
- Roll guards are attached to the bed frame (Fig. 14-2).
- Falls are prevented (Chapter 13).
- The person's furniture meets his or her needs (lower bed, reclining chair, rocking chair).
- Walls and furniture corners are padded.
- Observations and visits are made at least every 15 minutes. Or as often as noted in the care plan.
- The person is moved to a room close to the nurses' station.
- Procedures and care measures are explained.
- Frequent explanations are given about equipment or devices.
- Confused persons are oriented to person, time, and place. Calendars and clocks are provided.
- Light is adjusted to meet the person's basic needs and preferences.
- Staff assignments are consistent.
- Sleep is not interrupted.
- Noise levels are reduced.

RESTRAINT ALTERNATIVES

Often there are causes and reasons for harmful behaviors. Knowing and treating the cause can prevent restraint use. The nurse tries to find out what the behavior means. This is very important for persons who have speech or cognitive problems. The focus is on these questions:

- Is the person in pain, ill, or injured?
- Is the person short of breath? Are cells getting enough oxygen (Chapter 28)?
- Is the person afraid in a new setting?
- Does the person need to use the bathroom?
- Is a dressing tight or causing other discomfort (Chapter 35)?
- Is clothing tight or causing other discomfort?
- Is the person's position uncomfortable?

- Are body fluids, secretions, or excretions causing skin irritation?
- Is the person too hot or too cold?
- Is the person hungry or thirsty?
- What are the person's life-long habits at this time of day?
- Does the person have problems communicating?
- Is the person seeing, hearing, or feeling things that are not real (Chapter 43)?
- Is the person confused or disoriented (Chapter 44)?
- Are drugs causing the behaviors?

Restraint alternatives for the person are identified (Box 14-2). They become part of the care plan. Care plan changes are made as needed. Restraint alternatives may not protect the person. The doctor may need to order restraints. See Figure 14-3.

Fig. 14-1 Hip protector. *(Image courtesy Posey Company, Arcadia, Calif.)*

Fig. 14-2 Roll guard. *(Image courtesy Posey Company, Arcadia, Calif.)*

Date	Time	Nursing Margin	Other Depts Margin	
4–16	1340			Resident's chair alarm sounded as he tried to get out of his wheelchair.
				He repeated "I need to get up" over and over. I assisted him to the
				bathroom. He voided 275 mL. Then I pushed him around the enclosed
				garden for 15 minutes. He talked about the flowers he used to grow
				in his garden. After the walk, I positioned his wheelchair across from
				the nurses' station and locked the wheels. I told him to ask for help if he
				needs anything. He said "I will." I explained that to prevent him from
				falling, his chair alarm would sound if he tried to get up without help. I
				gave him a drink of water per his request. I gave him a magazine on
				gardening. He states "I'm OK." He appears calm and relaxed. I told him I
				would check on him in 15 minutes. I asked R. Carico, RN, and M. Herron
				at the nurses station to observe him. Lynn Larson, CNA

Fig. 14-3 Charting sample.

SAFE RESTRAINT USE

Restraints can cause serious injury and even death. CMS, OBRA, FDA, and TJC guidelines are followed. So are state laws. They are part of your center's policies and procedures for restraint use.

Restraints are not used to discipline a person. They are not used for staff convenience. Discipline is any action that punishes or penalizes a person. Convenience is any action that:

- Controls or manages the person's behavior
- Requires less effort by the center
- Is not in the person's best interests

Restraints are used only when necessary to treat a person's medical symptoms. The CMS defines a medical symptom as an indication or characteristic of a physical or psychological condition. Symptoms may relate to physical, emotional, or behavioral problems. Sometimes restraints are needed to protect the person or others. That is, a person may have violent or aggressive behaviors that are harmful to self or others.

OBRA-CMS OBRA-CMS OBRA-CMS

OBRA-CMS

Physical and Chemical Restraints

OBRA-CMS

According to the CMS, *physical restraints* include these points:

- May be any manual method, physical or mechanical device, material, or equipment
- Is attached to or next to the person's body
- Cannot be easily removed by the person
- Restricts freedom of movement or normal access to one's body

Physical restraints are applied to the chest, waist, elbows, wrists, hands, or ankles. They confine the person to a bed or chair. Or they prevent movement of a body part. Some furniture or barriers also prevent freedom of movement:

- A device used with a chair that the person cannot remove easily. The device prevents the person from rising. Trays, tables, bars, and belts are examples (Fig. 14-4).
- Any chair that prevents the person from rising.
- Any bed or chair placed so close to the wall that the person cannot get out of the bed or chair.
- Bed rails (Chapter 13) that prevent the person from getting out of bed. For example, four half-length bed rails are raised. They are restraints if the person cannot lower them.
- Tucking in or using Velcro to hold a sheet, fabric, or clothing so tightly that freedom of movement is restricted.

Drugs or drug dosages are *chemical restraints* if they:

- Control behavior or restrict movement
- Are not standard treatment for the person's condition

Drugs cannot be used for discipline or staff convenience. They cannot be used if not required for the person's treatment. They cannot be used if they affect physical or mental function.

Sometimes drugs can help persons who are confused or disoriented. They may be anxious, agitated, or aggressive. The doctor may order drugs to control these behaviors. The drugs should not make the person sleepy and unable to function at his or her highest level.

Complications of Restraint Use

Box 14-1 lists the many complications from restraints. Injuries occur as the person tries to get free of the restraint. Injuries also occur from using the wrong restraint, applying it wrong, or keeping it on too long. Cuts, bruises, and fractures are common. *The most serious risk is death from strangulation.*

There are also mental effects. Restraints affect dignity and self-esteem. See Box 14-1.

Restraints are medical devices. The Safe Medical Device Act applies if a restraint causes illness, injury, or death. Also, CMS requires the reporting of any death that occurs:

OBRA-CMS

- While a person is in a restraint.
- Within 24 hours after a restraint was removed.
- Within 1 week after a restraint was removed. This is done if the restraint may have contributed directly or indirectly to the person's death.

Legal Aspects

Laws applying to restraint use must be followed. Remember the following:

OBRA-CMS

- *Restraints must protect the person.* They are not used for staff convenience or to discipline a person. Restraining someone is not easier than properly supervising and observing the person. A restrained person requires more staff time for care, supervision, and observation. A restraint is used only when it is the best safety measure for the person. Restraints are not used to punish or penalize uncooperative persons.

OBRA-CMS

- *A doctor's order is required.* OBRA, CMS, state laws, FDA warnings, TJC, and other accrediting agencies protect persons from unnecessary restraint. If restraints are needed for medical reasons, a doctor's order is required. The doctor gives the reason for the restraint, what body part to restrain, what to use, and how long to use it. This information is on the care plan and your assignment sheet. In an emergency, the nurse can decide to apply restraints before getting a doctor's order.

Fig. 14-4 This lap-top tray is a restraint alternative. It is a restraint when used to prevent freedom of movement. *(Image courtesy Posey Company, Arcadia, Calif.)*

- *The least restrictive method is used.* It allows the greatest amount of movement or body access possible. Some restraints attach to the person's body and to a fixed (non-movable) object. It restricts freedom of movement or body access. Vest, jacket, ankle, wrist, hand, and some belt restraints are examples. Other restraints are near but not directly attached to the person's body (bed rails or wedge cushions). They do not totally restrict freedom of movement. They allow access to certain body parts and are the least restrictive.
- *Restraints are used only after other measures fail to protect the person (see Box 14-2).* Some people can harm themselves or others. The care plan must include measures to protect the person and prevent harm to others. Many fall prevention measures are restraint alternatives (Chapter 13).
- *Unnecessary restraint is false imprisonment (Chapter 4).* You must clearly understand the reason for the restraint and its risk. If not, politely ask about its use. If you apply an unneeded restraint, you could face false imprisonment charges.

- *Informed consent is required.* The person must understand the reason for the restraint. The person is told how the restraint will help the planned medical treatment. The person is told about the risks of restraint use. If the person cannot give consent, his or her legal representative is given the information. Either the person or the legal representative must give consent before a restraint can be used. The doctor or nurse provides the necessary information and obtains the consent.

See *Focus on Communication: Legal Aspects.*

Safety Guidelines

The restrained person must be kept safe. Follow the safety measures in Box 14-3, p. 172. Also remember these key points:

- *Observe for increased confusion and agitation.* Restraints can increase confusion and agitation. Whether confused or alert, people are aware of restricted movements. They may try to get out of the restraint or struggle or pull at it. Some restrained persons beg others to free or to help release them. These behaviors often are viewed as signs of confusion. Some people become more confused because they do not understand what is happening to them. Restrained persons need repeated explanations and reassurance. Spending time with them has a calming effect.

- *Protect the person's quality of life.* Restraints are used for as short a time as possible. The care plan must show how to reduce restraint use. The person's needs are met with as little restraint as possible. You must meet the person's physical, emotional, and social needs. Visit with the person and explain the reason for the restraints.
- *Follow the manufacturer's instructions.* They explain how to apply and secure the restraint for the person's safety. The restraint must be snug and firm, but not tight. Tight restraints affect circulation and breathing. The person must be comfortable and able to move the restrained part to a limited and safe extent. You could be negligent if you do not apply or secure a restraint properly.
- *Apply restraints with enough help to protect the person and staff from injury.* Persons in immediate danger of harming themselves or others are restrained quickly. Combative and agitated people can hurt themselves and the staff when restraints are applied. Enough staff members are needed to complete the task safely and quickly.
- *Observe the person at least every 15 minutes or as often as noted in the care plan.* Restraints are dangerous. Injuries and deaths can result from improper restraint use and poor observation. Prevent complications. Interferences with breathing and circulation are examples.
- *Remove or release the restraint, re-position the person, and meet basic needs at least every 2 hours or as often as noted in the care plan.* The restraint is removed or released for at least 10 minutes. Provide for food, fluid, comfort, safety, hygiene, and elimination needs and give skin care. Perform range-of-motion exercises or help the person walk (Chapter 26). Follow the care plan.

See *Focus on Communication: Safety Guidelines, p. 172.*
See *Teamwork and Time Management: Safety Guidelines, p. 172.*

Text continued on p. 176

FOCUS ON COMMUNICATION
Legal Aspects

You may not know the reason for a restraint. If so, politely ask the nurse why it is needed. For example:
- "Why does Mr. Reed need a restraint?"
- "I don't understand. Why did the doctor order the restraint?"

FOCUS ON COMMUNICATION
Safety Guidelines

Restraints can increase confusion. Remind the person why the restraint is necessary and to call for help when it is needed. Repeat the following as often as needed:

- "Dr. Monroe ordered this restraint so you don't hurt yourself. If you need to get up, please call for help. I'll check on you every 15 minutes. Other staff will check on you too."
- "How does the restraint feel? Is it too tight? Is it too loose?"
- "Please put your signal light on. I want to make sure that you can reach and use it with the restraint on."
- "Please call for help right away if the restraint is too tight."
- "Please call for help right away if you feel pain in your fingers or hands. Also call for me if you feel numbness or tingling."
- "Please call for help right away if you are having problems breathing."

TEAMWORK AND TIME MANAGEMENT
Safety Guidelines

You may not be assigned to a restrained person. However, you must still help the nursing team keep the person safe. Make sure you know who is restrained on your unit. Every time you walk past the person or the person's room, check to see if the person is safe and comfortable. Answer the person's signal light promptly.

Box 14-3   Safety Measures for Using Restraints

Before Applying Restraints
- Do not use sheets, towels, tape, rope, straps, bandages, Velcro, or other items to restrain a person.
- Apply a restraint only after being instructed about its proper use.
- Demonstrate proper application of the restraint before applying it.
- Use the restraint noted in the care plan. Use the correct size. Small restraints are tight. They cause discomfort and agitation. They also restrict breathing and circulation. Strangulation is a risk from big or loose restraints.
- Use only restraints that have manufacturer's instructions and warning labels.
- Read the manufacturer's warning labels. Note the front and back of the restraint.
- Follow the manufacturer's instructions. Some restraints are safe for bed, chair, and wheelchair use. Others are used only with certain equipment.
- Use intact restraints. Look for broken stitches, tears, cuts, or frayed fabric or straps. Look for missing or loose buckles, locks, hooks, loops, or straps or other damage. The restraint must hold securely.
- Test zippers, buckles, locks, hooks, and other closures. The device must fasten securely.
- Do not use a restraint near a fire, a flame, or smoking materials.

Applying Restraints
- Do not use restraints to position a person on a toilet.
- Do not use restraints to position a person on furniture that does not allow for correct application. Follow the manufacturer's instructions.
- Follow center policies and procedures.

Applying Restraints—cont'd
- Position the person in good alignment before applying the restraint (Chapter 16).
- Pad bony areas and the skin as instructed by the nurse. This prevents pressure and injury from the restraint.
- Secure the restraint. It should be snug but allow some movement of the restrained part. Follow the manufacturer's instructions to check for snugness. For example:
  - If applied to the chest or waist—Make sure that the person can breathe easily. A flat hand should slide between the restraint and the person's body (Fig. 14-5). Check with the nurse if you have very small or very large hands. Small or large hands could cause the restraint to be too tight or too loose.
  - For wrist and mitt restraints—You should be able to slide 1 finger under the restraint. Check with the nurse if you have very small or very large fingers. Small or large fingers could cause the restraint to be too tight or too loose.
- Criss-cross vest or jacket restraints in front (Fig. 14-6). Do not criss-cross restraints in the back unless part of the manufacturer's instructions (Fig. 14-7, p. 174). Criss-crossing vests or jackets in the back can cause death from strangulation.
- Buckle or tie restraints according to center policy. The policy should follow the manufacturer's instructions and allow for quick release in an emergency. Quick-release buckles or airline-type buckles are used (Fig. 14-8, p. 174). So are quick-release ties (Fig. 14-9, p. 174).
- Secure straps out of the person's reach.
- Leave 1 to 2 inches of slack in the straps (if directed to do so by the nurse). This allows some movement of the part.

Box 14-3 **Safety Measures for Using Restraints—cont'd**

Applying Restraints—cont'd

- Secure the restraint to the movable part of the bed frame at waist level (see Fig. 14-9, p. 174). The restraint will not tighten or loosen when the head or foot of the bed is raised or lowered. For chairs, secure straps under the seat of the wheelchair or chair (Fig. 14-10, p. 174).
- Make sure the straps cannot tighten, loosen, slip, or cause too much slack.
- Make sure that straps will not slide in any direction. If straps slide, they change the restraint's position. The person can get suspended off the mattress or chair (Figs. 14-11, p. 174 and 14-12, p. 175). Strangulation can result.
- Never secure restraints to the bed rails. The person can reach bed rails to release knots or buckles. Also, injury to the person is likely when raising or lowering bed rails.
- Use bed rail covers or gap protectors according to the nurse's instructions (Fig. 14-13, p. 175). They prevent entrapment between the rails or the bed rail bars (see Fig. 14-11, p. 174). Entrapment can occur between:
  - The bars of a bed rail
  - The space between half-length (split) bed rails
  - The bed rail and mattress
  - The head-board or foot-board and mattress
- Position the person in semi-Fowler's position (Chapter 16) when using a vest, jacket, or belt restraint.
- Position the person in a chair so the hips are well to the back of the chair.
- Apply a belt restraint at a 45-degree angle over the thighs (Fig. 14-14, p. 175).

After Applying Restraints

- Keep full bed rails up when using a vest, jacket, or belt restraint. Also use bed rail covers or gap protectors. Otherwise the person could fall off the bed and strangle on the restraint. If half-length bed rails are used, the person can get caught between them.
- Do not use back cushions when a person is restrained in a chair. If the cushion moves out of place, slack occurs in the straps. Strangulation could result if the person slides forward or down from the extra slack (see Fig. 14-12).
- Do not cover the person with a sheet, blanket, bedspread, or other covering. The restraint must be within plain view at all times.
- Check the person at least every 15 minutes for safety, comfort, and signs of injury.

After Applying Restraints—cont'd

- Check the person's circulation at least every 15 minutes if mitt, wrist, or ankle restraints are applied. You should feel a pulse at a pulse site below the restraint (Chapter 31). Fingers or toes should be warm and pink. Tell the nurse at once if:
  - You cannot feel a pulse.
  - Fingers or toes are cold, pale, or blue in color.
  - The person complains of pain, numbness, or tingling in the restrained part.
  - The skin is red or damaged.
- Check the person at least every 15 minutes if a belt, jacket, or vest restraint is used. The person should be able to breathe easily. Also check the position of the restraint, especially in the front and back.
- Monitor persons in the supine position constantly. They are at great risk for aspiration if vomiting occurs (Chapters 24 and 25). Call for the nurse at once.
- Keep scissors in your pocket. In an emergency, cutting the tie may be faster than untying a knot. Never leave scissors at the bedside where the person can reach them. Make sure the person cannot reach the scissors in your pocket.
- Remove or release the restraint and re-position the person every 2 hours or as often as noted in the care plan. The restraint is removed or released for at least 10 minutes. Meet the person's basic needs. You need to:
  - Measure vital signs.
  - Meet elimination needs.
  - Offer food and fluids.
  - Meet hygiene needs.
  - Give skin care.
  - Perform range-of-motion exercises or help the person walk. Follow the care plan.
  - Provide for physical and emotional comfort. (See the inside of the front book cover.)
- Keep the signal light within the person's reach. (Chart that this was done.)
- Complete a safety check before leaving the room. (See the inside of the front book cover.)
- Report to the nurse every time you checked the person and removed or released the restraint. Report your observations and the care given. Follow center policy for recording.

Fig. 14-5 A flat hand slides between the restraint and the person.

Fig. 14-6 The vest restraint criss-crosses in front. (NOTE: The bed rails are raised after the restraint is applied.)

Fig. 14-7 Never criss-cross vest or jacket straps in back. *(Image courtesy Posey Company, Arcadia, Calif.)*

Fig. 14-8 A, Quick-release buckle. B, Airline-type buckle. *(Image courtesy Posey Company, Arcadia, Calif.)*

How to Tie the Posey Quick-Release Tie

1. Wrap the strap once around a movable part of the bed frame leaving at least an 8″ (20 cm) tail. Fold the loose end in half to create a loop and cross it over the other end.
2. Insert the folded strap where the straps cross over each other, as if tying a shoelace. Pull on the loop to tighten.
3. Fold the loose end in half to create a second loop.
4. Insert the second loop into the first loop.
5. Pull on the loop to tighten. Test to make sure strap is secure and will not slide in any direction.
6. Repeat on other side. Practice quick-release ties to ensure the knot releases with one pull on the loose end of the strap.

Fig. 14-9 The Posey quick-release tie. *(Image courtesy Posey Company, Arcadia, Calif.)*

Fig. 14-10 The restraint straps are secured to the wheelchair frame. *(Image courtesy Posey Company, Arcadia, Calif.)*

Fig. 14-11 A, A person can get suspended and caught between bed rail bars. B, The person can get suspended and caught between half-length bed rails. *(Images courtesy Posey Company, Arcadia, Calif.)*

Straps to prevent sliding should always be over the thighs–NOT around the waist or chest. Straps should be at a 45° angle and secured to the chair under the seat, not behind the back. They should be snug but comfortable and not restrict breathing. If a belt or vest is too loose or applied around the waist, the person may slide partially off the seat– resulting in possible suffocation and death.

Tray tables (with or without a belt or vest) pose potential danger if the person should slide partly under the table and become caught. This could result in suffocation and death. Make sure the person's hips are positioned at the back of the chair– this may necessitate the use of an anti-slide material (Posey Grip), a pommel cushion, or a restrictive device if the person shows any tendency to slide forward.

Fig. 14-12 Strangulation could result if the person slides forward or down in the chair because of extra slack in the restraint. *(Images courtesy Posey Company, Arcadia, Calif.)*

Fig. 14-13 A, Bed rail protector. **B,** Guard rail pads. *(Images courtesy Posey Company, Arcadia, Calif.)*

Fig. 14-14 The safety belt is at a 45-degree angle over the thighs. *(Image courtesy Posey Company, Arcadia, Calif.)*

RESTRAINT RELEASE RECORD
(Reference tag: F221)

PLEASE NOTE: Restrained individuals must be checked at least every 15 minutes. In addition, restraints must be released for the purpose of exercise, toileting, etc. for at least 10 minutes at least every two hours.

REASON FOR RESTRAINT	RESTRAINT ORDERED (Circle)		REMOVAL REASON CODES	
Is nonweight bearing and attempts to rise when in W/C.	Waist Pelvic Siderails Wrist (Belt) 2 Full Geri Chair Vest 1 Full Ankle Bar 2 Half Other____ 1 Half		A- Supervised meals B- Supervised group activities C- Care provided by CNA D- One-to-one with volunteer E- One-to-one with social worker	F- 2-3 hrs. with periodic evaluation G- Total elimination of restraint H- *off when in bed* ____ I- ____ J- ____

DATE	15 MINUTE CHECK WHEN RESTRAINED			RELEASE EVERY TWO HOURS FOR PERSONAL CARE			TOTAL HOURS RELEASED PER SHIFT AND REASONS (USE REASON CODES ABOVE)			COMMENTS/ RESIDENT'S RESPONSE (Negative or Positive)
7/18	Shift Initials			Shift Initials						
Month/Year	11-7	7-3	3-11	11-7	7-3	3-11	11-7	7-3	3-11	
1	Lg	BG	MM	Lg	BG	MM	8(H)	4(A,B, C,H)	5(A,C, D,H)	No agitation – no falls no attempts to rise Joan Grieg, RN
2	Lg	BG	MM	Lg	BG	MM	8(H)	5(A,B, C,F,H)	6(A,C, F,H)	Doing well – no falls – Joan Grieg, RN
3	DL	RD	DL	ML	RD	ML	8(H)	6(A,B, C,F,H)	8(A,C, F,H)	No falls – Resident wants belt removed Ray Lopez, RN
4										
5										
6										

Fig. 14-15 Charting sample. *(Modified from Briggs Corp., Des Moines, Iowa.)*

Reporting and Recording

Information about restraints is recorded in the person's medical record (Fig. 14-15). You might apply restraints or care for a restrained person. Report and record the following:

- The type of restraint applied
- The body part or parts restrained
- The reason for the application
- Safety measures taken (for example, bed rails padded and up, signal light within reach)
- The time you applied the restraint
- The time you removed or released the restraint and for how long
- The person's vital signs
- The care given when the restraint was removed or released
- Skin color and condition
- Condition of the limbs
- The pulse felt in the restrained part
- Changes in the person's behavior
- Complaints of discomfort; a tight restraint; difficulty breathing; or pain, numbness, or tingling in the restrained part (Report these complaints to the nurse at once.)

Applying Restraints

Restraints are made of cloth or leather. Cloth restraints (soft restraints) are mitts, belts, straps, jackets, and vests. They are applied to the wrists, ankles, hands, waist, and chest. Leather restraints are applied to the wrists and ankles. Leather restraints are used for extreme agitation and combativeness.

Wrist Restraints Wrist restraints (limb holders) limit arm movement (Fig. 14-16). They may be used when a person continually tries to pull out tubes used for life-saving treatment (intravenous infusion, feeding tube). Or the person scratches at, pulls at, or peels the skin, a wound, or a dressing. This can damage the skin or the wound.

Mitt Restraints Hands are placed in mitt restraints. They prevent finger use. They allow hand, wrist, and arm movements. They are used for the same reasons as wrist restraints. Most mitts are padded (Fig. 14-17).

Belt Restraints The belt restraint (Fig. 14-18) is used when injuries from falls are risks or for positioning during a medical treatment. The person cannot get out of bed or out of a chair. However, a roll belt allows the person to turn from side to side or sit up in bed.

The belt is applied around the waist and secured to the bed or chair (lap belt). It is applied over a garment. The person can release the quick-release type. It is less restrictive than those that only staff members can release.

Fig. 14-16 Wrist restraint. The soft part is toward the skin. Note that 1 finger fits between the restraint and the wrist.

Fig. 14-17 Mitt restraint. *(Image courtesy Posey Company, Arcadia, Calif.)*

Fig. 14-18 Belt restraint. (NOTE: The bed rails are raised after the restraint is applied.)

Vest Restraints and Jacket Restraints Vest and jacket restraints are applied to the chest. They may be used to prevent injuries from falls. And they may be used for persons who need positioning for a medical treatment. The person cannot turn in bed or get out of a chair.

A jacket restraint is applied with the opening in the back (Fig. 14-19, p. 178). For a vest restraint, the vest crosses in front (see Fig. 14-6). *The straps of vest and jacket restraints always cross in the front.* They must *never* cross in the back. Vest and jacket restraints are never worn backward. Strangulation or other injury could occur if the person slides down in the bed or chair. The restraint is always applied over a garment. (NOTE: *A vest or jacket restraint may have a positioning slot in the back. Criss-cross the straps following the manufacturer's instructions.)*

Vest and jacket restraints have life-threatening risks. Death can occur from strangulation. If the person gets caught in the restraint, it can become so tight that the person's chest cannot expand to inhale air. The person quickly suffocates and dies. Correctly applying vest and jacket restraints is critical. You are advised to only assist the nurse in applying them. The nurse should assume full responsibility for applying a vest or jacket restraint.

See *Residents With Dementia: Applying Restraints,* p. 178.

See *Focus on Communication: Applying Restraints,* p. 178.

See *Delegation Guidelines: Applying Restraints,* p. 178.

See *Promoting Safety and Comfort: Applying Restraints,* p. 178.

Fig. 14-19 Jacket restraint. (NOTE: The bed rails are raised after the restraint is applied.)

DELEGATION GUIDELINES
Applying Restraints

Before applying a restraint, you need this information from the nurse and the care plan:
- Why the doctor ordered the restraint
- What type and size to use
- Where to apply the restraint
- How to safely apply the restraint (Have the nurse show you how to apply it. Then show correct application back to the nurse.)
- How to correctly position the person
- What bony areas to pad and how to pad them
- If bed rail covers or gap protectors are needed
- If bed rails are up or down
- What special equipment is needed
- If the person needs to be checked more often than every 15 minutes
- When to apply and release the restraint
- What observations to report and record (p. 176)
- When to report observations
- What specific resident concerns to report at once

RESIDENTS WITH DEMENTIA
Applying Restraints

Restraints may increase confusion and agitation in persons with dementia. They do not understand what you are doing. They may resist your efforts to apply a restraint. They may actively try to get free from the restraint. Serious injury and death are risks.

Never use force to apply a restraint. If a person is confused or agitated, ask a co-worker to help apply the restraint. Report problems to the nurse at once.

PROMOTING SAFETY AND COMFORT
Applying Restraints

Safety
Restraints can cause serious harm, even death. Always follow the manufacturer's instructions. Manufacturers have many types of restraints. The instructions for one type may not apply to another. Also, the manufacturer may have instructions for applying restraints on persons who are agitated.

Never use force to apply a restraint. Ask a co-worker to help apply a restraint on a person who is confused and agitated. Report problems to the nurse at once.

Check the person at least every 15 minutes or more often as instructed by the nurse and the care plan. Make sure the signal light is within reach. Ask the person to use the signal light at the first sign of problems or discomfort.

Never use a restraint as a seat belt in a car or other vehicle.

Comfort
The person's comfort is always important. It is more so when restraints are used. Remember, restraints limit movement. This affects position changes and reaching needed items. Position the person in good alignment before applying a restraint (Chapter 16). Also make sure the person can reach needed items—signal light, water, tissues, phone, bed controls, and so on.

FOCUS ON COMMUNICATION
Applying Restraints

The nurse may ask you to apply a restraint you have not used before. If you do not know how to apply a certain restraint, do not do so. Tell the nurse. Ask him or her to show you the correct application. You can say: "I've never applied a restraint like this before. Would you please show me how and then watch me apply it?" Then thank the nurse for helping you.

When applying a restraint, explain to the person what you are going to do. Then tell the person what you are doing step-by-step. Always check for safety and comfort. You can ask: "How does the restraint feel? Is it too tight? Is it too loose?"

Make sure the person can communicate with you after you leave the room. Place the signal light in reach. Make sure the person can use it with the restraint on. Remind the person to call if he or she becomes uncomfortable or if anything is needed.

APPLYING RESTRAINTS

QUALITY OF LIFE

Remember to:
- Knock before entering the person's room.
- Address the person by name.
- Introduce yourself by name and title.

- Explain the procedure to the person before beginning and during the procedure.
- Protect the person's rights during the procedure.
- Handle the person gently during the procedure.

PRE-PROCEDURE

1 Follow *Delegation Guidelines: Applying Restraints*. See *Promoting Safety and Comfort: Applying Restraints.*
2 Collect the following as instructed by the nurse:
- Correct type and size of restraints
- Padding for skin and bony areas
- Bed rail pads or gap protectors (if needed)

3 Practice hand hygiene.
4 Identify the person. Check the ID (identification) bracelet against the assignment sheet. Also call the person by name.
5 Provide for privacy.

PROCEDURE

6 Make sure the person is comfortable and in good alignment.
7 Put the bed rail pads or gap protectors (if needed) on the bed if the person is in bed. Follow the manufacturer's instructions.
8 Pad bony areas. Follow the nurse's instructions and the care plan.
9 Read the manufacturer's instructions. Note the front and back of the restraint.
10 *For wrist restraints:*
  a Apply the restraint following the manufacturer's instructions. Place the soft or foam part toward the skin.
  b Secure the restraint so it is snug but not tight. Make sure you can slide 1 finger under the restraint (see Fig. 14-16). Follow the manufacturer's instructions. Adjust the straps if the restraint is too loose or too tight. Check for snugness again.
  c Buckle or tie the straps to the movable part of the bed frame out of the person's reach. Use a quick-release tie.
  d Repeat steps 10 a, b, and c for the other wrist.
11 *For mitt restraints:*
  a Make sure the person's hands are clean and dry.
  b Apply the mitt restraint. Follow the manufacturer's instructions.
  c Secure the restraint to the bed if directed to do so by the nurse. Buckle or tie the straps to the movable part of the bed frame. Use a quick-release tie.
  d Make sure the restraint is snug. Slide 1 finger between the restraint and the wrist. Follow the manufacturer's instructions. Adjust the straps if the restraint is too loose or too tight. Check for snugness again.
  e Repeat steps 11 b, c, and d for the other hand.
12 *For a belt restraint:*
  a Assist the person to a sitting position.
  b Apply the restraint with your free hand. Follow the manufacturer's instructions.

  c Remove wrinkles or creases from the front and back of the restraint.
  d Bring the ties through the slots in the belt.
  e Position the straps at a 45-degree angle between the wheelchair seats and sides. Help the person lie down if he or she is in bed.
  f Make sure the person is comfortable and in good alignment.
  g Buckle or tie the straps to the movable part of the bed frame out of the person's reach. For a wheelchair, criss-cross and secure the straps as in Figure 14-10. Use a quick-release tie.
  h Make sure the belt is snug. Slide an open hand between the restraint and the person. Adjust the restraint if it is too loose or too tight. Check for snugness again.
13 *For a vest restraint:*
  a Assist the person to a sitting position.
  b Apply the restraint with your free hand. Follow the manufacturer's instructions. The "V" part of the vest crosses in front.
  c Bring the straps through the slots.
  d Position the straps at a 45-degree angle between the wheelchair seats and sides. (Omit this step if the person is in bed.)
  e Make sure the vest is free of wrinkles in the front and back.
  f Help the person lie down if he or she is in bed.
  g Make sure the person is comfortable and in good alignment.
  h Buckle or tie the straps to the movable part of the bed frame. Use a quick-release tie. The buckle or tie is out of the person's reach. For a wheelchair, criss-cross and secure the straps as in Figure 14-10.
  i Make sure the vest is snug. Slide an open hand between the restraint and the person. Adjust the restraint if it is too loose or too tight. Check for snugness again.

Continued

APPLYING RESTRAINTS—cont'd

PROCEDURE—cont'd

14 *For a jacket restraint:*
  a Assist the person to a sitting position.
  b Apply the restraint with your free hand. Follow the manufacturer's instructions. The jacket opening goes in the back.
  c Close the back with the zipper, ties, or hook and loop closures.
  d Make sure the side seams are under the arms. Remove any wrinkles in the front and back.
  e Position the straps at a 45-degree angle between the wheelchair seat and sides. Help the person lie down if he or she is in bed.

  f Make sure the person is comfortable and in good alignment.
  g Buckle or tie the straps to the movable part of the bed frame. Use a quick-release tie. The buckle or tie is out of the person's reach. For a wheelchair, criss-cross and secure straps as in Figure 14-10.
  h Make sure the jacket is snug. Slide an open hand between the restraint and the person. Adjust the restraint if it is too loose or too tight. Check for snugness again.

POST-PROCEDURE

15 Position the person as the nurse directs.
16 Provide for comfort. (See the inside of the front book cover.)
17 Place the signal light within the person's reach.
18 Raise or lower bed rails. Follow the care plan and the manufacturer's instructions for the restraint.
19 Unscreen the person.
20 Complete a safety check of the room. (See the inside of the front book cover.)
21 Decontaminate your hands.
22 Check the person and the restraint at least every 15 minutes. Report and record your observations:
  a For wrist or mitt restraints: check the pulse, color, and temperature of the restrained parts.
  b For a vest, jacket, or belt restraint: check the person's breathing. *Call for the nurse at once if the person is not breathing or is having problems breathing.* Make sure the restraint is properly positioned in the front and back.

23 Do the following at least every 2 hours for at least 10 minutes:
  a Remove or release the restraint.
  b Measure vital signs.
  c Re-position the person.
  d Meet food, fluid, hygiene, and elimination needs.
  e Give skin care.
  f Perform range-of-motion exercises or help the person walk. Follow the care plan.
  g Provide for physical and emotional comfort. (See the inside of the front book cover.)
  h Re-apply the restraints.
24 Complete a safety check of the room. (See the inside of the front book cover.)
25 Report and record your observations and the care given.

QUALITY OF LIFE

Restraints lessen the person's dignity. Therefore they are ordered only for a specific medical symptom. The restrained person depends on others for basic needs.
  Imagine the following:
• Your nose itches. But your hands and arms are restrained. You cannot scratch your nose.
• You need to use the bathroom. Your hands and arms are restrained. You cannot get up. You cannot reach your signal light. You soil yourself with urine or a bowel movement.
• Your phone is ringing. You cannot answer it because your hands and arms are restrained.
• You are not wearing your eyeglasses. You cannot identify people coming into and going out of your room. And you cannot speak because of a stroke. You have a vest restraint. You cannot move or turn in bed.

• You are thirsty. The water glass is within your reach but your hands and arms are restrained.
• You hear the fire alarm. You have on a restraint. You cannot get up to move to a safe place. You must wait until someone rescues you.
  What would you try to do? Would you calmly lie or sit there? Would you try to get free from the restraint? Would you cry out for help? What would the nursing staff think? Would they think that you are uncomfortable? Or would they think that you are agitated and uncooperative? Would they think your behavior is improving or getting worse? Would you feel anger, embarrassment, or humiliation?
  Try to put yourself in the person's situation. Then you can better understand how the person feels. Treat the person like you would want to be treated—with kindness, caring, respect, and dignity.

You can promote quality of life by:
- *Providing for comfort.* The person's comfort is always important. It is especially so when the person is restrained. The person must be in good alignment and in a comfortable position. The restraint must allow for some movement. It must be snug, but not tight. If tight, the restraint can interfere with breathing and circulation. Also make sure that any needed items are within the person's reach.
- *Meeting safety and security needs.* The signal light must always be within the person's reach. This safety measure also promotes physical and mental comfort. It promotes physical comfort because the person knows that he or she can call for help. Being able to call for help promotes mental comfort. So does knowing what is happening and why. The nurse explains the reason for the restraint to the person. You need to remind the person why the restraint is needed. When applying restraints, always explain what you are going to do. Tell the person what you are doing step-by-step. The person needs to feel safe and secure.

- *Promoting independence.* Mitt and hand restraints limit hand and arm use. Belt, vest, and jacket restraints allow hand and arm use. Make sure needed items are within the person's reach. Water, tissues, and bed and TV controls are examples. Let the person do as much for himself or herself as safely possible.
- *Allowing personal choice.* Restraints are removed at least every 2 hours. Food, fluid, hygiene, and elimination needs are met. The person walks or range-of-motion exercises are done. Let the person choose if he or she will use the bathroom first or walk first. Let the person choose where to walk and what to eat or drink. Allow choices that are safe for the person. Personal choices promote independence, dignity, and self-esteem.

REVIEW QUESTIONS

Circle T if the statement is TRUE. Circle F if the statement is FALSE.

1. T F Restraint alternatives fail to protect a person. You can apply a restraint.
2. T F A restraint restricts a person's freedom of movement.
3. T F Some drugs are restraints.
4. T F Restraints can be used for staff convenience.
5. T F A device is a restraint only if it is attached to the person's body.
6. T F Bed rails are restraints if the person cannot lower them.
7. T F Restraints are used only for a person's specific medical symptom.
8. T F Unnecessary restraint is false imprisonment.
9. T F You can apply restraints when you think they are needed.
10. T F You can use a vest restraint to position a person on the toilet.
11. T F Restraints are removed or released at least every 2 hours to re-position the person and give skin care.
12. T F Restraints are tied to bed rails.
13. T F Wrist restraints are used to prevent falls.
14. T F A vest restraint crosses in front.
15. T F Bed rails are left down when vest restraints are used.

Circle the BEST answer.

16. Which is *not* a restraint alternative?
    a Positioning the person's chair close to the wall
    b Answering signal lights promptly
    c Taking the person outside in nice weather
    d Padding walls and corners of furniture
17. Physical restraints
    a Can be removed easily by the person
    b Are not allowed by OBRA
    c Restrict freedom of movement
    d Are safer than chemical restraints

18. The following can occur because of restraints. Which is the *most* serious?
    a Fractures   c Pressure ulcers
    b Strangulation   d Urinary tract infections
19. A belt restraint is applied to a person in bed. Where should you secure the straps?
    a To the bed rails
    b To the head-board
    c To the movable part of the bed frame
    d To the foot-board
20. A person has a restraint. You should check the person and the position of the restraint at least every
    a 15 minutes   c Hour
    b 30 minutes   d 2 hours
21. A person has mitt restraints. Which of these is especially important to report to the nurse?
    a The heart rate
    b The respiratory rate
    c Why the restraints were applied
    d If you felt a pulse in the restrained extremities
22. The doctor ordered mitt restraints for a person. You need the following information from the nurse *except*
    a What size to use
    b What other equipment is needed
    c What drugs the person is taking
    d When to apply and release the restraints
23. A person has a vest restraint. It is not too tight or too loose if you can slide
    a A fist between the vest and the person
    b One finger between the vest and the person
    c An open hand between the vest and the person
    d Two fingers between the vest and the person
24. The correct way to apply any restraint is to follow the
    a Nurse's directions
    b Doctor's orders
    c Care plan
    d Manufacturer's instructions

Answers to these questions are on p. 719.

Preventing Infection

OBJECTIVES

- Define the key terms and key abbreviations listed in this chapter.
- Identify what microbes need to live and grow.
- List the signs and symptoms of infection.
- Explain the chain of infection.
- Describe healthcare-associated infections and the persons at risk.
- Describe the practices of medical asepsis.
- Describe disinfection and sterilization methods.
- Explain how to care for equipment and supplies.
- Describe Standard Precautions and Transmission-Based Precautions.
- Explain the Bloodborne Pathogen Standard.
- Explain the principles and practices of surgical asepsis.
- Perform the procedures described in this chapter.
- Explain how to promote quality of life.

KEY TERMS

asepsis Being free of disease-producing microbes

biohazardous waste Items contaminated with blood, body fluids, secretions, or excretions; *bio* means life, and *hazardous* means dangerous or harmful

carrier A human or animal that is a reservoir for microbes but does not have the signs and symptoms of infection

clean technique See "medical asepsis"

communicable disease A disease caused by pathogens that spreads easily; a contagious disease

contagious disease See "communicable disease"

contamination The process of becoming unclean

disinfection The process of destroying pathogens

germicide A disinfectant applied to the skin, tissues, or non-living objects

healthcare-associated infection (HAI) An infection that develops in a person cared for in any setting where health care is given; the infection is related to receiving health care

immunity Protection against a certain disease

infection A disease state resulting from the invasion and growth of microbes in the body

infection control Practices and procedures that prevent the spread of infection

medical asepsis Practices used to remove or destroy pathogens and to prevent their spread from one person or place to another person or place; clean technique

microbe See "microorganism"

microorganism A small *(micro)* living plant or animal *(organism)* seen only with a microscope; a microbe

non-pathogen A microbe that does not usually cause an infection

normal flora Microbes that live and grow in a certain area

pathogen A microbe that is harmful and can cause an infection

reservoir The environment in which a microbe lives and grows; host

KEY TERMS—cont'd

spore A bacterium protected by a hard shell
sterile The absence of *all* microbes
sterile field A work area free of *all* pathogens and non-pathogens (including spores)
sterile technique See "surgical asepsis"
sterilization The process of destroying *all* microbes

surgical asepsis The practices that keep items free of *all* microbes; sterile technique
vaccination Giving a vaccine to produce immunity against an infectious disease
vaccine A preparation containing dead or weakened microbes

KEY ABBREVIATIONS

AIIR Airborne infection isolation room
CDC Centers for Disease Control and Prevention
cm Centimeter
HAI Healthcare-associated infection
HBV Hepatitis B virus
HIV Human immunodeficiency virus
MDRO Multidrug-resistant organism

MRSA Methicillin-resistant *Staphylococcus aureus*
OPIM Other potentially infectious materials
OSHA Occupational Safety and Health Administration
PPE Personal protective equipment
TB Tuberculosis
VRE Vancomycin-resistant *Enterococcus*

An infection is a disease state resulting from the invasion and growth of microbes in the body. Infection is a major safety and health hazard. Minor infections cause short illnesses. Some infections are serious and can cause death. Older and disabled persons are at risk. The health team follows certain practices and procedures to prevent the spread of infection. Called infection control, such practices and procedures protect residents, visitors, and staff from infection.

MICROORGANISMS

A microorganism (microbe) is a small (*micro*) living plant or animal (*organism*). It is seen only with a microscope. Microbes are everywhere—in the mouth, nose, respiratory tract, stomach, and intestines. They are on the skin and in the air, soil, water, and food. They are on animals, clothing, and furniture.

Some microbes are harmful and can cause infections. They are called pathogens. Non-pathogens are microbes that do not usually cause an infection.

Types of Microbes

There are five types of microbes:
* *Bacteria*—plant life that multiplies rapidly. Often called *germs*, they are one cell. They can cause an infection in any body system.

* *Fungi*—plants that live on other plants or animals. Mushrooms, yeasts, and molds are common fungi. Fungi can infect the mouth, vagina, skin, feet, and other body areas.
* *Protozoa*—one-celled animals. They can infect the blood, brain, intestines, and other body areas.
* *Rickettsiae*—found in fleas, lice, ticks, and other insects. They are spread to humans by insect bites. Rocky Mountain spotted fever is an example. The person has fever, chills, headache, rash, and other signs and symptoms.
* *Viruses*—grow in living cells. They cause many diseases. The common cold, herpes, acquired immunodeficiency syndrome (AIDS), and hepatitis are examples.

Requirements of Microbes

Microbes need a reservoir to live and grow. The reservoir (host) is the environment in which a microbe lives and grows. People, plants, animals, the soil, food, and water are common reservoirs. Microbes need *water* and *nourishment* from the reservoir. Most need *oxygen* to live. A *warm* and *dark* environment is needed. Most grow best at body temperature. They are destroyed by heat and light.

Normal Flora

Normal flora are microbes that live and grow in a certain area. Certain microbes are in the respiratory tract, in the intestines, and on the skin. They are non-pathogens when in or on a natural reservoir. When a non-pathogen is transmitted from its natural site to another site or host, it becomes a pathogen. *Escherichia coli (E. coli)* is found in the colon. If it enters the urinary system, it can cause an infection.

Multidrug-Resistant Organisms

Multidrug-resistant organisms (MDROs) are microbes that can resist the effects of antibiotics. *Antibiotics* are drugs that kill microbes that cause infections. Some microbes can change their structures. This makes them harder to kill. They can survive in the presence of antibiotics. Therefore the infections they cause are hard to treat.

MDROs are caused by doctors prescribing antibiotics when they are not needed (over-prescribing). Not taking antibiotics for the length of time prescribed is another cause.

Two common MDROs are resistant to many antibiotics:

- *Methicillin-resistant Staphylococcus aureus (MRSA)*. Staphylococcus aureus ("staph") is a bacterium normally found in the nose and on the skin. MRSA is resistant to antibiotics often used for "staph" infections. It can cause serious wound and bloodstream infections and pneumonia.
- *Vancomycin-resistant Enterococci (VRE)*. Enterococcus is a bacterium normally found in the intestines and in feces. It can be transmitted to others by contaminated hands, toilet seats, care equipment, and other items that the hands touch. When not in their natural site (the intestines), enterococci can cause urinary tract, wound, pelvic, and other infections. Vancomycin is an antibiotic often used to treat such infections. Enterococci resistant to Vancomycin are called Vancomycin-resistant Enterococci (VRE).

INFECTION

A *local infection* is in a body part. A *systemic infection* involves the whole body. (Systemic means entire.) The person has some or all of the signs and symptoms listed in Box 15-1.

Infection in Older Persons

The immune system protects the body from disease and infection (Chapter 9). Like other body systems, changes occur in the immune system with aging. Therefore older persons are at risk for infection.

During an infection, an older person may not show the signs and symptoms listed in Box 15-1. The person may have only a slight fever or no fever at all. Redness and swelling may be very slight. The person may not complain of pain. Confusion and delirium may occur (Chapter 44).

An infection can become life-threatening before the older person has obvious signs and symptoms. You must be alert to the most minor changes in the person's behavior or condition. Report any concerns to the nurse at once.

Healing takes longer than when younger. Therefore an infection can prolong the rehabilitation process. Independence and quality of life are affected.

The Chain of Infection

The chain of infection (Fig. 15-1) is a process involving a:
- Source
- Reservoir
- Portal of exit
- Method of transmission
- Portal of entry
- Susceptible host

Box 15-1	**Signs and Symptoms of Infection**

- Fever (elevated body temperature)
- Chills
- Pulse rate: increased
- Respiratory rate: increased
- Pain or tenderness
- Fatigue and loss of energy
- Appetite: loss of *(anorexia)*
- Nausea
- Vomiting
- Diarrhea

- Rash
- Sores on mucous membranes
- Redness and swelling of a body part
- Discharge or drainage from the infected area
- Heat or warmth in a body part
- Limited use of a body part
- Headache
- Muscle aches
- Joint pain
- Confusion

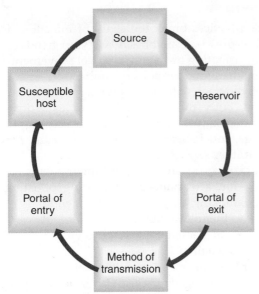

Fig. 15-1 The chain of infection. *(Redrawn from Potter PA, Perry AG: Fundamentals of nursing: concepts, process, and practice, ed 7, St Louis, 2009, Mosby.)*

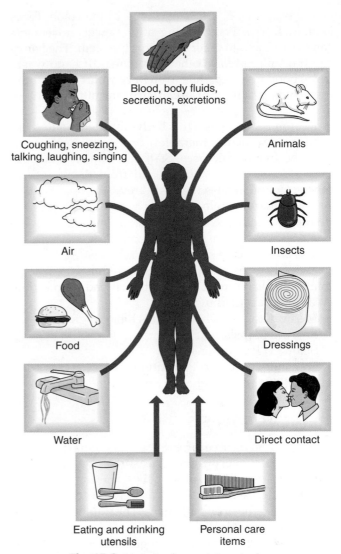

Fig. 15-2 Methods of transmitting microbes.

The *source* is a pathogen. It must have a *reservoir* where it can grow and multiply. Humans and animals are reservoirs. If they do not have signs and symptoms of infection, they are carriers. A **carrier** is a human or animal that is a reservoir for microbes but does not have the signs and symptoms of infection. Carriers can pass the pathogen to others. To leave the reservoir, the pathogen needs a *portal of exit*. Exits are the respiratory, gastro-intestinal (GI), urinary, and reproductive tracts; breaks in the skin; and the blood.

After leaving the reservoir, the pathogen must be *transmitted* to another host (Fig. 15-2). The pathogen enters the body through a *portal of entry*. Portals of entry and exit are the same (respiratory, GI, urinary, and reproductive tracts; breaks in the skin; blood). A *susceptible host* is needed for the microbe to grow and multiply. Susceptible hosts are persons at risk for infection. They include persons who:

- Are very young or who are older
- Are ill
- Were exposed to the pathogen
- Do not follow infection control practices

The human body can protect itself from infection. The ability to resist infection relates to age, nutrition, stress, fatigue, and health. Drugs, disease, and injury also are factors.

Healthcare-Associated Infection

A **healthcare-associated infection (HAI)** is an infection that develops in a person cared for in any setting where health care is given. The infection is related to receiving health care. Hospitals, nursing centers, clinics, and home care settings are examples. HAIs also are called *nosocomial infections*. (*Nosocomial* comes from the Greek word for hospital.) HAIs are caused by normal flora. Or they are caused by microbes transmitted to the person from other sources.

For example, *E. coli* is normally in the colon. Feces contain *E. coli*. Poor wiping after bowel movements can cause *E. coli* to enter the urinary system. The hands can transmit *E. coli* to other body areas. If hand washing is poor, *E. coli* spreads to any body part or anything the hands touch. It also can be transmitted to other people.

Microbes can enter the body through equipment used in treatments, therapies, and tests. Such items must be free of microbes. Staff can transfer microbes from one person to another and from themselves to others. Common sites for HAIs are:
- The urinary system
- The respiratory system
- Wounds
- The bloodstream

Older persons have a hard time fighting infections. The health team must prevent the spread of infection. HAIs are prevented by:
- Medical asepsis. This includes hand hygiene.
- Surgical asepsis.
- Standard Precautions.
- Transmission-Based Precautions.
- The Bloodborne Pathogen Standard.

MEDICAL ASEPSIS

Asepsis is being free of disease-producing microbes. Microbes are everywhere. Measures are needed to achieve asepsis. Medical asepsis (clean technique) is the practices used to:
- Remove or destroy pathogens. The number of pathogens is reduced.
- Prevent pathogens from spreading from one person or place to another person or place.

Microbes cannot be present during surgery or when instruments are inserted into the body. Open wounds (cuts, burns, incisions) require the absence of microbes. They are portals of entry for microbes. Surgical asepsis (sterile technique) is the practices that keep items free of *all* microbes. Sterile means the absence of *all* microbes—pathogens and non-pathogens. Sterilization is the process of destroying *all* microbes (pathogens and non-pathogens).

Contamination is the process of becoming unclean. In medical asepsis, an item or area is clean when it is free of pathogens. The item or area is contaminated if pathogens are present. A sterile item or area is contaminated when pathogens or non-pathogens are present.

Common Aseptic Practices

Aseptic practices break the chain of infection. To prevent the spread of microbes, wash your hands:
- After urinating or having a bowel movement.
- After changing tampons or sanitary pads.
- After contact with your own or another person's blood, body fluids, secretions, or excretions. This includes saliva, vomitus, urine, feces, vaginal discharge, mucus, semen, wound drainage, pus, and respiratory secretions.
- After coughing, sneezing, or blowing your nose.
- Before and after handling, preparing, or eating food.
- After smoking a cigarette, cigar, or pipe.
  Also do the following:
- Provide all persons with their own linens and personal care items.
- Cover your nose and mouth when coughing, sneezing, or blowing your nose. If tissues are not available, cough or sneeze into your upper arm. Do not cough or sneeze into your hands.
- Bathe, wash hair, and brush your teeth regularly.
- Wash fruits and raw vegetables before eating or serving them.
- Wash cooking and eating utensils with soap and water after use.

See *Residents With Dementia: Common Aseptic Practices.*

RESIDENTS WITH DEMENTIA
Common Aseptic Practices

Persons with dementia do not understand aseptic practices. Others must protect them from infection. Assist them with hand washing:
- After elimination
- After coughing, sneezing, or blowing the nose
- Before or after they eat or handle food
- Any time their hands are soiled
   Check and clean their hands and fingernails often. They may not or cannot tell you when soiling occurs.

Hand Hygiene

Hand hygiene is the easiest and most important way to prevent the spread of infection. Your hands are used for almost everything. They are easily contaminated. They can spread microbes to other persons or items. *Practice hand hygiene before and after giving care.* See Box 15-2 for the rules of hand hygiene.

See *Promoting Safety and Comfort: Hand Hygiene,* p. 188.

Box 15-2 Rules of Hand Hygiene

- Wash your hands (with soap and water) when they are visibly dirty or soiled with blood, body fluids, secretions, or excretions.
- Wash your hands (with soap and water) before eating and after using a restroom.
- Wash your hands (with soap and water) if exposure to the anthrax spore is suspected or proven.
- Use an alcohol-based hand rub to decontaminate your hands if they are not visibly soiled. (If an alcohol-based hand rub is not available, wash your hands with soap and water.) Follow this rule in the following situations:
  - Before having direct contact with a person.
  - After contact with the person's intact skin. Examples are after taking a pulse or blood pressure or after moving a person.
  - After contact with body fluids or excretions, mucous membranes, non-intact skin, and wound dressings if hands are not visibly soiled.
  - When moving from a contaminated body site to a clean body site during care activities.
  - After contact with objects (including equipment) in the person's care setting.
  - After removing gloves.
- Follow these rules for washing your hands with soap and water. See procedure: *Hand Washing*, p. 189.
  - Wash your hands under warm running water. Do not use hot water.
  - Stand away from the sink. Do not let your hands, body, or uniform touch the sink. The sink is contaminated. See Figure 15-3.
  - Do not touch the inside of the sink at any time.
  - Keep your hands and forearms lower than your elbows. Your hands are dirtier than your elbows and forearms. If you hold your hands and forearms up, dirty water runs from your hands to your elbows. Those areas become contaminated.
- Rub your palms together to work up a good lather (Fig. 15-4). The rubbing action helps remove microbes and dirt.
- Pay attention to areas often missed during hand washing—thumbs, knuckles, sides of the hands, little fingers, and under the nails.
- Clean fingernails by rubbing the fingertips against your palms (Fig. 15-5, p. 188).
- Use a nail file or orangewood stick to clean under fingernails (Fig. 15-6, p. 188). Microbes easily grow under the fingernails.
- Wash your hands for at least 15 to 20 seconds. Wash your hands longer if they are dirty or soiled with blood, body fluids, secretions, or excretions. Use your judgment and follow center policy.
- Use a clean, dry paper towel to dry your hands.
- Dry your hands starting at the fingertips. Work up to your forearms. You will dry the cleanest area first.
- Use a clean, dry paper towel for each faucet to turn the water off (Fig. 15-7, p. 188). Faucets are contaminated. The paper towels prevent clean hands from becoming contaminated again.
- Follow these rules when decontaminating your hands with an alcohol-based hand rub:
  - Apply the product to the palm of one hand. Follow the manufacturer's instructions for the amount to use.
  - Rub your hands together.
  - Make sure you cover all surfaces of your hands and fingers.
  - Continue rubbing your hands together until your hands are dry.
- Apply hand lotion or cream after hand hygiene. This prevents the skin from chapping and drying. Skin breaks can occur in chapped and dry skin. Skin breaks are portals of entry for microbes.

Modified from Centers for Disease Control and Prevention: Guideline for hand hygiene in health-care settings, Morbidity and Mortality Report 51*(RR-16), October 25, 2002.*

Fig. 15-3 The uniform does not touch the sink. Soap and water are within reach. Hands are lower than the elbows. Hands do not touch the inside of the sink.

Fig. 15-4 The palms are rubbed together to work up a good lather.

Fig. 15-5 The fingertips are rubbed against the palms to clean under the fingernails.

Fig. 15-6 A nail file is used to clean under the fingernails.

Fig. 15-7 A paper towel is used to turn off each faucet.

PROMOTING SAFETY AND COMFORT
Hand Hygiene

Safety

You use your hands in almost every task. They can pick up microbes from one person, place, or thing. Your hands transfer them to other people, places, and things. That is why hand hygiene is so very important. You must practice hand hygiene before and after giving care.

Comfort

You will practice hand hygiene very often during your shift. Hand lotions and hand creams help prevent chapping and dry skin. Apply hand lotion or cream as often as needed. Use a center-approved lotion or cream.

HAND WASHING

PROCEDURE

1 See *Promoting Safety and Comfort: Hand Hygiene.*
2 Make sure you have soap, paper towels, an orangewood stick or nail file, and a wastebasket. Collect missing items.
3 Push your watch up your arm 4 to 5 inches. If your uniform sleeves are long, push them up too.
4 Stand away from the sink so your clothes do not touch the sink. Stand so the soap and faucet are easy to reach (see Fig. 15-3). Do not touch the inside of the sink at any time.
5 Turn on and adjust the water until it feels warm.
6 Wet your wrists and hands. Keep your hands lower than your elbows. Be sure to wet the area 3 to 4 inches above your wrists.
7 Apply about 1 teaspoon of soap to your hands.
8 Rub your palms together and interlace your fingers to work up a good lather (see Fig. 15-4). This step should last at least 15 to 20 seconds. (NOTE: Some state competency tests require that you wash your hands for 20 to 30 seconds. Know what is required in your state.)

9 Wash each hand and wrist thoroughly. Clean well between the fingers.
10 Clean under the fingernails. Rub your fingertips against your palms (see Fig. 15-5).
11 Clean under the fingernails with a nail file or orangewood stick (see Fig. 15-6). This step is done for the first hand washing of the day and when your hands are highly soiled.
12 Rinse your wrists and hands well. Water flows from the arms to the hands.
13 Repeat steps 7 through 12, if needed.
14 Dry your wrists and hands with a clean, dry paper towel. Pat dry starting at your fingertips.
15 Discard the paper towel into the wastebasket.
16 Turn off faucets with clean, dry paper towels. This prevents you from contaminating your hands (see Fig. 15-7). Use a clean paper towel for each faucet.
17 Discard the paper towels into the wastebasket.

Supplies and Equipment

Most health care equipment is disposable. Single-use items are discarded after use. A person uses multi-use items many times. They include bedpans, urinals, wash basins, water pitchers, drinking cups, and glasses. Do not "borrow" them for another person. Disposable items help prevent the spread of infection.

Non-disposable items are cleaned and then disinfected. Then they are sterilized.

Cleaning Cleaning reduces the number of microbes present. It also removes organic matter such as blood, body fluids, secretions, and excretions. To clean equipment:

- Wear personal protective equipment (PPE) when cleaning items contaminated with blood, body fluids, secretions, or excretions. PPE includes gloves, a mask, a gown, and goggles or a face shield.
- Rinse the item to remove organic matter. Use cold water. Heat makes organic matter thick, sticky, and hard to remove.
- Wash the item with soap and hot water.
- Scrub thoroughly. Use a brush if necessary.
- Rinse the item in warm water.
- Dry the item.
- Disinfect or sterilize the item.
- Disinfect equipment and the sink used in the cleaning procedure.
- Discard PPE.
- Practice hand hygiene.

Nursing centers have "clean" and "dirty" utility rooms. Equipment is cleaned in the "dirty" utility room. Then it is disinfected or sterilized in the "clean" utility room.

Disinfection Disinfection is the process of destroying pathogens. Spores are not destroyed. Spores are bacteria protected by a hard shell. Spores are killed by very high temperatures.

Germicides are disinfectants applied to skin, tissues, and non-living objects. Alcohol is a common germicide.

Chemical disinfectants are used to clean surfaces. Counters, tubs, and showers are examples. They also are used to clean re-usable items. Such items include:

- Blood pressure cuffs
- Commodes and metal bedpans
- Wheelchairs and stretchers
- Furniture
  See *Promoting Safety and Comfort: Disinfection.*

PROMOTING SAFETY AND COMFORT
Disinfection

Safety
Chemical disinfectants can burn and irritate the skin. Wear utility gloves or rubber household gloves to prevent skin irritation. These gloves are *waterproof.* Do not wear disposable gloves.

Some chemical disinfectants have special measures for use and storage. Check the material safety data sheet (MSDS) before handling a disinfectant. See Chapter 12.

Sterilization Sterilizing destroys all non-pathogens and pathogens, including spores. Very high temperatures are used. Microbes are destroyed by heat.

Boiling water, radiation, liquid or gas chemicals, dry heat, and *steam under pressure* are sterilization methods. An *autoclave* (Fig. 15-8) is a pressure steam sterilizer. Glass, surgical items, and metal objects are autoclaved. High temperatures destroy plastic and rubber items. They are not autoclaved. Steam under pressure sterilizes objects in 30 to 45 minutes.

Other Aseptic Measures

Hand hygiene, cleaning, disinfection, and sterilization are important aseptic measures. So are the measures listed in Box 15-3. They are useful in home, work, and everyday life.

Fig. 15-8 An autoclave.

Box 15-3   Aseptic Measures

Controlling Reservoirs (Hosts—You or the Person)
- Provide for the person's hygiene needs (Chapter 20).
- Wash contaminated areas with soap and water. Feces, urine, and blood can contain microbes. So can body fluids, secretions, and excretions.
- Use leak-proof plastic bags for soiled tissues, linens, and other materials.
- Keep tables, counters, wheelchair trays, and other surfaces clean and dry.
- Label bottles with the person's name and the date the bottle was opened.
- Keep bottles and fluid containers tightly capped or covered.
- Keep drainage containers below the drainage site (Chapters 22 and 35).
- Empty drainage containers and dispose of drainage following center policy. Usually drainage containers are emptied every shift. Follow the nurse's directions.

Controlling Portals of Exit
- Cover your nose and mouth when coughing or sneezing.
- Provide the person with tissues to use when coughing or sneezing.
- Wear PPE as needed (p. 195).

Controlling Transmission
- Make sure all persons have their own personal care equipment. This includes wash basins, bedpans, urinals, commodes, and eating and drinking utensils.
- Do not take equipment from one person's room to use for another person. Even if the item is un-used, do not take it from one room to another.
- Hold equipment and linens away from your uniform (Fig. 15-9).
- Practice hand hygiene. See Box 15-2.

Controlling Transmission—cont'd
- Assist the person with hand washing:
  - Before and after eating
  - After elimination
  - After changing tampons, sanitary napkins, or other personal hygiene products
  - After contact with blood, body fluids, secretions, or excretions
- Prevent dust movement. Do not shake linens or equipment. Use a damp cloth for dusting.
- Clean from the cleanest area to the dirtiest. This prevents soiling a clean area.
- Clean away from your body. Do not dust, brush, or wipe toward yourself. Otherwise you transmit microbes to your skin, hair, and clothing.
- Flush urine and feces down the toilet. Avoid splatters and splashes.
- Pour contaminated liquids directly into sinks or toilets. Avoid splashing onto other areas.
- Do not sit on the person's bed. You will pick up microbes. You will transfer them to the next surface that you sit on.
- Do not use items that are on the floor. The floor is contaminated.
- Clean tubs, showers, and shower chairs after each use. Follow the center's disinfection procedures.
- Clean bedpans, urinals, and commodes after each use. Follow the center's disinfection procedures.
- Report pests—ants, spiders, mice, and so on.

Controlling Portals of Entry
- Provide for good skin care (Chapter 20). This promotes intact skin.
- Provide for good oral hygiene (Chapter 20). This promotes intact mucous membranes.

Box 15-3 Aseptic Measures—cont'd

Controlling Portals of Entry—cont'd

- Do not let the person lie on tubes or other items. This protects the skin from injury.
- Make sure linens are dry and wrinkle-free (Chapter 19). This protects the skin from injury.
- Turn and re-position the person as directed by the nurse and care plan (Chapters 16 and 17). This protects the skin from injury.
- Assist with or clean the genital area after elimination (Chapter 20). Wipe and clean from the urethra (the cleanest area) to the rectum (the dirtiest area). This helps prevent urinary tract infections.
- Make sure drainage tubes are properly connected. This prevents microbes from entering the drainage system.

Protecting the Susceptible Host

- Follow the care plan to meet hygiene needs. This protects the skin and mucous membranes.
- Follow the care plan to meet nutrition and fluid needs (Chapter 24). This helps prevent infection.
- Assist with deep-breathing and coughing exercises as directed (Chapter 28). This helps prevent respiratory infections.

Fig. 15-9 Hold equipment away from your uniform.

ISOLATION PRECAUTIONS

Blood, body fluids, secretions, and excretions can transmit pathogens. Sometimes barriers are needed to prevent their escape. The pathogens are kept within a certain area. Usually the area is the person's room. This requires isolation procedures.

The *Guideline for Isolation Precautions: Preventing Transmission of Infectious Agents in Healthcare Settings 2007* is followed. The guideline was issued by the Centers for Disease Control and Prevention (CDC).

Isolation precautions prevent the spread of communicable diseases (contagious diseases). They are diseases caused by pathogens that spread easily.

Isolation precautions are based on *clean* and *dirty*. *Clean* areas or objects are free of pathogens. They are not contaminated. *Dirty* areas or objects are contaminated with pathogens. If a *clean* area or object has contact with something *dirty*, the clean area is now dirty. *Clean* and *dirty* also depend on how the pathogen is spread.

The CDC's isolation precautions guideline has two tiers of precautions:
- Standard Precautions
- Transmission-Based Precautions

See *Focus on Communication: Isolation Precautions.*
See *Delegation Guidelines: Isolation Precautions.*
See *Promoting Safety and Comfort: Isolation Precautions,* p. 192.
See *Teamwork and Time Management: Isolation Precautions,* p. 192.

FOCUS ON COMMUNICATION
Isolation Precautions

Some centers require visitors to wear PPE when visiting a person needing isolation precautions. Visitors may question the need for PPE. They do not wear PPE around the person in his or her home or outside the center. They do not understand why it is needed. Some visitors ignore signs or requests to wear PPE. It is important to communicate with the person and visitors about PPE. You can politely say:
- "Your visitors will need to wear a gown and gloves while in your room."
- "Please wear this mask. It is our policy to protect you, your family member, and others."

Tell the nurse if the person or visitors have more questions. Also tell the nurse if someone refuses to follow isolation precautions.

DELEGATION GUIDELINES
Isolation Precautions

You may assist in the care of persons who require isolation precautions. If so, review the type used with the nurse. You also need this information from the nurse and the care plan:
- What PPE to use
- What special safety measures are needed

PROMOTING SAFETY AND COMFORT
Isolation Precautions

Safety

Preventing the spread of infection is important. Isolation precautions protect everyone—residents, visitors, staff, and you. If you are careless, everyone's safety is at risk.

Comfort

Persons requiring isolation precautions usually must stay in their rooms. The person may feel lonely, especially if visitors are few. You can help the person by:

- Remembering that the pathogen is undesirable, not the person
- Treating the person with respect, kindness, and dignity
- Providing newspapers, magazines, books, and other reading matter
- Providing hobby materials if possible
- Placing a clock in the room
- Urging the person to call family and friends
- Providing a current TV guide
- Organizing your work so you can stay to visit with the person
- Saying "hello" from the doorway often

Items brought into the person's room become contaminated. Disinfect or discard the items according to center policy.

TEAMWORK AND TIME MANAGEMENT
Isolation Precautions

Donning (putting on) and removing PPE take time and effort. Once you don PPE, you must remove it before leaving the room. Therefore you need to plan your time and work so that you do not need to leave the room. Meet the needs of other residents first. Ask a co-worker to answer their signal lights for you. Ask politely and thank your co-worker for helping you. Then gather the care items that you need to bring to the room. Before leaving the room, make sure the person's needs are met. Complete a safety check of the room. Also tell the person when you will return to the room.

Offer to help a co-worker if he or she will care for a person needing isolation. Bring items to the room as needed. Also answer signal lights for your co-worker. Be sure to tell the co-worker what you did for the person and what you observed.

known and unknown infections. *Standard Precautions are used for all persons whenever care is given.* They prevent the spread of infection from:

- Blood.
- All body fluids, secretions, and excretions (except sweat) even if blood is not visible. Sweat is not known to spread infection.
- Non-intact skin (skin with open breaks).
- Mucous membranes.

Transmission-Based Precautions

Some infections require Transmission-Based Precautions (Box 15-5, p. 194). You must understand how certain infections are spread (see Fig. 15-2). This helps you understand the types of Transmission-Based Precautions.

Standard Precautions

Standard Precautions are part of the CDC's isolation precautions (Box 15-4). They reduce the risk of spreading pathogens. They also reduce the risk of spreading

---

Box 15-4   Standard Precautions

Hand Hygiene
- Follow the rules for hand hygiene. See Box 15-2.
- Avoid unnecessary touching of surfaces close to the person. This prevents contamination of clean hands from environmental surfaces. It also prevents the transmission of pathogens from contaminated hands to other surfaces.
- Do not wear fake nails or nail extenders if you will have contact with persons at risk for infection or other adverse outcomes. (Note: Some centers do not allow fake nails or nail extenders.)

Personal Protective Equipment (PPE)
- Wear PPE when contact with blood or body fluids is likely.
- Do not contaminate your clothing or skin when removing PPE.
- Remove and discard PPE before leaving the person's room or care setting.

Gloves
- Wear gloves when contact with the following is likely:
  - Blood
  - Potentially infectious materials (body fluids, secretions, and excretions are examples)
  - Mucous membranes
  - Non-intact skin
  - Skin that may be contaminated (for example, a person is incontinent of feces or urine)
- Wear gloves that fit and are appropriate for the task:
  - Wear disposable gloves to provide direct care to the person.
  - Wear disposable gloves or utility gloves for cleaning equipment or care settings.

Modified from Siegel JD, Rhinehart E, Jackson M, Chiarello L, and the Healthcare Infection Control Practices Advisory Committee: Guideline for isolation precautions: preventing transmission of infectious agents in healthcare settings 2007, *Centers for Disease Control and Prevention, June 2007.*

Box 15-4 Standard Precautions—cont'd

Gloves cont'd

- Remove gloves after contact with the person or the person's care setting. The care setting includes equipment used in the person's care.
- Remove gloves after contact with care equipment.
- Do not wear the same pair of gloves to care for more than one person. Remove gloves after contact with a person and before going to another person.
- Do not wash gloves for re-use with different persons.
- Change gloves during care if your hands will move from a contaminated body site to a clean body site.

Gowns

- Wear a gown that is appropriate to the task.
- Wear a gown to protect your skin and clothing when contact with blood, body fluids, secretions, or excretions is likely.
- Wear a gown for direct contact with a person if he or she has uncontained secretions or excretions.
- Remove the gown and perform hand hygiene before leaving the person's room or care setting.
- Do not re-use gowns, even for repeat contacts with the same person.

Mouth, Nose, and Eye Protection

- Wear PPE—masks, goggles, face shields—for procedures and tasks that are likely to cause splashes and sprays of blood, body fluids, secretions, or excretions.
- Wear PPE—mask, goggles, face shield—appropriate for the procedure or task.
- Wear gloves, a gown, and one of the following for procedures that are likely to cause sprays of respiratory secretions:
  - A face shield that fully covers the front and sides of the face
  - A mask with attached shield
  - A mask and goggles

Respiratory Hygiene/Cough Etiquette

- Instruct persons with respiratory symptoms to:
  - Cover the nose and mouth when coughing or sneezing.
  - Use tissues to contain respiratory secretions.
  - Dispose of tissues in the nearest waste container after use.
  - Perform hand hygiene after contact with respiratory secretions.
- Provide visitors with masks according to center policy.

Care Equipment

- Wear appropriate PPE when handling care equipment that is visibly soiled with blood, body fluids, secretions, or excretions.
- Wear appropriate PPE when handling care equipment that may have been in contact with blood, body fluids, secretions, or excretions.
- Remove organic material before disinfection and sterilization procedures. Use cleaning agents according to center policy.

Care of the Environment

- Follow center policies and procedures for cleaning and maintaining surfaces. Environmental surfaces and care equipment are examples. Surfaces near the person may need more frequent cleaning and maintenance—door knobs, bed rails, overbed tables, toilet surfaces and areas, and so on.
- Clean and disinfect multi-use electronic equipment according to center policy. This includes:
  - Items used by residents
  - Items used to give care
  - Mobile devices that are moved in and out of resident rooms
- Follow these rules for toys used by children and toys in waiting areas:
  - Select toys that can be easily cleaned and disinfected.
  - Do not allow use of stuffed furry toys if they will be shared.
  - Clean and disinfect large stationary toys (for example, climbing equipment) at least weekly and whenever visibly soiled.
  - Rinse toys with water after disinfection if they are likely to be mouthed by children. Or wash them in a dishwasher.
  - Clean and disinfect a toy immediately when it requires cleaning. Or store the toy in a labeled container away from toys that are clean and ready for use.

Textiles and Laundry

- Handle used textiles and fabrics (linens) with minimum agitation. This is done to avoid contamination of air, surfaces, and other persons.

Worker Safety

- Protect yourself and others from exposure to bloodborne pathogens. This includes how to handle needles and other sharps. Follow federal and state standards and guidelines. See the Bloodborne Pathogen Standard (p. 203).
- Use a mouthpiece, resuscitation bag, or other ventilation device during resuscitation to prevent contact with the person's mouth and oral secretions. See Chapter 47.

Resident Placement

- A private room is preferred if the person is at risk for transmitting the infection to others.
- Follow the nurse's instructions if a private room is not available.

Box 15-5   Transmission-Based Precautions

Contact Precautions

- Used for persons with known or suspected infections or conditions that increase the risk of contact transmission.
- Resident placement:
  - A single room is preferred.
  - Do the following if a room is shared with another person who is not infected with the same agent:
    - Keep the privacy curtain between the beds closed.
    - Change PPE and perform hand hygiene between contact with persons in the same room. Do so regardless of whether one or both persons are on contact precautions.
- Gloves:
  - Don gloves upon entering the person's room or care setting.
  - Wear gloves whenever touching the person's intact skin.
  - Wear gloves whenever touching surfaces or items near the person.
- Gowns:
  - Wear a gown whenever clothing may have direct contact with the person.
  - Wear a gown whenever contact is likely with surfaces or equipment near the person.
  - Don the gown upon entering the person's room or care setting.
  - Remove the gown and perform hand hygiene before leaving the person's room or care setting.
  - Make sure your clothing and skin do not touch potentially contaminated surfaces after removing the gown.
- Resident transport:
  - Limit transport and movement of the person outside the room to medically-necessary purposes.
  - Cover the area of the person's body that is infected.
  - Remove and discard contaminated PPE and perform hand hygiene before transporting the person.
  - Don clean PPE to handle the person at the transport destination.
- Care equipment:
  - Follow Standard Precautions.
  - Use disposable equipment when possible. If possible, leave non-disposable equipment in the person's room.
  - Clean and disinfect non-disposable and multiple-use equipment before use on another person.

Droplet Precautions

- Used for persons known or suspected to be infected with pathogens transmitted by respiratory droplets. Such droplets are generated by a person who is coughing, sneezing, or talking.

Droplet Precautions—cont'd

- Resident placement:
  - A single room is preferred.
  - Do the following if a room is shared with another person who is not infected with the same agent:
    - Keep the privacy curtain between the beds closed.
    - Change PPE and perform hand hygiene between contact with persons in the same room. Do so regardless of whether one or both persons are on Droplet Precautions.
- Personal protective equipment:
  - Don a mask upon entering the person's room or care setting.
- Resident transport:
  - Limit transport and movement of the person outside the room to medically-necessary purposes.
  - Have the person wear a mask.
  - Instruct the person to follow Respiratory Hygiene/Cough Etiquette (see "Standard Precautions," Box 15-4).
  - No mask is required for health team members transporting the person.

Airborne Precautions

- Used for persons known or suspected to be infected with pathogens transmitted person-to-person by the airborne route. Tuberculosis (TB), measles, chickenpox, smallpox, and severe acute respiratory syndrome (SARS) are examples.
- The resident is placed in an airborne infection isolation room (AIIR). If one is not available, the person is transferred to an agency with an AIIR.
- Health team members susceptible to the infection are restricted from entering the room if immune staff members are available.
- Personal protective equipment:
  - An approved respirator is worn on entering the room or home of a person with TB.
  - Respiratory protection is recommended for all health team members when caring for persons with smallpox.
- Resident transport:
  - Limit transport and movement of the person outside the room to medically-necessary purposes.
  - Have the person wear a surgical mask.
  - Instruct the person to follow Respiratory Hygiene/Cough Etiquette (see "Standard Precautions," Box 15-4).
  - Cover skin lesions infected with the microbe.
  - No mask or respirator is required for health team members transporting the person.

Modified from Siegel JD, Rhinehart E, Jackson M, Chiarello L, and the Healthcare Infection Control Practices Advisory Committee: Guideline for isolation precautions: preventing transmission of infectious agents in healthcare settings 2007, *Centers for Disease Control and Prevention, June 2007.*

Box 15-6	Rules for Isolation Precautions

- Collect all needed items before entering the room.
- Prevent contamination of equipment and supplies. Floors are contaminated. So is any object on the floor or that falls to the floor.
- Use mops wetted with a disinfectant solution to clean floors. Floor dust is contaminated.
- Prevent drafts. Some microbes are carried in the air by drafts.
- Use paper towels to handle contaminated items.
- Remove items from the room in leak-proof plastic bags.
- Double-bag items if the outer part of the bag is or can be contaminated (p. 201).
- Follow center policy for removing and transporting disposable and re-usable items.
- Return re-usable dishes, drinking vessels, eating utensils, and trays to the food service (dietary) department. Discard disposable dishes, drinking vessels, eating utensils, and trays in the waste container in the person's room.
- Do not touch your hair, nose, mouth, eyes, or other body parts.
- Do not touch any clean area or object if your hands are contaminated.
- Wash your hands if they are visibly dirty or contaminated with blood, body fluids, secretions, or excretions.
- Place clean items on paper towels.
- Do not shake linens.
- Use paper towels to turn faucets on and off.
- Use a paper towel to open the door to the person's room. Discard it as you leave.
- Tell the nurse if you have any cuts, open skin areas, a sore throat, vomiting, or diarrhea.

Protective Measures

Center policies may differ from those in this text. The rules in Box 15-6 are a guide for giving safe care when using isolation precautions.

Isolation precautions involve wearing PPE—gloves, a gown, a mask, and goggles or a face shield.

Removing linens, trash, and equipment from the room may require double-bagging. Follow center procedures when collecting specimens and transporting persons.

See *Promoting Safety and Comfort: Protective Measures.*

PROMOTING SAFETY AND COMFORT
Protective Measures

Safety

The PPE needed for Standard Precautions depends on what tasks, procedures, and care measures you will do while in the room. The PPE needed also depends on the type of Transmission-Based Precautions ordered for the person. Sometimes only gloves are needed. The nurse tells you when other PPE are needed.

According to the CDC's isolation guideline, gloves are always worn when gowns are worn. Sometimes other PPE are needed when gowns are worn. The isolation guideline shows PPE donned and removed in the following order:

- Donning PPE (Fig. 15-10, A, p. 196):
  - Gown
  - Mask or respirator
  - Eyewear (goggles or face shield)
  - Gloves
- Removing PPE (removed at the doorway before leaving the person's room) (Fig. 15-10, B, p. 196):
  - Gloves
  - Goggles or face shield
  - Gown
  - Mask or respirator

SEQUENCE FOR DONNING PERSONAL PROTECTIVE EQUIPMENT (PPE)

The type of PPE used will vary based on the level of precautions required; e.g., Standard and Contact, Droplet or Airborne Infection Isolation.

1. GOWN
- Fully cover torso from neck to knees, arms to end of wrists, and wrap around the back
- Fasten in back of neck and waist

2. MASK OR RESPIRATOR
- Secure ties or elastic bands at middle of head and neck
- Fit flexible band to nose bridge
- Fit snug to face and below chin
- Fit-check respirator

3. GOGGLES OR FACE SHIELD
- Place over face and eyes and adjust to fit

4. GLOVES
- Extend to cover wrist of isolation gown

USE SAFE WORK PRACTICES TO PROTECT YOURSELF AND LIMIT THE SPREAD OF CONTAMINATION

- Keep hands away from face
- Limit surfaces touched
- Change gloves when torn or heavily contaminated
- Perform hand hygiene

SECUENCIA PARA PONERSE EL EQUIPO DE PROTECCIÓN PERSONAL (PPE)

El tipo de PPE que se debe utilizar depende del nivel de precaución que sea necesario; por ejemplo, equipo Estándar y de Contacto o de Aislamiento de infecciones transportadas por gotas o por aire.

1. BATA
- Cubra con la bata todo el torso desde el cuello hasta las rodillas, los brazos hasta la muñeca y dóblela alrededor de la espalda
- Átesela por detrás a la altura del cuello y la cintura

2. MÁSCARA O RESPIRADOR
- Asegúrese los cordones o la banda elástica en la mitad de la cabeza y en el cuello
- Ajústese la banda flexible en el puente de la nariz
- Acomódesela en la cara y por debajo del mentón
- Verifique el ajuste del respirador

3. GAFAS PROTECTORAS O CARETAS
- Colóquesela sobre la cara y los ojos y ajústela

4. GUANTES
- Extienda los guantes para que cubran la parte del puño en la bata de aislamiento

UTILICE PRÁCTICAS DE TRABAJO SEGURAS PARA PROTEGERSE USTED MISMO Y LIMITAR LA PROPAGACIÓN DE LA CONTAMINACIÓN

- Mantenga las manos alejadas de la cara
- Limite el contacto con superficies
- Cambie los guantes si se rompen o están demasiado contaminados
- Realice la higiene de las manos

A

SEQUENCE FOR REMOVING PERSONAL PROTECTIVE EQUIPMENT (PPE)

Except for respirator, remove PPE at doorway or in anteroom. Remove respirator after leaving patient room and closing door.

1. GLOVES
- Outside of gloves is contaminated!
- Grasp outside of glove with opposite gloved hand; peel off
- Hold removed glove in gloved hand
- Slide fingers of ungloved hand under remaining glove at wrist
- Peel glove off over first glove
- Discard gloves in waste container

2. GOGGLES OR FACE SHIELD
- Outside of goggles or face shield is contaminated!
- To remove, handle by head band or ear pieces
- Place in designated receptacle for reprocessing or in waste container

3. GOWN
- Gown front and sleeves are contaminated!
- Unfasten ties
- Pull away from neck and shoulders, touching inside of gown only
- Turn gown inside out
- Fold or roll into a bundle and discard

4. MASK OR RESPIRATOR
- Front of mask/respirator is contaminated — DO NOT TOUCH!
- Grasp bottom, then top ties or elastics and remove
- Discard in waste container

PERFORM HAND HYGIENE IMMEDIATELY AFTER REMOVING ALL PPE

SECUENCIA PARA QUITARSE EL EQUIPO DE PROTECCIÓN PERSONAL (PPE)

Con la excepción del respirador, quítese el PPE en la entrada de la puerta o en la antesala. Quítese el respirador después de salir de la habitación del paciente y de cerrar la puerta.

1. GUANTES
- ¡El exterior de los guantes está contaminado!
- Agarre la parte exterior del guante con la mano opuesta en la que todavía tiene puesto el guante y quíteselo
- Sostenga el guante que se quitó con la mano enguantada
- Deslice los dedos de la mano sin guante por debajo del otro guante que no se ha quitado todavía a la altura de la muñeca
- Quítese el guante de manera que acabe cubriendo el primer guante
- Arroje los guantes en el recipiente de deshechos

2. GAFAS PROTECTORAS O CARETA
- ¡El exterior de las gafas protectoras o de la careta está contaminado!
- Para quitárselas, tómelas por la parte de la banda de la cabeza o de las piezas de las orejas
- Colóquelas en el recipiente designado para reprocesar materiales o de materiales de deshecho

3. BATA
- ¡La parte delantera de la bata y las mangas están contaminadas!
- Desate los cordones
- Tocando solamente el interior de la bata, pásela por encima del cuello y de los hombros
- Voltee la bata al revés
- Dóblela o enróllela y deséchela

4. MÁSCARA O RESPIRADOR
- La parte delantera de la máscara o respirador está contaminada — ¡NO LA TOQUE!
- Primero agarre la parte de abajo, luego los cordones o banda elástica de arriba y por último quítese la máscara o respirador
- Arrójela en el recipiente de deshechos

EFECTÚE LA HIGIENE DE LAS MANOS INMEDIATAMENTE DESPUÉS DE QUITARSE CUALQUIER EQUIPO DE PROTECCIÓN PERSONAL

B

Fig. 15-10 A, Donning personal protective equipment. **B,** Removing personal protective equipment. *(From Centers for Disease Control and Prevention:* Guideline for isolation precautions: preventing transmission of infectious agents in healthcare settings 2007, *Atlanta, Ga, June 2004, Author.)*

Gloves The skin is a natural barrier. It prevents microbes from entering the body. Small skin breaks on the hands and fingers are common. Some are very small and hard to see. Disposable gloves act as a barrier. They protect you from pathogens in the person's blood, body fluids, secretions, and excretions. They also protect the person from microbes on your hands.

Wear gloves whenever contact with blood, body fluids, secretions, excretions, mucous membranes, or non-intact skin is likely. Contact may be direct. Or contact may be with items or surfaces contaminated with blood, body fluids, secretions, or excretions.

Wearing gloves is the most common protective measure used with Standard Precautions and Transmission-Based Precautions. Remember the following when using gloves:

- The outside of gloves is contaminated.
- Gloves are easier to put on when your hands are dry.
- Do not tear gloves when putting them on. Carelessness, long fingernails, and rings can tear gloves. Blood, body fluids, secretions, and excretions can enter the glove through the tear. This contaminates your hand.
- You need a new pair for every person.
- Remove and discard torn, cut, or punctured gloves at once. Practice hand hygiene. Then put on a new pair.
- Wear gloves once. Discard them after use.
- Put on clean gloves just before touching mucous membranes or non-intact skin.
- Put on new gloves whenever gloves become contaminated with blood, body fluids, secretions, or excretions. A task may require more than one pair of gloves.
- Change gloves whenever moving from a contaminated body site to a clean body site.
- Change gloves if interacting with the person involves touching portable computer keyboards or other mobile equipment that is transported from room to room.
- Put on gloves last when they are worn with other PPE.
- Make sure gloves cover your wrists. If you wear a gown, gloves cover the cuffs (Fig. 15-11).
- Remove gloves so the inside part is on the outside. The inside is *clean*.
- Decontaminate your hands after removing gloves. See *Promoting Safety and Comfort: Gloves.*

Fig. 15-11 The gloves cover the cuffs of the gown.

PROMOTING SAFETY AND COMFORT
Gloves

Safety

No special method is needed to put on non-sterile gloves. To remove gloves, see procedure: *Removing Gloves,* p. 198.

Some gloves are made of latex (a rubber product). Latex allergies are common. They can cause skin rashes. Asthma and shock are more serious problems. Report skin rashes and breathing problems to the nurse at once.

You may have a latex allergy. Some residents are allergic to latex. This information is on the care plan and your assignment sheet. Latex-free gloves are worn for latex allergies.

Comfort

Many nurses and nursing assistants wear gloves for every resident contact. Remember, gloves are needed whenever contact with blood, body fluids, secretions, excretions, mucous membranes, or non-intact skin is likely. You do not need to wear gloves when such contact is not likely. Back massages and brushing and combing hair are examples. Wearing gloves only when needed helps reduce exposure to latex.

REMOVING GLOVES

VIDEO   NNAAP™ Skill

PROCEDURE

1 See *Promoting Safety and Comfort: Gloves.* p. 197.
2 Make sure that glove touches only glove.
3 Grasp a glove just below the cuff (Fig. 15-12, *A*). Grasp it on the outside.
4 Pull the glove down over your hand so it is inside out (Fig. 15-12, *B*).
5 Hold the removed glove with your other gloved hand.

6 Reach inside the other glove. Use the first two fingers of the ungloved hand (Fig. 15-12, *C*).
7 Pull the glove down (inside out) over your hand and the other glove (Fig. 15-12, *D*).
8 Discard the gloves. Follow center policy.
9 Decontaminate your hands.

A   B   C   D

Fig. 15-12 Removing gloves. **A,** Grasp the glove below the cuff. **B,** Pull the glove down over the hand. The glove is inside out. **C,** Insert the fingers of the ungloved hand inside the other glove. **D,** Pull the glove down and over the other hand and glove. The glove is inside out.

 Gowns Gowns prevent the spread of microbes. They protect your clothes and body from contact with blood, body fluids, secretions, and excretions. They also protect against splashes and sprays.

Gowns must completely cover you from your neck to your knees. The long sleeves have tight cuffs. The gown opens at the back. It is tied at the neck and waist. The gown front and sleeves are considered to be *contaminated*.

Gowns are used once. A wet gown is contaminated. It is removed and a dry one put on. Disposable gowns are discarded after use.

DONNING AND REMOVING A GOWN

VIDEO · NNAAP™ Skill

PROCEDURE

1. Remove your watch and all jewelry.
2. Roll up uniform sleeves.
3. Practice hand hygiene.
4. Hold a clean gown out in front of you. Let it unfold. Do not shake the gown.
5. Put your hands and arms through the sleeves (see Fig. 15-10, *A*).
6. Make sure the gown covers you from your neck to your knees. It must cover your arms to the end of your wrists.
7. Tie the strings at the back of the neck (see Fig. 15-10, *A*).
8. Overlap the back of the gown. Make sure it covers your uniform. The gown should be snug, not loose.
9. Tie the waist strings. Tie them at the back or the side. Do not tie them in front.
10. Put on other PPE.
    a. Mask or respirator (if needed).
    b. Goggles or face shield (if needed).
    c. Gloves. Make sure the gloves cover the gown cuffs.
11. Provide care.
12. Remove and discard the gloves.
13. Remove and discard the goggles or face shield if worn.
14. Remove the gown. Do not touch the outside of the gown.
    a. Untie the neck and waist strings (see Fig. 15-10, *B*).
    b. Pull the gown down from each shoulder toward the same hand (see Fig. 15-10, *B*).
    c. Turn the gown inside out as it is removed. Hold it at the inside shoulder seams, and bring your hands together (Fig. 15-13).
15. Hold and roll up the gown away from you (see Fig. 15-10, *B*). Keep it inside out.
16. Discard the gown.
17. Remove and discard the mask if worn.
18. Decontaminate your hands.

Fig. 15-13 The gown is turned inside out as it is removed.

Fig. 15-14 Tuberculosis respirator.

Masks and Respiratory Protection You wear masks for these reasons:

- For protection from contact with infectious materials from the resident. Respiratory secretions and sprays of blood or body fluids are examples.
- During sterile procedures to protect the person from infectious agents carried in your mouth or nose.

Masks are disposable. A wet or moist mask is contaminated. Breathing can cause masks to become wet or moist. Apply a new mask when contamination occurs.

A mask fits snugly over your nose and mouth. Practice hand hygiene before putting on a mask. When removing a mask, touch only the ties or the elastic bands. The front of the mask is contaminated.

Tuberculosis respirators (Fig. 15-14) are worn when caring for persons with TB (Chapter 40).

DONNING AND REMOVING A MASK

VIDEO

PROCEDURE

1 Practice hand hygiene.
2 Put on a gown if required.
3 Pick up a mask by its upper ties. Do not touch the part that will cover your face.
4 Place the mask over your nose and mouth (Fig. 15-15, *A*).
5 Place the upper strings above your ears. Tie them at the back in the middle of your head (Fig. 15-15, *B*).
6 Tie the lower strings at the back of your neck (Fig. 15-15, *C*). The lower part of the mask is under your chin.
7 Pinch the metal band around your nose. The top of the mask must be snug over your nose. If you wear eyeglasses, the mask must be snug under the bottom of the eyeglasses.
8 Make sure the mask is snug over your face and under your chin.

9 Put on goggles or a face shield if needed and if not part of the mask.
10 Put on gloves.
11 Provide care. Avoid coughing, sneezing, and unnecessary talking.
12 Change the mask if it becomes wet or contaminated.
13 Remove the mask (see Fig. 15-10, *B*).
   a Remove the gloves.
   b Remove the goggles or face shield and gown if worn.
   c Untie the lower strings of the mask.
   d Untie the top strings.
   e Hold the top strings. Remove the mask.
14 Discard the mask.
15 Decontaminate your hands.

Fig. 15-15 Donning and removing a mask. NOTE: The mask has a face shield. **A,** The mask covers the nose and mouth. **B,** Upper strings are tied at the back of the head. **C,** Lower strings are tied at the back of the neck.

Goggles and Face Shields Goggles and face shields protect your eyes, mouth, and nose from splashing or spraying of blood, body fluids, secretions, and excretions (see Fig. 15-15). Splashes and sprays can occur when giving care, cleaning items, or disposing of fluids.

The front of goggles or a face shield is contaminated. The ties, ear pieces, or headband used to secure the device are considered "clean." Use them to remove the device after hand hygiene. They are safe to touch with bare hands.

Discard disposable goggles or face shields after use. Re-usable eyewear is cleaned before re-use. It is washed with soap and water. Then a disinfectant is used.

See *Promoting Safety and Comfort: Goggles and Face Shields.*

Bagging Items Contaminated items are bagged to remove them from the person's room. Leak-proof plastic bags are used. They have the *BIOHAZARD* symbol (Fig. 15-16). **Biohazardous waste** is items contaminated with blood, body fluids, secretions, or excretions. (*Bio* means life. *Hazardous* means dangerous or harmful.)

Bag and transport linens following center policy. Laundry bags with contaminated linen need a *BIOHAZARD* symbol. Melt-away bags are common. They dissolve in hot water. Once soiled linen is bagged, no one needs to handle it. Do not overfill the bag. Tie the bag securely. Then place it in a laundry hamper lined with a biohazard plastic bag.

Trash is placed in a container labeled with the *BIOHAZARD* symbol. Follow center policy for bagging and transporting trash, equipment, and supplies.

Usually one bag is needed. Double-bagging involves two bags. Double-bagging is not needed unless the outside of the bag is wet, soiled, or may be contaminated. Two staff members are needed:

* One is inside the room.
* The other is at the doorway outside the room.
* The person in the room places contaminated items into a bag. Then the bag is sealed.
* The person outside the room holds open another bag. This bag is clean. A wide cuff is made on the clean bag to protect the hands from contamination (Fig. 15-17).
* The contaminated bag is placed into the clean bag at the doorway.

PROMOTING SAFETY AND COMFORT
Goggles and Face Shields

Safety
Eyeglasses and contact lenses do not provide eye protection. If you wear eyeglasses, use a face shield that fits over your glasses with minimal gaps.

Goggles do not provide splash or spray protection to other parts of your face.

Fig. 15-16 *BIOHAZARD* symbol.

Fig. 15-17 Double-bagging. One nursing assistant is in the room by the doorway. The other is outside the doorway. The "dirty" bag is placed inside the "clean" bag.

Collecting Specimens Blood, body fluids, secretions, and excretions often require laboratory testing (Chapter 33). Specimens are transported to the laboratory in biohazard specimen bags. To collect a specimen:

- Label the specimen container and biohazard specimen bag. Apply warning labels according to center policy.
- Don PPE as required. Gloves are worn.
- Put the specimen container and lid in the person's bathroom. Put them on a paper towel.
- Collect the specimen. Do not contaminate the outside of the container. Also avoid contamination when transferring the specimen from the collecting vessel to the specimen container.
- Put the lid on securely.
- Remove the PPE. Decontaminate your hands.
- Use a paper towel to pick up and take the container outside the room.
- Put the container in the biohazard bag.
- Discard the paper towels.
- Follow center policy for storing the specimen.
- Decontaminate your hands.

Transporting Persons Persons on Transmission-Based Precautions usually do not leave their rooms. Sometimes they go to other areas for treatments or tests.

Transporting procedures vary among centers. Some require transport by bed. This prevents contaminating wheelchairs and stretchers. Others use wheelchairs and stretchers.

A safe transport means that other persons are protected from the infection. Follow center procedures and these guidelines:

- Have the person wear a clean gown or pajamas and an isolation gown.
- Have the person wear a mask as required by the Transmission-Based Precautions used.
- Cover any draining wounds.
- Give the person tissues and a leak-proof bag. Used tissues are placed in the bag.
- Wear PPE as required.
- Place an extra layer of sheets and absorbent pads on the stretcher or wheelchair. This protects against draining body fluids.
- Do not let anyone else on the elevator. This reduces exposure to infection.
- Alert staff in the receiving area about the Transmission-Based Precautions. They wear gloves and PPE as needed.
- Disinfect the stretcher or wheelchair after use.

Meeting Basic Needs

The person has love, belonging, and self-esteem needs. Often they are unmet when Transmission-Based Precautions are used. Visitors and staff often avoid the person. They may need to put on gowns, masks, goggles or face shields, and gloves. These tasks take extra effort before entering the room. Some are not sure what they can touch. They may fear getting the disease.

The person may feel lonely, unwanted, and rejected. Self-esteem suffers. The person knows the disease can be spread to others. He or she may feel dirty and undesirable. Without intending to, visitors and staff can make the person feel ashamed and guilty for having a contagious disease.

The nurse helps the person, visitors, and staff understand the need for Transmission-Based Precautions and how they affect the person. You can help meet love, belonging, and self-esteem needs. See *Promoting Safety and Comfort: Isolation Precautions*, p. 192.

Persons with poor vision need to know who you are. Let them see your face before you put on a mask or goggles or a face shield. State your name and explain what you are going to do. Then put on PPE.

See *Focus on Communication: Meeting Basic Needs.*
See *Residents With Dementia: Meeting Basic Needs.*

FOCUS ON COMMUNICATION
Meeting Basic Needs

Without intending to, people can make the person feel ashamed and guilty for having a contagious disease. Be careful what you say. For example, do *not* say:

- "What were you doing?"
- "How did you get that?"
- "I'm afraid to touch you."
- "Don't breathe on me."

Always treat the person with respect, kindness, and dignity.

RESIDENTS WITH DEMENTIA
Meeting Basic Needs

Persons with dementia do not understand the need for isolation precautions. Masks, gowns, goggles, and face shields may increase confusion and cause fear and agitation. These measures can help:

- Let the person see your face before putting on PPE.
- Tell the person who you are and what you are going to do.
- Use a calm, soothing voice.
- Do not hurry the person.
- Use touch to reassure the person.
- Follow the care plan and the nurse's instructions for other measures to help the person.
- Report signs of increased confusion or behavior changes.

Box 15-7 Bloodborne Pathogen Standard Terms

blood Human blood, human blood components, and products made from human blood

bloodborne pathogens Pathogens present in human blood and that can cause disease in humans; they include but are not limited to the hepatitis B virus (HBV) and human immunodeficiency virus (HIV)

contaminated The presence or reasonably anticipated presence of blood or other potentially infectious materials on an item or surface

contaminated laundry Laundry soiled with blood or other potentially infectious materials or that may contain sharps

contaminated sharps Any contaminated object that can penetrate the skin—needles, scalpels, broken glass, broken capillary tubes, exposed ends of dental wires, and so on

decontamination The use of physical or chemical means to remove, inactivate, or destroy bloodborne pathogens on a surface or item to the point where infectious particles can no longer be transmitted and the surface or item is safe for handling, use, or disposal

engineering controls Controls that isolate or remove the bloodborne pathogen hazard from the workplace (sharps disposal containers, self-sheathing needles)

exposure incident Eye, mouth, other mucous membrane, non-intact skin, or parenteral contact with blood or other potentially infectious materials that results from an employee's duties

hand washing facilities The adequate supply of running water, soap, single-use towels, or hot-air drying machines

HBV Hepatitis B virus

HIV Human immunodeficiency virus

occupational exposure Reasonably anticipated skin, eye, mucous membrane, or parenteral contact with blood or other potentially infectious materials that may result from an employee's duties

other potentially infectious materials (OPIM):
- Human body fluids—semen, vaginal secretions, cerebrospinal fluid, synovial fluid, pleural fluid, pericardial fluid, peritoneal fluid, amniotic fluid, saliva in dental procedures, any body fluid that is visibly contaminated with blood, and all body fluids when it is difficult or impossible to differentiate between them
- Any tissue or organ (other than intact skin) from a human (living or dead)
- HIV-containing cell or tissue cultures, organ cultures, and HIV- or HBV-containing culture medium or other solutions; blood, organs, or other tissues from experimental animals infected with HIV or HBV

parenteral Piercing mucous membranes or the skin barrier through needle-sticks, human bites, cuts, abrasions, and so on

personal protective equipment (PPE) The clothing or equipment worn by an employee for protection against a hazard

regulated waste:
- Liquid or semi-liquid blood or OPIM
- Contaminated items that would release blood or OPIM in a liquid or semi-liquid state if compressed
- Items caked with dried blood or OPIM that can release these materials during handling
- Contaminated sharps
- Pathological and microbiological wastes containing blood or OPIM

source individual Any person (living or dead) whose blood or OPIM may be a source of occupational exposure to employees; examples include but are not limited to:
- Hospital and clinic patients
- Clients in agencies for the developmentally disabled
- Trauma victims
- Clients of drug and alcohol treatment agencies
- Hospice and nursing center residents
- Human remains
- Persons who donate or sell blood or blood components

sterilize The use of a physical or chemical procedure to destroy all microbes, including spores

work practice controls Controls that reduce the likelihood of exposure by changing the way the task is performed

BLOODBORNE PATHOGEN STANDARD

The human immunodeficiency virus (HIV) and the hepatitis B virus (HBV) are major health concerns (Chapters 38 and 41). The health team is at risk for exposure to these viruses. The Bloodborne Pathogen Standard is intended to protect them from exposure. It is a regulation of the Occupational Safety and Health Administration (OSHA). See Box 15-7 for terms used in the standard.

HIV and HBV are found in the blood. They are bloodborne pathogens. They exit the body through blood. They are spread to others by blood. Other potentially infectious materials (OPIM) also spread the viruses (see Box 15-7).

Exposure Control Plan

The center must have an exposure control plan. It identifies staff at risk for exposure to blood or OPIM. All caregivers and the laundry, central supply, and housekeeping staffs are at risk. The plan includes actions to take for an exposure incident.

Staff at risk receive free training. Training occurs upon employment and yearly. Training is also required for new or changed tasks involving exposure to blood-borne pathogens. Training must include:

- An explanation of the standard and where to get a copy
- The causes, signs, and symptoms of bloodborne diseases
- How bloodborne pathogens are spread
- An explanation of the exposure control plan and where to get a copy
- How to know which tasks might cause exposure
- The use and limits of safe work practices, engineering controls, and PPE
- Information about the hepatitis B vaccination
- Who to contact and what to do in an emergency
- Information on reporting an exposure incident, postexposure evaluation, and follow-up
- Information on warning labels and color-coding

Preventive Measures

Preventive measures reduce the risk of exposure. Such measures follow.

Hepatitis B Vaccination   Hepatitis B is a liver disease. It is caused by the hepatitis B virus (HBV). HBV is spread by blood and sexual contact.

The hepatitis B vaccine produces immunity against hepatitis B. Immunity means that a person has protection against a certain disease. He or she will not get the disease.

A vaccination involves giving a vaccine to produce immunity against an infectious disease. A vaccine is a preparation containing dead or weakened microbes. The hepatitis B vaccination involves 3 injections (shots). The second injection is given 1 month after the first. The third injection is given 6 months after the second one. The vaccination can be given before or after exposure to HBV.

You can receive the hepatitis B vaccination within 10 working days of being hired. The center pays for it. You can refuse the vaccination. If so, you must sign a statement refusing the vaccine. You can have the vaccination at a later date.

Engineering and Work Practice Controls   *Engineering controls* reduce employee exposure in the workplace. Special containers for contaminated sharps (needles, broken glass) and specimens remove and isolate the hazard from staff. Containers are puncture-resistant, leak-proof, and color-coded in red. They have the *BIOHAZARD* symbol.

Work practice controls also reduce exposure risks. All tasks involving blood or OPIM are done in ways to limit splatters, splashes, and sprays. Producing droplets also is avoided. OSHA requires these work practice controls:

- Do not eat, drink, smoke, apply cosmetics or lip balm, or handle contact lenses in areas of occupational exposure.
- Do not store food or drinks where blood or OPIM are kept.
- Practice hand hygiene after removing gloves.
- Wash hands as soon as possible after skin contact with blood or OPIM.
- Never recap, bend, or remove needles by hand. When recapping, bending, or removing contaminated needles is required, use mechanical means (forceps) or a one-handed method.
- Never shear or break contaminated needles.
- Discard contaminated needles and sharp instruments (such as razors) in containers that are closable, puncture-resistant, and leak-proof. Containers are color-coded in red and have the *BIOHAZARD* symbol. Containers must be upright and not allowed to overfill.

Personal Protective Equipment (PPE)   This includes gloves, goggles, face shields, masks, laboratory coats, gowns, shoe covers, and surgical caps. Blood or OPIM must not pass through them. They protect your clothes, undergarments, skin, eyes, mouth, and hair.

PPE is free to employees. Correct sizes are available. The center makes sure that PPE is cleaned, laundered, repaired, replaced, or discarded. OSHA requires these measures for the safe handling and use of PPE:

- Remove PPE before leaving the work area.
- Remove PPE when a garment becomes contaminated.
- Place used PPE in marked areas or containers when being stored, washed, decontaminated, or discarded.
- Wear gloves when you expect contact with blood or OPIM.
- Wear gloves when handling or touching contaminated items or surfaces.
- Replace worn, punctured, or contaminated gloves.
- Never wash or decontaminate disposable gloves for re-use.
- Discard utility gloves that show signs of cracking, peeling, tearing, or puncturing. Utility gloves are decontaminated for re-use if the process will not ruin them.

Equipment Contaminated equipment is cleaned and decontaminated. Decontaminate work surfaces with a proper disinfectant:

- Upon completing tasks
- At once when there is obvious contamination
- After any spill of blood or OPIM
- At the end of the work shift when surfaces became contaminated since the last cleaning

Use a brush and dustpan or tongs to clean up broken glass. Never pick up broken glass with your hands, not even with gloves. Discard broken glass into a puncture-resistant container.

Waste Special measures are used to discard regulated waste:

- Liquid or semi-liquid blood or OPIM
- Items contaminated with blood or OPIM
- Items caked with blood or OPIM
- Contaminated sharps

Closable, puncture-resistant, and leak-proof containers are used. Containers are color-coded in red. They have the BIOHAZARD symbol.

Housekeeping The center must be kept clean and sanitary. A cleaning schedule is required. It includes decontamination methods and the tasks and procedures to be done.

Laundry OSHA requires these measures for contaminated laundry:

- Handle it as little as possible.
- Wear gloves or other needed PPE.
- Bag contaminated laundry where it is used.
- Mark laundry bags or containers with the BIOHAZARD symbol for laundry sent off-site.
- Place wet, contaminated laundry in leak-proof containers before transport. The containers are color-coded in red or have the BIOHAZARD symbol.

Exposure Incidents

An *exposure incident* is any eye, mouth, other mucous membrane, non-intact skin, or parenteral contact with blood or OPIM. *Parenteral* means piercing the mucous membranes or the skin barrier. Piercing occurs through needle-sticks, human bites, cuts, and abrasions.

Report exposure incidents at once. Medical evaluation, follow-up, and required tests are free. Your blood is tested for HIV and HBV. If you refuse testing, the blood sample is kept for at least 90 days. Testing is done later if you change your mind.

Confidentiality is important. You are told of the evaluation results. You also are told of any medical conditions that may need treatment. You receive a written opinion of the medical evaluation within 15 days after its completion.

The *source individual* is the person whose blood or body fluids are the source of an exposure incident. His or her blood is tested for HIV or HBV. The center informs you of laws affecting the source's identity and test results.

DELEGATION GUIDELINES
Assisting With Sterile Procedures

A nurse may ask you to assist with a sterile procedure. If so, you need this information from the nurse:

- The name of the procedure and the reason for it
- What gloves to wear—sterile or non-sterile
- What you are expected to do
- When to report observations
- What you can and cannot touch
- What specific resident concerns to report at once

PROMOTING SAFETY AND COMFORT
Assisting With Sterile Procedures

Safety
Do not perform a sterile procedure unless:

- Your state allows you to perform the procedure.
- The procedure is in your job description.
- You received the necessary education and training.
- You review the procedure with the nurse.
- A nurse is available for questions and guidance.

SURGICAL ASEPSIS

Surgical asepsis (sterile technique) is the practice that keeps equipment and supplies free of *all* microbes. Sterile means the absence of *all* microbes, including spores. Surgical asepsis is required any time the skin or sterile tissues are entered. If a break occurs in sterile technique, microbes can enter the body. Infection is a risk.

Assisting With Sterile Procedures

You can assist nurses with sterile procedures. Some states let nursing assistants perform certain sterile procedures. A sterile dressing change is an example.

See *Delegation Guidelines: Assisting With Sterile Procedures.*

See *Promoting Safety and Comfort: Assisting With Sterile Procedures.*

Principles of Surgical Asepsis

All items in contact with the person are kept sterile. If an item is contaminated, infection is a risk. A sterile field is needed. A sterile field is a work area free of *all* pathogens and non-pathogens (including spores). Box 15-8, p. 206 lists the principles and practices of surgical asepsis. Follow them to maintain a sterile field.

Box 15-8   Principles and Practices for Surgical Asepsis

- A sterile item can touch only another sterile item:
  - If a sterile item touches a clean item, the sterile item is contaminated.
  - If a clean item touches a sterile item, the sterile item is contaminated.
  - A sterile package that is open, torn, punctured, wet, or moist is contaminated.
  - A sterile package is contaminated when the expiration date has passed.
  - Place only sterile items on a sterile field.
  - Use sterile gloves or sterile forceps to handle other sterile items (Fig. 15-18).
  - Consider any item as contaminated if unsure of its sterility.
  - Do not use contaminated items. They are discarded or re-sterilized.
- A sterile field or sterile items are always kept within your vision and above your waist:
  - If you cannot see an item, the item is contaminated.
  - If the item is below your waist, the item is contaminated.
  - Keep sterile-gloved hands above your waist and within your sight.
  - Do not leave a sterile field unattended.
  - Do not turn your back on a sterile field.
- Airborne microbes can contaminate sterile items or a sterile field:
  - Prevent drafts. Close the door, and avoid extra movements. Ask other staff in the room to avoid extra movements.
  - Avoid coughing, sneezing, talking, or laughing over a sterile field. Turn your head away from the sterile field if you must talk.
  - Wear a mask if you need to talk during the procedure.
  - Do not perform or assist with sterile procedures if you have a respiratory infection.
  - Do not reach over a sterile field.

- Fluid flows downward, in the direction of gravity:
  - Hold wet items down (see Fig. 15-18). If held up, fluid flows down into a contaminated area. The contaminated fluid flows back into the sterile field when the item is held down.
- The sterile field is kept dry, unless the area below it is sterile:
  - The sterile field is contaminated if it gets wet and the area below it is not sterile.
  - Avoid spilling and splashing when pouring sterile fluids into sterile containers.
- The edges of a sterile field are contaminated:
  - A 1-inch (2.5 centimeter [cm]) margin around the sterile field is considered contaminated (Fig. 15-19).
  - Place all sterile items inside the 1-inch (2.5 cm) margin of the sterile field.
  - Items outside the 1-inch (2.5 cm) margin are contaminated.
- Honesty is essential to sterile technique:
  - You know when you contaminate an item or sterile field. Be honest with yourself even if other staff members are not present.
  - Remove the contaminated item, and correct the matter. If necessary, start over with sterile supplies.
  - Report the contamination to the nurse.

Fig. 15-18 Sterile forceps are used to handle sterile items.

Fig. 15-19 A 1-inch (2.5 cm) margin around the sterile field is considered contaminated. The shading and slash marks show that the 1-inch margin is contaminated.

✉ Sterile Gloving

You might need sterile gloves when assisting with a sterile procedure. The sterile field is set up first. Then sterile gloves are put on. After sterile gloves are on, you can handle sterile items within the sterile field. Do not touch anything outside the sterile field.

Sterile gloves are disposable. They come in many sizes so they fit snugly. The insides are powdered for ease in donning the gloves. The right and left gloves are marked on the package.

See *Promoting Safety and Comfort: Sterile Gloving.*

PROMOTING SAFETY AND COMFORT
Sterile Gloving

Safety
Always keep sterile gloved hands above your waist and within your vision. Touch only items within the sterile field. If you contaminate the gloves, remove them. Tell the nurse what happened. Decontaminate your hands, and put on a new pair. Replace gloves that are torn, cut, or punctured.

Comfort
If you or the nurse contaminate your gloves, they must be removed. This means leaving the bedside to get another pair. Care is delayed. The person's comfort is affected if the care is painful or involves an uncomfortable position. When collecting supplies, get an extra pair of gloves. The gloves are in the room if the first pair is contaminated. Care can continue with little delay.

 STERILE GLOVING

PROCEDURE

1 Follow *Delegation Guidelines: Assisting With Sterile Procedures,* p. 205. See *Promoting Safety and Comfort:*
  a *Assisting With Sterile Procedures,* p. 205
  b *Sterile Gloving*
2 Practice hand hygiene.
3 Inspect the package of sterile gloves for sterility.
  a Check the expiration date.
  b See if the package is dry.
  c Check for tears, holes, punctures, and watermarks.
4 Arrange a work surface.
  a Make sure you have enough room.
  b Arrange the work surface at waist level and within your vision.
  c Clean and dry the work surface.
  d Do not reach over or turn your back on the work surface.
5 Open the package. Grasp the flaps. Gently peel them back.
6 Remove the inner package. Place it on your work surface.
7 Read the manufacturer's instructions on the inner package. It may be labeled with *left, right, up,* and *down.*
8 Arrange the inner package for left, right, up, and down. The left glove is on your left. The right glove is on your right. The cuffs are near you with the fingers pointing away from you.
9 Grasp the folded edges of the inner package. Use the thumb and index finger of each hand.
10 Fold back the inner package to expose the gloves (Fig. 15-20, *A,* p. 208). Do not touch or otherwise contaminate the inside of the package or the gloves. The inside of the inner package is a sterile field.

11 Note that each glove has a cuff about 2 to 3 inches wide. The cuffs and insides of the gloves are *not considered sterile.*
12 Put on the right glove if you are right-handed. Put on the left glove if you are left-handed.
  a Pick up the glove with your other hand. Use your thumb and index and middle fingers (Fig. 15-20, *B,* p. 208).
  b Touch only the cuff and inside of the glove.
  c Turn the hand to be gloved palm side up.
  d Lift the cuff up. Slide your fingers and hand into the glove (Fig. 15-20, *C,* p. 208).
  e Pull the glove up over your hand. If some fingers get stuck, leave them that way until the other glove is on. *Do not use your ungloved hand to straighten the glove. Do not let the outside of the glove touch any non-sterile surface.*
  f Leave the cuff turned down.
13 Put on the other glove. Use your gloved hand.
  a Reach under the cuff of the second glove. Use the four fingers of your gloved hand (Fig. 15-20, *D,* p. 208). Keep your gloved thumb close to your gloved palm.
  b Pull on the second glove (Fig. 15-20, *E,* p. 208). Your gloved hand cannot touch the cuff or any surface. Hold the thumb of your first gloved hand away from the gloved palm.
14 Adjust each glove with the other hand. The gloves should be smooth and comfortable (Fig. 15-20, *F,* p. 208).
15 Slide your fingers under the cuffs to pull them up (Fig. 15-20, *G,* p. 208).
16 Touch only sterile items.
17 Remove the gloves. See Figure 15-12.
18 Decontaminate your hands.

Fig. 15-20 Sterile gloving. **A,** Open the inner wrapper to expose the gloves. **B,** Pick up the glove at the cuff with your thumb and index and middle fingers. **C,** Slide your fingers and hand into the glove. **D,** Reach under the cuff of the other glove with your fingers. **E,** Pull on the second glove. **F,** Adjust each glove for comfort. **G,** Slide your fingers under the cuffs to pull them up.

QUALITY OF LIFE

The health team must prevent the spread of microbes and infection. You must be very careful about your work. Staff and residents assume that you will practice medical asepsis. They also assume that you will follow Standard and Transmission-Based Precautions.

Even one careless act can spread microbes. It affects the person's safety. The reverse is also true. You can develop the person's infection. Practicing hand hygiene before and after resident contact greatly reduces the spread of microbes.

REVIEW QUESTIONS

Circle T if the statement is TRUE. Circle F if the statement is FALSE.

1 T F Microbes are pathogens in their natural sites.
2 T F A pathogen can cause an infection.
3 T F An infection results when microbes invade and grow in the body.
4 T F An item is sterile if non-pathogens are present.
5 T F You hold your hands and forearms up during hand washing.
6 T F Un-used items in the person's room are used for another person.
7 T F A person received the hepatitis B vaccine. The person will develop the disease.
8 T F The 1-inch edge around a sterile field is considered contaminated.
9 T F The inside and cuffs of sterile gloves are considered contaminated.

Circle the BEST answer.

10 Most pathogens need the following to grow *except*
  a Water   **c** Oxygen
  b Light   **d** Nourishment
11 Signs and symptoms of infection include the following *except*
  a Fever, nausea, vomiting, rash, and/or sores
  b Pain or tenderness, redness, and/or swelling
  c Fatigue, loss of appetite, and/or a discharge
  d A wound and/or bleeding
12 Which is *not* a portal of exit?
  a Respiratory tract   **c** Reproductive system
  b Blood   **d** Intact skin

13 Which does *not* prevent healthcare-associated infections?
  a Hand hygiene before and after giving care
  b Sterilizing all care items
  c Surgical asepsis
  d Standard Precautions

14 Your hands are soiled with blood. What should you do?
  a Wash your hands with soap and water.
  b Decontaminate your hands.
  c Rinse your hands.
  d Tell the nurse.

15 During care, you move from a contaminated body site to a clean body site. Your hands are not visibly soiled. What should you do?
  a Wash your hands.
  b Decontaminate your hands.
  c Rinse your hands.
  d Put on sterile gloves.

16 You are going to decontaminate your hands with an alcohol-based hand rub. Which action is *not* correct?
  a Wash your hands before applying the hand rub.
  b Rub your hands together.
  c Cover all surfaces of your hands and fingers.
  d Rub your hands together until your hands are dry.

17 When cleaning equipment, do the following *except*
  a Rinse the item in cold water before cleaning
  b Wash the item with soap and hot water
  c Use a brush if necessary
  d Work from dirty to clean areas

18 Isolation precautions
  a Prevent infection
  b Destroy pathogens
  c Keep pathogens within a certain area
  d Destroy all microbes

19 Standard Precautions
  a Are used for all persons
  b Prevent the spread of pathogens through the air
  c Require gowns, masks, gloves, and goggles
  d Require a doctor's order

20 You wear utility gloves for contact with
  a Blood
  b Body fluids
  c Secretions and excretions
  d Cleaning solutions

21 A mask
  a Can be re-used
  b Is clean on the inside
  c Is contaminated when moist
  d Should fit loosely for breathing

22 These statements are about PPE. Which is *false*?
  a Wash disposable gloves for re-use.
  b Remove PPE before leaving the work area.
  c Discard cracked or torn utility gloves.
  d Wear gloves when touching contaminated items or surfaces.

23 Contaminated surfaces are cleaned at the following times *except*
  a After completing a task
  b When there is obvious contamination
  c After blood is spilled
  d After removing gloves

24 Goggles or a face shield is worn
  a When using Standard Precautions
  b When splashing body fluids is likely
  c If you have an eye infection
  d When assisting with sterile procedures

25 According to the Bloodborne Pathogen Standard, you should *not*
  a Wear gloves
  b Discard sharp items into a biohazard container
  c Store food and blood in different places
  d Eat and drink in care settings

26 You were exposed to a bloodborne pathogen. Which is *true*?
  a You do not have to report the exposure.
  b You pay for required tests.
  c You can refuse HIV and HBV testing.
  d The source individual can refuse testing.

27 These statements are about surgical asepsis. Which is *false*?
  a A sterile item can touch only another sterile item.
  b Wet items are held up.
  c If you cannot see an item, it is considered contaminated.
  d Sterile items are kept above your waist.

28 You have on sterile gloves. You can touch
  a Anything on the sterile field
  b Anything on your work surface
  c Anything below your waist
  d Any part of your uniform

Answers to these questions are on p. 719.

CHAPTER 16

Body Mechanics

KEY TERMS

base of support The area on which an object rests

body alignment The way the head, trunk, arms, and legs are aligned with one another; posture

body mechanics Using the body in an efficient and careful way

dorsal recumbent position See "supine position"

ergonomics The science of designing a job to fit the worker

Fowler's position A semi-sitting position; the head of the bed is raised between 45 and 60 degrees

lateral position The person lies on one side or the other; side-lying position

posture See "body alignment"

prone position Lying on the abdomen with the head turned to one side

semi-prone side position See "Sims' position"

side-lying position See "lateral position"

Sims' position A left side-lying position in which the upper leg (right leg) is sharply flexed so it is not on the lower leg (left leg) and the lower arm (left arm) is behind the person; semi-prone side position

supine position The back-lying position; dorsal recumbent position

KEY ABBREVIATIONS

OSHA Occupational Safety and Health Administration

MSD Musculo-skeletal disorder

Body mechanics means using the body in an efficient and careful way. It involves good posture, balance, and using your strongest and largest muscles for work. Fatigue, muscle strain, and injury can result from the improper use and positioning of the body during activity or rest. Focus on the person's and your own body mechanics. Good body mechanics reduce the risk of injury.

PRINCIPLES OF BODY MECHANICS

Body alignment (posture) is the way the head, trunk, arms, and legs are aligned with one another. Good alignment lets the body move and function with strength and efficiency. Standing, sitting, and lying down require good alignment.

Base of support is the area on which an object rests. A good base of support is needed for balance (Fig. 16-1). When standing, your feet are your base of support.

Stand with your feet apart for a wider base of support and more balance.

Your strongest and largest muscles are in the shoulders, upper arms, hips, and thighs. Use these muscles to handle and move persons and heavy objects. Otherwise, you place strain and exertion on smaller and weaker muscles. This causes fatigue and injury. *Back injuries are a major risk.* For good body mechanics:

- Bend your knees and squat to lift a heavy object (Fig. 16-2, p. 212). Do not bend from your waist. Bending from the waist places strain on small back muscles.
- Hold items close to your body and base of support (see Fig. 16-2, p. 212). This involves upper arm and shoulder muscles. Holding objects away from your body places strain on small muscles in your lower arms.

All activities require good body mechanics. You must safely and efficiently handle and move persons and heavy objects. Follow the rules in Box 16-1, p. 212.

A   — Base of support —   B

Fig. 16-1 A, Anterior (front) view of an adult in good body alignment. The feet are apart for a wide base of support. **B,** Lateral (side) view of an adult with good posture and alignment.

Fig. 16-2 Picking up a box using good body mechanics.

Box 16-1   Rules for Body Mechanics

- Keep your body in good alignment with a wide base of support.
- Use an upright working posture. Bend your legs. Do not bend your back.
- Use the stronger and larger muscles in your shoulders, upper arms, thighs, and hips.
- Keep objects close to your body when you lift, move, or carry them (see Fig. 16-2).
- Avoid unnecessary bending and reaching. Raise the bed so it is close to your waist. Adjust the overbed table so it is at your waist level.
- Face your work area. This prevents unnecessary twisting.
- Push, slide, or pull heavy objects whenever you can rather than lifting them. Pushing is easier than pulling.
- Widen your base of support when pushing or pulling. Move your front leg forward when pushing. Move your rear leg back when pulling (Fig. 16-3).
- Use both hands and arms to lift, move, or carry objects.
- Turn your whole body when changing the direction of your movement. Move and turn your feet in the direction of the turn instead of twisting your body.
- Work with smooth and even movements. Avoid sudden or jerky motions.
- Do not lean over a person to give care.
- *Get help from a co-worker to move heavy objects. Do not lift or move them by yourself.*
- Bend your hips and knees to lift heavy objects from the floor (see Fig. 16-2). Straighten your back as the object reaches thigh level. Your leg and thigh muscles work to raise the item off the floor and to waist level.
- Do not lift objects higher than chest level. Do not lift above your shoulders. Use a step stool or ladder to reach an object higher than chest level.

Fig. 16-3 Move your rear leg back when pulling an item.

ERGONOMICS

Ergonomics is the science of designing the job to fit the worker. (*Ergo* means work. *Nomos* means law.) It involves changing the task, work station, equipment, and tools to help reduce stress on the worker's body. The goal is to eliminate a serious and disabling work-related musculo-skeletal disorder (MSD). MSDs are caused or made worse by the work setting.

Work-Related MSDs

MSDs are injuries and disorders of the muscles, tendons, ligaments, joints, and cartilage. They also can involve the nervous system. The arms and back are often affected. So are the hands, fingers, neck, wrists, legs, and shoulders. MSDs are painful and disabling. They can develop slowly over weeks, months, and years. Or they can occur from one event. Pain, numbness, tingling, stiff joints, difficulty moving, and muscle loss can occur. Sometimes there is paralysis.

MSDs are workplace health hazards. Early signs and symptoms include pain, limited joint movement, or soft tissue swelling. Time off work is often needed. According to the U.S. Department of Labor, nursing assistants are at great risk.

Always report a work-related injury as soon as possible. Early attention can help prevent the problem from becoming worse. Also, injuries are often less serious and less costly to treat if they receive early attention. In later stages, the problem can become more serious and harder and more costly to treat.

The following nursing tasks are known to be high risk for MSDs:
* Transfers—to and from beds, chairs, wheelchairs, Geri-chairs, toilets, stretchers, and bathtubs
* Trying to stop a person from falling
* Picking up a person from the floor to the bed
* Lifting alone
* Lifting persons who are confused or uncooperative
* Lifting persons who cannot support their own weight
* Lifting heavy persons
* Weighing a person
* Moving a person up in bed
* Re-positioning a person in a bed or in a chair
* Changing an incontinence product
* Making beds
* Dressing and undressing a person
* Feeding a person in bed
* Giving a bed bath
* Applying anti-embolism stockings

The Occupational Safety and Health Administration (OSHA) has identified risk factors for MSDs in nursing team members. The risk of an MSD increases if risk factors are combined. For example, a task involves both force and repeating actions.
* *Force*—the amount of physical effort needed to perform a task. Lifting or transferring heavy residents, preventing falls, and unexpected or sudden motions are examples.
* *Repeating action*—performing the same motion or series of motions continually or frequently. Repositioning residents and transfers to and from beds, chairs, and commodes without adequate rest breaks are examples. So is frequently cranking manual beds.
* *Awkward postures*—assuming positions that place stress on the body. Examples include reaching above shoulder height, kneeling, squatting, leaning over a bed, bending, or twisting the torso while lifting.
* *Heavy lifting*—manually lifting residents who cannot move themselves.

OSHA requires a safe work setting. The setting must be free of hazards that cause or are likely to cause death or serious physical harm to employees. The employer must make reasonable attempts to prevent or reduce the hazard. OSHA inspection teams enforce this law.

Back Injuries

Back injuries are major threats. Back injuries can occur from repeated activities or from one event. Signs and symptoms include:
* Pain when trying to assume a normal posture
* Decreased mobility
* Pain when standing or rising from a seated position

These and other factors can lead to back disorders:
* Reaching while lifting
* Poor posture when sitting or standing
* Staying in one position too long
* Poor body mechanics when lifting, pushing, pulling, or carrying objects
* Poor physical condition—not having the strength or endurance to perform tasks without strain
* Repeated lifting of awkward items, equipment, or persons
* Shifting weight when a person loses balance or strength while moving
* Twisting while lifting
* Bending while lifting
* Maintaining a bent posture such as leaning over a bed
* Reaching over raised bed rails
* Working in a confined, crowded, or cluttered area (rooms, bathrooms, hallways)
* Fatigue
* Poor footing such as on slippery floors
* Lifting with forceful movement

PROMOTING SAFETY AND COMFORT
Back Injuries

Safety

According to OSHA, these activities are associated with back injuries in nursing centers:

- Moving a person who totally depends on others for care
- Moving a person who is combative
- Transferring a person who is on the floor to the bed or a chair
- Re-positioning a person in bed or in a chair
- Transferring a person from bed to chair or from chair to bed
- Transferring a person from one chair to another (includes transfers to and from the wheelchair and toilet)
- Bending to bathe, dress, or feed a person
- Bending to make a bed or change linens
- Weighing a person
- Changing an incontinence product
- Trying to stop a person from falling

Use good body mechanics to protect yourself from injury. Do not work alone. Avoid lifting whenever possible.

Follow the rules in Box 16-1. They help prevent back injuries. Also, be extra careful when performing tasks associated with back injuries.

See *Promoting Safety and Comfort: Back Injuries.*

POSITIONING THE PERSON

The person must be properly positioned at all times. Regular position changes and good alignment promote comfort and well-being. Breathing is easier. Circulation is promoted. Pressure ulcers and contractures are prevented.

You move and turn when in bed or a chair for your comfort. Many residents do too. Some need reminding to adjust their positions. Other need help. Still others depend entirely on the nursing team for position changes.

Whether in bed or chair, the person is re-positioned at least every 2 hours. Some people are re-positioned more often. You must follow the nurse's instructions and the care plan. To safely position a person:

- Use good body mechanics.
- Ask a co-worker to help you if needed.
- Explain the procedure to the person.
- Be gentle when moving the person.
- Provide for privacy.

FOCUS ON COMMUNICATION
Positioning the Person

Moving is painful for many persons. Some older persons have painful joints. Most persons have pain after surgery or an injury. Make sure that you do not cause pain when positioning the person. Tell the person what you are going to do before and during the procedure. Move the person slowly and gently. Give the person time to tell you if a movement is painful. Make sure the person is comfortable. You can say:

- "Am I hurting you?"
- "Please tell me if I'm moving you too fast."
- "Please tell me if you feel pain or discomfort."
- "Do you need a pillow adjusted?"
- "Are you comfortable?"
- "How can I help make you more comfortable?"

DELEGATION GUIDELINES
Positioning the Person

You are often delegated tasks that involve positioning and re-positioning. You need this information from the nurse and the care plan:

- Position or positioning limits ordered by the doctor
- How often to turn and re-position the person
- How many staff members need to help you
- What assist devices to use (Chapter 17)
- What skin care measures to perform (Chapter 20)
- What range-of-motion exercises to perform (Chapter 26)
- Where to place pillows
- What positioning devices are needed and how to use them (Chapter 26)
- What observations to report and record
- When to report observations
- What specific resident concerns to report at once

- Use pillows as directed by the nurse for support and alignment.
- Provide for comfort after positioning. (See the inside of the front book cover.)
- Place the signal light within reach after positioning.
- Complete a safety check before leaving the room. (See the inside of the front book cover.)

See *Focus on Communication: Positioning the Person.*
See *Delegation Guidelines: Positioning the Person.*
See *Promoting Safety and Comfort: Positioning the Person.*

Fig. 16-4 Fowler's position.

Safety

Pressure ulcers (Chapter 36) are serious threats from lying or sitting too long in one place. Wet, soiled, and wrinkled linens are other causes. Whenever you re-position a person, make sure linens are clean, dry, and wrinkle-free. Change or straighten linens as needed.

Contractures can develop from staying in one position too long (Chapter 26). A *contracture* is the lack of joint mobility caused by abnormal shortening of a muscle. Re-positioning, exercise, and activity help prevent contractures.

Comfort

Pillows and positioning devices are used to position the person. They support body parts and keep the person in good alignment. This promotes comfort. Place pillows and positioning devices as directed by the nurse and the care plan.

Most older persons do not tolerate the prone position. They have limited range of motion in their necks. The Sims' position usually is not comfortable for them. Check with the nurse before placing any older person in the prone position or Sims' position.

Fowler's Position

Fowler's position is a semi-sitting position. The head of the bed is raised between 45 and 60 degrees (Fig. 16-4). The knees may be slightly elevated. For good alignment:

- The spine is straight.
- The head is supported with a small pillow.
- The arms are supported with pillows.

The nurse may ask you to place small pillows under the lower back, thighs, and ankles. Persons with heart and respiratory disorders usually breathe easier in Fowler's position.

Supine Position

The supine position (dorsal recumbent position) is the back-lying position (Fig. 16-5, p. 216). For good alignment:

- The bed is flat.
- The head and shoulders are supported on a pillow.
- Arms and hands are at the sides. You can support the arms with regular pillows. Or you can support the hands on small pillows with the palms down.

The nurse may ask you to place a folded or rolled towel under the lower back and a small pillow under the thighs. A pillow under the lower legs lifts the heels off of the bed. This prevents them from rubbing on the sheets.

Prone Position

A person in the prone position lies on the abdomen with the head turned to one side. For good alignment:

- The bed is flat.
- Small pillows are placed under the head, abdomen, and lower legs (Fig. 16-6, p. 216).
- Arms are flexed at the elbows with the hands near the head.

You also can position a person with the feet hanging over the end of the mattress (Fig. 16-7, p. 216). A pillow is not needed under the feet.

Lateral Position

A person in the lateral position (side-lying position) lies on one side or the other (Fig. 16-8, p. 216):

- The bed is flat.
- A pillow is under the head and neck.
- The upper leg is in front of the lower leg. (The nurse may ask you to position the upper leg behind the lower leg, not on top of it.)
- The ankle, upper leg, and thigh are supported with pillows.
- A small pillow is positioned against the person's back. The person rolls back against the pillow so that his or her back is at a 45-degree angle with the mattress.
- A small pillow is under the upper hand and arm.

Sims' Position

The Sims' position (semi-prone side position) is a left side-lying position. The upper leg (right leg) is sharply flexed so it is not on the lower leg (left leg). The lower arm (left arm) is behind the person (Fig. 16-9, p. 216). For good alignment:

- The bed is flat.
- A pillow is under the person's head and shoulder.
- The upper leg (right leg) is supported with a pillow.
- A pillow is under the upper arm (right arm) and hand (right hand).

Fig. 16-5 Supine position.

Fig. 16-6 Prone position.

Fig. 16-7 Prone position with the feet hanging over the edge of the mattress.

Fig. 16-8 Lateral position.

Fig. 16-9 Sims' position.

Fig. 16-10 The person is positioned in a chair. The person's feet are flat on the floor; the calves do not touch the chair. The back is straight and against the back of the chair.

Fig. 16-11 Elevated armrest. *(Image courtesy Posey Company, Arcadia, Calif.)*

Chair Position

Persons who sit in chairs must hold their upper bodies and heads erect. If not, poor alignment results. For good alignment:

- The person's back and buttocks are against the back of the chair.
- Feet are flat on the floor or wheelchair footplates. Never leave feet unsupported.
- Backs of the knees and calves are slightly away from the edge of the seat (Fig. 16-10).

The nurse may ask you to put a small pillow between the person's lower back and the chair. This supports the lower back. *Remember, a pillow is not used behind the back if restraints are used (Chapter 14).*

Paralyzed arms are supported on pillows. Some persons have positioners (Fig. 16-11). Ask the nurse about their proper use. Wrists are positioned at a slight upward angle.

Some people require postural supports if they cannot keep their upper bodies erect (Fig. 16-12). Postural supports help keep them in good alignment. The health team selects the best product for the person's needs. The person's safety, dignity, and function are considered.

Fig. 16-12 Postural supports. **A,** Posey Hugger. **B,** Torso support. *(Images courtesy Posey Company, Arcadia, Calif.)*

QUALITY OF LIFE

Nursing centers provide care in a manner that maintains and improves each person's quality of life, health, and safety. Proper body mechanics protect the person from injuries that could affect health and ability to function.

Remaining independent to the extent possible promotes dignity, self-esteem, and pride. Let the person help as much as safely possible. Let the person choose such things as bed positioning or where to place the chair or wheelchair. Talk with the person while moving him or her. Ask about his or her preferences. Doing so promotes comfort, independence, and social interaction.

REVIEW QUESTIONS

Circle the BEST answer.

1 Good body mechanics involve the following *except*
   a Good posture
   b Balance
   c Using the strongest and largest muscles
   d Having the job fit the worker

2 Good alignment means
   a The area on which an object rests
   b Having the head, trunk, arms, and legs aligned with one another
   c Using muscles, tendons, ligaments, and joints correctly
   d The back-lying or supine position

3 These actions are about body mechanics. Which action is *not* correct?
   a Hold objects away from your body when lifting, moving, or carrying them.
   b Face the direction you are working to prevent twisting.
   c Push, pull, or slide heavy objects.
   d Use both hands and arms to lift, move, or carry heavy objects.

4 Pulling is easier than pushing.
   a True
   b False

5 The purpose of ergonomics is to
   a Reduce stress on the worker's body
   b Safely position a person
   c Promote quality of life
   d Use good body mechanics

6 Risk factors for work-related musculo-skeletal disorders include the following *except*
   a Repeating actions
   b Awkward postures
   c Bending your hips and knees
   d Force

7 Residents are re-positioned at least every
   a 30 minutes
   b 1 hour
   c 2 hours
   d 3 hours

8 The back-lying position is called
   a Fowler's position
   b The supine position
   c The prone position
   d Sims' position

9 Breathing is usually easier in
   a Fowler's position
   b The supine position
   c The lateral position
   d Sims' position

10 For Fowler's position
   a The bed is flat
   b The head of the bed is raised between 45 and 60 degrees
   c The person's head is turned toward one side
   d The person's feet hang over the edge of the mattress

11 A pillow is placed against the person's back in
   a Fowler's position
   b The prone position
   c The lateral position
   d Sims' position

12 A person is positioned in a chair. The feet
   a Must be flat on the floor
   b Are positioned on footplates
   c Dangle
   d Are positioned on pillows

Answers to these questions are on p. 720.

Safe Resident Handling, Moving, and Transfers

OBJECTIVES

- Define the key terms and key abbreviations listed in this chapter.
- Identify comfort and safety measures for handling, moving, and transferring the person.
- Explain how to prevent work-related injuries when handling, moving, and transferring persons.

- Describe four levels of dependence.
- Identify the information needed from the nurse and care plan before handling, moving, and transferring persons.
- Perform the procedures described in this chapter.
- Explain how to promote quality of life.

KEY TERMS

friction The rubbing of one surface against another

logrolling Turning the person as a unit, in alignment, with one motion

shearing When skin sticks to a surface while muscles slide in the direction the body is moving

transfer Moving the person from one place to another

KEY ABBREVIATIONS

ID	Identification	**OSHA**	Occupational Safety and Health Administration

You will turn and re-position persons often. You move them in bed. You transfer them to and from beds, chairs, wheelchairs, stretchers, and toilets. To transfer a person means moving the person from one place to another. During these and other tasks, you must use your body correctly. This protects you and the person from injury.

See *Focus on Communication: Safe Resident Handling, Moving, and Transfers.*

See *Promoting Safety and Comfort: Safe Resident Handling, Moving, and Transfers.*

See *Teamwork and Time Management: Safe Resident Handling, Moving, and Transfers.*

FOCUS ON COMMUNICATION
Safe Resident Handling, Moving, and Transfers

Handling, moving, and transfers can be very painful following an injury or surgery. Many older persons have painful joints. The fears of pain and falling are common. Always explain what you are going to do before starting the procedure. Then explain what you are doing step-by-step. This promotes comfort. When giving step-by-step directions:

* Speak slowly and clearly.
* Talk loudly enough for the person to hear you.
* Give directions calmly and kindly. Do not yell at or insult the person.
* Face the person and use eye contact when possible.
* Give one direction at a time.

  You must make sure the person is comfortable and that you are not causing pain. You can say:
* "Am I hurting you?"
* "Please tell me when you feel pain or discomfort."
* "Do you need a pillow adjusted?"
* "Are you comfortable?"
* "How can I help make you more comfortable?"

TEAMWORK AND TIME MANAGEMENT
Safe Resident Handling, Moving, and Transfers

Residents need to be moved, turned, transferred, and re-positioned. These tasks and procedures are best done by at least 2 staff members.

Friendships are common among co-workers. And some working relationships are better than others. Do not just ask your friends or those with whom you work well to help you. Include all co-workers. Do not just help your friends or those with whom you work well. Assist anyone who asks for your help. This includes new staff members and those from other units.

PROMOTING SAFETY AND COMFORT
Safe Resident Handling, Moving, and Transfers

Safety

Many older persons have osteoporosis or arthritis (Chapter 39). They have fragile bones and joints. To prevent injuries:

* Follow the rules of body mechanics (Chapter 16).
* Always have help when moving a person.
* Be aware of equipment and tubings involved in the person's care. Urinary catheters and oxygen, intravenous, drainage, and naso-gastric tubes are examples.
* Move the person carefully to prevent injury or pain.
* Keep the person in good alignment.
* Position the person in good alignment after handling, moving, or transferring him or her.
* Make sure his or her face, nose, and mouth are not obstructed by a pillow or other device.

Comfort

To promote mental comfort when handling, moving, or transferring the person:

* Always explain what you are going to do and how the person can help.
* Always screen and cover the person to protect the right to privacy.

  To promote physical comfort:
* Keep the person in good alignment.
* Make sure the person's head does not hit the head-board when he or she is moved up in bed. If the person can be without a pillow, place it upright against the head-board.
* Use pillows to position the person as directed by the nurse and the care plan. If a pillow is allowed under the person's head, make sure it is under the head and shoulders.
* Use other positioning devices as directed by the nurse and the care plan.

PREVENTING WORK-RELATED INJURIES

You must prevent work-related injuries when handling, moving, and transferring residents. Follow the rules in Box 17-1. The Occupational Safety and Health Administration (OSHA) recommends that:
- Manual lifting be minimized in all cases.
- Manual lifting be eliminated when possible.

To safely handle, move, and transfer the person, the nurse and health team determine:
- *The person's dependence level.* Dependence levels relate to the ability to move without help. Some persons do not need help moving. Others totally depend on the staff. You need to know the person's dependence level before you handle, move, or transfer a person. See Box 17-2, p. 222.
- *The amount of assistance needed.* This depends on the person's height, weight, cognitive function, and dependence level. Some persons only need help from one staff member. Others need help from at least 2 or 3 staff members.

- *What procedure to use.* This chapter includes handling, moving, and transfer procedures. The nurse and care plan tell you what procedure to use.
- *The equipment needed.* Assist equipment and devices are useful to safely handle, move, and transfer persons. They are presented throughout this chapter. The nurse and care plan tell you what to use. Always follow the manufacturer's instructions. Ask for any needed training to use the equipment and devices safely.

See *Residents With Dementia: Preventing Work-Related Injuries,* p. 224.

See *Teamwork and Time Management: Preventing Work-Related Injuries,* p. 224.

See *Delegation Guidelines: Preventing Work-Related Injuries,* p. 224.

See *Promoting Safety and Comfort: Preventing Work-Related Injuries,* p. 224.

Text continued on p. 225

Box 17-1 Preventing Work-Related Injuries

General Guidelines
- Wear shoes that provide good traction. Avoid shoes with worn-down soles. Good traction can help prevent slips or falls.
- Use assist equipment and devices whenever possible instead of lifting and moving the person manually. Follow the person's care plan.
- Get help from other staff. The nurse and care plan tell you how many staff members are needed to complete the task.
- Plan and prepare for the task. For example, know what equipment you will need, where to place chairs or wheelchairs, and what side of the bed to work on.
- Schedule harder tasks early in your shift.
- Balance lighter and harder tasks. Plan your work so that you can complete a lighter task after a harder one.
- Lock bed wheels and wheelchair or stretcher wheels.
- Tell the person what he or she can do to help. Give clear, simple instructions. Give the person time to respond.
- Do not hold or grab the person under the underarms.
- Do not let the person hold or grasp you around your neck.

Manual Lifting
- Use good body mechanics.
  - Stand with good posture. Keep your back straight.
  - Bend your legs, not your back.
  - Use your legs to do the work.
  - Face the person.
  - Do not twist or turn. Pick up your feet, and pivot your whole body in the direction of the move.

Manual Lifting—cont'd
- Try to keep what you are moving close to you—the person, equipment, or supplies.
- Move the person toward you, not away from you.
- Use slides and lateral transfers instead of manual lifting.
- Use a wide, balanced base of support. Stand with one foot slightly ahead of the other.
- Lower the person slowly by bending your legs. Do not bend your back. Return to an erect position as soon as possible.
- Use smooth, even movements. Avoid jerking movements.
- Lift on the "count of 3" when lifting with others. Everyone should lift at the same time.

Lateral Transfers
- Position surfaces as close as possible to each other (bed and chair; bed and stretcher).
- Adjust surfaces so that they are at about waist height. The receiving surface should be slightly lower to take advantage of gravity. For example, when transferring the person from bed to a chair, the chair surface is lower than the bed.
- Make sure bed rails are down. Make sure side rails on stretchers are down.
- Use drawsheets, turning pads, large incontinence pads, or other friction-reducing devices. Such devices include slide boards, slide sheets, and low-friction mattress covers.
- Get a good hand-hold. Roll up drawsheets, turning pads, and incontinence pads. Or use assist devices with handles.

Modified from Cal/OSHA: A back injury prevention guide for health care providers, Sacramento, Calif, revised November 1997, and referenced in Ergonomics: guidelines for nursing homes, Occupational Safety and Health Administration, revised March 2009.

Continued

Box 17-1 Preventing Work-Related Injuries—cont'd

Lateral Transfers—cont'd
- Kneel on the bed or stretcher. This helps prevent extended reaches and bending the back.
- Have staff on both sides of the bed or other surface. Move the person on the "count of 3." Use a smooth, push-pull motion. Do not reach across the person.

Gait/Transfer Belts
- Keep the person as close to you as possible.
- Avoid bending, reaching, or twisting when:
  - Attaching or removing a belt
  - Lowering the person to a chair, the bed, toilet, or the floor
  - Assisting the person with ambulation
- Use a gentle rocking motion to assist the person to stand. The rocking motion gives strength and force as you pull the person to standing position.
- See Chapter 13.

Stand-Pivot Transfers
- Use assist devices as directed. Follow the care plan.
- Use a gait/transfer belt with handles.
- Keep your feet at least shoulder-width apart.
- Lower the bed so the person can place his or her feet on the floor.
- Plan the transfer so that the person moves his or her strong side first.
- Get the person close to the edge of the bed or the chair. Ask the person to lean forward as he or she stands.
- Block the person's weak leg with your legs or knees. If the position is awkward, do the following:
  - Use a transfer belt with handles.
  - Straddle your legs around the person's weak leg.
- Bend your legs. Do not bend your back.
- Pivot with your feet to turn.
- Use a gentle rocking motion to assist the person to stand. The rocking motion gives strength and force as you pull the person to a standing position.

Lifting or Moving the Person in Bed
- Adjust the height of the bed, stretcher, or other surface so that it is at waist level.
- Lower the bed rail or the stretcher side rail.
- Work on the side where the person will be closest to you.
- Place equipment or other items close to you and at waist level.
- Use drawsheets, turning pads, large incontinence pads, or slide sheets.

Transporting Residents and Equipment
- Push, do not pull.
- Keep the load close to your body.
- Use an upright posture.
- Push with your whole body, not just your arms.
- Move down the center of the hallway. This helps avoid collisions.
- Watch out for door handles and high thresholds on floors. These can cause abrupt stops.

Transferring the Person From the Floor
- Use a mechanical lift if possible (p. 244). If not, place a sling, blanket, drawsheet, cot, or other assist device under the person as directed by the nurse.
- Position at least two staff members on each side of the person. More staff is needed if the person is large.
- Bend at your knees, not your back. Do not twist.
- Roll the person onto his or her side to position the assist device. Do not reach across the person.
- Lower the boom (if using a mechanical lift) to attach the sling. The boom should be low enough so that you can easily attach the sling.
- Do the following for a manual lift:
  - Kneel on one knee.
  - Grasp the blanket, drawsheet, cot, or other device.
  - Lift smoothly with your legs as you stand on the "count of 3." Do not bend your back.

Box 17-2 Levels of Dependence

Code 4: Total Dependence. The person cannot help with the transfer. The task or procedure is done by the staff.
- The person should be lifted and transferred using a full-sling mechanical lift (Fig. 17-1). The mechanical lift is used for transfers between beds, chairs, and toilets. It is also used for transfers to and from bathtubs and weighing scales.

Code 3: Extensive Assistance. The person can bear some weight, can sit up with help, and may be able to pivot to transfer.
- The person should be lifted and transferred using a mechanical lift. The mechanical lift is used for transfers between beds, chairs, and toilets. It is also used for transfers to and from bathtubs and weighing scales. The type of lift to use is noted on the person's care plan—full-sling mechanical lift or stand-assist lift (Fig. 17-2).

Modified from Nelson AL: Patient care ergonomics resource guide: safe patient handling and movement, Patient Safety Center of Inquiry (Tampa, Fla), Veterans Health Administration and Department of Defense, August 2005.

Box 17-2   Levels of Dependence—cont'd

Code 2: Limited Assistance. The person is highly involved in the moving or transfer procedure. He or she needs some help moving the legs. The person can stand (bear weight). The person has upper body strength and can sit up. He or she is able to pivot to transfer.

- Stand-assist devices may be needed. These can be attached to the bed or chair (Fig. 17-3). Other stand-assist devices include walkers (Chapter 26) and gait/transfer belts with handles.
- Sliding boards are useful for transfers to and from beds and chairs (Fig. 17-4).

Code 1: Supervision. The staff needs to look after, encourage, or cue the person. To cue means to remind the person what to do.

- The devices for Code 2 may be needed.

Code 0: Independent. The person can walk without help. Sometimes the person may need limited assistance.

- Mechanical assistance is not normally required for transfers, lifting, or re-positioning.

Fig. 17-1 Full-sling mechanical lift. *(Courtesy ARJO, Inc., Roselle, Ill. [800]323-1245)*

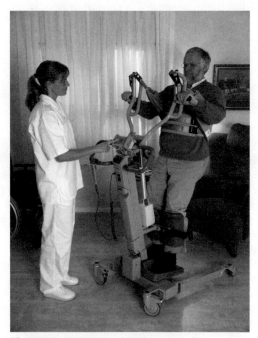

Fig. 17-2 Stand-assist lift. *(Courtesy ARJO, Inc., Roselle, Ill. [800]323-1245)*

Fig. 17-3 Stand-assist bed attachment.

Fig. 17-4 Slide board for transferring to and from surfaces.

RESIDENTS WITH DEMENTIA
Preventing Work-Related Injuries

Some older persons have dementia. They may not understand what you are doing. They may resist your handling, moving, and transfer efforts. The person may shout at you, grab you, or try to hit you. Always get a co-worker to help you. Do not force the person. The rules and guidelines in Box 17-1 apply. The person's care plan also has measures for providing safe care. For example:

- Proceed slowly.
- Use a calm, pleasant voice.
- Divert the person's attention. For example: let the person hold on to a washcloth or other soft object. This helps distract the person and keeps his or her hands busy.

Tell the nurse at once if you have problems handling, moving, or transferring the person.

TEAMWORK AND TIME MANAGEMENT
Preventing Work-Related Injuries

Some centers have "lift teams." These teams perform most of the lifting, moving, and transfer procedures. They use assist equipment and do not manually lift or move residents unless necessary.

The nurse advises the lift team of scheduled procedures. The team is called by beeper, pager, wireless phone, or other device for unscheduled transfers.

Do not assume that the lift team will lift, move, or transfer your assigned residents. Follow center policy for checking or adding to the lift team's schedule. Do not neglect or omit a procedure because the center has a lift team. If the person is on the team's schedule, always check to make sure that the procedure was done. Sometimes the team can get delayed because of unscheduled or unexpected events. Always thank the team for the work that they do. Their work protects residents and you from injury.

DELEGATION GUIDELINES
Preventing Work-Related Injuries

Many delegated tasks involve handling, moving, and transferring persons. Before doing so, you need this information from the nurse and the care plan:

- The person's height and weight.
- The person's dependence level (see Box 17-2).
- The person's physical abilities. For example, can the person sit up, stand up, or walk without help? Does the person have strength in his or her arms?
- If the person has a weak side. If yes, which side is weak?
- If the person has a medical condition that increases the risk of injury. Dizziness, confusion, hearing or vision problems, recent surgery, and fragile skin are examples.
- Any doctor's orders for handling, moving, or transferring the person.
- The person's ability to follow directions.
- If behavior problems are likely. Combative, agitated, uncooperative, and unpredictable behaviors are examples.
- The amount of assistance needed.
- How many staff members are needed to complete the task safely.
- What procedure to use.
- What equipment to use.

PROMOTING SAFETY AND COMFORT
Preventing Work-Related Injuries

Safety

Decide how to move the person before starting the procedure. If you need help from other staff members, ask them to help before you begin. Also plan how to protect drainage tubes or containers connected to the person.

Beds are raised to move persons in bed. This reduces bending and reaching. You must:

- Use the bed correctly.
- Protect the person from falling when the bed is raised.
- Follow the rules of body mechanics (Chapter 16).

Many delegated tasks involve moving the person in bed. Before moving a person, you need this information from the nurse and the care plan:
- What procedure to use
- How many workers are needed to safely move the person
- Position limits and restrictions
- How far you can lower the head of the bed
- Any limits in the person's ability to move or be re-positioned
- What pillows can be removed before moving the person
- What equipment is needed—trapeze, lift sheet, slide sheet, mechanical lift
- How to position the person
- If the person uses bed rails
- What observations to report and record:
  - Who helped you with the procedure
  - How much help the person needed
  - How the person tolerated the procedure
  - How you positioned the person
  - Complaints of pain or discomfort
- When to report observations
- What specific resident concerns to report at once

MOVING PERSONS IN BED

Some persons can move and turn in bed. Others need help from at least one person. Those who are weak, unconscious, paralyzed, or in casts need help. Sometimes 2 or 3 people or a mechanical lift is needed.
- A dependence level of *Code 4: Total Dependence*—use a mechanical lift or friction-reducing device and at least 2 staff members.
- A dependence level of *Code 3: Extensive Assistance*—use a mechanical lift or friction-reducing device and at least 2 staff members.
- The person weighs less than 200 pounds—2 to 3 staff members and a friction-reducing device are needed.
- If the person weighs more than 200 pounds—at least 3 staff members and a friction-reducing device are needed.

See *Delegation Guidelines: Moving Persons in Bed.*

Protecting the Skin

Older persons have fragile skin that is easily damaged. Protect their skin during handling, moving, and transfer procedures. Friction and shearing injure the skin. Both cause infection and pressure ulcers (Chapter 36).
- **Friction** is the rubbing of one surface against another. When moved in bed, the person's skin rubs against the sheet.
- **Shearing** is when the skin sticks to a surface while muscles slide in the direction the body is moving (Fig. 17-5). It occurs when the person slides down in bed or is moved in bed.

Reduce friction and shearing when moving the person in bed. Do so by:
- Rolling the person.
- Using friction-reducing devices. Such devices include a lift sheet (turning sheet). A cotton drawsheet (Chapter 19) serves as a lift sheet (turning sheet). Turning pads, large incontinence products, slide boards, and slide sheets are other friction-reducing devices.

▶ Raising the Person's Head and Shoulders

You may have to raise the person's head and shoulders to give care. Simply turning or removing a pillow requires this procedure. You can raise the person's head and shoulders easily and safely by locking arms with the person. *Do not pull on the person's arm or shoulder.* It is best to have help with older persons and with those who are heavy or hard to move. This protects the person and you from injury.

Fig. 17-5 Shearing. When the head of the bed is raised to a sitting position, skin on the buttocks stays in place. However, internal structures move forward as the person slides down in bed. This causes the skin to be pinched between the mattress and the hip bones.

RAISING THE PERSON'S HEAD AND SHOULDERS

QUALITY OF LIFE

Remember to:
- Knock before entering the person's room.
- Address the person by name.
- Introduce yourself by name and title.

- Explain the procedure to the person before beginning and during the procedure.
- Protect the person's rights during the procedure.
- Handle the person gently during the procedure.

PRE-PROCEDURE

1 Follow *Delegation Guidelines:*
   a *Preventing Work-Related Injuries*, p. 224
   b *Moving Persons in Bed*, p. 225
   See *Promoting Safety and Comfort:*
   a *Safe Resident Handling, Moving, and Transfers*, p. 220
   b *Preventing Work-Related Injuries*, p. 224
2 Ask a co-worker to assist if you need help.

3 Practice hand hygiene.
4 Identify the person. Check the ID (identification) bracelet against the assignment sheet. Also call the person by name.
5 Provide for privacy.
6 Lock the bed wheels.
7 Raise the bed for body mechanics. Bed rails are up if used.

PROCEDURE

8 Ask your co-worker to stand on the other side of the bed. Lower the bed rails if up.
9 Ask the person to put the near arm under your near arm and behind your shoulder. His or her hand rests on top of your shoulder. If you are standing on the right side, the person's right hand rests on your right shoulder (Fig. 17-6, *A*). The person does the same with your co-worker. The person's left hand rests on your co-worker's left shoulder (Fig. 17-7, *A*).
10 Put your arm nearest to the person under his or her arm. Your hand is on the person's shoulder. Your co-worker does the same.

11 Put your free arm under the person's neck and shoulders (Fig. 17-6, *B*). Your co-worker does the same (Fig. 17-7, *B*). Support the neck.
12 Help the person raise to a sitting or semi-sitting position on the "count of 3" (Figs. 17-6, *C*, and 17-7, *C*).
13 Use the arm and hand that supported the person's neck and shoulders to give care (Fig. 17-6, *D*). Your co-worker supports the person (Fig. 17-7, *D*).
14 Help the person lie down. Provide support with your locked arm. Support the person's neck and shoulders with your other arm. Your co-worker does the same.

POST-PROCEDURE

15 Provide for comfort. (See the inside of the front book cover.)
16 Place the signal light within reach.
17 Lower the bed to its lowest position.
18 Raise or lower bed rails. Follow the care plan.

19 Unscreen the person.
20 Complete a safety check of the room. (See the inside of the front book cover.)
21 Decontaminate your hands.
22 Report and record your observations.

Fig. 17-6 Raising the person's head and shoulders by locking arms with the person. **A,** The person's near arm is under the nursing assistant's near arm and behind the shoulder. **B,** The nursing assistant's far arm is under the person's neck and shoulders, with the near arm under the person's nearest arm. **C,** The person is raised to a semi-sitting position by locking arms. **D,** The nursing assistant lifts the pillow while the person is in a semi-sitting position.

Fig. 17-7 Raising the person's head and shoulders with a co-worker. **A,** Two nursing assistants lock arms with the person. **B,** The nursing assistants have their arms under the person's head and neck. **C,** The nursing assistants raise the person to a semi-sitting position. **D,** One nursing assistant supports the person in the semi-sitting position while the other gives care.

Moving the Person Up in Bed

When the head of the bed is raised, it is easy to slide down toward the middle and foot of the bed (Fig. 17-8). The person is moved up in bed for good alignment and comfort.

You can sometimes move lightweight adults up in bed alone if they can assist and use a trapeze. However, it is best to have help and to use an assist device—lift sheet, large incontinence product, slide sheet (p. 229). Two or more staff members are needed to move heavy, weak, and very old persons up in bed. Always protect the person and yourself from injury.

See *Promoting Safety and Comfort: Moving the Person Up in Bed.*

PROMOTING SAFETY AND COMFORT
Moving the Person Up in Bed

Safety
This procedure is best done with at least two staff members. Assist devices are used as directed by the nurse and the care plan.

Perform this procedure alone *only if:*
- The person is small in size.
- The person can follow directions.
- The person can assist with much of the moving.
- The person uses a trapeze.
- The person can push against the mattress with his or her feet.
- The nurse says it is safe to do so.
- You are comfortable doing so.

Follow the nurse's directions and the care plan. Ask any questions before you begin the procedure.

Fig. 17-8 A person in poor alignment after sliding down in bed.

MOVING THE PERSON UP IN BED

VIDEO

QUALITY OF LIFE

Remember to:
- Knock before entering the person's room.
- Address the person by name.
- Introduce yourself by name and title.

- Explain the procedure to the person before beginning and during the procedure.
- Protect the person's rights during the procedure.
- Handle the person gently during the procedure.

PRE-PROCEDURE

1 Follow *Delegation Guidelines:*
   a *Preventing Work-Related Injuries,* p. 224
   b *Moving Persons in Bed,* p. 225
   See *Promoting Safety and Comfort:*
   a *Safe Resident Handling, Moving, and Transfers,* p. 220
   b *Preventing Work-Related Injuries,* p. 224
   c *Moving the Person Up in Bed,* p. 227

2 Ask a co-worker to help you.
3 Practice hand hygiene.
4 Identify the person. Check the ID bracelet against the assignment sheet. Also call the person by name.
5 Provide for privacy.
6 Lock the bed wheels.
7 Raise the bed for body mechanics. Bed rails are up if used.

PROCEDURE

8 Lower the head of the bed to a level appropriate for the person. It is as flat as possible.
9 Stand on one side of the bed. Your co-worker stands on the other side.
10 Lower the bed rails if up.
11 Remove pillows as directed by the nurse. Place a pillow upright against the head-board if the person can be without it.
12 Stand with a wide base of support. Point the foot near the head of the bed toward the head of the bed. Face the head of the bed.
13 Bend your hips and knees. Keep your back straight.
14 Place one arm under the person's shoulder and one arm under the thighs. Your co-worker does the same. Grasp each other's forearms (Fig. 17-9).

15 Ask the person to grasp the trapeze.
16 Have the person flex both knees.
17 Explain the following:
   a You will count "1, 2, 3."
   b The move will be on "3."
   c On "3," the person pushes against the bed with the feet if able. And the person pulls up with the trapeze.
18 Move the person to the head of the bed on the count of "3." Shift your weight from your rear leg to your front leg (see Fig. 17-9). Your co-worker does the same.
19 Repeat steps 12 through 18 if necessary.

POST-PROCEDURE

20 Put the pillow under the person's head and shoulders. Straighten linens.
21 Position the person in good alignment. Raise the head of the bed to a level appropriate for the person.
22 Provide for comfort. (See the inside of the front book cover.)
23 Place the signal light within reach.

24 Lower the bed to its lowest position.
25 Raise or lower bed rails. Follow the care plan.
26 Unscreen the person.
27 Complete a safety check of the room. (See the inside of the front book cover.)
28 Decontaminate your hands.
29 Report and record your observations.

Fig. 17-9 A person is moved up in bed by two nursing assistants. Each has one arm under the person's shoulders and the other under the thighs. They have locked arms under the person. The person grasps the trapeze and flexes the knees. The nursing assistants shift their weight from the rear leg to the front leg as the person is moved up in bed.

Moving the Person Up in Bed With an Assist Device

Assist devices are used to move some persons up in bed. Such assist devices include a drawsheet (lift sheet), flat sheet folded in half, turning pad (Fig. 17-10), slide sheet (Fig. 17-11), and large incontinence product. With these devices, the person is moved more evenly. And the devices reduce shearing and friction.

The device is placed under the person from the head to above the knees or lower. At least two staff members are needed. This procedure is used for most residents. It is used:

- Following the guidelines for "Moving Persons in Bed," p. 225
- For persons recovering from spinal cord surgery or spinal cord injuries
- For older persons
  See *Promoting Safety and Comfort: Moving the Person Up in Bed With an Assist Device.*

PROMOTING SAFETY AND COMFORT
Moving the Person Up in Bed With an Assist Device

Safety

Not all incontinence products can be used as assist devices. Disposable, single-use underpads are not strong enough to hold the person's weight during the move. Reusable underpads are stronger. For safety, the underpad must:

- Be strong enough to support the person's weight
- Extend from under the person's head to above the knees or lower
- Be wide enough for you and other staff to get a firm grip for the lift

Check with the nurse to make sure the person's underpad is safe to use as an assist device.

If using a slide sheet, you will need to place it under the person. See procedure: *Making an Occupied Bed* in Chapter 19 for this step. After moving the person up in bed, remove the slide sheet. The person is in danger of sliding down in bed or off the bed if the slide sheet is not removed.

Fig. 17-10 Turning pad.

Fig. 17-11 Slide sheet.

MOVING THE PERSON UP IN BED WITH AN ASSIST DEVICE

QUALITY OF LIFE

Remember to:
- Knock before entering the person's room.
- Address the person by name.
- Introduce yourself by name and title.

- Explain the procedure to the person before beginning and during the procedure.
- Protect the person's rights during the procedure.
- Handle the person gently during the procedure.

PRE-PROCEDURE

1 Follow *Delegation Guidelines:*
   a *Preventing Work-Related Injuries,* p. 224
   b *Moving Persons in Bed,* p. 225
   See *Promoting Safety and Comfort:*
   a *Safe Resident Handling, Moving, and Transfers,* p. 220
   b *Preventing Work-Related Injuries,* p. 224
   c *Moving the Person Up in Bed,* p. 227
   d *Moving the Person Up in Bed With an Assist Device,* p. 229

2 Ask a co-worker to help you.
3 Practice hand hygiene.
4 Identify the person. Check the ID bracelet against the assignment sheet. Also call the person by name.
5 Provide for privacy.
6 Lock the bed wheels.
7 Raise the bed for body mechanics. Bed rails are up if used.

PROCEDURE

8 Lower the head of the bed to a level appropriate for the person. It is as flat as possible.
9 Stand on one side of the bed. Your co-worker stands on the other side.
10 Lower the bed rails if up.
11 Remove pillows as directed by the nurse. Place a pillow upright against the head-board if the person can be without it.
12 Stand with a broad base of support. Point the foot near the head of the bed toward the head of the bed. Face that direction.

13 Roll the sides of the assist device up close to the person. (NOTE: Omit this step if the device has handles.)
14 Grasp the rolled-up assist device firmly near the person's shoulders and hips (Fig. 17-12). Or grasp it by the handles. Support the head.
15 Bend your hips and knees.
16 Move the person up in bed on the count of "3." Shift your weight from your rear leg to your front leg.
17 Repeat steps 12 through 16 if necessary.
18 Unroll the assist device. (NOTE: Omit this step if the device has handles.)

POST-PROCEDURE

19 Put the pillow under the person's head and shoulders.
20 Position the person in good alignment. Raise the head of the bed to a level appropriate for the person.
21 Provide for comfort. (See the inside of the front book cover.)
22 Place the signal light within reach.
23 Lower the bed to its lowest position.

24 Raise or lower bed rails. Follow the care plan.
25 Unscreen the person.
26 Complete a safety check of the room. (See the inside of the front book cover.)
27 Decontaminate your hands.
28 Report and record your observations.

Fig. 17-12 A drawsheet is used to move the person up in bed. It extends from the person's head to above the knees. Rolled close to the person, the drawsheet is held near the shoulders and hips.

Moving the Person to the Side of the Bed

Re-positioning and care procedures require moving the person to the side of the bed. The person is moved to the side of the bed before turning. Otherwise, after turning, the person lies on the side of the bed—not in the middle.

Sometimes you have to reach over the person. Giving a bed bath is an example. You reach less if the person is close to you.

One method involves moving the person in segments (Fig. 17-13). Sometimes one person can do this. Use a mechanical lift (p. 244) or the assist device method:

- Following the guidelines for "Moving Persons in Bed," p. 225
- For older persons
- For persons with arthritis
- For persons recovering from spinal cord injuries or spinal cord surgery

Assist devices for this procedure include a draw-sheet (lift sheet), flat sheet folded in half, turning pad, slide sheet, slide board, and large incontinence product. Using an assist device helps prevent pain and skin damage. It also helps prevent injury to the bones, joints, and spinal cord.

See *Promoting Safety and Comfort: Moving the Person to the Side of the Bed.*

PROMOTING SAFETY AND COMFORT
Moving the Person to the Side of the Bed

Safety

Use the method and equipment that are best for the person. Get this information from the nurse and the care plan when delegated tasks involve moving the person to the side of the bed. Such tasks include re-positioning, bed-making, bathing, and range-of-motion exercises.

The wrong method could seriously injure a person. This is very important for persons who are very old, have arthritis, or have spinal cord involvement.

When using an assist device, you need at least 1 co-worker to help you. Depending on the person's size, 3 staff members may be needed. You will need to ask 2 co-workers to help you.

If using a slide board or slide sheet, you will need to place it under the person. After moving the person up in bed, remove the device.

To move the person in segments, move the person toward you, not away from you. This helps protect you from injury.

Comfort

After moving the person to the side of the bed, move the pillow too. Make sure the pillow is positioned correctly. It should be under the person's head and shoulders.

Fig. 17-13 Moving the person to the side of the bed in segments. **A,** The upper part of the body is moved. **B,** The lower part of the body is moved. **C,** The legs and feet are moved.

MOVING THE PERSON TO THE SIDE OF THE BED

QUALITY OF LIFE

Remember to:
- Knock before entering the person's room.
- Address the person by name.
- Introduce yourself by name and title.

- Explain the procedure to the person before beginning and during the procedure.
- Protect the person's rights during the procedure.
- Handle the person gently during the procedure.

PRE-PROCEDURE

1 Follow *Delegation Guidelines:*
  a *Preventing Work-Related Injuries,* p. 224
  b *Moving Persons in Bed,* p. 225
  See *Promoting Safety and Comfort:*
  a *Safe Resident Handling, Moving, and Transfers,* p. 220
  b *Preventing Work-Related Injuries,* p. 224
  c *Moving the Person to the Side of the Bed,* p. 231

2 Ask a co-worker to help you if using an assist device.
3 Practice hand hygiene.
4 Identify the person. Check the ID bracelet against the assignment sheet. Also call the person by name.
5 Provide for privacy.
6 Lock the bed wheels.
7 Raise the bed for body mechanics. Bed rails are up if used.

PROCEDURE

8 Lower the head of the bed to a level appropriate for the person. It is as flat as possible.
9 Stand on the side of the bed to which you will move the person.
10 Lower the bed rail near you if bed rails are used. (Both bed rails are lowered for step 15.)
11 Remove pillows as directed by the nurse.
12 Stand with your feet about 12 inches apart. One foot is in front of the other. Flex your knees.
13 Cross the person's arms over the person's chest.
14 *Method 1—Moving the person in segments:*
  a Place your arm under the person's neck and shoulders. Grasp the far shoulder.
  b Place your other arm under the mid-back.
  c Move the upper part of the person's body toward you. Rock backward and shift your weight to your rear leg (see Fig. 17-13, *A*).

  d Place one arm under the person's waist and one under the thighs.
  e Rock backward to move the lower part of the person toward you (see Fig. 17-13, *B*).
  f Repeat the procedure for the legs and feet (see Fig. 17-13, *C*). Your arms should be under the person's thighs and calves.
15 *Method 2—Moving the person with a drawsheet:*
  a Roll up the drawsheet close to the person (see Fig. 17-12).
  b Grasp the rolled-up drawsheet near the person's shoulders and hips. Your co-worker does the same. Support the person's head.
  c Rock backward on the count of "3," moving the person toward you. Your co-worker rocks backward slightly and then forward toward you while keeping the arms straight.
  d Unroll the drawsheet. Remove any wrinkles.

POST-PROCEDURE

16 Position the person in good alignment.
17 Provide for comfort. (See the inside of the front book cover.)
18 Place the signal light within reach.
19 Lower the bed to its lowest position.
20 Raise or lower bed rails. Follow the care plan.

21 Unscreen the person.
22 Complete a safety check of the room. (See the inside of the front book cover.)
23 Decontaminate your hands.
24 Report and record your observations.

TURNING PERSONS

Turning persons onto their sides helps prevent complications from bedrest (Chapter 26). Certain procedures and care measures also require the side-lying position. The person is turned toward you or away from you. The direction depends on the person's condition and the situation.

After the person is turned, position him or her in good alignment. Use pillows to support the person in the side-lying position.

Some persons can turn and re-position themselves in bed. Others need help. Some totally depend on the nursing staff for care. Make sure the person's face, nose, and mouth are not obstructed by a pillow or other device.

Many older persons suffer from arthritis in their spines, hips, and knees. When turning these persons, logrolling is preferred (p. 235). Logrolling may be less painful for these persons.

See *Delegation Guidelines: Turning Persons*.
See *Promoting Safety and Comfort: Turning Persons*.

DELEGATION GUIDELINES
Turning Persons

Before turning and re-positioning a person, you need this information from the nurse and the care plan:
- The person's dependency level (see Box 17-2)
- How much help the person needs
- How many staff members are needed to safely complete the procedure
- The person's comfort level and what body parts are painful
- Which procedure to use
- What assist devices to use
- What supportive devices are needed for positioning (Chapter 26)
- Where to place pillows
- What observations to report and record:
  - Who helped you with the procedure
  - How much help the person needed
  - How the person tolerated the procedure
  - How you positioned the person
  - Complaints of pain or discomfort
- When to report observations
- What specific resident concerns to report at once

PROMOTING SAFETY AND COMFORT
Turning Persons

Safety
Use good body mechanics when turning a person in bed (Chapter 16). Follow the rules in Box 17-1.

The person must be in good alignment. Otherwise, musculo-skeletal injuries, skin breakdown, or pressure ulcers could occur.

If using an assist device, ask a co-worker to help you.

Do not turn a person away from you with the far bed rail down. Raise the bed rail on the side near you. Then go to the other side of the bed. Lower that bed rail if up. Turn the person toward you.

Comfort
After turning, position the person in good alignment. Use pillows as directed to support the person in the side-lying position (Chapter 16).

 TURNING AND RE-POSITIONING THE PERSON

QUALITY OF LIFE

Remember to:
- Knock before entering the person's room.
- Address the person by name.
- Introduce yourself by name and title.

- Explain the procedure to the person before beginning and during the procedure.
- Protect the person's rights during the procedure.
- Handle the person gently during the procedure.

PRE-PROCEDURE

1 Follow *Delegation Guidelines:*
  a *Preventing Work-Related Injuries*, p. 224
  b *Moving Persons in Bed*, p. 225
  c *Turning Persons*
  See *Promoting Safety and Comfort:*
  a *Safe Resident Handling, Moving, and Transfers*, p. 220
  b *Preventing Work-Related Injuries*, p. 224
  c *Moving the Person to the Side of the Bed*, p. 231
  d *Turning Persons*

2 Practice hand hygiene.
3 Identify the person. Check the ID bracelet against the assignment sheet. Also call the person by name.
4 Provide for privacy.
5 Lock the bed wheels.
6 Raise the bed for body mechanics. Bed rails are up.

Continued

TURNING AND RE-POSITIONING THE PERSON—cont'd

PROCEDURE

7 Lower the head of the bed to a level appropriate for the person. It is as flat as possible.

8 Stand on the side of the bed opposite to where you will turn the person.

9 Lower the bed rail near you.

10 Move the person to the side near you. (See procedure: *Moving the Person to the Side of the Bed,* p. 232.)

11 Cross the person's arms over the person's chest. Cross the leg near you over the far leg.

12 *Turning the person away from you:*
   a   Stand with a wide base of support. Flex the knees.
   b   Place one hand on the person's shoulder. Place the other on the hip near you.
   c   Roll the person gently away from you toward the raised bed rail (Fig. 17-14, *A*). Shift your weight from your rear leg to your front leg.

13 *Turning the person toward you:*
   a   Raise the bed rail.
   b   Go to the other side of the bed. Lower the bed rail.
   c   Stand with a wide base of support. Flex your knees.
   d   Place one hand on the person's far shoulder. Place the other on the far hip.
   e   Roll the person toward you gently (Fig. 17-14, *B*).

14 Position the person. Follow the nurse's directions and the care plan. The following is common:
   a   Place a pillow under the head and neck.
   b   Adjust the shoulder. The person should not lie on an arm.
   c   Place a small pillow under the upper hand and arm.
   d   Position a pillow against the back.
   e   Flex the upper knee. Position the upper leg in front of the lower leg.
   f   Support the upper leg and thigh on pillows. Make sure the ankle is supported.

POST-PROCEDURE

15 Provide for comfort. (See the inside of the front book cover.)

16 Place the signal light within reach.

17 Lower the bed to its lowest position.

18 Raise or lower bed rails. Follow the care plan.

19 Unscreen the person.

20 Complete a safety check of the room. (See the inside of the front book cover.)

21 Decontaminate your hands.

22 Report and record your observations.

Fig. 17-14 Turning the person. **A,** Turning the person away from you, **B,** Turning the person toward you.
NOTE: Non-standard bed rails are used to show positioning and hand placement.

Logrolling

Logrolling is turning the person as a unit, in alignment, with one motion. The spine is kept straight. The procedure is used to turn:

- Older persons with arthritic spines or knees
- Persons recovering from hip fractures
- Persons with spinal cord injuries (the spine is kept straight at all times after spinal cord injury)
- Persons recovering from spinal surgery (the spine is kept straight at all times after spinal surgery)
  See *Promoting Safety and Comfort: Logrolling.*

PROMOTING SAFETY AND COMFORT
Logrolling

Safety

Two or three staff members are needed to logroll a person. Three are needed if the person is tall or heavy. Sometimes an assist device is needed—drawsheet, turning pad, large incontinence product, slide sheet.

Comfort

After spinal cord injury or surgery, the spine must be kept straight. This includes the person's neck. Therefore, *usually a pillow is not allowed under the head and neck.* Follow the nurse's directions and the care plan for positioning the person and using pillows.

LOGROLLING THE PERSON

QUALITY OF LIFE

Remember to:
- Knock before entering the person's room.
- Address the person by name.
- Introduce yourself by name and title.

- Explain the procedure to the person before beginning and during the procedure.
- Protect the person's rights during the procedure.
- Handle the person gently during the procedure.

PRE-PROCEDURE

1 Follow *Delegation Guidelines:*
  a *Preventing Work-Related Injuries,* p. 224
  b *Moving Persons in Bed,* p. 225
  c *Turning Persons,* p. 233
  See *Promoting Safety and Comfort:*
  a *Safe Resident Handling, Moving, and Transfers,* p. 220
  b *Preventing Work-Related Injuries,* p. 224
  c *Turning Persons,* p. 233
  d *Logrolling*

2 Ask a co-worker to help you.
3 Practice hand hygiene.
4 Identify the person. Check the ID bracelet against the assignment sheet. Also call the person by name.
5 Provide for privacy.
6 Lock the bed wheels.
7 Raise the bed for body mechanics. Bed rails are up if used.

PROCEDURE

8 Make sure the bed is flat.
9 Stand on the side opposite to which you will turn the person. Your co-worker stands on the other side.
10 Lower the bed rails if used.
11 Move the person as a unit to the side of the bed near you. Use the assist device. (If the person has a spinal cord injury, assist the nurse as directed.)
12 Place the person's arms across the chest. Place a pillow between the knees.
13 Raise the bed rail if used.
14 Go to the other side.
15 Stand near the shoulders and chest. Your co-worker stands near the hips and thighs.

16 Stand with a broad base of support. One foot is in front of the other.
17 Ask the person to hold his or her body rigid.
18 Roll the person toward you (Fig. 17-15, *A*, p. 236). Or use the assist device (Fig. 17-15, *B*, p. 236). Turn the person as a unit.
19 Position the person in good alignment. Use pillows as directed by the nurse and the care plan. The following is common (unless the spinal cord is involved):
  a One pillow against the back for support
  b One pillow under the head and neck if allowed
  c One pillow or a folded bath blanket between the legs
  d A small pillow under the upper arm and hand

POST-PROCEDURE

20 Provide for comfort. (See the inside of the front book cover.)
21 Place the signal light within reach.
22 Lower the bed to its lowest position.
23 Raise or lower bed rails. Follow the care plan.

24 Unscreen the person.
25 Complete a safety check of the room. (See the inside of the front book cover.)
26 Decontaminate your hands.
27 Report and record your observations.

Fig. 17-15 Logrolling. **A,** A pillow is between the person's legs. The arms are crossed on the chest. The person is on the far side of the bed. **B,** The assist device is used to logroll the person.

✉ SITTING ON THE SIDE OF THE BED (DANGLING)

Residents sit on the side of the bed *(dangle)* for many reasons. Many older persons become dizzy or faint when getting out of bed too fast. They may need to sit on the side of the bed for 1 to 5 minutes before walking or transferring. Some persons increase activity in stages—bedrest, to sitting on the side of the bed, and then to sitting in a chair. Walking is the next step.

While dangling the legs, the person coughs and deep breathes. He or she moves the legs back and forth in circles. This stimulates circulation.

Two staff members may be needed. Persons with balance and coordination problems need support. If dizziness or fainting occurs, lay the person down.

See *Delegation Guidelines: Dangling.*
See *Promoting Safety and Comfort: Dangling.*

PROMOTING SAFETY AND COMFORT
Dangling

Safety

This procedure is not used for persons with these dependence levels:
- Code 4: Total Dependence
- Code 3: Extensive Assistance

Problems with sitting and balance often occur after illness, injury, surgery, and bedrest. Some persons who are disabled also have problems sitting and with balance. Provide support when the person is sitting on the side of the bed. It is best to have a co-worker help you. This protects the person from falling and other injuries.

Comfort

Provide for the person's warmth during the dangling procedure. Help the person put on a robe. Or cover the person's shoulders and back with a bath blanket.

The person may want to perform simple hygiene measures while sitting on the side of the bed. Oral hygiene and washing the face and hands are examples. These measures refresh the person and stimulate circulation. Follow the nurse's directions and the care plan.

DELEGATION GUIDELINES
Dangling

The nurse may ask you to help a person sit on the side of the bed. The procedure is part of other tasks—assisting the person to stand, transferring from bed to chair, partial bath, and others. When delegated the dangling procedure or tasks that involve dangling, you need this information from the nurse and the care plan:
- Areas of weakness. For example, if the person's arms are weak, he or she cannot hold on to the side of the mattress for support. If the left side is weak, turn the person onto the stronger right side. The person can use the right arm to help move from the lying to sitting position.
- The person's dependence level (see Box 17-2).
- The amount of help the person needs.
- If you need a co-worker to help you.
- If the bed is raised or in its lowest position.
- How long the person needs to sit on the side of the bed.
- What exercises the person needs to perform while dangling:
  - Range-of-motion exercises (Chapter 26)
  - Deep-breathing and coughing exercises (Chapter 28)
- If the person will walk or transfer to a chair after dangling. If yes, the bed is in its lowest position.
- What observations to report and record (Fig. 17-16):
  - Pulse and respiratory rates (Chapter 31)
  - Pale or bluish skin color (cyanosis)
  - Complaints of dizziness, light-headedness, or difficulty breathing
  - Who helped you with the procedure
  - How well the activity was tolerated
  - The length of time the person dangled
  - The amount of help needed
  - Other observations and complaints
- When to report observations.
- What specific resident concerns to report at once.

Date	Time	Nursing Margin	Other Depts Margin	
9/9	0900			Assisted to sit on the side of the bed with assistance of one.
				Active leg exercises performed. Tolerated procedure without
				complaints of pain or discomfort. No c/o dizziness. BP-130/78 L
				arm sitting, P-74 regular rate and rhythm, R-20 unlabored. Color
				good. Assisted to lie down after 5 minutes. Positioned on L side.
				Bed in low position, signal light within reach. Adam Aims, CNA ———

Fig. 17-16 Charting sample.

SITTING ON THE SIDE OF THE BED (DANGLING)

QUALITY OF LIFE

Remember to:
- Knock before entering the person's room.
- Address the person by name.
- Introduce yourself by name and title.

- Explain the procedure to the person before beginning and during the procedure.
- Protect the person's rights during the procedure.
- Handle the person gently during the procedure.

PRE-PROCEDURE

1 Follow *Delegation Guidelines:*
  a *Preventing Work-Related Injuries,* p. 224
  b *Dangling*
  See *Promoting Safety and Comfort:*
  a *Safe Resident Handling, Moving, and Transfers,* p. 220
  b *Preventing Work-Related Injuries,* p. 224
  c *Dangling*
2 Ask a co-worker to help you if the person will dangle.

3 Practice hand hygiene.
4 Identify the person. Check the ID bracelet against the assignment sheet. Also call the person by name.
5 Provide for privacy.
6 Decide what side of the bed to use.
7 Move furniture to provide moving space.
8 Lock the bed wheels.
9 Raise the bed for body mechanics. Bed rails are up if used.

PROCEDURE

10 Lower the bed rail if up.
11 Position the person in a side-lying position facing you. The person lies on the strong side.
12 Raise the head of the bed to a sitting position.
13 Stand by the person's hips. Face the foot of the bed.
14 Stand with your feet apart. The foot near the head of the bed is in front of the other foot.
15 Slide one arm under the person's neck and shoulders. Grasp the far shoulder. Place your other hand over the thighs near the knees (Fig. 17-17, *A*, p. 238).
16 Pivot toward the foot of the bed while moving the person's legs and feet over the side of the bed. As the legs go over the edge of the mattress, the trunk is upright (Fig. 17-17, *B*, p. 238).
17 Ask the person to hold on to the edge of the mattress. This supports the person in the sitting position. If possible, raise a half-length bed rail for the person to grasp. Raise the bed rail on the person's strong side. Have your co-worker support the person at all times.

18 Do not leave the person alone. Provide support at all times.
19 Check the person's condition:
  a Ask how the person feels. Ask if the person feels dizzy or light-headed.
  b Check the pulse and respirations.
  c Check for difficulty breathing.
  d Note if the skin is pale or bluish in color *(cyanosis)*.
20 Reverse the procedure to return the person to bed. (Or prepare to transfer the person to a chair or wheelchair. Lower the bed to its lowest position so the person's feet are flat on the floor. Support the person at all times.)
21 Lower the head of the bed after the person returns to bed. Help him or her move to the center of the bed.
22 Position the person in good alignment.

POST-PROCEDURE

23 Provide for comfort. (See the inside of the front book cover.)
24 Place the signal light within reach.
25 Lower the bed to its lowest position.
26 Raise or lower bed rails. Follow the care plan.
27 Return furniture to its proper place.

28 Unscreen the person.
29 Complete a safety check of the room. (See the inside of the front book cover.)
30 Decontaminate your hands.
31 Report and record your observations.

Fig. 17-17 Helping the person sit on the side of the bed. **A,** The person's shoulders and thighs are supported. **B,** The person sits upright as the legs and feet are pulled over the edge of the bed.

TRANSFERRING PERSONS

Residents are moved to and from beds, chairs, wheelchairs, shower chairs, commodes, toilets, and stretchers. The amount of help needed and the method used vary with the person's dependency level (see Box 17-2). Some persons transfer by themselves or need little help. Some persons need help from at least 1, 2, or 3 people.

The rules of body mechanics apply to transfers (Chapter 16). So do guidelines in Box 17-1. Arrange the room so there is enough space for a safe transfer. Correct placement of the chair, wheelchair, or other device also is needed for a safe transfer.

See *Delegation Guidelines: Transferring Persons.*

See *Promoting Safety and Comfort: Transferring Persons.*

See *Teamwork and Time Management: Transferring Persons.*

DELEGATION GUIDELINES
Transferring Persons

When delegated transferring procedures, you need this information from the nurse and the care plan:

- What procedure to use.
- The person's dependency level (see Box 17-2).
- The amount of help the person needs.
- What equipment to use—transfer belt, wheelchair, mechanical assist device, positioning devices, wheelchair cushion, and so on.
- The person's height and weight.
- How many staff members are needed to complete the task safely.
- Areas of weakness. For example, if the person's arms are weak, the person cannot hold on to the mattress for support. If the person has a weak left side, he or she gets out of bed on the stronger right side. The person uses the right arm to help move from the lying to sitting position.
- What observations to report and record:
  - Pulse rate before and after the transfer (Chapter 31)
  - Complaints of light-headedness, pain, discomfort, difficulty breathing, weakness, or fatigue
  - The amount of help needed to transfer the person
  - Who helped you with the procedure
  - How the person helped with the transfer
  - How you positioned the person
- When to report observations.
- What specific resident concerns to report at once.

PROMOTING SAFETY AND COMFORT
Transferring Persons

Safety

The person wears non-skid footwear for transfers. Such footwear protects the person from falls. Slipping and sliding are prevented. Tie shoelaces securely. Otherwise the person can trip and fall.

Check the length of the person's gown or robe if necessary. Long gowns and robes can cause falls. Also, avoid robes with long ties. The person can trip and fall.

Lock bed and wheelchair wheels and wheels on other devices. This prevents the bed and the device from moving during the transfer. Otherwise, the person can fall. You also are at risk for injury.

Comfort

After the transfer, position the person in good alignment. Make sure needed items are within reach.

Mechanical assist devices are used to transfer some residents. After using such a device, return it to the storage area. It needs to be available for use by other staff. Do not leave a device in a person's room or other care setting. Your co-workers should not have to assume that an assist device is in use or take time looking for one.

Many mechanical assist devices are battery-operated. The battery must be charged for the device to work properly. Follow center policy for charging or replacing batteries.

You may need help from 1 or 2 co-workers to safely transfer a person. Politely ask co-workers to help you. Tell them what time you need the help and for how long. This helps them plan their own work. Always thank your co-workers for helping you. Willingly help them when asked.

Transfer Belts

Transfer belts were discussed in Chapter 13. Also called gait belts, they are used to support residents during transfers. They also are used to re-position persons in chairs and wheelchairs (p. 250).

Wider belts have padded handles. They are easier to grip and allow better control should the person fall.

Bed to Chair or Wheelchair Transfers

Safety is important for chair, wheelchair, commode, and shower chair transfers. Help the person out of bed on his or her strong side. If the left side is weak and the right side strong, get the person out of bed on the right side. In transferring, the strong side moves first. It pulls the weaker side along. Transfers from the weak side are awkward and unsafe.

The following stand and pivot transfers are used if:
* The person's legs are strong enough to bear some or all of his or her weight.
* The person is cooperative and can follow directions.
* The person can assist with the transfer.

See *Promoting Safety and Comfort: Bed to Chair or Wheelchair Transfers.*

Safety

The chair, wheelchair, or other device must support the person's weight. The number of staff members needed for a transfer depends on the person's abilities, condition, and size. For some persons, you will use mechanical assist devices (p. 244).

The person must not put his or her arms around your neck. Otherwise the person can pull you forward or cause you to lose your balance. Neck, back, and other injuries from falls are possible.

If not using a mechanical assist device, using a gait/transfer belt is the preferred method for chair or wheelchair transfers. It is safer for the person and you. Putting your arms around the person and grasping the shoulder blades is the other method. It can cause the person discomfort. And it can be stressful for you. Use this method *only* if instructed to do so by the nurse and the care plan.

Bed and wheelchair wheels are locked for a safe transfer. After the transfer, unlock the wheelchair wheels to position the wheelchair as the person prefers. After positioning the chair, lock the wheels or keep them unlocked according to the care plan. Locked wheels may be viewed as restraints if the person cannot unlock them to move the wheelchair (Chapter 14). However, falls and other injuries are risks if the person tries to stand when the wheelchair wheels are unlocked.

Comfort

Most wheelchairs and bedside chairs have vinyl seats and backs. Vinyl holds body heat. The person becomes warm and perspires more. You can cover the back and seat with a folded bath blanket. This increases the person's comfort in the chair. Some people have wheelchair cushions or positioning devices. Ask the nurse how to use and place the devices. Also follow the manufacturer's instructions.

TRANSFERRING THE PERSON TO A CHAIR OR WHEELCHAIR

QUALITY OF LIFE

Remember to:
- Knock before entering the person's room.
- Address the person by name.
- Introduce yourself by name and title.

- Explain the procedure to the person before beginning and during the procedure.
- Protect the person's rights during the procedure.
- Handle the person gently during the procedure.

PRE-PROCEDURE

1 Follow *Delegation Guidelines:*
  a *Preventing Work-Related Injuries,* p. 224
  b *Transferring Persons,* p. 238
  See *Promoting Safety and Comfort:*
  a *Transfer/Gait Belts* (Chapter 13)
  b *Safe Resident Handling, Moving, and Transfers,* p. 220
  c *Preventing Work-Related Injuries,* p. 224
  d *Transferring Persons,* p. 238
  e *Bed to Chair or Wheelchair Transfers,* p. 239
2 Collect:
  • Wheelchair or arm chair
  • Bath blanket

- Lap blanket
- Robe and non-skid footwear
- Paper or sheet
- Transfer belt (if needed)
- Seat cushion (if needed)

3 Practice hand hygiene.
4 Identify the person. Check the ID bracelet against the assignment sheet. Also call the person by name.
5 Provide for privacy.
6 Decide which side of the bed to use. Move furniture for a safe transfer.

PROCEDURE

7 Position the chair:
  a The chair is near the head of the bed on the person's strong side.
  b The chair faces the foot of the bed.
  c The arm of the chair almost touches the bed.
8 Place a folded bath blanket or cushion on the seat (if needed).
9 Lock the wheelchair wheels. Raise the footplates. Remove or swing the front rigging out of the way.
10 Lower the bed to its lowest position. Lock the bed wheels.
11 Fan-fold top linens to the foot of the bed.
12 Place the paper or sheet under the person's feet. (This protects the person's linens from the footwear.) Put footwear on the person.
13 Help the person sit on the side of the bed (p. 236). His or her feet touch the floor.
14 Help the person put on a robe.
15 Apply the transfer belt if needed (Chapter 13).
16 *Method 1: Using a transfer belt:*
  a Stand in front of the person.
  b Have the person hold on to the mattress.
  c Make sure the person's feet are flat on the floor.
  d Have the person lean forward.
  e Grasp the transfer belt at each side. Grasp the handles or grasp the belt from underneath. See Chapter 13.
  f Prevent the person from sliding or falling by doing one of the following:
    (1) Brace your knees against the person's knees (Fig. 17-18). Block his or her feet with your feet.

    (2) Use the knee and foot of one leg to block the person's weak leg or foot. Place your other foot slightly behind you for balance.
    (3) Straddle your legs around the person's weak leg.
  g Explain the following:
    (1) You will count "1, 2, 3."
    (2) The move will be on "3."
    (3) On "3," the person pushes down on the mattress and stands.
  h Ask the person to push down on the mattress and to stand on the count of "3." Pull the person to a standing position as you straighten your knees (Fig. 17-19).
17 *Method 2: No transfer belt:* (NOTE: Use this method only if directed by the nurse and the care plan.)
  a Follow steps 16, a-c.
  b Place your hands under the person's arms. Your hands are around the person's shoulder blades (Fig. 17-20).
  c Have the person lean forward.
  d Prevent the person from sliding or falling by doing one of the following:
    (1) Brace your knees against the person's knees. Block his or her feet with your feet.
    (2) Use the knee and foot of one leg to block the person's weak leg or foot. Place your other foot slightly behind you for balance.
    (3) Straddle your legs around the person's weak leg.
  e Explain the "count of 3." See step 16, g.
  f Ask the person to push down on the mattress and to stand on the count of "3." Pull the person up into a standing position as you straighten your knees.

TRANSFERRING THE PERSON TO A CHAIR OR WHEELCHAIR—cont'd

PROCEDURE—cont'd

18 Support the person in the standing position. Hold the transfer belt, or keep your hands around the person's shoulder blades. Continue to prevent the person from sliding or falling.

19 Turn the person so he or she can grasp the far arm of the chair. The legs will touch the edge of the chair (Fig. 17-21, p. 242).

20 Continue to turn the person until the other armrest is grasped.

21 Lower him or her into the chair as you bend your hips and knees. The person assists by leaning forward and bending the elbows and knees (Fig. 17-22, p. 242).

22 Make sure the hips are to the back of the seat. Position the person in good alignment.

23 Attach the wheelchair front rigging. Position the person's feet on the wheelchair footplates.

24 Cover the person's lap and legs with a lap blanket. Keep the blanket off the floor and the wheels.

25 Remove the transfer belt if used.

26 Position the chair as the person prefers. Lock the wheelchair wheels according to the care plan.

POST-PROCEDURE

27 Provide for comfort. (See the inside of the front book cover.)

28 Place the signal light and other needed items within reach.

29 Unscreen the person.

30 Complete a safety check of the room. (See the inside of the front book cover.)

31 Decontaminate your hands.

32 Report and record your observations.

33 See procedure: *Transferring the Person From a Chair or Wheelchair to Bed* (p. 243) to return the person to bed.

Fig. 17-18 The person's feet and knees are blocked by the nursing assistant's feet and knees. This prevents the person from sliding or falling.

Fig. 17-19 The person is pulled up to a standing position and supported by holding the transfer belt and blocking the person's knees and feet.

Fig. 17-20 The person is being prepared to stand. The hands are placed under the person's arms and around the shoulder blades.

Fig. 17-21 The person is supported as he or she grasps the far arm of the chair. The legs are against the chair.

Fig. 17-22 The person holds the armrests, leans forward, and bends the elbows and knees while being lowered into the chair.

Chair or Wheelchair to Bed Transfers

Chair or wheelchair to bed transfers have the same rules as bed to chair transfers. If the person is weak on one side, transfer the person so that the strong side moves first. Or the chair or wheelchair is positioned so the person's strong side is near the bed so it moves first.

For example, Mrs. Lee's right side is weak. Her left side is strong. To transfer her from bed to chair, the chair was on the left side of the bed. This allowed her left side (strong side) to move first. Now you will transfer Mrs. Lee back to bed. If the chair is on the left side of the bed, her right side—the weak side—is near the bed. It is not safe to move the weak side first. You need to move the chair to the other side of the bed or turn the chair around. Mrs. Lee's stronger left side will be near the bed. The stronger side moves first for a safe transfer.

Fig. 17-23 To transfer the person from chair to bed, the chair is positioned so the person's strong side is near the bed.

TRANSFERRING THE PERSON FROM A CHAIR OR WHEELCHAIR TO BED

QUALITY OF LIFE

Remember to:
- Knock before entering the person's room.
- Address the person by name.
- Introduce yourself by name and title.

- Explain the procedure to the person before beginning and during the procedure.
- Protect the person's rights during the procedure.
- Handle the person gently during the procedure.

PRE-PROCEDURE

1 Follow *Delegation Guidelines:*
  a *Preventing Work-Related Injuries*, p. 224
  b *Transferring Persons*, p. 238
  See *Promoting Safety and Comfort:*
  a *Transfer/Gait Belts* (Chapter 13)
  b *Safe Resident Handling, Moving, and Transfers*, p. 220
  c *Preventing Work-Related Injuries*, p. 224
  d *Transferring Persons*, p. 238
  e *Bed to Chair or Wheelchair Transfers*, p. 239

2 Collect a transfer belt if needed.
3 Practice hand hygiene.
4 Identify the person. Check the ID bracelet against the assignment sheet. Also call the person by name.
5 Provide for privacy.

PROCEDURE

6 Move furniture for moving space.
7 Raise the head of the bed to a sitting position. The bed is in the lowest position.
8 Move the signal light so it is on the strong side when the person is in bed.
9 Position the chair or wheelchair so the person's strong side is next to the bed (Fig. 17-23). Have a co-worker help you if necessary.
10 Lock the wheelchair and bed wheels.
11 Remove and fold the lap blanket.
12 Remove the person's feet from the footplates. Raise the footplates. Remove or swing the front rigging out of the way. (The person has on non-skid footwear.)
13 Apply the transfer belt (if needed).
14 Make sure the person's feet are flat on the floor.
15 Stand in front of the person.
16 Ask the person to hold on to the armrests. (If the nurse directs you to do so, place your arms under the person's arms. Your hands are around the shoulder blades.)
17 Have the person lean forward.
18 Grasp the transfer belt on each side if using it. Grasp underneath the belt.

19 Prevent the person from sliding or falling. Do one of the following:
  a Brace your knees against the person's knees. Block his or her feet with your feet.
  b Use the knee and foot of one leg to block the person's weak leg or foot. Place your other foot slightly behind you for balance.
  c Straddle your legs around the person's weak leg.
20 Explain the "count of 3." (See procedure: *Transferring the Person to a Chair or Wheelchair*, p. 240)
21 Ask the person to push down on the armrests on the count of "3." Pull the person into a standing position as you straighten your knees.
22 Support the person in the standing position. Hold the transfer belt, or keep your hands around the person's shoulder blades. Continue to prevent the person from sliding or falling.
23 Turn the person so he or she can reach the edge of the mattress. The legs will touch the mattress.
24 Continue to turn the person until he or she can reach the mattress with both hands.
25 Lower him or her onto the bed as you bend your hips and knees. The person assists by leaning forward and bending the elbows and knees.
26 Remove the transfer belt.
27 Remove the robe and footwear.
28 Help the person lie down.

POST-PROCEDURE

29 Provide for comfort. (See the inside of the front book cover.)
30 Place the signal light and other needed items within reach.
31 Raise or lower bed rails. Follow the care plan.
32 Arrange furniture to meet the person's needs.

33 Unscreen the person.
34 Complete a safety check of the room. (See the inside of the front book cover.)
35 Decontaminate your hands.
36 Report and record your observations.

Mechanical Lifts

Persons who cannot help themselves are transferred with mechanical lifts (Fig. 17-24). So are persons too heavy for the staff to transfer. The devices are used for transfers to and from beds, chairs, stretchers, tubs, shower chairs, toilets, commodes, whirlpools, or vehicles.

There are manual, battery-operated, and electric lifts. Some lifts are mounted on the ceiling.

Slings   The type of sling used depends on the person's size, condition, and other needs. Slings are padded, unpadded, or made of mesh.

- *Standard full sling*—used for normal transfers.
- *Extended length sling*—used for persons with extra large thighs.
- *Bathing sling*—used to transfer the person directly from the bed or chair into a bathtub. The sling is left in place and attached to the lift during the bath.
- *Toileting sling*—the sling bottom is open. For infection control, each person should have his or her own toileting sling.
- *Amputee sling*—used for the person who has had both legs amputated (double amputee).

Follow center policy and the manufacturer's instructions for washing slings. Also follow center policy for handling and washing contaminated slings. A sling is contaminated if it:

- Has any visible sign of blood, body fluids, secretions, or excretions
- Is used on a person's bare skin
- Is used to bathe a person

Using a Mechanical Lift   Before using a lift:

- You must be trained in its use.
- It must work.
- The sling, straps, hooks, and chains must be in good repair.
- The person's weight must not exceed the lift's capacity.
- At least two staff members are needed.

There are different types of mechanical lifts. Always follow the manufacturer's instructions. The following procedure is used as a guide.

See *Delegation Guidelines: Using a Mechanical Lift.*

See *Promoting Safety and Comfort: Using a Mechanical Lift.*

DELEGATION GUIDELINES
Using a Mechanical Lift

When delegated tasks that involve using a mechanical lift, you need this information from the nurse and the care plan:

- The person's dependency level (see Box 17-2)
- What lift to use
- What sling to use—full, extended length, bathing, toileting, amputee
- What size sling to use
- If you should use a padded, unpadded, or mesh sling
- How many staff members are needed to perform the task safely

---

PROMOTING SAFETY AND COMFORT
Using a Mechanical Lift

Safety

Always follow the manufacturer's instructions. Knowing how to use one lift does not mean that you know how to use others.

If you have questions, ask the nurse. If you have not used a certain lift before, ask for needed training. Ask the nurse to help you until you are comfortable using the lift.

Mechanical lifts must be in good working order. Tell the nurse when a lift needs repair or is not working properly.

Some mechanical lifts are powered by batteries. The batteries must be well-charged. Follow the manufacturer's instructions.

Comfort

The person will be lifted up and off the bed or chair. Falling from the lift is a common fear. To promote the person's mental comfort, always explain the procedure before you begin. Also show the person how the lift works.

Fig. 17-24 Parts of a mechanical lift.

TRANSFERRING THE PERSON USING A MECHANICAL LIFT

VIDEO

QUALITY OF LIFE

Remember to:
- Knock before entering the person's room.
- Address the person by name.
- Introduce yourself by name and title.

- Explain the procedure to the person before beginning and during the procedure.
- Protect the person's rights during the procedure.
- Handle the person gently during the procedure.

PRE-PROCEDURE

1 Follow *Delegation Guidelines:*
   a *Preventing Work-Related Injuries,* p. 224
   b *Transferring Persons,* p. 238
   c *Using a Mechanical Lift*
   See *Promoting Safety and Comfort:*
   a *Safe Resident Handling, Moving, and Transfers,* p. 220
   b *Preventing Work-Related Injuries,* p. 224
   c *Transferring Persons,* p. 238
   d *Using a Mechanical Lift*
2 Ask a co-worker to help you.

3 Collect:
   - Mechanical lift and sling
   - Arm chair or wheelchair
   - Footwear
   - Bath blanket or cushion
   - Lap blanket
4 Practice hand hygiene.
5 Identify the person. Check the ID bracelet against the assignment sheet. Also call the person by name.
6 Provide for privacy.

PROCEDURE

7 Raise the bed for body mechanics. Bed rails are up if used.
8 Lower the head of the bed to a level appropriate for the person. It is as flat as possible.
9 Stand on one side of the bed. Your co-worker stands on the other side.
10 Lower the bed rails if up.
11 Center the sling under the person (Fig. 17-25, *A,* p. 246). To position the sling, turn the person from side to side as if making an occupied bed (Chapter 19). Position the sling according to the manufacturer's instructions.
12 Position the person in semi-Fowler's position.
13 Place the chair at the head of the bed. It is even with the head-board and about 1 foot away from the bed. Place a folded bath blanket or cushion in the chair.
14 Lock the bed wheels. Lower the bed to its lowest position.
15 Raise the lift so you can position it over the person.
16 Position the lift over the person (Fig. 17-25, *B,* p. 246).
17 Lock the lift wheels in position.

18 Attach the sling to the sling hooks (Fig. 17-25, *C,* p. 246).
19 Raise the head of the bed to a sitting position.
20 Cross the person's arms over the chest.
21 Raise the lift high enough until the person and sling are free of the bed (Fig. 17-25, *D,* p. 246).
22 Have your co-worker support the person's legs as you move the lift and the person away from the bed (Fig. 17-25, *E,* p. 246).
23 Position the lift so the person's back is toward the chair.
24 Position the chair so you can lower the person into it.
25 Lower the person into the chair. Guide the person into the chair (Fig. 17-25, *F,* p. 246).
26 Lower the spreader bar to unhook the sling. Remove the sling from under the person unless otherwise indicated.
27 Put footwear on the person. Position the person's feet on the wheelchair footplates.
28 Cover the person's lap and legs with a lap blanket. Keep it off the floor and wheels.
29 Position the chair as the person prefers. Lock the wheelchair wheels according to the care plan.

POST-PROCEDURE

30 Provide for comfort. (See the inside of the front book cover.)
31 Place the signal light and other needed items within the person's reach.
32 Unscreen the person.

33 Complete a safety check of the room. (See the inside of the front book cover.)
34 Decontaminate your hands.
35 Report and record your observations.
36 Reverse the procedure to return the person to bed.

Fig. 17-25 Using a mechanical lift. **A,** The sling is positioned under the person. **B,** The lift is over the person. **C,** The sling is attached to the spreader bar. **D,** The lift is raised until the sling and person are off the bed. **E,** The person's legs are supported as the person and lift are moved away from the bed. **F,** The person is guided into a chair.

Transferring the Person to and From the Toilet

Using the bathroom for elimination promotes dignity, self-esteem, and independence. It also is more private than using a bedpan, urinal, or bedside commode. However, getting to the toilet is hard for persons who use wheelchairs. Bathrooms are often small. There is little room for you or a wheelchair. Therefore transfers involving wheelchairs and toilets are often hard. Falls and work-related injuries are risks.

Sometimes mechanical lifts are used to transfer the person to and from a toilet. A slide board (see Fig. 17-4) may be used if:

- The wheelchair armrests are removable.
- The person has upper body strength.
- The person has good sitting balance.
- There is enough room to position the wheelchair next to the toilet.

The following procedure can be used if the person can stand and pivot from the wheelchair to the toilet.

See *Promoting Safety and Comfort: Transferring the Person to and From the Toilet.*

PROMOTING SAFETY AND COMFORT
Transferring the Person to and From the Toilet

Safety

Make sure the person has a raised toilet seat. The toilet seat and wheelchair are at the same level.

Check the grab bars by the toilet. If they are loose, tell the nurse. Do not transfer the person to the toilet if the grab bars are not secure.

Follow Standard Precautions and the Bloodborne Pathogen Standard. Wear gloves if the person is incontinent of urine or feces.

TRANSFERRING THE PERSON TO AND FROM THE TOILET

QUALITY OF LIFE

Remember to:
- Knock before entering the person's room.
- Address the person by name.
- Introduce yourself by name and title.

- Explain the procedure to the person before beginning and during the procedure.
- Protect the person's rights during the procedure.
- Handle the person gently during the procedure.

PRE-PROCEDURE

1 Follow *Delegation Guidelines:*
  a *Preventing Work-Related Injuries,* p. 224
  b *Transferring Persons,* p. 238
  See *Promoting Safety and Comfort:*
  a *Transfer/Gait Belts* (Chapter 13)
  b *Safe Resident Handling, Moving, and Transfers,*
    p. 220

  c *Preventing Work-Related Injuries,* p. 224
  d *Transferring Persons,* p. 238
  e *Bed to Chair or Wheelchair Transfers,* p. 239
  f *Transferring the Person to and From the Toilet*
2 Practice hand hygiene.

PROCEDURE

3 Have the person wear non-skid footwear.
4 Position the wheelchair next to the toilet if there is enough room. If not, position the chair at a right angle (90-degree angle) to the toilet (Fig. 17-26, p. 248). It is best if the person's strong side is near the toilet.
5 Lock the wheelchair wheels.
6 Raise the footplates. Remove or swing the front rigging out of the way.
7 Apply the transfer belt.
8 Help the person unfasten clothing.
9 Use the transfer belt to help the person stand and to turn to the toilet. (See procedure: *Transferring the Person to a Chair or Wheelchair,* pp. 240-241.) The person uses the grab bars to turn to the toilet.
10 Support the person with the transfer belt while he or she lowers clothing. Or have the person hold on to the grab bars for support. Lower the person's pants and undergarments.
11 Use the transfer belt to lower the person onto the toilet seat. Make sure he or she is properly positioned on the toilet.
12 Remove the transfer belt.
13 Tell the person you will stay nearby. Remind the person to use the signal light or call for you when help is needed. Stay with the person if required by the care plan.

14 Close the bathroom door to provide for privacy.
15 Stay near the bathroom. Complete other tasks in the person's room. Check on the person every 5 minutes.
16 Knock on the bathroom door when the person calls for you.
17 Help with wiping, perineal care (Chapter 20), flushing, and hand washing as needed. Wear gloves and practice hand hygiene after removing the gloves.
18 Apply the transfer belt.
19 Use the transfer belt to help the person stand.
20 Help the person raise and secure clothing.
21 Use the transfer belt to transfer the person to the wheelchair. (See procedure: *Transferring the Person to a Chair or Wheelchair,* pp. 240-241).
22 Make sure the person's buttocks are to the back of the seat. Position the person in good alignment.
23 Position the person's feet on the footplates.
24 Remove the transfer belt.
25 Cover the person's lap and legs with a lap blanket. Keep the blanket off the floor and wheels.
26 Position the chair as the person prefers. Lock the wheelchair wheels according to the care plan.

POST-PROCEDURE

27 Provide for comfort. (See the inside of the front book cover.)
28 Place the signal light and other need items within the person's reach.
29 Unscreen the person.

30 Complete a safety check of the room. (See the inside of the front book cover.)
31 Practice hand hygiene.
32 Report and record your observations.

Fig. 17-26 The wheelchair is placed at a right angle (90-degree angle) to the toilet.

Moving the Person to a Stretcher

Stretchers (gurneys) are used to transport persons to other areas. They are used for persons who:
- Cannot sit up
- Must stay in a lying position
- Are seriously ill

The stretcher is covered with a folded flat sheet or bath blanket. A pillow and extra blankets are on hand. With the nurse's permission, raise the head of the stretcher to a Fowler's or semi-Fowler's position (Chapter 18). This increases the person's comfort.

A drawsheet, turning pad, large incontinence underpad, slide sheet, or slide board is used. At least 2 or 3 staff members are needed for a safe transfer. OSHA recommends the following:
- If the person weighs less than 100 pounds—use a lateral sliding aid and 2 staff members
- If the person weighs 100 to 200 pounds—use a lateral sliding aid or a friction-reducing device and 2 staff members
- If the person weighs more than 200 pounds, use one of the following:
  - A lateral sliding aid and 3 staff members
  - A friction-reducing device or lateral transfer device and 2 staff members
  - A mechanical lateral transfer device with a built-in slide board

Safety straps are used when the person is on the stretcher. The stretcher side rails are kept up during the transport. The stretcher is moved feet first. This is so the staff member at the head of the stretcher can watch the person's breathing and color during the transport. Never leave a person on a stretcher alone.

See *Promoting Safety and Comfort: Moving the Person to a Stretcher.*

> **PROMOTIONG SAFETY AND COMFORT**
> Moving the Person to a Stretcher
>
> **Safety**
> Protect yourself and the person from injury:
> - Position the stretcher and bed surfaces as close as possible to each other.
> - Avoid extended reaches and bending your back. You may need to kneel on the bed or stretcher.
> - Follow the rules for stretcher safety (Chapter 12).
> - Make sure the bed and stretcher wheels are locked.
> - Practice good body mechanics (Chapter 16) and follow the guidelines in Box 17-1.
> - Keep the person in good alignment.
> - Make sure you have enough help.
> - Hold the person securely. You must not drop the person onto the floor.

MOVING THE PERSON TO A STRETCHER

QUALITY OF LIFE

Remember to:
- Knock before entering the person's room.
- Address the person by name.
- Introduce yourself by name and title.

- Explain the procedure to the person before beginning and during the procedure.
- Protect the person's rights during the procedure.
- Handle the person gently during the procedure.

PRE-PROCEDURE

1 Follow *Delegation Guidelines:*
  a *Preventing Work-Related Injuries,* p. 224
  b *Transferring Persons,* p. 238
  See *Promoting Safety and Comfort:*
  a *Safe Resident Handling, Moving, and Transfers,* p. 220
  b *Preventing Work-Related Injuries,* p. 224
  c *Transferring Persons,* p. 238
  d *Moving the Person to a Stretcher*
2 Ask 1 or 2 staff members to help you.

3 Collect:
  - Stretcher covered with a sheet or bath blanket
  - Bath blanket
  - Pillow(s) if needed
  - Slide sheet, slide board, drawsheet, or other assist device
4 Practice hand hygiene.
5 Identify the person. Check the ID bracelet against the assignment sheet. Also call the person by name.
6 Provide for privacy.
7 Raise the bed and stretcher for body mechanics.

PROCEDURE

8 Position yourself and co-workers:
  a One or two workers stand on the side of the bed where the stretcher will be.
  b One worker stands on the other side of the bed.
9 Lower the head of the bed. It is as flat as possible.
10 Lower the bed rails if used.
11 Cover the person with a bath blanket. Fan-fold top linens to the foot of the bed.
12 Position the assist device. Or loosen the drawsheet on each side.
13 Use the assist device to move the person to the side of the bed. This is the side where the stretcher will be.
14 Protect the person from falling. Hold the far arm and leg.

15 Have your co-workers position the stretcher next to the bed. They stand behind the stretcher (Fig. 17-27, *A*).
16 Lock the bed and stretcher wheels.
17 Grasp the assist device (Fig. 17-27, *B*).
18 Transfer the person to the stretcher on the count of "3." Center the person on the stretcher.
19 Place a pillow or pillows under the person's head and shoulders if allowed. Raise the head of the stretcher if allowed.
20 Cover the person. Provide for comfort.
21 Fasten the safety straps. Raise the side rails.
22 Unlock the stretcher wheels. Transport the person.

POST-PROCEDURE

23 Decontaminate your hands.
24 Report and record:
  - The time of the transport
  - Where the person was transported to
  - Who went with him or her
  - How the transfer was tolerated

25 Reverse the procedure to return the person to bed.

Fig. 17-27 Transferring the person to a stretcher. **A,** The stretcher is against the bed and is held in place. **B,** A drawsheet is used to transfer the person from the bed to a stretcher.

RE-POSITIONING IN A CHAIR OR WHEELCHAIR

The person can slide down into the chair. For good alignment and safety, the person's back and buttocks must be against the back of the chair.

Some persons can help with re-positioning. Others need help. If the person cannot help, a mechanical lift is needed to re-position the person. Follow the nurse's directions and the care plan for the best way to re-position a person in a chair or wheelchair. *Do not pull the person from behind the chair or wheelchair.*

If the person's chair reclines, do the following:
- Ask a co-worker to help you.
- Lock the wheels.
- Recline the chair.
- Position a friction-reducing device (drawsheet or slide sheet) under the person.
- Use the device to move the person up. See procedure: *Moving the Person Up in Bed With an Assist Device*, p. 230.

The following method can be used if the person is alert and cooperative. The person must be able to follow directions. And the person must have the strength to help.
- Lock the wheelchair wheels.
- Remove or swing the front rigging out of the way.
- Position the person's feet flat on the floor.
- Apply a transfer belt.
- Position the person's arms on the armrests.
- Stand in front of the person. Block his or her knees and feet with your knees and feet.
- Grasp the transfer belt on each side while the person leans forward.
- Ask the person to push with his or her feet and arms on the count of "3."
- Move the person back into the chair on the count of "3" as the person pushes with his or her feet and arms (Fig. 17-28).

Fig. 17-28 Re-positioning the person in a wheelchair. A transfer belt is used to move the person to the back of the chair.

REVIEW QUESTIONS

Circle the BEST answer.

1 A person's skin rubs against the sheet. This is called
   a Shearing
   b Friction
   c Ergonomics
   d Posture

2 Which occurs when a person slides down in bed?
   a Shearing
   b Friction
   c Ergonomics
   d Posture

3 Which protects the skin when moving the person in bed?
   a Rolling the person
   b Sliding the person up in bed
   c Moving the mattress
   d Using ergonomics

4 Whenever you handle, move, or transfer a person, you must
   a Allow personal choice
   b Protect the person's privacy
   c Use pillows for support
   d Get help from a co-worker

5 You are delegated tasks that involve moving persons in bed. Which is *true*?
   a The nurse tells you how to position the person.
   b You decide which procedure to use.
   c Bed rails are used at all times.
   d Three workers are needed to complete the task safely.

6 You are using a drawsheet as an assist device. It is placed so that it
   a Covers the person's body
   b Is under the person from the head to above the knees
   c Extends from the mid-back to mid-thigh level
   d Covers the entire mattress

7 Before turning a person onto his or her side, you
   a Move the person to the side of the bed
   b Move the person to the middle of the bed
   c Lock arms with the person
   d Position pillows for comfort

8 The logrolling procedure
   a Is used after spinal cord injuries or surgeries
   b Requires a transfer belt
   c Requires a mechanical lift
   d Involves a stretcher and a drawsheet

9 When getting ready to dangle a person, you need to know
   a Which side is stronger
   b If bed rails are used
   c If a mechanical lift is needed
   d If a transfer belt is needed

10 For chair and wheelchair transfers, the person must
   a Wear non-skid footwear
   b Have the bed rails up
   c Use a mechanical lift
   d Have a drawsheet or other assist device

11 Before transferring a person to or from a bed, you must
   a Raise the bed rails
   b Lock the bed wheels
   c Apply a transfer belt
   d Position pillows for support

12 When transferring the person to bed, a chair, or the toilet
   a The person's strong side moves first
   b The weak side moves first
   c Pillows are used for support
   d The transfer belt is removed

13 You are going to use a mechanical lift. You must do the following *except*
   a Follow the manufacturer's instructions
   b Make sure the lift works
   c Compare the person's weight to the lift's weight limit
   d Use a transfer belt

14 To safely transfer a person with a mechanical lift, at least
   a 1 worker is needed
   b 2 workers are needed
   c 3 workers are needed
   d 4 workers are needed

15 These statements are about transfers to and from a toilet. Which is *false*?
   a The person wears non-skid footwear.
   b Wheelchair wheels must be locked.
   c The person uses the towel bars for support.
   d A transfer belt is used.

16 These statements are about transfers to and from a stretcher? Which is *false*?
   a The bed and stretcher wheels must be locked.
   b The stretcher's side rails are raised when the person is on the stretcher.
   c Once on the stretcher, the person can be left alone.
   d At least 2 workers are needed for a safe transfer.

Answers to these questions are on p. 720.

CHAPTER 18

The Resident's Unit

OBJECTIVES

- Define the key terms and key abbreviations listed in this chapter.
- Identify the room temperatures required by OBRA and the CMS.
- Describe how to protect the person from drafts.
- List ways to prevent or reduce odors and noise.
- Explain how lighting affects comfort.
- Describe the basic bed positions.
- Identify the persons at risk for entrapment in the hospital bed system.
- Identify hospital bed system entrapment zones.

- Explain how to use the furniture and equipment in the person's unit.
- Describe how a bathroom is equipped for the person's use.
- Describe how to provide for safety, privacy, and comfort in the person's unit.
- Explain how to maintain the person's unit.
- Describe OBRA and CMS requirements for resident rooms.
- Explain how to promote quality of life.

KEY TERMS

Fowler's position A semi-sitting position; the head of the bed is raised between 45 and 60 degrees

full visual privacy Having the means to be completely free from public view while in bed

high-Fowler's position A semi-sitting position, the head of the bed is raised 60 to 90 degrees

resident unit The personal space, furniture, and equipment provided for the person by the nursing center

reverse Trendelenburg's position The head of the bed is raised and the foot of the bed is lowered

semi-Fowler's position The head of the bed is raised 30 degrees; or the head of the bed is raised 30 degrees and the knee portion is raised 15 degrees

Trendelenburg's position The head of the bed is lowered and the foot of the bed is raised

KEY ABBREVIATIONS

CMS	Centers for Medicare & Medicaid Services	**OBRA**	Omnibus Budget Reconciliation Act of 1987
F	Fahrenheit		
FDA	Food and Drug Administration		

Fig. 18-1 Furniture and equipment in a resident's unit.

Nursing centers are designed to provide comfort, safety, and privacy. The intent is to have resident units as personal and home-like as possible. A **resident unit** is the personal space, furniture, and equipment provided for the person by the nursing center (Fig. 18-1).

Some residents have private rooms. Others share a room with another person. This area is private. It is treated like the person's home.

Residents bring some furniture and personal items from home. As space allows, the person chooses where to place personal items. This promotes dignity and self-esteem. However, a resident cannot take or use another person's space. Doing so violates the other person's rights.

COMFORT

Age, illness, and activity affect comfort. So do temperature, ventilation, noise, odors, and lighting. These factors are controlled to meet the person's needs.

Temperature and Ventilation

Heating and air conditioning systems maintain a comfortable temperature. Most healthy people are comfortable when the temperature is 68° F (Fahrenheit) to 74° F. This range may be too hot or too cold for others. Older persons and those who are ill may need higher temperatures for comfort. Nursing centers maintain a temperature range of 71° F to 81° F. This is a requirement of the Omnibus Budget Reconciliation Act of 1987 (OBRA) and the Centers for Medicare & Medicaid Services (CMS).

OBRA-CMS

Persons who are less active usually do not like cool areas. Nor do those who need help moving about. They must be dressed warmly. They also need warm room temperatures. You may find the rooms rather warm.

Stale room air and lingering odors affect comfort and rest. Ventilation systems provide fresh air and move room air. Drafts occur as air moves. Older persons and those who are ill are sensitive to drafts. To protect them from drafts:

- Make sure they wear the correct clothing.
- Make sure they wear enough clothing. Many wear sweaters during warm weather.
- Offer lap robes to those in chairs and wheelchairs. Lap robes cover the legs.
- Provide enough blankets for warmth.
- Cover them with bath blankets when giving care.
- Move them from drafty areas.

Odors

Many odors occur in nursing centers. Food aromas and flower scents are pleasant. Bowel movements and urine have embarrassing odors. So do draining wounds and vomitus. Body, breath, and smoking odors may offend others.

Some people are very sensitive to odors. They may become nauseated. Good nursing care, ventilation, and housekeeping practices help prevent odors. To reduce odors:

- Empty, clean, and disinfect bedpans, urinals, commodes, and kidney basins promptly.
- Check to make sure toilets are flushed.
- Check incontinent persons often (Chapters 22 and 23).
- Clean persons who are wet or soiled from urine, feces, vomitus, or wound drainage.
- Change wet or soiled linens and clothing promptly.
- Keep laundry containers closed.
- Follow center policy for wet or soiled linens and clothing.
- Dispose of incontinence and ostomy products promptly (Chapters 22 and 23).
- Provide good hygiene to prevent body and breath odors (Chapter 20).
- Use room deodorizers as needed and allowed by center policy. Sometimes odors remain after removing the cause. Do not use sprays around persons with breathing problems. Ask the nurse if you are unsure.

Smoke odors present special problems. Residents, visitors, and staff smoke only in the areas allowed. If you smoke, follow the center's policy. Practice hand washing after handling smoking materials and before giving care. Give careful attention to your uniforms, hair, and breath because of smoke odors.

The center is the person's home. Keep it free of unpleasant odors.

Noise

The CMS requires comfortable sound levels. A "comfortable" sound level:

- Does not interfere with a person's hearing.
- Promotes privacy when privacy is desired.
- Allows the person to take part in social activities.

Many older and ill persons are sensitive to noises and sounds. Common health care sounds may disturb them. Examples include:

- The clanging of equipment
- The clatter of dishes and meal trays
- Loud voices, TVs, radios, and so on
- Ringing phones
- Intercom systems and signal lights
- Equipment needing repair
- Wheels on stretchers, wheelchairs, carts, and other items needing oil
- Cleaning equipment

Loud talking and laughter in hallways and at the nurses' station are common. Residents may think that the staff are talking and laughing about them.

People want to know the cause and meaning of new sounds. This relates to safety and security needs. Residents may find sounds dangerous, frightening, or irritating. They may become upset, anxious, and uncomfortable. What is noise to one person may not be noise to another. For example, a teenager enjoys loud music. It may bother adults.

Nursing centers are designed to reduce noise. Window coverings, carpets, and acoustical tiles absorb noise. Plastic items make less noise than metal equipment (bedpans, urinals, wash basins). To decrease noise:

- Control your voice.
- Handle equipment carefully.
- Keep equipment in good working order.
- Answer phones, signal lights, and intercoms promptly.
  See *Residents With Dementia: Noise.*
  See *Focus on Communication: Noise.*

RESIDENTS WITH DEMENTIA
Noise

Persons with dementia do not understand what is happening around them. They do not react to common, everyday sounds as other people do. For example, a ringing phone may frighten a person with dementia. The person may not know or understand the sound. He or she may have an extreme reaction to the sound (Chapter 44). The reaction may be more severe at night. This is likely when the sound awakens the person suddenly. A dark, strange room can make the problem worse.

How do you feel when a strange sound wakes you? Do you feel safe and secure? Or are you afraid?

FOCUS ON COMMUNICATION
Noise

Reducing noise requires cooperation from all staff members. To reduce noise:

- Do not talk loudly in the hallways or nurses' station.
- If necessary, politely ask others to speak more softly.
- Avoid unnecessary conversation. Always be professional. Do not discuss inappropriate topics at work. Others may overhear and become offended.

RESIDENTS WITH DEMENTIA
Lighting

In dementia care units, lighting is adjusted to help control agitated and aggressive behaviors. Soft, non-glare lights are relaxing. They can decrease agitation. Brighter lighting may improve orientation. This is because the person can see surroundings more clearly.

Lighting

The CMS requires comfortable lighting. Such lighting:

- Lessens glares
- Allows the resident to control the intensity, location, and direction of light
- Allows persons who are visually impaired to maintain or increase independent functioning

Good lighting is needed for safety and comfort. Glares, shadows, and dull lighting can cause falls, headaches, and eyestrain. A bright room is cheerful. Dim light is better for relaxing and rest.

Adjust lighting to meet the person's changing needs. Window coverings are adjusted as needed. The over-bed light can provide soft, medium, or bright lighting. Some centers have ceiling lights. They provide soft to very bright light.

Persons with poor vision need bright light. This is very important at mealtime and when moving about in the room and center. Bright lighting also helps the staff perform procedures.

Always keep light controls within the person's reach. This protects the right to personal choice.

See *Residents With Dementia: Lighting.*

ROOM FURNITURE AND EQUIPMENT

Rooms are furnished and equipped to meet basic needs. The room has furniture and equipment for comfort, sleep, elimination, nutrition, hygiene, and activity. There is equipment to communicate with staff, family, and friends. The right to privacy is considered.

The Bed

Beds have electrical or manual controls. Beds are raised horizontally to give care. This reduces bending and reaching. The lowest horizontal position lets the person get out of bed with ease (Fig. 18-2). The head of the bed is flat or raised varying degrees.

Fig. 18-2 One bed is in the highest horizontal position. The other bed is in the lowest horizontal position.

Raises bed horizontally

Raises head of bed

Raises knee portion

Fig. 18-4 Manually operated bed.

A

B

Fig. 18-3 Controls for an electric bed. **A,** Controls in the bed rail. **B,** Hand-held bed control (see inset) can be attached to the bed rail.

PROMOTING SAFETY AND COMFORT
The Bed

Safety

Beds have bed rails and wheels. Bed wheels (Chapter 12) are locked at all times except when moving the bed. They must be locked when you:
• Give bedside care.
• Transfer the person to and from the bed. The person can be injured if the bed moves. So can you.

Use bed rails as the nurse and care plan direct. Otherwise the person could suffer injury or harm.

Comfort

Some persons spend a lot of time in bed. Make sure the bed is adjusted to meet the person's needs. Tell the nurse if the person complains about the bed or mattress.

Electric beds are common. Controls are on a side panel, bed rail, or the foot-board (Fig. 18-3, *A*). Some controls are hand-held devices (Fig. 18-3, *B*). Alert and oriented residents are taught to use the controls safely. They are warned not to raise the bed to the high position or to adjust the bed to harmful positions. They are told of any position limits or restrictions.

Most electric beds "lock" into any position by the staff. The person cannot adjust the bed to unsafe positions. Persons restricted to certain positions may need their beds locked. So may persons with confusion or dementia.

Manual beds have cranks at the foot of the bed (Fig. 18-4):
• Left crank—raises or lowers the head of the bed
• Right crank—adjusts the knee portion
• Center crank—raises or lowers the entire bed horizontally

The cranks are pulled up for use. They are kept down at all other times. Cranks in the "up" position are safety hazards. Anyone walking past may bump into them.

See *Promoting Safety and Comfort: The Bed.*

Fig. 18-5 Fowler's position.

Fig. 18-6 High-Fowler's position.

Fig. 18-7 Semi-Fowler's position.

Fig. 18-8 Trendelenburg's position.

Bed Positions The six basic bed positions are:

- *Flat*—This is the usual sleeping position. The position is used after spinal cord injury or surgery and for cervical traction.
- *Fowler's position*—**Fowler's position** is a semi-sitting position. The head of the bed is raised between 45 and 60 degrees (Fig. 18-5). See Chapter 16.
- *High-Fowler's position*—**High-Fowler's position** is a semi-sitting position. The head of the bed is raised 60 to 90 degrees (Fig. 18-6).
- *Semi-Fowler's position*—In **semi-Fowler's position,** the head of the bed is raised 30 degrees (Fig. 18-7). Some centers define semi-Fowler's position as when the head of the bed is raised 30 degrees and the knee portion is raised 15 degrees. This position is comfortable and prevents sliding down in bed. However, raising the knee portion can interfere with circulation in the legs. To give safe care, know the definition used by your center. Also check with the nurse before using this position.

- *Trendelenburg's position*—In **Trendelenburg's position,** the head of the bed is lowered and the foot of the bed is raised (Fig. 18-8). A doctor orders the position. Blocks are placed under the legs at the foot of the bed. Or the bed frame is tilted.
- *Reverse Trendelenburg's position*—In **reverse Trendelenburg's position,** the head of the bed is raised and the foot of the bed is lowered (Fig. 18-9). Blocks are placed under the legs at the head of the bed. Or the bed frame is tilted. This position requires a doctor's order.

Bed Safety Bed safety involves the *hospital bed system.* The Food and Drug Administration (FDA) defines the hospital bed system as the bed frame and its parts. The parts include the mattress, bed rails, headboards and foot-boards, and bed attachments. *Entrapment* within parts of the hospital bed system is a risk. That is, the person can get caught, trapped, or entangled in spaces created by bed rails, the mattress, the

Fig. 18-9 Reverse Trendelenburg's position.

bed frame, the head-board, or the foot-board. Serious injuries and deaths have occurred from head, neck, and chest entrapment. Arm and leg entrapment also can occur. Persons at greatest risk include persons who:

- Are older
- Are frail
- Are confused or disoriented
- Are restless
- Have uncontrolled body movements
- Have poor muscle control
- Are small in size
- Are restrained (Chapter 14)

Hospital bed systems have seven entrapment zones. See Figure 18-10. Also see Figure 18-11, p. 258. You may feel that a person is at risk for entrapment. Report your concerns to the nurse at once. Also, always check the person for entrapment. If a person is caught, trapped, or entangled in the bed or any of its parts, try to release the person. Also call for the nurse at once.

Zone 1: Within the rail

Zone 2: Between the top of the compressed mattress and the bottom of the rail, between the supports

Zone 3: Between the rail and the mattress

Zone 4: Between the top of the compressed mattress and the bottom of the rail, at the end of the rail

Zone 5: Between the split bed rails

Zone 6: Between the end of the rail and the side edge of the head-board or foot-board

Zone 7: Between the head- or foot-board and the mattress end

Fig. 18-10 Hospital bed system entrapment zones. *(Redrawn from* Guidance for industry and FDA staff: hospital bed system dimensional and assessment guidance to reduce entrapment, *March 10, 2006, Food and Drug Administration.)*

Fig. 18-11 Hospital bed system entrapment zones. **A,** *Zone 1:* Within the bed rail. **B,** *Zone 2:* Between the top of the compressed mattress and the bottom of the bed rail and between the rail supports. **C,** *Zone 3:* Between the bed rail and the mattress. **D,** *Zone 4:* Between the top of the compressed mattress and the bottom of the bed rail and at the end of the bed rail. **E,** *Zone 5:* Between the split bed rails. **F,** *Zone 6:* Between the end of the bed rail and the side edge of the head-board or foot-board. **G,** *Zone 7:* Between the head-board or foot-board and the end of the mattress. *(Redrawn from* Guidance for industry and FDA staff: hospital bed system dimensional and assessment guidance to reduce entrapment, *March 10, 2006, Food and Drug Administration.)*

The Overbed Table

The overbed table (see Fig. 18-1) is placed over the bed by sliding the base under the bed. It is raised or lowered for the person in bed or in a chair. Turn the handle or push the lever to adjust the table. It is used for meals, writing, reading, and other activities.

Many overbed tables have a storage area under the top. The storage area often is used for beauty, hair care, shaving, or other personal items. Many also have a flip-up mirror for grooming.

The nursing team uses the overbed table as a work area. Only clean and sterile items are placed on the table. Never place bedpans, urinals, or soiled linen on the overbed table. Clean the table after using it for a work surface. Also clean it before serving meal trays.

The Bedside Stand

The bedside stand is next to the bed. It is used to store personal items and personal care equipment. It has a top drawer and a lower cabinet with shelves or drawers (Fig. 18-12). The top drawer is used for money, eyeglasses, books, and other items.

The top shelf or middle drawer is used for the wash basin. The wash basin holds personal items—soap and soap dish, powder, lotion, deodorant, towels, washcloth, bath blanket, and sleepwear. An emesis basin or kidney basin (shaped like a kidney) holds oral hygiene items. The kidney basin is stored in the top drawer, middle drawer, or on the top shelf. The bedpan and its cover, the urinal, and toilet paper are stored on the lower shelf or in the bottom drawer.

The top of the stand is often used for tissues and other personal items. A radio, clock, photos, phone, flowers, cards, and gifts are examples. Some stands have a side or back rod for towels and washcloths.

Place only clean and sterile items on the bedside stand. Never place bedpans, urinals, or soiled linen on the top of the stand. Clean the bedside stand after using it for a work surface.

Chairs

The person's unit has at least one chair for personal and visitor use (see Fig. 18-1). The chair is usually upholstered with armrests. It must be comfortable and sturdy. It must not move or tip during transfers. The person should be able to get in and out of the chair with ease. It should not be too low or too soft. Nursing center residents may bring chairs from home.

Privacy Curtains

OBRA-CMS

OBRA and the CMS require that rooms are equipped and designed for full visual privacy. Full visual privacy is having the means to be completely free from public view while in bed. The privacy curtain helps provide full visual privacy. It extends around the bed.

The curtain is pulled around the bed to provide privacy for the person (Chapter 4). Rooms with more than one bed have a privacy curtain between the units. *Always pull the curtain completely around the bed before giving care.*

Privacy curtains prevent others from seeing the person. They do not block sound or voices. Others in the room can hear sounds or talking behind the curtain.

Personal Care Items

Personal care items are used for hygiene and elimination. A bedpan and urinal are provided. The center also provides a wash basin, kidney basin, water pitcher and cup, and soap and a soap dish (Fig. 18-13). Some provide powder, lotion, toothbrush, toothpaste, mouthwash, tissues, and a comb.

Often residents bring their own oral hygiene equipment, hair care supplies, and deodorant. Some also prefer their own soap, lotion, and powder. Respect the person's choices in personal care products.

Fig. 18-13 Personal care items.

Fig. 18-12 The bedside stand.

Fig. 18-14 The signal light button is pressed when help is needed. NOTE: There are different types of signal lights.

Fig. 18-15 A, Light above the room door. **B,** Light panel and intercom at the nurses' station.

The Call System

The CMS requires a resident call system. When in their rooms, using the toilet, or in a bathing area, residents must be able to contact the staff at the nurses' station. The call system lets the person signal for help. The signal light is at the end of a long cord (Fig. 18-14). In resident units, it attaches to the bed or chair. (See p. 261 for signal lights in bathrooms.) Always keep the signal light within the person's reach—in the room, bathroom, and shower or tub room.

To get help, the person presses a button at the end of the signal light. The signal light at the bedside (bathroom, shower or tub room) is connected to a light above the room door. The signal light also connects to a light panel or intercom system at the nurses' station (Fig. 18-15). These tell the staff that the person needs help. The staff member shuts off the light at the bedside when responding to the call for help.

An intercom system lets the staff talk with the person from the nurses' station. The person tells what is needed. Then the light is turned off at the station. Hard-of-hearing persons may have problems using an intercom. Be careful when using an intercom. Remember confidentiality. Persons nearby can hear what you and the person say.

Some signal lights are turned on by tapping with a hand or fist (Fig. 18-16). They are useful for persons with limited hand mobility.

Fig. 18-16 Signal light for a person with limited hand mobility.

The person is taught how to use the call system when admitted to the center. Some people cannot use signal lights. Examples are persons who are confused or in a coma. The care plan lists special communication measures. Check these persons often. Make sure their needs are met.

The phrase "signal light" is used in this book when referring to the call system. You must:

- Keep the signal light within the person's reach. Even if the person cannot use the signal light, keep it within reach for use by visitors and staff. They may need to signal for help.
- Place the signal light on the person's strong side.
- Remind the person to signal when help is needed.
- Answer signal lights promptly. The person signals when help is needed. For example, the person may have an urgent need to use the bathroom. Promptly helping the person to the bathroom prevents embarrassing problems. You also help prevent infection, skin breakdown, pressure ulcers, and falls.
- Answer bathroom and shower or tub room signal lights at once.

  See *Teamwork and Time Management: The Call System.*
  See *Focus on Communication: The Call System.*

The Bathroom

OBRA-CMS All resident rooms must be equipped with or near toilet facilities. Many centers have a bathroom in each room. Some have a bathroom between two rooms. A toilet, sink, call system, and mirror are standard equipment (Fig. 18-17, p. 262). Some bathrooms have showers.

Grab bars are by the toilet for safety. The person uses them for support when lowering to or raising from the toilet. Some bathrooms have raised toilet seats. The higher toilets make wheelchair transfers easier. They also are helpful for persons with joint problems.

TEAMWORK AND TIME MANAGEMENT
The Call System

Residents use their signal lights when they need help. A person may put on a signal light when you are with another person. The same may happen to another nursing team member. If nursing team members answer signal lights for each other, lights are answered promptly. Residents receive quality care. Everyone is responsible for answering signal lights even if not assigned to the person.

FOCUS ON COMMUNICATION
The Call System

You will answer signal lights for co-workers. You may not know their residents and they may not know you. To promote quality of life and promote safe care, you can say:
- "My name is Kate Hines. I'm a nursing assistant. How can I help you?"
- "Mrs. Janz, I'll need to check your care plan before I bring you more salt. I'll be right back, but is there anything else I can do before I leave?"
- "Mr. Duncan, I'll be happy to take your meal tray. I'll tell your nursing assistant what you ate."
- "Mrs. Palmer, do you use the bathroom or the bedpan?"

Sometimes a resident may use the signal light to ask for help often. Do not delay in meeting the person's needs. Never take the person's signal light away. This is not safe. Avoid statements that make the person feel as if he or she is a burden. For example, do not say:
- "I just helped you to the bathroom. Can't you wait?"
- "I was just in your room. What do you want now?"

Do not discourage the person from asking for help. The person may try to do something alone. This could cause injury. Tell the nurse. Your co-workers can help you meet the person's needs.

Towel racks, toilet paper, soap, paper towel dispenser, and a wastebasket are in the bathroom. They are placed within easy reach of the person.

Usually the signal light is next to the toilet. Pressing a button or pulling a cord turns on the signal light. When the bathroom signal light is used, the light flashes above the room door and at the nurses' station. The sound at the nurses' station is different from signal lights in rooms. These differences alert the staff that the person is in the bathroom. Someone must respond at once when a person needs help in a bathroom.

Fig. 18-17 Bathroom in a nursing center.

Fig. 18-18 The resident can reach items in his closet.

> **PROMOTING SAFETY AND COMFORT**
> Closet and Drawer Space
>
> **Safety**
> The nurse may ask you to inspect a person's closet, drawers, or personal items. If so, the person must be present. Also have a co-worker with you. Your co-worker is a witness to what you are doing. This protects you if the person claims that something was stolen or damaged.

> **PROMOTING SAFETY AND COMFORT**
> Other Equipment
>
> **Safety**
> The resident is allowed personal choice in arranging items. The choices must be safe and not cause falls or other accidents. Also, the person's choices must not interfere with the rights of others. You may have to help the person choose the best place for personal items.

Closet and Drawer Space

Closet and drawer space are provided for clothing. OBRA and the CMS require that nursing centers provide each person with closet space. The closet space must have shelves and a clothes rack (Fig. 18-18). The person must have free access to the closet and its contents.

Items in closets and drawers are the person's private property. You must have the person's permission to open or search closets or drawers.

Sometimes people hoard items—drugs, napkins, straws, food, sugar, salt, pepper, and so on. Hoarding can cause safety or health risks. Center staff can inspect a person's closet or drawers if hoarding is suspected. The person is informed of the inspection. He or she is present when it takes place.

See *Promoting Safety and Comfort: Closet and Drawer Space.*

Other Equipment

Nursing centers may allow residents to bring furniture and other items from home. TVs, radios, clocks, photos, and other small items help residents feel "at home" in their units. Phones and Internet access are available in some centers.

See *Promoting Safety and Comfort: Other Equipment.*
See *Focus on Rehabilitation: Other Equipment.*

GENERAL RULES

Everyone involved in the person's care must keep the unit clean, neat, safe, and comfortable. To maintain the person's unit, follow the rules in Box 18-1.

OBRA-CMS

FOCUS ON REHABILITATION
Other Equipment

Rehabilitation centers usually have more medical equipment and supplies to manage complex health care needs. Some rooms have blood pressure equipment mounted on the wall. Some beds have IV (intravenous) poles for IV therapy (Chapter 25). The poles are stored in the bed frame. If not part of the bed, an IV pole is brought to the bedside when needed. Some units have wall outlets for oxygen and suction.

Box 18-1 Maintaining the Person's Unit

- Keep the signal light within the person's reach at all times.
- Meet the needs of persons who cannot use the call system.
- Make sure the person can reach the overbed table and the bedside stand.
- Arrange personal items as the person prefers. Make sure they are easily reached.
- Make sure the person can reach the phone, TV, and bed and light controls.
- Provide the person with enough tissues and toilet paper.
- Adjust lighting, temperature, and ventilation for the person's comfort.
- Handle equipment carefully to prevent noise.
- Explain the causes of strange noises.
- Empty wastebaskets in the person's room and bathroom. Empty them every shift or at least once a day. Empty them more often if they become full.
- Respect the person's belongings. An item may not have importance or value to you. Yet it has great meaning for the person. Even a scrap of paper can have great meaning to the person.
- Do not throw away any items belonging to the person.
- Do not move furniture or the person's belongings. Persons with poor vision rely on memory or feel for the location of items.
- Straighten bed linens and towels as often as needed.
- Complete a safety check before leaving the room. (See the inside of the front book cover.)

Box 18-2 OBRA and CMS Requirements for Resident Rooms

- Rooms are designed for 1 to 4 persons.
- Rooms have a direct access to an exit corridor.
- Rooms are designed or equipped for full visual privacy—ceiling-suspended privacy curtain that extends around the bed, movable screens, window coverings, doors.
- Rooms have at least one window to the outside.
- Each person has closet space with racks and shelves.
- Toilet facilities are in the room or nearby (includes bathing facilities).
- Rooms, bathrooms, and bathing areas have a functioning call system.
- The person has a bed of proper height and size.
- The person has a clean, comfortable mattress.
- Bed and bath linens (towels and washcloths) are clean and in good condition.
- Bed linens are appropriate to the weather and climate.
- The room has furniture for clothing, personal items, and a chair for visitors.
- Rooms are clean and orderly.
- Room temperature levels are between 71° and 81° F.
- Ventilation, humidity, and odor levels are acceptable.
- Non-smoking areas are identified.
- Sound levels are comfortable.
- Lighting is adequate and comfortable with little glare.
- Rooms have clean, orderly drawers and shelves for personal items.
- The room is free of pests and rodents.
- Hand rails are in good repair.
- Floors are clean and dry.
- The person's setting is free of clutter.
- Personal supplies and items are labeled and stored appropriately.
- Items are within reach for use in bed or bathroom.
- There is space for wheelchair or walker use.
- A raised toilet seat is available (if needed).

QUALITY OF LIFE

Nursing center residents have left their homes. Each had furniture, appliances, a private bathroom, and many personal items and treasures. Now the person lives in a strange place. He or she probably has a roommate. Leaving one's home is a hard part of growing old with poor health. It is important to make the person's unit as home-like as possible.

Residents may bring some furniture and personal items from home. A chair, footstool, lamp, and small table are often allowed. They can bring photos, religious items, and books. Some have plants to care for. Personal choice is allowed in arranging items. You can help the person choose the best place for them. The health team must make sure that the person's choices:

- Are safe
- Will not cause falls or other accidents
- Do not interfere with the rights of others

The center is the person's home. You must help the person feel safe, secure, and comfortable. A home-like setting is important for quality of life. OBRA and the CMS serve to promote quality of life. Box 18-2 lists OBRA and CMS requirements for resident rooms.

REVIEW QUESTIONS

Circle the BEST answer.

1 Which temperature range is required by OBRA and the CMS?
  a 61° to 68° F
  b 68° to 74° F
  c 71° to 81° F
  d 76° to 81° F

2 Which does *not* protect a person from drafts?
  a Wearing enough clothing
  b Being covered with enough blankets
  c Being moved from a drafty area
  d Sitting by a fan

3 Which does *not* prevent or reduce odors?
  a Placing flowers in the room
  b Emptying bedpans promptly
  c Using room deodorizers
  d Practicing good hygiene

4 To prevent odors, you need to do the following *except*
  a Check incontinent persons often
  b Dispose of ostomy products at the end of your shift
  c Keep laundry containers closed
  d Clean persons who are wet or soiled

5 Which does *not* control noise?
  a Using plastic items
  b Handling dishes with care
  c Speaking softly
  d Talking with others in the hallway

6 Beds are raised horizontally to
  a Prevent bending and reaching when giving care
  b Let the person get in and out of bed with ease
  c Raise the head of the bed
  d Lock the bed in position

7 The head of the bed is raised 30 degrees. This is called
  a Fowler's position
  b Semi-Fowler's position
  c Trendelenburg's position
  d Reverse Trendelenburg's position

8 These statements are about hospital bed system entrapment. Which is *false?*
  a Serious injuries and death can occur.
  b Older, frail, and confused persons are at risk.
  c The head, neck, and chest are areas of entrapment.
  d Bed rails present the only risk for entrapment.

9 The overbed table is *not* used
  a For eating
  b As a working surface
  c For the urinal
  d To store shaving items

10 The bedpan is stored in the
  a Closet
  b Bedside stand
  c Overbed table
  d Bathroom

11 Signal lights are answered
  a When you have time
  b At the end of your shift
  c Promptly
  d When you are near the person's room

12 To maintain the person's unit, you can do the following *except*
  a Save items that do not look important
  b Provide enough tissues and toilet paper
  c Place personal items as you choose
  d Straighten bed linens as needed

Circle T if the statement is TRUE. Circle F if the statement is FALSE.

13 T F The person's unit is considered private.
14 T F Persons with dementia may have extreme reactions to strange sounds.
15 T F The privacy curtain prevents others from hearing conversations.
16 T F Soft, dim lighting is relaxing.
17 T F The signal light must always be within the person's reach.
18 T F The overbed table and bedside stand should be within the person's reach.
19 T F You should explain the cause of strange noises.
20 T F The person must be able to reach items in the closet.
21 T F You can adjust the person's room temperature for your comfort.
22 T F You can look through a person's closet and drawers.

Answers to these questions are on p. 720.

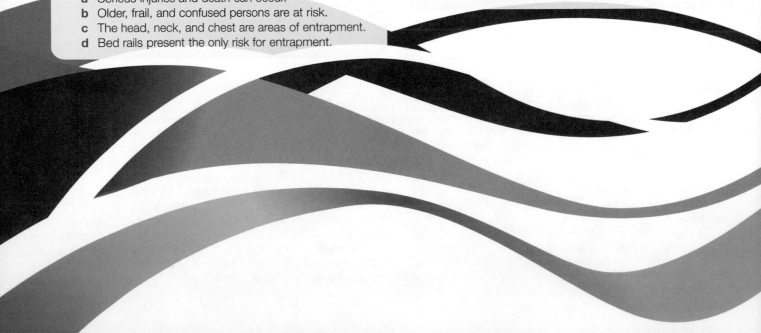

Bedmaking

OBJECTIVES

- Define the key terms listed in this chapter.
- Describe open, closed, occupied, and surgical beds.
- Explain when to change linens.
- Explain how to use drawsheets.

- Handle linens following the rules of medical asepsis.
- Perform the procedures described in this chapter.
- Explain how to promote quality of life.

KEY TERMS

cotton drawsheet A drawsheet made of cotton; it helps keep the mattress and bottom linens clean

drawsheet A small sheet placed over the middle of the bottom sheet

waterproof drawsheet A drawsheet made of plastic, rubber, or absorbent material used to protect the mattress and bottom linens from dampness and soiling

Most residents are up during the day. Some are always in bed. Food, fluid, hygiene, and elimination needs are met while in bed. Some persons are incontinent of urine or feces. Clean, dry, wrinkle-free linens are important for all residents to:

- Promote comfort
- Prevent skin breakdown and pressure ulcers

Beds are made every day. They are usually made in the morning after baths. Or they are made while the person is in the chair or out of the room. Beds are made and rooms straightened before visitors arrive.

To keep beds neat and clean:

- Straighten linens whenever loose or wrinkled.
- Straighten loose or wrinkled linens at bedtime.
- Check for and remove food and crumbs after meals.
- Check linens for dentures, eyeglasses, hearing aids, sharp objects, and other items.
- Change linens whenever they become wet, soiled, or damp.
- Follow Standard Precautions and the Bloodborne Pathogen Standard. Contact with blood, body fluids, secretions, or excretions is likely.

TYPES OF BEDS

Beds are made in these ways:

- A *closed bed* is not used until bedtime (Fig. 19-1). Or the bed is ready for a new resident. Top linens are not folded back.
- An *open bed* is in use. Top linens are fan-folded back so the person can get into bed. A closed bed becomes an open bed by fan-folding back the top linens (Fig. 19-2).
- An *occupied bed* is made with the person in it (Fig. 19-3).
- A *surgical bed* is made to transfer a person from a stretcher (Fig. 19-4). This bed also is made for persons who arrive by ambulance.

Fig. 19-2 Open bed. Top linens are fan-folded to the foot of the bed.

Fig. 19-3 Occupied bed.

Fig. 19-1 Closed bed.

Fig. 19-4 Surgical bed.

LINENS

In nursing centers, linens are not changed every day. The center is the person's home. People do not change linens every day at home. A complete linen change is usually done on the person's bath day. This may be once or twice a week. Pillowcases, top and bottom sheets, and drawsheets (if used) are changed twice a week. Linens are always changed if wet, damp, soiled, or very wrinkled.

Handling Linens

When handling linens and making beds, practice medical asepsis. Your uniform is considered dirty. Always hold linens away from your body and uniform. Never shake linens. Shaking spreads microbes. Place clean linens on a clean surface. Never put clean or dirty linens on the floor.

Collect enough linens. If the person has two pillows, get two pillowcases. The person may need extra blankets for warmth. Do not bring unneeded linens to a person's room. Once in the person's room, extra linen is considered contaminated. Do not use it for another person.

Collect linens in the order you will use them:
- Mattress pad (if needed)
- Bottom sheet (flat or fitted)
- Waterproof drawsheet or waterproof pad (if needed)
- Cotton drawsheet (if needed)
- Top sheet
- Blanket
- Bedspread
- Pillowcase(s)
- Bath towel(s)
- Hand towel
- Washcloth
- Gown or pajamas
- Bath blanket

Use one arm to hold the linens. Use your other hand to pick them up. The first item to use is at the bottom of your stack. (You picked up the mattress pad first. It is at the bottom. The bath blanket is on top.) You need the mattress pad first. To get it on top, place your arm over the bath blanket. Then turn the stack over onto the arm on the bath blanket (Fig. 19-5). The arm that held the linens is now free. Place the clean linen on a clean surface.

Remove dirty linen one piece at a time. Roll each piece away from you. The side that touched the person is inside the roll and away from you (Fig. 19-6).

Fig. 19-5 Collecting linens. Linens are held away from the body and uniform. **A,** The arm is placed over the top of the stack of linens. **B,** The stack of linens is turned onto the arm. Note that the linens are held away from the body.

Fig. 19-6 Roll dirty linen away from you.

Fig. 19-7 A, Waterproof pad. **B,** Disposable bed protector.

Drawsheets

A drawsheet is a small sheet placed over the middle of the bottom sheet.

- A cotton drawsheet is made of cotton. It helps keep the mattress and bottom linens clean.
- A waterproof drawsheet is made of plastic, rubber, or absorbent material. It protects the mattress and bottom linens from dampness and soiling. Some are rubber or plastic on one side—the waterproof side. The waterproof side is placed down, away from the person. The other side is cotton. It is placed up, toward the person. Other waterproof drawsheets are disposable. They are discarded when wet, soiled, or wrinkled.

The cotton drawsheet protects the person from contact with plastic or rubber and absorbs moisture. However, discomfort and skin breakdown may occur. Plastic and rubber retain heat. Waterproof drawsheets are hard to keep tight and wrinkle-free. Many centers use incontinence products (Chapter 22) to keep the person and linens dry. Others use waterproof pads or disposable bed protectors (Fig. 19-7).

Cotton drawsheets are often used without waterproof drawsheets. Plastic-covered mattresses cause some persons to perspire heavily. This causes discomfort. A cotton drawsheet reduces heat retention and absorbs moisture. Cotton drawsheets are often used as assist devices to move and transfer persons in bed (Chapter 17). If used as an assist device, do not tuck it in at the sides.

The procedures that follow include waterproof and cotton drawsheets. This is so you learn how to use them. Ask the nurse about the type used in your center.

MAKING BEDS

Safety and medical asepsis are important for bedmaking. Follow the rules in Box 19-1.

See *Delegation Guidelines: Making Beds.*
See *Promoting Safety and Comfort: Making Beds.*
See *Teamwork and Time Management: Making Beds.*

DELEGATION GUIDELINES
Making Beds

Before making a bed, you need this information from the nurse and the care plan:

- What type of bed to make—closed, open, occupied, or surgical.
- If you need to use a cotton drawsheet.
- If you need to use a waterproof drawsheet, waterproof pad, or incontinence product.
- Position restrictions or limits in the person's movement or activity.
- If the person uses bed rails.
- The person's treatment, therapy, and activity schedule. For example, Mr. Smith needs a treatment in bed. Change linens after the treatment. Make Mrs. Carter's bed while she is in physical therapy.
- How to position the person and the positioning devices needed.
- If the bed needs to be locked into a certain position (Chapter 18).
- When to report observations.
- What specific resident concerns to report at once.

Box 19-1 Rules for Bedmaking

- Use good body mechanics at all times (Chapter 16).
- Follow the rules in Chapter 17 to safely handle, move, and transfer the person.
- Follow the rules of medical asepsis.
- Follow Standard Precautions and the Bloodborne Pathogen Standard.
- Practice hand hygiene before handling clean linen.
- Practice hand hygiene after handling dirty linen.
- Bring enough linen to the person's room. Do not bring extra linens.
- Bring only the linens that you will need. You cannot use extra linen for another person.
- Place clean linen on a clean surface. Use the bedside chair, overbed table, or bedside stand. Place a barrier (towel, paper towels) between the clean surface and the linens if required by center policy.
- Do not use extra linen in the person's room for another resident. Extra linen is considered contaminated. Put it with the dirty laundry.
- Do not use torn or frayed linen.
- Never shake linens. Shaking spreads microbes.
- Hold linens away from your body and uniform. Do not let dirty or clean linen touch your uniform.
- Never put dirty linens on the floor or on clean linens. Follow center policy for dirty linen.
- Keep bottom linens tucked in and wrinkle-free.
- Cover a waterproof drawsheet with a cotton drawsheet. Plastic or rubber must not touch the person's body.
- Straighten and tighten loose sheets, blankets, and bedspreads as needed.
- Make as much of one side of the bed as possible before going to the other side. This saves time and energy.
- Change wet, damp, and soiled linens right away.

PROMOTING SAFETY AND COMFORT
Making Beds

Safety

You need to raise the bed for body mechanics. The bed also must be flat. If the bed is locked, unlock it. Then adjust the bed. Return the bed to the correct position when you are done. Then lock the bed.

Wear gloves when removing linen from the person's bed. Also follow other aspects of Standard Precautions and the Bloodborne Pathogen Standard. Linens may contain blood, body fluids, secretions, or excretions.

After making a bed, lower the bed to a level appropriate for the person. Follow the care plan. For an occupied bed, raise or lower bed rails according to the care plan.

Comfort

For an occupied bed, cover the person with a bath blanket before removing the top sheet. Do not leave the person uncovered when making the bed. The bath blanket provides for warmth and privacy.

If the person uses a pillow, adjust it as needed during the procedure. After the procedure, position the person as directed by the nurse and the care plan. Always make sure linens are straight and wrinkle-free.

TEAMWORK AND TIME MANAGEMENT
Making Beds

To save time and energy, make beds with a co-worker. Make one side of the bed while your co-worker makes the other.

Making beds with a co-worker is faster, easier, and safer for residents, you, and your co-worker. Always thank your co-worker for helping you. Also help your co-worker make beds when asked to do so.

The Closed Bed

Closed beds are made for:
- Residents who are up for most or all of the day. Top linens are folded back at bedtime. Clean linens are used as needed.
- For new residents. The bed is made after the bed frame and mattress are cleaned and disinfected. Clean linens are needed for the entire bed.

Text continued on p. 274

MAKING A CLOSED BED

QUALITY OF LIFE

Remember to:
- Knock before entering the person's room.
- Address the person by name.
- Introduce yourself by name and title.

- Explain the procedure to the person before beginning and during the procedure.
- Protect the person's rights during the procedure.
- Handle the person gently during the procedure.

PRE-PROCEDURE

1 Follow *Delegation Guidelines: Making Beds*, p. 268. See *Promoting Safety and Comfort: Making Beds*, p. 269.
2 Practice hand hygiene.
3 Collect clean linen:
   - Mattress pad (if needed)
   - Bottom sheet (flat sheet or fitted sheet)
   - Waterproof drawsheet or waterproof pad (if needed)
   - Cotton drawsheet (if needed)
   - Top sheet
   - Blanket
   - Bedspread
   - A pillowcase for each pillow

- Bath towel(s)
- Hand towel
- Washcloth
- Gown or pajamas
- Bath blanket
- Gloves
- Laundry bag
- Paper towels (if you need a barrier for clean linens)

4 Place linen on a clean surface. Use the paper towels as a barrier between the clean surface and clean linen if required by center policy.
5 Raise the bed for body mechanics. Bed rails are down.

PROCEDURE

6 Put on the gloves.
7 Remove linen. Roll each piece away from you. Place each piece in a laundry bag. (NOTE: Discard incontinence products or disposable bed protectors in the trash. Do not put them in the laundry bag.)
8 Clean the bed frame and mattress (if this is your job).
9 Remove and discard gloves. Decontaminate your hands.
10 Move the mattress to the head of the bed.
11 Put the mattress pad on the mattress. It is even with the top of the mattress.
12 Place the bottom sheet on the mattress pad (Fig. 19-8). Unfold it length-wise. Place the center crease in the middle of the bed. If using a flat sheet:
   a Position the lower edge even with the bottom of the mattress.
   b Place the large hem at the top and the small hem at the bottom.
   c Face hem-stitching downward, away from the person.
13 Open the sheet. Fan-fold it to the other side of the bed (Fig. 19-9).
14 Tuck the corners of a fitted sheet over the mattress at the top and then the foot of the bed. If using a flat sheet, tuck the top of the sheet under the mattress. The sheet is tight and smooth.
15 Make a mitered corner if using a flat sheet (Fig. 19-10, p. 272).
16 Place the waterproof drawsheet on the bed. It is in the middle of the mattress. Or put the waterproof pad on the bed.
17 Open the waterproof drawsheet. Fan-fold it to the other side of the bed.

18 Place a cotton drawsheet over the waterproof drawsheet. It covers the entire waterproof drawsheet (Fig. 19-11, p. 272).
19 Open the cotton drawsheet. Fan-fold it to the other side of the bed.
20 Tuck both drawsheets under the mattress. Or tuck each in separately.
21 Go to the other side of the bed.
22 Miter the top corner of the flat bottom sheet.
23 Pull the bottom sheet tight so there are no wrinkles. Tuck in the sheet.
24 Pull the drawsheets tight so there are no wrinkles. Tuck both in together or separately (Fig. 19-12, p. 272).
25 Go to the other side of the bed.
26 Put the top sheet on the bed. Unfold it length-wise. Place the center crease in the middle. Do the following if using a flat sheet:
   a Place the large hem even with the top of the mattress.
   b Open the sheet. Fan-fold it to the other side.
   c Face hem-stitching outward, away from the person.
   d Do not tuck the bottom in yet.
   e Never tuck top linens in on the sides.
27 Place the blanket on the bed:
   a Unfold it so the center crease is in the middle.
   b Put the upper hem about 6 to 8 inches from the top of the mattress.
   c Open the blanket. Fan-fold it to the other side.
   d If steps 33 and 34 are not done, turn the top sheet down over the blanket. Hem-stitching is down, away from the person.

MAKING A CLOSED BED—cont'd

PROCEDURE—cont'd

28 Place the bedspread on the bed:
  a Unfold it so the center crease is in the middle.
  b Place the upper hem even with the top of the mattress.
  c Open and fan-fold the bedspread to the other side.
  d Make sure the bedspread facing the door is even. It covers all top linens.
29 Tuck in top linens together at the foot of the bed so they are smooth and tight. Make a mitered corner.
30 Go to the other side.
31 Straighten all top linen. Work from the head of the bed to the foot.
32 Tuck in top linens together at the foot of the bed. Make a mitered corner.

33 Turn the top hem of the bedspread under the blanket to make a cuff (Fig. 19-13, p. 272).
34 Turn the top sheet down over the bedspread. Hem-stitching is down. (Steps 33 and 34 are not done in some centers. The bedspread covers the pillow. If so, tuck the bedspread under the pillow.)
35 Put the pillowcase on the pillow as in Figure 19-14, p. 273 or Figure 19-15, p. 273. Fold extra material under the pillow at the seam end of the pillowcase.
36 Place the pillow on the bed. The open end of the pillowcase is away from the door. The seam is toward the head of the bed.

POST-PROCEDURE

37 Provide for comfort. (See the inside of the front book cover.) NOTE: Omit this step if the bed is prepared for a new resident.
38 Attach the signal light to the bed. Or place it within the person's reach.
39 Lower the bed to its lowest position. Lock the bed wheels.

40 Put the towels, washcloth, gown or pajamas, and bath blanket in the bedside stand.
41 Complete a safety check of the room. (See the inside of the front book cover.)
42 Follow center policy for dirty linen.
43 Decontaminate your hands.

Fig. 19-8 The bottom sheet is on the bed with the center crease in the middle. The lower edge of the sheet is even with the bottom of the mattress.

Fig. 19-9 The bottom sheet is fan-folded to the other side of the bed.

A   B   C   D

Fig. 19-10 Making a mitered corner. **A,** The bottom sheet is tucked under the mattress at the head of the bed. The side of the sheet is raised onto the mattress. **B,** The remaining portion of the sheet is tucked under the mattress. **C,** The raised portion of the sheet is brought off the mattress. **D,** The entire side of the sheet is tucked under the mattress.

Cotton drawsheet

Waterproof drawsheet

Fig. 19-11 A cotton drawsheet is over the waterproof drawsheet. The cotton drawsheet completely covers the waterproof drawsheet.

Fig. 19-12 The drawsheet is pulled tight to remove wrinkles.

Top sheet

Blanket

Spread

Fig. 19-13 The top hem of the bedspread is turned under the top hem of the blanket to make a cuff.

Fig. 19-14 Putting a pillowcase on a pillow. **A,** Grasp the corners of the pillow at the seam end and form a "V" with the pillow. **B,** Open the pillowcase with your free hand. **C,** Guide the "V" end of the pillow into the pillowcase. **D,** Let the "V" end of the pillow fall into the corners of the pillowcase.

Fig. 19-15 Putting a pillowcase on a pillow. **A,** Grasp the closed end of the pillowcase. **B,** Using your other hand, gather up the pillowcase. The pillowcase should cover your hand holding the closed end. **C,** Grasp the pillow with the hand covered by the pillowcase. **D,** Pull the pillowcase down over the pillow with your other hand.

The Open Bed

A closed bed becomes an open bed by fan-folding back the top linen. The open bed lets the person get into bed with ease. Make this bed for:

- Newly admitted persons arriving by wheelchair
- Persons who are getting ready for bed
- Persons who are out of bed for a short time

MAKING AN OPEN BED

QUALITY OF LIFE

Remember to:
- Knock before entering the person's room.
- Address the person by name.
- Introduce yourself by name and title.

- Explain the procedure to the person before beginning and during the procedure.
- Protect the person's rights during the procedure.
- Handle the person gently during the procedure.

PROCEDURE

1 Follow *Delegation Guidelines: Making Beds,* p. 268. See *Promoting Safety and Comfort: Making Beds,* p. 269.
2 Practice hand hygiene.
3 Collect linen for a closed bed.
4 Make a closed bed. See procedure: *Making a Closed Bed,* p. 270.

5 Fan-fold top linens to the foot of the bed (see Fig. 19-2).
6 Attach the signal light to the bed.
7 Lower the bed to its lowest position.
8 Put towels, washcloth, gown or pajamas, and the bath blanket in the bedside stand.

POST-PROCEDURE

9 Provide for comfort. (See the inside of the front book cover.)
10 Place the signal light within the person's reach.
11 Complete a safety check of the room. (See the inside of the front book cover.)

12 Follow center policy for dirty linen.
13 Decontaminate your hands.

The Occupied Bed

You make an occupied bed when the person stays in bed. Keep the person in good alignment. Follow restrictions or limits in the person's movement or position.

Explain each procedure step to the person before it is done. This is important even if the person cannot respond to you or is in a coma.

See *Focus on Communication: The Occupied Bed.*
See *Promoting Safety and Comfort: The Occupied Bed.*

Text continued on p. 278

FOCUS ON COMMUNICATION
The Occupied Bed

After making an occupied bed, make sure the person is comfortable. You can ask:
- "Are you comfortable?"
- "How can I make you more comfortable?"
- "Are you warm enough?"
- "Can I adjust your pillow?"

After making the bed, thank the person for cooperating.

PROMOTING SAFETY AND COMFORT
The Occupied Bed

Safety
The person lies on one side of the bed and then the other. Protect the person from falling out of bed. If bed rails are used, the far bed rail is up. If the person does not use bed rails, have a co-worker help you. You work on one side of the bed. Your co-worker works on the other.

Comfort
To make an occupied bed, the person lies on his or her side. You tuck dirty bottom linens under the person. Then you put clean linens on the bed. These, too, are tucked under the person. The tucked linens create a "bump" in the middle of the bed. To make the other side, the person rolls over the "bump" to the other side of the bed. To promote comfort, make the "bump" as low as possible. Do this by fan-folding dirty and clean bottom linens neatly and flatly.

MAKING AN OCCUPIED BED

QUALITY OF LIFE

Remember to:
- Knock before entering the person's room.
- Address the person by name.
- Introduce yourself by name and title.

- Explain the procedure to the person before beginning and during the procedure.
- Protect the person's rights during the procedure.
- Handle the person gently during the procedure.

PRE-PROCEDURE

1 Follow *Delegation Guidelines: Making Beds*, p. 268. See *Promoting Safety and Comfort:*
   a *Making Beds*, p. 269
   b *The Occupied Bed*
2 Practice hand hygiene.
3 Collect the following:
   - Gloves
   - Laundry bag
   - Clean linen (see procedure: *Making a Closed Bed*, p. 270)
   - Paper towels (if you need a barrier for clean linens)

4 Place linen on a clean surface. Place the paper towels between the clean surface and clean linen if a barrier is required by center policy.
5 Identify the person. Check the ID (identification) bracelet against the assignment sheet. Also call the person by name.
6 Provide for privacy.
7 Remove the signal light.
8 Raise the bed for body mechanics. Bed rails are up if used. Bed wheels are locked.
9 Lower the head of the bed. It is as flat as possible.

PROCEDURE

10 Decontaminate your hands. Put on gloves.
11 Loosen top linens at the foot of the bed.
12 Lower the bed rail near you if up.
13 Remove the bedspread (Fig. 19-16, p. 276). Then remove the blanket in the same way. Place each over the chair.
14 Cover the person with a bath blanket. Use the blanket in the bedside stand.
   a Unfold the bath blanket over the top sheet.
   b Ask the person to hold onto the bath blanket. If he or she cannot, tuck the top part under the person's shoulders.
   c Grasp the top sheet under the bath blanket at the shoulders. Bring the sheet down to the foot of the bed. Remove the sheet from under the blanket (Fig. 19-17, p. 277).
15 Position the person on the side of the bed away from you. Adjust the pillow for comfort.
16 Loosen bottom linens from the head to the foot of the bed.
17 Fan-fold bottom linens one at a time toward the person. Start with the cotton drawsheet (Fig. 19-18, p. 277). If re-using the mattress pad, do not fan-fold it.
18 Place a clean mattress pad on the bed. Unfold it length-wise. The center crease is in the middle. Fan-fold the top part toward the person. If re-using the mattress pad, straighten and smooth any wrinkles.
19 Place the bottom sheet on the mattress pad. Hem-stitching is away from the person. Unfold the sheet so the crease is in the middle. If using a flat sheet, the small hem is even with the bottom of the mattress. Fan-fold the top part toward the person.
20 Tuck the corners of a fitted sheet over the mattress. If using a flat sheet, make a mitered corner at the head of the bed. Tuck the sheet under the mattress from the head to the foot.

21 Pull the waterproof drawsheet toward you over the bottom sheet. Tuck excess material under the mattress. Do the following for a clean waterproof drawsheet (Fig. 19-19, p. 277).
   a Place the waterproof drawsheet on the bed. It is in the middle of the mattress.
   b Fan-fold the top part toward the person.
   c Tuck in excess fabric.
22 Place the cotton drawsheet over the waterproof drawsheet. It covers the entire waterproof drawsheet. Fan-fold the top part toward the person. Tuck in excess fabric.
23 Explain to the person that he or she will roll over a "bump." Assure the person that he or she will not fall.
24 Help the person turn to the other side. Adjust the pillow for comfort.
25 Raise the bed rail. Go to the other side, and lower the bed rail.
26 Loosen bottom linens. Remove one piece at a time. Place each piece in the laundry bag. (NOTE: Discard disposable bed protectors and incontinence products in the trash. Do not put them in the laundry bag.)
27 Remove and discard the gloves. Decontaminate your hands.
28 Straighten and smooth the mattress pad.
29 Pull the clean bottom sheet toward you. Tuck the corners of a fitted sheet over the mattress. If using a flat sheet, make a mitered corner at the top. Tuck the sheet under the mattress from the head to the foot of the bed.
30 Pull the drawsheets tightly toward you. Tuck both under together or separately.
31 Position the person supine in the center of the bed. Adjust the pillow for comfort.
32 Put the top sheet on the bed. Unfold it length-wise. The crease is in the middle. The large hem is even with the top of the mattress. Hem-stitching is on the outside.

Continued

MAKING AN OCCUPIED BED—cont'd

PROCEDURE—cont'd

33 Ask the person to hold the top sheet so you can remove the bath blanket. Or tuck the top sheet under the person's shoulders. Remove and discard the bath blanket.

34 Place the blanket on the bed. Unfold it so the crease is in the middle and it covers the person. The upper hem is 6 to 8 inches from the top of the mattress.

35 Place the bedspread on the bed. Unfold it so the center crease is in the middle and it covers the person. The top hem is even with the mattress top.

36 Turn the top hem of the bedspread under the blanket to make a cuff.

37 Bring the top sheet down over the bedspread to form a cuff.

38 Go to the foot of the bed.

39 Make a toe pleat. Make a 2-inch pleat across the foot of the bed. The pleat is about 6 to 8 inches from the foot of the bed.

40 Lift the mattress corner with one arm. Tuck all top linens under the mattress. Make a mitered corner.

41 Raise the bed rail. Go to the other side, and lower the bed rail.

42 Straighten and smooth top linens.

43 Tuck all top linens under the mattress. Make a mitered corner.

44 Change the pillowcase(s).

POST-PROCEDURE

45 Provide for comfort. (See the inside of the front book cover.)

46 Place the signal light within reach.

47 Lower the bed to its lowest position. Bed wheels are locked.

48 Raise or lower bed rails. Follow the care plan.

49 Put the clean towels, washcloth, gown or pajamas, and bath blanket in the bedside stand.

50 Unscreen the person.

51 Complete a safety check of the room. (See the inside of the front book cover.)

52 Follow center policy for dirty linen.

53 Decontaminate your hands.

Fig. 19-16 Folding linen for re-use. **A,** Fold the top edge of the bedspread down to the bottom edge. **B,** Fold the bedspread from the far side of the bed to the near side. **C,** Fold the top edge of the bedspread down to the bottom edge again. **D,** Place the folded bedspread over the back of the chair.

Fig. 19-17 The person holds onto the bath blanket. The top sheet is removed from under the bath blanket.

Bath blanket over person
Old cotton drawsheet
Old waterproof drawsheet
Old bottom sheet
A

Old cotton drawsheet
Old waterproof drawsheet
Old mattress pad
Old bottom sheet
B

Fig. 19-18 Occupied bed. **A,** The cotton drawsheet is fan-folded and tucked under the person. **B,** All bottom linens are tucked under the person.

Old cotton drawsheet
Old waterproof drawsheet
Old bottom sheet and mattress pad
Clean bottom sheet and mattress pad
Clean waterproof drawsheet

Fig. 19-19 A clean bottom sheet and waterproof drawsheet are on the bed with both fan-folded and tucked under the person.

The Surgical Bed

The surgical bed also is called a *recovery bed* or *post-operative bed*. It is a form of the open bed. Top linens are folded to transfer the person from a stretcher to the bed. These beds are made for persons who:

- Arrive at the center by ambulance. A complete linen change is needed if the person is a new resident or is returning to the center from the hospital.
- Go by stretcher to treatment or therapy areas. A complete linen change is not needed.
- Use portable tubs. Because the person has a bath, a complete linen change is needed.

See *Promoting Safety and Comfort: The Surgical Bed.*

PROMOTING SAFETY AND COMFORT
The Surgical Bed

Safety
To safely transfer a person from a stretcher to a surgical bed, see procedure: (*Moving the Person to a Stretcher* Chapter 17). Also follow the rules for stretcher safety (Chapter 12). After the transfer, lower the bed to its lowest position. Make sure the bed wheels are locked. Raise or lower bed rails according to the care plan.

MAKING A SURGICAL BED

VIDEO

PROCEDURE

1. Follow *Delegation Guidelines: Making Beds*, p. 268. See *Promoting Safety and Comfort:*
   a. *Making Beds*, p. 269
   b. *The Surgical Bed*
2. Practice hand hygiene.
3. Collect the following:
   - Clean linen (see procedure: *Making a Closed Bed*, p. 270)
   - Gloves
   - Laundry bag
   - Equipment requested by the nurse
   - Paper towels (if you need a barrier for clean linens)
4. Place linen on a clean surface. Place the paper towels between the clean surface and clean linen if a barrier is required by center policy.
5. Remove the signal light.
6. Raise the bed for body mechanics.
7. Remove all linen from the bed. Wear gloves. Decontaminate your hands after removing them.
8. Make a closed bed (see procedure: *Making a Closed Bed*, p. 270). Do not tuck top linens under the mattress.
9. Fold all top linens at the foot of the bed back onto the bed. The fold is even with the edge of the mattress (Fig. 19-20, *A*).
10. Fan-fold linen length-wise to the side of the bed farthest from the door (Fig. 19-20, *B*).
11. Put the pillowcase(s) on the pillow(s).
12. Place the pillow(s) on a clean surface.
13. Leave the bed in its highest position.
14. Leave both bed rails down.
15. Put the clean towels, washcloth, gown or pajamas, and bath blanket in the bedside stand.
16. Move furniture away from the bed. Allow room for the stretcher and the staff.
17. Do not attach the signal light to the bed.
18. Complete a safety check of the room. (See the inside of the front book cover.)
19. Follow center policy for soiled linen.
20. Decontaminate your hands.

Fig. 19-20 Surgical bed. **A,** The bottom of the top linens is folded back onto the bed. The fold is even with the bottom edge of the mattress. **B,** Top linens are fan-folded length-wise to the opposite side of the bed.

QUALITY OF LIFE

The bed is the largest item in the resident's unit. The person, family, and visitors question the quality of care if the bed is unmade, messy, or dirty. They also question the person's quality of life. The bed must be neat, clean, and well made. It helps provide an orderly and pleasant setting. If the person stays in bed, straighten and tighten sheets and other linen as needed.

Some persons bring bedspreads, pillows, blankets, afghans, and quilts from home. Use these when making the bed. Such items are the person's property. Handle them with care and respect. Make sure they are labeled with the person's name. This protects them from loss. It also prevents them from becoming confused with the property of others.

Allow personal choice when possible. The center may use colored or printed linens. If so, let the person choose which linen to use. Also, let the person decide how many pillows or blankets to use. If possible, the person chooses when the bed is made. The more choices allowed, the greater the person's sense of control and quality of life.

REVIEW QUESTIONS

Circle T if the statement is TRUE. Circle F if the statement is FALSE.

1 T F In nursing centers, complete linen changes are required for closed beds and surgical beds.
2 T F Hem-stitching of the bottom sheet is placed away from the person.
3 T F To remove crumbs from the bed, you shake linens in the air.
4 T F The upper hem of the bedspread is even with the top of the mattress.
5 T F Top linens are fan-folded to the foot of the bed for an open bed.
6 T F A cotton drawsheet is used only with a waterproof drawsheet.
7 T F Residents can bring bed coverings from home.

Circle the BEST answer.

8 Which requires a linen change?
a The person will have visitors
b Wet linen
c Wrinkled linen
d Crumbs in the bed
9 You will transfer a person from a stretcher to the bed. Which bed should you make?
a A closed bed
b An open bed
c An occupied bed
d A surgical bed
10 When handling linens
a Put dirty linens on the floor
b Hold linens away from your body and uniform
c Shake linens to unfold them
d Take extra linen to another person's room
11 A resident is out of the bed most of the day. Which bed should you make?
a A closed bed
b An open bed
c An occupied bed
d A surgical bed
12 A complete linen change is done when
a The bottom linens are wet or soiled
b The bed is made for a new person
c The person will transfer from a stretcher to a bed
d Linens are loose or wrinkled
13 You are using a waterproof drawsheet. Which is *true*?
a A cotton drawsheet must completely cover the waterproof drawsheet.
b Waterproof pads are needed.
c The person's consent is needed.
d The plastic or rubber is in contact with the person's skin.
14 To make an occupied bed, you do the following *except*
a Cover the person with a bath blanket
b Screen the person
c Raise the far bed rail
d Fan-fold top linens to the foot of the bed
15 A surgical bed is kept
a In Fowler's position
b In the lowest position
c In the highest position
d In the supine position

Answers to these questions are on p. 720.

Hygiene

OBJECTIVES

- Define the key terms and key abbreviations listed in this chapter.
- Explain why personal hygiene is important.
- Describe the care given before and after breakfast, after lunch, and in the evening.
- Describe the rules for bathing.
- Identify safety measures for tub baths and showers.
- Explain the purposes of a back massage.
- Explain the purposes of perineal care.
- Identify the observations to report and record when assisting with hygiene.
- Perform the procedures described in this chapter.
- Explain how to promote quality of life.

KEY TERMS

AM care See "early morning care"

aspiration Breathing fluid, food, vomitus, or an object into the lungs

denture An artificial tooth or a set of artificial teeth

early morning care Care given before breakfast; AM care

evening care Care given in the evening at bedtime; PM care

morning care Care given after breakfast; hygiene measures are more thorough at this time

oral hygiene Mouth care

pericare See "perineal care"

perineal care Cleaning the genital and anal areas; pericare

plaque A thin film that sticks to the teeth; it contains saliva, microbes, and other substances

PM care See "evening care"

tartar Hardened plaque

KEY ABBREVIATIONS

C	Centigrade	ID	Identification
F	Fahrenheit		

Hygiene promotes comfort, safety, and health. The skin is the body's first line of defense against disease. Intact skin prevents microbes from entering the body and causing an infection. Likewise, mucous membranes of the mouth, genital area, and anus must be clean and intact. Besides cleansing, good hygiene prevents body and breath odors. It is relaxing and increases circulation.

Culture and personal choice affect hygiene. See *Caring About Culture: Personal Hygiene*. Some people take showers. Others take tub baths. Some bathe at bedtime. Others bathe in the morning. Bathing frequency also varies. Some bathe one or two times a day—before work and after work or exercise. Some people do not have water for bathing. Others cannot afford soap, deodorant, shampoo, toothpaste, or other hygiene products.

Many factors affect hygiene needs—perspiration, elimination, vomiting, drainage from wounds or body openings, bedrest, and activity. Illness and aging changes can affect self-care abilities. Some people need help with hygiene. The nurse uses the nursing process to meet the person's hygiene needs. Follow the nurse's directions and the care plan.

Some older persons resist your efforts to assist with hygiene. Illness, disability, dementia, and personal choice are common reasons. Follow the care plan to meet the person's needs.

See *Residents with Dementia: Hygiene*.
See *Focus on Communication: Hygiene*.
See *Focus on Rehabilitation: Hygiene*.

CARING ABOUT CULTURE
Personal Hygiene

Personal hygiene is very important to *East Indian Hindus*. Their religion requires at least one bath a day. Some believe bathing after a meal is harmful. Another belief is that a cold bath prevents a blood disease. Some believe that eye injuries can occur if a bath is too hot. Hot water can be added to cold water. However, cold water is not added to hot water. After bathing, the body is carefully dried with a towel.

From Giger JN, Davidhizar RE: Transcultural nursing: assessment and intervention, ed 5, St Louis, 2008, Mosby.

FOCUS ON COMMUNICATION
Hygiene

During hygiene procedures, make sure that the person is warm enough. You can ask:
- "Is the water warm enough?" "Is it too hot?" "Is it too cold?"
- "Are you warm enough?"
- "Do you need another bath blanket?"
- "Is the water starting to cool?"
- "Is the room warm enough?"

FOCUS ON REHABILITATION
Hygiene

Bending and reaching may be hard for older and disabled persons. Some have weak hand grips. They cannot hold soap or a washcloth. For independence, the person may use an adaptive device for hygiene (Fig. 20-1). Remember, let the person do as much for himself or herself as safely possible.

RESIDENTS WITH DEMENTIA
Hygiene

Persons with dementia may resist your efforts to assist with hygiene. Follow the care plan to meet the person's needs. Also see Chapter 44.

Fig. 20-1 Adaptive devices for hygiene. **A,** Tube squeezer for toothpaste. **B,** The wash mitt holds a bar of soap. **C,** A tap turner makes round knobs easy to turn. **D,** A long-handled sponge is used for hard-to-reach body parts. *(Courtesy ElderStore, Alpharetta, Ga.)*

DAILY CARE

Most people have hygiene routines and habits. For example, teeth are brushed and the face and hands washed after sleep. These and other hygiene measures are often done before and after meals and at bedtime.

Weak and disabled persons need help with hygiene. Routine care is given during the day and evening. You assist with hygiene whenever it is needed. You must protect the person's right to privacy and to personal choice.

Before Breakfast

Routine care given before breakfast is called early morning care or AM care. Night shift or day shift staff members give AM care. They get residents ready for breakfast or morning tests. AM care includes:

- Assisting with elimination
- Cleaning incontinent persons
- Changing wet or soiled linens and garments
- Assisting with hygiene—face and hand washing and oral hygiene
- Assisting with dressing and hair care
- Positioning persons for breakfast—dining room, bedside chair, or in bed
- Making beds and straightening units

After Breakfast

Morning care is given after breakfast. Hygiene measures are more thorough at this time. They usually involve:

- Assisting with elimination
- Cleaning incontinent persons
- Changing wet or soiled linens and garments
- Assisting with hygiene—face and hand washing, oral hygiene, bathing, back massage, and perineal care
- Assisting with grooming—hair care, shaving, dressing, and undressing
- Assisting with activity—range-of-motion exercises and ambulation
- Making beds and straightening units

Afternoon Care

Routine hygiene is done after lunch and before the evening meal. It is done before the person takes a nap, has visitors, or attends activity programs. Afternoon care involves:

- Assisting with elimination before and after naps
- Cleaning incontinent persons before and after naps
- Changing wet or soiled linens before and after naps
- Changing wet or soiled garments before and after naps

- Assisting with hygiene and grooming—face and hand washing, oral hygiene, and hair care
- Assisting with activity—range-of-motion exercises and ambulation
- Straightening beds and units

Evening Care

Care given in the evening at bedtime is called evening care or PM care. Evening care is relaxing and promotes comfort. Measures performed before sleep include:

- Assisting with elimination
- Cleaning incontinent persons
- Changing wet or soiled linens and garments
- Assisting with hygiene—face and hand washing, oral hygiene, and back massages
- Helping persons change into sleepwear
- Straightening beds and units

ORAL HYGIENE

Oral hygiene (mouth care) does the following:

- Keeps the mouth and teeth clean
- Prevents mouth odors and infections
- Increases comfort
- Makes food taste better
- Reduces the risk for cavities (dental caries) and periodontal disease

Periodontal disease (gum disease, pyorrhea) is an inflammation of tissues around the teeth. Plaque and tartar build up from poor oral hygiene. Plaque is a thin film that sticks to teeth. It contains saliva, microbes, and other substances. Plaque causes tooth decay (cavities). When plaque hardens, it is called tartar. Tartar builds up at the gum line near the neck of the tooth. Tartar buildup causes periodontal disease. The gums are red and swollen and bleed easily. As the disease progresses, bone is destroyed and teeth loosen. Tooth loss is common.

Illness, disease, and some drugs often cause:

- A bad taste in the mouth.
- A whitish coating in the mouth and on the tongue.
- Redness and swelling in the mouth and on the tongue.
- Dry mouth. Dry mouth also is common from oxygen, smoking, decreased fluid intake, and anxiety.

The nurse assesses the person's need for mouth care. The speech/language pathologist and the dietitian may also do so.

Flossing

Dental floss is a soft thread used to clean between the teeth. Flossing removes plaque and tartar from the teeth. These substances cause periodontal disease. Flossing also removes food from between the teeth. Usually done after brushing, it can be done at other times. Some people floss after meals. If done once a day, bedtime is the best time to floss.

You need to floss for persons who cannot do so themselves. Some older persons do not floss their teeth. Follow the care plan.

Equipment

A toothbrush, toothpaste, dental floss, and mouthwash are needed. A toothbrush with soft bristles is best. Persons with dentures need a denture cleaner, denture cup, and denture brush or toothbrush. Use only denture cleaning products. Otherwise, you could damage dentures.

Sponge swabs are used for persons with sore, tender mouths. They also are used for unconscious persons. Use sponge swabs with care. Check the foam pad to make sure it is tight on the stick. The person could choke on the foam pad if it comes off the stick.

You also need a kidney basin, water glass or cup, straw, tissues, towels, and gloves. Many persons bring oral hygiene equipment from home.

See *Delegation Guidelines: Oral Hygiene.*
See *Promoting Safety and Comfort: Oral Hygiene.*

DELEGATION GUIDELINES
Oral Hygiene

To assist with oral hygiene. You need this information from the nurse and the care plan:
- The type of oral hygiene to give. See procedures:
  - *Assisting the Person to Brush and Floss the Teeth*, p. 284
  - *Brushing and Flossing the Person's Teeth*, p. 285
  - *Providing Mouth Care for the Unconscious Person*, p. 287
  - *Providing Denture Care*, p. 289
- If flossing is needed
- What cleaning agent and equipment to use
- If lubricant is applied to the lips; if so, what lubricant to use
- How often to give oral hygiene
- How much help the person needs
- What observations to report and record:
  - Dry, cracked, swollen, or blistered lips
  - Mouth or breath odor
  - Redness, swelling, irritation, sores, or white patches in the mouth or on the tongue
  - Bleeding, swelling, or redness of the gums
  - Loose teeth
  - Rough, sharp, or chipped areas on dentures
- When to report observations
- What specific resident concerns to report at once

PROMOTING SAFETY AND COMFORT
Oral Hygiene

Safety
Follow Standard Precautions and the Bloodborne Pathogen Standard when giving oral hygiene. You have contact with the person's mucous membranes. Gums may bleed during mouth care. Also, the mouth has many microbes. Pathogens spread through sexual contact may be in the mouths of some persons.

Comfort
Assist with oral hygiene after sleep, after meals, and at bedtime. Many people practice oral hygiene before meals. Some persons need mouth care every 2 hours or more often. Always follow the care plan.

Brushing and Flossing Teeth

Many people perform oral hygiene themselves. Others need help gathering and setting up equipment for oral hygiene. You may have to perform oral hygiene for persons who:
- Are very weak
- Cannot move or use their arms
- Are too confused to brush their teeth

Text continued on p. 286

ASSISTING THE PERSON TO BRUSH AND FLOSS THE TEETH

QUALITY OF LIFE

Remember to:
- Knock before entering the person's room.
- Address the person by name.
- Introduce yourself by name and title.

- Explain the procedure to the person before beginning and during the procedure.
- Protect the person's rights during the procedure.
- Handle the person gently during the procedure.

PRE-PROCEDURE

1 Follow *Delegation Guidelines: Oral Hygiene*, p. 283. See *Promoting Safety and Comfort: Oral Hygiene*, p. 283.
2 Practice hand hygiene.
3 Collect the following:
- Toothbrush
- Toothpaste
- Mouthwash (or solution noted on the care plan)
- Dental floss (if used)
- Water glass with cool water
- Straw
- Kidney basin

- Hand towel
- Paper towels
- Gloves

4 Place the paper towels on the overbed table. Arrange items on top of them.
5 Identify the person. Check the ID (identification) bracelet against the assignment sheet. Also call the person by name.
6 Provide for privacy.
7 Lower the bed rail near you if up.

PROCEDURE

8 Position the person so he or she can brush with ease.
9 Place the towel over the person's chest. This protects garments and linens from spills.
10 Adjust the overbed table in front of the person.

11 Let the person perform oral hygiene. This includes brushing the teeth and tongue, rinsing the mouth, flossing, and using mouthwash or other solution.
12 Remove the towel when the person is done.
13 Move the overbed table to the side of the bed.

POST-PROCEDURE

14 Provide for comfort. (See the inside of the front book cover.)
15 Place the signal light within reach.
16 Raise or lower bed rails. Follow the care plan.
17 Clean and return items to their proper place. Wear gloves.
18 Wipe off the overbed table with the paper towels. Discard the paper towels.

19 Remove the gloves. Decontaminate your hands.
20 Unscreen the person.
21 Complete a safety check of the room. (See the inside of the front book cover.)
22 Follow center policy for dirty linen.
23 Decontaminate your hands.
24 Report and record your observations.

Fig. 20-2 Brushing teeth. **A,** The brush is held at a 45-degree angle to the gums. Teeth are brushed with short strokes. **B,** The brush is at a 45-degree angle against the inside of the front teeth. Teeth are brushed from the gum to the crown of the tooth with short strokes. **C,** The brush is held horizontally against the inner surfaces of the teeth. The teeth are brushed back and forth. **D,** The brush is positioned on the biting surfaces of the teeth. The teeth are brushed back and forth.

BRUSHING AND FLOSSING THE PERSON'S TEETH

QUALITY OF LIFE

Remember to:
- Knock before entering the person's room.
- Address the person by name.
- Introduce yourself by name and title.

- Explain the procedure to the person before beginning and during the procedure.
- Protect the person's rights during the procedure.
- Handle the person gently during the procedure.

PRE-PROCEDURE

1 Follow *Delegation Guidelines: Oral Hygiene*, p. 283. See *Promoting Safety and Comfort: Oral Hygiene*, p. 283.
2 Practice hand hygiene.
3 Collect the following:
- Toothbrush with soft bristles
- Toothpaste
- Mouthwash (or solution noted on the care plan)
- Dental floss (if used)
- Water glass with cool water
- Straw
- Kidney basin

- Hand towel
- Paper towels
- Gloves

4 Place the paper towels on the overbed table. Arrange items on top of them.
5 Identify the person. Check the ID bracelet against the assignment sheet. Also call the person by name.
6 Provide for privacy.
7 Raise the bed for body mechanics. Bed rails are up if used.

PROCEDURE

8 Lower the bed rail near you if up.
9 Assist the person to a sitting position or to a side-lying position near you.
10 Place the towel across the person's chest.
11 Adjust the overbed table so you can reach it with ease.
12 Decontaminate your hands. Put on the gloves.
13 Hold the toothbrush over the kidney basin. Pour some water over the brush.
14 Apply toothpaste to the toothbrush.
15 Brush the teeth gently (Fig. 20-2).
16 Brush the tongue gently.
17 Let the person rinse the mouth with water. Hold the kidney basin under the person's chin (Fig. 20-3, p. 286). Repeat this step as needed.
18 Floss the person's teeth (optional):
  a Break off an 18-inch piece of dental floss from the dispenser.
  b Hold the floss between the middle fingers of each hand (Fig. 20-4, *A*, p. 286).

  c Stretch the floss with your thumbs.
  d Start at the upper back tooth on the right side. Work around to the left side.
  e Move the floss gently up and down between the teeth (Fig. 20-4, *B*, p. 286). Move the floss up and down against the side of the tooth. Work from the top of the crown to the gum line.
  f Move to a new section of floss after every second tooth.
  g Floss the lower teeth. Use up and down motions as for the upper teeth. Start on the right side. Work around to the left side.
19 Let the person use mouthwash or other solution. Hold the kidney basin under the chin.
20 Wipe the person's mouth. Remove the towel.
21 Remove and discard the gloves. Decontaminate your hands.

POST-PROCEDURE

22 Provide for comfort. (See the inside of the front book cover.)
23 Place the signal light within reach.
24 Lower the bed to its lowest position.
25 Raise or lower bed rails. Follow the care plan.
26 Clean and return equipment to its proper place. Wear gloves.
27 Wipe off the overbed table with the paper towels. Discard the paper towels.

28 Unscreen the person.
29 Complete a safety check of the room. (See the inside of the front book cover.)
30 Follow center policy for dirty linen.
31 Remove the gloves. Decontaminate your hands.
32 Report and record your observations.

Fig. 20-3 The kidney basin is held under the person's chin.

Fig. 20-4 Flossing. **A,** Floss is wrapped around the middle fingers. **B,** Floss is moved in up-and-down motions between the teeth. Floss is moved up and down from the crown to the gum line.

Fig. 20-5 The unconscious person's head is turned well to the side to prevent aspiration. A padded tongue blade is used to keep the mouth open while cleaning the mouth with swabs.

Fig. 20-6 Making a padded tongue blade. **A,** Place two wooden tongue blades together. Wrap gauze around the top half. **B,** Tape the gauze in place.

✉ Mouth Care for the Unconscious Person

Unconscious persons cannot eat or drink. They may breathe with their mouths open. Many receive oxygen. These factors cause mouth dryness. They also cause crusting on the tongue and mucous membranes. Oral hygiene keeps the mouth clean and moist. It also helps prevent infection.

The care plan tells you what cleaning agent to use. Use sponge swabs to apply the cleaning agent. Apply a lubricant (check the care plan) to the lips after cleaning. It prevents cracking of the lips.

Unconscious persons usually cannot swallow. Protect them from choking and aspiration. **Aspiration** is breathing fluid, food, vomitus, or an object into the lungs. It can cause pneumonia and death. To prevent aspiration:

- Position the person on one side with the head turned well to the side (Fig. 20-5). In this position, excess fluid runs out of the mouth.
- Use only a small amount of fluid to clean the mouth.
- Do not insert dentures. Dentures are not worn when the person is unconscious.

Keep the person's mouth open with a padded tongue blade (Fig. 20-6). Do not use your fingers. The person can bite down on them. The bite breaks the skin and creates a portal of entry for microbes. Infection is a risk.

Unconscious persons cannot speak or respond to you. However, some can hear. Always assume that unconscious persons can hear. Explain what you are doing step-by-step. Also tell the person when you are done, when you are leaving the room, and when you will return.

Mouth care is given at least every 2 hours. Follow the nurse's directions and the care plan.

See *Promoting Safety and Comfort: Mouth Care for the Unconscious Person.*

PROMOTING SAFETY AND COMFORT
Mouth Care for the Unconscious Person

Safety
Use sponge swabs with care. Make sure the sponge pad is tight on the stick. The person could choke or aspirate on the sponge if it comes off the stick.

Comfort
Unconscious persons are re-positioned at least every 2 hours. To promote comfort, combine mouth care with skin care, re-positioning, and other comfort measures.

PROVIDING MOUTH CARE FOR THE UNCONSCIOUS PERSON

QUALITY OF LIFE

Remember to:
- Knock before entering the person's room.
- Address the person by name.
- Introduce yourself by name and title.
- Explain the procedure to the person before beginning and during the procedure.
- Protect the person's rights during the procedure.
- Handle the person gently during the procedure.

PRE-PROCEDURE

1 Follow *Delegation Guidelines: Oral Hygiene,* p. 283. See *Promoting Safety and Comfort:*
  a *Oral Hygiene,* p. 283
  b *Mouth Care for the Unconscious Person*
2 Practice hand hygiene.
3 Collect the following:
  - Cleaning agent (check the care plan)
  - Sponge swabs
  - Padded tongue blade
  - Water glass or cup with cool water
  - Hand towel
  - Kidney basin
  - Lip lubricant
  - Paper towels
  - Gloves
4 Place the towels on the overbed table. Arrange items on top of them.
5 Identify the person. Check the ID bracelet against the assignment sheet. Also call the person by name.
6 Provide for privacy.
7 Raise the bed for body mechanics. Bed rails are up if used.

PROCEDURE

8 Lower the bed rail near you if up.
9 Decontaminate your hands. Put on the gloves.
10 Position the person in a side-lying position near you. Turn his or her head well to the side.
11 Place the towel under the person's face.
12 Place the kidney basin under the chin.
13 Separate the upper and lower teeth. Use the padded tongue blade. Be gentle. Never use force. If you have problems, ask the nurse for help.
14 Clean the mouth using sponge swabs moistened with the cleaning agent (see Fig. 20-5).
  a Clean the chewing and inner surfaces of the teeth.
  b Clean the gums and outer surfaces of the teeth.
  c Swab the roof of the mouth, inside of the cheeks, and the lips.
  d Swab the tongue.
  e Moisten a clean swab with water. Swab the mouth to rinse.
  f Place used swabs in the kidney basin.
15 Remove the kidney basin and supplies.
16 Wipe the person's mouth. Remove the towel.
17 Apply lubricant to the lips.
18 Remove and discard the gloves. Decontaminate your hands.

Continued

POST-PROCEDURE

19 Provide for comfort. (See the inside of the front book cover.)
20 Place the signal light within reach.
21 Lower the bed to its lowest position.
22 Raise or lower bed rails. Follow the care plan.
23 Clean and return equipment to its proper place. Discard disposable items. (Wear gloves.)
24 Wipe off the overbed table with paper towels. Discard the paper towels.

25 Unscreen the person.
26 Complete a safety check of the room. (See the inside of the front book cover.)
27 Tell the person that you are leaving the room. Tell him or her when you will return.
28 Follow center policy for dirty linen.
29 Remove the gloves. Decontaminate your hands.
30 Report and record your observations.

Denture Care

A **denture** is an artificial tooth or a set of artificial teeth (Fig. 20-7). They are often called "false teeth." Dentures replace missing teeth. People lose teeth because of gum disease, tooth decay, or injury. Full and partial dentures are common:

- *Full denture.* The person has no upper or no lower natural teeth. Dentures replace the upper or lower teeth.
- *Partial denture.* The person has some natural teeth. The partial denture replaces the missing teeth.

Mouth care is given and dentures cleaned as often as natural teeth. Dentures are slippery when wet. They easily break or chip if dropped onto a hard surface (floors, sinks, counters). Hold them firmly when removing or inserting them. During cleaning, firmly hold them over a basin of water lined with a towel. This prevents them from falling onto a hard surface.

To use a cleaning agent, follow the manufacturer's instructions. They tell how to use the cleaning agent and what water temperature to use. Hot water causes dentures to lose their shape (warp). If not worn after cleaning, store dentures in a container with cool water or a denture soaking solution. Otherwise, they can dry out and warp.

Dentures are usually removed at bedtime. Some people do not wear their dentures. Others wear dentures for eating and remove them after meals. Remind them not to wrap dentures in tissues or napkins. Otherwise, they are easily discarded.

Many people clean their own dentures. Some need help collecting items used to clean dentures. They may need help getting to the bathroom. You clean dentures for those who cannot do so.

See *Promoting Safety and Comfort: Denture Care.*

Fig. 20-7 Dentures. **A,** Partial denture. **B,** Full denture.

PROMOTING SAFETY AND COMFORT
Denture Care

Safety

Dentures are the person's property. They are costly. Handle them very carefully. Label the denture cup with the person's name and room and bed number. Report lost or damaged dentures to the nurse at once. Losing or damaging dentures is negligent conduct.

Never carry dentures in your hands. Always use a denture cup or kidney basin. You could easily drop the dentures as you move from the bedside to the bathroom. Or you could drop them when moving from the bathroom to the bedside.

Comfort

Many people do not like being seen without their dentures. Privacy is important. Allow privacy when the person cleans dentures. If you clean dentures, return them to the person as quickly as possible.

Persons with dentures may have some natural teeth. They need to brush and floss the natural teeth. See procedure: *Assisting the Person to Brush and Floss the Teeth,* p. 284. Or see procedure: *Brushing and Flossing the Person's Teeth,* p. 285.

PROVIDING DENTURE CARE

QUALITY OF LIFE

Remember to:
- Knock before entering the person's room.
- Address the person by name.
- Introduce yourself by name and title.
- Explain the procedure to the person before beginning and during the procedure.
- Protect the person's rights during the procedure.
- Handle the person gently during the procedure.

PRE-PROCEDURE

1 Follow *Delegation Guidelines: Oral Hygiene,* p. 283. See *Promoting Safety and Comfort:*
  a *Oral Hygiene,* p. 283
  b *Denture Care*
2 Practice hand hygiene.
3 Collect the following:
  - Denture brush or toothbrush (for cleaning dentures)
  - Denture cup labeled with the person's name and room and bed number
  - Denture cleaning agent
  - Soft-bristled toothbrush or sponge swabs (for oral hygiene)
  - Toothpaste
  - Water glass with cool water
  - Straw
  - Mouthwash (or other noted solution)
  - Kidney basin
  - Two hand towels
  - Gauze squares
  - Paper towels
  - Gloves
4 Place the paper towels on the overbed table. Arrange items on top of them.
5 Identify the person. Check the ID bracelet against the assignment sheet. Also call the person by name.
6 Provide for privacy.
7 Raise the bed for body mechanics.

PROCEDURE

8 Lower the bed rail near you if used.
9 Decontaminate your hands. Put on the gloves.
10 Place a towel over the person's chest.
11 Ask the person to remove the dentures. Carefully place them in the kidney basin.
12 Remove the dentures if the person cannot do so. Use gauze squares to get a good grip on the slippery dentures.
  a Grasp the denture with your thumb and index finger (Fig. 20-8, p. 290). Move it up and down slightly to break the seal. Gently remove the denture. Place it in the kidney basin.
  b Grasp and remove the lower denture with your thumb and index finger. Turn it slightly, and lift it out of the person's mouth. Place it in the kidney basin.
13 Follow the care plan for raising bed rails.
14 Take the kidney basin, denture cup, denture brush, and denture cleaning agent to the sink.
15 Line the sink with a towel. Fill the sink half-way with water.
16 Rinse each denture under cool or warm running water. Follow center policy for water temperature.
17 Return dentures to the kidney basin or denture cup.
18 Apply the denture cleaning agent to the brush.
19 Brush the dentures as in Figure 20-9, p. 290. Brush the inner, outer, and chewing surfaces.
20 Rinse the dentures under running water. Use warm or cool water as directed by the cleaning agent manufacturer. (Some state competency tests require cool water.)
21 Rinse the denture cup and lid. Place dentures in the denture cup. Cover the dentures with cool or warm water. Follow center policy for water temperature.
22 Clean the kidney basin.
23 Take the denture cup and kidney basin to the overbed table.
24 Lower the bed rail if up.
25 Position the person for oral hygiene.
26 Clean the person's gums and tongue. Use toothpaste and the toothbrush (or sponge swabs).
27 Have the person use mouthwash (or noted solution). Hold the kidney basin under the chin.
28 Ask the person to insert the dentures. Insert them if the person cannot:
  a Hold the upper denture firmly with your thumb and index finger. Raise the upper lip with the other hand. Insert the denture. Gently press on the denture with your index fingers to make sure it is in place.
  b Hold the lower denture with your thumb and index finger. Pull the lower lip down slightly. Insert the denture. Gently press down on it to make sure it is in place.
29 Place the denture cup in the top drawer of the bedside stand if the dentures are not worn. The dentures must be in water or in a denture soaking solution.
30 Wipe the person's mouth. Remove the towel.
31 Remove the gloves. Decontaminate your hands.

Continued

PROVIDING DENTURE CARE—cont'd

VIDEO CLIP | VIDEO | ⊙ | NNAAP™ Skill

POST-PROCEDURE

32 Assist with hand washing.
33 Provide for comfort. (See the inside of the front book cover.)
34 Place the signal light within reach.
35 Lower the bed to its lowest position.
36 Raise or lower bed rails. Follow the care plan.
37 Remove the towel from the sink. Drain the sink.
38 Clean and return equipment to its proper place. Discard disposable items. Wear gloves for this step.

39 Wipe off the overbed table with the paper towels. Discard the paper towels.
40 Unscreen the person.
41 Complete a safety check of the room. (See the inside of the front book cover.)
42 Follow center policy for dirty linen.
43 Remove the gloves. Decontaminate your hands.
44 Report and record your observations.

Fig. 20-8 Remove the upper denture by grasping it with the thumb and index finger of one hand. Use a piece of gauze to grasp the slippery denture.

Fig. 20-9 Cleaning dentures. **A,** Brush the outer surfaces of the denture with back-and-forth motions. The denture is held over the sink. The sink is filled half-way with water and is lined with a towel. **B,** Position the brush vertically to clean the inner surfaces of the denture. Use upward strokes.

BATHING

Bathing cleans the skin. It also cleans the mucous membranes of the genital and anal areas. Microbes, dead skin, perspiration, and excess oils are removed. A bath is refreshing and relaxing. Circulation is stimulated and body parts exercised. Observations are made, and you have time to talk to the person.

Complete or partial baths, tub baths, or showers are given. The method depends on the person's condition, self-care abilities, and personal choice. In nursing centers, bathing usually occurs after breakfast or the evening meal. The person's choice of bath time is respected whenever possible.

Bathing frequency is a personal matter. Some people bathe daily. Others bathe once or twice a week. Personal choice, weather, activity, and illness affect bathing frequency. Ill persons may have fevers and perspire heavily. They need frequent bathing. Other illnesses and dry skin may limit bathing to every 2 or 3 days.

Dry skin occurs with aging. Soap also dries the skin. Dry skin is easily damaged. Therefore older persons usually need a complete bath or shower twice a week. Partial baths are taken the other days. Some bathe daily but not with soap. Thorough rinsing is needed when using soap. Lotions and oils help keep the skin soft.

The rules for bed baths, showers, and tub baths are listed in Box 20-1. Table 20-1 describes common skin care products.

See *Focus on Communication: Hygiene,* p. 281.
See *Residents With Dementia: Bathing,* p. 292.
See *Delegation Guidelines: Bathing,* p. 292.
See *Promoting Safety and Comfort: Bathing,* p. 293.

Box 20-1 Rules for Bathing

- Follow the care plan for bathing method and skin care products.
- Allow personal choice whenever possible.
- Follow Standard Precautions and the Bloodborne Pathogen Standard.
- Collect needed items before starting the procedure.
- Provide for privacy. Screen the person. Close doors and window coverings—drapes, shades, blinds, shutters, and so on.
- Assist the person with elimination. Bathing stimulates the need to urinate. Comfort and relaxation increase if urination needs are met.
- Cover the person for warmth and privacy.
- Reduce drafts. Close doors and windows.
- Protect the person from falling.
- Use good body mechanics at all times.
- Follow the rules to safely handle, move, and transfer the person (Chapter 17).

- Know what water temperature to use. See *Delegation Guidelines: Bathing*, p. 292.
- Keep bar soap in the soap dish between latherings. This prevents soapy water. It also reduces the chances of slipping and falls in showers and tubs.
- Wash from the cleanest areas to the dirtiest areas.
- Encourage the person to help as much as is safely possible.
- Rinse the skin thoroughly. You must remove all soap.
- Pat the skin dry to avoid irritating or breaking the skin. Do not rub the skin.
- Dry under the breasts, between skin folds, in the perineal area, and between the toes.
- Bathe skin when urine or feces are present. This prevents skin breakdown and odors.

Table 20-1 Skin Care Products

Type	Purpose	Care Considerations
Soaps	• Clean the skin • Remove dirt, dead skin, skin oil, some microbes, and perspiration	• Tend to dry and irritate the skin • Dry skin is easily injured and causes itching and discomfort • Skin must be thoroughly rinsed to remove all soap • Not needed for every bath; plain water can clean the skin • Plain water is often used for older persons due to dry skin • People with dry skin may use soaps containing bath oils • Not used if a person has very dry skin
Bath oils	• Keep the skin soft • Prevent dry skin	• Some soaps contain bath oil • Liquid bath oil can be added to bath water • Showers and tubs become slippery from bath oils; safety measures are needed to prevent falls
Creams and lotions	• Protect the skin from the drying effect of air and evaporation	• Do not feel greasy but leave an oily film on the skin • Lotion applied to body areas after bathing to prevent skin breakdown (back, elbows, knees, and heels) • Lotion used for back massages • Most are scented
Powders	• Absorb moisture • Prevent friction when two skin surfaces rub together	• Usually applied under the breasts, under the arms, and in the groin area, and sometimes between the toes • Applied to dry skin in a thin, even layer • Excessive amounts cause caking and crusts that can irritate the skin
Deodorants	• Mask and control body odors	• Applied to the underarms • Not applied to irritated skin • Do not take the place of bathing
Antiperspirants	• Reduce the amount of perspiration	• Applied to the underarms • Not applied to irritated skin • Do not take the place of bathing

RESIDENTS WITH DEMENTIA
Bathing

Bathing procedures can threaten persons with dementia. They do not understand what is happening or why. And they may fear harm or danger. Confusion can increase. Therefore they may resist care and become agitated and combative. They may shout at you and cry out for help. You must be calm, patient, and soothing.

The nurse assesses the person's behaviors and routines. The person may be calmer and less confused or agitated during a certain time of the day. Bathing is scheduled for the person's calm times. The nurse decides if a bed bath, tub bath, shower, or towel bath (p. 297) is best for the person.

The rules in Box 20-1 apply when bathing these persons. The care plan also includes measures to help the person through the bath. Such measures may include:

- Use terms such as "cleaned up" or "washed" rather than "shower" or "bath."
- Complete pre-procedure activities. For example, ready supplies and linens. Make sure you have everything that you need.
- Provide for warmth. Increase the room temperature before starting the bath or shower. Have extra towels and a robe nearby.
- Play soft music to help the person relax.
- Provide for safety:
  - Use a hand-held shower nozzle.
  - Have the person use a shower chair or shower bench.
  - Do not use bath oil. It can make the tub or shower slippery. And it may cause a urinary tract infection.
  - Do not leave the person alone in the tub or shower.
- Draw bath water ahead of time. Test the water temperature. Add warm or cold water as necessary.
- Tell the person what you are doing step-by-step. Use clear, simple statements.
- Let the person help as much as possible. For example, give the person a washcloth. Ask him or her to wash the arms. If the person does not know what to do, still let the person hold the washcloth if it is safe to do so.
- Put a towel over the person's shoulder or lap (tub or shower). This helps the person feel less exposed.
- Do not rush the person.
- Use a calm, pleasant voice.
- Divert the person's attention if necessary.
- Calm the person.
- Handle the person gently.
- Try giving a partial bath if a shower or tub bath agitates the person.
- Try the bath later if the person continues to resist care.

Persons with dementia may respond well to a *towel bath*. An over-sized towel is used. It covers the body from the neck to the feet. The towel is wet with a solution—water, cleaning agent, and skin-softening agent. It also has a drying agent so the person's body dries fast. The nurse and care plan tell you when to use a towel bath. To give a towel bath, follow center policy.

DELEGATION GUIDELINES
Bathing

To assist with bathing, you need this information from the nurse and the care plan:

- What bath to give—complete bed bath, partial bath, tub bath, shower, towel bath, or bag bath.
- How much help the person needs.
- The person's activity or position limits.
- What water temperature to use. Bath water cools rapidly. Heat is lost to the bath basin, overbed table, washcloth, and your hands. Therefore water temperature for complete bed baths and partial bed baths is usually between 110° and 115° F (Fahrenheit) (43.3° and 46.1° C [centigrade]) for adults. Older persons have fragile skin. They need lower water temperatures.
- What skin care products to use and what the person prefers.
- What observations to report and record:
  - The color of the skin, lips, nail beds, and sclera (whites of the eyes)
  - The location and description of rashes
  - Dry skin
  - Bruises or open skin areas
  - Pale or reddened areas, particularly over bony parts
  - Drainage or bleeding from wounds or body openings
  - Swelling of the feet and legs
  - Corns or calluses on the feet
  - Skin temperature
  - Complaints of pain or discomfort
- When to report observations.
- What specific resident concerns to report at once.

PROMOTING SAFETY AND COMFORT
Bathing

Safety

Hot water can burn delicate and fragile skin. Measure water temperature according to center policy. If unsure if the water is too hot, ask the nurse to check it.

Protect the person from falls and other injuries. Practice the safety measures presented in Chapters 12 and 13. Also protect the person from drafts.

Use caution when applying powder. Do not use powders near persons with respiratory disorders. Inhaling powder can irritate the airway and lungs. Before applying powder, check with the nurse and the care plan. Do not shake or sprinkle powder onto the person. To safely apply powder:

- Turn away from the person.
- Sprinkle a small amount of powder onto your hands or a cloth.
- Apply the powder in a thin layer.
- Make sure powder does not get on the floor. Powder is slippery and can cause falls.

Beds are made after baths. After making the bed, lower the bed to its lowest position. Then lock the bed wheels. For an occupied bed, raise or lower bed rails according to the care plan.

Protect the person and yourself from infection. When giving baths and making beds, contact with blood, body fluids, secretions, and excretions is likely. Follow Standard Precautions and the Bloodborne Pathogen Standard.

Comfort

Before bathing, allow the person to meet elimination needs (Chapters 22 and 23). Bathing stimulates the need to urinate. The person is more comfortable if his or her bladder is empty. Also, bathing is not interrupted.

Many people perform oral hygiene as part of their bathing routine. Some do so before the bathing procedure; others do so after. Allow personal choice and follow the person's care plan.

Provide for warmth. Cover the person with a bath blanket. Make sure the water is warm enough for the person. Cool water causes chilling.

Remove the person's gown or pajamas after washing the eyes, face, ears, and neck. Waiting to remove sleepwear at this time helps the person feel less exposed and more comfortable with the bath. If the person prefers, you can remove the sleepwear before washing the eyes, face, ears, and neck.

The Complete Bed Bath

The *complete bed bath* involves washing the person's entire body in bed. You give complete bed baths to persons who cannot bathe themselves. Bed baths are usually needed by persons who are:

- Unconscious
- Paralyzed
- In casts or traction
- Weak from illness or surgery

A bed bath is new to some people. Some are embarrassed to have others see their bodies. Some fear exposure. Explain how the bed bath is given. Also explain how you cover the body for privacy.

Text continued on p. 297

GIVING A COMPLETE BED BATH

QUALITY OF LIFE

Remember to:
- Knock before entering the person's room.
- Address the person by name.
- Introduce yourself by name and title.
- Explain the procedure to the person before beginning and during the procedure.
- Protect the person's rights during the procedure.
- Handle the person gently during the procedure.

PRE-PROCEDURE

1 Follow *Delegation Guidelines: Bathing*, p. 292. See *Promoting Safety and Comfort: Bathing*, p. 293.
2 Practice hand hygiene.
3 Identify the person. Check the ID bracelet against the assignment sheet. Also call the person by name.
4 Collect clean linen for a closed bed. See procedure: *Making a Closed Bed* in Chapter 19. Place linen on a clean surface.
5 Collect the following:
   - Wash basin
   - Soap
   - Bath thermometer
   - Orangewood stick or nail file
   - Washcloth
   - Two bath towels and two hand towels

- Bath blanket
- Clothing or sleepwear
- Lotion
- Powder
- Deodorant or antiperspirant
- Brush and comb
- Other grooming items as requested
- Paper towels
- Gloves

6 Cover the overbed table with paper towels. Arrange items on the overbed table. Adjust the height as needed.
7 Provide for privacy.
8 Raise the bed for body mechanics. Bed rails are up if used.

PROCEDURE

9 Remove the signal light.
10 Decontaminate your hands. Put on gloves.
11 Cover the person with a bath blanket. Remove top linens (see procedure: *Making an Occupied Bed* in Chapter 19).
12 Lower the head of the bed. It is as flat as possible. The person has at least one pillow.
13 Fill the wash basin ⅔ (two-thirds) full with water. Follow the care plan for water temperature. Water temperature is usually 110° to 115° F (43.3° to 46.1° C) for adults. Measure water temperature. Use the bath thermometer. Or test the water by dipping your elbow or inner wrist into the basin.
14 Lower the bed rail near you if up.
15 Ask the person to check the water temperature. Adjust the water temperature if it is too hot or too cold. Raise the bed rail before leaving the bedside. Lower it when you return.
16 Place the basin on the overbed table.
17 Remove the sleepwear. Do not expose the person.
18 Place a hand towel over the person's chest.
19 Make a mitt with the washcloth (Fig. 20-10). Use a mitt for the entire bath.
20 Wash around the person's eyes with water. Do not use soap.
   a Clean the far eye. Gently wipe from the inner to the outer aspect of the eye with a corner of the mitt (Fig. 20-11, p. 296).
   b Clean around the eye near you. Use a clean part of the washcloth for each stroke.
21 Ask the person if you should use soap to wash the face.
22 Wash the face, ears, and neck. Rinse and pat dry with the towel on the chest.

23 Help the person move to the side of the bed near you.
24 Expose the far arm. Place a bath towel length-wise under the arm. Apply soap to the washcloth.
25 Support the arm with your palm under the person's elbow. His or her forearm rests on your forearm.
26 Wash the arm, shoulder, and underarm. Use long, firm strokes (Fig. 20-12, p. 296). Rinse and pat dry.
27 Place the basin on the towel. Put the person's hand into the water (Fig. 20-13, p. 296). Wash it well. Clean under the fingernails with an orangewood stick or nail file.
28 Have the person exercise the hand and fingers.
29 Remove the basin. Dry the hand well. Cover the arm with the bath blanket.
30 Repeat steps 24 to 29 for the near arm.
31 Place a bath towel over the chest cross-wise. Hold the towel in place. Pull the bath blanket from under the towel to the waist. Apply soap to the washcloth.
32 Lift the towel slightly, and wash the chest (Fig. 20-14, p. 296). Do not expose the person. Rinse and pat dry, especially under the breasts.
33 Move the towel length-wise over the chest and abdomen. Do not expose the person. Pull the bath blanket down to the pubic area. Apply soap to the washcloth.
34 Lift the towel slightly, and wash the abdomen (Fig. 20-15, p. 296). Rinse and pat dry.
35 Pull the bath blanket up to the shoulders, covering both arms. Remove the towel.
36 Change soapy or cool water. Measure bath water temperature as in step 13. If bed rails are used, raise the bed rail near you before leaving the bedside. Lower it when you return.

GIVING A COMPLETE BED BATH—cont'd

PROCEDURE—cont'd

37 Uncover the far leg. Do not expose the genital area. Place a towel length-wise under the foot and leg. Apply soap to the washcloth.

38 Bend the knee, and support the leg with your arm. Wash it with long, firm strokes. Rinse and pat dry.

39 Place the basin on the towel near the foot.

40 Lift the leg slightly. Slide the basin under the foot.

41 Place the foot in the basin (Fig. 20-16, p. 297). Use an orangewood stick or nail file to clean under toenails if necessary. If the person cannot bend the knees:

  a Wash the foot. Carefully separate the toes. Rinse and pat dry.

  b Clean under the toenails with an orangewood stick or nail file if necessary.

42 Remove the basin. Dry the leg and foot. Apply lotion to the foot if directed by the nurse and care plan. Cover the leg with the bath blanket. Remove the towel.

43 Repeat steps 37 to 42 for the near leg.

44 Change the water. Measure water temperature as in step 13. If bed rails are used, raise the bed rail near you before leaving the bedside. Lower it when you return.

45 Turn the person onto the side away from you. The person is covered with the bath blanket.

46 Uncover the back and buttocks. Do not expose the person. Place a towel length-wise on the bed along the back. Apply soap to the washcloth.

47 Wash the back. Work from the back of the neck to the lower end of the buttocks. Use long, firm, continuous strokes (Fig. 20-17, p. 297). Rinse and dry well.

48 Give a back massage (p. 302). The person may want the back massage after the bath.

49 Turn the person onto his or her back.

50 Change the water for perineal care (p. 305). For water temperature, see step 14 in procedure: *Giving Female Perineal Care*, p. 307. (Some state competency tests also require changing gloves and hand hygiene at this time.) If bed rails are used, raise the bed rail near you before leaving the bedside. Lower it when you return.

51 Let the person wash the genital area. Adjust the overbed table so he or she can reach the wash basin, soap, and towels with ease. Place the signal light within reach. Ask the person to signal when finished. Make sure the person understands what to do.

52 Remove the gloves. Decontaminate your hands.

53 Answer the signal light promptly. Knock before entering the room. Provide perineal care if the person cannot do so (p. 305). (Decontaminate your hands and wear gloves for perineal care.)

54 Give a back massage if you have not already done so.

55 Apply deodorant or antiperspirant. Apply lotion and powder as requested. See *Promoting Safety and Comfort: Bathing*, p. 293.

56 Put clean garments on the person.

57 Comb and brush the hair (Chapter 21).

58 Make the bed.

POST-PROCEDURE

59 Provide for comfort. (See the inside of the front book cover.)

60 Place the signal light within reach.

61 Lower the bed to its lowest position.

62 Raise or lower bed rails. Follow the care plan.

63 Put on clean gloves.

64 Empty, clean, and dry the wash basin. Return it and other supplies to their proper place.

65 Wipe off the overbed table with paper towels. Discard the paper towels.

66 Unscreen the person.

67 Complete a safety check of the room. (See the inside of the front book cover.)

68 Follow center policy for dirty linen.

69 Remove the gloves. Decontaminate your hands.

70 Report and record your observations.

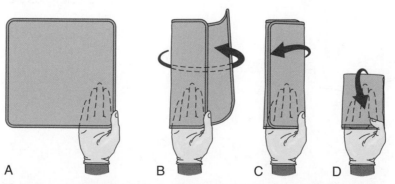

Fig. 20-10 Making a mitted washcloth. **A,** Grasp the near side of the washcloth with your thumb. **B,** Bring the washcloth around and behind your hand. **C,** Fold the side of the washcloth over your palm as you grasp it with your thumb. **D,** Fold the top of the washcloth down and tuck it under next to your palm.

Fig. 20-12 The person's arm is washed with firm, long strokes using a mitted washcloth.

Fig. 20-11 Wash the person's eyes with a mitted washcloth. Wipe from the inner to the outer aspect of the eye.

Fig. 20-13 The person's hand is washed by placing the wash basin on the bed.

Fig. 20-14 The person's breasts are not exposed during the bath. A bath towel is placed horizontally over the chest area. The towel is lifted slightly to reach under to wash the breasts and chest.

Fig. 20-15 The bath towel is turned so that it is vertical to cover the breasts and abdomen. The towel is lifted slightly to bathe the abdomen. The bath blanket covers the pubic area.

Fig. 20-16 The foot is washed by placing it in the wash basin on the bed.

Fig. 20-17 The back is washed with long, firm, continuous strokes. Note that the person is in a side-lying position. A towel is placed length-wise on the bed to protect the linens from water.

Towel Baths

For a towel bath, an over-sized towel is used. It covers the body from the neck to the feet. The towel is completely wet with a solution—water and cleaning, skin-softening, and drying agents. The drying agent promotes fast drying of the person's body. The nurse and care plan tell you when to use a towel bath. To give a towel bath, follow center policy.

See *Residents With Dementia: Towel Baths.*

Bag Baths

Bag baths are commercially prepared or prepared at the center. A plastic bag has 8 to 10 washcloths. They are moistened with a cleaning agent that does not need rinsing. To give a towel bath:

- Warm the washcloths in a microwave oven. Follow the manufacturer's instructions for what microwave setting to use.
- Use a new washcloth for each body part.
- Let the skin air-dry. You do not need towels.

The Partial Bath

The *partial bath* involves bathing the face, hands, axillae (underarms), back, buttocks, and perineal area. Odors or discomfort occurs if these areas are not clean. Some persons bathe themselves in bed or at the sink. You assist as needed. Most need help washing the back. You give partial baths to persons who cannot bathe themselves.

The rules for bathing apply (see Box 20-1). So do the complete bed bath considerations.

 ASSISTING WITH THE PARTIAL BATH   VIDEO CLIP   VIDEO

QUALITY OF LIFE

Remember to:
- Knock before entering the person's room.
- Address the person by name.
- Introduce yourself by name and title.

- Explain the procedure to the person before beginning and during the procedure.
- Protect the person's rights during the procedure.
- Handle the person gently during the procedure.

PRE-PROCEDURE

1 Follow *Delegation Guidelines: Bathing*, p. 292. See *Promoting Safety and Comfort: Bathing*, p. 293.

2 Follow steps 2 through 7 in procedure: *Giving a Complete Bed Bath*, p. 294.

Continued

ASSISTING WITH THE PARTIAL BATH—cont'd

PROCEDURE

3 Make sure the bed is in the lowest position.
4 Decontaminate your hands. Put on gloves.
5 Cover the person with a bath blanket. Remove top linens.
6 Fill the wash basin ⅔ (two-thirds) full with water. Water temperature is usually 110° to 115° F (43.3° to 46.1° C) or as directed by the nurse. Measure water temperature with the bath thermometer. Or test bath water by dipping your elbow or inner wrist into the basin.
7 Ask the person to check the water temperature. Adjust the water temperature if it is too hot or too cold.
8 Place the basin on the overbed table.
9 Position the person in Fowler's position. Or assist him or her to sit at the bedside.
10 Adjust the overbed table so the person can reach the basin and supplies.
11 Help the person undress. Provide for privacy and warmth with the bath blanket.
12 Ask the person to wash easy-to-reach body parts (Fig. 20-18). Explain that you will wash the back and areas the person cannot reach.
13 Place the signal light within reach. Ask him or her to signal when help is needed or bathing is complete.

14 Decontaminate your hands. Then leave the room.
15 Return when the signal light is on. Knock before entering. Decontaminate your hands.
16 Change the bath water. Measure bath water temperature as in step 6.
17 Raise the bed for body mechanics. The far bed rail is up if used.
18 Ask what was washed. Put on gloves. Wash and dry areas the person could not reach. The face, hands, underarms, back, buttocks, and perineal area are washed for the partial bath.
19 Remove the gloves. Decontaminate your hands.
20 Give a back massage (p. 302).
21 Apply lotion, powder, and deodorant or antiperspirant as requested.
22 Help the person put on clean garments.
23 Assist with hair care and other grooming needs.
24 Assist the person to a chair. (Lower the bed if the person transfers to a chair.) Or turn the person onto the side away from you.
25 Make the bed. (Raise the bed for body mechanics.)

POST-PROCEDURE

26 Provide for comfort. (See the inside of the front book cover.)
27 Place the signal light within reach.
28 Lower the bed to its lowest position.
29 Raise or lower bed rails. Follow the care plan.
30 Put on clean gloves.
31 Empty, clean, and dry the bath basin. Return the basin and supplies to their proper place.

32 Wipe off the overbed table with the paper towels. Discard the paper towels.
33 Unscreen the person.
34 Complete a safety check of the room. (See the inside of the front book cover.)
35 Follow center policy for dirty linen.
36 Remove the gloves. Decontaminate your hands.
37 Report and record your observations.

Fig. 20-18 The person is bathing himself while sitting on the side of the bed. Necessary equipment is within his reach.

Tub Baths and Showers

Some people like tub baths. Others like showers. Falls, burns, and chilling from water are risks. Safety is important (Box 20-2). The measures in Box 20-1 also apply. If other measures are needed, follow the nurse's directions and the care plan.

Some bathrooms have showers. If not, reserve the shower or tub room for the person.

Tub Baths Tub baths are relaxing. A tub bath can make a person feel faint, weak, or tired. These are great risks for persons who were on bedrest. A tub bath lasts no longer than 20 minutes.

The person may need one of these devices to get in and out of the tub:

- Transfer bench (Fig. 20-19, p. 300).
- A tub with a side entry door (Fig. 20-20, p. 300).
- Wheelchair or stretcher lift. The person is transferred to the tub room by wheelchair or stretcher. Then the device and person are lifted into the tub (Fig. 20-21, p. 300).
- Mechanical lift (Chapter 17).

Whirlpool tubs have a cleansing action. You wash the upper body. Carefully wash under the breasts and between skin folds. Also wash the perineal area. Pat dry the person with towels after the bath.

Showers Some people can stand and use a regular shower. They use the grab bars for support during the shower. Like tubs, showers have non-skid surfaces. If not, a bath mat is used. Never let weak or unsteady persons stand in the shower. They need to use one of the following:

- *Shower chairs.* Water drains through an opening (Fig. 20-22, p. 300). You use the chair to transport the person to and from the shower. Lock the wheels during the shower to prevent the chair from moving.
- *Shower stalls or cabinets.* The person walks into the device or is wheeled in on a wheelchair (Fig. 20-23, p. 300). Use the hand-held nozzle.
- *Shower trolleys (portable tubs).* The person has a shower lying down (Fig. 20-24, p. 300). You lower the sides to transfer the person from the bed to the trolley. Raise the side rails after the transfer. Then transport the person to the tub or shower room. Use the hand-held nozzle to give the shower in the usual manner.

Some shower rooms have two or more stations. Provide for privacy. The person has the right not to have his or her body seen by others. Properly screen and cover the person. Also close doors and the shower curtain.

See *Delegation Guidelines: Tub Baths and Showers,* p. 301.

See *Promoting Safety and Comfort: Tub Baths and Showers,* p. 301.

See *Teamwork and Time Management: Tub Baths and Showers,* p. 301.

Text continued on p. 302

Box 20-2 Safety Measures for Tub Baths and Showers

- Know what water temperature to use. See *Delegation Guidelines: Tub Baths and Showers,* p. 301.
- Clean and disinfect the tub or shower before and after use.
- Dry the tub or shower room floor.
- Check handrails, grab bars, hydraulic lifts, and other safety aids. They must be in working order.
- Place a bath mat in the tub or on the shower floor. This is not needed if there are non-skid strips or a non-skid surface.
- Cover the person for warmth and privacy. This includes during transport to and from the shower or tub room.
- Place needed items within the person's reach.
- Place the signal light within the person's reach.
- Show the person how to use the signal light in the shower or tub room.
- Have the person use the grab bars when getting in and out of the tub. The person must not use towel bars for support.
- Turn cold water on first, then hot water. Turn hot water off first, then the cold water.
- Adjust water temperature and pressure to prevent chilling or burns. Do this before the person gets into the shower. If a shower chair is used, position it first.

- Direct water away from the person while adjusting water temperature and pressure.
- Fill the tub before the person gets into it.
- Measure the water temperature. For showers and tub baths, use the digital display. Or you can use a bath thermometer for a tub bath.
- Keep the water spray directed toward the person during the shower. This helps keep him or her warm. (NOTE: Do not direct the water spray toward the person's face. This can frighten the person.)
- Keep bar soap in the soap dish between latherings. This prevents soapy water. It reduces the risk of slipping and falls in showers and tubs.
- Avoid using bath oils. They make tub and shower surfaces slippery.
- Do not leave weak or unsteady persons unattended.
- Stay within hearing distance if the person can be left alone. Wait outside the shower curtain or door. You will be nearby if the person calls for you or has an accident.
- Drain the tub before the person gets out of the tub. Turn off the shower before the person gets out of the shower. Cover him or her to provide privacy and prevent chilling.

Fig. 20-19 A transfer bench is positioned for the person's use in getting into and out of the tub. A floor mat is in front of the tub.

Fig. 20-20 Tub with a side entry door. *(Courtesy ARJO, Inc., Roselle, Ill. [800]323-1245)*

Fig. 20-21 The stretcher and person are lowered into the tub.

Fig. 20-22 A shower chair in a shower stall.

Fig. 20-23 A shower cabinet.

Fig. 20-24 Shower trolley. The sides are lowered for transfers into and out of the trolley. *(Courtesy ARJO, Inc., Roselle, Ill. [800]323-1245)*

DELEGATION GUIDELINES
Tub Baths and Showers

Before assisting with a tub bath or shower, you need this information from the nurse and the care plan:

- If the person takes a tub bath or shower
- What water temperature to use (usually 105° F; 40.5° C)
- What equipment is needed—shower chair, shower cabinet, shower trolley, and so on
- How much help the person needs
- If the person can bathe himself or herself
- What observations to report and record:
  - Dizziness
  - Light-headedness
  - See *Delegation Guidelines: Bathing,* p. 292
- When to report observations
- What specific resident concerns to report at once

TEAMWORK AND TIME MANAGEMENT
Tub Baths and Showers

Most centers do not have tub and shower equipment for each person. You need to reserve the room and needed equipment for the person. Your co-workers do the same for their residents. Consider the needs of others. For example, you reserve the shower room from 0945 to 1030. Do your very best to follow the schedule. Make sure the shower room is clean and ready for the next person. Or you and a co-worker schedule something for the same time. Plan a new schedule with your co-worker.

All bed linens are changed on the person's bath or shower day. Ask co-workers to make the person's bed while you assist with the tub bath or shower. Also ask them to straighten the person's unit. The person returns to a clean bed and unit. Return the favor when your co-workers are assisting with tub baths, showers, or other care measures.

PROMOTING SAFETY AND COMFORT
Tub Baths and Showers

Safety
Some persons are very weak. At least two persons are needed to safely assist them with tub baths and showers. If the person is heavy, 3 staff members may be needed.

The person may use a tub with a side entry door, a shower chair, a shower trolley, or other device. Always follow the manufacturer's instructions.

Protect the person from falls, chilling, and burns. Follow the safety measures in Chapters 12 and 13. Remember to measure water temperature.

Clean and disinfect the tub or shower before and after use. This prevents the spread of microbes and infection.

Comfort
Warmth and privacy promote comfort during tub baths and showers. You need to:
- Make sure the tub or shower room is warm.
- Provide for privacy. Close the room door, screen the person, and close window coverings.
- Make sure water temperature is warm enough for the person.
- Have the person remove his or her clothing or robe and footwear just before getting into the tub or shower. Do not let the person remain exposed longer than necessary.
- Leave the room if the person can be alone.

 ## ASSISTING WITH A TUB BATH OR SHOWER

QUALITY OF LIFE

Remember to:
- Knock before entering the person's room.
- Address the person by name.
- Introduce yourself by name and title.

- Explain the procedure to the person before beginning and during the procedure.
- Protect the person's rights during the procedure.
- Handle the person gently during the procedure.

PRE-PROCEDURE

1 Follow *Delegation Guidelines:*
   a *Bathing,* p. 292
   b *Tub Baths and Showers*
   See *Promoting Safety and Comfort:*
   a *Bathing,* p. 292
   b *Tub Baths and Showers*
2 Reserve the bathtub or shower.
3 Practice hand hygiene.
4 Identify the person. Check the ID bracelet against the assignment sheet. Also call the person by name.

5 Collect the following:
- Washcloth and two bath towels
- Soap
- Bath thermometer (for a tub bath)
- Clothing or sleepwear
- Grooming items as requested
- Robe and non-skid footwear
- Rubber bath mat if needed
- Disposable bath mat
- Gloves
- Wheelchair, shower chair, transfer bench, and so on as needed

Continued

ASSISTING WITH A TUB BATH OR SHOWER—cont'd

PROCEDURE

6 Place items in the tub or shower room. Use the space provided or a chair.
7 Clean and disinfect the tub or shower.
8 Place a rubber bath mat in the tub or on the shower floor. Do not block the drain.
9 Place the disposable bath mat on the floor in the front of the tub or shower.
10 Put the OCCUPIED sign on the door.
11 Return to the person's room. Provide for privacy. Decontaminate your hands.
12 Help the person sit on the side of the bed.
13 Help the person put on a robe and non-skid footwear. Or the person can leave on clothing.
14 Assist or transport the person to the tub room or shower.
15 Have the person sit on a chair if he or she walked to the tub or shower room.
16 Provide for privacy.
17 *For a tub bath:*
 a Fill the tub half-way with warm water (usually 105° F; 40.5° C). Follow the care plan for water temperature.
 b Measure water temperature. Use the bath thermometer or check the digital display.
 c Ask the person to check the water temperature. Adjust the water temperature if it is too hot or too cold.
18 *For a shower:*
 a Turn on the shower.
 b Adjust water temperature and pressure. Check the digital display.
 c Ask the person to check the water temperature. Adjust the water temperature if it is too hot or too cold.

19 Help the person undress and remove footwear.
20 Help the person into the tub or shower. Position the shower chair, and lock the wheels.
21 Assist with washing as necessary. Wear gloves.
22 Ask the person to use the signal light when done or when help is needed. Remind the person that a tub bath lasts no longer than 20 minutes.
23 Place a towel across the chair.
24 Leave the room if the person can bathe alone. If not, stay in the room or nearby. Remove the gloves and decontaminate your hands if you will leave the room.
25 Check the person at least every 5 minutes.
26 Return when he or she signals for you. Knock before entering. Decontaminate your hands.
27 Turn off the shower, or drain the tub. Cover the person while the tub drains.
28 Help the person out of the shower or tub and onto the chair.
29 Help the person dry off. Pat gently. Dry under the breasts, between skin folds, in the perineal area, and between the toes.
30 Assist with lotion and other grooming items as needed.
31 Help the person dress and put on footwear.
32 Help the person return to the room. Provide for privacy.
33 Assist the person to a chair or into bed.
34 Provide a back massage if the person returns to bed.
35 Assist with hair care and other grooming needs.

POST-PROCEDURE

36 Provide for comfort. (See the inside of the front book cover.)
37 Place the signal light within reach.
38 Raise or lower bed rails. Follow the care plan.
39 Unscreen the person.
40 Complete a safety check of the room. (See the inside of the front book cover.)

41 Clean and disinfect the tub or shower. Remove soiled linen. Wear gloves.
42 Discard disposable items. Put the UNOCCUPIED sign on the door. Return supplies to their proper place.
43 Follow center policy for dirty linen.
44 Remove the gloves. Decontaminate your hands.
45 Report and record your observations.

THE BACK MASSAGE

The back massage (back rub) relaxes muscles and stimulates circulation. You give back massages after baths and showers and with evening care. You also give them at other times. Examples include after re-positioning or helping the person to relax.

Back massages last 3 to 5 minutes. Observe the skin before the massage. Look for breaks in the skin, bruises, reddened areas, and other signs of skin breakdown.

Lotion reduces friction during the massage. It is warmed before being applied. To warm lotion, do one of the following:

• Rub some lotion between your hands.
• Place the bottle in the bath water.
• Hold the bottle under warm water.

Use firm strokes. Also keep your hands in contact with the person's skin. After the massage, apply some lotion to the elbows, knees, and heels. This keeps the skin soft. These bony areas are at risk for skin breakdown.

See *Delegation Guidelines: The Back Massage.*
See *Promoting Safety and Comfort: The Back Massage.*

DELEGATION GUIDELINES
The Back Massage

Before giving a back massage, you need this information from the nurse and the care plan:
- If the person can have a back massage (see *Promoting Safety and Comfort: The Back Massage*)
- How to position the person
- If the person has position limits
- When the person is to receive a back massage
- If the person needs frequent back massages for comfort and to relax

- What observations to report and record:
  - Breaks in the skin
  - Bruising
  - Reddened areas
  - Signs of skin breakdown
- When to report observations
- What specific resident concerns to report at once

PROMOTING SAFETY AND COMFORT
The Back Massage

Safety

Back massages are dangerous for persons with certain heart and kidney diseases, back injuries, back and other surgeries, skin diseases, and lung disorders. Check with the nurse and the care plan before giving back massages to persons with these conditions.

Do not massage reddened bony areas. Reddened areas signal skin breakdown and pressure ulcers. Massage can lead to more tissue damage.

Wear gloves if the person's skin is not intact. Always follow Standard Precautions and the Bloodborne Pathogen Standard.

Comfort

The prone position is best for a massage. The side-lying position is often used. Older and disabled persons usually find the side-lying position more comfortable.

The back massage involves stroking down the back and over the buttocks. Some persons may not want the buttocks exposed and touched for massage. Explain the procedure to the person. Obtain the person's consent to expose and touch the buttocks. If the person does not give consent, modify the procedure as in step 14 in procedure: *Giving a Back Massage*.

 GIVING A BACK MASSAGE

QUALITY OF LIFE

Remember to:
- Knock before entering the person's room.
- Address the person by name.
- Introduce yourself by name and title.

- Explain the procedure to the person before beginning and during the procedure.
- Protect the person's rights during the procedure.
- Handle the person gently during the procedure.

PRE-PROCEDURE

1 Follow *Delegation Guidelines: The Back Massage*. See *Promoting Safety and Comfort: The Back Massage*.
2 Practice hand hygiene.
3 Identify the person. Check the ID bracelet against the assignment sheet. Also call the person by name.

4 Collect the following:
- Bath blanket
- Bath towel
- Lotion
5 Provide for privacy.
6 Raise the bed for body mechanics. Bed rails are up if used.

Continued

GIVING A BACK MASSAGE—cont'd

PROCEDURE

7 Lower the bed rail near you if up.

8 Position the person in the prone or side-lying position. The back is toward you.

9 Expose the back, shoulders, upper arms, and buttocks. Cover the rest of the body with the bath blanket. Expose the buttocks only if the person gives consent.

10 Lay the towel on the bed along the back. Do this if the person is in a side-lying position.

11 Warm the lotion.

12 Explain that the lotion may feel cool and wet.

13 Apply lotion to the lower back area.

14 Stroke up from the buttocks to the shoulders. Then stroke down over the upper arms. Stroke up the upper arms, across the shoulders, and down the back to the buttocks (Fig. 20-25). Use firm strokes. Keep your hands in contact with the person's skin. If the person does not want the buttocks exposed, stroke down the back to the waist and up the back to the shoulders.

15 Repeat step 14 for at least 3 minutes.

16 Knead the back (Fig. 20-26):
  a Grasp the skin between your thumb and fingers.
  b Knead half of the back. Start at the buttocks and move up to the shoulder. Then knead down from the shoulder to the buttocks.
  c Repeat on the other half of the back.

17 Apply lotion to bony areas. Use circular motions with the tips of your index and middle fingers. (Do not massage reddened bony areas.)

18 Use fast movements to stimulate. Use slow movements to relax the person.

19 Stroke with long, firm movements to end the massage. Tell the person you are finishing.

20 Straighten and secure clothing or sleepwear.

21 Cover the person. Remove the towel and bath blanket.

POST-PROCEDURE

22 Provide for comfort. (See the inside of the front book cover.)

23 Place the signal light within reach.

24 Lower the bed to its lowest position.

25 Raise or lower bed rails. Follow the care plan.

26 Return lotion to its proper place.

27 Unscreen the person.

28 Complete a safety check of the room. (See the inside of the front book cover.)

29 Follow center policy for dirty linen.

30 Decontaminate your hands.

31 Report and record your observations.

Fig. 20-25 The person lies in the prone position for a back massage. Stroke upward from the buttocks to the shoulders, down over the upper arms, back up the upper arms, across the shoulders, and down the back to the buttocks.

Fig. 20-26 Kneading is done by picking up tissue between the thumb and fingers.

PERINEAL CARE

Perineal care (pericare) involves cleaning the genital and anal areas. These areas provide a warm, moist, and dark place for microbes to grow. Cleaning prevents infection and odors, and it promotes comfort.

Perineal care is done daily during the bath. It also is done whenever the area is soiled with urine or feces. Perineal care is very important for persons who:

- Have urinary catheters (Chapter 22).
- Have had rectal or genital surgery.
- Are menstruating (Chapter 9).
- Are incontinent of urine or feces.
- Are uncircumcised. Being *circumcised* means that the fold of skin (foreskin) covering the head of the penis was surgically removed. Being *uncircumcised* means that the person has foreskin covering the head of the penis.

The person does perineal care if able. Otherwise, it is given by the nursing staff. This procedure embarrasses many people and nursing staff, especially when it involves the other sex.

Perineal and *perineum* are not common terms. Most people understand *privates, private parts, crotch, genitals,* or the *area between the legs.* Use terms the person understands. The term must be in good taste professionally.

Standard Precautions, medical asepsis, and the Bloodborne Pathogen Standard are followed. Work from the cleanest area to the dirtiest. This is commonly called cleaning from "front to back." The urethral area (the front) is the cleanest. The anal area (the back) is the dirtiest. Therefore clean from the urethra to the anal area. This prevents the transmission of bacteria from the anal area to the vagina and urinary system.

The perineal area is delicate and easily injured. Use warm water, not hot. Use washcloths, towelettes, cotton balls, or swabs according to center policy. Rinse thoroughly. Pat dry after rinsing. This reduces moisture and promotes comfort.

See *Focus on Communication: Perineal Care.*
See *Delegation Guidelines: Perineal Care.*
See *Promoting Safety and Comfort: Perineal Care,* p. 306.

Text continued on p. 309

FOCUS ON COMMUNICATION
Perineal Care

Talking to the person about perineal care may be difficult. You may be embarrassed. However, you must explain the procedure to the person.

When a person performs his or her own perineal care, you can say:

- "Mrs. Bell, I'll give you some privacy while you finish your bath. Can you reach everything you need? Please call me if you need help. Here is your signal light."
- "Mr. Monroe, I'll give you time to finish your bath. Please wash your genital and rectal areas. Signal for me when you're done or need help."

If you provide perineal care for the person, you can say:

- "Mrs. Allan, next I'll clean between your legs. I'll keep you covered with the bath blanket. I'll tell you before I touch you. Please tell me if you feel any pain or discomfort."
- "Mr. Scott, I'll clean your private parts now. Please let me know if you feel any pain or discomfort."

DELEGATION GUIDELINES
Perineal Care

Before giving perineal care, you need this information from the nurse and the care plan:

- When to give perineal care.
- What terms the person understands—perineum, privates, private parts, crotch, genitals, area between the legs, and so on.
- How much help the person needs.
- What water temperature to use—usually 105° to 109° F (40.5° to 42.7° C). Water in a basin cools rapidly.
- What cleaning agent to use.
- Any position restrictions or limits.
- What observations to report and record:
  - Odors
  - Redness, swelling, discharge, bleeding, or irritation
  - Complaints of pain, burning, or other discomfort
  - Signs of urinary or fecal incontinence
- When to report observations.
- What specific resident concerns to report at once.

PROMOTING SAFETY AND COMFORT
Perineal Care

Safety

Hot water can burn delicate perineal tissues. To prevent burns, measure water temperature according to center policy. If the water seems too hot, ask the nurse to check it.

Protect yourself and the person from infection. Contact with blood, body fluids, secretions, or excretions is likely during perineal care. Follow Standard Precautions and the Bloodborne Pathogen Standard.

Persons who are incontinent need perineal care. Protect the person and dry garments and linens from the wet or soiled items. After cleaning and drying the perineal area, remove the wet or soiled incontinence products, garments, and linen. Then apply clean, dry ones.

Comfort

To avoid embarrassment, it is best if the person does perineal care. If you provide this care, explain how privacy is protected. Act in a professional manner at all times.

Perineal care involves touching the genital and anal areas. The person may prefer that someone of the same sex provide this care. Or the person may fear sexual assault. Always obtain the person's consent before providing perineal care. For mental comfort, the person may want a family member or another staff member present to witness the procedure. Ask if he or she wants someone present and that person's name.

Fig. 20-27 Draping for perineal care. **A,** Position the bath blanket like a diamond: one corner is at the neck, there is a corner at each side, and one corner is between the person's legs. **B,** Wrap the blanket around the leg by bringing the corner around under the leg and over the top. Tuck the corner under the hip.

Fig. 20-28 Separate the labia with one hand. Use a mitted washcloth to cleanse between the labia with downward strokes.

Fig. 20-29 The rectal area is cleaned by wiping from the vagina to the anus. The side-lying position allows the anal area to be cleaned more thoroughly.

GIVING FEMALE PERINEAL CARE

QUALITY OF LIFE

Remember to:
- Knock before entering the person's room.
- Address the person by name.
- Introduce yourself by name and title.

- Explain the procedure to the person before beginning and during the procedure.
- Protect the person's rights during the procedure.
- Handle the person gently during the procedure.

PRE-PROCEDURE

1 Follow *Delegation Guidelines: Perineal Care*, p. 305. See *Promoting Safety and Comfort: Perineal Care*.
2 Practice hand hygiene.
3 Collect the following:
- Soap or other cleaning agent as directed
- At least 4 washcloths
- Bath towel
- Bath blanket
- Bath thermometer
- Wash basin
- Waterproof pad
- Gloves
- Paper towels

4 Cover the overbed table with paper towels. Arrange items on top of them.
5 Identify the person. Check the ID bracelet against the assignment sheet. Also call the person by name.
6 Provide for privacy.
7 Raise the bed for body mechanics. Bed rails are up if used.

PROCEDURE

8 Lower the bed rail near you if up.
9 Decontaminate your hands. Put on gloves.
10 Cover the person with a bath blanket. Move top linens to the foot of the bed.
11 Position the person on the back.
12 Drape the person as in Figure 20-27.
13 Raise the bed rail if used.
14 Fill the wash basin. Water temperature is usually 105° to 109° F (40.5° to 42.7° C). Follow the care plan for water temperature. Measure water temperature according to center policy.
15 Ask the person to check the water temperature. Adjust the water temperature if it is too hot or too cold. Raise the bed rail before leaving the bedside. Lower it when you return.
16 Place the basin on the overbed table.
17 Lower the bed rail if up.
18 Help the person flex her knees and spread her legs. Or help her spread her legs as much as possible with the knees straight.
19 Place a waterproof pad under her buttocks. Protect the person and dry linen from the wet or soiled incontinence product.
20 Fold the corner of the bath blanket between her legs onto her abdomen.
21 Wet the washcloths.
22 Squeeze out excess water from a washcloth. Make a mitted washcloth. Apply soap.
23 Separate the labia. Clean downward from front to back with one stroke (Fig. 20-28).

24 Repeat steps 22 and 23 until the area is clean. Use a clean part of the washcloth for each stroke. Use more than one washcloth if needed.
25 Rinse the perineum with a clean washcloth. Separate the labia. Stroke downward from front to back. Repeat as necessary. Use a clean part of the washcloth for each stroke. Use more than one washcloth if needed.
26 Pat the area dry with the towel. Dry from front to back.
27 Fold the blanket back between her legs.
28 Help the person lower her legs and turn onto her side away from you.
29 Apply soap to a mitted washcloth.
30 Clean the rectal area. Clean from the vagina to the anus with one stroke (Fig. 20-29).
31 Repeat steps 29 and 30 until the area is clean. Use a clean part of the washcloth for each stroke. Use more than one washcloth if needed.
32 Rinse the rectal area with a washcloth. Stroke from the vagina to the anus. Repeat as necessary. Use a clean part of the washcloth for each stroke. Use more than one washcloth if needed.
33 Pat the area dry with the towel. Dry from front to back.
34 Remove any wet or soiled incontinence product. Remove the waterproof pad.
35 Remove and discard the gloves. Decontaminate your hands. Put on clean gloves.
36 Provide clean and dry linens and incontinence products as needed.

Continued

GIVING FEMALE PERINEAL CARE—cont'd

POST-PROCEDURE

37 Cover the person. Remove the bath blanket.
38 Provide for comfort. (See the inside of the front book cover.)
39 Place the signal light within reach.
40 Lower the bed to its lowest position.
41 Raise or lower bed rails. Follow the care plan.
42 Empty, clean, and dry the wash basin.
43 Return the basin and supplies to their proper place.

44 Wipe off the overbed table with the paper towels. Discard the paper towels.
45 Unscreen the person.
46 Complete a safety check of the room. (See the inside of the front book cover.)
47 Follow center policy for dirty linen.
48 Remove the gloves. Decontaminate your hands.
49 Report and record your observations.

GIVING MALE PERINEAL CARE

QUALITY OF LIFE

Remember to:
- Knock before entering the person's room.
- Address the person by name.
- Introduce yourself by name and title.

- Explain the procedure to the person before beginning and during the procedure.
- Protect the person's rights during the procedure.
- Handle the person gently during the procedure.

PROCEDURE

1 Follow steps 1 through 17 in procedure: *Giving Female Perineal Care*, p. 307. Drape the person as in Figure 20-27.
2 Place a waterproof pad under his buttocks. Protect the person and dry linen from the wet or soiled incontinence product.
3 Retract the foreskin if the person is uncircumcised (Fig. 20-30).
4 Grasp the penis.
5 Clean the tip. Use a circular motion. Start at the meatus of the urethra, and work outward (Fig. 20-31). Repeat as needed. Use a clean part of the washcloth each time.
6 Rinse the area with another washcloth.
7 Return the foreskin to its natural position immediately after rinsing.
8 Clean the shaft of the penis. Use firm downward strokes. Rinse the area.

9 Help the person flex his knees and spread his legs. Or help him spread his legs as much as possible with his knees straight.
10 Clean the scrotum. Rinse well. Observe for redness and irritation of the skin folds.
11 Pat dry the penis and the scrotum. Use the towel.
12 Fold the bath blanket back between his legs.
13 Help him lower his legs and turn onto his side away from you.
14 Clean the rectal area (see procedure: *Giving Female Perineal Care*, p. 307). (NOTE: For males, clean from the scrotum to the anus.) Rinse and dry well.
15 Remove any wet or soiled incontinence product. Remove the waterproof pad.
16 Remove and discard the gloves. Decontaminate your hands. Put on clean gloves.
17 Provide clean and dry linens and incontinence products.

POST-PROCEDURE

18 Follow steps 37 through 49 in procedure: *Giving Female Perineal Care*.

Fig. 20-30 The foreskin of the uncircumcised male is pulled back for perineal care. It is returned to the normal position immediately after cleaning and rinsing.

Fig. 20-31 The penis is cleaned with circular motions starting at the meatus.

REPORTING AND RECORDING

You make many observations while assisting with hygiene. Report the following at once:

- Bleeding
- Signs of skin breakdown
- Discharge from the vagina or urinary tract
- Unusual odors
- Changes from prior observations

Also report and record the care given (Fig. 20-32). If care is not recorded, it is assumed that care was not given. This can cause serious legal problems.

Activities-of-Daily-Living Flow Sheet

JAN FEB MAR APR MAY JUN JUL AUG SEP (OCT) NOV DEC

ORDER/INSTRUCTION	TIME	1	2	3	4	5	6	7	8	9	10	11	12	13	14	15	16	17	18	19	20	21	22	23	24	25	26	27	28	29	30	31
Oral Care	11-7																																
Own/Dentures/None I=Independent S=Set up	7-3	S	S	S																													
A=Assist	3-11	S	S	S																													
Hygiene, Washing Face	11-7	/	/	/																													
and Hands I=Independent S=Set up	7-3	/	/	/																													
A=Assist T=Total Care	3-11	/	/	/																													
Bath and Shampoo every	11-7																																
Monday and _Thurs_ on __7-3__ shift	7-3	T																															
T=Tub S=Shower B=Bed bath	3-11																																
Back massage daily	11-7																																
	7-3																																
	3-11	√	√	√																													
Pericare	11-7	A	A	A																													
I=Independent S=Set up A=Assist T=Total Care	7-3																																
	3-11	A	A	A																													

Fig. 20-32 Charting sample.

QUALITY OF LIFE

Residents' rights serve to improve the person's quality of life, health, and safety. You must provide hygiene in a way that maintains or improves the person's quality of life, health, and safety. You must protect the person's rights when giving care.

To protect the right to privacy:

- Do not expose the person.
- Ask visitors to leave the room before you give care. A family member or friend may want to help. The person must consent to this.
- Close doors, privacy curtains, and window coverings.
- Expose only the body part involved in the procedure.
- Cover persons who are taken to and from tub or shower rooms. In some centers, residents wear their clothes to the shower or tub room. They put on clean clothes in the shower or tub room after the procedure.
- Protect the person from exposure when others are present. Some centers have more than one shower station.

Residents have the right to personal choice. They have the right to be involved in planning care and treatment. Hygiene is a very personal matter. Residents have a voice about when and how hygiene is done. Personal choice is allowed in such matters as bath time, products used, what to wear, and hair styling.

Residents have the right to keep and use personal items. You will handle the person's property during hygiene procedures. Protect dentures and eyeglasses from loss or breakage. If jewelry or religious items are removed for care, protect them from loss, damage, or theft.

Freedom from restraint is another resident right. Sometimes bed rails are restraints (Chapter 14). Follow the person's care plan for bed rail use.

REVIEW QUESTIONS

Circle T if the statement is TRUE. Circle F if the statement is FALSE.

1 T F   Hygiene is needed for comfort, safety, and health.
2 T F   After lunch, Mrs. Bell asks for a back massage. You can give the back massage.
3 T F   A toothbrush with hard bristles is good for oral hygiene.
4 T F   Unconscious persons are supine for mouth care.
5 T F   You use your fingers to keep an unconscious person's mouth open for oral hygiene.
6 T F   A person has a lower denture. You clean it over a counter.
7 T F   Bath oils cleanse and soften the skin.
8 T F   Powders absorb moisture and prevent friction.
9 T F   Deodorants reduce the amount of perspiration.
10 T F   A tub bath lasts 30 minutes.
11 T F   You can give permission for showers but not tub baths.
12 T F   Weak persons are left alone in the shower if they are sitting.
13 T F   A back massage relaxes muscles and stimulates circulation.
14 T F   Perineal care helps prevent infection.
15 T F   Foreskin is returned to its normal position immediately after cleaning.

Circle the BEST answer.

16 Oral hygiene does the following *except*
  a Prevent mouth odors
  b Prevent infection
  c Increase comfort
  d Coat and dry the mouth

17 You brush a person's teeth and note the following. Which is *not* reported to the nurse?
  a Bleeding, swelling, or redness of the gums
  b Irritations, sores, or white patches in the mouth or on the tongue
  c Lips that are dry, cracked, swollen, or blistered
  d Food between the teeth

18 Which is *not* a purpose of bathing?
  a Increasing circulation
  b Promoting drying of the skin
  c Exercising body parts
  d Refreshing and relaxing the person

19 Soaps do the following *except*
  a Remove dirt and dead skin
  b Soften the skin
  c Remove skin oil
  d Dry the skin

20 Which action is *wrong* when bathing a person?
  a Covering the person for warmth and privacy
  b Rinsing the skin thoroughly to remove all soap
  c Washing from the dirtiest to the cleanest area
  d Patting the skin dry

21 Water for a complete bed bath is at least
  a 100° F
  b 105° F
  c 110° F
  d 120° F

22 You are going to give a back massage. Which is *false*?
  a It should last 3 to 5 minutes.
  b Lotion is warmed before being applied.
  c Your hands are always in contact with the skin.
  d The side-lying position is best.

Answers to these questions are on p. 720.

Grooming

OBJECTIVES

- Define the key terms and key abbreviations listed in this chapter.
- Explain why grooming is important.
- Identify the factors that affect hair care.
- Explain how to care for matted and tangled hair.
- Describe how to shampoo hair.
- Describe the measures practiced when shaving a person.

- Explain why nail and foot care are important.
- Describe the rules for changing clothing and gowns.
- Perform the procedures described in this chapter.
- Explain how to promote quality of life.

KEY TERMS

alopecia Hair loss

anticoagulant A drug that prevents or slows down *(anti)* blood clotting *(coagulate)*

dandruff Excessive amounts of dry, white flakes from the scalp

hirsutism Excessive body hair

lice See "pediculosis"

mite A very small spider-like organism

pediculosis Infestation with wingless insects; lice

pediculosis capitis Infestation of the scalp *(capitis)* with lice; head lice

pediculosis corporis Infestation of the body *(corporis)* with lice

pediculosis pubis Infestation of the pubic *(pubis)* hair with lice

KEY ABBREVIATIONS

C	Centigrade	ID	Identification
F	Fahrenheit	IV	Intravenous

Hair care, shaving, and nail and foot care are important to many residents. Like hygiene, these grooming measures prevent infection and promote comfort. They also affect love, belonging, and self-esteem needs.

People differ in their grooming measures. Some want only clean hair. Others want a certain hair style. Some want only clean hands. Others want clean, manicured, and polished nails. Many men shave and groom their beards. Likewise, many women shave their legs and underarms. Some women have facial hair. They may shave or use other hair removal methods.

See *Focus on Rehabilitation: Grooming.*

See *Teamwork and Time Management: Grooming.*

FOCUS ON REHABILITATION
Grooming

As with hygiene, the person should tend to grooming measures to the extent possible. This promotes the person's independence and quality of life. The person may use adaptive devices for hair care and dressing. See Figure 21-1 for examples.

TEAMWORK AND TIME MANAGEMENT
Grooming

Some equipment for grooming procedures is shared among residents. Shampoo trays, electric shavers, and whirlpool foot baths are examples. Let other team members know when you need to use an item. Schedule use of the item following center policy. After the procedure, clean and promptly return the item to its proper place. Do not make your co-workers look for or clean an item.

HAIR CARE

How the hair looks and feels affects mental well-being. Some people cannot perform hair care. You assist with hair care whenever needed.

The nursing process reflects the person's culture, personal choice, skin and scalp condition, health history, and self-care ability. Many nursing centers have beauty and barber shops for residents (Fig. 21-2). Residents can have their hair shampooed, cut, and styled. Men also can have their mustaches and beards groomed.

Fig. 21-1 Grooming aids. **A,** Long-handled combs and brushes are used for hair care. **B,** A button hook is used to button and zip clothing. **C,** A sock assist is used to pull on socks and stockings. **D,** A shoe remover is used to take off shoes. *(From North Coast Medical Inc., Morgan Hill, Calif.)*

Fig. 21-2 Beauty shop in a nursing center.

Skin and Scalp Conditions

Skin and scalp conditions include hair loss, excessive body hair, dandruff, lice, and scabies.

See *Focus on Communication: Skin and Scalp Conditions.*

Alopecia, Hirsutism, and Dandruff Alopecia means hair loss. Hair loss may be complete or partial. Male pattern baldness occurs with aging. It results from heredity. Hair also thins in some women with aging. Cancer treatments (radiation therapy to the head and chemotherapy) often cause alopecia in males and females. Skin disease is another cause. Stress, poor nutrition, pregnancy, some drugs, and hormone changes are other causes. Except for hair loss from aging, hair usually grows back.

Hirsutism is excessive body hair. It can occur in women and children. It results from heredity and abnormal amounts of male hormones.

Dandruff is the excessive amount of dry, white flakes from the scalp. Itching often occurs. Sometimes eyebrows and ear canals are involved. Medicated shampoos correct the problem.

Lice Pediculosis (lice) is the infestation with wingless insects (*lice*). See Figure 21-3. *Infestation* means being in or on a host. Lice attach their eggs (*nits*) to hair shafts. Nits are oval and yellow to white in color. They hatch in about one week.

After hatching, lice feed on blood to live. Therefore they bite the scalp or skin. Adult lice are about the size of a sesame seed. They are tan to grayish-white in color. Lice bites cause severe itching in the affected body area.

- Pediculosis capitis is the infestation of the scalp (*capitis*) with lice. It is commonly called "head lice."
- Pediculosis pubis is the infestation of the pubic (*pubis*) hair with lice. This form of lice is also called "crabs."
- Pediculosis corporis is the infestation of the body (*corporis*) with lice.

Lice easily spread to others through clothing, head coverings, furniture, beds, towels, bed linen, and sexual

Fig. 21-3 Head lice. *(Redrawn from MedlinePlus: Head lice. Bethesda, Md, National Institutes of Health.)*

contact. They also are spread by sharing combs and brushes. Lice are treated with medicated shampoos, lotions, and creams. Thorough bathing is needed. So is washing clothing and linens in hot water.

Report signs and symptoms of lice to the nurse at once:

- Complaints of a tickling feeling or something moving in the hair
- Itching
- Irritability
- Sores on the head or body caused by scratching
- Rash

Scabies Scabies is a skin disorder caused by a female mite (Fig. 21-4, p. 314). A mite is a very small spider-like organism (Fig. 21-5, p. 314). The female mite burrows into the skin and lays eggs. When the eggs hatch, the females produce more eggs. The person becomes infested with mites.

The person has a rash and intense itching. Common sites are between the fingers, around the wrists, in the underarm area, on the thighs, and in the genital area. Other sites include the breasts, waist, and buttocks.

Scabies is highly contagious. It is transmitted to others by close contact. Persons living in crowded living settings are at risk. So are persons with weakened immune systems. Special creams are ordered to kill the mites. The person's room is cleaned. Clothing and linens are washed in hot water.

Fig. 21-4 Scabies. *(From Lookingbill and Marks' Principles of dermatology, ed. 4, St. Louis, 2006, Saunders.)*

Fig. 21-5 Dust mite. *(From Adkinson NF: Middleton's Allergy: Principles and Practice, ed. 7, St. Louis, 2008, Mosby.)*

Brushing and Combing Hair

Brushing and combing hair are part of early morning care, morning care, and afternoon care. And they are done whenever needed. Some people also brush and comb hair at bedtime. Make sure you complete hair care before visitors arrive.

Encourage residents to do their own hair care. Assist as needed. Perform hair care for those who cannot do so. The person chooses how to brush, comb, and style hair.

Brushing increases blood flow to the scalp. And it brings scalp oils along the hair shaft. Scalp oils help keep hair soft and shiny. Brushing and combing prevent tangled and matted hair. When brushing and combing hair, start at the scalp. Then brush or comb to the hair ends.

Long hair easily mats and tangles. Daily brushing and combing prevent the problem. So does braiding. You need the person's consent to braid hair. *Never cut matted or tangled hair. Never cut hair for any reason.* Tell the nurse if the person has matted or tangled hair. The nurse may have you comb or brush through the matting and tangling.

Special measures are needed for curly, coarse, and dry hair. Use a wide-tooth comb for curly hair. Start at the neckline. Working upward, lift and fluff hair outward. Continue to the forehead. Wet hair or apply conditioner or petroleum jelly as directed. This makes combing easier.

The person may have certain hair care practices and hair care products. They are part of the care plan. Also, let the person guide you when giving hair care.

See *Caring About Culture: Brushing and Combing Hair.*

See *Delegation Guidelines: Brushing and Combing Hair.*

See *Promoting Safety and Comfort: Brushing and Combing Hair.*

CARING ABOUT CULTURE
Brushing and Combing Hair

Styling hair in small braids is a common practice of some cultural groups. The braids are left intact for shampooing. To undo these braids, the nurse obtains the person's consent.

DELEGATION GUIDELINES
Brushing and Combing Hair

To brush and comb hair, you need this information from the nurse and the care plan:

- How much help the person needs
- What to do if hair is matted or tangled
- What to do for curly, coarse, or dry hair
- What hair care products to use
- The person's preferences and routine hair care measures
- What observations to report and record:
  - Scalp sores
  - Flaking
  - Itching
  - The presence of nits or lice
    - Nits (lice eggs attached to hair shafts)—oval and yellow to white in color
    - Lice—about the size of a sesame seed and grayish-white in color
  - Patches of hair loss
  - Hair falling out in patches
  - Very dry or very oily hair
  - Matted or tangled hair
- When to report observations
- What specific resident concerns to report at once

PROMOTING SAFETY AND COMFORT
Brushing and Combing Hair

Safety

Sharp bristles can injure the scalp. So can a comb with sharp or broken teeth. Tell the nurse if you have concerns about the person's brush or comb.

Comfort

When giving hair care, place a towel across the person's back and shoulders to protect garments from falling hair. If the person is in bed, give hair care before changing linens and the pillowcase. If done after a linen change, place a towel across the pillow to collect falling hair.

 BRUSHING AND COMBING THE PERSON'S HAIR

QUALITY OF LIFE

Remember to:

- Knock before entering the person's room.
- Address the person by name.
- Introduce yourself by name and title.

- Explain the procedure to the person before beginning and during the procedure.
- Protect the person's rights during the procedure.
- Handle the person gently during the procedure.

PRE-PROCEDURE

1 Follow *Delegation Guidelines: Brushing and Combing Hair.* See *Promoting Safety and Comfort: Brushing and Combing Hair.*
2 Practice hand hygiene.
3 Identify the person. Check the ID (identification) bracelet against the assignment sheet. Also call the person by name.

4 Ask the person how to style hair.
5 Collect the following:
   - Comb and brush
   - Bath towel
   - Other hair care items as requested
6 Arrange items on the bedside stand.
7 Provide for privacy.

PROCEDURE

8 Lower the bed rail if up.
9 Help the person to the chair. The person puts on a robe and non-skid footwear when up. (If the person is in bed, raise the bed for body mechanics. Bed rails are up if used. Lower the bed rail near you. Assist the person to a semi-Fowler's position if allowed.)
10 Place a towel across the person's back and shoulders or across the pillow.
11 Ask the person to remove eyeglasses. Put them in the eyeglass case. Put the case inside the bedside stand.

12 *Brush and comb hair that is __not__ matted or tangled:*
   a Use the comb to part the hair.
      (1) Part hair down the middle into 2 sides (Fig. 21-6, *A*, p. 316).
      (2) Divide one side into 2 smaller sections (Fig. 21-6, *B*, p. 316).
   b Brush one of the small sections of hair. Start at the scalp, and brush toward the hair ends (Fig. 21-7, p. 316). Do the same for the other small section of hair.
   c Repeat steps 12, a(2) and 12, b for the other side.

Continued

BRUSHING AND COMBING THE PERSON'S HAIR—cont'd

PROCEDURE—cont'd

13 *Brush and comb matted and tangled hair:*
  a Take a small section of hair near the ends.
  b Comb or brush through to the hair ends.
  c Add small sections of hair as you work up to the scalp.
  d Comb or brush through each longer section to the hair ends.
  e Brush or comb from the scalp to the hair ends.

14 Style the hair as the person prefers.
15 Remove the towel.
16 Let the person put on the eyeglasses.

POST-PROCEDURE

17 Provide for comfort. (See the inside of the front book cover.)
18 Place the signal light within reach.
19 Lower the bed to its lowest position.
20 Raise or lower bed rails. Follow the care plan.
21 Clean and return hair care items to their proper place.

22 Unscreen the person.
23 Complete a safety check of the room. (See the inside of the front book cover.)
24 Follow center policy for dirty linen.
25 Decontaminate your hands.

Fig. 21-6 Part hair. **A,** Part hair down the middle. Divide it into two sides. **B,** Then part one side into two smaller sections.

Fig. 21-7 Brush hair by starting at the scalp. Brush down to the hair ends.

🔹 SHAMPOOING

Oil gland secretion decreases with aging. Therefore older persons have dry hair. Shampooing frequency depends on the person's needs and preferences. Usually shampooing is done weekly on the person's bath day.

Some persons use certain shampoos and conditioners. Others used medicated products ordered by the doctor.

Residents usually need help with shampooing. If a woman's hair is done by a hairdresser, do not shampoo her hair. She wears a shower cap during the tub bath or shower.

The shampoo method depends on the person's condition, safety factors, and personal choice. The health team decides on the method to use.

- *Shampoo during the shower or tub bath.* The person shampoos in the shower. You use a hand-held nozzle for those using shower chairs or taking tub baths. You direct a spray of water at the hair.
- *Shampoo at the sink.* The person sits facing away from the sink. A folded towel is placed over the sink edge to protect the neck. The person's head is tilted back over the edge of the sink. You use a water pitcher or hand-held nozzle to wet and rinse the hair.
- *Shampoo on a stretcher.* The stretcher is in front of the sink. A towel is placed under the neck. The head is tilted over the edge of the sink (Fig. 21-8). You use a water pitcher or hand-held nozzle to wet and rinse the hair.
- *Shampoo in bed.* The person's head and shoulders are moved to the edge of the bed if possible. A shampoo tray is placed under the head to protect the linens and mattress from water. The tray drains into a basin placed on a chair by the bed (Fig. 21-9). You use a water pitcher to wet and rinse the hair. This method is used for persons who need complete bed baths. It also is used for persons who cannot use a chair, wheelchair, or stretcher.

Dry and style hair as quickly as possible after the shampoo. Women may want hair curled or rolled up before drying. Check with the nurse before doing so.

See *Delegation Guidelines: Shampooing.*

See *Promoting Safety and Comfort: Shampooing,* p. 318.

Fig. 21-8 Shampooing while the person is on a stretcher. The stretcher is in front of the sink.

Fig. 21-9 A shampoo tray is used to shampoo a person in bed. The tray is directed to the side of the bed so water drains into a collecting basin.

DELEGATION GUIDELINES
Shampooing

Before shampooing a person, you need this information from the nurse and the care plan:
- When to shampoo the person's hair
- What method to use
- What shampoo and conditioner to use
- The person's position restrictions or limits
- What water temperature to use—usually 105° F (Fahrenheit) (40.5° C [centigrade])
- If hair is curled or rolled up before drying
- What observations to report and record:
  - Scalp sores
  - Flaking
  - Itching
  - The presence of nits or lice
  - Patches of hair loss
  - Hair falling out in patches
  - Very dry or very oily hair
  - Matted or tangled hair
  - How the person tolerated the procedure
- When to report observations
- What specific resident concerns to report at once

PROMOTING SAFETY AND COMFORT
Shampooing

Safety

Keep shampoo away from and out of the eyes. Have the person hold a washcloth over the eyes. When rinsing, cup your hand at the person's forehead. This keeps soapy water from running down the person's forehead and into the eyes.

Return medicated products to the nurse. Never leave them at the bedside unless instructed to do so.

Wear gloves if the person has scalp sores. Follow Standard Precautions and the Bloodborne Pathogen Standard.

For a shampoo on a stretcher, follow the rules for stretcher use (Chapter 12). To safely transfer the person to and from the stretcher, see procedure: *Moving the Person to a Stretcher* (Chapter 17). Lock the stretcher wheels and use the safety straps and side rails. The far side rail is raised during the procedure.

Some people can shampoo themselves during a tub bath or shower. Place an extra towel, shampoo, and hair conditioner within the person's reach. Assist as needed.

Comfort

When shampooing during the tub bath or shower, the person tips his or her head back to keep shampoo and water out of the eyes. Support the back of the person's head with one hand. Shampoo with your other hand. Some persons cannot tip their heads back. They lean forward and hold a folded washcloth over the eyes. Support the forehead with one hand as you shampoo with the other. Make sure that the person can breathe easily.

Many people have limited range of motion in their necks. They are not shampooed at the sink or on a stretcher.

 SHAMPOOING THE PERSON'S HAIR

QUALITY OF LIFE

Remember to:
- Knock before entering the person's room.
- Address the person by name.
- Introduce yourself by name and title.

- Explain the procedure to the person before beginning and during the procedure.
- Protect the person's rights during the procedure.
- Handle the person gently during the procedure.

PRE-PROCEDURE

1 Follow *Delegation Guidelines: Shampooing*, p. 317. See *Promoting Safety and Comfort: Shampooing*.
2 Practice hand hygiene.
3 Collect the following:
   - Two bath towels
   - Washcloth
   - Shampoo
   - Hair conditioner (if requested)
   - Bath thermometer
   - Pitcher or hand-held nozzle (if needed)
   - Shampoo tray (if needed)
   - Basin or pan (if needed)
   - Waterproof pad (if needed)
   - Gloves (if needed)
   - Comb and brush
   - Hair dryer
4 Arrange items nearby.
5 Identify the person. Check the ID bracelet against the assignment sheet. Also call the person by name.
6 Provide for privacy.
7 Raise the bed for body mechanics for a shampoo in bed. Bed rails are up if used.
8 Decontaminate your hands.

PROCEDURE

9 Lower the bed rail near you if up.
10 Cover the person's chest with a bath towel.
11 Brush and comb the hair to remove snarls and tangles.
12 Position the person for the method you will use. To shampoo the person in bed:
   a Lower the head of the bed and remove the pillow.
   b Place the waterproof pad and shampoo tray under the head and shoulders.
   c Support the head and neck with a folded towel if necessary.
13 Raise the bed rail if used.

14 Obtain water. Water temperature is usually 105° F (40.5° C). Test water temperature according to center policy. Also ask the person to check the water. Adjust water temperature as needed. Raise the bed rail before leaving the bedside.
15 Lower the bed rail near you if up.
16 Put on gloves (if needed).
17 Ask the person to hold a washcloth over the eyes. It should not cover the nose and mouth. (NOTE: A damp washcloth is easier to hold. It will not slip. However, some state competency tests require a dry washcloth.)

SHAMPOOING THE PERSON'S HAIR—cont'd

PROCEDURE—cont'd

18 Use the pitcher or nozzle to wet the hair.
19 Apply a small amount of shampoo.
20 Work up a lather with both hands. Start at the hairline. Work toward the back of the head.
21 Massage the scalp with your fingertips. Do not scratch the scalp.
22 Rinse the hair until the water runs clear.
23 Repeat steps 19 through 22.
24 Apply conditioner. Follow directions on the container.
25 Squeeze water from the person's hair.
26 Cover the hair with a bath towel.

27 Remove the shampoo tray, basin, and waterproof pad.
28 Dry the person's face with the towel. Use the towel on the person's chest.
29 Help the person raise the head if appropriate. For the person in bed, raise the head of the bed.
30 Rub the hair and scalp with the towel. Use the second towel if the first one is wet.
31 Comb the hair to remove snarls and tangles.
32 Dry and style hair as quickly as possible.
33 Remove and discard the gloves (if used). Decontaminate your hands.

POST-PROCEDURE

34 Provide for comfort. (See the inside of the front book cover.)
35 Place the signal light within reach.
36 Lower the bed to its lowest position.
37 Raise or lower bed rails. Follow the care plan.
38 Unscreen the person.
39 Complete a safety check of the room. (See the inside of the front book cover.)

40 Clean, dry, and return equipment to its proper place. Remember to clean the brush and comb. Discard disposable items.
41 Follow center policy for dirty linen.
42 Decontaminate your hands.
43 Report and record your observations.

SHAVING

Many men shave for comfort and mental well-being. Many women shave their legs and underarms. Women with coarse facial hair may shave. Or they may use other hair removal methods. See Box 21-1 for shaving rules.

Safety razors or electric shavers are used (Fig. 21-10, p. 320). Usually residents are required to have their own electric shavers. If the center's shaver is used, clean it after every use. Follow the manufacturer's instructions for brushing out whiskers. Also follow center policy for cleaning electric shavers.

Safety razors (blade razors) involve razor blades. They can cause nicks and cuts. Older persons with wrinkled skin are at risk for nicks and cuts. Therefore safety razors are not used on persons who have healing problems or for those who take anticoagulant drugs. An **anticoagulant** is a drug that prevents or slows down (*anti*) blood clotting (*coagulate*). Bleeding occurs easily and is hard to stop. A nick or cut can cause serious bleeding. Electric shavers are used.

Box 21-1 Rules for Shaving

- Use electric shavers for persons taking anticoagulant drugs. Never use safety razors.
- Protect bed linens. Place a towel under the part being shaved. Or place a towel across the person's chest and shoulders to protect clothing.
- Soften the skin before shaving. Apply a wet washcloth or towel to the face for a few minutes.
- Encourage the person to do as much as safely possible.
- Hold the skin taut as needed.
- Shave in the correct direction:
  - Shaving the face with a safety razor—shave in the direction of hair growth.
  - Shaving the underarms with a safety razor—shave in the direction of hair growth.
  - Shaving the legs with a safety razor—shave up from the ankles. This is against hair growth.
  - Using an electric shaver—shave against the direction of hair growth. If using a rotary-type shaver, move the shaver in small circles over the face.
- Do not cut, nick, or irritate the skin.
- Rinse the body part thoroughly.
- Apply direct pressure to nicks or cuts (Chapter 47).
- Report nicks, cuts, or irritation to the nurse at once.

Soften the beard before using an electric shaver or safety razor. Do so by applying a moist, warm wash-cloth or towel for a few minutes. Then pat dry the face and apply talcum powder if using an electric shaver. If using a safety razor, lather the face with soap and water or shaving cream.

See *Residents With Dementia: Shaving*.
See *Delegation Guidelines: Shaving*.
See *Promoting Safety and Comfort: Shaving*.

RESIDENTS WITH DEMENTIA
Shaving

Safety razors are not used to shave persons with dementia. They may not understand what you are doing. They may resist care and move suddenly. Serious nicks and cuts can occur. Use electric shavers for these persons.

DELEGATION GUIDELINES
Shaving

Before shaving a person, you need this information from the nurse and the care plan:
* What shaver to use—electric or safety
* If the person takes anticoagulant drugs
* When to shave the person
* What facial hair to shave
* The location of tender or sensitive areas on the person's face
* What observations to report and record:
  * Nicks (report at once)
  * Cuts (report at once)
  * Bleeding (report at once)
  * Irritation
* When to report observations
* What specific resident concerns to report at once

PROMOTING SAFETY AND COMFORT
Shaving

Safety
Safety razors are very sharp. Protect the person and yourself from nicks or cuts. Prevent contact with blood. If using an electric shaver, follow safety measures for electrical equipment (Chapter 12).

Rinse the safety razor often during the shaving procedure. Rinsing removes whiskers and lather. Then wipe the razor. To protect yourself from cuts:
* Place several thicknesses of tissues or paper towels on the overbed table. Do not hold them in your hand.
* Wipe the razor on the tissues or paper towels.

Follow Standard Precautions and the Bloodborne Pathogen Standard. Discard used razor blades and disposable shavers in the sharps container. Do not recap the razor.

Comfort
Some men have tender and sensitive skin. Usually the neck area below the jaw is tender and sensitive. Some electric shavers become very warm or hot while in use. Such heat can irritate the skin. Shave tender areas first while the shaver is cool. Then move to the other areas of the face.

Some people apply lotion or after-shave to the skin after shaving. Lotion softens the skin. After-shave closes skin pores. Heat is applied before shaving to soften the skin. It also opens pores.

Fig. 21-10 Electric shaver (top) and safety razor (bottom).

Fig. 21-11 Shave in the direction of hair growth. Use longer strokes on the larger areas of the face. Use short strokes around the chin and lips.

SHAVING THE PERSON'S FACE WITH A SAFETY RAZOR `VIDEO`

QUALITY OF LIFE

Remember to:
- Knock before entering the person's room.
- Address the person by name.
- Introduce yourself by name and title.

- Explain the procedure to the person before beginning and during the procedure.
- Protect the person's rights during the procedure.
- Handle the person gently during the procedure.

PRE-PROCEDURE

1 Follow *Delegation Guidelines: Shaving.* See *Promoting Safety and Comfort: Shaving.*
2 Practice hand hygiene.
3 Collect the following:
- Wash basin
- Bath towel
- Hand towel
- Washcloth
- Safety razor
- Mirror
- Shaving cream, soap, or lotion
- Shaving brush
- After-shave or lotion
- Tissues or paper towels
- Paper towels
- Gloves

4 Arrange paper towels and supplies on the overbed table.
5 Identify the person. Check the ID bracelet against the assignment sheet. Also call the person by name.
6 Provide for privacy.
7 Raise the bed for body mechanics. Bed rails are up if used.

PROCEDURE

8 Fill the wash basin with warm water.
9 Place the basin on the overbed table.
10 Lower the bed rail near you if up.
11 Decontaminate your hands. Put on gloves.
12 Assist the person to semi-Fowler's position if allowed or to the supine position.
13 Adjust lighting to clearly see the person's face.
14 Place the bath towel over the person's chest and shoulders.
15 Adjust the overbed table for easy reach.
16 Tighten the razor blade to the shaver if necessary.
17 Wash the person's face. Do not dry.
18 Wet the washcloth or towel. Wring it out.
19 Apply the washcloth or towel to the face for a few minutes.

20 Apply shaving cream with your hands. Or use a shaving brush to apply lather.
21 Hold the skin taut with one hand.
22 Shave in the direction of hair growth. Use shorter strokes around the chin and lips (Fig. 21-11).
23 Rinse the razor often. Wipe it with tissues or paper towels.
24 Apply direct pressure to any bleeding areas (Chapter 47).
25 Wash off any remaining shaving cream or soap. Pat dry with a towel.
26 Apply after-shave or lotion if requested. (If there are nicks or cuts, do not apply after-shave or lotion.)
27 Remove the towel and gloves. Decontaminate your hands.

POST-PROCEDURE

28 Provide for comfort. (See the inside of the front book cover.)
29 Place the signal light within reach.
30 Lower the bed to its lowest position.
31 Raise or lower bed rails. Follow the care plan.
32 Clean and return equipment and supplies to their proper place. Discard a razor blade or a disposable razor into the sharps container. Discard other disposable items. Wear gloves.

33 Wipe off the overbed table with paper towels. Discard the paper towels.
34 Unscreen the person.
35 Complete a safety check of the room. (See the inside of the front book cover.)
36 Follow center policy for dirty linen.
37 Remove the gloves. Decontaminate your hands.
38 Report nicks, cuts, irritation, or bleeding to the nurse at once. Also report and record other observations.

Caring for Mustaches and Beards

Mustaches and beards need daily care. Food can collect in the whiskers. So can mouth and nose drainage. Daily washing and combing are needed. Ask the person how to groom his mustache or beard. *Never trim a mustache or beard without the person's consent.*

Shaving Legs and Underarms

Many women shave their legs and underarms. This practice varies among cultures. Some women shave only the lower legs. Others shave to mid-thigh or the entire leg.

Legs and underarms are shaved after bathing. The skin is soft at this time. Soap and water, shaving cream, or lotion is used for lather. Collect shaving items with bath items. Use the kidney basin to rinse the razor. Do not use the bath water. Follow the rules in Box 21-1.

NAIL AND FOOT CARE

Nail and foot care prevents infection, injury, and odors. Hangnails, ingrown nails (nails that grow in at the side), and nails torn away from the skin cause skin breaks. These breaks are portals of entry for microbes. Long or broken nails can scratch skin or snag clothing.

The feet are easily infected and injured. Dirty feet, socks, or stockings harbor microbes and cause odors. Shoes and socks provide a warm, moist environment for microbes to grow. Injuries occur from stubbing toes, stepping on sharp objects, or being stepped on. Shoes that fit poorly cause blisters.

Poor circulation prolongs healing. Diabetes and vascular diseases are common causes of poor circulation. Infections or foot injuries are very serious for older persons and persons with circulatory disorders. Gangrene and amputation are serious complications (Chapter 39). Trimming and clipping toenails can easily cause injuries.

Nails are easier to trim and clean right after soaking or bathing. Use nail clippers to cut fingernails. *Never use scissors.* Use extreme caution to prevent damage to nearby tissues.

Some centers do not let nursing assistants cut or trim toenails. Follow center policy.

See *Delegation Guidelines: Nail and Foot Care.*

See *Promoting Safety and Comfort: Nail and Foot Care.*

See *Teamwork and Time Management: Nail and Foot Care.*

DELEGATION GUIDELINES
Nail and Foot Care

Before giving nail and foot care, you need this information from the nurse and the care plan:
- What water temperature to use
- How long to soak fingernails (usually 5 to 10 minutes)
- How long to soak feet (usually 15 to 20 minutes)
- What observations to report and record:
  - Reddened, irritated, or calloused areas
  - Breaks in the skin
  - Corns (Chapter 35) on top of and between the toes
  - Very thick nails
  - Loose nails
- When to report observations
- What specific resident concerns to report at once

PROMOTING SAFETY AND COMFORT
Nail and Foot Care

Safety
You do not cut or trim toenails if a person:
- Has diabetes
- Has poor circulation to the legs and feet
- Takes drugs that affect blood clotting
- Has very thick nails or ingrown toenails

The RN or podiatrist (foot *[pod]* doctor) cuts toenails and provides foot care for these persons.

Check between the toes for cracks and sores. These areas are often overlooked. If left untreated, a serious infection could occur.

The feet are easily burned. Persons with decreased sensation or circulatory problems may not feel hot temperatures.

After soaking, apply lotion or petroleum jelly to the feet. This can cause slippery feet. Help the person put on non-skid footwear before you transfer the person or let the person walk.

Breaks in the skin and bleeding can occur. Follow Standard Precautions and the Bloodborne Pathogen Standard.

Comfort
Sometimes just the fingernails are trimmed. Sometimes just foot care is given. Sometimes both are done. When both are done, the person sits at the overbed table (Fig. 21-12). Make sure the person is warm and comfortable.

Promote your own comfort when giving nail and foot care. Sit in front of the overbed table when cleaning and trimming fingernails. When giving foot care, rest the person's lower leg and foot on your lap. Or you can kneel on the floor. Lay a towel across your lap or on the floor to protect your uniform. Remember to use good body mechanics. However you position yourself, you must support the person's foot and ankle when giving foot care.

TEAMWORK AND TIME MANAGEMENT
Nail and Foot Care

Use your time well when giving nail and foot care. The fingernails soak for 5 to 10 minutes. The feet soak for 15 to 20 minutes. You can make the person's bed or straighten the person's unit while the fingernails and feet soak. Or you could assist with brushing and combing hair. Check your assignment sheet for other ways to meet the person's needs.

Fig. 21-12 Nail and foot care. The feet soak in a whirlpool foot bath. The fingers soak in a kidney basin.

 GIVING NAIL AND FOOT CARE

QUALITY OF LIFE

Remember to:
- Knock before entering the person's room.
- Address the person by name.
- Introduce yourself by name and title.
- Explain the procedure to the person before beginning and during the procedure.
- Protect the person's rights during the procedure.
- Handle the person gently during the procedure.

PRE-PROCEDURE

1 Follow *Delegation Guidelines: Nail and Foot Care*. See *Promoting Safety and Comfort: Nail and Foot Care*.
2 Practice hand hygiene.
3 Collect the following:
- Wash basin or whirlpool foot bath
- Soap
- Bath thermometer
- Bath towel
- Hand towel
- Washcloth
- Kidney basin
- Nail clippers
- Orangewood stick
- Emery board or nail file
- Lotion for the hands
- Lotion or petroleum jelly for the feet
- Paper towels
- Bath mat
- Gloves
4 Arrange paper towels and other items on the overbed table.
5 Identify the person. Check the ID bracelet against the assignment sheet. Also call the person by name.
6 Provide for privacy.
7 Assist the person to the bedside chair. Place the signal light within reach.

Continued

GIVING NAIL AND FOOT CARE—cont'd

PROCEDURE

8 Place the bath mat under the feet.

9 Fill the wash basin or whirlpool foot bath ⅔ (two-thirds) full with water. The nurse tells you what water temperature to use. (Measure water temperature with a bath thermometer. Or test it by dipping your elbow or inner wrist into the basin. Follow center policy.) Also ask the person to check the water temperature. Adjust the water temperature as needed.

10 Place the basin or foot bath on the bath mat.

11 Put on gloves.

12 Help the person put the feet into the basin or foot bath. Make sure both feet are completely covered by water.

13 Adjust the overbed table in front of the person.

14 Fill the kidney basin ⅔ (two-thirds) full with water. See step 9 for water temperature.

15 Place the kidney basin on the overbed table.

16 Place the person's fingers into the basin. Position the arms for comfort (see Fig. 21-12).

17 Let the fingers soak for 5 to 10 minutes. Let the feet soak for 15 to 20 minutes. Re-warm water as needed.

18 Remove the kidney basin.

19 Clean under the fingernails with the flat end of the orangewood stick. Use a towel to wipe the orangewood stick after each nail.

20 Dry the hands and between the fingers thoroughly.

21 Clip fingernails straight across with the nail clippers (Fig. 21-13).

22 Shape nails with an emery board or nail file. Nails are smooth with no rough edges. Check each nail for smoothness. File as needed.

23 Push cuticles back with the orangewood stick or a washcloth (Fig. 21-14).

24 Apply lotion to the hands. Warm lotion before applying it.

25 Move the overbed table to the side.

26 Lift a foot out of the water. Support the foot and ankle with one hand. With your other hand, wash the foot and between the toes with soap and a washcloth. Return the foot to the water for rinsing. Make sure you rinse between the toes.

27 Repeat step 26 for the other foot.

28 Remove the feet from the basin or foot bath. Dry thoroughly, especially between the toes.

29 Apply lotion or petroleum jelly to the tops and soles of the feet. Do not apply between the toes. Warm lotion or petroleum jelly before applying it. Remove excess lotion or petroleum jelly with a towel.

30 Remove and discard the gloves. Decontaminate your hands.

31 Help the person put on non-skid footwear.

POST-PROCEDURE

32 Provide for comfort. (See the inside of the front book cover.)

33 Place the signal light within reach.

34 Raise or lower bed rails. Follow the care plan.

35 Clean, dry, and return equipment and supplies to their proper place. Discard disposable items. Wear gloves for this step.

36 Unscreen the person.

37 Complete a safety check of the room. (See the inside of the front book cover.)

38 Follow center policy for dirty linen.

39 Remove the gloves. Decontaminate your hands.

40 Report and record your observations.

Fig. 21-13 Clip fingernails straight across. Use a nail clipper.

Fig. 21-14 Push the cuticle back with an orangewood stick.

CHANGING CLOTHING AND HOSPITAL GOWNS

Residents change from sleepwear into clothing after morning care. They undress and put on sleepwear at bedtime. Garments are changed whenever wet or soiled. These activities are easier for those who can move their arms and legs. You may need to assist with changing clothes and hospital gowns. Follow these rules:

- Provide for privacy. Do not expose the person.
- Encourage the person to do as much as possible.
- Let the person choose what to wear. Make sure the right undergarments are chosen.
- Remove clothing from the strong or "good" side first. This is often call the *unaffected side*.
- Put clothing on the weak side first. This is often called the *affected side*.
- Support the arm or leg when removing or putting on a garment.

See *Residents With Dementia: Changing Clothing and Hospital Gowns*.

✉ Dressing and Undressing

Most residents wear street clothes during the day. Some dress and undress themselves. Others need help. Personal choice is a resident right. Let the person choose what to wear. Follow the rules for changing clothing and hospital gowns.

See *Focus on Communication: Dressing and Undressing*.

See *Delegation Guidelines: Dressing and Undressing*.

Text continued on p. 330

FOCUS ON COMMUNICATION
Dressing and Undressing

Allow for personal choice and independence when assisting with dressing and undressing. You can ask:
- "What would you like to wear today?"
- "There's a concert today in the lounge. Do you want to wear something special?"
- "Can I help you with those buttons?"
- "Would you like me to help you with that zipper?"

RESIDENTS WITH DEMENTIA
Changing Clothing and Hospital Gowns

Persons with dementia may not want to change clothes. Or they may not know how. For example, a person may try to put slacks on over his or her head. The Alzheimer's Disease Education and Referral Center (ADEAR) suggests the following:
- Try to assist with dressing and undressing at the same time each day. The person learns to expect these tasks as a part of his or her daily routine.
- Let the person dress himself or herself to the extent possible. Allow extra time for this task. Do not rush the person.
- Let the person choose what to wear from 2 or 3 outfits. If the person has a favorite outfit, the family may buy several of the same outfit. This makes dressing easier if the person insists on wearing the same outfit.
- Choose clothes that are comfortable to wear and easy to get on and off. Garments with elastic waistbands and Velcro closures are examples. The person does not have to handle zippers, buttons, hooks, snaps, or other closures.
- Stack clothes in the order that they are put on. The person sees one item at a time. For example, underpants or undershorts are put on first. The item is on top of the stack.
- Give clear, simple, step-by-step directions.

DELEGATION GUIDELINES
Dressing and Undressing

Before assisting with dressing and undressing, you need this information from the nurse and the care plan:
- How much help the person needs
- Which side is the person's strong side
- If the person needs to wear certain garments
- What observations to report and record:
  - How much help was given
  - How the person tolerated the procedure
  - Any complaints by the person
  - Any changes in the person's behavior
- When to report observations
- What specific resident concerns to report at once

UNDRESSING THE PERSON

QUALITY OF LIFE

Remember to:
- Knock before entering the person's room.
- Address the person by name.
- Introduce yourself by name and title.

- Explain the procedure to the person before beginning and during the procedure.
- Protect the person's rights during the procedure.
- Handle the person gently during the procedure.

PRE-PROCEDURE

1 Follow *Delegation Guidelines: Dressing and Undressing,* p. 325.
2 Practice hand hygiene.
3 Collect a bath blanket and clothing requested by the person.
4 Identify the person. Check the ID bracelet against the assignment sheet. Also call the person by name.

5 Provide for privacy.
6 Raise the bed for body mechanics. Bed rails are up if used.
7 Lower the bed rail on the person's weak side.
8 Position him or her supine.
9 Cover the person with a bath blanket. Fan-fold linens to the foot of the bed.

PROCEDURE

10 Remove garments that open in the back.
  a Raise the head and shoulders. Or turn him or her onto the side away from you.
  b Undo buttons, zippers, ties, or snaps.
  c Bring the sides of the garment to the sides of the person (Fig. 21-15). If he or she is in a side-lying position, tuck the far side under the person. Fold the near side onto the chest (Fig. 21-16).
  d Position the person supine.
  e Slide the garment off the shoulder on the strong side. Remove it from the arm (Fig. 21-17).
  f Remove the garment from the weak side.
11 Remove garments that open in the front:
  a Undo buttons, zippers, ties, or snaps.
  b Slide the garment off the shoulder and arm on the strong side.
  c Assist the person to sit up or raise the head and shoulders. Bring the garment over to the weak side (Fig. 21-18).
  d Lower the head and shoulders. Remove the garment from the weak side.
  e If you cannot raise the head and shoulders:
    (1) Turn the person toward you. Tuck the removed part under the person.
    (2) Turn him or her onto the side away from you.
    (3) Pull the side of the garment out from under the person. Make sure he or she will not lie on it when supine.
    (4) Return the person to the supine position.
    (5) Remove the garment from the weak side.

12 Remove pullover garments:
  a Undo any buttons, zippers, ties, or snaps.
  b Remove the garment from the strong side.
  c Raise the head and shoulders. Or turn the person onto the side away from you. Bring the garment up to the person's neck (Fig. 21-19).
  d Remove the garment from the weak side.
  e Bring the garment over the person's head.
  f Position him or her in the supine position.
13 Remove pants or slacks:
  a Remove footwear and socks.
  b Position the person supine.
  c Undo buttons, zippers, ties, snaps, or buckles.
  d Remove the belt.
  e Ask the person to lift the buttocks off the bed. Slide the pants down over the hips and buttocks (Fig. 21-20). Have the person lower the hips and buttocks.
  f If the person cannot raise the hips off the bed:
    (1) Turn the person toward you.
    (2) Slide the pants off the hip and buttock on the strong side (Fig. 21-21, p. 328).
    (3) Turn the person away from you.
    (4) Slide the pants off the hip and buttock on the weak side (Fig. 21-22, p. 328).
  g Slide the pants down the legs and over the feet.
14 Dress the person. See procedure: *Dressing the Person,* p. 328.

POST-PROCEDURE

15 Provide for comfort. (See the inside of the front book cover.)
16 Place the signal light within reach.
17 Lower the bed to its lowest position.
18 Raise or lower bed rails. Follow the care plan.
19 Unscreen the person.

20 Complete a safety check of the room. (See the inside of the front book cover.)
21 Follow center policy for soiled clothing.
22 Decontaminate your hands.
23 Report and record your observations.

Fig. 21-15 The sides of the garment are brought from the back to the sides of the person. (Note that the "weak" side is *indicated by slash marks.*)

Fig. 21-16 A garment that opens in the back is removed from the person in the side-lying position. The far side of the garment is tucked under the person. The near side is folded onto the person's chest. (Note that the "weak" side is *indicated by slash marks.*)

Fig. 21-17 The garment is removed from the strong side first. (Note that the "weak" side is *indicated by slash marks.*)

Fig. 21-18 A front-opening garment is removed with the person's head and shoulders raised. The garment is removed from the strong side first. Then it is brought around the back to the weak side. (Note that the "weak" side is *indicated by slash marks.*)

Fig. 21-19 A pullover garment is removed from the strong side first. Then the garment is brought up to the person's neck so that it can be removed from the weak side. (Note that the "weak" side is *indicated by slash marks.*)

Fig. 21-20 The person lifts the hips and buttocks for removing the pants. The pants are slid down over the hips and buttocks. (Note that the "weak" side is *indicated by slash marks.*)

Fig. 21-21 Pants are removed in the side-lying position. They are removed from the strong side first. They are slid over the hip and buttock. (Note that the "weak" side is *indicated by slash marks.*)

Fig. 21-22 The person is turned onto the strong side. The pants are removed from the weak side. (Note that the "weak" side is *indicated by slash marks.*)

DRESSING THE PERSON

QUALITY OF LIFE

Remember to:
- Knock before entering the person's room.
- Address the person by name.
- Introduce yourself by name and title.

- Explain the procedure to the person before beginning and during the procedure.
- Protect the person's rights during the procedure.
- Handle the person gently during the procedure.

PRE-PROCEDURE

1 Follow *Delegation Guidelines: Dressing and Undressing,* p. 325.
2 Practice hand hygiene.
3 Ask the person what he or she would like to wear.
4 Get a bath blanket and clothing requested by the person.
5 Identify the person. Check the ID bracelet against the assignment sheet. Also call the person by name.
6 Provide for privacy.

7 Raise the bed for body mechanics. Bed rails are up if used.
8 Lower the bed rail (if up) on the person's strong side.
9 Position the person supine.
10 Cover the person with a bath blanket. Fan-fold linens to the foot of the bed.
11 Undress the person. (See procedure: *Undressing the Person,* p. 326.)

PROCEDURE

12 Put on garments that open in the back:
  a Slide the garment onto the arm and shoulder of the weak side.
  b Slide the garment onto the arm and shoulder of the strong side.
  c Raise the person's head and shoulders.
  d Bring the sides to the back.
  e If you cannot raise the person's head and shoulders:
    (1) Turn the person toward you.
    (2) Bring one side of the garment to the person's back (Fig. 21-23, *A*).
    (3) Turn the person away from you.
    (4) Bring the other side to the person's back (Fig. 21-23, *B*).
  f Fasten buttons, zippers, snaps, or other closures.
  g Position the person supine.

13 Put on garments that open in the front:
  a Slide the garment onto the arm and shoulder on the weak side.
  b Raise the head and shoulders. Bring the side of the garment around to the back. Lower the person down. Slide the garment onto the arm and shoulder of the strong arm.
  c If the person cannot raise the head and shoulders:
    (1) Turn the person away from you.
    (2) Tuck the garment under him or her.
    (3) Turn the person toward you.
    (4) Pull the garment out from under him or her.
    (5) Turn the person back to the supine position.
    (6) Slide the garment over the arm and shoulder of the strong arm.
  d Fasten buttons, zippers, ties, snaps, or other closures.

DRESSING THE PERSON—cont'd

PROCEDURE—cont'd

14 Put on pullover garments:
  a Position the person supine.
  b Bring the neck of the garment over the head.
  c Slide the arm and shoulder of the garment onto the weak side.
  d Raise the person's head and shoulders.
  e Bring the garment down.
  f Slide the arm and shoulder of the garment onto the strong side.
  g If the person cannot assume a semi-sitting position:
    (1) Turn the person away from you.
    (2) Tuck the garment under the person.
    (3) Turn the person toward you.
    (4) Pull the garment out from under him or her.
    (5) Position the person supine.
    (6) Slide the arm and shoulder of the garment onto the strong side.
  h Fasten buttons, zippers, ties, snaps, or other closures.

15 Put on pants or slacks:
  a Slide the pants over the feet and up the legs.
  b Ask the person to raise the hips and buttocks off the bed.
  c Bring the pants up over the buttocks and hips.
  d Ask the person to lower the hips and buttocks.
  e If the person cannot raise the hips and buttocks:
    (1) Turn the person onto the strong side.
    (2) Pull the pants over the buttock and hip on the weak side.
    (3) Turn the person onto the weak side.
    (4) Pull the pants over the buttock and hip on the strong side.
    (5) Position the person supine.
  f Fasten buttons, zippers, ties, snaps, a belt buckle, or other closures.
16 Put socks and non-skid footwear on the person. Make sure socks are up all the way and smooth.
17 Help the person get out of bed. If the person will stay in bed, cover the person. Remove the bath blanket.

POST-PROCEDURE

18 Provide for comfort. (See the inside of the front book cover.)
19 Place the signal light within reach.
20 Lower the bed to its lowest position.
21 Raise or lower bed rails. Follow the care plan.
22 Unscreen the person.

23 Complete a safety check of the room. (See the inside of the front book cover.)
24 Follow center policy for soiled clothing.
25 Decontaminate your hands.
26 Report and record your observations.

Fig. 21-23 Dressing a person. **A,** The side-lying position can be used to put on garments that open in the back. Turn the person toward you after the garment is put on the arms. The side of the garment is brought to the person's back. **B,** Then turn the person away from you. The other side of the garment is brought to the back and fastened. (Note that the "weak" side is *indicated by slash marks.*)

Changing Hospital Gowns

Some residents wear hospital gowns. Gowns are usually worn for IV (intravenous) therapy (Chapter 25). Some centers have special gowns for IV therapy. They open along the sleeve and close with ties, snaps, or Velcro. Sometimes standard gowns are used.

If there is injury or paralysis, the gown is removed from the strong arm first. Support the weak arm while removing the gown. Put the clean gown on the weak arm first and then on the strong arm.

See *Delegation Guidelines: Changing Hospital Gowns.*

See *Promoting Safety and Comfort: Changing Hospital Gowns.*

DELEGATION GUIDELINES
Changing Hospital Gowns

Before changing a gown, you need this information from the nurse and the care plan:
- Which arm has the IV
- If the person has an IV pump (see *Promoting Safety and Comfort: Changing Hospital Gowns*)

PROMOTING SAFETY AND COMFORT
Changing Hospital Gowns

Safety
IV pumps control how fast fluid enters a vein. This is called the *flow rate.* If the person has an IV pump and a standard gown, do not use the following procedure. The arm with the IV is not put through the sleeve.

If the person has an IV, changing the gown can cause the flow rate to change. Always ask the nurse to check the flow rate after you change a gown.

Do not disconnect or remove any part of the IV set-up.

Comfort
Some hospital gowns are secured with ties at the upper back. The back and buttocks are exposed when the person stands. Other gowns overlap in the back and tie at the side. These gowns provide more privacy. Because they tie at the side, uncomfortable bows and knots at the back are avoided.

Fig. 21-24 Changing a gown. **A,** The gown is removed from the arm with no IV. The sleeve on the arm with the IV is gathered up, slipped over the IV site and tubing, and removed from the arm and hand. **B,** The gathered sleeve is slipped along the IV tubing to the bag. **C,** The IV bag is removed from the pole and passed through the sleeve. **D,** The gathered sleeve of the clean gown is slipped over the IV bag at the shoulder part of the gown.

CHANGING THE GOWN OF THE PERSON WITH AN IV   `VIDEO`

QUALITY OF LIFE

Remember to:
- Knock before entering the person's room.
- Address the person by name.
- Introduce yourself by name and title.

- Explain the procedure to the person before beginning and during the procedure.
- Protect the person's rights during the procedure.
- Handle the person gently during the procedure.

PRE-PROCEDURE

1 Follow *Delegation Guidelines: Changing Hospital Gowns.* See *Promoting Safety and Comfort: Changing Hospital Gowns.*
2 Practice hand hygiene.
3 Get a clean gown and a bath blanket.

4 Identify the person. Check the ID bracelet against the assignment sheet. Also call the person by name.
5 Provide for privacy.
6 Raise the bed for body mechanics. Bed rails are up if used.

PROCEDURE

7 Lower the bed rail near you (if up).
8 Cover the person with a bath blanket. Fan-fold linens to the foot of the bed.
9 Untie the gown. Free parts that the person is lying on.
10 Remove the gown from the arm with *no IV.*
11 Gather up the sleeve of the arm *with the IV.* Slide it over the IV site and tubing. Remove the arm and hand from the sleeve (Fig. 21-24, *A*).
12 Keep the sleeve gathered. Slide your arm along the tubing to the bag (Fig. 21-24, *B*).
13 Remove the bag from the pole. Slide the bag and tubing through the sleeve (Fig. 21-24, *C*). Do not pull on the tubing. Keep the bag above the person.

14 Hang the IV bag on the pole.
15 Gather the sleeve of the clean gown that will go on the arm with the IV infusion.
16 Remove the bag from the pole. Slip the sleeve over the bag at the shoulder part of the gown (Fig. 21-24, *D*). Hang the bag.
17 Slide the gathered sleeve over the tubing, hand, arm, and IV site. Then slide it onto the shoulder.
18 Put the other side of the gown on the person. Fasten the gown.
19 Cover the person. Remove the bath blanket.

POST-PROCEDURE

20 Provide for comfort. (See the inside of the front book cover.)
21 Place the signal light within reach.
22 Lower the bed to its lowest position.
23 Raise or lower bed rails. Follow the care plan.
24 Unscreen the person.

25 Complete a safety check of the room. (See the inside of the front book cover.)
26 Follow center policy for dirty linen.
27 Decontaminate your hands.
28 Ask the nurse to check the flow rate.
29 Report and record your observations.

QUALITY OF LIFE

Grooming measures promote comfort. They also help the person's body image and esteem needs. Clean hair, nails, and garments all help mental well-being. So does a clean-shaven face or a well-groomed beard or mustache.

The person may not have energy for some procedures. The nurse tells you what care to give and when to give it. Encourage and allow personal choice whenever possible. Grooming practices vary from person to person. Always assist as needed.

Carefully handle the person's grooming products, shaver, hair dryer, brush and comb, perfumes, and other personal care items. Garments also need your attention. Do not break zippers, tear clothing, lose buttons, or cause other damage. Treat the person's property with care and respect.

Sometimes family members want to help with grooming. For example, they want to help style the person's hair. Or they want to apply lotion to the person's hands and feet. With the person's permission, allow family members to assist with grooming measures as much as safely possible. This promotes social interaction. It also involves the family in the person's care.

Report your observations to the nurse. Also record your observations and the care given according to center policy (Fig. 21-25, p. 332). This information is needed to meet the person's needs.

Activities-of-Daily-Living Flow Sheet

JAN   FEB   (MAR)   APR   MAY   JUN   JUL   AUG   SEP   OCT   NOV   DEC

ORDER/INSTRUCTION	TIME	1	2	3	4	5	6	7	8	9	10	11	12	13	14	15	16	17	18	19	20	21	22	23	24	25	26	27	28	29	30	31
Dressing	11-7																																
I=Independent S=Set up A=Assist T=Total Care	7-3	*SS*	*SS*	*BG*																													
	3-11																																
Grooming, Combing Hair	11-7																																
I=Independent S=Set up A=Assist T=Total Care	7-3	*SS*	*SS*	*BG*																													
	3-11																																
Shave Men Daily	11-7																																
Shave Women every ___2___ days	7-3	*SS*		*BG*																													
	3-11																																
Trim Fingernails Weekly	11-7																																
	7-3																																
	3-11	*MB*																															

Fig. 21-25 Charting sample.

REVIEW QUESTIONS

Circle the BEST answer.

1 A person has alopecia. This is
  a Excessive body hair
  b Dry, white flakes from the scalp
  c An infestation with lice
  d Hair loss

2 Which prevents hair from matting and tangling?
  a Bedrest
  b Daily brushing and combing
  c Daily shampooing
  d Cutting hair

3 A person's hair is not matted or tangled. When brushing hair, start at
  a The forehead and brush backward
  b The hair ends
  c The scalp
  d The back of the neck and brush forward

4 Brushing keeps the hair
  a Soft and shiny
  b Clean
  c Free of lice
  d Long

5 A person requests a shampoo. You should
  a Shampoo the hair during the person's shower
  b Shampoo hair at the sink
  c Shampoo the person in bed
  d Follow the care plan

6 When shaving a person's face, do the following *except*
  a Practice Standard Precautions
  b Follow the Bloodborne Pathogen Standard
  c Shave in the direction of hair growth
  d Shave when the skin is dry

7 A person is nicked during shaving. Your first action is to
  a Wash your hands
  b Apply direct pressure
  c Tell the nurse
  d Apply a bandage

8 Fingernails are cut with
  a An emery board
  b Scissors
  c A nail file
  d Nail clippers

9 Fingernails are trimmed
  a Before soaking
  b After soaking
  c Before trimming toenails
  d After trimming toenails

Circle T if the statement is TRUE. Circle F if the statement is FALSE.

10 T F Mr. Polk has a mustache and beard. To promote his comfort, you can shave his beard and mustache.

11 T F Clothing is removed from the strong side first.

12 T F The person chooses what to wear.

13 T F A person has poor circulation in the legs and feet. You can cut and trim the person's toenails.

14 T F You can cut matted hair.

Answers to these questions are on p. 720.

Urinary Elimination

OBJECTIVES

- Define the key terms and key abbreviations listed in this chapter.
- Describe normal urine.
- Describe the rules for normal urinary elimination.
- Identify the observations to report to the nurse.
- Describe urinary incontinence and the care required.
- Describe straight, indwelling, and condom catheters.

- Explain why catheters are used.
- Explain how to care for persons with catheters.
- Describe two methods of bladder training.
- Perform the procedures described in this chapter.
- Explain how to promote quality of life.

KEY TERMS

catheter A tube used to drain or inject fluid through a body opening

catheterization The process of inserting a catheter

dysuria Painful or difficult *(dys)* urination *(uria)*

Foley catheter See "indwelling catheter"

functional incontinence The person has bladder control but cannot use the toilet in time

hematuria Blood *(hemat)* in the urine *(uria)*

indwelling catheter A catheter left in the bladder so urine drains constantly into a drainage bag; retention or Foley catheter

micturition See "urination"

mixed incontinence The combination of stress incontinence and urge incontinence

nocturia Frequent urination *(uria)* at night *(noct)*

oliguria Scant amount *(olig)* of urine *(uria);* less than 500 mL in 24 hours

overflow incontinence Small amounts of urine leak from a full bladder

polyuria Abnormally large amounts *(poly)* of urine *(uria)*

reflex incontinence Urine is lost at predictable intervals when the bladder is full

retention catheter See "indwelling catheter"

straight catheter A catheter that drains the bladder and then is removed

stress incontinence When urine leaks during exercise and certain movements that cause pressure on the bladder

transient incontinence Temporary or occasional incontinence that is reversed when the cause is treated

urge incontinence The loss of urine in response to a sudden, urgent need to void; the person cannot get to a toilet in time

urinary frequency Voiding at frequent intervals

urinary incontinence The involuntary loss or leakage of urine

urinary urgency The need to void at once

urination The process of emptying urine from the bladder; micturition or voiding

voiding See "urination"

KEY ABBREVIATIONS

C	Centigrade	**IV**	Intravenous
CMS	Centers for Medicare & Medicaid Services	**mL**	Milliliter
F	Fahrenheit	**OBRA**	Omnibus Budget Reconciliation Act of 1987
ID	Identification	**UTI**	Urinary tract infection

Eliminating waste is a physical need. The respiratory, digestive, integumentary, and urinary systems remove body wastes. The digestive system rids the body of solid wastes. The lungs remove carbon dioxide. Sweat contains water and other substances. Blood contains waste products from body cells burning food for energy. The urinary system removes waste products from the blood. It also maintains the body's water balance.

NORMAL URINATION

The healthy adult produces about 1500 mL (milliliters) or 3 pints of urine a day. Many factors affect urine production. They include age, disease, the amount and kinds of fluid ingested, dietary salt, body temperature, perspiration, and drugs. Some substances increase urine production—coffee, tea, alcohol, and some drugs. A diet high in salt causes the body to retain water. When water is retained, less urine is produced.

Urination, micturition, and voiding mean the process of emptying urine from the bladder. The amount of fluid intake, habits, and available toilet facilities affect frequency. So do activity, work, and illness. People usually void at bedtime, after sleep, and before meals. Some people void every 2 to 3 hours. The need to void at night disturbs sleep.

Some persons need help getting to the bathroom. Others use bedpans, urinals, or commodes. Follow the rules in Box 22-1 and the person's care plan.

See *Focus on Communication: Normal Urination.*

See *Teamwork and Time Management: Normal Urination.*

Box 22-1   Rules for Normal Urination

- Practice medical asepsis.
- Follow Standard Precautions and the Bloodborne Pathogen Standard.
- Provide fluids as the nurse and care plan direct.
- Follow the person's voiding routines and habits. Check with the nurse and the care plan.
- Help the person to the bathroom when the request is made. Or provide the commode, bedpan, or urinal. The need to void may be urgent.
- Help the person assume a normal position for voiding if possible. Women sit or squat. Men stand.
- Warm the bedpan or urinal.
- Cover the person for warmth and privacy.
- Provide for privacy. Pull the curtain around the bed, close room and bathroom doors, and close window coverings. Leave the room if the person can be alone.
- Tell the person that running water, flushing the toilet, or playing music can mask voiding sounds. Voiding with others close by embarrasses some people.
- Stay nearby if the person is weak or unsteady.
- Place the signal light and toilet tissue within reach.
- Allow enough time. Do not rush the person.
- Promote relaxation. Some people like to read.
- Run water in a sink if the person cannot start the stream. Or place the person's fingers in warm water.
- Provide perineal care as needed (Chapter 20).
- Assist with hand washing after voiding. Provide a wash basin, soap, washcloth, and towel.
- Assist the person to the bathroom or offer the bedpan, urinal, or commode at regular times. Some people are embarrassed or are too weak to ask for help.

FOCUS ON COMMUNICATION
Normal Urination

Residents may not use "voiding" or "urinating" terms. The person may not understand what you are saying. Instead you can ask these questions:
- "Do you need to use the bathroom?"
- "Do you need to use the bedpan?"
- "Do you need to pass urine?"
- "Do you need to pee?"

TEAMWORK AND TIME MANAGEMENT
Normal Urination

The need to void may be urgent. Answer signal lights promptly. Also answer signal lights for co-workers. Otherwise incontinence may result. The person is wet and embarrassed. He or she is at risk for skin breakdown and infection. Your co-worker has extra work—changing linens and garments. You like help when you are busy. So do your co-workers.

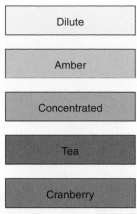

Fig. 22-1 Color chart for urine.

Dilute
Amber
Concentrated
Tea
Cranberry

Fig. 22-2 Standard bedpan *(left)* and the fracture pan *(right)*.

Table 22-1	Urinary Elimination Problems	
Problem	**Definition**	**Causes**
Dysuria	Painful or difficult *(dys)* urination *(uria)*	Urinary tract infection (UTI), trauma, urinary tract obstruction
Hematuria	Blood *(hemat)* in the urine *(uria)*	Kidney disease, UTI, trauma
Nocturia	Frequent urination *(uria)* at night *(noct)*	Excess fluid intake, kidney disease, prostate disease
Oliguria	Scant amount *(olig)* of urine *(uria)*; less than 500 mL in 24 hours	Poor fluid intake, shock, burns, kidney disease, heart failure
Polyuria	Abnormally large amounts *(poly)* of urine *(uria)*	Drugs, excess fluid intake, diabetes, hormone imbalance
Urinary frequency	Voiding at frequent intervals	Excess fluid intake, UTI, pressure on the bladder, drugs
Urinary incontinence	The involuntary loss or leakage of urine	Trauma, disease, UTI, reproductive or urinary tract surgeries, aging, fecal impaction, constipation, not getting to the bathroom in time
Urinary urgency	The need to void at once	UTI, fear of incontinence, full bladder, stress

Observations

Normal urine is pale yellow, straw-colored, or amber (Fig. 22-1). It is clear with no particles. A faint odor is normal. Observe urine for color, clarity, odor, amount, and particles.

Some foods affect urine color. Red food dyes, beets, blackberries, and rhubarb cause red-colored urine. Carrots and sweet potatoes cause bright yellow urine. Certain drugs change urine color. Asparagus causes a urine odor.

Ask the nurse to observe urine that looks or smells abnormal. Report complaints of urgency, burning on urination, or painful or difficult urination. Also report the problems in Table 22-1. The nurse uses the information for the nursing process.

Bedpans

Bedpans are used by persons who cannot be out of bed. Women use bedpans for voiding and bowel movements. Men use them for bowel movements.

The *standard bedpan* is shown in Figure 22-2. A *fracture pan* has a thin rim. It is only about ½-inch deep at one end (see Fig. 22-2). The smaller end is placed under the buttocks (Fig. 22-3, p. 336). Fracture pans are used:
- By persons with casts
- By persons in traction
- By persons with limited back motion
- After spinal cord injury or surgery
- After a hip fracture
- After hip replacement surgery

See *Delegation Guidelines: Bedpans*, p. 336.
See *Promoting Safety and Comfort: Bedpans*, p. 336.

Bladder   Urethra

Colon   Anus

Fig. 22-3 A person positioned on a fracture pan. The small end is under the buttocks.

DELEGATION GUIDELINES
Bedpans

Before assisting with a bedpan, you need this information from the nurse and the care plan:

- What bedpan to use—standard bedpan or fracture pan
- Position or activity limits
- If you can leave the room or if you need to stay with the person
- If the nurse needs to observe the results before disposing of the contents
- What observations to report and record:
  - Urine color, clarity, and odor
  - Amount
  - Presence of particles
  - Blood in the urine
  - Cloudy urine
  - Complaints of urgency, burning, dysuria, or other problems (see Table 22-1)
  - For bowel movements, see Chapter 23
- When to report observations
- What specific resident concerns to report at once

PROMOTING SAFETY AND COMFORT
Bedpans

Safety

Urine and bowel movements may contain blood and microbes. Microbes can live and grow in dirty bedpans. Follow Standard Precautions and the Bloodborne Pathogen Standard when handling bedpans and their contents. Thoroughly clean and disinfect bedpans after use.

Remember to raise the bed as needed for good body mechanics. Lower the bed before leaving the room. Raise or lower the bed rails according to the care plan.

Comfort

Some older persons have fragile bones from osteoporosis or painful joints from arthritis (Chapter 39). Fracture pans provide more comfort for them than standard bedpans.

Most bedpans are made of plastic. Some are made of metal. Metal bedpans are often cold. Warm them with warm water and then dry them before use.

The person must not sit on a bedpan for a long time. Bedpans are uncomfortable. And they can lead to pressure ulcers from prolonged pressure (Chapter 36).

Fig. 22-4 The person raises the buttocks off the bed with help. The bedpan is slid under the person.

GIVING THE BEDPAN

QUALITY OF LIFE

Remember to:
- Knock before entering the person's room.
- Address the person by name.
- Introduce yourself by name and title.

- Explain the procedure to the person before beginning and during the procedure.
- Protect the person's rights during the procedure.
- Handle the person gently during the procedure.

PRE-PROCEDURE

1 Follow *Delegation Guidelines: Bedpans.* See *Promoting Safety and Comfort: Bedpans.*
2 Provide for privacy.
3 Practice hand hygiene.
4 Put on gloves.
5 Collect the following:
   - Bedpan
   - Bedpan cover
   - Toilet tissue
   - Waterproof pad (if required by the center)
6 Arrange equipment on the chair or bed.

PROCEDURE

7 Lower the bed rail near you if up.
8 Position the person supine. Raise the head of the bed slightly.
9 Fold the top linens and gown out of the way. Keep the lower body covered.
10 Ask the person to flex the knees and raise the buttocks by pushing against the mattress with his or her feet.
11 Slide your hand under the lower back. Help raise the buttocks. If using a waterproof pad, place it under the person's buttocks.
12 Slide the bedpan under the person (Fig. 22-4).
13 If the person cannot assist in getting on the bedpan:
   a Place the waterproof pad under the person's buttocks if using one.
   b Turn the person onto the side away from you.
   c Place the bedpan firmly against the buttocks (Fig. 22-5, *A*, p. 338).
   d Push the bedpan down and toward the person (Fig. 22-5, *B*, p. 338).
   e Hold the bedpan securely. Turn the person onto his or her back.
   f Make sure the bedpan is centered under the person.
14 Cover the person.
15 Raise the head of the bed so the person is in a sitting position (Fowler's position) if the person uses a standard bedpan. (NOTE: Some state competency tests require that you remove gloves and wash your hands before raising the head of the bed.)
16 Make sure the person is correctly positioned on the bedpan (Fig. 22-6, p. 338).
17 Raise the bed rail if used.
18 Place the toilet tissue and signal light within reach.
19 Ask the person to signal when done or when help is needed.
20 Remove the gloves. Practice hand hygiene.
21 Leave the room, and close the door.
22 Return when the person signals. Or check on the person every 5 minutes. Knock before entering.
23 Practice hand hygiene. Put on gloves.
24 Raise the bed for body mechanics. Lower the bed rail (if used) and lower the head of the bed.
25 Ask the person to raise the buttocks. Remove the bedpan. Or hold the bedpan and turn him or her onto the side away from you.
26 Clean the genital area if the person cannot do so. Clean from front (urethra) to back (anus) with toilet tissue. Use fresh tissue for each wipe. Provide perineal care if needed. Remove and discard the waterproof pad if using one.
27 Cover the bedpan. Take it to the bathroom. Raise the bed rail (if used) before leaving the bedside.
28 Note the color, amount, and character of urine or feces.
29 Empty the bedpan contents into the toilet and flush.
30 Rinse the bedpan. Pour the rinse into the toilet and flush.
31 Clean the bedpan with a disinfectant.
32 Remove soiled gloves. Practice hand hygiene, and put on clean gloves.
33 Return the bedpan and clean cover to the bedside stand.
34 Help the person with hand washing. (Wear gloves for this step.)
35 Remove the gloves. Practice hand hygiene.

POST-PROCEDURE

36 Provide for comfort. (See the inside of the front book cover.)
37 Place the signal light within reach.
38 Lower the bed to its lowest position.
39 Raise or lower bed rails. Follow the care plan.
40 Unscreen the person.
41 Complete a safety check of the room. (See the inside of the front book cover.)
42 Follow center policy for soiled linen.
43 Practice hand hygiene.
44 Report and record your observations.

Fig. 22-5 Giving a bedpan. **A,** Position the person on one side. Place the bedpan firmly against the buttocks. **B,** Push downward on the bedpan and toward the person.

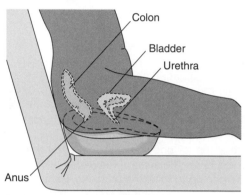

Fig. 22-6 The person is positioned on the bedpan so the urethra and anus are directly over the opening.

Fig. 22-7 Male urinal.

 Urinals

Men use urinals to void (Fig. 22-7). Plastic urinals have caps and hook-type handles. The urinal hooks to the bed rail within the man's reach. He stands to use the urinal if possible. Or he sits on the side of the bed or lies in bed to use it. Some men need support when standing. You may have to place and hold the urinal for some men.

After voiding, the urinal cap is closed. This prevents urine spills. Remind men to hang urinals on bed rails and to use the signal light after using them. Remind them not to place urinals on overbed tables and bedside stands. The overbed table is used for eating and as a work surface. Bedside stands are used for supplies. These surfaces must not be contaminated with urine.

Some beds may not have bed rails. Follow center policy for where to place urinals.

See *Focus on Communication: Urinals*
See *Delegation Guidelines: Urinals.*
See *Promoting Safety and Comfort: Urinals.*

FOCUS ON COMMUNICATION
Urinals

Some men cannot use a urinal on their own. You may need to assist them. You may need to stay with the person. For the person's comfort, explain why you must help him. You can say:
- "Mr. Turner, I'll help you use your urinal. I need to stay with you to make sure you don't fall."
- "Mr. Gomez, I'll help you place and remove your urinal so it doesn't spill."

DELEGATION GUIDELINES
Urinals

Before assisting with urinals, you need this information from the nurse and the care plan:

- How the urinal is used—standing, sitting, or lying in bed
- If help is needed with placing or holding the urinal
- If the man needs support to stand (If yes, how many staff members are needed)
- If you can leave the room or if you need to stay with the person
- If the nurse needs to observe the urine before its disposal
- What observations to report and record (see *Delegation Guidelines: Bedpans*, p. 336)
- When to report observations
- What specific resident concerns to report at once

PROMOTING SAFETY AND COMFORT
Urinals

Safety
Urine may contain microbes and blood. Follow Standard Precautions and the Bloodborne Pathogen Standard when handling urinals and their contents. Empty them promptly to prevent odors and the spread of microbes. A filled urinal spills easily, causing safety hazards. Also, it is an unpleasant sight and a source of odor. Urinals are cleaned and disinfected like bedpans.

Comfort
You may have to place the urinal for some men. This means that you have to place the penis in the urinal. This may embarrass both the person and you. Act in a professional manner at all times.

 ## GIVING THE URINAL   `VIDEO`

QUALITY OF LIFE

Remember to:
- Knock before entering the person's room.
- Address the person by name.
- Introduce yourself by name and title.

- Explain the procedure to the person before beginning and during the procedure.
- Protect the person's rights during the procedure.
- Handle the person gently during the procedure.

PRE-PROCEDURE

1 Follow *Delegation Guidelines: Urinals.* See *Promoting Safety and Comfort: Urinals.*
2 Provide for privacy.
3 Determine if the man will stand, sit, or lie in bed.
4 Practice hand hygiene.

5 Put on gloves.
6 Collect the following:
- Urinal
- Non-skid footwear if the person will stand to void

PROCEDURE

7 Give him the urinal if he is in bed. Remind him to tilt the bottom down to prevent spills.
8 If he is going to stand:
   a Help him sit on the side of the bed.
   b Put non-skid footwear on him.
   c Help him stand. Provide support if he is unsteady.
   d Give him the urinal.
9 Position the urinal if necessary. Position his penis in the urinal if he cannot do so.
10 Place the signal light within reach. Ask him to signal when done or when he needs help.
11 Provide for privacy.
12 Remove the gloves. Practice hand hygiene.
13 Leave the room, and close the door.

14 Return when he signals for you. Or check on him every 5 minutes. Knock before entering.
15 Practice hand hygiene. Put on gloves.
16 Close the cap on the urinal. Take it to the bathroom.
17 Note the color, amount, and clarity of urine.
18 Empty the urinal into the toilet and flush.
19 Rinse the urinal with cold water. Pour rinse into the toilet and flush.
20 Clean the urinal with a disinfectant.
21 Return the urinal to its proper place.
22 Remove soiled gloves. Practice hand hygiene, and put on clean gloves.
23 Assist with hand washing.
24 Remove the gloves. Practice hand hygiene.

POST-PROCEDURE

25 Provide for comfort. (See the inside of the front book cover.)
26 Place the signal light within reach.
27 Raise or lower bed rails. Follow the care plan.
28 Unscreen him.

29 Complete a safety check of the room. (See the inside of the front book cover.)
30 Follow center policy for soiled linen.
31 Practice hand hygiene.
32 Report and record your observations.

✉ Commodes

A commode is a chair or wheelchair with an opening for a container (Fig. 22-8). Persons unable to walk to the bathroom often use commodes. The commode allows a normal position for elimination. The commode arms and back provide support and help prevent falls.

Some commodes are wheeled into bathrooms and placed over toilets. They are useful for persons who need support when sitting. The container is removed if the commode is used with the toilet. Wheels are locked after the commode is positioned over the toilet.

See *Delegation Guidelines: Commodes.*
See *Promoting Safety and Comfort: Commodes.*

Fig. 22-8 A, The commode has a toilet seat with a container. The container slides out from under the seat for emptying. **B,** The container is removed. The commode chair is placed over the toilet.

DELEGATION GUIDELINES
Commodes

You need this information from the nurse and care plan when assisting with commodes:
- If the commode is used at the bedside or over the toilet
- How much help the person needs
- If you can leave the room or if you need to stay with the person
- If the nurse needs to observe urine or bowel movements
- What observations to report and record (see *Delegation Guidelines: Bedpans,* p. 336)
- When to report observations
- What specific resident concerns to report at once

PROMOTING SAFETY AND COMFORT
Commodes

Safety
For commode use, transfer the person from the bed, chair, or wheelchair to the commode. Practice safe transfer procedures (Chapter 17). Use the transfer belt, and lock the wheels. Remember to remove the transfer belt after the transfer. See "Transfer/Gait Belts" in Chapter 13.

Urine and feces may contain blood and microbes. Follow Standard Precautions and the Bloodborne Pathogen Standard. Thoroughly clean and disinfect the commode container after use. Clean and disinfect the seat and other commode parts if necessary.

Comfort
After the person transfers to the commode, cover his or her lap and legs with a bath blanket. This provides warmth and promotes privacy.

HELPING THE PERSON TO THE COMMODE | VIDEO |

QUALITY OF LIFE

Remember to:
- Knock before entering the person's room.
- Address the person by name.
- Introduce yourself by name and title.

- Explain the procedure to the person before beginning and during the procedure.
- Protect the person's rights during the procedure.
- Handle the person gently during the procedure.

PRE-PROCEDURE

1 Follow *Delegation Guidelines: Commodes.* See *Promoting Safety and Comfort: Commodes.*
2 Provide for privacy.
3 Practice hand hygiene.
4 Put on gloves.

5 Collect the following:
- Commode
- Toilet tissue
- Bath blanket
- Transfer belt
- Robe and non-skid footwear

PROCEDURE

6 Bring the commode next to the bed. Remove the chair seat and container lid.
7 Help the person sit on the side of the bed. Lower the bed rail if used.
8 Help him or her put on a robe and non-skid footwear.
9 Assist the person to the commode. Use the transfer belt.
10 Remove the transfer belt. Cover the person with a bath blanket for warmth.
11 Place the toilet tissue and signal light within reach.
12 Ask him or her to signal when done or when help is needed. (Stay with the person if necessary. Be respectful. Provide as much privacy as possible.)
13 Remove the gloves. Practice hand hygiene.
14 Leave the room. Close the door.
15 Return when the person signals. Or check on the person every 5 minutes. Knock before entering.
16 Decontaminate your hands. Put on the gloves.
17 Help the person clean the genital area as needed. Remove the gloves, and practice hand hygiene.

18 Apply the transfer belt. Help the person back to bed using the transfer belt. Remove the transfer belt, robe, and footwear. Raise the bed rail if used.
19 Put on clean gloves. Remove and cover the commode container. Clean the commode.
20 Take the container to the bathroom.
21 Observe urine and feces for color, amount, and character.
22 Empty the container contents into the toilet and flush.
23 Rinse the container. Pour the rinse into the toilet and flush.
24 Clean and disinfect the container.
25 Return the container to the commode. Return other supplies to their proper place.
26 Remove soiled gloves. Practice hand hygiene, and put on clean gloves.
27 Assist with hand washing.
28 Remove the gloves. Practice hand hygiene.

POST-PROCEDURE

29 Provide for comfort. (See the inside of the front book cover.)
30 Place the signal light within reach.
31 Raise or lower bed rails. Follow the care plan.
32 Unscreen the person.

33 Complete a safety check of the room. (See the inside of the front book cover.)
34 Follow center policy for dirty linen.
35 Practice hand hygiene.
36 Report and record your observations.

URINARY INCONTINENCE

Urinary incontinence is the involuntary loss or leakage of urine. While it occurs in some older persons, it is not a normal part of aging. However, older persons are at risk for incontinence because of changes in the urinary tract, medical and surgical conditions, and drug therapy.

Incontinence may be temporary or permanent. The basic types of incontinence are:

- **Stress incontinence.** Urine leaks during exercise and certain movements that cause pressure on the bladder. Urine loss is small (less than 50 mL). Often called dribbling, it occurs with laughing, sneezing, coughing, lifting, or other activities. Obesity and late pregnancy also are causes. The problem is common in women and may begin during menopause. Pelvic muscles weaken from pregnancies and with aging.
- **Urge incontinence.** Urine is lost in response to a sudden, urgent need to void. The person cannot get to a toilet in time. Urinary frequency, urinary urgency, and night-time voidings are common. Causes include UTIs, Alzheimer's disease, nervous system disorders, bladder cancer, and an enlarged prostate.
- **Overflow incontinence.** Small amounts of urine leak from a full bladder. The person feels like the bladder is not empty. The person only dribbles or has a weak urine stream. Diabetes, enlarged prostate, and some drugs are causes. So are spinal cord injuries.
- **Functional incontinence.** The person has bladder control but cannot use the toilet in time. Immobility, restraints, unanswered signal lights, no signal light within reach, and not knowing where to find the bathroom are causes. So is difficulty removing clothing. Confusion and disorientation are other causes.
- **Reflex incontinence.** Urine is lost at predictable intervals when the bladder is full. The person does not feel the need to void. Nervous system disorders and injuries are common causes.
- **Mixed incontinence.** The person has a combination of stress incontinence and urge incontinence. Many older women have this type.
- **Transient incontinence.** *Transient* means for a *short time*. Transient incontinence refers to temporary or occasional incontinence that is reversed when the cause is treated. Common causes are delirium (Chapter 44), UTI, some drugs, increased urine production, restricted mobility, and fecal impaction (Chapter 23).

Sometimes incontinence results from intestinal, rectal, and reproductive system surgeries. Incontinence may result from a physical illness or drugs. Some causes of incontinence can be reserved. Others cannot. If incontinence is a new problem, tell the nurse at once.

The Centers for Medicare & Medicaid Services (CMS) require appropriate treatment and services for persons who are incontinent. The goals are to:

- Prevent UTIs.
- Restore as much normal bladder function as possible.

Incontinence is embarrassing. Garments get wet, and odors develop. The person is uncomfortable. Skin irritation, infection, and pressure ulcers are risks. Falling is a risk when trying to get to the bathroom quickly. Pride, dignity, and self-esteem are affected. Social isolation, loss of independence, and depression are common. Quality of life suffers.

The person's care plan may include some of the measures listed in Box 22-2. *Good skin care and dry garments and linens are essential.* Promoting normal urinary elimination prevents incontinence in some people (see Box 22-1). Others need bladder training (p. 353). Sometimes catheters are needed (p. 344).

Incontinence products help keep the person dry (Fig. 22-9). They have two layers and a waterproof back. Fluid passes through the first layer. It is absorbed by the lower layer. The nurse selects products that best meet the person's needs. Follow the manufacturer's instructions and center procedures when using them.

Incontinence is linked to abuse, mistreatment, and neglect. Persons who are incontinent need frequent care. They may wet again right after skin care and changing wet garments and linens. Remember, incontinence is beyond the person's control. It is not something the person chooses to do. Be patient. The person's needs are great. If you are becoming short-tempered and impatient, talk to the nurse at once. The person has the right to be free from abuse, mistreatment, and neglect. Kindness, empathy, understanding, and patience are needed.

See *Residents With Dementia: Urinary Incontinence.*

Box 22-2   Nursing Measures for Persons With Urinary Incontinence

- Record the person's voidings. This includes incontinent times and successful use of the toilet, commode, bedpan, or urinal.
- Answer signal lights promptly. The need to void may be urgent.
- Promote normal urinary elimination (see Box 22-1).
- Promote normal bowel elimination (Chapter 23).
- Assist with elimination after sleep, before and after meals, and at bedtime.
- Follow the person's bladder training program (p. 353).
- Make sure the person has a clear pathway to the bathroom.
- Have the person wear easy-to-remove clothing. Incontinence can occur while trying to deal with buttons, zippers, other closures, and undergarments.
- Encourage the person to do pelvic muscle exercises as instructed by the nurse.
- Check the person often to make sure he or she is clean and dry.
- Help prevent UTIs:
  - Promote fluid intake as the nurse directs.
  - Have the person wear cotton underwear.
  - Keep the perineal area clean and dry.
- Decrease fluid intake at bedtime.

- Provide good skin care.
- Apply a barrier cream or moisturizer (cream, lotion, paste) as directed by the nurse. The cream prevents irritation and skin damage.
- Provide dry garments and linens.
- Observe for signs of skin breakdown (Chapters 35 and 36).
- Use incontinence products as the nurse directs. Follow the manufacturer's instructions.
- Do not leave urinals in place to catch urine in men who are incontinent.
- Keep the perineal area clean and dry (Chapter 20). Remember to:
  - Use soap and water or a no-rinse incontinence cleanser (perineal rinse). Follow the care plan. If using soap and water, remember to use a safe and comfortable water temperature and to rinse thoroughly.
  - Follow Standard Precautions and the Bloodborne Pathogen Standard.
  - Protect the person and dry garments and linen from the wet incontinence product.
  - Expose only the perineal area.
  - Dry the perineal area and buttocks.
  - Remove wet incontinence products, garments, and linen. Apply clean, dry ones.

RESIDENTS WITH DEMENTIA
Urinary Incontinence

Persons with dementia may develop incontinence. They may void in the wrong places. Trash cans, planters, heating vents, and closets are examples. Some persons remove incontinence products and throw them on the floor or in the toilet. Other persons resist staff efforts to keep them clean and dry.

You must provide safe care for these persons. The care plan lists needed measures. The care plan may include these measures recommended by the Alzheimer's Disease Education and Referral Center (ADEAR):

- Follow the person's bathroom routine as closely as possible. For example, take the person to the bathroom every 2 to 3 hours during the day. Do not wait for the person to ask.
- Observe for signs that the person may need to void. Restlessness and pulling at clothes are examples. Respond quickly.

- Stay calm when the person is incontinent. Re-assure the person if he or she becomes upset.
- Tell the nurse when the person is incontinent. Report the time, what the person was doing, and other observations. A pattern may emerge to the person's incontinence. If so, measures are planned to prevent the problem.
- Prevent episodes of incontinence during sleep. Limit the type and amount of fluids in the evening. Follow the care plan.
- Plan ahead if the person will leave the center. Have the person wear clothing that is easy to remove. Pack an extra set of clothing. Know where to find restrooms.

You may need a co-worker's help to keep the person clean and dry. If you have questions, ask the nurse for help.

Remember, everyone has the right to safe care. They also have the right to be treated with dignity and privacy.

Fig. 22-9 Disposable garment protectors. **A,** Complete incontinence brief. **B,** Pant liner and undergarment.

✉ CATHETERS

A catheter is a tube used to drain or inject fluid through a body opening. Inserted through the urethra into the bladder, a urinary catheter drains urine.

- A straight catheter drains the bladder and then is removed.
- An indwelling catheter (retention or Foley catheter) is left in the bladder. Urine drains constantly into a drainage bag. A balloon near the tip is inflated with sterile water after the catheter is inserted. The balloon prevents the catheter from slipping out of the bladder (Fig. 22-10). Tubing connects the catheter to the drainage bag.

Catheterization is the process of inserting a catheter. It is done by a doctor or nurse. With the proper education and supervision, some states and centers let nursing assistants insert and remove catheters.

Catheters often are used before, during, and after surgery. They keep the bladder empty. This reduces the risk of bladder injury during surgery. After surgery, a full bladder causes pressure on nearby organs. Such pressure can lead to pain or discomfort.

Some people are too weak or disabled to use the bedpan, urinal, commode, or toilet. Dying persons are examples. For them, catheters can promote comfort and prevent incontinence. Catheters can protect wounds and pressure ulcers from contact with urine. They also allow hourly urinary output measurements. However, they are a last resort for incontinence. Catheters do not treat the cause of incontinence.

Catheters also are used to:

- Collect sterile urine specimens.
- Measure the amount of urine left in the bladder after the person voids. This is called *residual urine*.

You will care for persons with indwelling catheters. The risk of UTI is high. Follow the rules in Box 22-3 to promote safety and comfort.

CMS surveyors will determine if the person is receiving appropriate treatment and services. The surveyor may ask you questions about:

- Your understanding of the person's bladder management program
- Your training related to handling catheters, catheter tubing, drainage bags, catheter care, UTIs, catheter-related injuries, dislodgement, and skin breakdown
- What observations to report, when to report them, and to whom you should report observations

See *Delegation Guidelines: Catheters.*
See *Promoting Safety and Comfort: Catheters.*

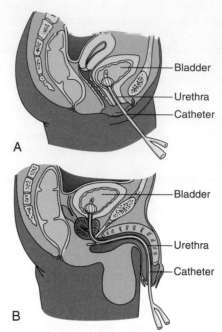

Fig. 22-10 Indwelling catheter. **A,** Indwelling catheter in the female bladder. The inflated balloon at the tip prevents the catheter from slipping out through the urethra. **B,** Indwelling catheter with the balloon inflated in the male bladder.

Fig. 22-11 Securing catheters. **A,** The drainage tube is coiled on the bed and secured to the bottom linens. The catheter is secured to the inner thigh with tape. Drainage tubing is secured to bottom linens with tape. **B,** The catheter is secured to the man's abdomen with a tube holder. Drainage tubing is secured to bottom linens with a clamp.

Box 22-3   Caring for Persons With Indwelling Catheters

- Follow the rules of medical asepsis.
- Follow Standard Precautions and the Bloodborne Pathogen Standard.
- Allow urine to flow freely through the catheter or tubing. Tubing should not have kinks. The person should not lie on the tubing.
- Keep the catheter connected to the drainage tubing. Follow the measures on p. 347 if the catheter and drainage tube are disconnected.
- Keep the drainage tube below the bladder. This prevents urine from flowing backward into the bladder.
- Move the bag to the other side of the bed when the person is turned and re-positioned on his or her other side.
- Attach the drainage bag to the bed frame, back of the chair, or lower part of an IV (intravenous) pole. *Never attach the drainage bag to the bed rail.* Otherwise it is higher than the bladder when the bed rail is raised.
- Do not let the drainage bag rest on the floor. This can contaminate the system.
- Coil the drainage tubing on the bed. Secure it to the bottom linen (Fig. 22-11). Follow center policy. Use a clip, bed sheet clamp, tape, safety pin with rubber band, or other device as directed by the nurse. Tubing must not loop below the drainage bag.
- Secure the catheter to the inner thigh (see Fig. 22-11). Or secure it to the man's abdomen. This prevents excess catheter movement and friction at the insertion site. Secure the catheter with a tube holder, tape, or other devices as the nurse directs.
- Check for leaks. Check the site where the catheter connects to the drainage bag. Report any leaks to the nurse at once.
- Provide catheter care according to the care plan—daily, twice a day, after bowel movements, or when vaginal discharge is present. (See procedure: *Giving Catheter Care,* p. 346). Some centers consider perineal care to be sufficient. Follow the care plan.
- Provide perineal care daily or twice a day, after bowel movements, and when there is vaginal drainage. Follow the care plan.
- Empty the drainage bag at the end of the shift or as the nurse directs. Measure and record the amount of urine (see procedure: *Emptying a Urinary Drainage Bag,* p. 350). Report an increase or decrease in the amount of urine.
- Use a separate measuring container for each person. This prevents the spread of microbes from one person to another.
- Do not let the drain on the drainage bag touch any surface.
- Encourage fluid intake as directed by the nurse and the care plan.
- Report complaints to the nurse at once—pain, burning, the need to void, or irritation. Also report the color, clarity, and odor of urine and the presence of particles.
- Observe for signs and symptoms of a UTI. Report the following at once:
  - Fever
  - Chills
  - Flank pain or tenderness (The flank area is in the back between the ribs and the hip.)
  - Change in the urine—blood, foul smell, particles, cloudiness, oliguria
  - Change in mental or functional status—confusion, decreased appetite, falls, decreased activity, tiredness, and so on
  - Urine leakage around the catheter

DELEGATION GUIDELINES
Catheters

The nurse may delegate catheter care to you. If so, you need this information from the nurse and the care plan:
- When to give catheter care—daily, twice a day, after bowel movements, or when vaginal discharge is present
- Where to secure the catheter—thigh or abdomen
- How to secure the catheter—tube holder, tape, or other device
- How to secure drainage tubing—clip, bed sheet clamp, tape, safety pin with rubber band, or other device
- What observations to report and record:
  - Complaints of pain, burning, irritation, or the need to void (report at once)
  - Crusting, abnormal drainage, or secretions
  - The color, clarity, and odor of urine
  - Particles in the urine
  - Blood in the urine
  - Cloudy urine
  - Urine leaking at the insertion site
  - Drainage system leaks
- When to report observations
- What specific resident concerns to report at once

PROMOTING SAFETY AND COMFORT
Catheters

Safety

Urine may contain microbes and blood. Follow Standard Precautions and the Bloodborne Pathogen Standard.

Be very careful when using a safety pin and rubber band to secure the drainage tubing to the bottom linens:
- Check the safety pin and rubber band:
  - The safety pin must work properly. It must not be stretched out of shape.
  - The rubber band must be intact. It should not be frayed or over-stretched.
- Do not insert the pin through the catheter.
- Point the pin away from the person.

Comfort

The catheter must not pull at the insertion site. This causes discomfort and irritation. Hold the catheter securely during catheter care. Then properly secure the catheter. Make sure the tubing is not under the person. Besides obstructing urine flow, lying on the tubing is uncomfortable. It can also cause skin breakdown. To promote comfort, see Box 22-3.

GIVING CATHETER CARE

QUALITY OF LIFE

Remember to:
- Knock before entering the person's room.
- Address the person by name.
- Introduce yourself by name and title.

- Explain the procedure to the person before beginning and during the procedure.
- Protect the person's rights during the procedure.
- Handle the person gently during the procedure.

PRE-PROCEDURE

1 Follow *Delegation Guidelines:*
  a *Perineal Care* (Chapter 20)
  b *Catheters,* p. 345
  See *Promoting Safety and Comfort:*
  a *Perineal Care* (Chapter 20)
  b *Catheters,* p. 345
2 Practice hand hygiene.
3 Collect the following:
  - Items for perineal care (Chapter 20)
  - Gloves
  - Bath blanket
4 Cover the overbed table with paper towels. Arrange items on top of them.

5 Identify the person. Check the ID (identification) bracelet against the assignment sheet. Also call the person by name.
6 Provide for privacy.
7 Fill the wash basin. Water temperature is about 105° F (Fahrenheit) (40.5° C [centigrade]). Measure water temperature according to center policy. Ask the person to check the water temperature. Adjust water temperature as needed.
8 Raise the bed for body mechanics. Bed rails are up if used.

PROCEDURE

9 Lower the bed rail near you if up.
10 Decontaminate your hands. Put on the gloves.
11 Cover the person with a bath blanket. Fan-fold top linens to the foot of the bed.
12 Drape the person for perineal care (Chapter 20).
13 Fold back the bath blanket to expose the genital area.
14 Place the waterproof pad under the buttocks. Ask the person to flex the knees and raise the buttocks off the bed.
15 Separate the labia (female). In an uncircumcised male, retract the foreskin (Fig. 22-12). Check for crusts, abnormal drainage, or secretions.
16 Give perineal care (Chapter 20).
17 Apply soap to a clean, wet washcloth.
18 Hold the catheter near the meatus.
19 Clean the catheter from the meatus down the catheter about 4 inches (Fig. 22-13). Clean downward, away from the meatus with 1 stroke. Do not tug or pull on the catheter. Repeat as needed with a clean area of the washcloth. Use a clean washcloth if needed.

20 Rinse the catheter with a clean washcloth. Rinse from the meatus down the catheter about 4 inches. Rinse downward, away from the meatus with 1 stroke. Do not tug or pull on the catheter. Repeat as needed with a clean area of the washcloth. Use a clean washcloth if needed.
21 Dry the catheter with a towel. Dry from the meatus down the catheter about 4 inches. Do not tug or pull on the catheter.
22 Pat dry the perineal area. Dry from front to back.
23 Return the foreskin to its natural position.
24 Secure the catheter. Coil and secure tubing (see Fig. 22-11).
25 Remove the waterproof pad.
26 Cover the person. Remove the bath blanket.
27 Remove the gloves. Practice hand hygiene.

POST-PROCEDURE

28 Provide for comfort. (See the inside of the front book cover.)
29 Place the signal light within reach.
30 Lower the bed to its lowest position.
31 Raise or lower bed rails. Follow the care plan.
32 Clean, dry, and return equipment to its proper place. Discard disposable items. (Wear gloves for this step.)

33 Unscreen the person.
34 Complete a safety check of the room. (See the inside of the front book cover.)
35 Follow center policy for soiled linen.
36 Remove the gloves. Practice hand hygiene.
37 Report and record your observations (Fig. 22-14).

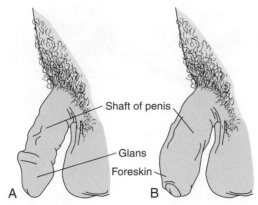

Fig. 22-12 **A,** Circumcised male. **B,** Uncircumcised male.

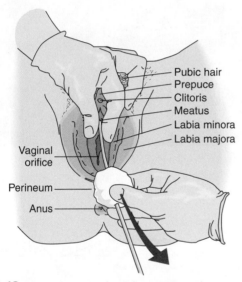

Fig. 22-13 The catheter is cleaned starting at the meatus. About 4 inches of the catheter are cleaned.

Date	Time	Nursing Margin	Other Depts Margin
12/21	0900	Catheter care given. No drainage from around the catheter. Resident denies discomfort. Clear amber urine flowing freely. Catheter secured to abdomen with tape. Drainage tubing attached to bed with clip. Resident positioned on L side. Bed in low position. Signal light within reach. Adam Aims, CNA ———	

Fig. 22-14 Charting sample.

Drainage Systems

A closed drainage system is used for indwelling catheters. Nothing can enter the system from the catheter to the drainage bag. The urinary system is sterile. Infection can occur if microbes enter the drainage system. The microbes travel up the tubing or catheter into the bladder and kidneys. A UTI can threaten health and life.

The drainage system has drainage tubing and a drainage bag (see Fig. 22-11). Tubing attaches at one end to the catheter. At the other end, it attaches to the drainage bag.

The bag hangs from the bed frame, chair, or wheelchair. It must not touch the floor. The bag is always kept lower than the person's bladder (see Fig. 22-11). Some people wear leg bags when up. The leg bag attaches to the thigh or calf (p. 351).

Microbes can grow in urine. If the drainage bag is higher than the bladder, urine can flow back into the bladder. A UTI can occur. *Therefore do not hang the drainage bag on a bed rail.* Otherwise when the bed rail is raised, the bag is higher than bladder level. When the person walks, the bag is held lower than the bladder.

Sometimes drainage systems are disconnected accidentally. If that happens, tell the nurse at once. Do not touch the ends of the catheter or tubing. Do the following:

* Practice hand hygiene. Put on gloves.
* Wipe the end of the tube with an antiseptic wipe.
* Wipe the end of the catheter with another antiseptic wipe.
* Do not put the ends down. Do not touch the ends after you clean them.
* Connect the tubing to the catheter.
* Discard the wipes into a biohazard bag.
* Remove the gloves. Practice hand hygiene.

Leg bags are changed to drainage bags when the person is in bed. This drainage bag stays lower than bladder level. You need to open the closed drainage system. You must prevent microbes from entering the system.

Drainage bags are emptied and urine is measured:

- At the end of every shift
- When changing from a leg bag to a drainage bag
- When changing from a drainage to a leg bag
- When the bag is becoming full

See *Delegation Guidelines: Drainage Systems.*
See *Promoting Safety and Comfort: Drainage Systems.*

DELEGATION GUIDELINES
Drainage Systems

Your delegated tasks may involve urinary drainage systems. If so, you need this information from the nurse and the care plan:

- When to empty the drainage bag
- If the person uses a leg bag
- When to switch a drainage bag and leg bag
- If you should clean or discard the drainage bag
- What observations to report and record:
  - The amount of urine measured
  - The color, clarity, and odor of urine
  - Particles in the urine
  - Blood in the urine
  - Cloudy urine
  - Complaints of pain, burning, irritation, or the need to urinate
  - Drainage system leaks
- When to report observations
- What specific resident concerns to report at once

PROMOTING SAFETY AND COMFORT
Drainage Systems

Safety
Urine may contain microbes and blood. Follow Standard Precautions and the Bloodborne Pathogen Standard.

For the procedure: *Changing a Leg Bag to a Drainage Bag,* you will open sterile packages. You must keep sterile items free from contamination. Review "Surgical Asepsis" in Chapter 15.

A leg bag attaches to the thigh or calf (p. 351). Leg bags hold less than 1000 mL of urine. Most standard drainage bags hold at least 2000 mL of urine. Therefore leg bags fill faster than standard drainage bags. Check leg bags often. Empty the leg bag if it is becoming half full. Measure the contents.

Comfort
Having urine in a drainage bag embarrasses some people. Visitors can see the urine when they are with the person. To promote mental comfort, have visitors sit on the side away from the drainage bag. Sometimes you can empty the bag before visitors arrive. Make sure you measure, report, and record the amount of urine.

Some centers provide drainage bag holders. The drainage bag is placed inside the holder. Urine cannot be seen.

Fig. 22-15 The clamped catheter prevents urine from draining out of the bladder. The clamp is applied directly to the catheter—not to the drainage tube.

Fig. 22-16 Sterile cap and catheter plug. The inside of the cap is sterile. Touch only the end of the plug.

Fig. 22-17 Sterile plug inserted into the end of the catheter. The sterile cap is on the end of the drainage tube.

CHANGING A LEG BAG TO A DRAINAGE BAG

QUALITY OF LIFE

Remember to:
- Knock before entering the person's room.
- Address the person by name.
- Introduce yourself by name and title.

- Explain the procedure to the person before beginning and during the procedure.
- Protect the person's rights during the procedure.
- Handle the person gently during the procedure.

PRE-PROCEDURE

1 Follow *Delegation Guidelines: Drainage Systems.* See *Promoting Safety and Comfort: Drainage Systems.*
2 Practice hand hygiene.
3 Collect the following:
- Gloves
- Drainage bag and tubing
- Antiseptic wipes
- Waterproof pad
- Sterile cap and plug
- Catheter clamp
- Paper towels
- Bedpan
- Bath blanket

4 Arrange paper towels and equipment on the overbed table.
5 Identify the person. Check the ID bracelet against the assignment sheet. Also call the person by name.
6 Provide for privacy.

PROCEDURE

7 Have the person sit on the side of the bed.
8 Practice hand hygiene. Put on the gloves.
9 Expose the catheter and leg bag.
10 Clamp the catheter (Fig. 22-15). This prevents urine from draining from the catheter into the drainage tubing.
11 Let urine drain from below the clamp into the drainage tubing. This empties the lower end of the catheter.
12 Help the person lie down.
13 Raise the bed rails if used. Raise the bed for body mechanics.
14 Lower the bed rail near you if up.
15 Cover the person with a bath blanket. Fan-fold top linens to the foot of the bed. Expose the catheter and leg bag.
16 Place the waterproof pad under the person's leg.
17 Open the antiseptic wipes. Set them on the paper towels.
18 Open the package with the sterile cap and plug. Set the package on the paper towels. Do not let anything touch the sterile cap or plug (Fig. 22-16).
19 Open the package with the drainage bag and tubing.
20 Attach the drainage bag to the bed frame.

21 Disconnect the catheter from the drainage tubing. Do not let anything touch the ends.
22 Insert the sterile plug into the catheter end (Fig. 22-17). Touch only the end of the plug. Do not touch the part that goes inside the catheter. (If you contaminate the end of the catheter, wipe the end with an antiseptic wipe. Do so before you insert the sterile plug.)
23 Place the sterile cap on the end of the leg bag drainage tube (see Fig. 22-17). (If you contaminate the tubing end, wipe the end with an antiseptic wipe. Do so before you put on the sterile cap.)
24 Remove the cap from the new drainage tubing.
25 Remove the sterile plug from the catheter.
26 Insert the end of the drainage tubing into the catheter.
27 Remove the clamp from the catheter.
28 Loop the drainage tubing on the bed. Secure the tubing to the bottom linens.
29 Remove the leg bag. Place it in the bedpan.
30 Remove and discard the waterproof pad.
31 Cover the person. Remove the bath blanket.
32 Take the bedpan to the bathroom.
33 Remove the gloves. Practice hand hygiene.

POST-PROCEDURE

34 Provide for comfort. (See the inside of the front book cover.)
35 Place the signal light within reach.
36 Lower the bed to its lowest position.
37 Raise or lower bed rails. Follow the care plan.
38 Unscreen the person.
39 Put on clean gloves. Discard disposable items.
40 Empty the drainage bag. See procedure: *Emptying a Urinary Drainage Bag,* p. 350.
41 Discard the drainage tubing and bag following center policy. Or clean the bag following center policy.

42 Clean and disinfect the bedpan. Place it in a clean cover.
43 Return the bedpan and other supplies to their proper place.
44 Remove the gloves. Practice hand hygiene.
45 Complete a safety check of the room. (See the inside of the front book cover.)
46 Follow center policy for soiled linen.
47 Practice hand hygiene.
48 Report and record your observations.

EMPTYING A URINARY DRAINAGE BAG   VIDEO

QUALITY OF LIFE

Remember to:
- Knock before entering the person's room.
- Address the person by name.
- Introduce yourself by name and title.

- Explain the procedure to the person before beginning and during the procedure.
- Protect the person's rights during the procedure.
- Handle the person gently during the procedure.

PRE-PROCEDURE

1 Follow *Delegation Guidelines: Drainage Systems*, p. 348. See *Promoting Safety and Comfort: Drainage Systems*, p. 348.
2 Collect the following:
- Graduate (measuring container)
- Gloves
- Paper towels

3 Practice hand hygiene.
4 Identify the person. Check the ID bracelet against the assignment sheet. Call the person by name.
5 Provide for privacy.

PROCEDURE

6 Put on the gloves.
7 Place a paper towel on the floor. Place the graduate on top of it.
8 Position the graduate under the collection bag.
9 Open the clamp on the drain.
10 Let all urine drain into the graduate. Do not let the drain touch the graduate (Fig. 22-18).
11 Close and position the clamp (see Fig. 22-11).
12 Measure urine.
13 Remove and discard the paper towel.

14 Empty the contents of the graduate into the toilet and flush.
15 Rinse the graduate. Empty the rinse into the toilet and flush.
16 Clean and disinfect the graduate.
17 Return the graduate to its proper place.
18 Remove the gloves. Practice hand hygiene.
19 Record the time and amount on the intake and output (I&O) record (Chapter 24).

POST-PROCEDURE

20 Provide for comfort. (See the inside of the front book cover.)
21 Place the signal light within reach.
22 Unscreen the person.

23 Complete a safety check of the room. (See the inside of the front book cover.)
24 Report and record the amount and other observations.

Fig. 22-18 The clamp on the drainage bag is opened. The drain is directed into the graduate. The drain must not touch the inside of the graduate. *(From Potter PA, Perry AF: Fundamentals of Nursing, ed 7, St. Louis, 2009, Mosby)*

Condom Catheters

Condom catheters are often used for incontinent men. They also are called *external catheters, Texas catheters,* and *urinary sheaths.* A condom catheter is a soft sheath that slides over the penis. Tubing connects the condom catheter and the drainage bag. Many men prefer leg bags (Fig. 22-19).

Condom catheters are changed daily after perineal care. To apply a condom catheter, follow the manufacturer's instruction. Thoroughly wash the penis with soap and water. Then dry it before applying the catheter.

Some condom catheters are self-adhering. Adhesive inside the catheter adheres to the penis. Other catheters are secured in place with elastic tape. Use the elastic tape packaged with the catheter. Elastic tape expands when the penis changes size. This allows blood flow to the penis. *Only use elastic tape. Never use adhesive or other tape to secure catheters. They do not expand. Blood flow to the penis is cut off, injuring the penis.*

See *Delegation Guidelines: Condom Catheters.*

See *Promoting Safety and Comfort: Condom Catheters.*

Fig. 22-19 Condom catheter attached to a leg bag.

DELEGATION GUIDELINES
Condom Catheters

Before removing or applying a condom catheter, you need this information from the nurse and the care plan:
- What size to use—small, medium, or large
- When to remove the catheter and apply a new one
- If a leg bag or standard drainage system is used
- What observations to report and record:
  - Reddened or open areas on the penis
  - Swelling of the penis
  - Color, clarity, and odor of urine
  - Particles in the urine
  - Blood in the urine
  - Cloudy urine
- When to report observations
- What specific resident concerns to report at once

PROMOTING SAFETY AND COMFORT
Condom Catheters

Safety

Do not apply a condom catheter if the penis is red, irritated, or shows signs of skin breakdown. Report your observations to the nurse at once.

If you do not know how to use the condom catheters used at your center, ask the nurse to show you the correct application. Then ask the nurse to observe you applying the catheter.

Blood must flow to the penis. If tape is needed, use the elastic tape packaged with the catheter. Apply it in a spiral fashion.

Urine may contain microbes and blood. Follow Standard Precautions and the Bloodborne Pathogen Standard.

Comfort

To apply a condom catheter, you need to touch and handle the penis. This can embarrass the man. Some men become sexually aroused. Always act in a professional manner. If necessary, allow the man some privacy. Provide for his safety and place the urinal within reach. Tell him when you will return, and then leave the room. Knock before entering the room again.

APPLYING A CONDOM CATHETER

VIDEO

QUALITY OF LIFE

Remember to:
- Knock before entering the person's room.
- Address the person by name.
- Introduce yourself by name and title.

- Explain the procedure to the person before beginning and during the procedure.
- Protect the person's rights during the procedure.
- Handle the person gently during the procedure.

PRE-PROCEDURE

1 Follow *Delegation Guidelines:*
  a *Perineal Care* (Chapter 20)
  b *Condom Catheters,* p. 351
  See *Promoting Safety and Comfort:*
  a *Perineal Care* (Chapter 20)
  b *Condom Catheters,* p. 351
2 Practice hand hygiene.
3 Collect the following:
- Condom catheter
- Elastic tape
- Drainage bag or leg bag
- Cap for the drainage bag
- Basin of warm water
- Soap
- Towel and washcloths

- Bath blanket
- Gloves
- Waterproof pad
- Paper towels

4 Cover the overbed table with paper towels. Arrange items on top of them.
5 Identify the person. Check the ID bracelet against the assignment sheet. Also call the person by name.
6 Provide for privacy.
7 Fill the wash basin. Water temperature is about 105° F (40.5° C). Measure water temperature according to center policy. Ask the person to check the water temperature. Adjust water temperature as needed.
8 Raise the bed for body mechanics. Bed rails are up if used.

PROCEDURE

9 Lower the bed rail near you if up.
10 Practice hand hygiene. Put on the gloves.
11 Cover the person with a bath blanket. Lower top linens to the knees.
12 Ask the person to raise his buttocks off the bed. Or turn him onto his side away from you.
13 Slide the waterproof pad under his buttocks.
14 Have the person lower his buttocks. Or turn him onto his back.
15 Secure the drainage bag to the bed frame. Or have a leg bag ready. Close the drain.
16 Expose the genital area.
17 Remove the condom catheter.
  a Remove the tape. Roll the sheath off the penis.
  b Disconnect the drainage tubing from the condom. Cap the drainage tube.
  c Discard the tape and condom.
18 Provide perineal care (Chapter 20). Observe the penis for reddened areas, skin breakdown, and irritation.
19 Remove the gloves, and practice hand hygiene. Put on clean gloves.

20 Remove the protective backing from the condom. This exposes the adhesive strip.
21 Hold the penis firmly. Roll the condom onto the penis. Leave a 1-inch space between the penis and the end of the catheter (Fig. 22-20).
22 Secure the condom.
  a For a self-adhering condom: press the condom to the penis.
  b For a condom secured with elastic tape: apply elastic tape in a spiral fashion. See Figure 22-20. Do not apply tape completely around the penis.
23 Make sure the penis tip does not touch the condom. Make sure the condom is not twisted.
24 Connect the condom to the drainage tubing. Coil and secure excess tubing on the bed. Or attach a leg bag.
25 Remove the waterproof pad and gloves. Discard them. Practice hand hygiene.
26 Cover the person. Remove the bath blanket.

POST-PROCEDURE

27 Provide for comfort. (See the inside of the front book cover.)
28 Place the signal light within reach.
29 Lower the bed to its lowest position.
30 Raise or lower bed rails. Follow the care plan.
31 Unscreen the person.
32 Practice hand hygiene. Put on clean gloves.

33 Measure and record the amount of urine in the bag. Clean or discard the collection bag.
34 Clean, dry, and return the wash basin and other equipment. Return items to their proper place.
35 Remove the gloves. Practice hand hygiene.
36 Complete a safety check of the room. (See the inside of the front book cover.)
37 Report and record your observations.

Fig. 22-20 A condom catheter applied to the penis. A 1-inch space is between the penis and the end of the catheter. Elastic tape is applied in a spiral fashion to secure the condom catheter to the penis.

BLADDER TRAINING

Bladder training helps some persons with urinary incontinence. Some persons need bladder training after indwelling catheter removal. Control of urination is the goal. Bladder control promotes comfort and quality of life. It also increases self-esteem. You assist with bladder training as directed by the nurse and the care plan. Successful bladder training may take several weeks.

The rules for normal elimination are followed. The normal position for urination is assumed if possible. Privacy is important. The person's care plan may include one of the following:

- *Bladder retraining (bladder rehabilitation)*. This requires that the person:
  - Resist or ignore the strong desire to urinate
  - Postpone or delay voiding
  - Urinate following a schedule rather than the urge to void

  The time between voidings may be increased as bladder retraining progresses.
- *Prompted voiding*. The person uses the toilet, commode, bedpan, or urinal at scheduled times. The person is taught to:
  - Recognize when the bladder is full
  - Recognize the need to void
  - Ask for help
  - Respond when prompted to void

- *Habit training/scheduled voiding*. Voiding is scheduled at regular times to match the person's voiding habits. This is usually every 3 to 4 hours while awake. The person does not delay or resist voiding. Timed-voiding is based on the person's usual voiding pattern.
- *Catheter clamping*. The catheter is clamped to prevent urine flow from the bladder (see Fig. 22-15). It is usually clamped for 1 hour at first. Over time, it is clamped for 3 to 4 hours. Urine drains when the catheter is unclamped. When the catheter is removed, voiding is encouraged every 3 to 4 hours or as directed by the nurse and the care plan.

QUALITY OF LIFE

People do not usually void in front of others. Illness, disease, and aging can affect this private act. Residents often depend on the nursing staff to assist with elimination needs. Some are very weak and disabled. They cannot use the bathroom, commode, bedpan, or urinal alone.

You must protect the person's privacy. Pull privacy curtains and close doors and window coverings. If you must stay in the room, allow as much privacy as possible. Stand just outside the bathroom door in case the person needs you. Or stand on the other side of the privacy curtain if safe to do so. The nurse helps you with ways to protect the person's privacy.

Some persons can place bedpans and urinals themselves. Some can get on and off bedside commodes themselves. Other persons need some help but can be left alone to void. Allow persons to do as much as safely possible.

To safely promote independence, keep devices within reach for persons who use them without help. For persons who need some help, check on them often. Do not leave a person sitting on a bedpan or commode for a long time. Discomfort, odors, and skin breakdown are likely. Also, the person may think you forgot about him or her. The person may try to get off of the bedpan or commode alone. He or she may be harmed. Make sure the signal light is within reach. Respond promptly when a person calls for help.

Empty urinals, bedpans, and commodes promptly. Leaving urine-filled devices in the person's room does not respect the person's right to a neat and clean setting. It also may cause embarrassment. Do your best to promote comfort, dignity, and respect when assisting with elimination needs.

Privacy and confidentiality are important for persons who are incontinent. Incontinence is embarrassing. It affects the person's pride, dignity, and self-esteem. Only those involved in the person's care need to know about incontinence. Patience and understanding are important. Incontinence is not something the persons wants or chooses.

REVIEW QUESTIONS

Circle the BEST answer.

1 Which is *false?*
   a Urine is normally clear and yellow or amber in color.
   b Urine normally has an ammonia odor.
   c Micturition usually occurs before going to bed and after sleep.
   d A person normally voids 1500 mL a day.

2 Which is *not* a rule for normal elimination?
   a Help the person assume a normal position for voiding.
   b Provide for privacy.
   c Help the person to the bathroom or commode. Or provide the bedpan or urinal as soon as requested.
   d Stay with the person who uses the bedpan.

3 The person using a standard bedpan is in
   a Fowler's position
   b The supine position
   c The prone position
   d The side-lying position

4 After using the urinal, the man should
   a Put it on the bedside stand
   b Use the signal light
   c Put it on the overbed table
   d Empty it

5 After a person uses a commode, you should
   a Clean and disinfect the container, seat, and commode parts
   b Return the commode to the supply area
   c Get a new container
   d Get a new commode

6 Urinary incontinence
   a Is always permanent
   b Requires good skin care
   c Is treated with a catheter
   d Requires bladder training

7 Which is *not* a cause of functional incontinence?
   a Unanswered signal light
   b No signal light within reach
   c Problems removing clothing
   d UTI

8 A person has an indwelling catheter. Which is *not* correct?
   a Keep the drainage bag above the level of the bladder.
   b Keep drainage tubing free of kinks.
   c Coil the drainage tubing on the bed.
   d Secure the catheter according to center policy.

9 A person has an indwelling catheter. Which is *not* correct?
   a Tape any leaks at the connection site.
   b Follow Standard Precautions and the Bloodborne Pathogen Standard.
   c Empty the drainage bag at the end of your shift.
   d Report complaints of pain, burning, the need to void, or irritation at once.

10 A person has an indwelling catheter. You are going to turn the person from the left side to the right side. What should you do with the drainage bag?
   a Move it to the right side.
   b Keep it on the left side.
   c Hang it from an IV pole.
   d Remove the catheter and the drainage bag.

11 When giving catheter care, you clean the catheter
   a From the meatus down the catheter about 4 inches
   b From the meatus down the entire catheter
   c From the drainage tube connection up the catheter to the meatus
   d From the drainage tube connection up the catheter about 4 inches

12 Mr. Cooper has a condom catheter. You apply elastic tape
   a Completely around the penis
   b To the inner thigh
   c To the abdomen
   d In a spiral fashion

13 The goal of bladder training is to
   a Remove the catheter
   b Clamp the catheter
   c Allow the person to walk to the bathroom
   d Gain control of urination

14 A person is taught to ignore the urge to void. This type of bladder training is called
   a Bladder retraining
   b Prompted voiding
   c Habit training
   d Scheduled voiding

Answers to these questions are on p. 720.

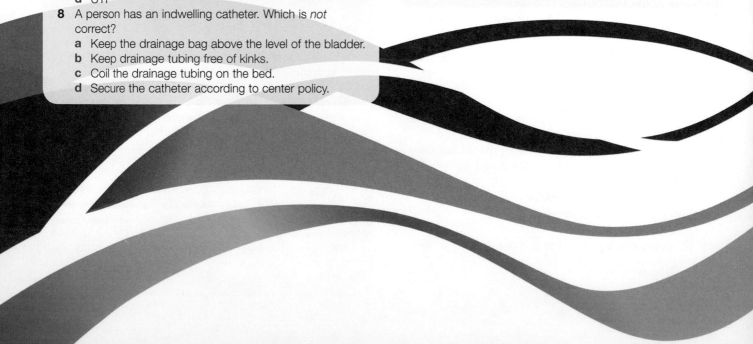

Bowel Elimination

OBJECTIVES

- Define the key terms and key abbreviations listed in this chapter.
- Describe normal defecation.
- List the observations to make about defecation.
- Identify the factors that affect bowel elimination.
- Describe the common bowel elimination problems.
- Explain how to promote comfort and safety during defecation.

- Describe bowel training.
- Explain why enemas are given.
- Describe the common enema solutions.
- Describe the rules for giving enemas.
- Describe how to care for a person with an ostomy.
- Perform the procedures described in this chapter.
- Explain how to promote quality of life.

KEY TERMS

colostomy A surgically created opening *(stomy)* between the colon *(colo)* and abdominal wall

constipation The passage of a hard, dry stool

defecation The process of excreting feces from the rectum through the anus; a bowel movement

dehydration The excessive loss of water from tissues

diarrhea The frequent passage of liquid stools

enema The introduction of fluid into the rectum and lower colon

fecal impaction The prolonged retention and buildup of feces in the rectum

fecal incontinence The inability to control the passage of feces and gas through the anus

feces The semi-solid mass of waste products in the colon that is expelled through the anus

flatulence The excessive formation of gas or air in the stomach and intestines

flatus Gas or air passed through the anus

ileostomy A surgically created opening *(stomy)* between the ileum (small intestine *[ileo]*) and the abdominal wall

ostomy A surgically created opening for the elimination of body wastes; see "colostomy" and "ileostomy"

peristalsis The alternating contraction and relaxation of intestinal muscles

stoma An opening that can be seen through the abdominal wall; see "colostomy" and "ileostomy"

stool Excreted feces

suppository A cone-shaped, solid drug that is inserted into a body opening; it melts at body temperature

KEY ABBREVIATIONS

BM	Bowel movement	**IV**	Intravenous
C	Centigrade	**mL**	Milliliter
F	Fahrenheit	**oz**	Ounce
GI	Gastro-intestinal	**SSE**	Soapsuds enema
ID	Identification		

Bowel elimination is a basic physical need. It is the excretion of wastes from the gastro-intestinal system (GI) (Chapter 9). Many factors affect bowel elimination. They include privacy, habits, age, diet, exercise and activity, fluids, and drugs. Problems easily occur. Promoting normal bowel elimination is important. You assist residents in meeting elimination needs.

NORMAL BOWEL ELIMINATION

Foods and fluids are partially digested in the stomach. The partially digested food and fluids are called *chyme*. Chyme passes from the stomach into the small intestine. It enters the large intestine (large bowel or colon) where fluid is absorbed. Chyme becomes less fluid and more solid in consistency. Feces refers to the semi-solid mass of waste products in the colon that is expelled through the anus.

Feces move through the intestines by peristalsis. Peristalsis is the alternating contraction and relaxation of intestinal muscles. The feces move through the large intestine to the rectum. Feces are stored in the rectum until excreted from the body. Defecation (bowel movement [BM]) is the process of excreting feces from the rectum through the anus. Stool refers to excreted feces.

Some people have a BM every day. Others have one every 2 to 3 days. Some people have 2 or 3 BMs a day. Many people have a BM after breakfast. Others do so in the evening. Many older persons expect to have a BM every day. They are very concerned if they do not do so. The nurse teaches them about normal elimination.

Stools are normally brown. Bleeding in the stomach and small intestine causes black or tarry stools. Bleeding in the lower colon and rectum causes red-colored stools. So do beets, tomato juice or soup, red Jell-O, and foods with red food coloring. A diet high in green vegetables can cause green stools. Diseases and infection can cause clay-colored or white, pale, orange-colored, or green-colored stools.

Stools are normally soft, formed, moist, and shaped like the rectum. They have a normal odor caused by bacterial action in the intestines. Certain foods and drugs also cause odors.

Observations

Your observations are used for the nursing process. Carefully observe stools before disposing of them. Ask the nurse to observe abnormal stools. Observe and report the following to the nurse. If allowed to chart, also record the following:

- Color
- Amount
- Consistency
- Presence of blood or mucus
- Odor
- Shape
- Frequency of BMs
- Complaints of pain or discomfort
  See *Focus on Communication: Observations.*

FACTORS AFFECTING BOWEL ELIMINATION

These factors affect stool frequency, consistency, color, and odor. The nurse considers them when using the nursing process to meet the person's elimination needs. Normal, regular elimination is the goal.

FOCUS ON COMMUNICATION
Observations

Many residents tend to their own bowel elimination needs. However, information is still needed for the person's record and the nursing process. You may need to ask these questions:

- "Did you have a bowel movement today?"
- "Please tell me about your bowel movement."
- "When did you have a bowel movement?"
- "What was the amount?"
- "Were the stools formed or loose?"
- "What was the color?"
- "Did you have any bleeding, pain, or problems having a bowel movement?"
- "Did you pass any gas?"
- "How much gas did you pass?"
- "Do you need to pass more gas?"
- "Do you need help cleaning yourself?"

- *Privacy.* Bowel elimination is a private act. Odors and sounds are embarrassing. Lack of privacy can prevent a BM despite having the urge. Some people ignore the urge when others are present.
- *Habits.* Many people have a BM after breakfast. Some drink a hot beverage, read, or take a walk. These activities are relaxing. A BM is easier when a person is relaxed, not tense.
- *Diet—high-fiber foods.* High-fiber foods leave a residue for needed bulk. Fruits, vegetables, and whole grain cereals and breads are high in fiber. Many people do not eat enough fruits and vegetables. Some cannot chew these foods. They may not have teeth. Or dentures may fit poorly. Some people think that they cannot digest fruits and vegetables. So they refuse to eat them. In nursing centers, bran may be added to cereal, prunes, or prune juice. These foods provide fiber and prevent constipation.
- *Diet—other foods.* Milk and milk products can cause constipation or diarrhea. Chocolate and other foods cause similar reactions. Spicy foods can irritate the intestines. Frequent stools or diarrhea can result. Gas-forming foods stimulate peristalsis, which aids a BM. Such foods include onions, beans, cabbage, cauliflower, radishes, and cucumbers.
- *Fluids.* Feces contain water. Stool consistency depends on the amount of water absorbed in the colon. The amount of fluid intake, urine output, and vomiting are factors. Feces harden and dry when large amounts of water are absorbed or when fluid intake is poor. Hard, dry feces move slowly through the colon. Constipation can occur. Drinking 6 to 8 glasses of water daily promotes normal bowel elimination. Warm fluids—coffee, tea, hot cider, warm water—increase peristalsis.
- *Activity.* Exercise and activity maintain muscle tone and stimulate peristalsis. Irregular elimination and constipation often occur from inactivity and bedrest. Inactivity may result from disease, surgery, injury, and aging.
- *Drugs.* Drugs can prevent constipation or control diarrhea. Other drugs have diarrhea or constipation as side effects. Drugs for pain relief often cause constipation. Antibiotics (used to fight or prevent infections) often cause diarrhea. Diarrhea occurs when the antibiotics kill normal flora in the colon. Normal flora is needed to form feces.
- *Disability.* Some people cannot control bowel movements. They have a BM whenever feces enter the rectum. A bowel training program is needed (p. 359).
- *Aging.* Aging causes changes in the GI tract. Feces pass through the intestines at a slower rate. Constipation is a risk. Some older persons lose bowel control. Older persons may not completely empty the rectum. They often need to have another BM about 30 to 45 minutes after the first BM. Older persons are at risk for intestinal tumors and disorders.

Box 23-1 Safety and Comfort During Bowel Elimination

- Follow Standard Precautions and the Bloodborne Pathogen Standard.
- Provide for privacy. Ask visitors to leave the room. Close doors, privacy curtains, and window coverings.
- Help the person to the toilet or commode. Or provide the bedpan as soon as requested.
- Wheel the person into the bathroom on the commode if possible. Place the commode over the toilet. This provides privacy. Remember to lock the commode wheels.
- Make sure the bedpan is warm.
- Position the person in a normal sitting or squatting position.
- Cover the person for warmth and privacy.
- Allow enough time for a BM.
- Place the signal light and toilet tissue within reach.
- Leave the room if the person can be alone. Check on the person every 5 minutes.
- Stay nearby if the person is weak or unsteady.
- Provide perineal care.
- Dispose of stools promptly. This reduces odors and prevents the spread of microbes.
- Assist the person with hand washing after elimination.
- Follow the care plan if the person has fecal incontinence. The care plan tells you when to assist with elimination.

TEAMWORK AND TIME MANAGEMENT
Safety and Comfort

The need to have a BM may be urgent. Answer signal lights promptly. Also help co-workers answer signal lights. Residents must not be left sitting on toilets, commodes, or bedpans. They must not be left sitting or lying in stools.

Safety and Comfort

The care plan includes measures to meet the person's elimination needs. It may involve diet, fluids, and exercise. Follow the measures in Box 23-1 to promote safety and comfort.

See *Teamwork and Time Management: Safety and Comfort.*

COMMON PROBLEMS

Common problems include constipation, fecal impaction, diarrhea, fecal incontinence, and flatulence.

Constipation

Constipation is the passage of a hard, dry stool. The person usually strains to have a BM. Stools are large or marble-size. Large stools cause pain as they pass through the anus. Constipation occurs when feces move slowly through the bowel. This allows more time for water absorption. Common causes of constipation include:

- A low-fiber diet
- Ignoring the urge to have a BM
- Decreased fluid intake
- Inactivity
- Drugs
- Aging
- Certain diseases

Dietary changes, fluids, and activity prevent or relieve constipation. So do drugs and enemas.

Fecal Impaction

A **fecal impaction** is the prolonged retention and build-up of feces in the rectum. Feces are hard or putty-like. Fecal impaction results if constipation is not relieved. The person cannot defecate. More water is absorbed from the already hard feces. Liquid feces pass around the hardened fecal mass in the rectum. The liquid feces seep from the anus.

The person tries many times to have a BM. Abdominal discomfort, abdominal distention (swelling), nausea, cramping, and rectal pain are common. Older persons may have poor appetite or confusion. Some persons may have a fever. Report these signs and symptoms to the nurse.

The nurse does a digital (finger) exam to check for an impaction. A lubricated, gloved finger is inserted into the rectum to feel for a hard mass (Fig. 23-1). The mass is felt in the lower rectum. Sometimes it is higher in the colon and out of reach. The digital exam often causes the urge to have a BM. The doctor may order drugs and enemas to remove the impaction.

Sometimes the nurse removes the fecal mass with a gloved finger. This is called *digital removal of an impaction.*

Diarrhea

Diarrhea is the frequent passage of liquid stools. Feces move through the intestines rapidly. This reduces the time for fluid absorption. The need for a BM is urgent. Some people cannot get to a bathroom in time. Abdominal cramping, nausea, and vomiting may occur.

Causes of diarrhea include infections, some drugs, irritating foods, and microbes in food and water. Diet and drugs are ordered to reduce peristalsis. You need to:

- Assist with elimination needs promptly.
- Dispose of stools promptly. This prevents odors and the spread of microbes.
- Give good skin care. Liquid stools irritate the skin. So does frequent wiping with toilet tissue. Skin breakdown and pressure ulcers are risks.

Fluid lost through diarrhea is replaced. Otherwise dehydration occurs. **Dehydration** is the excessive loss of water from tissues. The person has pale or flushed skin, dry skin, and a coated tongue. The urine is dark and scant in amount (oliguria). Thirst, weakness, dizziness, and confusion also occur. Falling blood pressure and increased pulse and respirations are serious signs. Death can occur. The nursing process is used to meet the person's fluid needs. The doctor may order IV (intravenous) fluids in severe cases (Chapter 25).

Microbes can cause diarrhea. Preventing the spread of infection is important. Always follow Standard Precautions and the Bloodborne Pathogen Standard when in contact with stools.

See *Promoting Safety and Comfort: Diarrhea.*

Fecal Incontinence

Fecal incontinence is the inability to control the passage of feces and gas through the anus. Causes include:

- Intestinal diseases
- Nervous system diseases and injuries
- Fecal impaction
- Diarrhea
- Some drugs
- Chronic illness
- Aging
- Mental health problems or dementia (Chapters 43 and 44)—the person may not recognize the need for or act of having a BM
- Not answering signal lights when help is needed with elimination
- Not getting to the bathroom in time
- Not finding the bathroom when in a new setting

Fig. 23-1 A gloved index finger is used to check for a fecal impaction.

Safety
Death is a risk when dehydration is not recognized and treated. Older persons are at risk for dehydration. The amount of body water decreases with aging. Therefore diarrhea is very serious in older persons. Report signs of diarrhea at once. Ask the nurse to observe the stool.

Clostridium difficile
Clostridium difficile (*C. difficile* [CDI]) is a microbe that causes diarrhea and intestinal infections. It can cause death. Persons at risk include persons who are older, ill, or need the prolonged use of antibiotics. Signs and symptoms include:
- Watery diarrhea with a foul odor
- Fever
- Loss of appetite
- Nausea
- Abdominal pain or tenderness

The microbe is found in feces. A person becomes infected by touching items or surfaces contaminated with feces and then touching his or her mouth or mucous membranes. You can spread the microbe if your contaminated hands or gloves:
- Touch a person
- Contaminate surfaces

You must practice good hand hygiene. Alcohol-based hand rubs are not effective against *C. difficile*. You must wash your hands with soap and water. Also follow Standard Precautions.

Persons with dementia may smear stools on themselves, furniture, and walls. Some are not aware of having BMs. Some resist care. Follow the person's care plan. The measures for urinary incontinence (Chapter 22) may be part of the care plan. Be patient. Ask for help from co-workers. Talk to the nurse if you have problems keeping the person clean.

Fecal incontinence affects the person emotionally. Frustration, embarrassment, anger, and humiliation are common. The person may need:
- Bowel training
- Help with elimination after meals and every 2 to 3 hours
- Incontinence products to keep garments and linens clean
- Good skin care

See *Residents With Dementia: Fecal Incontinence*.

Flatulence

Gas and air are normally in the stomach and intestines. They are expelled through the mouth (burping, belching, eructating) and anus. Gas or air passed through the anus is called flatus. Flatulence is the excessive formation of gas or air in the stomach and intestines. Causes include:
- Swallowing air while eating and drinking. This includes chewing gum, eating fast, drinking through a straw, and drinking carbonated beverages. Tense or anxious people may swallow large amounts of air when drinking.
- Bacterial action in the intestines.
- Gas-forming foods (onions, beans, cabbage, cauliflower, radishes, and cucumbers).
- Constipation.
- Bowel and abdominal surgeries.
- Drugs that decrease peristalsis.

If flatus is not expelled, the intestines distend. That is, they swell or enlarge from the pressure of gases. Abdominal cramping or pain, shortness of breath, and a swollen abdomen occur. "Bloating" is a common complaint. Exercise, walking, moving in bed, and the left-side lying position often produce flatus. Doctors may order enemas and drugs to relieve flatulence.

BOWEL TRAINING

Bowel training has two goals:
- To gain control of bowel movements.
- To develop a regular pattern of elimination. Fecal impaction, constipation, and fecal incontinence are prevented.

Meals, especially breakfast, stimulate the urge for a BM. The person's usual time of day for a BM is noted on the care plan. So is toilet, commode, or bedpan use. Offer help with elimination at the times noted. Factors that promote elimination are part of the care plan and bowel training program. These include a high-fiber diet, increased fluids, warm fluids, activity, and privacy. The nurse tells you about a person's bowel training program.

The doctor may order a suppository to stimulate a BM. A suppository is a cone-shaped, solid drug that is inserted into a body opening. It melts at body temperature. A nurse inserts a rectal suppository into the rectum (Fig. 23-2, p. 360). A BM occurs about 30 minutes later.

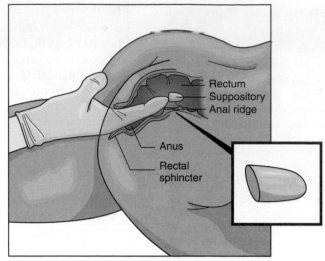

Fig. 23-2 The suppository *(inset)* is inserted into the rectum.

ENEMAS

An **enema** is the introduction of fluid into the rectum and lower colon. Doctors order enemas:

- To remove feces
- To relieve constipation, fecal impaction, or flatulence
- To clean the bowel of feces before certain surgeries and diagnostic procedures

Safety and comfort measures for bowel elimination are practiced when giving an enema (see Box 23-1). So are the rules in Box 23-2.

The doctor orders the enema solution. The solution depends on the enema's purpose:

- *Tap water enema*—is obtained from a faucet.
- *Saline enema*—is a solution of salt and water. For adults, add 1 to 2 teaspoons of table salt to 500 to 1000 mL (milliliters) of tap water.
- *Soapsuds enema (SSE)*—for adults, add 3 to 5 mL of castile soap to 500 to 1000 mL of tap water.
- *Small-volume enema*—the adult size contains about 120 mL (4 ounces [oz]) of solution. The commercially prepared enema is ready to use.
- *Oil-retention enema*—has mineral, olive, or cotton-seed oil. The adult size contains about 120 mL (4 oz) of solution. The commercially prepared enema is ready to use.

Other enema solutions may be ordered. Consult with the nurse and use the center's procedure manual to safely prepare and give enemas. You do not give enemas that contain drugs. Nurses give them.

See *Delegation Guidelines: Enemas.*

See *Promoting Safety and Comfort: Enemas.*

Box 23-2 Safety and Comfort Measures for Giving Enemas

- Have the person void first. This increases the person's comfort during the enema procedure.
- Measure solution temperature with a bath thermometer. See *Delegation Guidelines: Enemas.*
- Give the amount of solution ordered.
- Position the person as the nurse directs. The Sims' position or the left side-lying position is preferred.
- Ask the nurse and check the procedure manual for how far to insert the enema tubing. It is usually inserted 2 to 4 inches in adults.
- Lubricate the enema tip before inserting it.
- Stop tube insertion if you feel resistance, the person complains of pain, or bleeding occurs.
- Ask the nurse how high to raise the enema bag. For adults, it is usually held 12 inches above the anus.
- Give the solution slowly. Usually it takes 10 to 15 minutes to give 750 to 1000 mL.
- Hold the enema tube in place while giving the solution.
- Ask the nurse how long the person should retain the solution. The length of time depends on the amount and type of solution.
- Make sure the bathroom will be vacant when the person needs to defecate. Make sure that another person will not use the bathroom. If the person uses the commode, have the commode ready.
- Ask the nurse to observe the enema results.

DELEGATION GUIDELINES
Enemas

Some states and centers let nursing assistants give enemas. Others do not. Before giving an enema, make sure that:

- Your state allows you to perform the procedure.
- The procedure is in your job description.
- You have the necessary education and training.
- You review the procedure with the nurse.
- A nurse is available to answer questions and to supervise you.

If the above conditions are met, you need this information from the nurse:

- What type of enema to give—cleansing, small-volume, or oil-retention
- What size enema tube to use
- When to give the enema
- How many times to repeat the enema
- The amount of solution ordered by the doctor—usually 500 to 1000 mL for a cleansing enema (for adults)
- How much castile soap to use for an SSE
- How much salt to use for a saline enema
- What the solution temperature should be—usually body temperature (98.6° F [Fahrenheit] or 37° C [centigrade]); sometimes warmer temperatures (105° F [40.5° C]) are used for adults
- How to position the person—Sims' or the left side-lying position
- How far to insert the enema tubing—usually 2 to 4 inches for adults
- How high to hold the solution container—usually 12 inches above the anus
- How fast to give the solution—750 to 1000 mL are usually given over 10 to 15 minutes
- How long the person should try to retain the solution
- What to report and record:
  - The amount of solution given
  - If you noted bleeding or resistance when inserting the tube
  - How long the person retained the enema solution
  - Color, amount, consistency, shape, and odor of stools
  - Complaints of cramping, pain, or discomfort
  - Complaints of nausea or weakness
  - How the person tolerated the procedure
- When to report observations
- What specific resident concerns to report at once

PROMOTING SAFETY AND COMFORT
Enemas

Safety

Enemas are usually safe procedures. Many people give themselves enemas at home. However, enemas are dangerous for older persons and those with certain heart and kidney diseases.

Contact with stools is likely when giving enemas. They contain microbes and may contain blood. Follow Standard Precautions and the Bloodborne Pathogen Standard.

Comfort

Before starting the procedure, make sure that the bathroom is ready for the person's use. If the person will use the commode or bedpan, make sure the device is ready. Always keep a bedpan nearby in case the person starts to expel the enema solution and stools. Mental comfort is promoted when the person knows that the bathroom, commode, or bedpan is ready for use.

Make sure the person is comfortable in the Sims' or left side-lying position. When comfortable, it is easier for the person to tolerate the procedure.

To prevent cramping:

- Use the correct water temperature. Cool water causes cramping.
- Give the solution slowly.

The Cleansing Enema

Cleansing enemas clean the bowel of feces and flatus. They relieve constipation and fecal impaction. They are needed before certain surgeries and diagnostic procedures. Cleansing enemas take effect in 10 to 20 minutes.

The doctor orders a tap water, saline, or soapsuds enema. The doctor may order *enemas until clear.* This means that enemas are given until the return solution is clear and free of stools. Ask the nurse how many enemas to give. Center policy may allow repeating enemas 2 or 3 times.

Tap water enemas can be dangerous. The colon may absorb some of the water into the bloodstream. This creates a fluid imbalance. *Only one tap water enema is given. Do not repeat the enema.* Repeated enemas increase the risk of excessive fluid absorption.

The *saline enema* solution is similar to body fluid. However, some of the salt solution may be absorbed. This too can cause a fluid imbalance. When excess salt is in the body, the body retains water.

Soapsuds enemas irritate the bowel's mucous lining. Repeated enemas can damage the bowel. So can using more than 3 to 5 mL of castile soap or stronger soaps.

VIDEO

QUALITY OF LIFE

Remember to:
- Knock before entering the person's room.
- Address the person by name.
- Introduce yourself by name and title.
- Explain the procedure to the person before beginning and during the procedure.
- Protect the person's rights during the procedure.
- Handle the person gently during the procedure.

PRE-PROCEDURE

1 Follow *Delegation Guidelines: Enemas,* p. 361. See *Promoting Safety and Comfort: Enemas,* p. 361.
2 Practice hand hygiene.
3 Collect the following before going to the person's room:
- Disposable enema kit as directed by the nurse (enema bag, tube, clamp, and waterproof pad)
- Bath thermometer
- Waterproof pad (if not in the enema kit)
- Water-soluble lubricant
- 3 to 5 mL (1 teaspoon) of castile soap or 1 to 2 teaspoons of salt
- IV pole
- Gloves
4 Arrange items in the person's room and bathroom.

5 Decontaminate your hands.
6 Identify the person. Check the ID (identification) bracelet against the assignment sheet. Also call the person by name.
7 Put on gloves.
8 Collect the following:
- Commode or bedpan and cover
- Toilet tissue
- Bath blanket
- Robe and non-skid footwear
- Paper towels
9 Provide for privacy.
10 Raise the bed for body mechanics. Bed rails are up if used.

PROCEDURE

11 Remove the gloves, and decontaminate your hands. Put on clean gloves.
12 Lower the bed rail near you if up.
13 Cover the person with a bath blanket. Fan-fold top linens to the foot of the bed.
14 Position the IV pole so the enema bag is 12 inches above the anus. Or it is at the height directed by the nurse.
15 Raise the bed rail if used.
16 Prepare the enema:
  a Close the clamp on the tube.
  b Adjust water flow until it is lukewarm.
  c Fill the enema bag for the amount ordered.
  d Measure water temperature with the bath thermometer. The nurse tells you what temperature to use.
  e Prepare the solution as directed by the nurse:
    (1) Tap water: add nothing
    (2) Saline enema: add salt as directed
    (3) SSE: add castile soap as directed
  f Stir the solution with the bath thermometer. Scoop off any suds (SSE).
  g Seal the bag.
  h Hang the bag on the IV pole.
17 Lower the bed rail near you if up.
18 Position the person in Sims' position or in a left side-lying position.
19 Place a waterproof pad under the buttocks.
20 Expose the anal area.
21 Place the bedpan behind the person.
22 Position the enema tube in the bedpan. Remove the cap from the tubing.
23 Open the clamp. Let solution flow through the tube to remove air. Clamp the tube.
24 Lubricate the tube 2 to 4 inches from the tip.
25 Separate the buttocks to see the anus.

26 Ask the person to take a deep breath through the mouth.
27 Insert the tube gently 2 to 4 inches into the adult's rectum (Fig. 23-4). Do this when the person is exhaling. Stop if the person complains of pain, you feel resistance, or bleeding occurs.
28 Check the amount of solution in the bag.
29 Unclamp the tube. Give the solution slowly (Fig. 23-5).
30 Ask the person to take slow deep breaths. This helps the person relax.
31 Clamp the tube if the person needs to have a BM, has cramping, or starts to expel solution. Also clamp the tube if the person is sweating or complains of nausea or weakness. Unclamp when symptoms subside.
32 Give the amount of solution ordered. Stop if the person cannot tolerate the procedure.
33 Clamp the tube before it is empty. This prevents air from entering the bowel.
34 Hold toilet tissue around the tube and against the anus. Remove the tube.
35 Discard toilet tissue into the bedpan.
36 Wrap the tubing tip with paper towels. Place it inside the enema bag.
37 Assist the person to the bathroom or commode. The person wears a robe and non-skid footwear when up. The bed is in the lowest position. Or help the person onto the bedpan. Raise the head of the bed. Raise or lower bed rails according to the care plan.
38 Place the signal light and toilet tissue within reach. Remind the person not to flush the toilet.
39 Discard disposable items.
40 Remove the gloves. Practice hand hygiene.
41 Leave the room if the person can be left alone.
42 Return when the person signals. Or check on the person every 5 minutes. Knock before entering the room or bathroom.

PROCEDURE—cont'd

43 Decontaminate your hands, and put on gloves. Lower the bed rail if up.
44 Observe enema results for amount, color, consistency, shape, and odor. Call the nurse to observe the results.
45 Provide perineal care as needed.
46 Remove the waterproof pad.

47 Empty, clean, and disinfect equipment. Flush the toilet after the nurse observes the results.
48 Return equipment to its proper place.
49 Remove the gloves, and practice hand hygiene.
50 Assist with hand washing. Wear gloves for this step.
51 Cover the person. Remove the bath blanket.

POST-PROCEDURE

52 Provide for comfort. (See the inside of the front book cover.)
53 Place the signal light within reach.
54 Lower the bed to its lowest position.
55 Raise or lower bed rails. Follow the care plan.
56 Unscreen the person.

57 Complete a safety check of the room. (See the inside of the front book cover.)
58 Follow center policy for dirty linen and used supplies.
59 Practice hand hygiene.
60 Report and record your observations (Fig. 23-3).

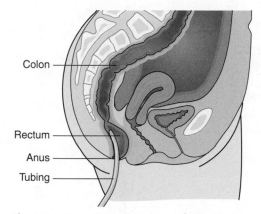

Colon

Rectum

Anus

Tubing

Fig. 23-4 Enema tubing inserted into the adult rectum.

Fig. 23-5 Giving an enema. The person is in Sims' position. The enema bag hangs from an IV pole. The bag is 12 inches above the anus and 18 inches above the mattress.

	Date	Time	Nursing Margin	Other Depts Margin	
7/8	1700			750 mL tap water enema given with the resident in the L side-lying position.	
				The resident was asked to retain the enema for at least 15 minutes. Bed in low	
				position. Signal light within reach. No resident complaints at this time. Resident	
				informed that I would check on her in 5 minutes or when the signal light was used.	
				Angie Martinez, CNA	
	1715			Assisted resident to the bedside commode. Privacy curtain pulled. Signal light and	
				toilet tissue within reach. Resident reminded to signal when finished expelling the	
				enema or if she needs assistance. Angie Martinez, CNA	

Fig. 23-3 Charting sample.

The Small-Volume Enema

Small-volume enemas irritate and distend the rectum. This causes a BM. They are often ordered for constipation or when the bowel does not need complete cleansing.

These enemas are ready to give. The solution is usually given at room temperature. To give the enema, squeeze and roll up the plastic bottle from the bottom.

Do not release pressure on the bottle. Otherwise, solution is drawn from the rectum back into the bottle.

Urge the person to retain the solution until there is a need to have a BM. This usually takes about 5 to 10 minutes. Staying in the Sims' or left side-lying position helps retain the enema.

GIVING A SMALL-VOLUME ENEMA

QUALITY OF LIFE

Remember to:
- Knock before entering the person's room.
- Address the person by name.
- Introduce yourself by name and title.

- Explain the procedure to the person before beginning and during the procedure.
- Protect the person's rights during the procedure.
- Handle the person gently during the procedure.

PRE-PROCEDURE

1 Follow *Delegation Guidelines: Enemas*, p. 361. See *Promoting Safety and Comfort: Enemas*, p. 361.
2 Practice hand hygiene.
3 Collect the following before going to the person's room:
   - Small-volume enema
   - Waterproof pad
   - Gloves
4 Arrange items in the person's room.
5 Practice hand hygiene.
6 Identify the person. Check the ID bracelet against the assignment sheet. Also call the person by name.

7 Put on gloves.
8 Collect the following:
   - Commode or bedpan
   - Waterproof pad
   - Toilet tissue
   - Robe and non-skid footwear
   - Bath blanket
9 Provide for privacy.
10 Raise the bed for body mechanics. Bed rails are up if used.

PROCEDURE

11 Remove the gloves, and practice hand hygiene. Put on clean gloves.
12 Lower the bed rail near you if up.
13 Cover the person with a bath blanket. Fan-fold top linens to the foot of the bed.
14 Position the person in Sims' or a left side-lying position.
15 Place the waterproof pad under the buttocks.
16 Expose the anal area.
17 Position the bedpan near the person.
18 Remove the cap from the enema tip.
19 Separate the buttocks to see the anus.

20 Ask the person to take a deep breath through the mouth.
21 Insert the enema tip 2 inches into the adult's rectum (Fig. 23-6). Do this when the person is exhaling. Insert the tip gently. Stop if the person complains of pain, you feel resistance, or bleeding occurs.
22 Squeeze and roll the bottle gently. Release pressure on the bottle after you remove the tip from the rectum.
23 Put the bottle into the box, tip first.

GIVING A SMALL-VOLUME ENEMA—cont'd | VIDEO |

PROCEDURE—cont'd

24 Assist the person to the bathroom or commode when he or she has the urge to have a BM. The person wears a robe and non-skid footwear when up. The bed is in the lowest position. Or help the person onto the bedpan, and raise the head of the bed. Raise or lower bed rails according to the care plan.
25 Place the signal light and toilet tissue within reach. Remind the person not to flush the toilet.
26 Discard disposable items.
27 Remove the gloves. Practice hand hygiene.
28 Leave the room if the person can be left alone.
29 Return when the person signals. Or check on the person every 5 minutes. Knock before entering the room or bathroom.
30 Practice hand hygiene. Put on gloves.
31 Lower the bed rail if up.
32 Observe enema results for amount, color, consistency, shape, and odor. Call the nurse to observe the results.
33 Provide perineal care as needed.
34 Remove the waterproof pad.
35 Empty, clean, and disinfect equipment. Flush the toilet after the nurse observes the results.
36 Return equipment to its proper place.
37 Remove the gloves, and practice hand hygiene.
38 Assist with hand washing. Wear gloves for this step.
39 Cover the person. Remove the bath blanket.

POST-PROCEDURE

40 Provide for comfort. (See the inside of the front book cover.)
41 Place the signal light within reach.
42 Lower the bed to its lowest position.
43 Raise or lower bed rails. Follow the care plan.
44 Unscreen the person.
45 Complete a safety check of the room. (See the inside of the front book cover.)
46 Follow center policy for dirty linen and used supplies.
47 Practice hand hygiene.
48 Report and record your observations.

Fig. 23-6 The small-volume enema tip is inserted 2 inches into the rectum.

The Oil-Retention Enema

Oil-retention enemas relieve constipation and fecal impactions. The oil is retained for 30 to 60 minutes or longer (1 to 3 hours). Retaining oil softens feces and lubricates the rectum. This lets feces pass with ease. Most oil-retention enemas are commercially prepared.

See *Promoting Safety and Comfort: The Oil-Retention Enema.*

PROMOTING SAFETY AND COMFORT
The Oil-Retention Enema

Safety
The oil-retention enema is retained for at least 30 to 60 minutes. Leave the room after giving the enema. Make sure you check on the person often. After checking on the person, tell him or her when you will return. Remind the person to signal for you if he or she needs help.

GIVING AN OIL-RETENTION ENEMA

QUALITY OF LIFE

Remember to:
- Knock before entering the person's room.
- Address the person by name.
- Introduce yourself by name and title.

- Explain the procedure to the person before beginning and during the procedure.
- Protect the person's rights during the procedure.
- Handle the person gently during the procedure.

PRE-PROCEDURE

1 Follow *Delegation Guidelines: Enemas*, p. 361. See *Promoting Safety and Comfort:*
  a *Enemas*, p. 361
  b *The Oil-Retention Enema*, p. 365
2 Practice hand hygiene.
3 Collect the following before going to the person's room:
- Oil-retention enema
- Waterproof pads
4 Arrange items in the person's room.
5 Practice hand hygiene.

6 Identify the person. Check the ID bracelet against the assignment sheet. Also call the person by name.
7 Put on gloves.
8 Collect the following:
- Gloves
- Bath blanket
9 Provide for privacy.
10 Raise the bed for body mechanics. Bed rails are up if used.

PROCEDURE

11 Follow steps 11 through 23 in procedure: *Giving a Small-Volume Enema*, p. 364.
12 Cover the person. Leave him or her in the Sims' or left side-lying position.

13 Encourage him or her to retain the enema for the time ordered.
14 Place more waterproof pads on the bed if needed.
15 Remove the gloves. Practice hand hygiene.

POST-PROCEDURE

16 Provide for comfort. (See the inside of the front book cover.)
17 Place the signal light within reach.
18 Lower the bed to its lowest position.
19 Raise or lower bed rails. Follow the care plan.
20 Unscreen the person.

21 Complete a safety check of the room. (See the inside of the front book cover.)
22 Follow center policy for dirty linen and used supplies.
23 Practice hand hygiene.
24 Report and record your observations.
25 Check the person often.

THE PERSON WITH AN OSTOMY

Sometimes part of the intestines is removed surgically. Cancer, bowel disease, and trauma (stab or bullet wounds) are common reasons. An ostomy is sometimes necessary. An ostomy is a surgically created opening for the elimination of body wastes. The opening that can be seen through the abdominal wall is called a stoma. The person wears a pouch over the stoma to collect stools and flatus.

Colostomy

A colostomy is a surgically created opening (*stomy*) between the colon (*colo*) and abdominal wall. Part of the colon is brought out onto the abdominal wall and a stoma is made. Feces and flatus pass through the stoma instead of the anus.

Colostomies are temporary or permanent. If permanent, the diseased part of the colon is removed. A temporary colostomy gives the diseased or injured bowel

time to heal. After healing, surgery is done to reconnect the bowel.

The colostomy site depends on the site of disease or injury (Fig. 23-7). Stool consistency—liquid to formed—depends on the colostomy site. The more colon remaining to absorb water, the more solid and formed the stool. If the colostomy is near the start of the colon, stools are liquid. A colostomy near the end of the colon results in formed stools.

Stools irritate the skin. Skin care prevents skin breakdown around the stoma. The skin is washed and dried. Then a skin barrier is applied around the stoma. It prevents stools from having contact with the skin. The skin barrier is part of the pouch or a separate device.

Ileostomy

An ileostomy is a surgically created opening (*stomy*) between the ileum (*small intestine [ileo]*) and the abdominal wall. Part of the ileum is brought out onto the

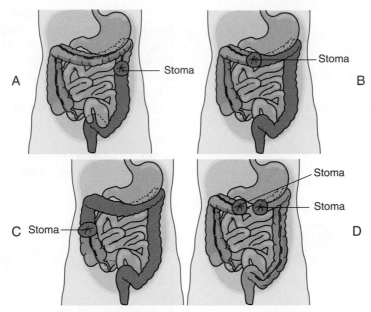

Fig. 23-7 Colostomy sites. *Shading for A, B, and C* shows the part of the bowel surgically removed. **A,** Sigmoid or descending colostomy. **B,** Transverse colostomy. **C,** Ascending colostomy. **D,** Double-barrel colostomy has two stomas. One allows for the excretion of feces. The other is for the introduction of drugs to help the bowel heal. This type of colostomy is usually temporary.

Fig. 23-8 An ileostomy. The entire large intestine is surgically removed.

Fig. 23-9 The ostomy pouch is secured to an ostomy belt. The pouch is emptied by directing it into the toilet and opening the end.

abdominal wall, and a stoma is made. The entire colon is removed (Fig. 23-8).

Liquid stools drain constantly from an ileostomy. Water is not absorbed because the colon was removed. Feces in the small intestine contain digestive juices that are very irritating to the skin. The ileostomy pouch must fit well. Stools must not touch the skin. Good skin care is required.

Ostomy Pouches

The pouch has an adhesive backing that is applied to the skin. Sometimes pouches are secured to ostomy belts (Fig. 23-9).

Many pouches have a drain at the bottom that close with a clip, clamp, or wire closure. The drain is opened to empty the pouch. The pouch is emptied when stools are present. It is opened when it balloons or bulges with flatus. The drain is wiped with toilet tissue before it is closed.

The pouch is changed every 3 to 7 days and when it leaks. Frequent pouch changes can damage the skin.

Odors are prevented by:

- Good hygiene
- Emptying the pouch
- Avoiding gas-forming foods
- Putting deodorants into the pouch (The nurse tells you what to use.)

The person wears normal clothes. However, tight garments can prevent feces from entering the pouch. Also, bulging from stools and flatus can be seen with tight clothes.

Peristalsis increases after eating and drinking. Therefore stomas are usually quiet after sleep. That is, expelling feces is less likely at this time. If the person showers or bathes with the pouch off, it is best done before breakfast. Showers and baths are delayed for 1 to 2 hours after applying a new pouch. This gives the adhesive time to seal to the skin.

Do not flush pouches down the toilet. Follow center policy for disposing of them.

See *Delegation Guidelines: Ostomy Pouches.*
See *Promoting Safety and Comfort: Ostomy Pouches.*

DELEGATION GUIDELINES
Ostomy Pouches

Many people manage their own ostomies. Others need help. When the nurse delegates changing an ostomy pouch to you, make sure that:

- Your state allows you to perform the procedure.
- The procedure is in your job description.
- You have the necessary education and training.
- You review the procedure with the nurse.
- The nurse is available to answer questions and to supervise you.

   If the above conditions are met, you need this information from the nurse and the care plan:

- If the person has a colostomy or ileostomy
- When to change the pouch
- What equipment and supplies to use
- What soap or cleaning agent to use
- Drying time for the skin barrier (usually 1 to 2 minutes)
- What pouch deodorant to use
- What observations to report and record:
  - Signs of skin breakdown (the normal stoma is red like a mucous membrane)
  - Color, amount, consistency, and odor of stools
  - Complaints of pain or discomfort
- When to report observations
- What specific resident concerns to report at once

PROMOTING SAFETY AND COMFORT
Ostomy Pouches

Safety
When changing an ostomy pouch, contact with stools and the stoma is likely. Stools contain microbes and may contain blood. The stoma may bleed slightly when washed. Follow Standard Precautions and the Bloodborne Pathogen Standard.

Comfort
The stoma does not have sensation. Touching the stoma does not cause pain or discomfort.

QUALITY OF LIFE

Remember to:

- Knock before entering the person's room.
- Address the person by name.
- Introduce yourself by name and title.
- Explain the procedure to the person before beginning and during the procedure.
- Protect the person's rights during the procedure.
- Handle the person gently during the procedure.

PRE-PROCEDURE

1 Follow *Delegation Guidelines: Ostomy Pouches.* See *Promoting Safety and Comfort: Ostomy Pouches.*
2 Practice hand hygiene.
3 Collect the following before going to the person's room:
   - Clean pouch with skin barrier
   - Pouch clamp, clip, or wire closure
   - Clean ostomy belt (if used)
   - Gauze pads or washcloths
   - Adhesive remover wipes
   - Skin paste (optional)
   - Pouch deodorant
   - Disposable bag
4 Arrange your work area.
5 Practice hand hygiene.
6 Identify the person. Check the ID bracelet against the assignment sheet. Also call the person by name.
7 Put on gloves.
8 Collect the following:
   - Bedpan with cover
   - Waterproof pad
   - Bath blanket
   - Wash basin with warm water
   - Paper towels
   - Gloves
9 Provide for privacy.
10 Raise the bed for body mechanics. Bed rails are up if used.

PROCEDURE

11 Remove the gloves, and practice hand hygiene. Put on clean gloves.
12 Lower the bed rail near you if up.
13 Cover the person with a bath blanket. Fan-fold linens to the foot of the bed.
14 Place the waterproof pad under the buttocks.
15 Disconnect the pouch from the belt if one is worn. Remove the belt.
16 Remove and place the pouch and skin barrier in the bedpan. Gently push the skin down and lift up on the barrier. Use the adhesive remover wipes if necessary.
17 Wipe the stoma and around it with a gauze pad. This removes excess stool and mucous. Discard the gauze pad into the disposable bag.
18 Wet the gauze pads or the washcloth.
19 Wash the stoma and the skin around it with a gauze pad or washcloth. Wash gently. Do not scrub or rub the skin.
20 Pat dry with a gauze pad or the towel.
21 Observe the stoma and the skin around the stoma. Report bleeding, skin irritation, or skin breakdown to the nurse.
22 Remove the backing from the new pouch.
23 Apply a thin layer of paste around the pouch opening. Let it dry following the manufacturer's instructions.
24 Pull the skin around the stoma taut. The skin must be wrinkle-free.
25 Center the pouch over the stoma. The drain points downward.
26 Press around the pouch and skin barrier so it seals to the skin. Apply gentle pressure with your fingers. Start at the bottom and work up around the sides to the top.
27 Maintain the pressure for 1 to 2 minutes. Follow the manufacturer's instructions.
28 Tug downward on the pouch gently. Make sure the pouch is secure.
29 Add deodorant to the pouch.
30 Close the pouch at the bottom. Use a clamp, clip, or wire closure.
31 Attach the ostomy belt if used. The belt should not be too tight. You should be able to slide 2 fingers under the belt.
32 Remove the waterproof pad.
33 Discard disposable supplies into the disposable bag.
34 Remove the gloves. Practice hand hygiene.
35 Cover the person. Remove the bath blanket.

POST-PROCEDURE

36 Provide for comfort. (See the inside of the front book cover.)
37 Place the signal light within reach.
38 Lower the bed to its lowest position.
39 Raise or lower bed rails. Follow the care plan.
40 Unscreen the person.
41 Practice hand hygiene. Put on gloves.
42 Take the bedpan and disposable bag into the bathroom.
43 Empty the pouch and bedpan into the toilet. Observe the color, amount, consistency, and odor of stools. Flush the toilet.
44 Discard the pouch into the disposable bag. Discard the disposable bag.
45 Empty, clean, and disinfect equipment. Return equipment to its proper place.
46 Remove the gloves. Practice hand hygiene.
47 Complete a safety check of the room. (See the inside of the front book cover.)
48 Follow center policy for dirty linens.
49 Practice hand hygiene.
50 Report and record your observations.

QUALITY OF LIFE

The "Quality of Life" described for urinary elimination (Chapter 22) applies for bowel elimination. As always, protect the person's rights. Assist with bowel elimination as directed by the nurse and the care plan.

Bowel elimination is a very private act. People want and need privacy. Do all you can to protect the person's right to privacy. Otherwise, normal bowel elimination can be affected. Constipation and fecal impaction can result.

Odors and sounds often occur with BMs. You must control your verbal and non-verbal responses. Act in a professional manner at all times. Do not laugh at or make fun of another person. Such reactions are unprofessional. They lessen the person's dignity and self-esteem.

Bowel control is important to people. Physical and mental well-being are related to normal bowel function. Personal BM habits also affect well-being. Good hygiene is needed after BMs.

Normal bowel elimination is not always possible. Constipation, fecal impaction, diarrhea, fecal incontinence, and flatulence are common problems. The doctor may order diet changes, drugs, or enemas to relieve the problem. The nurse may ask you to give an enema. You must completely understand the nurse's instructions and the procedure.

Residents have the right to personal choice. Persons with ostomies manage their own care if able. Some have had ostomies for a long time. They have their own routines and care measures. Their choices in ostomy care are followed.

REVIEW QUESTIONS

Circle the BEST answer.

1 Which is *false*?
   a A person must have a BM every day.
   b Stools are normally brown, soft, and formed.
   c Diarrhea occurs when feces move rapidly through the bowels.
   d Constipation results when feces move slowly through the colon.

2 The prolonged retention and accumulation of feces in the rectum is called
   a Constipation
   b Fecal impaction
   c Diarrhea
   d Fecal incontinence

3 Which does *not* promote comfort and safety for bowel elimination?
   a Asking visitors to leave the room
   b Helping the person to a sitting position
   c Offering the bedpan after meals
   d Telling the person that you will return very soon

4 Bowel training is aimed at
   a Bowel control and regular elimination
   b Ostomy control
   c Preventing fecal impaction, constipation, and fecal incontinence
   d Preventing bleeding

5 Which is *not* used for a cleansing enema?
   a Castile soap
   b Salt
   c Oil
   d Tap water

6 These statements are about enemas. Which is *false*?
   a The solution should be cool.
   b The Sims' position is used.
   c The enema bag is held 12 inches above the anus.
   d The solution is given slowly.

7 In adults, the enema tube is inserted
   a 2 to 4 inches
   b 4 to 6 inches
   c 6 to 8 inches
   d 8 to 10 inches

8 The oil-retention enema is retained for at least
   a 10 to 15 minutes
   b 15 to 30 minutes
   c 30 to 60 minutes
   d 60 to 90 minutes

9 These statements are about ostomies. Which is *false*?
   a Good skin care around the stoma is needed.
   b Deodorants can control odors.
   c The person wears a pouch.
   d Stools are liquid.

10 An ostomy pouch is usually emptied
   a Every 4 to 6 hours
   b Every shift
   c Every 3 to 7 days
   d When stools are present

Answers to these questions are on p. 720.

Nutrition and Fluids

OBJECTIVES

- Define the key terms and key abbreviations listed in this chapter.
- Explain the purpose and use of the MyPlate symbol.
- Explain how to use the *Dietary Guidelines for Americans*.
- Describe the functions and sources of nutrients.
- Explain how to read and use food labels.
- Describe the factors that affect eating and nutrition.
- Describe the OBRA requirements for serving food.
- Describe the special diets and between-meal snacks.
- Identify the signs, symptoms, and precautions for aspiration.

- Describe fluid requirements and the causes of dehydration.
- Explain what to do when the person has special fluid orders.
- Explain the purpose of intake and output records.
- Identify what is counted as fluid intake.
- Explain how to assist with food and fluid needs.
- Explain how to assist with calorie counts.
- Explain how to safely provide drinking water.
- Explain how to prevent foodborne illnesses.
- Perform the procedures described in this chapter.
- Explain how to promote quality of life.

KEY TERMS

anorexia The loss of appetite

aspiration Breathing fluid, food, vomitus, or an object into the lungs

calorie The fuel or energy value of food

Daily Value (DV) How a serving fits into the daily diet; expressed in a percent (%) based on a daily diet of 2000 calories

dehydration A decrease in the amount of water in body tissues

dysphagia Difficulty *(dys)* swallowing *(phagia)*

edema The swelling of body tissues with water

graduate A measuring container for fluid

intake The amount of fluid taken in

nutrient A substance that is ingested, digested, absorbed, and used by the body

nutrition The processes involved in the ingestion, digestion, absorption, and use of foods and fluids by the body

output The amount of fluid lost

KEY ABBREVIATIONS

CMS	Centers for Medicare & Medicaid Services	**mL**	Milliliter
DV	Daily Value	**NPO**	Non per os; nothing by mouth
F	Fahrenheit	**OBRA**	Omnibus Budget Reconciliation Act of 1987
GI	Gastro-intestinal		
ID	Identification	**oz**	Ounce
I&O	Intake and output	**USDA**	United States Department of Agriculture
mg	Milligram		

Food and water are physical needs. They are necessary for life. The person's diet affects physical and mental well-being. A poor diet and poor eating habits:

- Increase the risk for infection
- Increase the risk of acute and chronic diseases
- Cause chronic illnesses to become worse
- Cause healing problems
- Affect physical and mental function, increasing the risk for accidents and injuries

Eating and drinking provide pleasure. They often are part of social times with family and friends. A friendly, social setting for meals is important. Otherwise, the person may eat poorly.

Many factors affect dietary practices. They include culture, finances, and personal choice. See *Caring About Culture: Meal Time Practices.* Dietary practices also include selecting, preparing, and serving food. The health team considers these factors when planning to meet the person's nutrition needs.

The Centers for Medicare & Medicaid Services (CMS) require that the health team assess the resident's nutritional status. This will include:

- Drugs that affect taste or cause dry mouth, nausea, confusion, and so on
- Weight and height (Chapter 34)
- Appearance
- Food intake (p. 396) and fluid intake (p. 388)
- Factors affecting eating and nutrition (p. 381)

CARING ABOUT CULTURE

Meal Time Practices

Many cultural groups have their main meal at mid-day. The *Austrians* do so. They eat light meals in the evening. Persons from *Brazil* also eat their main meal at noon. They have a light meal in the evening. A main meal at lunch also is common in *Finland*, *Germany*, and *Greece*. In *Iran*, the most important meal is eaten at mid-day.

Modified from D'Avanzo CE: Pocket guide to cultural health assessment, ed 4, St Louis, 2008, Mosby.

The health team then must develop a care plan to meet the person's nutritional needs. CMS surveyors may ask you about the following. You will learn how to answer their questions as you study this chapter.

- How the person's food and fluid intake is observed and reported.
- How the person's eating ability is observed and reported.
- How the person's weight is measured and reported.
- What measures are taken to prevent or meet changes in the person's nutritional needs. Snacks and frequent meals are examples.
- The goals for nutrition in the person's care plan.

BASIC NUTRITION

Nutrition is the processes involved in the ingestion, digestion, absorption, and use of foods and fluids by the body. Good nutrition is needed for growth, healing, and body functions. A well-balanced diet and correct calorie intake are needed. A high-fat and high-calorie diet causes weight gain and obesity. Weight loss occurs with a low-calorie diet.

Foods and fluids contain nutrients. A nutrient is a substance that is ingested, digested, absorbed, and used by the body. Nutrients are grouped into fats, proteins, carbohydrates, vitamins, minerals, and water.

Fats, proteins, and carbohydrates give the body fuel for energy. The amount of energy provided by a nutrient is measured in calories. A calorie is the fuel or energy value of food:

- 1 gram of fat—9 calories
- 1 gram of protein—4 calories
- 1 gram of carbohydrate—4 calories

Older persons need fewer calories than younger people. Energy and activity levels are lower.

Dietary Guidelines

The *Dietary Guidelines for Americans, 2010* (Box 24-1) is for persons 2 years of age and older. It is also for persons at risk for chronic disease. Certain diseases are linked to poor diet and lack of physical activity. They include cardiovascular disease, hypertension (high blood pressure), diabetes, obesity, osteoporosis, and some cancers. The Dietary Guidelines help people:

- Attain and maintain a healthy weight
- Reduce the risk of chronic disease
- Promote over-all health

The Dietary Guidelines focus on:
- Consuming fewer calories
- Making informed food choices
- Being physically active

Box 24-1 **Key Recommendations from Dietary Guidelines 2010**

Balancing Calories To Manage Weight

- Prevent and/or reduce overweight and obesity through improved eating and physical activity behaviors.
- Control total calorie intake to manage body weight. For people who are overweight or obese, this will mean consuming fewer calories from foods and beverages.
- Increase physical activity and reduce time spent in sedentary behaviors.
- Maintain appropriate calorie balance during each stage of life—childhood, adolescence, adulthood, pregnancy and breastfeeding, and older age.

Food And Food Components To Reduce

- Reduce daily sodium intake to less than 2300 milligrams (mg) and further reduce intake to 1500 mg among persons who are 51 and older and those of any age who are African-American or have hypertension, diabetes, or chronic kidney disease. The 1500 mg recommendation applies to about half of the U.S. population, including children and the majority of adults.

- Consume less than 10% of calories from saturated fatty acids by replacing them with monounsaturated and polyunsaturated fatty acids.
- Consume less than 300 mg per day of dietary cholesterol.
- Keep *trans* fatty acid consumption as low as possible by limiting foods that contain synthetic sources of *trans* fats, such as partially hydrogenated oils, and by limiting other solid fats.
- Reduce the intake of calories from solid fats and added sugars.
- Limit the consumption of foods that contain refined grains, especially refined grain foods that contain solid fats, added sugars, and sodium.
- If alcohol is consumed, it should be consumed in moderation—up to one drink per day for women and two drinks per day for men—and only by adults of legal drinking age.[*]

From Dietary Guidelines for Americans, 2010, United States Department of Agriculture
For complete information go to http://www.cnpp.usda.gov/publications/dietaryguidelines/2010/policydoc/execsumm.pdf

Continued

Box 24-1   Key Recommendations from Dietary Guidelines 2010—cont'd

Food And Nutrients To Increase

Individuals should meet the following recommendations as part of a healthy eating pattern while staying within their calorie needs.

- Increase vegetable and fruit intake.
- Eat a variety of vegetables, especially dark-green, red, and orange vegetables and beans and peas.
- Consume at least half of all grains as whole grains (Fig. 24-1). Increase whole-grain intake by replacing refined grains with whole grains.
- Increase intake of fat-free or low-fat milk and milk products, such as milk, yogurt, cheese, or fortified soy beverages.*
- Choose a variety of protein foods, which include seafood, lean meat, and poultry, eggs, beans, and peas, soy products, and unsalted nuts and seeds.
- Increase the amount and variety of seafood consumed by choosing seafood in place of meat and poultry.
- Replace protein foods that are higher in solid fats with choices that are lower in solid fats and calories and/or are sources of oils.
- Use oils to replace solid fats where possible.
- Choose foods that provide more potassium, dietary fiber, calcium, and vitamin D, which are nutrients of concern in American diets. These foods include vegetables, fruits, whole grains, and milk and milk products.

Recommendations for specific population groups

Women capable of becoming pregnant*

- Choose foods that supply heme iron, which is more readily absorbed by the body, additional iron sources, and enhancers of iron absorption such as vitamin C-rich foods.
- Consume 400 micrograms (mcg) per day of synthetic folic acid (from fortified foods and/or supplements) in addition to food forms of folate from a varied diet.*

Women who are pregnant or breastfeeding*

- Consume 8 to 12 ounces of seafood per week from a variety of seafood types.
- Due to their high methyl mercury content, limit white (albacore) tuna to 6 ounces per week and do not eat the following four types of fish: tilefish, shark, swordfish, and king mackerel.
- If pregnant, take an iron supplement, as recommended by an obstetrician or other health care provider.

Individuals ages 50 years and older

- Consume foods fortified with vitamin B_{12}, such as fortified cereals, or dietary supplements.

Building Healthy Eating Patterns

- Select an eating pattern that meets nutrient needs over time at an appropriate calorie level.
- Account for all foods and beverages consumed and assess how they fit within a total healthy eating pattern.
- Follow food safety recommendations when preparing and eating foods to reduce the risk of foodborne illnesses (Fig. 24-2).

From Dietary Guidelines for Americans, 2010, *United States Department of Agriculture*
For complete information go to http://www.cnpp.usda.gov/publications/dietaryguidelines/2010/policydoc/execsumm.pdf

Fig. 24-1 A, The amount of whole grain that equals a 1-ounce slice of bread. **B,** A 3 ounce-equivalent serving of whole grain.

Fig. 24-2 Food temperature guide. *(Redrawn from U.S. Department of Health and Human Services and U.S. Department of Agriculture:* Finding your way to a healthier you: based on the dietary guidelines for Americans, *updated April 5, 2005.)*

MyPlate

The MyPlate symbol (Fig. 24-3) encourages healthy eating from 5 food groups. MyPlate, issued by the United States Department of Agriculture (USDA), helps you make wise food choices by:

- Balancing calories
  - Eating less
  - Avoiding over-sized portions
- Increasing certain foods
  - Making half of your plate fruits and vegetables
  - Making at least half of your grains whole grains
  - Drinking fat-free or low-fat (1%) milk
- Reducing certain foods
  - Choosing low-sodium foods
  - Drinking water instead of sugary drinks

The amount needed from each food group depends on age, sex, and physical activity (Table 24-1).

Activity should be moderate or vigorous (Box 24-2). The USDA recommends that adults do at least one of the following:

- 2 hours and 30 minutes each week of moderate physical activity
- 1 hour and 15 minutes each week of vigorous physical activity

Physical activity at least 3 days a week is best. Each activity should be for at least 10 minutes at a time. Adults should also do strengthening activities at least 2 days a week. Push-ups, sit-ups, and weight-lifting are examples.

Fig. 24-3 The MyPlate symbol. *(Courtesy U.S. Department of Agriculture, Center for Nutrition and Policy Promotion, 2011.)*

Box 24-2	Moderate and Vigorous Physical Activities

Moderate Physical Activities
- Walking briskly (about 3½ miles per hour)
- Bicycling (less than 10 miles per hour)
- Gardening (raking, trimming bushes)
- Dancing
- Golf (walking and carrying clubs)
- Water aerobics
- Canoeing
- Tennis (doubles)

Vigorous Physical Activities
- Running and jogging (5 miles per hour)
- Walking very fast (4½ miles per hour)
- Bicycling (more than 10 miles per hour)
- Heavy yard work (chopping wood)
- Swimming (freestyle laps)
- Aerobics
- Basketball (competitive)
- Tennis (singles)

From What is Physical Activity?, *U.S. Department of Agriculture, June 4, 2011.*

Table 24-1	MyPlate Serving Sizes	
Group	**Daily Servings**	**Serving Sizes**
Grains	• Adult women: 5 to 6 ounces (oz); at least 3 oz from whole grains • Adult men: 6 to 8 oz; at least 3 to 4 oz from whole grains	1 oz = 1 slice of bread 1 oz = 1 cup of breakfast cereal 1 oz = ½ cup of cooked rice, cereal, or pasta
Vegetables	• Adult women: 2 to 2 ½ cups • Adult men: 2 ½ to 3 cups	1 cup = 1 cup of raw or cooked vegetables or vegetable juice 1 cup = 2 cups of raw leafy greens
Fruits	• Adult women: 1 ½ to 2 cups • Adult men: 2 cups	1 cup = 1 cup fruit 1 cup = 1 cup fruit juice 1 cup = ½ cup dried fruit
Dairy	• Adult women: 3 cups • Adult men: 3 cups	1 cup = 1 cup milk or yogurt 1 cup = 1½ oz natural cheese 1 cup = 2 oz processed cheese
Protein food	• Adult women: 5 to 5 ½ oz • Adult men: 5 ½ to 6 ½ oz	1 oz = 1 oz of lean meat, poultry, or fish 1 oz = 1 egg 1 oz = 1 tablespoon peanut butter 1 oz = ¼ cup cooked dry beans 1 oz = ½ oz of nuts or seeds

Modified from MyPlate, U.S. Department of Agriculture, June 2011.

Grains Group Food made from wheat, rice, oats, cornmeal, barley, or other cereal grain is a grain product. Bread, pasta, oatmeal, breakfast cereals, tortillas, and grits are examples. The two types of grains are:
• *Whole grains* contain the entire grain kernel. Whole-wheat flour, bulgur (cracked wheat), oatmeal, whole cornmeal, and brown rice are examples.
• *Refined grains* were processed to remove the grain kernel. These grains have a fine texture. White flour, white bread, and white rice are examples. They have less dietary fiber than whole grains.

Grains have these health benefits:
• Reduce the risk of coronary artery disease.
• May prevent constipation.
• May help with weight management.
• May prevent certain birth defects.
• Contain these nutrients—dietary fiber, several B vitamins (thiamine, riboflavin, niacin, folate), and minerals (iron, magnesium, and selenium).

Vegetable Group Vegetables can be eaten raw or cooked. They may be fresh, frozen, canned, dried, or juice. You can eat them whole, cut-up, or mashed. The 5 vegetable subgroups are:

- *Dark green vegetables*—bok choy, broccoli, collard greens, dark green leafy lettuce, kale, mesclun, mustard greens, romaine lettuce, spinach, turnips, watercress
- *Red and orange vegetables*—acorn, butternut, and hubbard squashes; carrots; pumpkin; red peppers; sweet potatoes; tomatoes; tomato juice
- *Beans and peas*—black beans, black-eyed peas, garbanzo beans (chickpeas), kidney beans, lentils, navy beans, pinto beans, soy beans, split peas, and white beans
- *Starchy vegetables*—corn, green bananas, green peas, green lima beans, plantains, potatoes, taro, water chestnuts
- *Other vegetables*—artichokes, asparagus, avocado, bean sprouts, beets, Brussels sprouts, cabbage, cauliflower, celery, cucumbers, eggplant, green beans, green peppers, iceberg (head) lettuce, mushrooms, okra, onions, parsnips, turnips, wax beans, zucchini

Vegetables have these health benefits:

- May reduce the risk for stroke, coronary artery disease, other cardiovascular diseases, and type 2 diabetes.
- Protect against certain cancers. Cancers of the mouth, stomach, and colon-rectum are examples.
- May reduce the risk of developing kidney stones.
- May reduce the risk of bone loss.
- May help lower calorie intake. Most vegetables are naturally low in fat and calories.
- Contain no cholesterol.
- Contain these nutrients—potassium, dietary fiber, folate (folic acid), vitamins A and C.

Fruit Group Any fruit or 100% fruit juice counts as part of the fruit group. Fruit choices should vary. Fresh, frozen, canned, or dried fruits are best. Avoid fruits canned in syrup. Syrup contains added sugar. Choose fruits canned in 100% fruit juice or water.

Fruits have these health benefits:

- May reduce the risk for stroke, coronary artery disease, other cardiovascular diseases, and type 2 diabetes.
- Protect against certain cancers. Cancers of the mouth, stomach, and colon-rectum are examples.
- May reduce the risk of developing kidney stones.
- May reduce the risk of bone loss.
- May help lower calorie intake. Most fruits are naturally low in fat and calories.
- Contain no cholesterol.

- Are naturally low in sodium.
- Contain these nutrients—potassium, dietary fiber, vitamin C, and folate (folic acid).

Dairy Group All fluid milk products are part of the dairy group. So are many foods made from milk. Low-fat or fat-free choices are best. The milk group includes all fluid milk, yogurt, and cheese. (Cream, cream cheese, and butter are not part of the group.)

Milk has these health benefits:

- Helps build and maintain bone mass throughout the life-span. This may reduce the risk of osteoporosis.
- Improves the overall quality of the diet.
- Contains these nutrients—calcium, potassium, and vitamin D.

Protein Foods Group This group includes all foods made from meat, poultry, seafood, beans and peas, eggs, processed soy products, nuts, and seeds.

When selecting foods from this group, remember:

- To choose lean or low-fat meat and poultry. Higher fat choices include regular ground beef (75 to 80% lean) and chicken with skin.
- Using fat for cooking increases the calories. Fried chicken and eggs fried in butter are examples.
- Salmon, trout, and herring are rich in substances that may reduce the risk of heart disease.
- Liver and other organ meats are high in cholesterol.
- Egg yolks are high in cholesterol. Egg whites are cholesterol-free.
- Processed meats have added sodium (salt). They include ham, sausage, frankfurters, and luncheon and deli meats.

Many protein foods are high in fat and cholesterol. Heart disease is a major risk. However, this group provides nutrients needed for health and body maintenance:

- Protein
- B vitamins (niacin, thiamin, riboflavin, and B_6) and vitamin E
- Iron, zinc, and magnesium

Oils Oils are fats that are liquid at room temperature. Vegetable oils for cooking are examples. They include canola oil, corn oil, and olive oil. Oils come from plants and fish. Because they have nutrients, the USDA includes oils in food patterns. However, *oils are not a food group.*

Adult women are allowed 5 to 6 teaspoons of oils daily. Adult men are allowed 6 to 7 teaspoons daily. Some foods are high in oil—nuts, olives, some fish, and avocados. When making oil choices, remember:

- Oils are high in calories.
- The best oil choices come from fish, nuts, and vegetable oils.

- Some foods are mainly oil. Mayonnaise, certain salad dressings, and soft margarine (tub or squeeze) are examples.
- Oils from plant sources do not contain cholesterol.
- *Solid fats* are solid at room temperature. Common solid fats include butter, beef fat (tallow, suet), chicken fat, pork fat (lard), stick margarine, and shortening.

Oils contain some fatty acids that are essential for health. Oils also are a major source of vitamin E.

Nutrients

No food or food group has every essential nutrient. A well-balanced diet ensures an adequate intake of essential nutrients.

- *Protein*—is the most important nutrient. It is needed for tissue growth and repair. Sources include meat, fish, poultry, eggs, milk and milk products, cereals, beans, peas, and nuts. Protein is needed for tissue growth and repair. The diets of some older persons may lack protein. High-protein foods are costly.
- *Carbohydrates*—provide energy and fiber for bowel elimination. They are found in fruits, vegetables, breads, cereals, and sugar. Carbohydrates break down into sugars during digestion. The sugars are absorbed into the bloodstream. Fiber is not digested. It provides the bulky part of chyme for elimination.
- *Fats*—provide energy. They add flavor to food and help the body use certain vitamins. Sources include meats, lard, butter, shortening, oils, milk, cheese, egg yolks, and nuts. Dietary fat not needed by the body is stored as body fat (*adipose tissue*).
- *Vitamins*—are needed for certain body functions. They do not provide calories. The body stores vitamins A, D, E, and K. Vitamin C and the B complex vitamins are not stored. They must be ingested daily. The lack of a certain vitamin results in signs and symptoms of an illness. See Table 24-2.
- *Minerals*—are used for many body processes. Bone and tooth formation, nerve and muscle function, and fluid balance are examples. Foods containing calcium help prevent musculo-skeletal changes. See Table 24-3, p. 380.
- *Water*—is needed for all body processes (p. 388).

Table 24-2	Functions and Sources of Common Vitamins	
Vitamin	**Major Functions**	**Sources**
Vitamin A	Growth; vision; healthy hair, skin, and mucous membranes; resistance to infection	Liver, spinach, green leafy and yellow vegetables, yellow fruits, fish liver oils, egg yolks, butter, cream, whole milk
Vitamin B₁ (thiamine)	Muscle tone, nerve function, digestion, appetite, normal elimination, carbohydrate use	Pork, fish, poultry, eggs, liver, breads, pastas, cereals, oatmeal, potatoes, peas, beans, soybeans, peanuts
Vitamin B₂ (riboflavin)	Growth, healthy eyes, protein and carbohydrate metabolism, healthy skin and mucous membranes	Milk and milk products, liver, green leafy vegetables, eggs, breads, cereals
Vitamin B₃ (niacin)	Protein, fat, and carbohydrate metabolism; nervous system function; appetite; digestive system function	Meat, pork, liver, fish, peanuts, breads and cereals, green vegetables, dairy products
Vitamin B₁₂	Formation of red blood cells, protein metabolism, nervous system function	Liver, meats, poultry, fish, eggs, milk, cheese
Folate (folic acid)	Formation of red blood cells, intestinal function, protein metabolism	Liver, meats, fish, poultry, green leafy vegetables, whole grains
Vitamin C (ascorbic acid)	Formation of substances that hold tissues together; healthy blood vessels, skin, gums, bones, and teeth; wound healing; prevention of bleeding; resistance to infection	Citrus fruits, tomatoes, potatoes, cabbage, strawberries, green vegetables, melons
Vitamin D	Absorption and metabolism of calcium and phosphorus, healthy bones	Fish liver oils, milk, butter, liver, exposure to sun light
Vitamin E	Normal reproduction, formation of red blood cells, muscle function	Vegetable oils, milk, eggs, meats, cereals, green leafy vegetables
Vitamin K	Blood clotting	Liver, green leafy vegetables, egg yolks, cheese

Table 24-3 **Functions and Sources of Common Minerals**

Mineral	Major Functions	Sources
Calcium	Formation of teeth and bones, blood clotting, muscle contraction, heart function, nerve function	Milk and milk products, green leafy vegetables, whole grains, egg yolks, dried peas and beans, nuts
Phosphorus	Formation of bones and teeth; use of proteins, fats, and carbohydrates; nerve and muscle function	Meat, fish, poultry, milk and milk products, nuts, egg yolks, dried peas and beans
Iron	Allows red blood cells to carry oxygen	Liver, meat, eggs, green leafy vegetables, breads and cereals, dried peas and beans, nuts
Iodine	Thyroid gland function, growth, metabolism	Iodized salt, seafood, shellfish
Sodium	Fluid balance, nerve and muscle function	Almost all foods
Potassium	Nerve function, muscle contraction, heart function	Fruits, vegetables, cereals, meats, dried peas and beans

Food Labels

Most foods have labels (Fig. 24-4). They are used to make informed food choices for a healthy diet. Figure 24-5 shows how to use a food label. Food labels contain information about:

- Serving size and the number of servings in each package.
- Calories and calories from fat. The number of servings eaten determines the number of calories of that food. For example: 1 cup of macaroni and cheese contains 250 calories with 110 of them from fat. If you eat 2 cups, you consume 500 calories—220 from fat.
- Nutrients—total fat (saturated fat and *trans* fat), cholesterol, sodium, carbohydrate (dietary fibers and sugar), protein, vitamins A and C, calcium, and iron.

How a serving fits into the daily diet is called the **Daily Value (DV)**. The DV is expressed in a percent (%). The percent is based on a daily diet of 2000 calories. The % DV helps you decide if a food is high or low in a nutrient. According to the Food and Drug Administration (FDA), a 5% DV is low. A DV of 20% or more is high. In Figure 24-5, a serving of macaroni and cheese is low in dietary fiber, vitamins A and C, and iron. It is high in sodium and calcium.

Fig. 24-4 Food labels. The labels are required by the Nutrition Labeling and Education Act of 1990.

Fig. 24-5 Nutrition Facts label. *(From U.S. Food and Drug Administration, November 2004.)*

FACTORS AFFECTING EATING AND NUTRITION

Poor nutrition is common in persons needing long-term care. They need good nutrition to correct or prevent health problems. A team approach is needed to meet a person's nutritional needs. The nursing team, doctor, dietitian, speech-language pathologist, and occupational therapist are involved. The person is involved. So is the family if necessary. The person's likes, dislikes, and life-long habits are part of his or her nutritional care plan.

Some of the following factors begin during infancy and continue throughout life. Others develop later.

Culture and Religion

Culture influences dietary practices, food choices, and food preparation. Frying, baking, smoking, or roasting food and eating raw food are cultural practices. So is the use of sauces, herbs, and spices. See *Caring About Culture: Food Practices*.

CARING ABOUT CULTURE
Food Practices

Food practices vary among cultural groups. Rice, corn, and beans are protein sources in *Mexico*. In the *Philippines*, rice is a main food. And fish, vegetables, and native fruits are preferred. A diet high in sugar and animal fat is common in *Poland*. In *China*, a meal of rice with meat, fish, and vegetables is common. High sodium content is from the use of soy sauce and dried and preserved foods.

Eating beef is common in the *United States*. In *India*, Hindus do not eat beef.

Modified from D'Avanzo CE: Pocket guide to cultural health assessment, *ed 4, St Louis, 2008, Mosby.*

Selecting, preparing, and eating food often involve religious practices (Box 24-3). A person may follow all, some, or none of the dietary practices of his or her faith. You must respect the person's religious practices.

Box 24-3 **Religion and Dietary Practices**

Church of Jesus Christ of Latter Day Saints (Mormon)
- Alcohol, beverages containing caffeine (coffee, tea, colas), and chocolate are avoided.
- Fruits, vegetables, grains, and nuts take the place of meats.
- Meats, sugar, cheeses, and spices are avoided.
- Fasting is practiced.

Greek Orthodox
- Fasting is required during the Great Lent and before other holy days.
- Meat, fish, and dairy products are not eaten during a fast.

Hinduism
- Pork, fowl, ducks, snails, and crabs are avoided.
- No beef is eaten. The cow is a sacred animal to Hindus.
- Products from cows—milk, yogurt, and butter—are allowed.
- Days of fast include Hindu holidays, Sundays, birthdays, and marriage and death anniversaries.

Islam
- All pork and pork products are forbidden.
- Tea and coffee are discouraged.
- Alcohol is not allowed.
- Fasting is practiced on Mondays and Thursdays, for six days during the Shawwal (the tenth month of the Islamic calendar), and during the entire month of Ramadan (the ninth month of the Islamic calendar). Fasting means no food or drink from sunrise to sunset.

Judaism (Jewish Faith)
- Foods must be kosher. (*Kosher* means fit, proper, or correct.) Food must be prepared according to Jewish law.
- Meat of kosher animals can be eaten—cows, goats, and lambs.
- Chickens, ducks, and geese are kosher fowl.
- Kosher fish have scales and fins—tuna, sardines, carp, salmon, herring, whitefish, and so on. Lobster, shrimp, and clams are not allowed.
- Milk, milk products, and eggs from kosher animals and fowl are allowed.
- Meat and milk cannot be cooked together.
- Meat and milk products cannot be eaten at the same meal. They cannot be served on the same plate.
- Meat and milk products are not prepared or served with the same utensils and dishes. Two sets of utensils and dishes are needed. They are washed and stored separately.
- Fermented grain products are not consumed during Passover—cookies, noodles, alcohol, and so on.

Roman Catholic
- Fasting from meat is required on Ash Wednesday, Good Friday, and all Fridays during Lent.
- Not eating food is required for 1 hour before receiving Holy Communion. Water and drugs are allowed.

Seventh-Day Adventist
- Coffee, tea, and alcohol are avoided.
- Beverages with caffeine (colas) are avoided.
- Some groups have restrictions about meat, fish, and fowl.
- A vegetarian diet is encouraged.

Finances

People with limited incomes often buy the cheaper carbohydrate foods. Their diets often lack protein and certain vitamins and minerals.

Appetite

Appetite relates to the desire for food. When hungry, a person seeks food. He or she eats until the appetite is satisfied. Aromas and thoughts of food can stimulate the appetite. However, loss of appetite (anorexia) can occur. Causes include illness, drugs, anxiety, pain, and depression. Unpleasant sights, thoughts, and smells are other causes.

Personal Choice

Food likes and dislikes are personal. They begin in childhood. They are influenced by foods served in the home. As children grow older, they try new foods at school and social events. Food choices depend on how food looks, how it is prepared, its smell, and ingredients. Usually food likes expand with age and social experiences.

Sometimes resident groups plan holiday and birthday meals. They also plan picnics, pizza parties, ice cream socials, and other events. Remember, residents have the right to personal choice.

Body Reactions and Illness

People usually avoid foods that cause allergic reactions. They also avoid foods that cause nausea, vomiting, diarrhea, indigestion, gas, or headaches.

Appetite usually decreases during illness and recovery from injuries. However, nutritional needs are increased. The body must fight infection, heal tissue, and replace lost blood cells. Nutrients lost through vomiting and diarrhea need replacement.

Many drugs can affect nutrition. They can cause loss of appetite, confusion, nausea, constipation, impaired taste, or changes in gastro-intestinal (GI) function. They can cause inflammation of the mouth, throat, esophagus, and stomach.

Chewing and Swallowing Problems

Mouth, teeth, and gum problems can affect chewing. Examples include oral pain, dry or sore mouth, gum disease (Chapter 20), and dentures that fit poorly. Broken, decayed, or missing teeth also affect chewing, especially protein foods (the meat group).

Foods providing soft bulk are often ordered for persons with chewing problems. These foods include whole-grain cereals and cooked fruits and vegetables.

Some people have to avoid high-fiber foods needed for bowel elimination. High-fiber foods are hard to chew and can irritate the intestines. Such foods include apricots, celery, and fruits and vegetables with skins and seeds.

Many health problems can affect swallowing. They include stroke, pain, confusion, dry mouth, and diseases of the mouth, throat, and esophagus. See "The Dysphagia Diet" on p. 386.

Disability

Disease or injury can affect the hands, wrists, and arms. Assistive devices let the person eat independently (Fig. 24-6). The speech-language pathologist and occupational therapist teach the person how to use them. Make sure each person has needed devices.

Impaired cognitive function may affect the person's ability to use eating utensils. And it may affect eating, chewing, and swallowing. Follow the care plan to assist the person.

Age

With aging, changes occur in the GI system:

- Taste and smell dull. Good oral hygiene and denture care improve taste.
- Appetite decreases.
- Secretion of digestive juices decreases. Therefore fried and fatty foods are hard to digest. They may cause indigestion. Dry, fried, and fatty foods are avoided. This helps digestion and swallowing problems (p. 386).

OBRA DIETARY REQUIREMENTS

OBRA-CMS

The Omnibus Budget Reconciliation Act of 1987 (OBRA) and the CMS have requirements for food served in nursing centers:

- Each person's nutritional and dietary needs are met.
- The person's diet is well-balanced. It is nourishing and tastes good. Food is well-seasoned. It is not too salty or too sweet.
- Food is appetizing. It has an appealing aroma and is attractive.
- The foods served vary in color and texture.
- Food is served at the correct temperature. Hot food is served hot. Cold food is served cold. Food servers keep food at the correct temperature.
- Food is served promptly. Otherwise, hot food cools and cold food warms.
- Food is prepared to meet each person's needs. Some people need food cut, ground, or chopped. Others have special diets ordered by the doctor.
- Other foods are offered to residents who refuse the food served. Substituted food must have a similar nutritional value to the first foods served.
- Each person receives at least 3 meals a day.
- A bedtime snack is offered.
- The center provides assistive devices and utensils (see Fig. 24-6).

Fig. 24-6 Eating utensils for persons with special needs. **A,** The fork and spoon are angled. Fingers are inserted through the opening or wrapped around the handle. **B,** The utensils can be adjusted for the person's grip strength. **C,** Eating utensils have tapered and angled handles. The knife cuts with slicing and rocking motions. **D,** The thumb grips on the cup help prevent spilling. **E,** The plate guard helps keep food on the plate. *(Courtesy ElderStore, Alpharetta, Ga.)*

SPECIAL DIETS

Doctors may order special diets for a nutritional deficiency or a disease (Table 24-4, p. 384). They also order them for weight control (gain or loss) or to eliminate or decrease certain substances in the diet. The doctor, nurses, and dietitian work together to meet the person's nutritional needs. They consider the need for dietary changes, personal choices, religion, culture, and eating problems. They also consider food allergies and sensitivities. The nurse and dietitian teach the person and family about the diet.

Regular diet, general diet, and *house diet* mean no dietary limits or restrictions. Persons with diseases of the heart, kidneys, gallbladder, liver, stomach, or intestines often need special diets. Persons with wounds or pressure ulcers need high-protein diets for healing. Some persons may have bran added to their food. It provides fiber for bowel elimination. Allergies, excess weight, and other disorders also require special diets.

The sodium-controlled diet is often ordered. So is a diabetes meal plan. Persons with difficulty swallowing may need a dysphagia diet.

The Sodium-Controlled Diet

The average amount of sodium in the daily diet is 3000 to 5000 mg. The body needs no more than 2400 mg a day. Healthy people excrete excess sodium in the urine.

Heart, liver, and kidney diseases and certain drugs cause the body to retain extra sodium. A sodium-controlled diet is often needed. Sodium causes the body to retain water. If there is too much sodium, the body retains more water. Tissues swell with water. There is excess fluid in the blood vessels. The heart has to work harder. That is, the workload of the heart increases. With heart disease, the extra workload can cause serious problems or death.

Sodium control decreases the amount of sodium in the body. The body retains less water. Less water in the tissues and blood vessels reduces the heart's workload.

The doctor orders the amount of sodium allowed. Sodium-controlled diets involve:

- Omitting high-sodium foods (Box 24-4, p. 385)
- Not adding salt to food at the table
- Limiting the amount of salt used in cooking
- Diet planning

Text continued on p. 386

Table 24-4 Special Diets

Diet	Use	Foods Allowed
Clear liquid—foods liquid at body temperature and that leave small amounts of residue; non-irritating and non–gas forming	Post-operatively, acute illness, infection, nausea and vomiting, and to prepare for GI exams	Water, tea, and coffee (without milk or cream); carbonated drinks; gelatin; clear fruit juices (apple, grape, cranberry); fat-free clear broth; hard candy, sugar, and Popsicles
Full-liquid—foods liquid at room temperature or melt at body temperature	Advance from clear-liquid diet post-operatively; for stomach irritation, fever, nausea, and vomiting; for persons unable to chew, swallow, or digest solid foods	Foods on the clear-liquid diet; custard; eggnog; strained soups; strained fruit and vegetable juices; milk and milk shakes; strained, cooked cereals; plain ice cream and sherbet; pudding; yogurt
Mechanical soft—semi-solid foods that are easily digested	Advance from full-liquid diet, chewing or swallowing problems, GI disorders, and infections	All liquids; eggs (not fried); broiled, baked, or roasted meat, fish, or poultry that is chopped or shredded; mild cheeses (American, Swiss, cheddar, cream, cottage); strained fruit juices; refined bread (no crust) and crackers; cooked cereal; cooked or pureed vegetables; cooked or canned fruit without skin or seeds; pudding; plain cakes and soft cookies without fruit or nuts
Fiber- and residue-restricted—food that leaves a small amount of residue in the colon	Diseases of the colon and diarrhea	Coffee, tea, milk, carbonated drinks, strained fruit juices; refined bread and crackers; creamed and refined cereal; rice; cottage and cream cheese; eggs (not fried); plain puddings and cakes; gelatin; custard; sherbet and ice cream; strained vegetable juices; canned or cooked fruit without skin or seeds; potatoes (not fried); strained cooked vegetables; plain pasta; *no raw fruits or vegetables*
High-fiber—foods that increase the amount of residue and fiber in the colon to stimulate peristalsis	Constipation and GI disorders	All fruits and vegetables; whole-wheat bread; whole-grain cereals; fried foods; whole-grain rice; milk, cream, butter, and cheese; meats
Bland—foods that are mechanically and chemically non-irritating and low in roughage; foods served at moderate temperatures; no strong spices or condiments	Ulcers, gallbladder disorders, and some intestinal disorders; after abdominal surgery	Lean meats; white bread; creamed and refined cereals; cream or cottage cheese; gelatin; plain puddings, cakes, and cookies; eggs (not fried); butter and cream; canned fruits and vegetables without skin and seeds; strained fruit juices; potatoes (not fried); pastas and rice; strained or soft cooked carrots, peas, beets, spinach, squash, and asparagus tips; creamed soups from allowed vegetables; no fried foods
High-calorie—calorie intake is increased to about 3000 to 4000 daily; includes 3 full meals and between-meal snacks	Weight gain and some thyroid imbalances	Dietary increases in all foods; large portions of regular diet with 3 between-meal snacks
Calorie-controlled—provides adequate nutrients while controlling calories to promote weight loss and reduce body fat	Weight reduction	Foods low in fats and carbohydrates and lean meats; avoid butter, cream, rice, gravies, salad oils, noodles, cakes, pastries, carbonated and alcoholic drinks, candy, potato chips, and similar foods
High-iron—foods that are high in iron	Anemia, following blood loss, for women during the reproductive years	Liver and other organ meats, lean meats, egg yolks, shellfish, dried fruits, dried beans, green leafy vegetables, lima beans, peanut butter, enriched breads and cereals
Fat-controlled (low cholesterol)—foods low in fat and prepared without adding fat	Heart disease, gallbladder disease, disorders of fat digestion, liver disease, diseases of the pancreas	Skim milk (fat-free) or buttermilk; cottage cheese (no other cheeses allowed); gelatin; sherbet; fruit; lean meat, poultry, and fish (baked, broiled, or roasted); fat-free broth; soups made with skim milk (fat-free); margarine; rice, pasta, breads, and cereals; vegetables; potatoes

Table 24-4	Special Diets—cont'd	
Diet	**Use**	**Foods Allowed**
High-protein—aids and promotes tissue healing	For burns, high fever, infection, and some liver diseases	Meat, milk, eggs, cheese, fish, poultry; breads and cereals; green leafy vegetables
Sodium-controlled—a certain amount of sodium is allowed	Heart disease, fluid retention, liver disease, and some kidney diseases	Fruits and vegetables and unsalted butter are allowed; adding salt at the table is not allowed; highly salted foods and foods high in sodium are not allowed; the use of salt during cooking may be restricted
Diabetes meal plan—the same amounts of carbohydrates, protein, and fat are eaten at the same time each day	Diabetes	Determined by nutritional and energy requirements

Box 24-4 High-Sodium Foods

Grains
- Baked goods—biscuits, muffins, cakes, cookies, pies, pastries, sweet rolls, donuts, and so on
- Breads and rolls
- Cereals—cold, instant hot
- Noodle mixes
- Pancakes
- Salted snack foods—pretzels, corn chips, popcorn, crackers, chips, and so on
- Stuffing mixes
- Waffles

Vegetables
- Canned vegetables
- Olives
- Pickles and other pickled vegetables
- Relish
- Sauerkraut
- Tomato sauce or paste
- Vegetable juices—tomato, V-8, bloody Mary mixes
- Vegetables with sauces, creams, or seasonings

Fruits
- None—fruits are not high in sodium

Dairy Group
- Buttermilk
- Cheese
- Commercial dips made with sour cream

Protein Foods Group
- Bacon
- Canadian bacon
- Canned meats and fish—chicken, tuna, salmon, anchovies, sardines
- Caviar
- Chipped and corned beef
- Dried beef and other meats
- Dried fish
- Ham

Protein Foods Group—cont'd
- Herring
- Hot dogs (frankfurters)
- Liverwurst
- Lox
- Luncheon meats—turkey, ham, bologna, salami
- Mackerel
- Pastrami
- Pepperoni
- Salt pork
- Sausages
- Scrapple
- Shellfish—shrimp, crab, clams, oysters, scallops, lobster
- Smoked salmon

Other
- Asian foods—Chinese, Japanese, East Indian, Thai, Vietnamese
- Baking soda and baking powder
- Catsup (ketchup)
- Mayonnaise
- Salad dressings
- Cocoa mixes
- Commercially prepared dinners—frozen, canned, boxed, and so on
- Mexican foods
- Mustard
- Pasta dishes—lasagna, manicotti, ravioli
- Peanut butter
- Pizzas
- Pot pies
- Salted nuts or seeds
- Sauces—soy, teriyaki, Worcestershire, steak, barbecue, pasta, chili, cocktail
- Seasoning salts—garlic, onion, celery, meat tenderizers, monosodium glutamate (MSG), and so on
- Soups—canned, packaged, instant, dried, bouillon

Diabetes Meal Plan

Diabetes is a chronic illness in which the body cannot produce or use insulin properly (Chapter 41). The pancreas produces and secretes insulin. Insulin lets the body use sugar. Without enough insulin, sugar builds up in the bloodstream. It is not used by cells for energy. Diabetes is usually treated with insulin or other drugs, diet, and exercise.

The dietitian and person develop a meal plan for healthy eating. Consistency is key. It involves:

- The person's food preferences (likes, eating habits, meal times, culture, and life-style). It may involve limiting the amount of food or changing how it is prepared.
- Calories needed. The same amounts of carbohydrates, protein, and fat are eaten each day.
- Eating meals and snacks at regular times. The person eats at the same time every day.

Serve meals and snacks on time. The person eats at regular times to maintain a certain blood sugar level.

Always check what was eaten. Report what the person did and did not eat. If all food was not eaten, a between-meal snack is needed (p. 396). The nurse tells you what to give the person. It makes up for what was not eaten at the meal. The amount of insulin given also depends on daily food intake. Report changes in the person's eating habits.

The Dysphagia Diet

Dysphagia means difficulty (*dys*) swallowing (*phagia*). Food thickness is changed to meet the person's needs (Box 24-5). The doctor, speech-language pathologist, occupational therapist, dietitian, and nurse choose the right food thickness.

A *slow swallow* means the person has difficulty getting enough food and fluids for good nutrition and fluid balance. An *unsafe swallow* means that food enters the airway (aspiration). **Aspiration** is breathing fluid, food, vomitus, or an object into the lungs (Chapter 25).

You may need to feed a person with dysphagia. To promote safety and comfort, you must:

- Know the signs and symptoms of dysphagia (Box 24-6).
- Feed the person according to the care plan (Fig. 24-7).
- Follow aspiration precautions (Box 24-7).
- Report changes in how the person eats.
- Observe for signs and symptoms of aspiration: choking, coughing, difficulty breathing during or after meals, and abnormal breathing or respiratory sounds. Report these observations at once.

Box 24-5 **Dysphagia Diet**

Consistency	Description
Thickened liquid	No lumps. Pureed with milk, gravy, or broth to thickness of baby food. Thickener is added to some pureed foods as needed. Does not mound on a plate. May be called *creamy* or a *sauce*. Stir before serving if the food settles. Use a spoon.
Medium thick	The thickness of *nectar* or *V-8 juice* (does not hold its shape). Stir right before serving.
Extra thick	Thick like *honey*. Mounds a bit on a spoon. Can drink from a cup. Stir before serving.
Yogurt-like	Thick like *yogurt* or *pudding*. Holds its shape. Served with a spoon.
Puree	No lumps; mounds on a plate. May be thick like mashed potatoes.

Box 24-6 **Signs and Symptoms of Dysphagia**

- The person avoids food that needs chewing.
- The person avoids food with certain textures and temperatures.
- The person tires during a meal.
- Food spills out of the person's mouth while eating.
- Food "pockets" or is "squirreled" in the person's cheeks. This means that food remains or is hidden in the mouth.
- The person eats slowly, especially solid foods.
- The person complains that food will not go down or that the food is stuck.
- The person frequently coughs or chokes before, during, or after swallowing.
- The person regurgitates food after eating (Chapter 25).
- The person spits out food suddenly and almost violently.
- Food comes up through the person's nose.
- The person is hoarse—especially after eating.
- After swallowing, the person makes gargling sounds while talking or breathing.
- The person has a runny nose, sneezes, or has excessive drooling of saliva.
- The person complains of frequent heartburn.
- Appetite is decreased.

Box 24-7 **Aspiration Precautions**

- Help the person with meals and snacks. Follow the care plan.
- Position the person in Fowler's position or upright in a chair for meals and snacks.
- Support the upper back, shoulders, and neck with a pillow. Follow the care plan.
- Observe for signs and symptoms of aspiration during meals and snacks (Chapter 25).

- Check the person's mouth after eating for pocketing. Check inside the cheeks, under the tongue, and on the roof of the mouth. Remove any food.
- Position the person in a chair or in semi-Fowler's position after eating. The person maintains this position for at least 1 hour after eating. Follow the care plan.
- Provide mouth care after eating.
- Report and record your observations.

Fig. 24-7 Sections of a swallowing guide. (*Excerpted from "Swallowguide™." Courtesy Interactive Therapeutics, Inc., Stow, Ohio. For information regarding the entire form, call 800-253-5111.*)

Box 24-8	Common Causes of Dehydration

- Bleeding
- Coma
- Dementia
- Diarrhea
- Drug therapy
- Fever
- Fluid intake: poor
- Fluid restriction
- Fluids: refusing
- Functional impairments: difficulty drinking, reaching fluids, communicating fluid needs
- Sweating: excess
- Urine production: increased
- Vomiting

FLUID BALANCE

Water is needed to live. Death can result from too much or too little water. Water is ingested through fluids and foods. Water is lost through urine, feces, and vomit. It is also lost through the skin (perspiration) and the lungs (expiration).

Fluid balance is needed for health. The amount of fluid taken in (intake) and the amount of fluid lost (output) must be equal. If fluid intake exceeds fluid output, body tissues swell with water. This is called edema. Edema is common in people with heart and kidney diseases. Dehydration is a decrease in the amount of water in body tissues. Fluid output exceeds intake. Common causes of dehydration are listed in Box 24-8.

Normal Fluid Requirements

An adult needs 1500 mL (milliliters) of water daily to survive. About 2000 to 2500 mL are needed for normal fluid balance. The water requirement increases with hot weather, exercise, fever, illness, and excess fluid losses.

The amount of body water decreases with age. Older persons also are at risk for diseases that affect fluid balance. Examples include heart disease, kidney disease, cancer, and diabetes. Some drugs cause the body to lose fluids. Others cause the body to retain water. The older person is at risk for dehydration and edema.

Older persons may have a decreased sense of thirst. Their bodies need water, but they may not feel thirsty. Offer water and other fluids often. Some persons have special fluid orders.

Special Fluid Orders

The doctor may order the amount of fluid a person can have during a 24-hour period. This is done to maintain fluid balance. Found in the care plan and in the Kardex, common orders are:

- *Encourage fluids.* The person drinks an increased amount of fluid. The order states the amount to ingest. Intake records are kept. The person is given a variety of fluids allowed on the diet. They are kept within the person's reach. They are served at the correct temperature. Fluids are offered regularly to persons who cannot feed themselves.
- *Restrict fluids.* Fluids are limited to a certain amount. They are offered in small amounts and in small containers. The water pitcher is removed from the room or kept out of sight. Intake records are kept. The person needs frequent oral hygiene. It helps keep mucous membranes of the mouth moist.
- *Nothing by mouth.* The person cannot eat or drink anything. *NPO* is the abbreviation for *non per os.* It means nothing (*non*) by (*per*) mouth (*os*). NPO often is ordered before and after surgery, before some laboratory tests and diagnostic procedures, and in treating certain illnesses. An NPO sign is posted above the bed. The water pitcher and glass are removed. Frequent oral hygiene is needed, but the person must not swallow any fluid. The person is NPO for 6 to 8 hours before surgery and before some laboratory tests and diagnostic procedures.
- *Thickened liquids.* All fluids are thickened, including water. The thickness depends on the person's ability to swallow (see Box 24-5). Thickener is added before fluids are served. Or commercial fluids are used. They are already thickened.

Intake and Output Records

The doctor or nurse may order intake and output (I&O) measurements. I&O records are kept. They are used to evaluate fluid balance and kidney function. They help in planning medical treatment. They also are kept when the person has special fluid orders.

All fluids taken by mouth are measured and recorded—water, milk, coffee, tea, juices, soups, and soft drinks. So are foods that melt at room temperature—ice cream, sherbet, custard, pudding, gelatin, and Popsicles. The nurse measures and records intravenous (IV) fluids and tube feedings (Chapter 25). Output includes urine, vomitus, diarrhea, and wound drainage.

Measuring Intake and Output Intake and output are measured in milliliters (mL). You need to know these amounts:

- 1 oz equals 30 mL.
- 1 pint is about 500 mL.
- 1 quart is about 1000 mL.

You also need to know the serving sizes of bowls, dishes, cups, pitchers, glasses, and other containers. This information may be on the I&O record (Fig. 24-8).

A measuring container for fluid is called a graduate. It is used to measure left-over fluids, urine, vomitus, and drainage from suction. Like a measuring cup, the graduate is marked in ounces and milliliters (Fig. 24-9, p. 390). Plastic urinals and kidney basins also have amounts marked. The measuring device is held at eye level to read the amount.

OSF
ST. JOSEPH MEDICAL CENTER
Bloomington, Illinois

DATE _6/15_

FLUID BALANCE CHART

Water Glass	250mL		Ice Cream	120mL
Styrofoam Cup	180mL		Ice Chips	1/2 amt. of
Cup (coffee)	250mL			mL's in cup
Milk Carton	240mL		Pitcher	
Pop (1 can)	360mL		(Yellow)	1000mL
Broth-Soup	175mL			
Juice Carton	120mL			
Juice Glass	120mL			
Jello	120mL			

	INTAKE				OUTPUT					
		Parenteral		Amt. mL Absbd.	URINE		OTHER		CONT. IRRIGATION	
TIME	ORAL				Method Collected	Amt. (mL)	Method Collected	Amt. (mL)	In	Out
2400-0100		mL from previous shift			V	150				
0100-0200							Vom.	150		
0200-0300										
0300-0400										
0400-0500										
0500-0600	125				V	200				
0600-0700										
0700-0800										
	125	8 - hour Sub-total			8-hr T	350	8-hr T	150		
0800-0900	400	mL from previous shift			V	250				
0900-1000	100									
1000-1100										
1100-1200										
1200-1300	400				V	250				
1300-1400										
1400-1500	200									
1500-1600										
	1100	8 - hour Sub-total			8-hr T	500	8-hr T			
1600-1700		mL from previous shift			V	270				
1700-1800	350									
1800-1900	50									
1900-2000	200									
2000-2100					V	400				
2100-2200										
2200-2300										
2300-2400										
	600	8 - hour Sub-total			8-hr T	670	8-hr T			
	1825	24 - hour Sub-total			24-hr T	1520	24-hr T	150		

310' Marie Mills

Source Key:		Source Key:	
URINE		OTHER	
V	- Voided	G.I.T.	- Gastric Intestinal Tube
C	- Catheter	T.T.	- T. Tube
INC	- Incontinent	Vom.	- Vomitus
U.C.	- Ureteral Catheter	Liq S.	- Liquid Stool
		H.V.	- Hemovac

Form No. MF36722 (Rev. 5/97)   **MFI**

Fig. 24-8 An intake and output record. *(Modified from OSF St. Joseph Medical Center, Bloomington, Ill.)*

Fig. 24-9 A graduate marked in ounces and milliliters.

An I&O record is kept at the bedside. When intake or output is measured, the amount is recorded in the correct column (see Fig. 24-8). Amounts are totaled at the end of the shift. The totals are recorded in the person's chart. They also are shared during the end-of-shift report.

The purpose of measuring I&O and how to help are explained to the person. Some persons measure and record their intake. Family members may help. The urinal, commode, bedpan, or specimen pan is used for voiding. Remind the person not to void in the toilet. Also remind the person not to put toilet tissue into the receptacle.

See *Delegation Guidelines: Intake and Output.*
See *Promoting Safety and Comfort: Intake and Output.*

DELEGATION GUIDELINES
Intake and Output

When measuring I&O, you need this information from the nurse and the care plan:
* If the person has a special fluid order—encourage fluids, restrict fluids, NPO, or thickened fluids
* When to report measurements—hourly or end-of-shift
* What the person uses for voiding—urinal, bedpan, commode, or specimen pan (Chapter 22)
* If the person has a catheter
* What specific resident concerns to report at once

PROMOTING SAFETY AND COMFORT
Intake and Output

Safety
Urine may contain microbes or blood. Microbes can grow in urinals, commodes, bedpans, specimen pans, and drainage systems. Follow Standard Precautions and the Bloodborne Pathogen Standard when handling such equipment. Thoroughly clean the item after it is used. Use a disinfectant for cleaning.

Comfort
Promptly measure the contents of urinals, bedpans, commodes, and specimen pans. This helps prevent or reduce odors. Odors can disturb the person.

 MEASURING INTAKE AND OUTPUT

QUALITY OF LIFE

Remember to:
* Knock before entering the person's room.
* Address the person by name.
* Introduce yourself by name and title.

* Explain the procedure to the person before beginning and during the procedure.
* Protect the person's rights during the procedure.
* Handle the person gently during the procedure.

PRE-PROCEDURE

1 Follow *Delegation Guidelines: Intake and Output.* See *Promoting Safety and Comfort: Intake and Output.*
2 Practice hand hygiene.

3 Collect the following:
* I&O record
* Graduates
* Gloves

MEASURING INTAKE AND OUTPUT—cont'd

PROCEDURE

4 Put on gloves.

5 Measure intake as follows:

  a Pour liquid remaining in the container into the graduate.

  b Measure the amount at eye level or on a flat surface. Keep the container level.

  c Check the serving amount on the I&O record.

  d Subtract the remaining amount from the full serving amount. Note the amount.

  e Pour fluid in the graduate back into the container.

  f Repeat steps 5a through 5e for each liquid.

  g Add the amounts from each liquid together.

  h Record the time and amount on the I&O record.

6 Measure output as follows:

  a Pour the fluid into the graduate used to measure output.

  b Measure the amount at eye level or on a flat surface. Keep the container level.

  c Dispose of fluid in the toilet. Avoid splashes.

7 Clean and rinse the graduates. Dispose of rinse into the toilet. Return the graduates to their proper place.

8 Clean and rinse the voiding receptacle or drainage container. Dispose of the rinse into the toilet. Return the item to its proper place.

9 Remove the gloves. Practice hand hygiene.

10 Record the output amount on the I&O record.

POST-PROCEDURE

11 Provide for comfort. (See the inside of the front book cover.)

12 Make sure the signal light is within reach.

13 Complete a safety check of the room. (See the inside of the front book cover.)

14 Report and record your observations.

MEETING FOOD AND FLUID NEEDS

Weakness, illness, and confusion can affect appetite and ability to eat. So can unpleasant odors, sights, and sounds. An uncomfortable position, the need for oral hygiene, the need to eliminate, and pain also affect appetite.

See *Focus on Communication: Meeting Food and Fluid Needs.*

FOCUS ON COMMUNICATION
Meeting Food and Fluid Needs

The person may not eat or drink all the food and fluids served. You need to find out why and tell the nurse. Ask the person to explain the answer.

- "Please tell me why you didn't eat everything."
- "Was there something wrong with your food?"
- "Did your food taste okay?"
- "Was there something you didn't like?"
- "Was your food too hot or too cold?"
- "Would you like something else?"
- "Weren't you hungry?"

Dining Programs

Some residents are alert and oriented. They enjoy being together for meals. Others like eating in their rooms. Others are confused and noisy at meal time. Some persons are incontinent or have odor problems. Some are too weak or ill to leave their rooms for meals.

The following dining programs are common in nursing centers:

- *Social dining.* Four to six residents are seated at a dining room table (Fig. 24-10, p. 392). Food is served as in a restaurant. This program is for persons who are oriented and can feed themselves. Sometimes quietly confused persons are included. They must be able to feed themselves and not disrupt others.
- *Family dining.* This is like social dining. However, food is served in bowls and on platters. Residents serve themselves as at home.
- *Low-stimulation dining.* Meal time distractions are prevented. The health team decides on the best place for each person to sit.
- *Restaurant-style menus.* The person selects food from a menu. This program allows more food choices. The person is served as in a restaurant.
- *Open-dining.* A buffet is open for several hours. A breakfast buffet is an example. Residents can eat any time while the buffet is open.

Some centers have areas where residents can dine privately with guests. The person can have a meal with a partner, children, and other family or friends. They can celebrate holidays, birthdays, anniversaries, or other events. Food is provided by guests or the dietary department.

Fig. 24-10 These residents are eating in the dining room.

Preparing for Meals

Preparing residents for meals promotes their comfort. To promote comfort:

* Assist with elimination needs.
* Provide oral hygiene. Make sure dentures are in place.
* Make sure eyeglasses and hearing aids are in place.
* Make sure incontinent persons are clean and dry.
* Position the person in a comfortable position.
* Assist the person with hand washing.
  See *Delegation Guidelines: Preparing for Meals.*
  See *Promoting Safety and Comfort: Preparing for Meals.*

PREPARING THE PERSON FOR A MEAL

QUALITY OF LIFE

Remember to:
- Knock before entering the person's room.
- Address the person by name.
- Introduce yourself by name and title.
- Explain the procedure to the person before beginning and during the procedure.
- Protect the person's rights during the procedure.
- Handle the person gently during the procedure.

PRE-PROCEDURE

1 Follow *Delegation Guidelines: Preparing for Meals.* See *Promoting Safety and Comfort: Preparing for Meals.*
2 Practice hand hygiene.
3 Collect the following:
   - Equipment for oral hygiene
   - Bedpan and cover, urinal, commode, or specimen pan
   - Toilet tissue
   - Wash basin
   - Soap
   - Washcloth
   - Towel
   - Gloves
4 Provide for privacy.

PROCEDURE

5 Make sure eyeglasses and hearing aids are in place.
6 Assist with oral hygiene. Make sure dentures are in place. Wear gloves, and decontaminate your hands after removing them.
7 Assist with elimination. Make sure the incontinent person is clean and dry. Wear gloves, and practice hand hygiene after removing them.
8 Assist with hand washing. Wear gloves, and practice hand hygiene after removing them.
9 Do the following if the person will eat in bed:
   a Raise the head of the bed to a comfortable position. Fowler's position is preferred.
   b Remove items from the overbed table. Clean the overbed table.
   c Adjust the overbed table in front of the person.
10 Do the following if the person will sit in a chair:
   a Position the person in a chair or wheelchair.
   b Remove items from the overbed table. Clean the table.
   c Adjust the overbed table in front of the person.
11 Assist the person to the dining area. (This step is for the person who eats in a dining area.)

POST-PROCEDURE

12 Provide for comfort. (See the inside of the front book cover.)
13 Place the signal light within reach.
14 Empty, clean, and disinfect equipment. Return equipment to its proper place. Wear gloves, and practice hand hygiene after removing them.
15 Straighten the room. Eliminate unpleasant noise, odors, or equipment.
16 Unscreen the person.
17 Complete a safety check of the room. (See the inside of the front book cover.)
18 Decontaminate your hands.

 Serving Meals

Food is served in containers that keep foods at the correct temperature. Hot food is kept hot. Cold food is kept cold. OBRA requires that food be at the correct temperature when the person receives it.

You serve meals after preparing residents for meals. You can serve meals promptly if residents are ready to eat. Prompt serving keeps food at the correct temperature.

Serve meals in the assigned order. Residents seated at tables are served at the same time.

If food is not served within 15 minutes, re-check food temperatures. Follow center policy. If not at the correct temperature, get fresh food. Temperature guides and food thermometers are in dining rooms and in nursing unit kitchens. Some centers allow re-heating in microwave ovens.

See *Delegation Guidelines: Serving Meals,* p. 394.
See *Promoting Safety and Comfort: Serving Meals,* p. 394.
See *Teamwork and Time Management: Serving Meals,* p. 394.

OBRA-CMS

DELEGATION GUIDELINES
Serving Meals

Before serving meal trays, you need this information from the nurse and the care plan:

- What assistive devices the person uses
- If the person needs help opening cartons, cutting food, buttering bread, and so on
- If the person's intake is measured (p. 389)
- If calorie counts are done (p. 396)
- When to report observations
- What specific resident concerns to report at once

TEAMWORK AND TIME MANAGEMENT
Serving Meals

Meal trays are served in the order set by the health team. You will serve trays to your residents and to those assigned to other nursing assistants. Your co-workers will do the same. The goal is to serve trays as fast as possible. This keeps food at the desired temperature.

PROMOTING SAFETY AND COMFORT
Serving Meals

Safety
Always check food temperature after re-heating. Food that is too hot can cause burns.

Comfort
Check the person's position when serving a meal. The position may have changed after the person was prepared to eat. Provide other comfort measures as needed. See the inside of the front book cover for comfort measures.

SERVING MEAL TRAYS

VIDEO

QUALITY OF LIFE

Remember to:
- Knock before entering the person's room.
- Address the person by name.
- Introduce yourself by name and title.

- Explain the procedure to the person before beginning and during the procedure.
- Protect the person's rights during the procedure.
- Handle the person gently during the procedure.

PRE-PROCEDURE

1 Follow *Delegation Guidelines: Serving Meals.* See *Promoting Safety and Comfort: Serving Meals.*

2 Practice hand hygiene.

PROCEDURE

3 Make sure the tray is complete. Check items on the tray with the dietary card. Make sure assistive devices are included.

4 Identify the person. Check the ID (identification) bracelet against the dietary card. Also call the person by name.

5 Place the tray within the person's reach. Adjust the overbed table as needed.

6 Remove food covers. Open cartons, cut food into bite-size pieces, butter bread, and so on as needed (Fig. 24-11). Season food as the person prefers and is allowed on the care plan.

7 Place the napkin, clothes protector, assistive devices, and eating utensils within reach.

8 Place the signal light within reach.

9 Do the following when the person is done eating:
   a Measure and record intake if ordered (p. 389).
   b Note the amount and type of foods eaten. (See "Calorie Counts" on p. 396.)
   c Check for and remove any food in the person's mouth (pocketing). Wear gloves. Decontaminate your hands after removing them.
   d Remove the tray.
   e Clean spills. Change soiled linen and clothing.
   f Help the person return to bed if needed.
   g Assist with oral hygiene and hand washing. Wear gloves. Decontaminate your hands after removing the gloves.

SERVING MEAL TRAYS—cont'd

VIDEO

POST-PROCEDURE

10 Provide for comfort. (See the inside of the front book cover.)

11 Place the signal light within reach.

12 Raise or lower bed rails. Follow the care plan.

13 Complete a safety check of the room. (See the inside of the front book cover.)

14 Follow center policy for soiled linen.

15 Decontaminate your hands.

16 Report and record your observations.

Fig. 24-11 Cartons and containers are opened for the person.

Fig. 24-12 The numbers on a clock are used to help a visually impaired person locate food.

📨 Feeding the Person

Weakness, paralysis, casts, confusion, and other limits may make self-feeding impossible. These persons are fed.

Serve food and fluids in the order the person prefers. Offer fluids during the meal. Fluids help the person chew and swallow.

Use teaspoons to feed the person. They are less likely to cause injury than forks. The teaspoon should only be one-third full. This portion is chewed and swallowed easily. Some people need smaller portions. Follow the care plan.

Persons who need to be fed are often angry, humiliated, and embarrassed. Some are depressed or resentful or refuse to eat. Let them do as much as possible. Some can manage "finger foods" (bread, cookies, crackers). If strong enough, let them hold milk or juice cups (never hot drinks). Do not exceed activity limits ordered by the doctor. Provide support. Encourage them to try, even if food is spilled.

Visually impaired persons are often very aware of food aromas. They may know the food served. Always tell the person what is on the tray. When feeding visually impaired persons, describe what you are offering. For persons who feed themselves, describe foods and fluids and their place on the tray. Use the numbers on a clock for the location of foods (Fig. 24-12).

Many people pray before eating. Allow time and privacy for prayer. This shows respect and caring.

Meals provide social contact with others. Engage the person in pleasant conversation. However, allow time for chewing and swallowing. Also, sit facing the person. Sitting is more relaxing. It shows that you have time for the person. By facing the person, you can see how well the person is eating. You can also see if the person has problems swallowing.

See *Residents With Dementia: Feeding the Person,* p. 396.

See *Delegation Guidelines: Feeding the Person,* p. 396.

See *Promoting Safety and Comfort: Feeding the Person,* p. 396.

RESIDENTS WITH DEMENTIA
Feeding the Person

Residents with dementia may become distracted during meals. Some persons cannot sit long enough for a meal. Others forget how to use eating utensils. Some persons resist your efforts to assist them with eating. A confused person may throw or spit food.

The Alzheimer's Disease Education and Referral Center (ADEAR) recommends the following. The measures may be part of the person's care plan.

- Provide a calm, quiet setting for eating. Limit noise and other distractions. This helps the person focus on the meal.
- Limit the number of food choices.
- Offer several small meals throughout the day instead of larger ones.
- Use straws or cups with lids. These make drinking easier.
- Provide finger foods if the person has problems with utensils. A bowl may be easier to use than a plate.
- Provide healthy snacks. Keep snacks where the person can see them.

You must be patient. Talk to the nurse if you feel upset or impatient. Remember, the person has the right to be treated with dignity and respect.

DELEGATION GUIDELINES
Feeding the Person

Before feeding a person, you need this information from the nurse and the care plan:
- Why the person needs help
- How much help the person needs
- If the person can manage finger foods
- What the person's activity limits are
- What the person's dietary restrictions are
- What size portion to feed the person—⅓ teaspoonful or less
- What safety measures are needed if the person has dysphagia
- If the person can use a straw
- What observations to report and record:
  - The amount and kind of food eaten
  - Complaints of nausea or dysphagia
  - Signs and symptoms of dysphagia
  - Signs and symptoms of aspiration
- When to report observations
- What specific resident concerns to report at once

PROMOTING SAFETY AND COMFORT
Feeding the Person

Safety
Check food temperature. Very hot foods can burn the person.

Prevent aspiration. Check the person's mouth before offering more food or fluids. The person's mouth must be empty between bites and swallows.

Comfort
The person will eat better if not rushed. Sit to show the person that you have time for him or her. Standing communicates that you are in a hurry.

Wipe the person's hands, face, and mouth as needed during the meal. Use the napkin. If necessary, use a wet washcloth. Then dry the person with a towel.

Between-Meal Snacks

Many special diets involve between-meal snacks. Common snacks are crackers, milk, juice, a milkshake, cake, wafers, a sandwich, gelatin, and custard.

Snacks are served upon arrival on the nursing unit. Provide needed utensils, a straw, and a napkin. Follow the same considerations and procedures for serving meals and feeding persons.

Calorie Counts

Calorie records are kept for some people. On a flow sheet, note what the person ate and how much. For example, a chicken breast, rice, beans, a roll, pudding, and two pats of butter were served. The person ate all the chicken, half the rice, and the roll. One pat of butter was used. The beans and pudding were not eaten. Note these on the flow sheet. A nurse or dietitian converts these portions into calories. The nurse tells you which persons need calorie counts.

Fig. 24-13 A spoon is used to feed the person. The spoon is one-third full.

FEEDING THE PERSON

QUALITY OF LIFE

Remember to:
- Knock before entering the person's room.
- Address the person by name.
- Introduce yourself by name and title.

- Explain the procedure to the person before beginning and during the procedure.
- Protect the person's rights during the procedure.
- Handle the person gently during the procedure.

PRE-PROCEDURE

1 Follow *Delegation Guidelines: Feeding the Person.* See *Promoting Safety and Comfort: Feeding the Person.*
2 Practice hand hygiene.

3 Position the person in a comfortable position for eating—usually sitting or Fowler's.
4 Get the tray. Place it on the overbed table or dining table.

PROCEDURE

5 Identify the person. Check the ID bracelet against the dietary card. Also call the person by name.
6 Drape a napkin across the person's chest and underneath the chin.
7 Tell the person what foods and fluids are on the tray.
8 Prepare food for eating. Cut food into bite-size pieces. Season foods as the person prefers and is allowed on the care plan.
9 Place the chair where you can sit comfortably. Sit facing the person.
10 Serve foods in the order the person prefers. Identify foods as you serve them. Alternate between solid and liquid foods. Use a spoon for safety (Fig. 24-13). Allow enough time for chewing and swallowing. Do not rush the person. Also offer water, coffee, tea, or other beverage on the tray.
11 Check the person's mouth before offering more food or fluids. Make sure the person's mouth is empty between bites and swallows.
12 Use straws for liquids if the person cannot drink out of a glass or cup. Have one straw for each liquid. Provide short straws for weak persons.

13 Wipe the person's hands, face, and mouth as needed during the meal. Use the napkin.
14 Follow the care plan if the person has dysphagia. (Some persons with dysphagia do not use straws.) Give thickened liquid with a spoon.
15 Converse with the person in a pleasant manner.
16 Encourage him or her to eat as much as possible.
17 Wipe the person's mouth with a napkin. Discard the napkin.
18 Note how much and which foods were eaten. See "Calorie Counts."
19 Measure and record intake if ordered (p. 389).
20 Remove the tray.
21 Take the person back to his or her room (if in a dining area).
22 Assist with oral hygiene and hand washing. Wear gloves. Provide for privacy. Decontaminate your hands after removing the gloves.

POST-PROCEDURE

23 Provide for comfort. (See the inside of the front book cover.)
24 Place the signal light within reach.
25 Raise or lower bed rails. Follow the care plan.
26 Complete a safety check of the room. (See the inside of the front book cover.)

27 Return the food tray to the food cart.
28 Decontaminate your hands.
29 Report and record your observations.

Providing Drinking Water

Residents need fresh drinking water each shift. They also need water whenever the pitcher is empty.

Some centers do not use the procedure that follows. Each person's pitcher is filled as needed. The pitcher is taken to an ice and water dispenser. If so, fill the pitcher with ice first. Then add water to the pitcher. Follow the center's procedure for providing fresh drinking water.

See *Delegation Guidelines: Providing Drinking Water.*

See *Promoting Safety and Comfort: Providing Drinking Water,* p. 398.

DELEGATION GUIDELINES
Providing Drinking Water

Before providing water, you need this information from the nurse and the care plan:
- The person's fluid orders
- If the person can have ice
- If the person uses a straw

PROMOTING SAFETY AND COMFORT
Providing Drinking Water

Safety

Water cups and pitchers can spread microbes. To prevent the spread of microbes:

- Make sure the pitcher is labeled with the person's name and room and bed number.
- Do not touch the rim or inside of the cup or pitcher.
- Do not let the ice scoop touch the rim or inside of the cup or pitcher.

- Do not put the ice scoop in the ice container or dispenser. Place it in the scoop holder or on a towel for the scoop.
- Make sure the person's pitcher and cup are clean. Also check for cracks and chips. Provide a new pitcher or cup as needed.

 PROVIDING DRINKING WATER

QUALITY OF LIFE

Remember to:
- Knock before entering the person's room.
- Address the person by name.
- Introduce yourself by name and title.

- Explain the procedure to the person before beginning and during the procedure.
- Protect the person's rights during the procedure.
- Handle the person gently during the procedure.

PRE-PROCEDURE

1 Follow *Delegation Guidelines: Providing Drinking Water,* p. 397. See *Promoting Safety and Comfort: Providing Drinking Water.*
2 Obtain a list of persons who have special fluid orders from the nurse. Or use your assignment sheet.
3 Practice hand hygiene.
4 Collect the following:
   - Cart
   - Ice chest filled with ice
   - Cover for the ice chest
   - Scoop
   - Water cups
   - Straws
   - Paper towels
   - Water pitchers for resident use
   - Large water pitcher filled with cold water (optional, depending on center procedure)
   - Towel for the scoop
5 Cover the cart with paper towels. Arrange equipment on top of the paper towels.

PROCEDURE

6 Take the cart to the person's room door. Do not take the cart into the room.
7 Check the person's fluid orders. Use the list from the nurse.
8 Identify the person. Check the ID bracelet against the fluid orders sheet or your assignment sheet. Also call the person by name.
9 Take the pitcher from the person's overbed table. Empty it into the bathroom sink.
10 Determine if a new pitcher is needed.
11 Use the scoop to fill the pitcher with ice (Fig. 24-14). Do not let the scoop touch the rim or inside of the pitcher.
12 Place the ice scoop on the towel.
13 Fill the pitcher with water. Get water from the bathroom or use the larger water pitcher on the cart.
14 Place the pitcher, cup, and straw (if used) on the overbed table. Fill the cup with water. Do not let the water pitcher touch the rim or inside of the cup.
15 Make sure the pitcher, cup, and straw (if used) are within the person's reach.

POST-PROCEDURE

16 Provide for comfort. (See the inside of the front book cover.)
17 Place the signal light within reach.
18 Complete a safety check of the room. (See the inside of the front book cover.)
19 Decontaminate your hands.
20 Repeat steps 6 through 19 for each person.

Fig. 24-14 Providing drinking water.

FOODBORNE ILLNESSES

A foodborne illness (food poisoning) is caused by pathogens in food and fluids. Report the signs and symptoms listed in Box 24-9 to the nurse at once.

Food is not sterile. Therefore pathogens are present in food. Cooked and ready-to-eat foods can become contaminated from other food. For example, meat juices can spill or splash onto other food. Food handlers with poor hygiene can contaminate the food.

Pathogens grow rapidly between 40° and 140° F (Fahrenheit). This range is called the "danger zone" by the United States Department of Agriculture (USDA). You must keep food out of the "danger zone." To do so, keep cold food cold and hot food hot.

To keep food safe, the USDA recommends these 4 safety tips:

- *Clean.* Wash hands, utensils, and counter tops often.
- *Separate.* Avoid cross-contamination. Do not let raw meat, poultry, or their juices touch other foods that will not be cooked.
- *Cook.* Cook food to a safe internal temperature (see Fig. 24-2). Use a food thermometer to check the internal temperature. When re-heating cooked food, re-heat to 165° F.
- *Chill.* Refrigerate or freeze food within 2 hours. If the air is 90° F or above, chill food within 1 hour.

Box 24-9   Signs and Symptoms of Foodborne Illnesses

- Abdominal cramps or pain
- Backache
- Breathing problems
- Chills
- Diarrhea (may be bloody)
- Eyelids: droopy
- Fever
- Headache
- Muscle pain
- Nausea
- Speaking problems
- Swallowing problems
- Vision: double
- Vomiting

QUALITY OF LIFE

OBRA serves to promote the person's quality of life. Nutrition and fluid balance are important for quality of life.

The right to personal choice is important in meeting food and fluid needs. Everyone has a life-time of likes and dislikes. These do not change when in a nursing center. Cultural, social, religious, medical, and personal factors affect food choices. Persons often express their food likes and dislikes. A person may say that the food is too cold. Or it is too bland. Or the food tastes bad.

Residents have the right to express their preferences. Do not become angry or upset. Do not make the person feel as if he or she is complaining or being picky. Learning the person's likes and dislikes can improve nutrition. It also shows interest and concern for the person. Respect the person's right to express personal food choices. Share this information with the nurse. With the person's help, the dietitian plans healthy meals that include personal choices.

Persons with dementia may require special measures to meet their nutritional needs. Be patient. Provide a quiet and calm meal time. Treat the person with dignity and respect.

Sometimes families and friends bring food from home. This helps meet love and belonging needs. Sometimes the center cannot provide everything the person likes. Residents are usually pleased to receive home-made food. Holidays have food traditions. Holidays mean more when life-long traditions are shared. Gifts of food are common. Tell the nurse when the person receives food. The food must not interfere with the person's diet.

OBRA requires that food be served correctly. Hot food must be hot. Cold food must be cold. Cold mashed potatoes are not very good. You would not eat them. The person should not have to. Serve meals promptly. If a meal is delayed, tell the person why. Then get fresh food. Provide needed help with eating. This includes providing eating devices and utensils.

REVIEW QUESTIONS

Circle the BEST answer.

1 Nutrition is
   a Fats, proteins, carbohydrates, vitamins, and minerals
   b The many processes involved in the ingestion, digestion, absorption, and use of food and fluids by the body
   c The MyPlate symbol
   d The balance between calories taken in and used by the body

2 MyPlate encourages the following *except*
   a The same diet for everyone
   b Balancing calories
   c Increasing the amount of fruits and vegetables
   d Choosing low-sodium foods

3 On a 2000-calorie a day diet, what is the amount of grains needed for an adult woman?
   a 6 oz   c 2 to 4 oz
   b 4 to 5 oz   d 3 oz

4 On a 2000-calorie a day diet, what is the amount of protein foods needed by an adult man?
   a 2½ oz   c 4 to 5 oz
   b 3 to 4 oz   d 5½ to 6½ oz

5 Which food group contains the *most* fat?
   a Grains   c Milk
   b Vegetables   d Meat and beans

6 These statements are about oils. Which is *false*?
   a Oils are high in calories.
   b The best oil choices come from fish, nuts, and vegetable oils.
   c Oils from plant sources contain cholesterol.
   d Mayonnaise, certain salad dressings, and soft margarine are mainly oil.

7 Protein is needed for
   a Tissue growth and repair
   b Energy and the fiber for bowel elimination
   c Body heat and to protect organs from injury
   d Improving the taste of food

8 Which foods provide the *most* protein?
   a Butter and cream   c Meats and fish
   b Tomatoes and potatoes   d Corn and lettuce

9 The sodium-controlled diet involves
   a Omitting high-sodium foods
   b Adding salt to food at the table
   c Using 2400 mg of salt in cooking
   d A sodium-intake flow sheet

10 A person on a sodium-controlled diet wants a salt shaker. You should
   a Provide the salt
   b Salt the person's food
   c Explain that added salt is not allowed on the diet
   d Ignore the request

11 Diabetes meal planning involves the following *except*
   a Food the person likes
   b Eating the same amount of carbohydrates, protein, and fat each day
   c Eating at regular times
   d Sodium control

12 OBRA requires the following *except*
   a Offering 24-hour meal service
   b Serving hot food hot; serving cold food cold
   c Providing needed eating devices
   d Serving food promptly

13 OBRA requires
   a 2 regular meals
   b 3 regular meals
   c 4 regular meals and a bedtime snack
   d Meals every 6 hours

14 Adult fluid requirements for normal fluid balance are about
   a 1000 to 1500 mL daily
   b 1500 to 2000 mL daily
   c 2000 to 2500 mL daily
   d 2500 to 3000 mL daily

15 A person is NPO. You should
   a Provide a variety of fluids
   b Offer fluids in small amounts and in small containers
   c Remove the water pitcher and cup from the room
   d Remove oral hygiene equipment from the room

16 Which are *not* counted as liquid foods?
   a Coffee, tea, juices, and soft drinks
   b Butter, sauces, and melted cheese
   c Ice cream, sherbet, custard, pudding
   d Jell-O, Popsicles, and creamed cereals

17 Residents are eating in the dining room. They serve themselves from bowls and platters on their tables. This is
   a A social dining program
   b A family dining program
   c A low-stimulation feeding program
   d An open-dining program

18 Persons with dysphagia
   a Use straws for all liquids
   b Have a regular diet
   c Are fed according to the care plan
   d Eat alone in their rooms

19 Which is *not* a sign of a swallowing problem?
   a Drooling   c Pocketing
   b Coughing while eating   d Edema

20 You are feeding a person. Which action is *not correct*?
   a Ask if he or she wants to pray before eating.
   b Use a fork to feed the person.
   c Ask the person the order in which to serve food and fluids.
   d Engage the person in a pleasant conversation.

21 Before providing fresh drinking water, you need to know the person's
   a I&O   c Fluid orders
   b Diet   d Preferred beverages

22 You are re-heating cooked food. The food temperature should be
   a 40° F   c 140° F
   b 90° F   d 165° F

Answers to these questions are on p. 720.

Nutritional Support and IV Therapy

OBJECTIVES

- Define the key terms and key abbreviations listed in this chapter.
- Identify the reasons for nutritional support and IV therapy.
- Explain how tube feedings are given.
- Describe scheduled and continuous feedings.
- Explain how to prevent aspiration.
- Describe the comfort measures for the person with a feeding tube.
- Describe parenteral nutrition.

- Describe the IV therapy sites.
- Identify the equipment used in IV therapy.
- Describe how to assist with the IV flow rate.
- Identify the safety measures for IV therapy.
- Identify the observations to report when a person has nutritional support or IV therapy.
- Explain how to assist with nutritional support and IV therapy.
- Explain how to promote quality of life.

KEY TERMS

aspiration Breathing fluid, food, vomitus, or an object into the lungs

enteral nutrition Giving nutrients into the gastrointestinal (GI) tract *(enteral)* through a feeding tube

flow rate The number of drops per minute *(gtt/min)*

gastrostomy tube A tube inserted through a surgically created opening *(stomy)* in the stomach *(gastro)*; stomach tube

gavage The process of giving a tube feeding

intravenous (IV) therapy Giving fluids through a needle or catheter inserted into a vein; IV and IV infusion

jejunostomy tube A feeding tube inserted into a surgically created opening *(stomy)* in the *jejunum* of the small intestine

naso-enteral tube A feeding tube inserted through the nose *(naso)* into the small bowel *(enteral)*

naso-gastric (NG) tube A feeding tube inserted through the nose *(naso)* into the stomach *(gastro)*

parenteral nutrition Giving nutrients through a catheter inserted into a vein; *para* means beyond; *enteral* relates to the bowel

percutaneous endoscopic gastrostomy (PEG) tube A feeding tube inserted into the stomach *(gastro)* through a small incision *(stomy)* made through *(per)* the skin *(cutaneous)*; a lighted instrument *(scope)* is used to see inside a body cavity or organ *(endo)*

regurgitation The backward flow of stomach contents into the mouth

KEY ABBREVIATIONS

GI	Gastro-intestinal	**NG**	Naso-gastric
gtt	Drops	**NPO**	Nothing by mouth
gtt/min	Drops per minute	**oz**	Ounce
IV	Intravenous	**PEG**	Percutaneous endoscopic gastrostomy
mL	Milliliter	**TPN**	Total parenteral nutrition

Many persons cannot eat or drink because of illness, surgery, or injury. They may have chewing or swallowing problems. Aspiration is a risk. Aspiration is breathing fluid, food, vomitus, or an object into the lungs. Some persons have problems eating or refuse to eat or drink. Others cannot eat enough to meet their nutritional needs. The doctor may order nutritional support or intravenous (IV) therapy to meet food and fluid needs.

ENTERAL NUTRITION

Some persons cannot or will not ingest, chew, or swallow food. Or food cannot pass from the mouth into the esophagus and into the stomach or small intestine. Poor nutrition results. Common causes are:

- Cancer, especially cancers of the head, neck, and esophagus
- Trauma to the face, mouth, head, or neck
- Coma
- Dysphagia
- Dementia
- Eating disorders
- Nervous system disorders (Chapter 39)
- Prolonged vomiting
- Major trauma or surgery
- Acquired immunodeficiency syndrome (AIDS)
- Illnesses and disorders affecting eating and nutrition

Enteral nutrition is giving nutrients into the gastro-intestinal (GI) tract (enteral) through a feeding tube. Gavage is the process of giving a tube feeding. Tube feedings replace or supplement normal nutrition.

Types of Feeding Tubes

These feeding tubes are common:

- **Naso-gastric (NG) tube.** A feeding tube is inserted through the nose (naso) into the stomach (gastro) (Fig. 25-1). A doctor or an RN inserts the tube.
- **Naso-enteral tube.** A feeding tube is inserted through the nose (naso) into the small bowel (enteral) (Fig. 25-2). A doctor or RN inserts the tube.
- **Gastrostomy tube.** Also called a *stomach tube*, it is inserted into the stomach (Fig. 25-3). A doctor surgically creates an opening (stomy) in the stomach (gastro).
- **Jejunostomy tube.** A feeding tube inserted into a surgically created opening (stomy) in the jejunum of the small intestine (Fig. 25-4).
- **Percutaneous endoscopic gastrostomy (PEG) tube.** The doctor inserts the feeding tube with an endoscope. An endoscope is a lighted instrument (scope) used to see inside a body cavity or organ (endo). The tube is inserted through the mouth and esophagus and into the stomach. The doctor makes a small incision (stomy) through (per) the skin (cutaneous) and into the stomach (gastro). A tube is inserted into the stomach through the incision (Fig. 25-5). The endoscope allows the doctor to see correct tube placement in the stomach.

NG and naso-enteral tubes are used for short-term nutritional support—usually less than 6 weeks. Gastrostomy, jejunostomy, and PEG tubes are used for long-term nutritional support—usually longer than 6 weeks.

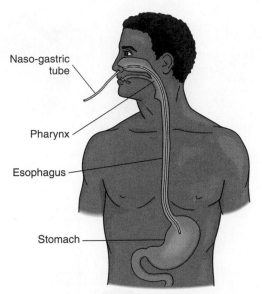

Fig. 25-1 A naso-gastric (NG) tube is inserted through the nose and esophagus and into the stomach.

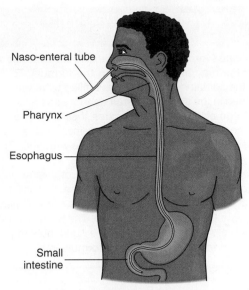

Fig. 25-2 A naso-enteral tube is inserted through the nose and into the small intestine.

Fig. 25-3 A gastrostomy tube.

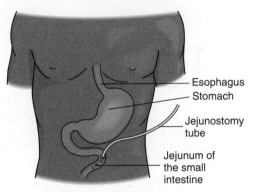

Fig. 25-4 A jejunostomy tube.

Fig. 25-5 A percutaneous endoscopic gastrostomy (PEG) tube.

TEAMWORK AND TIME MANAGEMENT

Formulas

Refrigerated formula needs to warm to room temperature. The nurse may ask you to warm the formula. To do so, place the container in a wash basin filled with warm water. If warmed in the sink, other staff cannot use the sink. They need to go elsewhere. This wastes their time and energy. Or someone may remove the container to use the sink. The container does not warm in a timely manner. That affects you, the nurse, and the resident.

The nurse and manufacturer's instructions tell you how long formula can hang. Check the time that the feeding started. Remind the nurse when the time limit is near. For example, a feeding started at 0800. The formula can hang for 8 hours. At 1530 or 1545, tell the nurse how much time is left. Also report the amount of formula left.

Fig. 25-6 A, A tube feeding is given with a syringe. **B,** Formula drips from a feeding bag into the feeding tube.

Formulas

The doctor orders the type of formula, the amount to give, and when to give tube feedings. Most formulas contain protein, carbohydrates, fat, vitamins, and minerals. Commercial formulas are common.

A nurse gives formula through the feeding tube. Formula is given at room temperature. Cold fluids can cause cramping.

Opened formula can remain at room temperature for about 8 hours. Microbes can grow in warm formula. See *Teamwork and Time Management: Formulas.*

Feeding Times

Tube feedings are given at certain times (scheduled feedings). Or they are given over a 24-hour period (continuous feedings).

Scheduled Feedings Such feedings also are called intermittent feedings. (*Intermittent* means to start, stop, and then start again.) Feeding times are scheduled. Four or more feedings are given each day. Usually 8 to 12 ounces (oz) (240 to 360 milliliters [mL]) are given over about 30 minutes. The frequency, amount, and time are like a normal eating pattern.

The nurse uses a syringe or a feeding bag (Fig. 25-6). The syringe attaches to the feeding tube. Connecting tubing connects the feeding bag to the tube. Formula is added to the syringe or to the feeding bag. Then it slowly flows through the feeding tube into the stomach.

The nurse removes the syringe or connecting tubing after the feeding. Then the nurse clamps and covers the end of the feeding tube with a cap or gauze. Gauze is secured in place with a rubber band. Clamping prevents air from entering the tube. It also prevents fluid from leaking out of the tube. Covering the end of the tube also prevents leaking.

Continuous Feedings These feedings are usually given over 24 hours. A feeding pump is used (Fig. 25-7). Formula drips into the feeding tube at a certain rate per minute. The person receives a certain amount every hour.

A pump alarm sounds if something is wrong. When you hear an alarm, tell the nurse.

Observations

Diarrhea, constipation, delayed stomach emptying, and aspiration are risks. Report the following at once:

- Nausea
- Discomfort during the feeding
- Vomiting
- Distended (enlarged and swollen) abdomen
- Coughing
- Complaints of indigestion or heartburn
- Redness, swelling, drainage, odor, or pain at the ostomy site
- Fever
- Signs and symptoms of respiratory distress (Chapter 28)
- Increased pulse rate (Chapter 31)
- Complaints of flatulence (Chapter 23)
- Diarrhea (Chapter 23)

Fig. 25-7 Feeding pump. *(From Potter PA, Perry AG: Fundamentals of nursing, ed 7, St Louis, 2009, Mosby.)*

Preventing Aspiration

Aspiration is a major risk from tube feedings. It can cause pneumonia and death. Aspiration can occur:

- *During insertion.* NG tubes and naso-enteral tubes are passed through the esophagus and then into the stomach or small intestine. The tube can slip into the airway. An x-ray is taken after insertion to check tube placement.
- *From tube movement out of place.* Coughing, sneezing, vomiting, suctioning, and poor positioning are common causes. A tube can move from the stomach or intestines into the esophagus and then into the airway. The RN checks tube placement before every scheduled tube feeding. With continuous feedings, the RN checks tube placement every 4 hours. To do so, the RN attaches a syringe to the tube. GI secretions are withdrawn through the syringe. Then the pH of the secretions is measured (Chapter 33). *You never check feeding tube placement.*
- *From regurgitation.* **Regurgitation** is the backward flow of stomach contents into the mouth. Delayed stomach emptying and over-feeding are common causes.

To help prevent regurgitation and aspiration:

- Position the person in Fowler's or semi-Fowler's position before the feeding. Follow the care plan and the nurse's directions.
- Maintain Fowler's or semi-Fowler's position after the feeding. It allows formula to move through the GI tract. The position is required for 1 to 2 hours after the feeding or at all times. Follow the care plan and the nurse's directions.
- Avoid the left side-lying position. When the person lays on the left side, the stomach cannot empty into the small intestine.

Persons with NG or gastrostomy tubes are at great risk for regurgitation. The risk is less with intestinal tubes. Formula passes directly into the small intestine. Also, formula is given at a slow rate. During digestion, food slowly passes from the stomach into the small intestine. The stomach handles larger amounts of food at one time than does the small intestine.

Digestion slows with aging. Stomach emptying also slows. Older persons are at risk for regurgitation and aspiration. Less formula and longer feeding times prevent over-feeding.

Comfort Measures

Persons with feeding tubes usually are not allowed to eat or drink. They are NPO—nothing by mouth (Chapter 24). Dry mouth, dry lips, and sore throat cause discomfort. Sometimes hard candy or gum is allowed. These measures are common:

- Oral hygiene every 2 hours while the person is awake
- Lubricant for the lips every 2 hours while the person is awake
- Mouth rinses every 2 hours while the person is awake

Feeding tubes can irritate and cause pressure on the nose. They can change the shape of the nostrils or cause pressure ulcers. These measures are common:

- Clean the nose and nostrils every 4 to 8 hours.
- Secure the tube to the nose (Fig. 25-8, p. 406). Use tape or a tube holder. Tube holders have foam cushions that prevent pressure on the nose. Re-taping is not needed. Re-taping irritates the nose. Do not use safety pins.
- Secure the tube to the person's garment at the shoulder area. This prevents the tube from pulling or dangling. Both can cause pressure on the nose. These methods are common. Follow center policy.
  - Loop a rubber band around the tube. Then pin the rubber band to the garment with a safety pin.
  - Tape the tube to the garment.

Fig. 25-8 The feeding tube is secured to the nose.

Giving Tube Feedings

You assist the nurse with tube feedings. In some states and centers, nursing assistants give tube feedings and remove NG tubes. *Remember, you never insert feeding tubes or check their placement. They are the RN's responsibility.*

See *Delegation Guidelines: Giving Tube Feedings.*

See *Promoting Safety and Comfort: Giving Tube Feedings.*

DELEGATION GUIDELINES
Giving Tube Feedings

Before giving tube feedings or removing an NG tube, make sure that:

- Your state allows you to perform the procedure.
- The procedure is in your job description.
- You have had the necessary education and training.
- You know how to use the center's equipment and supplies.
- You review the procedure in the center's procedure manual.
- You review the procedure with the nurse.
- A nurse is available to answer questions and to supervise you.
- An RN has identified and labeled all other tubes, catheters, and needles.
- An RN checks tube placement.

If the above conditions are met, you need this information from the nurse and the care plan:

- The type of tube—NG, naso-enteral, gastrostomy, PEG, or jejunostomy
- What feeding method to use—syringe, feeding bag, or feeding pump
- What size syringe to use—usually 30 or 60 mL for an adult

- How to position the person for the feeding—Fowler's or semi-Fowler's
- How to position the person after the feeding—Fowler's or semi-Fowler's
- What formula to use
- How much formula to give
- How high to raise the syringe or hang the feeding bag (usually 18 inches above the stomach or intestines)
- The amount of flushing solution to use—usually 30 to 60 mL (1 to 2 oz) of water for an adult
- How fast to give the feeding if using a syringe—usually over 30 minutes
- The flow rate if a feeding bag is used (Flow rate is the number of drops per minute. See p. 410.)
- The flow rate if a feeding pump is used
- If ice is kept around the bag for a continuous feeding
- If you are to remove an NG tube, when to remove the tube
- What observations to report and record—see p. 404
- When to report observations
- What specific resident concerns to report at once

Safety

The person may have an IV (p. 408), a breathing tube (Chapter 29), and drainage tubes (Chapter 35). You must know the purpose of each tube. Ask the nurse to label each tube to identify its purpose. *Formula must enter only the feeding tube.* Otherwise, the person can die.

Before giving a tube feeding, always:

- Turn on the light if the room is dark. Do so even if the person is sleeping.
- Check and inspect the feeding tube and label with the nurse.
- Make sure an RN checks for tube placement.
- Make sure every tube, catheter, and needle is labeled.
- Trace the feeding tube back to the insertion site. Start at the end of the feeding tube. Trace the tube backward. For example, if the person has an NG tube, you will end at the nose. If the person has a gastrostomy tube, you will end at the abdomen. *If you do not end at the correct place, do not give the tube feeding. Call for the nurse.*

Nasal secretions may contain blood or microbes. So can drainage at an ostomy site. Wear gloves. Follow Standard Precautions and the Bloodborne Pathogen Standard.

Remind visitors to call for a nurse if any tube becomes disconnected. They could connect the wrong tubes together.

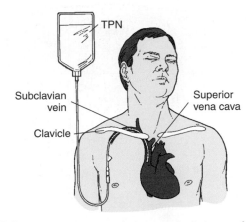

Fig. 25-9 Parenteral nutrition. *(From* Mosby's dictionary of medicine, nursing, and health professions, *ed 8, St Louis, 2009, Mosby.)*

PARENTERAL NUTRITION

Parenteral nutrition is giving nutrients through a catheter inserted into a vein (Fig. 25-9). (*Para* means beyond. *Enteral* relates to the bowel). A nutrient solution is given directly into the bloodstream. Nutrients do not enter the GI tract. Parenteral nutrition is often called *total parenteral nutrition (TPN)* or *hyperalimentation.* (*Hyper* means high or *excessive. Alimentation* means *nourishment.*)

The solution contains water, proteins, carbohydrates, vitamins, and minerals. It drips through a catheter inserted into a large vein (p. 408). TPN is used when the person cannot receive oral or enteral feedings. Or it is used when oral or enteral feedings are not enough to meet the person's needs.

Common reasons for TPN include:

- Disease, injury, or surgery to the GI tract
- Severe trauma, infection, or burns
- Being NPO for more than 5 to 7 days
- GI side effects from cancer treatments (Chapter 38)
- Prolonged coma
- Prolonged anorexia (loss of appetite)

Observations

TPN risks include infection, fluid imbalances, and blood sugar imbalances. Report these signs and symptoms to the nurse at once:

- Fever, chills, and other signs and symptoms of infection (Chapter 15)
- Signs and symptoms of sugar imbalances (see "Diabetes" in Chapter 41)
- Chest pain
- Difficulty breathing or shortness of breath
- Cough
- Nausea and vomiting
- Diarrhea
- Thirst
- Rapid heart rate or an irregular heartbeat
- Weakness or fatigue
- Sweating
- Pallor (pale skin)
- Trembling
- Confusion or behavior changes

Assisting With TPN

The nurse is responsible for all aspects of TPN. You assist by carefully observing the person. You also assist with the person's basic needs and activities of daily living. Persons receiving TPN may be NPO. Provide frequent oral hygiene, lubricant to the lips, and mouth rinses as the nurse and care plan direct (p. 405). Also follow other aspects of the person's care plan.

Many aspects of IV therapy apply to TPN. See p. 408.

IV bag

Drip chamber

IV tube

Clamp

IV catheter

Fig. 25-10 Equipment for IV therapy.

IV THERAPY

Intravenous (IV) therapy is giving fluids through a needle or catheter inserted into a vein (Fig. 25-10). Fluid flows directly into the bloodstream. *IV* and *IV infusion* also refer to IV therapy. Doctors order IV therapy to:

- Provide fluids when they cannot be taken by mouth
- Replace minerals and vitamins lost because of illness or injury
- Provide sugar for energy
- Give drugs and blood

RNs are responsible for IV therapy. They start and maintain the infusion according to the doctor's orders. RNs also give IV drugs and administer blood. State laws vary about the role of LPNs/LVNs and nursing assistants in IV therapy.

IV Sites

Peripheral and central venous sites are used. Peripheral means around *(peri)* a boundary *(pheral)*. The boundary is the center of the body near the heart. *Peripheral IV sites* are away from the center of the body. For adults, the back of the hand and inner forearm are useful sites (Fig. 25-11).

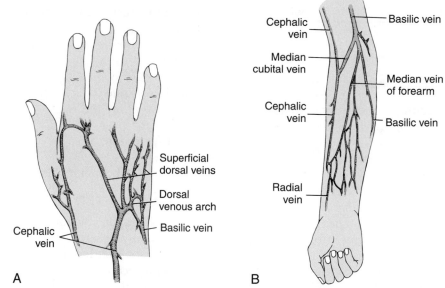

Superficial dorsal veins

Dorsal venous arch

Cephalic vein

Basilic vein

Cephalic vein

Median cubital vein

Cephalic vein

Radial vein

Basilic vein

Median vein of forearm

Basilic vein

A

B

Fig. 25-11 Peripheral IV sites. **A,** Back of the hand. **B,** Inner forearm. *(From Potter PA, Perry AG: Fundamentals of nursing, ed 7, St Louis, 2009, Mosby.)*

The subclavian vein and the internal jugular vein are *central venous sites.* They are close to the heart. A catheter is threaded into the right atrium or superior vena cava (Fig. 25-12, *A* and *B*). The catheter is called a *central venous catheter* or a *central line.* The cephalic and basilic veins in the arm also are used. Catheters inserted into these sites are called *peripherally inserted central catheters (PICCs).* The catheter is threaded into the subclavian vein or the superior vena cava (Fig. 25-12, *C*).

Central venous sites are used:

- For parenteral nutrition
- To give large amounts of fluid
- For long-term IV therapy
- To give drugs that irritate peripheral veins

IV Equipment

The basic equipment used in IV therapy is shown in Figure 25-10:

- The solution container is a plastic bag. It is called the *IV bag.*
- A *catheter* or *needle* is inserted into a vein (Fig. 25-13).
- The *IV tube* or *infusion tubing* connects the IV bag to the catheter or needle. Fluid drips from the bag into the *drip chamber.* The *clamp* is used to regulate the flow rate.
- The IV bag hangs from an IV pole (IV standard) or ceiling hook.

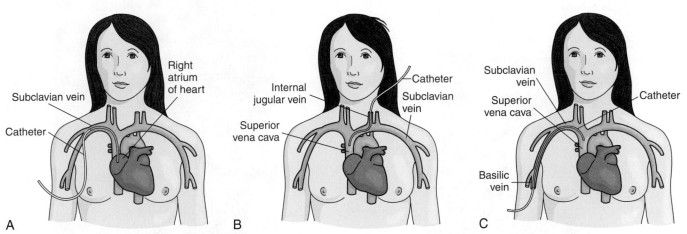

Fig. 25-12 Central venous sites. **A,** Subclavian vein. The catheter tip is in the right atrium. **B,** Internal jugular vein. The catheter tip is in the superior vena cava. **C,** Basilic vein. This is a peripherally inserted central catheter (PICC).

Fig. 25-13 A, Intravenous catheter. **B,** Butterfly needle.

Flow Rate

The doctor orders the amount of fluid to give (infuse) and the amount of time to give it in. With this information, the RN figures the flow rate. The **flow rate** is the number of drops per minute *(gtt/min)*. The abbreviation *gtt* means drops. The Latin word *guttae* means drops.

The RN sets the clamp for the flow rate. Or an electronic pump is used to control the flow rate (Fig. 25-14). An alarm sounds if something is wrong. Tell the nurse at once if you hear an alarm. *Never change the position of the clamp or adjust any controls on IV pumps.*

You can check the flow rate. The RN tells you the number of drops per minute (gtt/min). To check the flow rate, count the number of drops in 1 minute (Fig. 25-15). Tell the RN at once if:

- No fluid is dripping.
- The rate is too fast.
- The rate is too slow.

The time tape shows how much fluid to give over a period of time (Fig. 25-16). For example, the doctor orders 1000 mL of fluid over 8 hours. The RN marks the tape in 8 one-hour intervals. To check if the infusion is on time, compare the fluid line with the time line on the tape. If the fluid line is above or below the time line, the flow rate is too slow or too fast. Tell the RN at once if too much or too little fluid was given.

See *Promoting Safety and Comfort: Flow Rate.*

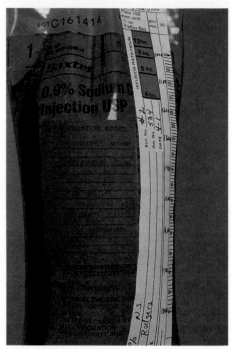

Fig. 25-16 Time tape applied to an IV bag. *(From Elkin MK, Perry AG, Potter PA: Nursing interventions and clinical skills, ed 4, St Louis, 2007, Mosby.)*

Fig. 25-14 Electronic IV pump. *(Courtesy Baxter Healthcare Corp., Round Lake, Ill.)*

Fig. 25-15 The flow rate is checked by counting the number of drops per minute.

PROMOTING SAFETY AND COMFORT
Flow Rate

Safety

The person can suffer serious harm if the flow rate is too fast or too slow. The flow rate can change from position changes. Kinked tubes and lying on the tube also affect the flow rate.

Never change the position of the clamp or adjust any controls on infusion pumps. Tell the nurse at once if there is a problem with the flow rate.

Assisting With IV Therapy

You help meet the safety, hygiene, and activity needs of persons with IVs. Follow the safety measures in Box 25-1. Report any of the signs and symptoms listed in Box 25-2, p. 412 at once.

Your state and center may allow you to change dressings at peripheral IV sites. They also may let you discontinue a peripheral IV.

You never start or maintain IV therapy. Nor do you regulate the flow rate or change IV bags. You never give blood or IV drugs.

See *Teamwork and Time Management: Assisting With IV Therapy*, p. 412.

See *Delegation Guidelines: Assisting With IV Therapy*, p. 412.

Box 25-1   Safety Measures for IV Therapy

- Follow Standard Precautions and the Bloodborne Pathogen Standard.
- Do not move the needle or catheter. Needle or catheter position must be maintained. If the needle or catheter is moved, it may come out of the vein. Then fluid flows into tissues (infiltration). Or the flow stops.
- Follow the safety measures for restraints (Chapter 14). The nurse may splint or restrain the extremity to prevent movement (Fig. 25-17). Or the nurse may apply a protective device (Fig. 25-18). This helps prevent the needle or catheter from moving.
- Protect the IV bag, tubing, and needle or catheter when the person walks. Portable IV standards are rolled along next to the person (Fig. 25-19).
- Assist the person with turning and re-positioning. Move the IV bag to the side of the bed on which the person is lying. Always allow enough slack in the tubing. The needle or catheter can move from pressure on the tube.
- Tell the nurse at once if bleeding occurs from the insertion site. Follow Standard Precautions and the Bloodborne Pathogen Standard.
- Tell the nurse at once of any signs and symptoms listed in Box 25-2.

Fig. 25-18 I.V. House protective device. *(Courtesy I.V. House, St Louis, Mo.)*

Fig. 25-19 A person walking with an IV.

Fig. 25-17 An armboard prevents movement at an IV site. *(From Elkin MK, Perry AG, Potter PA:* Nursing interventions and clinical skills, *ed 4, St Louis, 2007, Mosby.)*

Box 25-2   Signs and Symptoms of IV Therapy Complications

Local—At the IV Site
- Bleeding
- Puffiness, swelling, or leaking fluid
- Pale or reddened skin
- Complaints of pain at or above the IV site
- Hot or cold skin near the site

Systemic—Involving the Whole Body
- Fever
- Itching
- Drop in blood pressure
- Pulse rate greater than 100 beats per minute
- Irregular pulse
- Cyanosis
- Confusion or changes in mental function
- Loss of consciousness
- Difficulty breathing
- Shortness of breath
- Decreasing or no urine output
- Chest pain
- Nausea

TEAMWORK AND TIME MANAGEMENT
Assisting With IV Therapy

If a person's care is part of your assignment, you must know the IV flow rate. When you are with the person, always check the flow rate. Report any problems to the nurse at once.

Also check the amount of fluid in the bag. Tell the nurse at once if the bag is empty or almost empty.

Residents cared for by other staff may have IVs. When you are near the person or walking past the person's room, always make sure the IV is dripping. Also check the amount of fluid in the bag. Report any problems to a nurse at once.

DELEGATION GUIDELINES
Assisting With IV Therapy

Before changing a peripheral IV dressing or discontinuing a peripheral IV, make sure that:
- Your state lets nursing assistants perform the procedure.
- The procedure is in your job description.
- You have the necessary education and training.
- You know how to use the center's supplies and equipment.
- You review the procedure in the center's procedure manual.
- You review the procedure with the nurse.
- A nurse is available to answer questions and to supervise you.
- An RN has identified and labeled all other tubes, catheters, and needles.

If the above conditions are met, you need this information from the nurse and the care plan:
- When to change the IV dressing
- If the person has an IV needle or catheter
- When to discontinue the IV
- If the person has more than one IV, which IV to discontinue
- What supplies to use
- What observations to report and record (see Box 25-2)
- When to report observations
- What specific resident concerns to report at once

QUALITY OF LIFE

Persons needing nutritional support or IV therapy are often very ill. Their care needs may be great and take a lot of time. Do not take short cuts or omit care. Doing so is unethical. It could also cause great harm. At all times, you must give quality care and protect the person's rights.

Sometimes decisions are made to stop nutritional support or IV therapy. The person is allowed to die. The person may make the decision. Or the family does so after talking to the doctor. (See Chapter 48.) You may agree or disagree with such choices. The choice may or may not be within your religious or cultural beliefs and values. The person's or family's wishes and doctor's orders must be followed. The person must receive quality care. Talk to the nurse if you have problems with the decision. The nurse may need to change your assignment.

REVIEW QUESTIONS

Circle the BEST answer.

1 Enteral nutrition
   a Requires an NG tube
   b Is given into a central venous site
   c Is given into the GI tract
   d Requires an IV

2 The process of giving a tube feeding is called
   a Gavage
   b Parenteral nutrition
   c Aspiration
   d Regurgitation

3 For a tube feeding, the person is positioned in
   a Fowler's or semi-Fowler's position
   b The left side-lying position
   c The right side-lying position
   d The supine position

4 Formula for a tube feeding is given
   a At body temperature
   b At room temperature
   c Hot
   d Cold

5 Continuous feedings are given with a
   a Syringe
   b Feeding bag
   c PEG tube
   d Feeding pump

6 The nurse checks feeding tube placement to prevent
   a Aspiration
   b Regurgitation
   c Over-feeding
   d Cramping

7 Which position prevents regurgitation after a tube feeding?
   a Fowler's or semi-Fowler's position
   b The supine position
   c The left or right side-lying position
   d The prone position

8 The risk of regurgitation is the greatest with
   a NG and gastrostomy tubes
   b A PEG tube
   c Naso-enteral tubes
   d A jejunostomy tube

9 A person with a feeding tube is NPO. You should do the following *except*
   a Give the person hard candy or gum
   b Provide oral hygiene
   c Provide mouth rinses
   d Apply lubricant to the lips

10 A person has an NG tube. The care plan includes the following measures to prevent nasal irritation. Which measure should you question?
   a Clean the nose and nostrils every 4 hours.
   b Tape the tube to the nose.
   c Remove the tube every 4 hours.
   d Secure the tube to the person's gown.

11 A nurse asks you to give a tube feeding. The procedure is not in your job description. What should you do?
   a Refuse to perform the task.
   b Give the tube feeding.
   c Tell the director of nursing.
   d Ask another nurse what you should do.

12 A person is receiving TPN. The person complains of chest pain and difficulty breathing. What should you do?
   a Position the person in Fowler's position.
   b Call for the nurse.
   c Stop the TPN.
   d Provide oral hygiene.

13 A person is receiving TPN. You know that TPN
   a Involves a nutrient solution
   b Is given through a feeding tube
   c Can cause pressure ulcers on the nose
   d Requires that the person be NPO

14 Which is a peripheral IV site?
   a Subclavian vein
   b Superior vena cava
   c Jugular vein
   d A vein on the back of the hand

15 A nurse asks you to check an IV flow rate. What should you do?
   a Count the drops in 30 seconds; multiply the number by 2.
   b Count the drops for 1 minute.
   c Check if the fluid is dripping too fast or slow.
   d Measure the amount of fluid.

16 The IV flow rate is
   a The number of gtt/mL
   b The number of gtt/min
   c The amount of fluid given in 1 hour
   d The amount of fluid in the IV bag

17 You note that an IV bag is almost empty. What should you do?
   a Clamp the IV tubing.
   b Tell the nurse.
   c Discontinue the IV.
   d Adjust the flow rate.

18 You note bleeding from an IV insertion site. What should you do?
   a Tell the nurse.
   b Move the needle or catheter.
   c Discontinue the IV.
   d Clamp the IV tubing.

Answers to these questions are on p. 720.

Exercise and Activity

OBJECTIVES

- Define the key terms and key abbreviations listed in this chapter.
- Describe bedrest.
- Explain how to prevent the complications from bedrest.
- Describe the devices used to support and maintain body alignment.

- Explain the purpose of a trapeze.
- Describe range-of-motion exercises.
- Describe four walking aids.
- Perform the procedures described in this chapter.
- Explain how to promote quality of life.

KEY TERMS

abduction Moving a body part away from the midline of the body

adduction Moving a body part toward the midline of the body

ambulation The act of walking

atrophy The decrease in size or the wasting away of tissue

contracture The lack of joint mobility caused by abnormal shortening of a muscle

deconditioning The loss of muscle strength from inactivity

dorsiflexion Bending the toes and foot up at the ankle

extension Straightening a body part

external rotation Turning the joint outward

flexion Bending a body part

footdrop The foot falls down at the ankle; permanent plantar flexion

hyperextension Excessive straightening of a body part

internal rotation Turning the joint inward

orthostatic hypotension Abnormally low *(hypo)* blood pressure when the person suddenly stands up *(ortho* and *static);* postural hypotension

plantar flexion The foot *(plantar)* is bent *(flexion);* bending the foot down at the ankle

postural hypotension See "orthostatic hypotension"

pronation Turning the joint downward

range of motion (ROM) The movement of a joint to the extent possible without causing pain

rotation Turning the joint

supination Turning the joint upward

syncope A brief loss of consciousness; fainting

KEY ABBREVIATIONS

ADL	Activities of daily living	**OBRA**	Omnibus Budget Reconciliation Act of 1987
CMS	Centers for Medicare & Medicaid Services	**PT**	Physical therapist
ID	Identification	**ROM**	Range of motion

Being active is important for physical and mental well-being. Most people move about and function without help. Illness, surgery, injury, pain, and aging cause weakness and some activity limits. Some people are in bed for a long time. Some are paralyzed. Some disorders worsen over time. They cause decreases in activity. Examples include arthritis and nervous system and muscular disorders (Chapter 39). Inactivity, whether mild or severe, affects every body system. It also affects mental well-being.

Deconditioning is the loss of muscle strength from inactivity. When not active, older persons become deconditioned quickly. Nurses use the nursing process to promote exercise and activity in all persons to the extent possible. The care plan and your assignment sheet include the person's activity level and needed exercises.

See *Residents With Dementia: Exercise and Activity*.

BEDREST

The doctor orders bedrest to treat a health problem. It may be a nursing measure if the person's condition changes. Generally bedrest is ordered to:

- Reduce physical activity
- Reduce pain
- Encourage rest
- Regain strength
- Promote healing

These types of bedrest are common:

- *Strict bedrest.* Everything is done for the person. No activities of daily living (ADL) are allowed.
- *Bedrest.* Some ADL are allowed. Self-feeding, oral hygiene, bathing, shaving, and hair care are often allowed.
- *Bedrest with commode privileges.* The person uses the commode for elimination.
- *Bedrest with bathroom privileges (bedrest with BRP).* The person uses the bathroom for elimination.

The person's care plan and your assignment sheet tell you the activities allowed. Always ask the nurse what bedrest means for each person. Check with the nurse if you have questions about a person's activity limits.

RESIDENTS WITH DEMENTIA
Exercise and Activity

Persons with dementia may resist exercise and activity. They do not understand what is happening and may fear harm. They may become agitated and combative. Some cry out for help. Do not force the person to exercise or take part in activities. Stay calm, and ask the nurse for help. Follow the care plan.

Complications From Bedrest

Bedrest and lack of exercise and activity can cause serious complications. Every system is affected. Pressure ulcers, constipation, and fecal impaction can result. Urinary tract infections and renal calculi (kidney stones) can occur. So can blood clots (thrombi) and pneumonia (inflammation and infection of the lung).

The musculo-skeletal system is affected by lack of exercise and activity. These complications must be prevented to maintain normal movement:

- A contracture is the lack of joint mobility caused by abnormal shortening of a muscle. The contracted muscle is fixed into position, is deformed, and cannot stretch (Fig. 26-1, p. 416). Common sites are the fingers, wrists, elbows, toes, ankles, knees, and hips. They can also occur in the neck and spine. The person is permanently deformed and disabled.
- Atrophy is the decrease in size or the wasting away of tissue. Tissues shrink in size. Muscle atrophy is a decrease in size or a wasting away of muscle (Fig. 26-2, p. 416).

Orthostatic hypotension and blood clots (Chapter 35) occur in the circulatory system. Orthostatic hypotension is abnormally low *(hypo)* blood pressure when the person suddenly stands up *(ortho* and *static)*. When a person moves from lying or sitting to a standing position, the blood pressure drops. The person is dizzy and weak and has spots before the eyes. Syncope can occur. Syncope (fainting) is a brief loss of consciousness. (Syncope comes from the Greek word *synkoptein*. It means to cut short.) Orthostatic hypotension also is called **postural hypotension**. (*Postural* relates to posture or standing.) Box 26-1 lists the measures that prevent orthostatic hypotension. Slowly changing positions is key.

Good nursing care prevents complications from bedrest. Good alignment, range-of-motion exercises (p. 419), and frequent position changes are important measures. These are part of the care plan.

See *Focus on Communication: Complications of Bedrest.*

Fig. 26-1 A contracture.

Fig. 26-2 Muscle atrophy.

FOCUS ON COMMUNICATION
Complications of Bedrest

Orthostatic hypotension can occur when the person moves from lying to sitting or standing. Fainting is a risk. To check for orthostatic hypotension, ask these questions:
- "Do you feel weak?"
- "Do you feel dizzy?"
- "Do you see spots before your eyes?"
- "Do you feel like fainting?"

Box 26-1   Preventing Orthostatic Hypotension

- Measure blood pressure, pulse, and respirations with the person supine.
- Position the person in Fowler's position. Raise the head of the bed slowly.
  - Ask the person about weakness, dizziness, or spots before the eyes. Lower the head of the bed if symptoms occur.
  - Measure blood pressure, pulse, and respirations.
  - Keep the person in Fowler's position for a short while. Ask about weakness, dizziness, or spots before the eyes.
- Help the person sit on the side of the bed (Chapter 17).
  - Ask about weakness, dizziness, or spots before the eyes. Help the person to Fowler's position if symptoms occur.
  - Measure blood pressure, pulse, and respirations.
  - Have the person sit on the side of the bed for a short while.
- Help the person stand.
  - Ask about weakness, dizziness, or spots before the eyes. Help the person sit on the side of the bed if any symptoms occur.
  - Measure blood pressure, pulse, and respirations.
- Help the person sit in a chair or walk as directed by the nurse.
  - Ask about weakness, dizziness, or spots before the eyes. If the person is walking, help the person to sit if symptoms occur.
  - Measure blood pressure, pulse, and respirations.
- Report blood pressure, pulse, and respirations to the nurse. Also report other symptoms or complaints.

Positioning

Body alignment and positioning were discussed in Chapter 16. Supportive devices are often used to support and maintain the person in a certain position:

- *Bed-boards*—are placed under the mattress. They prevent the mattress from sagging (Fig. 26-3). Usually made of plywood, they are covered with canvas or other material. There are two sections so the head of the bed can be raised. One section is for the head of the bed. The other is for the foot of the bed.
- *Foot-boards*—are placed at the foot of mattresses (Fig. 26-4). They prevent plantar flexion that can lead to footdrop. In **plantar flexion,** the foot (*plantar*) is bent (*flexion*). **Footdrop** is when the foot falls down at the ankle (permanent plantar flexion). The foot-board is placed so the soles of the feet are flush against it. The feet are in good alignment as when standing. Foot-boards also serve as bed cradles. They prevent pressure ulcers by keeping top linens off the feet and toes.
- *Trochanter rolls*—prevent the hips and legs from turning outward (external rotation) (Fig. 26-5). A bath blanket is folded to the desired length and rolled up. The loose end is placed under the person from the hip to the knee. Then the roll is tucked alongside the body. Pillows or sandbags also keep the hips and knees in alignment.
- *Hip abduction wedges*—keep the hips abducted (apart) (Fig. 26-6). The wedge is placed between the person's legs. These are common after hip replacement surgery.
- *Hand rolls or hand grips*—prevent contractures of the thumb, fingers, and wrist (Fig. 26-7, p. 418). Foam rubber sponges, rubber balls, and finger cushions (Fig. 26-8, p. 418) also are used.
- *Splints*—keep the elbows, wrists, thumbs, fingers, ankles, and knees in normal position. They are usually secured in place with Velcro (Fig. 26-9, p. 418).
- *Bed cradles*—keep the weight of top linens off the feet and toes (Fig. 26-10, p. 418). The weight of top linens can cause footdrop and pressure ulcers.

Fig. 26-4 A foot-board. Feet are flush with the board to keep them in normal alignment.

Fig. 26-5 A trochanter roll is made from a bath blanket. It extends from the hip to the knee.

Fig. 26-3 Bed-boards. **A,** Mattress sagging without bed-boards. **B,** Bed-boards are under the mattress. No sagging occurs.

Fig. 26-6 Hip abduction wedge.

Fig. 26-7 Hand grip. *(Image courtesy J. T. Posey Co., Arcadia, Calif.)*

Fig. 26-8 Finger cushion. *(Image courtesy J. T. Posey Co., Arcadia, Calif.)*

Fig. 26-9 A splint.

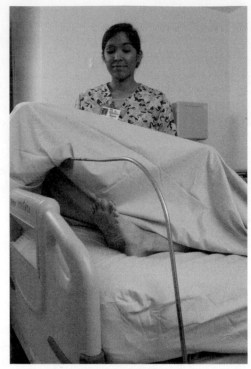

Fig. 26-10 A bed cradle.

Fig. 26-11 A trapeze is used to strengthen arm muscles.

Exercise

Exercise helps prevent contractures, muscle atrophy, and other complications from bedrest. Some exercise occurs with ADL and when turning and moving in bed without help. Other exercises are needed for muscles and joints. (See "Range-of-Motion Exercises" and "Ambulation," p. 424.)

A trapeze is used for exercises to strengthen arm muscles. The trapeze hangs from an overbed frame (Fig. 26-11). The person grasps the bar with both hands to lift the trunk off the bed. The trapeze is also used to move up and turn in bed.

See *Focus on Rehabilitation: Exercise.*

FOCUS ON REHABILITATION
Exercise

The person works closely with physical and occupational therapists to improve strength and endurance. Care plan goals for exercise and ambulation (p. 424) may change daily. The goal may be to improve the person's independence so he or she can go home. Or the goal may be to attain the highest level of function possible. The health team works with the person to meet rehabilitation goals. Follow the care plan carefully.

🏊 RANGE-OF-MOTION EXERCISES

The movement of a joint to the extent possible without causing pain is the **range of motion (ROM)** of that joint. Range-of-motion exercises involve moving the joints through their complete range of motion (Box 26-2). They are usually done at least 2 times a day.

* *Active* range-of-motion exercises—are done by the person himself or herself.
* *Passive* range-of-motion exercises—you move the joints through their range of motion.
* *Active-assistive* range-of-motion exercises—the person does the exercises with some help.

Bathing, hair care, eating, reaching, dressing and undressing, and walking all involve joint movements. Persons on bedrest need more frequent ROM exercises. So do those who cannot walk, turn, or transfer themselves because of illness or injury. The doctor or nurse may order ROM exercises.

The Omnibus Budget Reconciliation Act of 1987 (OBRA) and the Centers for Medicare & Medicaid Services (CMS) require an assessment and care planning process focused on a person's ROM. The intent is that the person reach or maintain his or her highest level of ROM. Or the focus is on preventing a decline in ROM. The goal may be one of the following:

* Prevent loss in range of motion
* Increase range of motion
* Prevent further decrease in range of motion

During a survey, CMS surveyors may observe you performing ROM exercises.

See *Focus on Communication: Range-of-Motion Exercises.*

See *Delegation Guidelines: Range-of-Motion Exercises.*

See *Promoting Safety and Comfort: Range-of-Motion Exercises,* p. 420.

Box 26-2 Joint Movements

Abduction—moving a body part away from the midline of the body
Adduction—moving a body part toward the midline of the body
Extension—straightening a body part
Flexion—bending a body part
Hyperextension—excessive straightening of a body part
Dorsiflexion—bending the toes and foot up at the ankle
Rotation—turning the joint
Internal rotation—turning the joint inward
External rotation—turning the joint outward
Plantar flexion—bending the foot down at the ankle
Pronation—turning the joint downward
Supination—turning the joint upward

FOCUS ON COMMUNICATION
Range-of-Motion Exercises

You must not force a joint beyond its present ROM or to the point of pain. Ask the person to tell you if he or she:
* Feels that the joint cannot move any farther
* Feels pain or discomfort in the joint

DELEGATION GUIDELINES
Range-of-Motion Exercises

When delegated ROM exercises, you need this information from the nurse and the care plan:
* The kind of ROM ordered—active, passive, active-assistive
* Which joints to exercise
* How often the exercises are done
* How many times to repeat each exercise
* What observations to report and record:
  * The time the exercises were performed
  * The joints exercised
  * The number of times the exercises were performed on each joint
  * Complaints of pain or signs of stiffness or spasm
  * The degree to which the person took part in the exercises
* When to report observations
* What specific resident concerns to report at once

PROMOTING SAFETY AND COMFORT
Range-of-Motion Exercises

Safety
Range-of-motion exercises can cause injury if not done properly. Muscle strain, joint injury, and pain are possible. Practice the rules in Box 26-3 when performing or assisting with ROM exercises.

ROM exercises to the neck can cause serious injury if not done properly. Some centers require that nursing assistants have special training before doing such exercises. Other centers do not let nursing assistants do them. Know your center's policy. *Perform ROM exercises to the neck only if allowed by your center and if the nurse instructs you to do so.*

Comfort
To promote physical comfort during ROM exercises, follow the rules in Box 26-3. Also cover the person with a bath blanket. Expose only the part being exercised. Providing for privacy promotes physical and mental comfort.

Box 26-3   Performing Range-of-Motion Exercises

- Exercise only the joints the nurse tells you to exercise.
- Expose only the body part being exercised.
- Use good body mechanics.
- Support the part being exercised.
- Move the joint slowly, smoothly, and gently.
- Do not force a joint beyond its present range of motion.
- Do not force a joint to the point of pain.
- Ask the person if he or she has pain or discomfort.
- *Perform range-of-motion exercises to the neck only if allowed by center policy.* In some centers, only physical or occupational therapists do neck exercises. This is because of the danger of neck injuries.

Flexion   Extension   Hyperextension   Rotation   Lateral flexion

Fig. 26-12 Range-of-motion exercises for the neck.

Flexion   Abduction   Adduction   External rotation   Internal rotation   Extension   Hyperextension

Fig. 26-13 Range-of-motion exercises for the shoulder.

Flexion   Extension

Fig. 26-14 Range-of-motion exercises for the elbow.

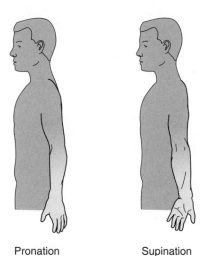

Pronation   Supination

Fig. 26-15 Range-of-motion exercises for the forearm.

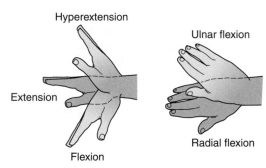

Hyperextension   Ulnar flexion   Extension   Flexion   Radial flexion

Fig. 26-16 Range-of-motion exercises for the wrist.

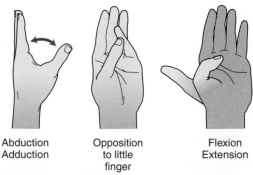

Abduction Adduction   Opposition to little finger   Flexion Extension

Fig. 26-17 Range-of-motion exercises for the thumb.

QUALITY OF LIFE

Remember to:
- Knock before entering the person's room.
- Address the person by name.
- Introduce yourself by name and title.

- Explain the procedure to the person before beginning and during the procedure.
- Protect the person's rights during the procedure.
- Handle the person gently during the procedure.

PRE-PROCEDURE

1 Follow *Delegation Guidelines: Range-of-Motion Exercises*, p. 419. See *Promoting Safety and Comfort: Range-of-Motion Exercises.*
2 Practice hand hygiene.
3 Identify the person. Check the ID (identification) bracelet against the assignment sheet. Also call the person by name.

4 Obtain a bath blanket.
5 Provide for privacy.
6 Raise the bed for body mechanics. Bed rails are up if used.

PROCEDURE

7 Lower the bed rail near you if up.
8 Position the person supine.
9 Cover the person with a bath blanket. Fan-fold top linens to the foot of the bed.
10 Exercise the neck *if allowed by your center and if the nurse instructs you to do so* (Fig. 26-12):
  a Place your hands over the person's ears to support the head. Support the jaws with your fingers.
  b Flexion—bring the head forward. The chin touches the chest.
  c Extension—straighten the head.
  d Hyperextension—bring the head backward until the chin points up.
  e Rotation—turn the head from side to side.
  f Lateral flexion—move the head to the right and to the left.
  g Repeat flexion, extension, hyperextension, rotation, and lateral flexion 5 times—or the number of times stated on the care plan.
11 Exercise the shoulder (Fig. 26-13):
  a Grasp the wrist with one hand. Grasp the elbow with the other hand.
  b Flexion—raise the arm straight in front and over the head.
  c Extension—bring the arm down to the side.
  d Hyperextension—move the arm behind the body. (Do this if the person sits in a straight-backed chair or is standing.)
  e Abduction—move the straight arm away from the side of the body.
  f Adduction—move the straight arm to the side of the body.
  g Internal rotation—bend the elbow. Place it at the same level as the shoulder. Move the forearm down toward the body.
  h External rotation—move the forearm toward the head.
  i Repeat flexion, extension, hyperextension, abduction, adduction, and internal and external rotation 5 times—or the number of times stated on the care plan.

12 Exercise the elbow (Fig. 26-14):
  a Grasp the person's wrist with one hand. Grasp the elbow with your other hand.
  b Flexion—bend the arm so the same-side shoulder is touched.
  c Extension—straighten the arm.
  d Repeat flexion and extension 5 times—or the number of times stated on the care plan.
13 Exercise the forearm (Fig. 26-15):
  a Continue to support the wrist and elbow.
  b Pronation—turn the hand so the palm is down.
  c Supination—turn the hand so the palm is up.
  d Repeat pronation and supination 5 times—or the number of times stated on the care plan.
14 Exercise the wrist (Fig. 26-16):
  a Hold the wrist with both of your hands.
  b Flexion—bend the hand down.
  c Extension—straighten the hand.
  d Hyperextension—bend the hand back.
  e Radial flexion—turn the hand toward the thumb.
  f Ulnar flexion—turn the hand toward the little finger.
  g Repeat flexion, extension, hyperextension, radial flexion, and ulnar flexion 5 times—or the number of times stated on the care plan.
15 Exercise the thumb (Fig. 26-17):
  a Hold the person's hand with one hand. Hold the thumb with your other hand.
  b Abduction—move the thumb out from the inner part of the index finger.
  c Adduction—move the thumb back next to the index finger.
  d Opposition—touch each fingertip with the thumb.
  e Flexion—bend the thumb into the hand.
  f Extension—move the thumb out to the side of the fingers.
  g Repeat abduction, adduction, opposition, flexion, and extension 5 times—or the number of times stated on the care plan.

Continued

PERFORMING RANGE-OF-MOTION EXERCISES—cont'd

PROCEDURE—cont'd

16 Exercise the fingers (Fig. 26-18):
   a Abduction—spread the fingers and the thumb apart.
   b Adduction—bring the fingers and thumb together.
   c Flexion—make a fist.
   d Extension—straighten the fingers so the fingers, hand, and arm are straight.
   e Repeat abduction, adduction, flexion, and extension 5 times—or the number of times stated on the care plan.

17 Exercise the hip (Fig. 26-19):
   a Support the leg. Place one hand under the knee. Place your other hand under the ankle.
   b Flexion—raise the leg.
   c Extension—straighten the leg.
   d Abduction—move the leg away from the body.
   e Adduction—move the leg toward the other leg.
   f Internal rotation—turn the leg inward.
   g External rotation—turn the leg outward.
   h Repeat flexion, extension, abduction, adduction, and internal and external rotation 5 times—or the number of times stated on the care plan.

18 Exercise the knee (Fig. 26-20):
   a Support the knee. Place one hand under the knee. Place your other hand under the ankle.
   b Flexion—bend the knee.
   c Extension—straighten the knee.
   d Repeat flexion and extension of the knee 5 times—or the number of times stated on the care plan.

19 Exercise the ankle (Fig. 26-21):
   a Support the foot and ankle. Place one hand under the foot. Place your other hand under the ankle.
   b Dorsiflexion—pull the foot upward. Push down on the heel at the same time.
   c Plantar flexion—turn the foot down. Or point the toes.
   d Repeat dorsiflexion and plantar flexion 5 times—or the number of times stated on the care plan.

20 Exercise the foot (Fig. 26-22):
   a Continue to support the foot and ankle.
   b Pronation—turn the outside of the foot up and the inside down.
   c Supination—turn the inside of the foot up and the outside down.
   d Repeat pronation and supination 5 times—or the number of times stated on the care plan.

21 Exercise the toes (Fig. 26-23):
   a Flexion—curl the toes.
   b Extension—straighten the toes.
   c Abduction—spread the toes apart.
   d Adduction—pull the toes together.
   e Repeat flexion, extension, abduction, and adduction 5 times—or the number of times stated on the care plan.

22 Cover the leg. Raise the bed rail if used.
23 Go to the other side. Lower the bed rail near you if up.
24 Repeat steps 11 through 21.

POST-PROCEDURE

25 Provide for comfort. (See the inside of the front book cover.)
26 Remove the bath blanket.
27 Place the signal light within reach.
28 Lower the bed to its lowest level.
29 Raise or lower bed rails. Follow the care plan.

30 Fold and return the bath blanket to its proper place.
31 Unscreen the person.
32 Complete a safety check of the room. (See the inside of the front book cover.)
33 Decontaminate your hands.
34 Report and record your observations.

Abduction

Adduction

Flexion

Extension

Fig. 26-18 Range-of-motion exercises for the fingers.

Flexion

Extension   Abduction   Adduction

Internal rotation

External rotation

Fig. 26-19 Range-of-motion exercises for the hip.

Flexion

Extension

Fig. 26-20 Range-of-motion exercises for the knee.

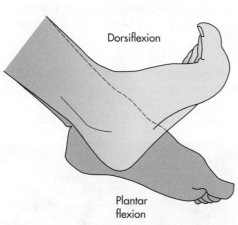

Dorsiflexion

Plantar flexion

Fig. 26-21 Range-of-motion exercises for the ankle.

Supination

Pronation

Fig. 26-22 Range-of-motion exercises for the foot.

Flexion   Extension   Abduction   Adduction

Fig. 26-23 Range-of-motion exercises for the toes.

✉ AMBULATION

Ambulation is the act of walking. Some people are weak and unsteady from bedrest, illness, surgery, or injury. They may need help walking. Some become strong enough to walk alone. Others will always need help.

After bedrest, activity increases slowly and in steps. First the person sits on the side of the bed (dangles). Sitting in a bedside chair follows. Next the person walks in the room and then in the hallway. To walk, contractures and muscle atrophy must be prevented. Proper positioning and exercises are needed during bedrest.

Regular walking helps prevent deconditioning. Some persons who use wheelchairs can walk with help. Follow the care plan when helping a person walk. Use a gait (transfer) belt if the person is weak or unsteady. The person also uses hand rails along the wall. Always check for orthostatic hypotension (p. 415).

See *Focus on Communication: Ambulation.*
See *Delegation Guidelines: Ambulation.*
See *Promoting Safety and Comfort: Ambulation.*

FOCUS ON COMMUNICATION
Ambulation

Before ambulating, talk with the person about the activity. Doing so promotes comfort and reduces fear. Explain to the person:
- How far to walk
- What assistive devices are used
- How you will assist
- What the person is to report to you
- How you will help if the person begins to fall
  For example, you can say:

  "Mr. Owens, I am going to help you walk from your bed to the doorway and back. This belt helps support you while you walk. I will be at your side and hold the belt at all times. Tell me right away if you feel unsteady, dizzy, or weak. Also tell me if you feel any pain or discomfort. If you begin to fall, I will use the belt to pull you close to me and gently lower you to the floor. Do you have any questions?"

DELEGATION GUIDELINES
Ambulation

Before helping with ambulation, you need this information from the nurse and the care plan:
- How much help the person needs
- If the person uses a cane, walker, crutches, or a brace
- Areas of weakness—right arm or leg, left arm or leg
- How far to walk the person
- What observations to report and record:
  - How well the person tolerated the activity
  - Shuffling, sliding, limping, or walking on tip-toes
  - Complaints of pain or discomfort
  - Complaints of orthostatic hypotension—weakness, dizziness, spots before the eyes, feeling faint
  - The distance walked
- When to report observations
- What specific resident concerns to report at once

PROMOTING SAFETY AND COMFORT
Ambulation

Safety
Practice the safety measures to prevent falls (Chapter 13). Use a gait belt to help the person stand. Also use it during ambulation.

Comfort
The fear of falling affects mental comfort. Explain the purpose of the gait belt. Also explain how you will help the person if he or she starts to fall (Chapter 13).

Fig. 26-24 The nursing assistant walks at the person's side and slightly behind her.

QUALITY OF LIFE

Remember to:
- Knock before entering the person's room.
- Address the person by name.
- Introduce yourself by name and title.
- Explain the procedure to the person before beginning and during the procedure.
- Protect the person's rights during the procedure.
- Handle the person gently during the procedure.

PRE-PROCEDURE

1. Follow *Delegation Guidelines: Ambulation*. See *Promoting Safety and Comfort: Ambulation.*
2. Practice hand hygiene.
3. Collect the following:
   - Robe and non-skid shoes
   - Paper or sheet to protect bottom linens
   - Gait (transfer) belt
4. Identify the person. Check the ID bracelet against the assignment sheet. Also call the person by name.
5. Provide for privacy.

PROCEDURE

6. Lower the bed to its lowest position. Lock the bed wheels. Lower the bed rail if up.
7. Fan-fold top linens to the foot of the bed.
8. Place the paper or sheet under the person's feet. Put the shoes on the person. Fasten the shoes.
9. Help the person sit on the side of the bed. (See procedure: *Sitting on the Side of the Bed [Dangling]*, Chapter 17.)
10. Help the person put on the robe.
11. Make sure the person's feet are flat on the floor.
12. Apply the gait belt. (See procedure: *Applying a Transfer/Gait Belt,* Chapter 13.)
13. Help the person stand. (See procedure: *Transferring the Person to a Chair or Wheelchair,* Chapter 17.) Grasp the gait belt at each side. If no gait belt, place your arms under the person's arms around to the shoulder blades.
14. Stand at the person's weak side while he or she gains balance. Hold the belt at the side and back. If not using a gait belt, have one arm around the back and the other at the elbow to support the person.
15. Encourage the person to stand erect with the head up and back straight.
16. Help the person walk. Walk to the side and slightly behind the person on the person's weak side. Provide support with the gait belt (Fig. 26-24). If not using a gait belt, have one arm around the back and the other at the elbow to support the person. Encourage the person to use the hand rail on his or her strong side.
17. Encourage the person to walk normally. The heel strikes the floor first. Discourage shuffling, sliding, or walking on tip-toes.
18. Walk the required distance if the person tolerates the activity. Do not rush the person.
19. Help the person return to bed. Remove the gait belt. (See procedure: *Transferring the Person From a Chair or Wheelchair to Bed,* Chapter 17.)
20. Lower the head of the bed. Help the person to the center of the bed.
21. Remove the shoes. Remove and discard the paper or sheet over the bottom sheet.

POST-PROCEDURE

22. Provide for comfort. (See the inside of the front book cover.)
23. Place the signal light within reach.
24. Raise or lower bed rails. Follow the care plan.
25. Return the robe and shoes to their proper place.
26. Unscreen the person.
27. Complete a safety check of the room. (See the inside of the front book cover.)
28. Decontaminate your hands.
29. Report and record your observations (Fig. 26-25).

Date	Time	Nursing Margin	Other Depts Margin
10/10	1400	Ambulated 25 feet in the hallway c̄ assist of one and use of a gait belt.	
		Reminded not to shuffle her feet. Showed no signs of distress or discomfort.	
		Denied feeling dizzy, lightheaded, or weak. No c/o pain. Assisted to her recliner	
		chair and elevated her feet after ambulating. BP-132/84 L arm sitting. P-76	
		regular rate and rhythm. R-20 and unlabored. Overbed table c̄ water pitcher	
		and glass within reach. Signal light within reach. Adam Aims, CNA ———	

Fig. 26-25 Charting sample.

Walking Aids

Walking aids support the body. The doctor, nurse, or physical therapist (PT) orders them. The need may be temporary or permanent. The type ordered depends on the person's condition, the amount of support needed, and the type of disability. Older persons often need walkers or canes for safety. The PT measures and teaches the person to use the device.

Crutches Crutches are used when the person cannot use one leg or when one or both legs need to gain strength. Some persons with permanent leg weakness can use crutches. They usually use forearm crutches (Fig. 26-26). Underarm crutches extend from the underarm to the ground (Fig. 26-27).

The person learns to crutch walk, use stairs, and sit and stand. Safety is important. The person on crutches is at risk for falls. Follow these safety measures:

- Check the crutch tips. They must not be worn down, torn, or wet. Replace worn or torn crutch tips. Dry wet tips with a towel or paper towels.
- Check crutches for flaws. Check wooden crutches for cracks and metal crutches for bends.
- Tighten all bolts.
- Have the person wear street shoes. They must be flat and have non-skid soles.
- Make sure clothes fit well. Loose clothes may get caught between the crutches and underarms. Loose clothes and long skirts can hang forward and block the person's view of the feet and crutch tips.
- Practice safety rules to prevent falls (Chapter 13).
- Keep crutches within the person's reach. Put them by the person's chair or against a wall.
- Know which crutch gait the person uses:
  - Four-point gait (Fig. 26-28)
  - Three-point gait (Fig. 26-29)
  - Two-point gait (Fig. 26-30)
  - Swing-to gait (Fig. 26-31)
  - Swing-through gait (Fig. 26-32)

Fig. 26-26 Forearm crutches. *(From Elkin MK, Perry AG, Potter PA: Nursing interventions & clinical skills, ed 2, St Louis, 2000, Mosby.)*

Fig. 26-27 Underarm crutches.

Fig. 26-28 The four-point gait. The person uses both legs. The right crutch is moved forward and then the left foot. Then the left crutch is moved forward followed by the right foot.

Fig. 26-29 The three-point gait. One leg is used. Both crutches are moved forward. Then the good foot is moved forward.

Fig. 26-30 The two-point gait. The person bears some weight on each foot. The left crutch and right foot are moved forward at the same time. Then the right crutch and left foot are moved forward.

Fig. 26-31 Swing-to gait. The person bears some weight on each leg. Both crutches are moved forward. Then the person lifts both legs and *swings to* the crutches.

Fig. 26-32 Swing-through gait. The person bears some weight on each leg. Both crutches are moved forward. Then the person lifts both legs and *swings through* the crutches.

Canes Canes are used for weakness on one side of the body. They help provide balance and support. Single-tip and four-point (quad) canes are common (Fig. 26-33). A cane is held on the *strong side* of the body. (If the left leg is weak, the cane is held in the right hand.) Four-point canes give more support than single-tip canes. However, they are harder to move.

The cane tip is about 6 to 10 inches to the side of the foot. It is about 6 to 10 inches in front of the foot on the strong side. The grip is level with the hip. The person walks as follows:

- *Step A:* The cane is moved forward 6 to 10 inches (Fig. 26-34, *A*).
- *Step B:* The weak leg (opposite the cane) is moved forward even with the cane (Fig. 26-34, *B*).
- *Step C:* The strong leg is moved forward and ahead of the cane and the weak leg (Fig. 26-34, *C*).

Fig. 26-33 A, Single-tip cane. **B,** Four-point cane.

Fig. 26-34 Walking with a cane. **A,** The cane is moved forward about 6 to 10 inches. **B,** The leg opposite the cane (weak leg) is brought forward even with the cane. **C,** The leg on the cane side (strong side) is moved ahead of the cane and the weak leg.

Walkers A walker gives more support than a cane. Wheeled walkers are common (Fig. 26-35). They have wheels on the front legs and rubber tips on the back legs. The person pushes the walker about 6 to 8 inches in front of his or her feet. Rubber tips on the back legs prevent the walker from moving while the person is standing. Some have a braking action when weight is applied to the walker's back legs.

Baskets, pouches, and trays attach to the walker. They are used for needed items. This allows more independence. They also free the hands to grip the walker.

Braces Braces support weak body parts. They also prevent or correct deformities or prevent joint movement. Metal, plastic, or leather is used for braces. A brace is applied over the ankle, knee, or back (Fig. 26-36). An ankle-foot orthosis (AFO) is placed in the shoe (Fig. 26-37). Then the foot is inserted. The AFO is secured in place with a Velcro strap. This type of brace is common after a stroke.

Keep skin and bony points under braces clean and dry. This prevents skin breakdown. Report redness or signs of skin breakdown at once. Also report complaints of pain or discomfort. The nurse assesses the skin under braces every shift. The care plan tells you when to apply and remove a brace.

RECREATIONAL ACTIVITIES

OBRA requires activity programs for residents. Recreational activities are important for an older person's physical and mental well-being. Joints and muscles are exercised. Circulation is stimulated. Recreational activities also are social events and are mentally stimulating. A good activity program improves a person's quality of life.

Activities must meet each person's interests and physical, mental, and psycho-social needs. Bingo, movies, dances, exercise groups, shopping trips, museum trips, concerts, guest speakers, and gardening activities are common.

The right to personal choice is protected. Well-being is promoted when the person attends activities of personal choice. The person is not forced to do things that do not interest him or her.

Some persons need help getting to an activity. Some also need help taking part in them. You must assist as needed.

Activity ideas are always welcome. Residents may share ideas with you or tell you about favorite pastimes. Or you may have ideas. Share these with the health team. They are given to the resident group that plans activities. Remember, OBRA also requires that persons be allowed to take part in resident group activities.

See *Teamwork and Time Management: Recreational Activities.*

Fig. 26-35 Wheeled walker.

Fig. 26-36 Leg brace.

Fig. 26-37 Ankle-foot orthosis (AFO).

TEAMWORK AND TIME MANAGEMENT
Recreational Activities

Some persons need help getting to activity programs. Some also need help with activities. When you can, help co-workers assist residents to and from and with activity programs. For example, you have 1 or 2 people who need help. A co-worker has 4 to 5 persons needing help.

QUALITY OF LIFE

You assist residents with exercise and activity. You must protect the rights to privacy and personal choice. Privacy is protected. During ROM, cover the person with a bath blanket. Expose only the body part being exercised. The person is properly clothed when walking. The person's body is not exposed. Remember, privacy promotes dignity and mental comfort.

Personal choice in walking is encouraged. The person may want to walk outside. The person may prefer to walk in the morning, afternoon, or evening. Or the person may want to wait until a visitor arrives or leaves. Such choices are allowed whenever safe and possible. Be sure to get the nurse's approval.

Disease, injury, pain, and aging affect a person's activities. Even with such limits, you can promote activity, exercise, and well-being. You can:

- Encourage the person to be as active as possible.
- Resist the urge to do things for the person that he or she can safely do alone or with some help.
- Focus on the person's abilities.
- Tell the person when he or she is doing well or making progress.
- Tell the person you are proud of what he or she did or tried to do.

REVIEW QUESTIONS

Circle the BEST answer.

1 The purpose of bedrest is to
  a Prevent orthostatic hypotension
  b Reduce pain and promote healing
  c Prevent pressure ulcers, constipation, and blood clots
  d Cause contractures and muscle atrophy

2 Which helps prevent plantar flexion?
  a Bed-boards
  b A foot-board
  c A trochanter roll
  d Hand rolls

3 Which prevents the hip from turning outward?
  a Bed-boards
  b A foot-board
  c A trochanter roll
  d A leg brace

4 A contracture is
  a The loss of muscle strength from inactivity
  b The lack of joint mobility from shortening of a muscle
  c A decrease in the size of a muscle
  d A blood clot in the muscle

5 A trapeze is used to
  a Prevent footdrop
  b Prevent contractures
  c Strengthen arm muscles
  d Strengthen leg muscles

6 Passive ROM exercises are performed by
  a The person
  b Someone else
  c The person with the help of another
  d The person with the use of a trapeze

7 ROM exercises are ordered. You do the following *except*
  a Support the part being exercised
  b Move the joint slowly, smoothly, and gently
  c Force the joint through its full range of motion
  d Exercise only the joints indicated by the nurse

8 Flexion involves
  a Bending the body part
  b Straightening the body part
  c Moving the body part toward the body
  d Moving the body part away from the body

9 When ambulating a person
  a A gait belt is used if the person is weak or unsteady
  b The person can shuffle or slide when walking after bedrest
  c Walking aids are needed
  d You walk on the person's strong side

10 You are getting a person ready to crutch walk. You should do the following *except*
  a Check the crutch tips
  b Have the person wear non-skid shoes
  c Get a pair of crutches from physical therapy
  d Tighten the bolts on the crutches

11 A single-tip cane is used
  a At waist level
  b On the strong side
  c On the weak side
  d On either side

Circle T if the statement is TRUE. Circle F if the statement is FALSE.

12 T F   A walker and a four-point cane give the same support.

13 T F   When using a cane, the feet are moved first.

14 T F   When using a walker, the walker is pushed in front of the person's feet.

15 T F   A person has a brace. Bony areas need protection from skin breakdown.

Answers to these questions are on p. 720.

Comfort, Rest, and Sleep

OBJECTIVES

- Define the key terms and key abbreviations listed in this chapter.
- Explain why comfort, rest, and sleep are important.
- List the OBRA room requirements for comfort, rest, and sleep.
- Describe four types of pain and the factors affecting pain.
- Explain why pain is personal.
- List the signs and symptoms of pain.
- List the nursing measures that relieve pain.
- Explain why meeting basic needs is important for rest.

- Identify when rest is needed.
- Explain how circadian rhythm affects sleep.
- Describe the stages of sleep.
- Know the sleep requirements for each age-group.
- Describe the factors that affect sleep.
- Describe the common sleep disorders.
- List the nursing measures that promote rest and sleep.
- Explain how dementia affects sleep.
- Explain how to promote quality of life.

KEY TERMS

acute pain Pain that is felt suddenly from injury, disease, trauma, or surgery

chronic pain Pain that continues for a long time (months or years) or occurs off and on; persistent pain

circadian rhythm Daily rhythm based on a 24-hour cycle; the day-night cycle or body rhythm

comfort A state of well-being; the person has no physical or emotional pain and is calm and at peace

discomfort See "pain"

distraction To change the person's center of attention

enuresis Urinary incontinence in bed at night

guided imagery Creating and focusing on an image

insomnia A chronic condition in which the person cannot sleep or stay asleep all night

NREM sleep The phase of sleep when there is *no rapid eye movement*; non-REM sleep

pain To ache, hurt, or be sore; discomfort

persistent pain See "chronic pain"

phantom pain Pain felt in a body part that is no longer there

radiating pain Pain felt at the site of tissue damage and in nearby areas

relaxation To be free from mental and physical stress

REM sleep The phase of sleep when there is *rapid eye movement*

rest To be calm, at ease, and relaxed; no anxiety or stress

sleep A state of unconsciousness, reduced voluntary muscle activity, and lowered metabolism

Comfort, rest, and sleep are needed for well-being. The total person—the physical, emotional, social, and spiritual—is affected by comfort, rest, and sleep problems. Discomfort and pain can be physical or emotional. Whatever the cause, they affect rest and sleep. They also decrease function and quality of life.

Rest and sleep restore energy and well-being. Illness and injury increase the need for rest and sleep. The body needs more energy for healing and repair. And more energy is needed for daily functions.

COMFORT

Comfort is a state of well-being. The person has no physical or emotional pain. He or she is calm and at peace. Age, illness, and activity affect comfort. So do temperature, ventilation, noise, odors, and lighting. Such factors are controlled to meet the person's needs (Chapter 18).

See *Focus on Communication: Comfort*.

OBRA Requirements

The Omnibus Budget Reconciliation Act of 1987 (OBRA) and the Centers for Medicare & Medicaid Services (CMS) require care that promotes well-being. Comfort, rest, and sleep are needed for physical, emotional, and mental well-being. Rooms are designed and equipped for comfort.

- No more than 4 persons in a room
- A suspended curtain that goes around the bed for privacy
- A bed of proper height and size for the person
- A clean, comfortable mattress
- Linens (sheets, blankets, spreads) that suit the weather and climate
- A clean and orderly room
- An odor-free room
- A room temperature between 71° and 81° F (Fahrenheit)
- A comfortable sound level
- Adequate ventilation and room humidity
- Adequate and comfortable lighting

FOCUS ON COMMUNICATION
Comfort

Do not assume that a person is comfortable. Ask the following:

- "Are you comfortable?"
- "How can I help you be more comfortable?"
- "Are you warm enough?"
- "Do you need another blanket?"
- "Do you need another pillow?"
- "Should I adjust your pillow?"

PAIN

Pain or **discomfort** means to ache, hurt, or be sore. It is unpleasant. Comfort and discomfort are subjective (Chapter 7). That is, you cannot see, hear, touch, or smell pain or discomfort. You must rely on what the person says. Report complaints to the nurse for the nursing process.

Pain differs for each person. What *hurts* to one person may *ache* to another. What one person calls *sore*, another may call *aching*. If a person complains of pain or discomfort, the person *has* pain or discomfort. Believe the person. You cannot see, hear, feel, or smell the person's pain or discomfort.

Pain is a warning from the body. Often called the fifth vital sign (Chapter 31), pain signals tissue damage. Pain often causes the person to seek health care.

See *Focus on Communication: Pain*.

FOCUS ON COMMUNICATION
Pain

Communicating with persons about pain promotes comfort. You can say:

- "I want you to be comfortable. Please tell me if you are having any pain."
- "I will tell the nurse about your pain."

If a person complains of pain, the person has pain. You must rely on what the person tells you. Promptly report any complaints of pain to the nurse.

Box 27-3 Nursing Measures to Promote Comfort and Relieve Pain

- Position the person in good alignment. Use pillows for support.
- Keep bed linens tight and wrinkle-free.
- Make sure the person is not lying on tubes.
- Assist with elimination needs.
- Adjust the room temperature to meet the person's needs.
- Provide blankets for warmth and to prevent chilling.
- Use correct handling, moving, and turning procedures.
- Wait 30 minutes after pain drugs are given before giving care or starting activities.
- Give a back massage.
- Provide soft music to distract the person.
- Talk softly and gently.
- Use touch to provide comfort.

- Allow family and friends at the b̶̶ ... the person.
- Avoid sudden or jarring movements ...
- Handle the person gently.
- Practice safety measures if the person ta̶̶ drugs or sedatives:
  - Keep the bed in the low position.
  - Raise bed rails as directed. Follow the care p̶̶ ...
  - Check on the person every 10 to 15 minutes.
  - Provide help when the person needs to get up an̶̶ when he or she is up and about.
- Apply warm or cold applications as directed by the nurse (Chapter 35).
- Provide a calm, quiet, darkened setting.

Fig. 27-5 Measures are implemented to relieve pain. The person is positioned in good alignment with pillows used for comfort. The room is darkened. Blankets provide warmth.

Fig. 27-6 A comforting pet can distract attention away from pain.

Nursing Measures

The nurse uses the nursing process to promote comfort and relieve pain. The care plan may include the measures in Box 27-3. See Figure 27-5.

Other measures are often needed. They include distraction, relaxation, and guided imagery. If asked to assist, the nurse tells you what to do.

Distraction means to change the person's center of attention. Attention is moved away from the pain. Music, games, singing, praying, TV, and needlework can distract attention (Fig. 27-6).

Relaxation means to be free from mental and physical stress. This state reduces pain and anxiety. The person is taught relaxation methods. The person is taught to breathe deeply and slowly and to contract and relax

muscle groups. A comfortable position is important. So is a quiet room.

Guided imagery is creating and focusing on an image. The person is asked to create a pleasant scene. This is noted on the care plan so all staff members use the same image with the person. A calm, soft voice is used to help the person focus on the image. Soft music, a blanket for warmth, and a darkened room may help. The person is coached to focus on the image and then to practice relaxation exercises.

Doctors often order drugs to control or relieve pain. Nurses give these drugs. Such drugs can cause orthostatic hypotension (Chapter 26). They also can cause drowsiness, dizziness, and coordination problems. Protect the person from injury, falls, and fractures. The nurse and care plan alert you to needed safety measures.

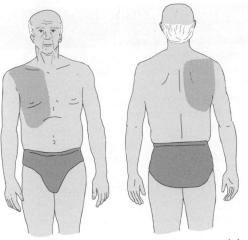

Fig. 27-1 Gallbladder pain may radiate to the right upper abdomen, the back, and the right shoulder.

Types of Pain

There are different types of pain:

- **Acute pain** is felt suddenly from injury, disease, trauma, or surgery. It may signal a new injury or a life-threatening event. There is tissue damage. Acute pain lasts a short time. It lessens with healing.
- **Chronic pain (persistent pain)** continues for a long time (months or years) or occurs off and on. There is no longer tissue damage. Chronic pain remains long after healing. Arthritis is a common cause.
- **Radiating pain** is felt at the site of tissue damage and in nearby areas. Pain from a heart attack is often felt in the left chest, left jaw, left shoulder, and left arm. Gallbladder disease can cause pain in the right upper abdomen, the back, and the right shoulder (Fig. 27-1).
- **Phantom pain** is felt in a body part that is no longer there. A person with an amputated leg may still sense leg pain.

Factors Affecting Pain

A person may handle pain well one time and poorly the next time. Many factors affect reactions to pain.

Past Experience We learn from past experiences. They help us know what to do or what to expect. Whether it is going to school, driving, taking a test, shopping, having a baby, or caring for children, the past prepares us for like events at another time. We also learn from the experiences of family and friends.

A person may have had pain before. The severity of pain, its cause, how long it lasted, and if relief occurred all affect the current response to pain. Knowing what to expect can help or hinder how the person handles pain.

Some people have not had pain. When it occurs, pain can cause fear and anxiety. They can make pain worse.

Anxiety Anxiety relates to feelings of fear, dread, worry, and concern. The person is uneasy and tense. The person may feel troubled or threatened. Or the person may sense danger. Something is wrong but the person does not know what or why.

Pain and anxiety are related. Pain can cause anxiety. Anxiety increases how much pain is felt. Reducing anxiety helps lessen pain. For example, the nurse explains to Mr. Smith about pain after surgery. The nurse also explains that drugs are given for pain relief. Mr. Smith knows the cause of pain and what to expect. This helps lessen anxiety and therefore the amount of pain felt.

Rest and Sleep Rest and sleep restore energy. They reduce body demands. The body repairs itself. Lack of needed rest and sleep affects thinking and coping with daily life. Sleep and rest needs increase with illness and injury. Pain seems worse when tired or restless. Also, the person tends to focus on pain when tired and unable to rest or sleep.

Attention The more a person thinks about the pain, the worse it seems. Sometimes severe pain is all the person thinks about. Even mild pain can seem worse if the person thinks about it all the time.

Pain often seems worse at night. Activity is less, and it is quiet. There are no visitors. The radio or TV is off. Others are asleep. When unable to sleep, the person has time to think about the pain.

Personal and Family Duties Personal and family duties affect pain responses. Often pain is ignored when there are children to care for. Some people go to work with pain. Others deny pain if a serious illness is feared. The illness can interfere with a job, going to school, or caring for children, a partner, or ill parents.

The Value or Meaning of Pain To some people, pain is a sign of weakness. It may mean a serious illness and the need for painful tests and treatments. Therefore pain is ignored or denied. Sometimes pain gives pleasure. The pain of childbirth is one example.

For some persons, pain means not having to work or assume daily routines. Pain is used to avoid certain people or things. The pain is useful. Some people like doting and pampering by others. The person values and wants such attention.

Support From Others Dealing with pain is often easier when family and friends offer comfort and support. The pain of childbirth is easier when a loving father gives support and encouragement. A child bears pain much better when comforted by a caring parent or family member. The use of touch by a valued person is very comforting. Just being nearby also helps.

Some people do not have caring family or friends. They deal with pain alone. Being alone can increase anxiety. The person has more time to think about the pain. Facing pain alone is hard for everyone, especially children and older persons.

CARING ABOUT CULTURE

Pain Reactions

People of *Mexico* and the *Phillippines* may appear stoic in reaction to pain. In the *Phillippines*, pain is viewed as the will of God. It is believed that God will give strength to bear the pain.

In *Vietnam*, pain may be severe before pain-relief measures are requested. The people of *India* accept pain quietly. They accept pain-relief measures.

In *China*, showing emotion is a weakness of character. Therefore pain is often suppressed.

From D'Avanzo CE, Geissler EM: Pocket guide to cultural health assessment, ed 4, St Louis, 2008, Mosby.

RESIDENTS WITH DEMENTIA

Factors Affecting Pain—Age

Persons with dementia may not be able to tell you about their pain. Changes in usual behavior may signal pain. A person who normally moans and groans may become quiet and withdrawn. A person who is friendly and outgoing may become agitated and aggressive. One who is nonverbal and quiet may become restless and cry easily. Loss of appetite also signals pain.

Report any changes in a person's usual behavior to the nurse. All persons have the right to correct pain management. The nurse does a pain assessment when behavior changes.

Culture Culture affects pain responses. In some cultures, the person in pain is *stoic*. To be stoic means to show no reaction to joy, sorrow, pleasure, or pain. Strong verbal and nonverbal reactions to pain are seen in other cultures. See *Caring About Culture: Pain Reactions.*

OBRA-CMS — OBRA requires that the care planning process reflect the person's culture. Non–English-speaking persons may have problems describing pain. The center must know who these persons are. Someone must be available to interpret the person's needs. All persons have the right to be comfortable and as pain-free as possible.

Illness Some diseases cause decreased pain sensations. Central nervous system disorders are examples. The person may not feel pain. Or it may not feel severe. The person is at risk for undetected disease or injury. Pain occurs with tissue damage. The pain signals illness or injury. If pain is not felt, the person does not know to seek health care.

Age Some older persons have many painful health problems. Chronic pain may mask new pain. Older persons may ignore or deny new pain. They may think it relates to a known health problem. Older persons often deny or ignore pain because of what it may mean.

Older persons may have decreased pain sensations. They may not feel pain. Or it may not feel severe. The person is at risk for undetected disease or injury. Pain occurs with tissue damage. The pain signals illness or injury. If pain is not felt, the person does not know to seek health care.

Thinking and reasoning are affected in some older persons. Some cannot verbally communicate pain. Increased confusion, grimacing, or restlessness may signal pain. So may changes in usual behavior. You must be alert for the signs of pain. Always report changes in the person's behavior.

See *Residents With Dementia: Factors Affecting Pain—Age.*

Signs and Symptoms

You cannot see, hear, feel, or smell the person's pain. You must rely on what the person tells you. Promptly report any information you collect about pain. Write down what the person says. Use the person's exact words when reporting and recording. The nurse needs this information to assess the person's pain:

- *Location.* Where is the pain? Ask the person to point to the area of pain (Fig. 27-2). Pain can radiate. Ask the person if the pain is anywhere else and to point to those areas.
- *Onset and duration.* When did the pain start? How long has it lasted?
- *Intensity.* Is the pain mild, moderate, or severe? Ask the person to rate the pain on a scale of 1 to 10, with 10 as the most severe (Fig. 27-3). Or use the Wong-Baker Faces Pain Rating Scale (Fig. 27-4). Designed for children, the scale is useful for persons of all ages. To use the scale, tell the person that each face shows how a person is feeling. Read the description for each face. Then ask the person to choose the face that best describes how he or she feels.
- *Description.* Ask the person to describe the pain. If the person cannot describe the pain, offer some of the words listed in Box 27-1.
- *Factors causing pain.* These are called *precipitating* factors. To "precipitate" means "to cause." Such factors include moving or turning in bed, coughing or deep breathing, and exercise. Ask what the person was doing before the pain started and when it started.
- *Factors affecting pain.* Ask the person what makes the pain better. Also ask what makes it worse.
- *Vital signs.* Measure the person's pulse, respirations, and blood pressure (Chapter 31). Increases in these vital signs often occur with acute pain. Vital signs may be normal with chronic pain.
- *Other signs and symptoms.* Does the person have other symptoms? Box 27-2 lists the signs and symptoms that often occur with pain.

Fig. 27-2 The person points to the area of pain.

Box 27-1   Words Used to Describe Pain

- Aching
- Burning
- Cramping
- Crushing
- Discomfort
- Dull
- Gnawing
- Heaviness
- Hurting
- Knife-like
- Numbness
- Piercing
- Pins and needles
- Pressure
- Radiating
- Ripping
- Sharp
- Shooting
- Soreness
- Spasms
- Squeezing
- Stabbing
- Tearing
- Tenderness
- Throbbing
- Tingling
- Vise-like

PAIN: Ask patient to rate pain on scale of 0-10										
No pain									Worst pain imaginable	
0	1	2	3	4	5	6	7	8	9	10

Fig. 27-3 Pain rating scale *(From deWit SC: Fundamental concepts and skills for nursing, ed 3, St Louis, 2009, Saunders.)*

0	1	2	3	4	5
No hurt	Hurts little bit	Hurts little more	Hurts even more	Hurts whole lot	Hurts worst

Fig. 27-4 Wong-Baker Faces Pain Rating Scale. *(From Hockenberry MJ and others: Wong's nursing care of infants and children, ed 8, St Louis, 2007, Mosby.)*

Box 27-2   Signs and Symptoms of Pain

Body Responses
- Appetite: changes in
- Dizziness
- Nausea
- Numbness
- Pulse, respirations, and blood pressure: increased
- Skin: pale (pallor)
- Sleep: difficulty with
- Sweating (diaphoresis)
- Tingling
- Vomiting
- Weakness
- Weight loss

Behaviors
- Clenching of the jaw
- Crying
- Frowning
- Gait: changes in; limping

Behaviors—cont'd
- Gasping
- Grimacing
- Groaning
- Grunting
- Holding the affected body part (splinting; guarding)
- Irritability
- Moaning
- Mood: changes in; depressed
- Pacing
- Positioning: maintaining one position; refusing to move
- Quietness
- Resisting care
- Restlessness
- Rubbing a body part or area
- Screaming
- Speech: slow or rapid; loud or quiet
- Whimpering

REST

Rest means to be calm, at ease, and relaxed. The person has no anxiety or stress. Rest may involve inactivity. Or the person does things that are calming and relaxing. Examples include reading, music, TV, needlework, and prayer. Some people garden, bake, golf, walk, or do woodworking.

Promote rest by meeting physical needs. Thirst, hunger, and elimination needs can affect rest. So can pain or discomfort. A comfortable position and good alignment are important. A quiet setting promotes rest. So does a clean, dry, and wrinkle-free bed. Some people rest easier in a clean, neat, and uncluttered room.

Meet safety and security needs. The person must feel safe from falling or other injuries. The person is secure with the signal light within reach. Understanding the reasons for care also helps the person feel safe. So does knowing how care is given. That is why you always explain procedures before doing them.

Many people have rituals or routines before resting. These may include going to the bathroom, brushing teeth, and washing the face and hands. Some people pray. Some have a snack or beverage, lock doors, or make sure loved ones are safe at home. The person may want a certain blanket or afghan. Follow routines and rituals whenever possible.

Love and belonging promote rest. Visits or calls from family and friends may relax the person. The person knows that others care and are concerned. Reading cards and letters may also help the person relax and rest (Fig. 27-7).

Self-esteem needs relate to feeling good about oneself. Some people find hospital gowns embarrassing. Others fear exposure. Many persons rest better in their own sleepwear. Hygiene and grooming also affect self-esteem. This includes hair care and being clean and odor-free. Hygiene and grooming measures help people feel good about themselves. If esteem needs are met, the person may rest easier.

Some people are refreshed after a 15- or 20-minute rest. Others need more time. Health care routines usually allow time for afternoon rest.

Ill or injured persons need to rest more often. Some rest during or after a procedure. For example, a bath tires a person. So does getting dressed. The person needs to rest before you make the bed. Some people need a few hours for hygiene and grooming. Others need to rest after meals. Do not push the person beyond his or her limits. Allow rest when needed. Do not rush the person.

Distraction, relaxation, and guided imagery also promote rest. So does a back massage. Plan and organize care to allow uninterrupted rest.

The doctor may order bedrest for a person. Bedrest is presented in Chapter 26.

Fig. 27-7 The resident reads cards and letters from family and friends.

SLEEP

Sleep is a state of unconsciousness, reduced voluntary muscle activity, and lowered metabolism. An unconscious person is not aware of his or her setting. He or she cannot respond to people and things. There are no voluntary arm or leg movements. *Metabolism* is the burning of food to produce energy for the body. Less energy is needed during sleep. Thus metabolism is reduced during sleep. The sleep state is temporary. People wake up from sleep.

Sleep is a basic need. It lets the mind and body rest. The body saves energy. Body functions slow. Vital signs are lower than when awake. Tissue healing and repair occur. Sleep lowers stress, tension, and anxiety. It refreshes and renews the person. The person regains energy and mental alertness. The person thinks and functions better after sleep.

Circadian Rhythm

Sleep is part of circadian rhythm. (*Circa* means *about*. *Dies* means *day*.) Circadian rhythm is a daily rhythm based on a 24-hour cycle. It is called the *day-night cycle* or *body rhythm*. It affects functioning. Some people function better in the morning. They are more alert and active. They think and react better. Others do better in the evening.

Circadian rhythm includes a sleep-wake cycle. The person's *biological clock* signals when to sleep and when to wake up. You sleep and wake up at certain times. You may awaken before the alarm clock goes off. That is part of your biological clock. Health care often interferes with a person's circadian rhythm and the sleep-wake cycle. Sleep problems easily occur.

Many people work evening and night shifts. Their bodies must adjust to changes in the sleep-wake cycle.

Sleep Cycle

There are two phases of sleep (Box 27-4). **NREM sleep** *(non-REM sleep)* is the phase of sleep where there is *no rapid eye movement.* NREM sleep has 4 stages. Sleep goes from light to deep as the person moves through the four stages.

The *rapid eye movement* phase is called **REM sleep.** The person is hard to arouse. Mental restoration occurs. Events and problems of the day are thought to be reviewed. The person prepares for the next day.

There are usually 4 to 6 cycles of NREM and REM sleep during 7 to 8 hours of sleep. Stage 1 of NREM is usually not repeated (Fig. 27-8).

Sleep Requirements

Sleep needs vary for each age-group. The amount needed decreases with age (Table 27-1). Infants need more sleep than toddlers. Toddlers need more than preschool children. School-age children need more than teenagers. Older persons need less sleep than middle-age adults.

Box 27-4　Sleep Cycle

Stage 1: NREM Sleep
- Lightest sleep level
- Lasts a few minutes
- Gradual decrease in vital signs
- Gradual lowering of metabolism
- Person feels drowsy and relaxed
- Person is easily aroused
- Daydreaming feeling after being aroused

Stage 2: NREM Sleep
- Sound sleep
- Relaxation increases
- Still easy to arouse
- Lasts 10 to 20 minutes
- Body functions continue to slow

Stage 3: NREM Sleep
- First stage of deep sleep
- Hard to arouse the person
- Person rarely moves
- Muscles relax completely
- Vital signs decrease
- Lasts 15 to 30 minutes

Stage 4: NREM Sleep
- Deepest stage of sleep
- Hard to arouse the person
- Body rests and is restored
- Vital signs much lower than when awake
- Lasts about 15 to 30 minutes
- Sleepwalking may occur
- **Enuresis** (urinary incontinence in bed at night) may occur

REM Sleep
- Vivid, full-color dreaming
- Usually starts 50 to 90 minutes after sleep has begun
- Rapid eye movements
- Blood pressure, pulse, and respirations may fluctuate
- Voluntary muscles are relaxed
- Mental restoration occurs
- Hard to arouse the person
- Lasts about 20 minutes

Modified from Potter PA, Perry AG: Fundamentals of nursing, *ed 7, St Louis, 2009, Mosby.*

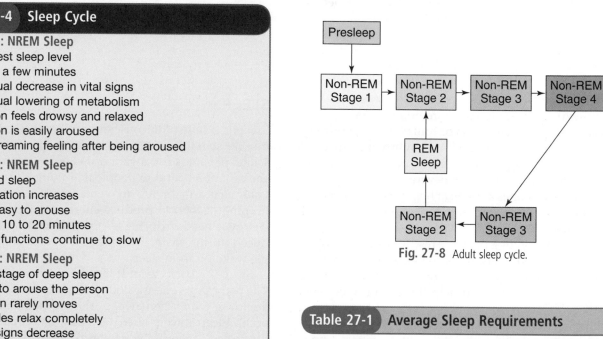

Fig. 27-8 Adult sleep cycle.

Table 27-1　Average Sleep Requirements

Age-Group	Hours per Day
Newborns (birth to 4 weeks)	14 to 18
Infants (4 weeks to 1 year)	12 to 14
Toddlers (1 to 3 years)	11 to 12
Preschoolers (3 to 6 years)	11 to 12
Middle and late childhood (6 to 12 years)	10 to 11
Adolescents (12 to 18 years)	8 to 9
Young adults (18 to 40 years)	7 to 8
Middle-age adults (40 to 65 years)	7
Older adults (65 years and older)	5 to 7

Factors Affecting Sleep

Many factors affect the amount and quality of sleep. Quality relates to how well the person slept. It also involves getting needed amounts of NREM and REM sleep.

- *Illness.* Illness increases the need for sleep. However, signs and symptoms of illness can interfere with sleep. They include pain, nausea, vomiting, coughing, difficulty breathing, diarrhea, frequent voiding, and itching. Treatments and therapies can also interfere with sleep. Often residents are awakened for treatments or drugs. Care devices can cause uncomfortable positions. The emotional effects of illness can affect sleep. These include fear, anxiety, and worry.
- *Nutrition.* Sleep needs increase with weight gain. They decrease with weight loss. Some foods affect sleep. Those with caffeine (chocolate, coffee, tea, or colas) prevent sleep. The protein *tryptophan* tends to help sleep. It is found in protein sources—milk, cheese, red meat, fish, poultry, and peanuts.
- *Exercise.* Exercise improves health and fitness. Exercise requires energy. People usually feel good after exercising. Eventually they tire. Being tired helps them sleep well. Exercise before bedtime interferes with sleep. Exercise causes the release of substances into the bloodstream that stimulate the body. Exercise is avoided 2 hours before bedtime.
- *Environment.* People adjust to their usual sleep settings. They get used to such things as the bed, pillows, noises, lighting, and a sleeping partner. Any change in the usual setting can affect the amount and quality of sleep.
- *Drugs and other substances.* Sleeping pills promote sleep. Drugs for anxiety, depression, and pain may cause the person to sleep. However, these drugs and sleeping pills reduce the length of REM sleep. Mental restoration occurs during REM sleep. Behavior problems and sleep deprivation can occur. Alcohol is a drug. It causes drowsiness and sleep. However, it interferes with REM sleep. Those under the influence of alcohol may awaken during sleep. Difficulty returning to sleep is common. Some drugs contain caffeine. Caffeine is a stimulant and prevents sleep. Besides drugs, caffeine is found in coffee, tea, chocolate, and colas. The side effects of some drugs cause frequent voiding and nightmares.
- *Life-style changes.* Life-style relates to a person's daily routines and way of living. Work, school, play, and social events are all part of life-style. Life-style changes can affect sleep. Travel, vacation, and social events often affect usual sleep and wake times. Children usually stay up later during school holidays. They may sleep later, too. If work hours change, sleep hours may change. Such changes affect normal sleep-wake cycles and the circadian rhythm.
- *Emotional problems.* Fear, worry, depression, and anxiety affect sleep. Causes include work, personal, or family problems. Loss of a loved one or friend is another cause. Money problems are stressful. People may have problems falling asleep, or they awaken often. Some have problems getting back to sleep.

Sleep Disorders

Sleep disorders involve repeated sleep problems. The amount and quality of sleep are affected. Sleep disorders affect life-style. Box 27-5 lists the signs and symptoms that occur.

Insomnia Insomnia is a chronic condition in which the person cannot sleep or stay asleep all night. There are three forms of insomnia:

- Cannot fall asleep
- Cannot stay asleep
- Early awakening and cannot fall back asleep

Emotional problems are common causes of insomnia. The fear of dying during sleep is another cause. Some people are afraid of not waking up. This may occur with heart disease or when told of a terminal illness. The fear of not being able to sleep is another cause. The physical and emotional discomforts of illness can also cause insomnia.

The nurse plans measures to promote sleep. However, the emotional or physical problems causing the insomnia also are treated.

Box 27-5 Signs and Symptoms of Sleep Disorders

- Agitation
- Attention: decreased
- Coordination: problems with
- Disorientation
- Eyes: red, puffy, dark circles under the eyes
- Fatigue
- Hallucinations (Chapters 43 and 44)
- Irritability
- Memory: reduced word memory; problems finding the right word
- Mood: moodiness; mood swings
- Pulse: irregular
- Reasoning and judgment: decreased
- Responses to questions, conversations, or situations: slowed
- Restlessness
- Sleepiness
- Speech: slurred
- Tremors: in the hands

TEAMWORK AND TIME MANAGEMENT
Sleepwalking

You may find a person sleepwalking. Help him or her back to bed even if you are not assigned to provide the person's care. Provide for the person's comfort. Then tell the nurse what happened and what you did.

Sleep Deprivation With sleep deprivation, the amount and quality of sleep are decreased. Sleep is interrupted. NREM and REM sleep stages are not completed. Illness, pain, and hospital care are common causes. Factors that affect sleep can also lead to sleep deprivation. The signs and symptoms in Box 27-5 may occur.

Sleepwalking The person leaves the bed and walks about. The person is not aware of sleepwalking. He or she has no memory of the event on awakening. Children sleepwalk more than adults. The event may last 3 to 4 minutes or longer.

Stress, fatigue, and some drugs are common causes. Protect the person from injury. Falling is a risk. Care tubings (intravenous, catheters, naso-gastric) can cause injury. They can be pulled out of the body when the person gets out of bed. Guide sleepwalkers back to bed. They startle easily. Awaken them gently.

See *Teamwork and Time Management: Sleepwalking.*

Promoting Sleep

The nurse assesses the person's sleep patterns. Report any of the signs and symptoms listed in Box 27-5. Measures are planned to promote sleep (Box 27-6). Follow the care plan. Also report your observations about how the person slept. This helps the nurse evaluate if the person has a regular sleep pattern.

Many people have rituals and routines before bedtime. They are important to the person. They are allowed if safe. The person may perform personal hygiene in a certain order. A bedtime snack may be important. Some watch certain TV shows in bed. Others read religious writings, pray, or say a rosary before going to sleep.

Older persons have less energy than younger people. They may nap during the day. Let the person sleep. Plan the person's care to allow uninterrupted naps.

The person is involved in planning care. The person chooses when to nap or go to bed. The person chooses the measures that promote comfort, rest, and sleep. Follow the care plan and the person's wishes.

See *Residents With Dementia: Promoting Sleep.*

Box 27-6   Nursing Measures to Promote Sleep

- Plan care for uninterrupted rest.
- Avoid physical activity before bedtime.
- Encourage the person to avoid business or family matters before bedtime.
- Allow a flexible bedtime. Bedtime is when the person is tired, not a certain time.
- Provide a comfortable room temperature.
- Let the person take a warm bath or shower.
- Provide a bedtime snack.
- Avoid caffeine (coffee, tea, colas, chocolate).
- Avoid alcoholic beverages.
- Have the person void before going to bed.
- Make sure incontinent persons are clean and dry.
- Follow bedtime routines.
- Have the person wear loose-fitting sleepwear.
- Provide for warmth (blankets, socks) for those who tend to be cold.
- Reduce noise.
- Darken the room—close window coverings and the privacy curtain. Shut off or dim lights.
- Dim lights in hallways and the nursing unit.
- Make sure linens are clean, dry, and wrinkle-free.
- Position the person in good alignment and in a comfortable position.
- Support body parts as ordered.
- Give a back massage.
- Provide measures to relieve pain.
- Let the person read. Or read to the person if he or she wants you to.
- Let the person listen to music or watch TV.
- Assist with relaxation exercises as ordered.
- Sit and talk with the person.

RESIDENTS WITH DEMENTIA
Promoting Sleep

Sleep problems are common in persons with Alzheimer's disease and other dementias. Night wandering is common. Restlessness and confusion often increase at night. This increases the risk of falls. It may help to quietly and calmly direct the person to his or her room. Night-time wandering in a safe and supervised setting is the best approach for some persons. The measures listed in Box 27-6 are tried. Follow the care plan.

QUALITY OF LIFE

Comfort, rest, and sleep are needed for quality of life and well-being. OBRA and the CMS require measures that promote comfort, rest, and sleep. They relate to the bed, mattress, room temperature, noise level, lighting, linens, odors, and the number of persons in each room. The right to personal choice and taking part in planning care also promote comfort, rest, and sleep.

Comfort involves more than physical needs alone. Emotional, spiritual, and social needs must also be met. Time spent with friends and family provides comfort for residents. For some, religious ceremonies or rituals promote peace and healing. Allow time and privacy for these needs.

Residents have the right to have pain assessed and managed. Untreated pain decreases quality of life. You must report signs and symptoms of pain. This helps the nurse meet the person's needs.

REVIEW QUESTIONS

Circle the BEST answer.

1 These statements are about pain. Which is *false?*
 a Pain can be seen, heard, smelled, or felt.
 b Pain is a warning from the body.
 c Pain differs for each person.
 d Pain is used to make diagnoses.

2 A person has pain in the left chest, the left jaw, and the left shoulder and arm. This is
 a Acute pain
 b Chronic pain
 c Radiating pain
 d Phantom pain

3 A person complains of pain. You should ask the person to do the following *except*
 a Point to where the pain is felt
 b Tell you when the pain started
 c Describe the pain
 d Let you look at the pain

4 The nurse gives a person a drug for pain relief. When should you give scheduled care?
 a Before the drug is given
 b Right after the drug is given
 c 30 minutes after the drug was given
 d The next day

5 A drug was given for pain relief. To promote safety, you should do the following *except*
 a Keep the bed in the high position
 b Raise bed rails as directed
 c Check on the person every 10 to 15 minutes
 d Provide help if the person needs to get up

6 Which measure will *not* help relieve pain?
 a Providing blankets as needed
 b Keeping lights on in the room
 c Providing soft music
 d Giving a back massage

7 A person's care plan has these measures. Which will *not* promote rest or sleep?
 a Voiding before rest or sleep
 b Positioning in a comfortable position
 c Having the person walk before rest or sleep
 d Letting the person choose sleepwear

8 A person tires easily. Morning care includes a bath, hair care, getting dressed, and making the bed. When should the person rest?
 a After you complete morning care
 b After the bath and before hair care
 c After you make the bed
 d When the person needs to

9 These statements are about sleep. Which is *false?*
 a Tissue healing and repair occur during sleep.
 b Voluntary muscle activity increases during sleep.
 c Sleep refreshes and renews the person.
 d Sleep lowers stress, tension, and anxiety.

10 A person was awake several nights. Which is *false?*
 a Circadian rhythm may be affected.
 b NREM and REM sleep are affected.
 c The person's biological clock still tells when to sleep and wake up.
 d Functioning may be affected.

11 A healthy 70-year-old person needs about
 a 12 to 14 hours of sleep per day
 b 8 to 9 hours of sleep per day
 c 7 to 8 hours of sleep per day
 d 5 to 7 hours of sleep per day

12 Which prevents sleep?
 a Chocolate
 b Cheese
 c Milk
 d Beef

13 These measures for sleep are in the person's care plan. Which should you question?
 a Let the person choose the bedtime.
 b Provide hot tea and a cheese sandwich at bedtime.
 c Position the person in good alignment.
 d Follow the person's bedtime rituals.

Circle T if the statement is TRUE. Circle F if the statement is FALSE.

14 T F Changes in usual behavior may signal pain.
15 T F Persons with dementia usually sleep well at night.
16 T F A person's culture may affect how he or she reacts to pain.

Answers to these questions are on p. 720.

Oxygen Needs

OBJECTIVES

- Define the key terms and key abbreviations listed in this chapter.
- Describe the factors affecting oxygen needs.
- List the signs and symptoms of hypoxia and altered respiratory function.
- Describe the tests used to diagnose respiratory problems.

- Explain the measures that promote oxygenation.
- Describe the devices used to give oxygen.
- Explain how to safely assist with oxygen therapy.
- Perform the procedures described in this chapter.
- Explain how to promote quality of life.

KEY TERMS

allergy A sensitivity to a substance that causes the body to react with signs and symptoms

apnea The lack or absence *(a)* of breathing *(pnea)*

Biot's respirations Rapid and deep respirations followed by 10 to 30 seconds of apnea

bradypnea Slow *(brady)* breathing *(pnea)*; respirations are fewer than 12 per minute

Cheyne-Stokes respirations Respirations gradually increase in rate and depth and then become shallow and slow; breathing may stop *(apnea)* for 10 to 20 seconds

cyanosis Bluish color to the skin, lips, mucous membranes, and nail beds

dyspnea Difficult, labored, or painful *(dys)* breathing *(pnea)*

hemoptysis Bloody *(hemo)* sputum *(ptysis* means *to spit)*

hyperventilation Respirations *(ventilation)* are rapid *(hyper)* and deeper than normal

hypoventilation Respirations *(ventilation)* are slow *(hypo)*, shallow, and sometimes irregular

hypoxemia A reduced amount *(hypo)* of oxygen *(ox)* in the blood *(emia)*

hypoxia Cells do not have enough *(hypo)* oxygen *(oxia)*

Kussmaul respirations Very deep and rapid respirations

orthopnea Breathing *(pnea)* deeply and comfortably only when sitting *(ortho)*

orthopneic position Sitting up *(ortho)* and leaning over a table to breathe *(pneic)*

oxygen concentration The amount (percent) of hemoglobin containing oxygen

pollutant A harmful chemical or substance in the air or water

respiratory arrest When breathing stops

respiratory depression Slow, weak respirations at a rate of fewer than 12 per minute

sputum Mucus from the respiratory system that is expectorated *(expelled)* through the mouth

tachypnea Rapid *(tachy)* breathing *(pnea)*; respirations are more than 20 per minute

KEY ABBREVIATIONS

CO_2	Carbon dioxide	RBC	Red blood cell
ID	Identification	SpO_2	Saturation of peripheral oxygen (pulse oximetry)
L/min	Liters per minute		
O_2	Oxygen		

Oxygen (O_2) is a gas. It has no taste, odor, or color. It is a basic need required for life. Death occurs within minutes if breathing stops. Brain damage and serious illness can occur without enough oxygen. Illness, surgery, and injuries affect the amount of oxygen in the blood and cells.

You assist in the care of persons with oxygen needs. You must give safe and effective care.

FACTORS AFFECTING OXYGEN NEEDS

The respiratory and circulatory systems must function properly for cells to get enough oxygen. Any disease, injury, or surgery involving these systems affects the intake and use of oxygen. Body systems depend on each other. Altered function of any system (for example, the nervous, musculo-skeletal, or urinary system) affects oxygen needs. Oxygen needs are affected by:

- *Respiratory system.* Structures must be intact and function properly. An open *(patent)* airway is needed. Alveoli (air sacs) must exchange O_2 and carbon dioxide (CO_2).
- *Circulatory system.* Blood must flow to and from the heart. Narrowed vessels affect blood flow. Capillaries and cells must exchange O_2 and CO_2.
- *Red blood cell count.* Red blood cells (RBCs) contain hemoglobin. Hemoglobin picks up O_2 in the lungs and carries it to the cells. The bone marrow must produce enough RBCs. Poor diet, chemotherapy, and leukemia affect bone marrow function. Blood loss also reduces the number of RBCs.
- *Nervous system.* Nervous system diseases and injuries can affect respiratory muscles. Breathing may be difficult or impossible. Brain damage affects respiratory rate, rhythm, and depth. Narcotics and depressant drugs affect the brain. They slow respirations. O_2 and CO_2 blood levels also affect brain function. Respirations increase to bring in more O_2. They also increase to rid the body of excess CO_2.
- *Aging.* Respiratory muscles weaken. Lung tissue is less elastic. Strength for coughing decreases. The person must cough and remove secretions from the upper airway. Otherwise, *pneumonia* (inflammation and infection of the lung) can develop. Respiratory complications are risks after surgery.

- *Exercise.* O_2 needs increase with exercise. Respiratory rate and depth increase to bring in O_2. Persons with heart and respiratory diseases may have enough oxygen at rest. However, even slight activity can increase O_2 needs. Their bodies may not be able to bring in O_2 and carry it to the cells.
- *Fever.* O_2 needs increase. Respiratory rate and depth increase to meet the body's needs.
- *Pain.* O_2 needs increase. Respirations increase to meet this need. Chest and abdominal injuries and surgeries often involve respiratory muscles. It hurts to breathe in and out.
- *Drugs.* Some drugs depress the respiratory center in the brain. **Respiratory depression** means slow, weak respirations at a rate of fewer than 12 per minute. Respirations are too shallow to bring enough O_2 into the lungs. **Respiratory arrest** is when breathing stops. Narcotics (morphine, Demerol, and others) can have these effects. (Narcotic comes from the Greek word *narkoun*. It means *stupor* or *to be numb*.) In safe amounts, these drugs relieve severe pain. Substance abusers are at risk for respiratory depression and respiratory arrest from drug over-doses.
- *Smoking.* Smoking causes lung cancer and chronic obstructive pulmonary disease (COPD). It is a risk factor for coronary artery disease.
- *Allergies.* An **allergy** is a sensitivity to a substance that causes the body to react with signs and symptoms. Runny nose, wheezing, and congestion are common. Mucous membranes in the upper airway swell. With severe swelling, the airway closes. Shock and death are risks. Pollens, dust, foods, drugs, insect bites, and cigarette smoke often cause allergies. Chronic bronchitis and asthma are risks.
- *Pollutant exposure.* A **pollutant** is a harmful chemical or substance in the air or water. Examples are dust, fumes, toxins, asbestos, coal dust, and sawdust. They damage the lungs. Pollutant exposure occurs in home, work, and public settings.
- *Nutrition.* The body needs iron and vitamins (vitamin B_{12}, vitamin C, and folate) to produce RBCs.
- *Alcohol.* Alcohol depresses the brain. Excessive amounts reduce the cough reflex and increase the risk of aspiration. Obstructed airway and pneumonia are risks from aspiration.

Box 28-1   Signs and Symptoms of Hypoxia

- Restlessness
- Dizziness
- Disorientation
- Confusion
- Behavior and personality changes
- Concentrating and following directions: problems with
- Apprehension
- Anxiety
- Fatigue
- Agitation
- Pulse rate: increased
- Respirations: increased rate and depth
- Sitting position: often leaning forward
- Cyanosis (bluish color to the skin, lips, mucous membranes, and nail beds)
- Dyspnea

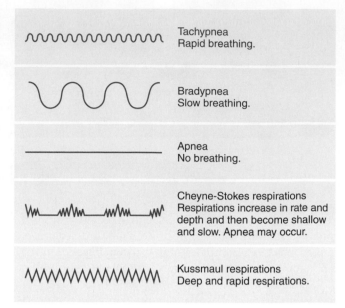

Tachypnea
Rapid breathing.

Bradypnea
Slow breathing.

Apnea
No breathing.

Cheyne-Stokes respirations
Respirations increase in rate and depth and then become shallow and slow. Apnea may occur.

Kussmaul respirations
Deep and rapid respirations.

Fig. 28-1 Some abnormal breathing patterns. *(Modified from Talbot L, Meyers-Marquardt M: Pocket guide to critical care assessment, ed 3, St Louis, 1997, Mosby.)*

ALTERED RESPIRATORY FUNCTION

Respiratory function involves three processes. Respiratory function is altered if even one process is affected.
- Air moves into and out of the lungs.
- O_2 and CO_2 are exchanged at the alveoli.
- The blood carries O_2 to the cells and removes CO_2 from them.

Hypoxia

Hypoxia means that cells do not have enough *(hypo)* oxygen *(oxia)*. Without enough oxygen, cells cannot function properly. Anything affecting respiratory function can cause hypoxia. The brain is very sensitive to inadequate O_2. Restlessness is an early sign. So are dizziness and disorientation. Report the signs and symptoms in Box 28-1 at once.

Hypoxia threatens life. All organs need oxygen to function. Oxygen is given. The cause of hypoxia is treated.

Abnormal Respirations

Normal adult respirations are 12 to 20 per minute. They are quiet, effortless, and regular. Both sides of the chest rise and fall equally. These breathing patterns are abnormal (Fig. 28-1):
- **Tachypnea**—rapid *(tachy)* breathing *(pnea)*. Respirations are more than 20 per minute. Fever, exercise, pain, pregnancy, airway obstruction, and hypoxemia are common causes. **Hypoxemia** is a reduced amount *(hypo)* of oxygen *(ox)* in the blood *(emia)*.
- **Bradypnea**—slow *(brady)* breathing *(pnea)*. Respirations are fewer than 12 per minute. Drug over-dose and nervous system disorders are common causes.
- **Apnea**—lack or absence *(a)* of breathing *(pnea)*. It occurs in sudden cardiac arrest and respiratory arrest. Sleep apnea is another type of apnea.
- **Hypoventilation**—respirations *(ventilation)* are slow *(hypo)*, shallow, and sometimes irregular. Lung disorders affecting the alveoli are common causes. Pneumonia is an example. Other causes include obesity, airway obstruction, and drug side effects. Nervous system and musculo-skeletal disorders affecting the respiratory muscles also are causes.
- **Hyperventilation**—respirations *(ventilation)* are rapid *(hyper)* and deeper than normal. Causes include asthma, emphysema, infection, fever, nervous system disorders, hypoxia, anxiety, pain, and some drugs.
- **Dyspnea**—difficult, labored, or painful *(dys)* breathing *(pnea)*. Heart disease and anxiety are common causes.
- **Cheyne-Stokes respirations**—respirations gradually increase in rate and depth. Then they become shallow and slow. Breathing may stop *(apnea)* for 10 to 20 seconds. Drug over-dose, heart failure, renal failure, and brain disorders are common causes. Cheyne-Stokes are common when death is near.
- **Orthopnea**—breathing *(pnea)* deeply and comfortably only when sitting *(ortho)*. Common causes are emphysema, asthma, pneumonia, angina, and other heart and respiratory disorders.
- **Biot's respirations**—rapid and deep respirations followed by 10 to 30 seconds of apnea. They occur with nervous system disorders.
- **Kussmaul respirations**—very deep and rapid respirations. They signal diabetic coma.

Box 28-2 Signs and Symptoms of Altered Respiratory Function

- Hypoxia: signs and symptoms of (see Box 28-1)
- Breathing pattern: abnormal
- Shortness of breath or complaints of being "winded" or "short-winded"
- Cough (note frequency and time of day)
  - Dry and hacking
  - Harsh and barking
  - Productive (produces sputum) or non-productive
- Sputum (mucus from the respiratory system)
  - Color: clear, white, yellow, green, brown, or red
  - Odor: none or foul odor
  - Consistency: thick, watery, or frothy (with bubbles or foam)
  - Hemoptysis: bloody (hemo) sputum (ptysis means to spit); note if the sputum is bright red, dark red, blood-tinged, or streaked with blood
- Respirations: noisy
  - Wheezing
  - Wet-sounding
  - Crowing sounds
- Chest pain (note location)
  - Constant or comes and goes
  - Person's description (stabbing, knife-like, aching)
  - What makes it worse (movement, coughing, yawning, sneezing, sighing, deep breathing)
- Cyanosis (bluish color)
  - Skin
  - Mucous membranes
  - Lips
  - Nail beds
- Vital signs: changes in
- Position
  - Sitting upright
  - Leaning forward or hunched over a table

FOCUS ON COMMUNICATION
Assisting With Assessment and Diagnostic Tests

The questions you ask the person aid the nurse in the assessment step of the nursing process. For example:
- "Do you need more pillows?"
- "Do you want the head of your bed raised more?"
- "How often are you coughing?"
- "Are you coughing anything up?"
- "Please use a tissue when you cough up mucus, then put on your signal light. The nurse needs to observe the mucus."

ASSISTING WITH ASSESSMENT AND DIAGNOSTIC TESTS

Altered respiratory function may be an acute or chronic problem. Report your observations promptly and accurately (Box 28-2). Quick action is needed to meet the person's oxygen needs. Measures are taken to correct the problem and to prevent it from becoming worse.

See Focus on Communication: Assisting With Assessment and Diagnostic Tests.

The doctor orders tests to find the cause of the problem. These tests are commonly done in hospitals:

- *Chest x-ray (CXR).* An x-ray is taken of the chest to study lung changes.
- *Lung scan.* The lungs are scanned to see what areas are not getting air or blood. The person inhales radioactive gas. *Radioactive* means to give off radiation. A radioisotope is injected into a vein. A *radioisotope* is a substance that gives off radiation. Lung tissue getting air and blood flow "take up" the substance.

- *Bronchoscopy.* A scope *(scopy)* is passed into the trachea and bronchi *(broncho)*. Airway structures are checked for bleeding and tumors. Tissue samples *(biopsies)* are taken. Or mucous plugs and foreign objects are removed. The person is NPO (non per os; nothing by mouth) for 6 to 8 hours before the procedure. This reduces the risks of vomiting and aspiration. An anesthetic is given. After the procedure, the person is NPO and observed carefully until the gag and swallow reflexes return. This can take about 2 hours.
- *Thoracentesis.* The pleura *(thora)* is punctured. Air or fluid is removed *(centesis)* from it. The doctor inserts a needle through the chest wall into the pleural sac (Fig. 28-2, p. 446). Injury or disease can cause the sac to fill with air, blood, or fluid. Anti-cancer drugs can be injected into the pleural sac. The procedure takes a few minutes. Vital signs are taken. Then a local anesthetic is given. The person sits up and leans forward. He or she must not talk, cough, or move suddenly. Afterward a dressing is applied to the puncture site. Vital signs are taken. A chest x-ray is taken to detect lung damage. The person is observed for shortness of breath, dyspnea, cough, sputum, chest pain, cyanosis, vital sign changes, and other respiratory signs and symptoms.
- *Pulmonary function tests.* These measure the amount of air moving into and out of the lungs *(volume)*. They also measure how much air the lungs can hold *(capacity)*. The person takes as deep a breath as possible. Using a mouthpiece, the person blows into a machine (Fig. 28-3, p. 446). The tests help assess the risk for lung diseases or post-operative lung complications. They also measure the progress of lung disease and its treatment. Fatigue is common after the tests. The person needs to rest.
- *Arterial blood gases (ABGs).* A radial, femoral, or brachial artery is punctured to obtain arterial blood. Laboratory tests measure the amount of O_2 in the blood. Bleeding from the artery must be prevented. Pressure is applied to the artery for at least 5 minutes after the procedure. Pressure is applied longer if there are blood-clotting problems.

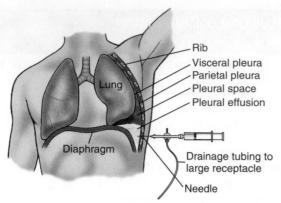

Fig. 28-2 Thoracentesis. *(Modified from Monahan FD, Neighbors M: Foundations for clinical practice, ed 2, Philadelphia, 1998, Saunders.)*

Rib
Visceral pleura
Parietal pleura
Pleural space
Pleural effusion
Lung
Diaphragm
Drainage tubing to large receptacle
Needle

Fig. 28-3 Pulmonary function testing.

Fig. 28-4 A pulse oximetry sensor is attached to a finger.

Pulse Oximetry

Pulse oximetry measures *(metry)* the oxygen *(oxi)* concentration in arterial blood. **Oxygen concentration** is the amount (percent) of hemoglobin containing O_2. Measurements are used to prevent and treat hypoxia. The normal range is 95% to 100%. For example, if 97% of all hemoglobin (100%) carries O_2, tissues get enough oxygen. If only 90% contains O_2, tissues do not get enough oxygen. As low as 85% may be normal for persons with some chronic diseases.

A sensor attaches to a finger, toe, earlobe, nose, or forehead (Fig. 28-4). Light beams on one side of the sensor pass through the tissues. A detector on the other side measures the amount of light passing through the tissues. With this information, the oximeter measures the O_2 concentration. The value and pulse rate are shown. Oximeter alarms are set when continuous monitoring is needed. An alarm sounds if:

- O_2 concentration is low
- The pulse is too fast or slow
- Other problems occur

A good sensor site is needed. Avoid swollen sites and sites with skin breaks. Aging and vascular disease often cause poor circulation. Sometimes blood flow to the fingers or toes is poor. Then the earlobe, nose, and forehead sites are used.

Bright light, nail polish, fake nails, and movements affect measurements. Place a towel over the sensor to block bright light. Remove nail polish, or use another site. Do not use a finger site if the person has fake nails. Movements from shivering, seizures, or tremors affect finger sensors. The earlobe is a better site for such problems. Blood pressure cuffs affect blood flow. If using a finger site, do not measure blood pressure on that side.

Report and record oxygen concentration accurately according to center policy. A center may use:

- Pulse oximetry or pulse ox
- O_2 saturation or O_2 sat
- SpO_2 (saturation of peripheral oxygen)
  See *Promoting Safety and Comfort: Pulse Oximetry.*
  See *Delegation Guidelines: Pulse Oximetry.*

PROMOTING SAFETY AND COMFORT
Pulse Oximetry

Safety
The person's condition can change rapidly. Pulse oximetry does not lessen the need for good observations. Observe for signs and symptoms of hypoxia (see Box 28-1) and altered respiratory system function (see Box 28-2).

Comfort
A clip-on sensor feels like a clothespin when applied. It should not hurt or cause discomfort. Ask the person to tell you at once if it causes pain, discomfort, or too much pressure. Change the sensor site when the nurse tells you to do so.

Delegation Guidelines
Pulse Oximetry

When assisting with pulse oximetry, you need this information from the nurse and the care plan:
- What site to use
- How to use the equipment
- What sensor to use
- What type of tape to use
- The normal SpO$_2$ range for the person
- Alarm limits for SpO$_2$ and pulse rate for continuous monitoring:
  - Tell the nurse at once if the SpO$_2$ goes below the alarm limit (usually 95%)
  - Tell the nurse at once if the pulse rate goes above or below the alarm limit
- When to do the measurement

- What pulse site to use: apical or radial
- How often to check the sensor site (usually every 2 hours)
- What observations to report and record:
  - The date and time
  - The SpO$_2$ and display pulse rate
  - Apical or radial pulse rate
  - What the person was doing at the time
  - Oxygen flow rate (p. 453) and the device used (p. 452)
  - Reason for the measurement: routine or condition change
- When to report observations
- What specific resident concerns to report at once

USING A PULSE OXIMETER

VIDEO

QUALITY OF LIFE

Remember to:
- Knock before entering the person's room.
- Address the person by name.
- Introduce yourself by name and title.

- Explain the procedure to the person before beginning and during the procedure.
- Protect the person's rights during the procedure.
- Handle the person gently during the procedure.

PRE-PROCEDURE

1 Follow *Delegation Guidelines: Pulse Oximetry*. See *Promoting Safety and Comfort: Pulse Oximetry*.
2 Practice hand hygiene.
3 Collect the following before going to the person's room:
   - Oximeter and sensor
   - Tape
   - Towel

4 Arrange your work area.
5 Decontaminate your hands.
6 Identify the person. Check the identification (ID) bracelet against your assignment sheet. Also call the person by name.
7 Provide for privacy.

PROCEDURE

8 Provide for comfort.
9 Dry the site with a towel.
10 Clip or tape the sensor to the site.
11 Turn on the oximeter.
12 Set the high and low alarm limits for SpO$_2$ and pulse rate. Turn on audio and visual alarms. (This step is for continuous monitoring.)

13 Check the person's pulse (apical or radial) with the pulse on the display. The pulses should be about the same. Note both pulse rates on your assignment sheet.
14 Read the SpO$_2$ on the display. Note the value on the flow sheet and your assignment sheet.
15 Leave the sensor in place for continuous monitoring. Otherwise, turn off the device and remove the sensor.

POST-PROCEDURE

16 Provide for comfort. (See the inside of the front book cover.)
17 Place the signal light within reach.
18 Unscreen the person.
19 Complete a safety check of the room. (See the inside of the front book cover.)

20 Return the device to its proper place (unless monitoring is continuous).
21 Decontaminate your hands.
22 Report and record the SpO$_2$, the pulse rates, and your other observations.

Sputum Specimens

Respiratory disorders cause the lungs, bronchi, and trachea to secrete mucus. Mucus from the respiratory system is called **sputum** when expectorated *(expelled)* through the mouth. Sputum specimens are studied for blood, microbes, and abnormal cells. See Chapter 33.

PROMOTING OXYGENATION

To get enough oxygen, air must move deep into the lungs. Air must reach the alveoli where O_2 and CO_2 are exchanged. Disease and injury can prevent air from reaching the alveoli. Pain and immobility interfere with deep breathing and coughing. So do narcotics. Therefore secretions collect in the airway and lungs. They interfere with air movement and lung function. Secretions also provide a place for microbes to grow and multiply. Infection is a threat.

Oxygen needs must be met. The following measures are common in care plans.

Positioning

Breathing is usually easier in semi-Fowler's and Fowler's positions. Persons with difficulty breathing often prefer sitting up and leaning over a table to breathe. This is called the **orthopneic position**. (*Ortho* means *sitting* or *standing*. *Pneic* means *breathing*.) Place a pillow on the table to increase the person's comfort (Fig. 28-5).

Frequent position changes are needed. Unless the doctor limits positioning, the person must not lie on one side for a long time. Secretions pool. The lungs cannot expand on that side. Position changes are needed at least every 2 hours. Follow the care plan.

Fig. 28-5 The person is in the orthopneic position. A pillow is on the overbed table for the person's comfort.

Deep Breathing and Coughing

Deep breathing moves air into most parts of the lungs. Coughing removes mucus. Deep-breathing and coughing exercises promote oxygenation. They are done after surgery or injury and during bedrest. The exercises are painful after surgery or injury. Breaking an incision open while coughing is a fear.

Deep breathing and coughing help prevent pneumonia and atelectasis. *Atelectasis* is the collapse of a portion of the lung. It occurs when mucus collects in the airway. Air cannot get to a part of the lung. The lung collapses. Atelectasis is a risk after surgery. Bedrest, lung diseases, and paralysis are other risk factors.

Deep breathing and coughing are usually done every 2 hours while the person is awake. Sometimes they are done every hour while the person is awake.

See *Focus on Communication: Deep Breathing and Coughing.*

See *Delegation Guidelines: Deep Breathing and Coughing.*

See *Promoting Safety and Comfort: Deep Breathing and Coughing.*

FOCUS ON COMMUNICATION
Deep Breathing and Coughing

To encourage cough etiquette (Chapter 15), you can say: "Please remember to cover your nose and mouth when coughing. I'll put these tissues where you can reach them. Here is a waste container to dispose of your tissues. Where would you like me to place it? Also, please remember to disinfect or wash your hands often. Let me know if you need help."

DELEGATION GUIDELINES
Deep Breathing and Coughing

When delegated deep-breathing and coughing exercises, you need this information from the nurse and the care plan:

- When to do them
- How many deep breaths and coughs the person needs to do
- What observations to report and record:
  - The number of deep breaths and coughs
  - How the person tolerated the procedure
- When to report observations
- What specific resident concerns to report at once

PROMOTING SAFETY AND COMFORT
Deep Breathing and Coughing

Safety

Respiratory hygiene and cough etiquette are needed if the person has a productive cough (Chapter 15). The person needs to:

- Cover the nose and mouth when coughing or sneezing.
- Use tissues to contain respiratory secretions.
- Dispose of tissues in the nearest waste container after use.
- Wash his or her hands after coughing or contact with respiratory secretions.

Fig. 28-6 The hands are over the rib cage for deep breathing.

ASSISTING WITH DEEP-BREATHING AND COUGHING EXERCISES | VIDEO

QUALITY OF LIFE

Remember to:
- Knock before entering the person's room.
- Address the person by name.
- Introduce yourself by name and title.

- Explain the procedure to the person before beginning and during the procedure.
- Protect the person's rights during the procedure.
- Handle the person gently during the procedure.

PRE-PROCEDURE

1 Follow *Delegation Guidelines: Deep Breathing and Coughing.* See *Promoting Safety and Comfort: Deep Breathing and Coughing.*
2 Practice hand hygiene.

3 Identify the person. Check the ID bracelet against the assignment sheet. Also call the person by name.
4 Provide for privacy.

PROCEDURE

5 Lower the bed rail if up.
6 Help the person to a comfortable sitting position: sitting on the side of the bed, semi-Fowler's, or Fowler's.
7 Have the person deep breathe:
  a Have the person place the hands over the rib cage (Fig. 28-6).
  b Have the person take a deep breath. It should be as deep as possible. Remind the person to inhale through the nose.
  c Ask the person to hold the breath for 2 to 3 seconds.
  d Ask the person to exhale slowly through pursed lips (Fig. 28-7, p. 450). Ask the person to exhale until the ribs move as far down as possible.
  e Repeat this step 4 more times.

8 Ask the person to cough:
  a Have the person place both hands over the incision. One hand is on top of the other (Fig. 28-8, *A,* p. 450). The person can hold a pillow or folded towel over the incision (Fig. 28-8, *B,* p. 450).
  b Have the person take in a deep breath as in step 7.
  c Ask the person to cough strongly twice with the mouth open.

POST-PROCEDURE

9 Provide for comfort. (See the inside of the front book cover.)
10 Place the signal light within reach.
11 Raise or lower bed rails. Follow the care plan.
12 Unscreen the person.

13 Complete a safety check of the room. (See the inside of the front book cover.)
14 Decontaminate your hands.
15 Report and record your observations (Fig. 28-9, p. 450).

Fig. 28-7 The person inhales through the nose and exhales through pursed lips during the deep-breathing exercise.

Fig. 28-8 The person supports an incision for the coughing exercises. **A,** The hands are over the incision. **B,** A pillow is held over the incision.

Date	Time	Nursing Margin	Other Depts Margin
3/15	0830	Assisted resident with deep-breathing and coughing exercises.	
		Resident performed exercises x2. He states "It is getting easier every	
		day." Denied pain or discomfort. Requested to sit in his chair after	
		the exercises. Tray table with water pitcher and glass, tissues, and	
		a book within reach. Signal light within reach. Jean Hein, CNA	

Fig. 28-9 Charting sample.

Incentive Spirometry

Incentive means to encourage. A *spirometer* is a machine that measures the amount *(volume)* of air inhaled. With incentive spirometry, the person is encouraged to inhale until reaching a preset volume of air. Balls or bars in the machine let the person see air movement when inhaling (Fig. 28-10).

Incentive spirometry also is called *sustained maximal inspiration (SMI)*. Sustained means constant. *Maximal* means the most or the greatest. And *inspiration* relates to breathing in. SMI means inhaling as deeply as possible and holding the breath for a certain time. The breath is usually held for at least 3 seconds.

The goal is to improve lung function. Atelectasis is prevented or treated. Like yawning or sighing, breathing is long, slow, and deep. This moves air deep into the lungs. Secretions loosen. O_2 and CO_2 exchange occurs between the alveoli and the capillaries.

The device is used as follows:

1. The spirometer is placed upright.
2. The person exhales normally.
3. He or she seals the lips around a mouthpiece.
4. A slow, deep breath is taken until the balls rise to the desired height.
5. The breath is held for 3 to 6 seconds to keep the balls floating.
6. The person removes the mouthpiece and exhales slowly. The person may cough at this time.
7. After some normal breaths, the device is used again.

See *Delegation Guidelines: Incentive Spirometry.*

Fig. 28-10 The person uses a spirometer.

DELEGATION GUIDELINES
Incentive Spirometry

Before assisting a person with incentive spirometry, you need this information from the nurse and the care plan:
- How often the person needs incentive spirometry
- How many breaths the person needs to take
- The desired height of the floating balls
- How to clean the mouthpiece
- When to replace the mouthpiece
- What observations to report and record:
  - How many breaths the person took
  - The height of the floating balls
  - If the person coughed after using the spirometer
  - How the person tolerated the incentive spirometry
- When to report observations
- What specific resident concerns to report at once

ASSISTING WITH OXYGEN THERAPY

Disease, injury, and surgery often interfere with breathing. The amount of O_2 in the blood may be less than normal (hypoxemia). If so, the doctor orders oxygen therapy.

Oxygen is treated as a drug. The doctor orders the amount of oxygen to give, the device to use, and when to give it. Some people need oxygen constantly. Others need it for symptom relief—chest pain or shortness of breath. Oxygen helps relieve chest pain. Persons with respiratory diseases may have enough oxygen at rest. With mild exercise or activity, they become short of breath. Oxygen helps to relieve shortness of breath.

You do not give oxygen. The nurse and respiratory therapist start and maintain oxygen therapy. You assist the nurse in providing safe care.

Oxygen Sources

Oxygen is supplied as follows:
- *Wall outlet.* O_2 is piped into each person's unit (Fig. 28-11).
- *Oxygen tank.* The oxygen tank is placed at the bedside. Small tanks are used during emergencies and transfers. They also are used by persons who walk or use wheelchairs (Fig. 28-12). A gauge tells how much oxygen is left (Fig. 28-13, p. 452).
- *Oxygen concentrator.* The machine removes oxygen from the air (Fig. 28-14, p. 452). A power source is needed. If the machine is not portable, the person stays near it. A portable oxygen tank is needed for power failures and mobility.
- *Liquid oxygen system.* A portable unit is filled from a stationary unit. The portable unit has enough oxygen for about 8 hours of use. A dial shows the amount of oxygen in the unit. The portable unit can be worn over the shoulder (Fig. 28-15, p. 452). This allows the person to be mobile.

See *Promoting Safety and Comfort: Oxygen Sources,* p. 452.

See *Teamwork and Time Management: Oxygen Sources,* p. 452.

Fig. 28-11 Wall oxygen outlet.

Fig. 28-12 A portable oxygen tank is used when walking.

Fig. 28-13 The gauge shows the amount of oxygen in the tank.

Fig. 28-14 Oxygen concentrator.

Fig. 28-15 A portable liquid oxygen unit is worn over the shoulder. *(Image used by permission from Nellcor Puritan Bennet LLC, Boulder, Colo; part of Covidien.)*

Oxygen Devices

The doctor orders the device for giving oxygen. These devices are common:

- *Nasal cannula* (Fig. 28-16). The prongs are inserted into the nostrils. A band goes behind the ears and under the chin to keep the device in place. A cannula allows eating and drinking. Tight prongs can irritate the nose. Pressure on the ears and cheekbones is possible.
- *Simple face mask* (Fig. 28-17). It covers the nose and mouth. The mask has small holes in the sides. CO_2 escapes when exhaling.
- *Partial-rebreather mask* (Fig. 28-18). A bag is added to the simple face mask. The bag is for exhaled air. When breathing in, the person inhales oxygen and some exhaled air. Some room air also is inhaled. The bag should not totally deflate when inhaling.
- *Non-rebreather mask* (Fig. 28-19). Exhaled air and room air cannot enter the bag. Exhaled air leaves through holes in the mask. When inhaling, only oxygen from the bag is inhaled. The bag must not totally collapse during inhalation.
- *Venturi mask* (Fig. 28-20). Precise amounts of oxygen are given. Color-coded adapters show the amount of oxygen given.

Talking and eating are hard to do with a mask. Listen carefully. Moisture can build up under the mask. Keep the face clean and dry. This helps prevent irritation from the mask. Masks are removed for eating. Usually oxygen is given by cannula during meals.

Fig. 28-16 Nasal cannula.

Fig. 28-17 Simple face mask.

Fig. 28-18 Partial-rebreather mask.

Fig. 28-19 Non-rebreather mask.

Fig. 28-20 Venturi mask.

Fig. 28-21 The flowmeter is used to set the oxygen flow rate.

Oxygen Flow Rates

The *flow rate* is the amount of oxygen given. It is measured in liters per minute (L/min). The doctor orders 2 to 15 liters of O_2 per minute. The nurse or respiratory therapist sets the flow rate (Fig. 28-21).

The nurse and care plan tell you the person's flow rate. When giving care and checking the person, always check the flow rate. Tell the nurse at once if it is too high or too low. A nurse or respiratory therapist will adjust the flow rate. Some states and centers let nursing assistants adjust O_2 flow rates. Know your center's policy.

✉ Oxygen Administration Set-Up

Oxygen is a dry gas. If not humidified (made moist), oxygen dries the airway's mucous membranes. Distilled water is added to the humidifier (Fig. 28-22). (Distilled water is pure. Dissolved salts were removed by a chemical process.)

When added to the humidifier, the distilled water creates water vapor. Oxygen picks up the water vapor as it flows into the system. Bubbling in the humidifier means that water vapor is being produced. Low flow rates (1 to 2 L/min) by cannula are not usually humidified.

See *Delegation Guidelines: Oxygen Administration Set-Up.*

See *Promoting Safety and Comfort: Oxygen Administration Set-Up.*

See *Teamwork and Time Management: Oxygen Administration Set-Up.*

Fig. 28-22 Oxygen administration system with humidifier.

DELEGATION GUIDELINES
Oxygen Administration Set-Up

If setting up oxygen is delegated to you, you need this information from the nurse:
• The person's name and room and bed number
• What oxygen device was ordered
• If humidification was ordered

PROMOTING SAFETY AND COMFORT
Oxygen Administration Set-Up

Safety
You do not give oxygen. Tell the nurse when the oxygen administration system is set up. The nurse turns on the oxygen, sets the flow rate, and applies the oxygen device.
    Practice medical asepsis. Do not let the connecting tubing hang on the floor.

TEAMWORK AND TIME MANAGEMENT
Oxygen Administration Set-Up

As you walk past the room of any person receiving oxygen, always check the humidifier. Make sure the humidifier is bubbling. Also make sure it has enough water. Tell the nurse if:
• There is no bubbling.
• The water level is low.

Oxygen Safety

You assist the nurse with oxygen therapy. You do not give oxygen. You do not adjust the flow rate unless allowed by your state and center. However, you must give safe care. Follow the rules in Box 28-3. Also follow the rules for fire and the use of oxygen (Chapter 12).

SETTING UP FOR OXYGEN ADMINISTRATION

QUALITY OF LIFE

Remember to:
- Knock before entering the person's room.
- Address the person by name.
- Introduce yourself by name and title.

- Explain the procedure to the person before beginning and during the procedure.
- Protect the person's rights during the procedure.
- Handle the person gently during the procedure.

PRE-PROCEDURE

1. Follow *Delegation Guidelines: Oxygen Administration Set-Up.* See *Promoting Safety and Comfort: Oxygen Administration Set-Up.*
2. Practice hand hygiene.
3. Collect the following before going to the person's room:
   - Oxygen device with connecting tubing
   - Flowmeter

   - Humidifier (if ordered)
   - Distilled water (if using a humidifier)
4. Arrange your work area.
5. Decontaminate your hands.
6. Identify the person. Check the ID bracelet against the assignment sheet. Also call the person by name.

PROCEDURE

7. Make sure the flowmeter is in the *OFF* position.
8. Attach the flowmeter to the wall outlet or to the tank.
9. Fill the humidifier with distilled water.
10. Attach the humidifier to the bottom of the flowmeter.
11. Attach the oxygen device and connecting tubing to the humidifier. *Do not set the flowmeter. Do not apply the oxygen device on the person.*

12. Place the cap securely on the distilled water. Store the water according to center policy.
13. Discard the packaging from the oxygen device and connecting tubing.

POST-PROCEDURE

14. Provide for comfort. (See the inside of the front book cover.)
15. Place the signal light within reach.
16. Decontaminate your hands.
17. Complete a safety check of the room. (See the inside of the front book cover.)

18. Tell the nurse when you are done. *The nurse will:*
    a. *Turn on the oxygen and set the flow rate.*
    b. *Apply the oxygen device on the person.*

Box 28-3 | Safety Rules for Oxygen Therapy

- Never remove the oxygen device.
- Make sure the oxygen device is secure but not tight.
- Check for signs of irritation from the device. Check behind the ears, under the nose (cannula), and around the face (mask). Also check the cheekbones.
- Keep the face clean and dry when a mask is used.
- Never shut off the oxygen flow.
- Do not adjust the flow rate unless allowed by your state and center.
- Tell the nurse at once if the flow rate is too high or too low.
- Tell the nurse at once if the humidifier is not bubbling.
- Secure tubing in place. Tape or pin it to the person's garment following center policy.

- Make sure there are no kinks in the tubing.
- Make sure the person does not lie on any part of the tubing.
- Make sure the oxygen tank is secure in its holder.
- Report signs and symptoms of hypoxia, respiratory distress, or abnormal breathing patterns to the nurse at once (see Boxes 28-1 and 28-2).
- Give oral hygiene as directed. Follow the care plan.
- Make sure the oxygen device is clean and free of mucus.
- Maintain an adequate water level in the humidifier.

QUALITY OF LIFE

Residents have the right to safe care. Perform only procedures that you understand. Do not perform unfamiliar procedures.

You do not give oxygen. You assist in providing safe care to persons receiving oxygen. You need to understand oxygen therapy and its safety rules. Careful observation is needed. Promptly report observations and complaints. Some treatments and procedures have severe side effects and complications. Every sign, symptom, or complaint is important.

Protect the right to privacy. Do all you can to provide privacy. Screening with the privacy curtain is not enough. If possible, provide care when the roommate is out of the room. Close doors and window coverings.

REVIEW QUESTIONS

Circle the BEST answer.

1 Alcohol and narcotics affect oxygen needs because they
   a Depress the brain
   b Are pollutants
   c Cause allergies
   d Cause infection

2 Hypoxia is
   a Not enough oxygen in the blood
   b The amount of hemoglobin that affects oxygen
   c Not enough oxygen in the cells
   d The lack of carbon dioxide

3 An early sign of hypoxia is
   a Cyanosis
   b Increased pulse and respiratory rates
   c Restlessness
   d Dyspnea

4 A person can breathe deeply and comfortably only while sitting. This is called
   a Biot's respirations
   b Orthopnea
   c Bradypnea
   d Kussmaul respirations

5 The nurse tells you that a person has tachypnea. The person's respirations are
   a Slow
   b Rapid
   c Absent
   d Difficult or painful

6 The person needs to rest after
   a A chest x-ray
   b A lung scan
   c Arterial blood gases
   d Pulmonary function tests

7 A person's pulse oximeter measurement is 98%. Which is *true?*
   a The pulse oximeter is wrong.
   b The pulse is 98 beats per minute.
   c The measurement is within normal range.
   d The person has respiratory depression.

8 Which is *not* a site for a pulse oximetry sensor?
   a Toe
   b Finger
   c Earlobe
   d Upper arm

9 You are assisting with deep breathing and coughing. Which is *false?*
   a The person inhales through pursed lips.
   b The person sits in a comfortable sitting position.
   c The person inhales deeply through the nose.
   d The person holds a pillow over an incision.

10 Deep-breathing and coughing exercises are ordered. The person has a productive cough. You need to remind the person to
   a Cover the nose and mouth when coughing
   b Use a face mask
   c Provide a sputum specimen
   d Inhale through the mouth

11 Which is useful for deep breathing?
   a Pulse oximeter
   b Incentive spirometry
   c Simple face mask
   d Partial-rebreather mask

12 When assisting with oxygen therapy, you can
   a Turn the oxygen on and off
   b Start the oxygen
   c Decide what device to use
   d Keep connecting tubing secure and free of kinks

Answers to these questions are on p. 720.

Respiratory Support and Therapies

OBJECTIVES

- Define the key terms and key abbreviations listed in this chapter.
- Explain how to assist in the care of persons with artificial airways.
- Describe the principles and safety measures for suctioning.

- Explain how to assist in the care of persons on mechanical ventilation.
- Explain how to assist in the care of persons with chest tubes.
- Explain how to promote quality of life.

KEY TERMS

hemothorax Blood *(hemo)* in the pleural space *(thorax)*

intubation Inserting an artificial airway

mechanical ventilation Using a machine to move air into and out of the lungs

patent Open and unblocked

pleural effusion The escape and collection of fluid *(effusion)* in the pleural space

pneumothorax Air *(pneumo)* in the pleural space *(thorax)*

suction The process of withdrawing or sucking up fluid *(secretions)*

tracheostomy A surgically created opening *(stomy)* into the trachea *(tracheo)*

KEY ABBREVIATIONS

CO_2	Carbon dioxide	O_2	Oxygen
ET	Endotracheal		

Some persons need artificial airways, suctioning, mechanical ventilation, and chest tubes. Needing respiratory rehabilitation, often they are very ill. They need to recover from problems affecting the airway and lungs. They need complex procedures and equipment.

The nurse may ask you to assist in their care. The center must teach and train you to provide needed care. The goals of care are to help the person:

- Reach his or her highest level of function
- Live as independently as possible
- Return home

ARTIFICIAL AIRWAYS

Artificial airways keep the airway **patent** (open and unblocked). They are needed:

- When disease, injury, secretions, or aspiration obstructs the airway
- For mechanical ventilation (p. 461)
- By some persons who are semi-conscious or unconscious

Intubation means inserting an artificial airway. Such airways are usually plastic and disposable. They come in various sizes. These airways are common:

- *Oropharyngeal airway*—inserted through the mouth and into the pharynx (Fig. 29-1, *A*). A nurse or respiratory therapist inserts the airway.
- *Endotracheal (ET) tube*—inserted through the mouth or nose and into the trachea (Fig. 29-1, *B*). A doctor inserts it using a lighted scope. Some RNs and respiratory therapists are trained to insert ET tubes. A cuff is inflated to keep the airway in place.
- *Tracheostomy tube*—inserted through a surgically created opening *(stomy)* into the trachea *(tracheo)* (Fig. 29-1, *C*). Cuffed tubes are common. The cuff is inflated to keep the tube in place. Doctors perform tracheostomies.

Vital signs are checked often. Observe for hypoxia and other signs and symptoms. If an airway comes out or is dislodged, tell the nurse at once. Frequent oral hygiene is needed. Follow the care plan.

Gagging and choking feelings are common. Imagine something in your mouth, nose, or throat. Comfort and reassure the person. Remind the person that the airway helps breathing. Use touch to show you care.

Persons with ET tubes cannot speak. Some tracheostomy tubes allow speech. Paper and pencils, Magic Slates, and communication boards are ways to communicate. Hand signals, nodding the head, and hand squeezes are common for simple "yes" and "no" questions. Follow the care plan. *Always keep the signal light within reach.*

Tracheostomies

A **tracheostomy** is a surgically created opening *(stomy)* into the trachea *(tracheo)*. Tracheostomies are temporary or permanent for mechanical ventilation (p. 461). They are permanent when airway structures are surgically removed. Cancer, severe airway trauma, or brain damage may require a permanent tracheostomy.

A tracheostomy tube is made of plastic, silicone, or metal. It has three parts (Fig. 29-2):

- The *obturator* has a round end. It is used to guide the insertion of the outer cannula (tube). Then it is removed. The obturator is placed within easy reach in case the tracheostomy tube falls out and needs reinsertion. It is taped to the wall or bedside stand.
- The *inner cannula* is inserted and locked in place. It fits inside the outer cannula. It is removed for cleaning and mucus removal. This keeps the airway patent. Some inner cannulas are disposable. Other tracheostomy tubes do not have inner cannulas.
- The *outer cannula* is secured in place with ties around the neck or a Velcro collar. The outer cannula is not removed. It keeps the tracheostomy patent.

Outer cannula

Flange

Inner cannula

Obturator

Fig. 29-2 Parts of a tracheostomy tube.

Fig. 29-1 Artificial airways. **A,** Oropharyngeal airway. **B,** Endotracheal tube. **C,** Tracheostomy tube.

The cuffed tracheostomy tube provides a seal between the cannula and the trachea (see Fig. 29-1, C). This prevents air from leaking around the tube. It also prevents aspiration. A nurse or respiratory therapist inflates and deflates the cuff.

The tube must not come out (*extubation*). If not secure, it could come out with coughing or if pulled on. A loose tube moves up and down. It can damage the trachea. *Call the nurse if the outer cannula comes out.*

The tube must remain patent. If able, the person coughs up secretions. Otherwise suctioning is needed. *Call for the nurse if you note signs and symptoms of hypoxia or respiratory distress.*

Nothing must enter the stoma. Otherwise the person can aspirate. These safety measures are needed:

- Dressings do not have loose gauze or lint.
- The stoma or tube is covered when outdoors. The person wears a stoma cover, scarf, or shirt or blouse that buttons at the neck. The cover prevents dust, insects, and other small particles from entering the stoma.
- The stoma is not covered with plastic, leather, or similar materials. They prevent air from entering the stoma. The person cannot breathe.
- Tub baths are taken. If showers are taken, a shower guard is worn. A hand-held nozzle is used to direct water away from the stoma.
- The person is assisted with shampooing. Water must not enter the stoma.
- The stoma is covered when shaving.
- Swimming is not allowed. Water will enter the tube or stoma.
- Medical-alert jewelry is worn. The person carries a medical-alert ID card.

The nurse may ask you to assist with tracheostomy care. The care is done daily or every 8 to 12 hours. It also is done as needed for excess secretions, soiled ties or collar, or soiled or moist dressings. The care involves:

- Cleaning the inner cannula to remove mucus and keep the airway patent. Disposable inner cannulas are discarded after one use. A new one is inserted. Re-usable inner cannulas are cleaned with a small bottle brush or a pipe cleaner. The nurse tells you what cleaning agent to use—usually hydrogen peroxide or a mild soap.
- Cleaning the stoma to prevent infection and skin breakdown.
- Applying clean ties or a Velcro collar to prevent infection. Clean ties are applied before removing the dirty ones. Hold the outer cannula in place when the nurse changes the ties or collar. Continue to do so until the nurse secures the new ties or collar. The ties or collar must be secure but not tight. For an adult, a finger should slide under the ties or collar (Fig. 29-3). See *Promoting Safety and Comfort: Tracheostomies.*

Fig. 29-3 For an adult, a finger is inserted under the ties.

PROMOTING SAFETY AND COMFORT
Tracheostomies

Safety
Mucus may contain microbes or blood. Follow Standard Precautions and the Bloodborne Pathogen Standard.

SUCTIONING THE AIRWAY

Secretions can collect in the airway. Retained secretions:

- Obstruct air flow into and out of the airway
- Provide an environment for microbes
- Interfere with oxygen (O_2) and carbon dioxide (CO_2) exchange

Hypoxia can occur. Usually coughing removes secretions. Some persons cannot cough, or the cough is too weak to remove secretions. They need suctioning.

Suction is the process of withdrawing or sucking up fluid (*secretions*). A suction source is needed—wall outlet or suction machine. A tube connects to a suction source at one end and to a suction catheter at the other end. The catheter is inserted into the airway. Secretions are withdrawn through the catheter.

The nose, mouth, and pharynx make up the upper airway. The trachea and bronchi make up the lower airway. These routes are used to suction the airway:

- *Oropharyngeal.* The mouth (*oro*) and pharynx (*pharyngeal*) are suctioned. A suction catheter is passed through the mouth and into the pharynx. The Yankauer suction catheter is often used for thick secretions (Fig. 29-4, p. 460).
- *Nasopharyngeal.* The nose (*naso*) and pharynx (*pharyngeal*) are suctioned. The suction catheter is passed through the nose into the pharynx.
- *Lower airway.* The suction catheter is passed through an ET or tracheostomy tube.

Fig. 29-4 The Yankauer suction catheter is often used when there are large amounts of thick secretions.

Fig. 29-5 The Ambu bag is squeezed with two hands.

The person's lungs are hyperventilated before suctioning an ET or a tracheostomy tube. *Hyperventilate* means to give extra *(hyper)* breaths *(ventilate)*. An Ambu bag is used (Fig. 29-5). The Ambu bag is attached to an oxygen source. Then the oxygen delivery device is removed from the ET or tracheostomy tube. The Ambu bag is attached to the ET or tracheostomy tube. To give a breath, the bag is squeezed with both hands. The nurse or respiratory therapist gives 3 to 5 breaths.

Oxygen is treated like a drug. You do not give drugs. Check if your state and center allow you to use an Ambu bag attached to an oxygen source.

See *Promoting Safety and Comfort: Suctioning.*

PROMOTING SAFETY AND COMFORT
Suctioning

Safety

If not done correctly, suctioning can cause serious harm. Suctioning removes oxygen from the airway. The person does not get oxygen during suctioning. Hypoxia and life-threatening problems can occur. They arise from the respiratory, cardiovascular, and nervous systems. Cardiac arrest can occur. Infection and airway injury are possible.

You can assist the nurse with suctioning (Box 29-1). However, you do not perform the suctioning procedure.

Always keep needed suction equipment and supplies at the bedside. When suctioning is needed, you do not have time to collect items from the supply area.

Mucus may contain microbes or blood. Follow Standard Precautions and the Bloodborne Pathogen Standard.

Box 29-1 Assisting With Suctioning: Safety Measures

- Review the procedure with the nurse. Know what the nurse wants you to do.
- Report coughing and the signs and symptoms of respiratory distress (Chapter 28). They signal the need for suctioning. Suctioning is done as needed, not on a schedule.
- Standard Precautions and the Bloodborne Pathogen Standard are followed. Secretions may contain blood and are potentially infectious.
- Sterile technique is used (Chapter 15). This helps prevent microbes from entering the airway.
- The nurse tells you the catheter type and size needed. If too large, it can injure the airway.
- Needed suction supplies and equipment are kept at the bedside. They are ready when the person needs suctioning.
- Suction is *not* applied while inserting the catheter. When suction is applied, air is sucked out of the airway.
- The catheter is inserted smoothly. This helps prevent injury to mucous membranes.

- A suction cycle for adults takes no more than 10 to 15 seconds. A suction cycle involves:
  - Inserting the catheter
  - Suctioning
  - Removing the catheter
- The catheter is cleared with sterile water or saline between suction cycles.
- The nurse waits 20 to 30 seconds between each suction cycle. Some centers require waiting 60 seconds.
- The suction catheter is passed (inserted) no more than 3 times. Injury and hypoxia are risks each time the suction catheter is passed.
- Check the person's pulse, respirations, and pulse oximeter measurements (Chapter 28) before, during, and after the procedure. Also observe the person's level of consciousness. Tell the nurse at once if any of these occur:
  - A drop in pulse rate or a pulse rate less than 60 beats per minute.
  - Irregular pulse rhythms.
  - A drop or rise in blood pressure.
  - Respiratory distress.
  - A drop in oxygen saturation. Normal range is 95% to 100%. See Chapter 28.

Fig. 29-6 A mechanical ventilator. *(Courtesy VIASYS Respiratory Care, Yorba Linda, Calif.)*

MECHANICAL VENTILATION

Weak muscle effort, obstructed airway, and damaged lung tissue cause hypoxia. Nervous system diseases and injuries can affect the respiratory center in the brain. Nerve damage interferes with messages between the lungs and the brain. Drug over-dose depresses the brain. With severe problems, the person cannot breathe. Or normal blood oxygen levels are not maintained. Often mechanical ventilation is needed.

Mechanical ventilation is using a machine to move air into and out of the lungs (Fig. 29-6). Oxygen enters the lungs. Carbon dioxide leaves them. An ET or tracheostomy tube is needed.

Mechanical ventilation is started in the hospital. Some people need it for a few hours or days. Others need it longer. They may require long-term care. Often the person needs *weaning* from the ventilator. That is, the person needs to breathe without the machine. The respiratory therapist and RN plan the weaning process. Weaning can take many weeks.

Box 29-2 Care of Persons on Mechanical Ventilation

- Keep the signal light within reach.
- Make sure hoses and connecting tubing have slack. They must not pull on the artificial airway.
- Answer signal lights promptly. The person depends on others for basic needs.
- Explain who you are and what you are going to do. Do this whenever you enter the room.
- Give the day, date, and time every time you give care.
- Report signs of respiratory distress or discomfort at once.
- Do not change settings on the machine or reset alarms.
- Follow the care plan for communication. The person cannot talk. Use agreed-upon hand or eye signals for "yes" and "no." For effective communication, everyone must use the same signals. Some persons can use paper and pencils, Magic Slates, communication boards, and hand signals.
- Ask questions that have simple answers. It may be hard to write long responses.
- Watch what you say and do. This includes when you are near and away from the person and family. They pay close attention to your verbal and non-verbal communication. Do not say or do anything that could upset the person.
- Use touch to comfort and reassure the person. Also tell the person about the weather, pleasant news events, and gifts and cards.
- Meet basic needs. Follow the care plan.
- Tell the person when you are leaving the room and when you will return.
- Complete a safety check before leaving the room. (See the inside of the front book cover.)

Alarms sound when something is wrong. One alarm means the person is disconnected from the ventilator. The nurse shows you how to reconnect the ET or tracheostomy tube. *When any alarm sounds, first check to see if the tube is attached to the ventilator. If not, attach it to the ventilator. The person can die if not attached to the ventilator.* Then tell the nurse at once about the alarm. Do not reset alarms.

Persons needing mechanical ventilation are often very ill. Other problems and injuries are common. Some persons are confused, disoriented, or cannot think clearly. The machine and fear of dying frighten many. Some are relieved to get enough oxygen. Many fear needing the machine for life. Mechanical ventilation can be painful for those with chest injuries or chest surgery. Tubes and hoses restrict movement. This causes more discomfort.

The nurse may ask you to assist with the person's care. See Box 29-2.

CHEST TUBES

Air, blood, or fluid can collect in the pleural space (sac or cavity). This occurs when the chest is entered because of injury or surgery.

- **Pneumothorax** is air *(pneumo)* in the pleural space *(thorax)*.
- **Hemothorax** is blood *(hemo)* in the pleural space *(thorax)*.
- **Pleural effusion** is the escape and collection of fluid *(effusion)* in the pleural space.

Pressure occurs when air, blood, or fluid collects in the pleural space. The pressure collapses the lung. Air cannot reach affected alveoli. O_2 and CO_2 are not exchanged. Respiratory distress and hypoxia result. Pressure on the heart affects the heart's ability to pump blood.

Hospital care is required. The doctor inserts chest tubes to remove the air, blood, or fluid (Fig. 29-7). The sterile procedure is done in surgery, in the emergency room, or at the bedside. A nurse assists.

Chest tubes attach to a drainage system (Fig. 29-8). The system must be airtight so air does not enter the pleural space. Water-seal drainage keeps the system airtight. The bottles in Figure 29-9 show how the system works:

- A chest tube attaches to connecting tubing.
- Connecting tubing attaches to a tube in the drainage container.
- The tube in the drainage container extends under water. The water prevents air from entering the chest tube and then the pleural space.

See Box 29-3 for care of the person with chest tubes.

Fig. 29-8 Chest tubes attached to a disposable water-seal drainage system. Chest tubes are inserted into the pleural space. *(From Perry AG, Potter PA: Clinical nursing skills and techniques, ed 7, St Louis, 2010, Mosby.)*

Fig. 29-9 Water-seal drainage system. *(From Lewis SM and others: Medical-surgical nursing: assessment and management of clinical problems, ed 6, St Louis, 2004, Mosby.)*

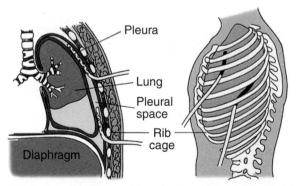

Fig. 29-7 Chest tubes inserted into the pleural space. *(Modified from Perry AG, Potter PA: Clinical nursing skills and techniques, ed 7, St Louis, 2010, Mosby.)*

QUALITY OF LIFE

Respiratory support and therapies involve complex care. Serious problems can occur from the wrong care. Know your limits. Follow the nurse's directions when assisting with care measures. Remember your legal and ethical responsibilities. You have the right to refuse a function or task. Do not function beyond your legal scope, preparation, and skill level.

REVIEW QUESTIONS

Circle the BEST answer.

1 A person has a tracheostomy. Which is *false?*
   a The person must not cough.
   b The obturator is taped to the wall or bedside stand.
   c The nurse removes the inner cannula for cleaning.
   d The outer cannula must be secured in place.

2 A person with a tracheostomy *cannot*
   a Shampoo
   b Shave
   c Shower with a hand-held nozzle
   d Swim

3 The nurse is changing tracheostomy ties. You must
   a Remove the inner cannula
   b Clean the stoma
   c Remove the dressing
   d Hold the outer cannula in place

4 A person has a tracheostomy. You cannot slide a finger under the ties. This means that the ties
   a Are secure
   b Are too tight
   c Need to be replaced
   d Need to be removed

5 Which signals the need for suctioning?
   a A pulse rate of 90 beats per minute
   b Signs and symptoms of respiratory distress
   c The orthopneic position
   d Being unable to speak

6 Suctioning requires
   a Sterile technique
   b Mechanical ventilation
   c An artificial airway
   d Chest tubes

7 You are assisting the nurse with suctioning. You must
   a Insert the catheter no more than 3 times
   b Suction for no more than 10 to 15 minutes
   c Clear the suction catheter with water
   d Keep needed suction supplies at the bedside

8 You note the following while assisting with suctioning. Which should you report at once?
   a A pulse rate of 82 beats per minute
   b A regular heart rhythm
   c Oxygen saturation of 92%
   d Thick secretions

9 A person requires mechanical ventilation. Which is *false?*
   a The person has an ET or tracheostomy tube.
   b The signal light must always be within reach.
   c Touch provides comfort and reassurance.
   d You can reset alarms on the ventilator.

10 An alarm sounds on a person's ventilator. What should you do *first?*
   a Reset the alarm.
   b Check to see if the airway is attached to the machine.
   c Call the nurse at once.
   d Ask the person what is wrong.

11 A person has a pneumothorax. This is
   a Fluid in the pleural space
   b Blood in the pleural space
   c Air in the pleural space
   d Secretions in the pleural space

12 Chest tubes are attached to water-seal drainage. You should do the following *except*
   a Tell the nurse if bubbling increases, decreases, or stops
   b Make sure tubing is not kinked
   c Keep the drainage system below the chest
   d Hang tubing in loops

Answers to these questions are on p. 720.

Assisted Living

OBJECTIVES

- Define the key terms and key abbreviations listed in this chapter.
- Identify the purpose of assisted living.
- Identify the person's rights.
- Identify the types of assisted living residences and the living areas offered.
- Describe the physical and environmental requirements for assisted living.
- Describe the requirements for assisted living staff.

- Describe the requirements for persons who want to live in an assisted living residence.
- Explain the purpose of a service plan.
- Explain how to assist with housekeeping and laundry.
- Identify food safety measures.
- Explain how to assist with drugs.
- Identify the reasons for transferring, discharging, or evicting a person.
- Explain how to promote quality of life.

KEY TERMS

assisted living A housing option for older persons who need help with activities of daily living yet wish to remain independent as long as possible

medication reminder Reminding the person to take drugs, observing them being taken as prescribed, and charting that they were taken

service plan A written plan listing the services needed by the person, how much help is needed, and who provides the services

KEY ABBREVIATIONS

AD	Alzheimer's disease	**ALR**	Assisted living residence
ADL	Activities of daily living		

Many older people cannot or do not want to live alone. Some need help with self-care. Some have physical or cognitive problems and disabilities (Chapter 44). Still others need help taking drugs. Yet these people do not need constant care.

Assisted living offers quality of life with independence, companionship, and social involvement. Assisted living is a housing option for older persons who need help with activities of daily living (ADL) yet wish to remain independent as long as possible. Little or no medical care is provided. Housing, personal care, support services, health care, and social activities are provided in a home-like setting. Assisted living usually offers these services:

- 3 meals a day
- Help with ADL—bathing, dressing, grooming, toileting, eating, walking
- Housekeeping and maintenance
- Linen and personal laundry
- A 24-hour emergency communication system to use for an emergency or to call for help
- 24-hour security
- 24-hour supervision
- Transportation arrangements
- Social, educational, recreational, and spiritual services
- Help with shopping, banking, and money management
- Some health services
- Exercise and wellness programs
- Medication (drug) management or help taking drugs
- Supervision for persons with Alzheimer's disease (AD), dementia, and other disabilities

Living areas vary. A small apartment has a bedroom, bathroom, living area, kitchen, and laundry area (Figs. 30-1 and 30-2). Some people just want a bedroom and bathroom. Box 30-1 lists the requirements and features of assisted living units. Box 30-2, p. 466 lists environment requirements.

Fig. 30-1 A living area in an assisted living apartment.

Fig. 30-2 A kitchen in an assisted living apartment.

Box 30-1 **Requirements and Features of Assisted Living Units**

- A door that locks; the person keeps a key
- A telephone jack
- A 24-hour emergency communication system in the person's room
- A window or door that provides natural light
- Wheelchair access
- Lighted common areas
- A window or door that allows safe exit in an emergency
- A mailbox for each person
- A bathroom that provides privacy:
  - A sink in the bathroom or in the next room (sink is not used for food preparation)
  - A bathtub or shower that has a shower curtain and non-slip surfaces
  - Ventilation or a window that opens
  - Grab bars for the toilet and bathtub or shower
  - Other assistive devices needed for safety and identified in the service plan (p. 468)

- Smoke detectors
- A fire sprinkler system
- A bed (frame and mattress) that is clean and in good repair
- Adequate general and task lighting
- An easy chair
- A table and chair for meals
- Adjustable window covers that provide privacy
- A dresser or storage space for clothing and personal items
- Appliances for food—sink, stove, refrigerator with freezer, and storage for food and cooking items

> **Box 30-2   Environment Requirements**
>
> - The ALR is clean, safe, orderly, odor-free, and in good repair.
> - The ALR is free of insects and rodents.
> - Garbage is stored in covered containers lined with plastic bags. Bags are removed from the ALR at least once a week.
> - Hot water temperatures are between 95° F (Fahrenheit) and 120° F in areas used by residents.
> - The hot and cold water supply meets hygiene needs.
> - Common bathrooms have toilet paper, soap, and cloth towels, paper towels, or a dryer.
> - Clean linens are handled, transported, and stored to prevent contamination.
> - Soiled linen and clothing are stored in closed containers away from food, kitchen, and dining areas.
> - Oxygen containers are stored according to the manufacturer's instructions.
> - Cleaning solutions, insecticides, and other hazardous substances are stored in their original containers. They are in locked cabinets in rooms separate from food, dining areas, and drugs.
> - Pets or animals are controlled to protect residents and maintain sanitation.
> - Employees have access to a first aid kit.

PROMOTING SAFETY AND COMFORT
Assisted Living

Safety

Residents have the same diseases and illnesses as persons at home, in hospitals, and in nursing centers. They are at risk for infections. This includes sexually transmitted and other communicable diseases. Follow Standard Precautions and the Bloodborne Pathogen Standard when contact with blood, body fluids, secretions, excretions, or potentially contaminated items and surfaces is likely.

Assisted living residences (ALRs) also are called *assisted living facilities (ALFs)*. Some are part of retirement communities. Others are separate facilities. State laws and licensing requirements for ALRs vary. Resident's rights are part of such laws.

See *Promoting Safety and Comfort: Assisted Living.*

PURPOSE

People choose assisted living for many reasons. People are living longer, and there are more older people than before. Men and women lose life partners through death or divorce. Some remarry; others do not. Some persons have never married. Today's older persons had some birth control options. Many had small families. And the United States is a mobile society. Children grow up and move away from their families. For these reasons, many older persons live alone. Often there is no family nearby to help them.

ALR RESIDENTS

ALR residents usually need some help with one or more ADL:
- Personal care—bathing, dressing, grooming, elimination
- Meals—cooking, eating
- Taking drugs
- Housekeeping
- Personal safety
- Transportation

ALR residents do not need 24-hour nursing care. And they are not bedridden. Some persons have chronic illnesses or are cognitively impaired.

Mobility is often a requirement. The person walks or uses a wheelchair or motor scooter. The person must be able to leave the building in an emergency. Stable health is another requirement. Only limited health care or treatment is needed.

RESIDENT RIGHTS

ALR residents have rights and liberties as United States citizens. They also gain special rights under state laws and rules (Box 30-3). If unable to exercise his or her rights, family members, legal representatives, or ombudsmen act on the person's behalf.

Box 30-3 Assisted Living Residents' Rights

Quality of Life—Residents have the right to:
- Receive a list of current resident rights when accepted into an ALR. Language barriers or disabilities will not interfere with becoming aware of one's rights.
- Current phone numbers of state and local agencies protecting the rights of older persons. Adult Protective Services and a long-term care ombudsman are examples.
- Be treated with dignity and respect.
- Make choices about how to live one's everyday life.
- Make choices about how to receive care.
- Receive the care and services needed to attain or maintain the highest level of physical, mental, and social well-being.
- Take part in deciding what services he or she will receive.

Self-Determination—Residents have the right to:
- Live in a setting that promotes and supports dignity, individuality, independence, self-determination, privacy, and choice.
- Exercise free choice in selecting a primary care provider, pharmacy, or other service provider and assume costs resulting from such choices.
- Submit grievances to employees and outside agencies.
- Take part in developing a written service plan (p. 468).
- Receive a copy of service plans.
- Receive services specified in the service plan.
- Review and revise the service plan at any time.
- Refuse services, unless:
  - Such services are court-ordered
  - Refusing services endangers the health, safety, or welfare of others
- Free choice in selecting activities, schedules, and daily routines.
- Have the same civil and human rights as other persons.
- Terminate living at an ALR without notice if a government agency has proven:
  - Neglect
  - Exploitation
  - Conditions that are an immediate threat to life, health, or safety
- Terminate living at an ALR after giving 14 days written notice if documentation shows that the ALR failed to comply with the service plan or residency agreement.
- Receive written notice from the ALR when it terminates the person's residency. The notice shall include:
  - The effective date
  - The right to submit a grievance
  - The grievance procedure
  - The ALR's refund policy

Transfer and Discharge—Residents have the right to:
- Request to locate or refuse to relocate within the ALR.
- Understand the reasons why the ALR may terminate residency.
  - Without notice:
    - If behavior is an immediate threat to the health and safety of others in the ALR
    - For urgent medical or health needs requiring immediate transfer to another health care agency
    - If care and service needs exceed the level of care provided by the ALR
  - Within 14 days of written notice for:
    - Failure to pay fees or charges
    - Not complying with the residency agreement or ALR requirements

Personal and Privacy Rights—Residents have the right to:
- Take part in or refuse to take part in social, recreational, rehabilitative, religious, political, or community activities.
- Perform or refuse to perform work for the ALR.
- Privacy in correspondence, communication, visits, and financial and personal matters.
- Privacy in hygiene and health-related services.
- Receive visitors.
- Make private phone calls.
- Maintain and use personal items, unless the health, safety, or welfare of others is affected.
- Have financial and other records kept in confidence. Release of such records requires written consent except when required by law.
- Be treated with consideration and respect.
- Have access to common areas in the ALR.

Rights Against Restraints and Abuse—Residents have the right to:
- Be free from physical, mental, and sexual abuse and sexual assault.
- Be free from involuntary seclusion.
- Not be deprived of the care and services needed to maintain physical or mental health.
- Not have one's resources used for another's profit or advantage.
- Be free from the use of physical restraints used for discipline or staff convenience.
- Be free from chemical restraints used to control behavior.
- Be free from discrimination in regard to race, color, national origin, sex, sexual orientation, and religion.

Right to Information—Residents have the right to:
- Review the ALR's most recent survey conducted by the state. This includes any plan of correction in effect.
- Review a copy of the state's administrative code for ALRs.
- Be informed, in writing, of any change to a fee or charge at least 30 days before the change. The exception is a change in one's service plan.
- Review one's records during normal business hours or at an agreed upon time.

Modified from Assisted Living Residents' Rights, Arizona Administrative Code R9-Chapter 10-Article 7.

STAFF REQUIREMENTS

Staff requirements vary among states. Some require that the staff complete a nursing assistant training and competency evaluation program. Others require training in these areas:

- The needs and goals of ALR residents
- Promoting dignity, independence, and resident rights
- Using service plans
- Ethics, privacy, and confidentiality of records and information
- Hygiene and infection control
- Nutrition and menu planning
- Food preparation, service, and storage
- Housekeeping and sanitation
- Preventing and reporting abuse and neglect
- Incident reports
- Fire, emergency, and disaster plans
- Assisting with drugs
- Early signs of illness and the need for health care
- Safety measures
- Communication skills
- Special needs of persons with AD and other dementias
- Cardiopulmonary resuscitation and first aid (Chapter 47)

Criminal background and fingerprint checks are common requirements. The ALR cannot employ a person with a criminal record.

SERVICE PLAN

A service plan is a written plan listing:
- The services needed by the person
- How much help is needed
- Who provides the services

The plan relates to ADL, activities and social services, dietary needs, taking drugs, and special needs. Health services are included.

For example, a person needs help getting dressed. The service plan states that you will assist the person. The service plan also states that a nurse will replace the person's catheter. The person needs physical therapy after a hip fracture. The service plan states a physical therapist will visit. And the person needs help taking drugs. A family member will assist the person.

The plan is reviewed when the person's condition, wants, or service needs change. Services are added or reduced as the person's needs change.

Meals

Three meals a day and snacks are provided. Usually there are no more than 14 hours between the evening meal and breakfast. It can be longer if there is a nutritious evening snack. Special dietary needs are met. Menus are posted for residents to see.

Residents are encouraged to eat in the dining room with others. Or they can eat in their rooms. Assistive devices are provided as needed. So is help with eating, opening cartons, buttering bread, cutting meat, and so on (Chapter 24).

Housekeeping

The following housekeeping measures help prevent infection. And they keep living units neat and clean.
- Dust furniture at least weekly.
- Vacuum floors at least weekly and as needed.
- Wipe up spills right away.
- Use a dust mop or broom to sweep. Use a dustpan to collect dust and crumbs.
- Sweep daily or more often as needed.
- Make sure toilets are flushed after each use.
- Rinse the sink after washing, shaving, or oral hygiene.
- Clean the tub or shower after each use.
- Remove and dispose of hair from the sink, tub, or shower.
- Hang towels to dry. Or place them in a hamper.
- Clean bathroom surfaces every day. Use a disinfectant or water and detergent to clean all surfaces. They include:
  - The toilet bowl, seat, and outside areas of the toilet
  - The floor
  - The sides, walls, and curtain or door of the tub or shower
  - Towel racks and toilet tissue, toothbrush, and soap holders
  - The sink and mirror
  - Windowsills
- Mop or vacuum the bathroom floor every day.
- Empty bathroom wastebaskets every day.
- Put out clean towels and washcloths every day.
- Wash bath mats, the wastebasket, and laundry hamper every week.
- Replace toilet and facial tissue as needed.
- Open bathroom windows for a short time. Also use air fresheners.

Fig. 30-3 Safe handling instructions for meat and poultry. They are required by the U.S. Department of Agriculture.

Food Safety

Certain measures are needed when handling, preparing, and storing food. They protect against infection. See Chapter 24. Also practice these measures:

- Handle meat and poultry safely. Follow the safe handling instructions on food labels (Fig. 30-3).
- Protect left-over foods. Place left-over food in small containers. Cover containers with lids, foil, or plastic wrap. Date and refrigerate containers as soon as possible.
- Use left-over food within 2 or 3 days.
- Use liquid detergent and hot water to wash eating and cooking items. Wash glasses and cups first. Follow with silverware, plates, bowls, and then pots and pans. Rinse well with hot water.
- Place washed eating and cooking items in a drainer to dry. Air-drying is more aseptic than towel drying.
- Rinse dishes before loading them into a dishwasher. Use dishwasher soap.
- Do not wash pots and pans and cast iron, wood, and some plastic items in a dishwasher.
- Clean appliances, counters, tables, and other surfaces after each meal. Use hot, soapy water and paper towels or clean cloths.
- Remove grease spills and splashes. Use a liquid surface cleaner.
- Clean sinks with a sink cleaner.
- Dispose of garbage, left-overs, and other soiled supplies after each meal. A garbage disposal is best for food and liquid garbage. Do not put bones in the garbage disposal.
- Recycle paper, boxes, cans, and plastic containers according to the ALR policy.
- Empty garbage at least once a day.

Laundry

Laundry services include providing clean linens. Residents can use a washing machine, dryer, iron, and ironing board for personal laundry. When assisting with laundry:

- Wear gloves when handling soiled laundry (see *Promoting Safety and Comfort: Assisted Living*, p. 466).
- Follow the person's preferences.
- Follow care label directions.
- Sort items by color and fabric. Separate white, colored, and dark items. Separate sturdy and delicate fabrics.
- Empty pockets.
- Fasten buttons, zippers, snaps, hooks, and other closures.
- Wash heavily soiled items separately.
- Follow detergent directions.
- Select the correct wash cycle and water temperature. Follow care label directions and the person's preferences.
- Select the correct drying temperature and cycle. Follow care label directions and the person's preferences.
- Fold, hang, or iron clothes as the person prefers. See *Teamwork and Time Management: Laundry*.

TEAMWORK AND TIME MANAGEMENT
Laundry

Residents may share washers and dryers. If assisting with laundry, remove clothes from washers and dryers promptly. Other residents and staff may want to use them. You may find someone's laundry left in a washer or dryer when you are ready to use the machine. First, try to find the person who left the laundry. Politely tell the person that the washer or dryer is done and that you are ready to use the machine. Offer to remove laundry if the other person is busy. If you cannot find that person, do the following:

- If left in a washer—place the wet laundry on a clean surface. Do not put it in the dryer. Some items may need to dry flat or hang to dry. Some fabrics may need certain dryer settings. Or the resident may have drying preferences.
- If left in a dryer—fold the laundry. Then place it on a clean surface.

While laundry is in the washer or dryer, use the time for other tasks. Assist with ADL, do housekeeping tasks, prepare meals, and so on.

Nursing Services

Some ALRs provide limited nursing services. The nurse assesses each person and monitors health. The nurse supervises tasks delegated to you. If a person cannot manage his or her own drugs, the nurse gives them.

Medication Assistance

Drugs must be taken as prescribed. The six rights of drug administration are:

* The right drug
* The right dose (amount)
* The right route (by mouth, injection, applied to the skin, inhalation, vaginally, or rectally)
* The right time
* The right person
* The right documentation

Your role in assisting with drugs depends on your state's laws, ALR policy, and your training and education. It may involve one or more of the following. *Remember, you do not give drugs* (Chapter 3). *Also remember that the person has the right to refuse to take prescribed drugs.*

* Reminding the person it is time to take a drug
* Reading the drug label to the person
* Opening containers for persons who cannot do so
* Checking the dosage against the drug label
* Providing water, juice, milk, crackers, applesauce, or other food and fluids as needed
* Making sure the person takes the right drug, the right amount, at the right time, and in the right way
* Charting that the person took or refused to take the drug (right documentation)
* Storing drugs

Residents manage and take their own drugs if able. This is called *self-directed medication management*. The person knows drugs by name, color, or shape. The person knows what drugs to take, the correct doses, and when and how to take them. The person is able to question changes in the usual drug routine. For example, the person comments that a pill is not broken in half. Or the person says that a pill looks different. Report comments or questions to the nurse.

Pill organizers (Fig. 30-4) have sections for days and times. Some are for a week. Others are for a month. The person, a family member or legal representative, or a nurse prepares the pill organizer. The person then takes the drugs on the right day and at the right time.

You may need to remind some people. A **medication reminder** means reminding the person to take drugs, observing them being taken as prescribed, and charting that they were taken.

See *Focus on Communication: Medication Assistance.*

Fig. 30-4 Pill organizer.

FOCUS ON COMMUNICATION
Medication Assistance

Your role may include assisting the person with drugs. To remind a person to take his or her drugs, you can say:

* "Ms. Parks, it's time to take your 8 o'clock pills."
* "Mr. Ladd, you'll need to take your pills in about 10 minutes."
* "Mrs. Young, are you ready to take your medicine?"
  To read a drug label to a person, read the following:
* The name of the person on the drug label
* The name of the drug
* How to take the drug (by mouth, with food, with a full glass of water, apply to the skin, rectally, and so on)
* The dosage
* When to take the drug (before meals, with meals, after meals, and so on)
* How often to take the drug
* Warnings and other information on the drug label

Medication Record A medication record is kept for each person needing help with drugs. The record includes:

- The person's name
- Drug name, dose, directions, and route of administration
- Date and time to take the drug
- Date and time help was given
- Signature or initials of the person assisting

Drug Errors Report any drug error to the nurse. Also complete an incident report. An error means one or more of the following:

- Taking another person's drugs
- Taking the wrong drug
- Taking the wrong dose
- Taking an extra dose
- Missing or skipping a dose
- Taking a drug at the wrong time
- Taking a drug by the wrong route
- Not taking a drug when ordered
- Not recording that a drug was taken

Storing Drugs Drugs are kept in a secure place. This prevents others from taking them. If the ALR stores the drugs, they are kept in a locked container, cabinet, or area.

Some persons store their own drugs. This is on the service plan. If sharing a room, each person's ability to safely have drugs is assessed. Drugs are kept in a locked container if safety is a factor.

Drugs must have the original pharmacy label. They are stored as directed on the label. For example, some drugs are refrigerated. Others are kept away from light. The label also has an expiration date. The ALR has procedures for disposing of expired or discontinued drugs.

Activities and Recreation

Residents are urged to take part in activity and recreational programs. Social, physical, and community activities promote well-being and independence. An activities director plans, organizes, and conducts the ALR's activity program. These activities are on a weekly or monthly calendar. The calendar also tells about community events and activities.

Special Services and Safety Needs

Sometimes emergencies occur. Some people need help getting out of bed or transferring to a wheelchair. Then they can leave the building with little or no help.

Other people cannot walk or use a wheelchair or motor scooter. They need attendants. If an attendant is needed, the ALR and the person agree on how and who will meet the person's needs. An attendant is needed 24 hours a day.

TRANSFER, DISCHARGE, AND EVICTION

Residents can be transferred, discharged, or evicted. State laws require that the ALR tell the person about the action. Reasons for such action are:

- The ALR can no longer meet the person's health needs. The person is a threat to the health and safety of self or others. Or the ALR cannot provide needed care.
- The person fails to pay for services as agreed upon.
- The person fails to comply with ALR policies or rules.
- The person wants to transfer.
- The ALR closes.

QUALITY OF LIFE

ALR residents have rights. Federal and state laws protect their rights as citizens. State laws usually protect the rights listed in Box 30-3. You need to protect those rights.

People choose assisted living for many reasons. Most need some help. But they want to live independently with dignity and respect. You can help them by following their service plans. Assist them as needed while allowing as much privacy and personal choice as possible.

REVIEW QUESTIONS

Circle the BEST answer.

1 ALRs provide the following *except*
   a 24-hour nursing care
   b Housing
   c Help with ADL
   d Support services

2 These statements are about ALRs. Which is *false?*
   a Each person has a private apartment.
   b Some residents have Alzheimer's disease.
   c 24-hour security is provided.
   d Three meals a day are provided.

3 Which statement is *false?*
   a Residents can refuse care.
   b Residents must plan and organize their own activities.
   c Residents are able to lock their doors.
   d An emergency communication system is provided.

4 Which of these violates an ALR resident's rights?
   a Covering the person during personal care
   b Giving the person unopened mail
   c Keeping information confidential
   d Choosing activities for the person

5 A person wants to attend a concert. Which statement is *true?*
   a The ALR must approve the concert.
   b The person must return by 10 PM.
   c An attendant must go with the person.
   d The ALR must respect the person's choice.

6 Assisted living staff must
   a Complete a nursing assistant training and competency evaluation program
   b Meet state requirements
   c Assist with drugs
   d Provide transportation

7 ALRs often require the following *except*
   a That persons be mobile
   b That persons have stable health
   c That persons require only limited care
   d That persons speak English

8 A service plan
   a Describes nursing care needs
   b Describes the services needed and who provides them
   c Lists the drugs the person needs to take
   d Lists service fees and charges

9 ALR residents are encouraged to eat
   a In their rooms
   b In the dining room
   c At home
   d At community events

10 You assist with housekeeping. Which is *false?*
   a Dusting and vacuuming are done at least weekly.
   b Spills are wiped up right away.
   c Bathroom surfaces are cleaned daily.
   d Spills and splashes are wiped up after meals.

11 You assist with food. Which is *false?*
   a Safe handling instructions are followed.
   b Left-over food is used in 3 to 5 days.
   c Garbage is emptied at least once a day.
   d Pots and pans are washed by hand.

12 You assist with laundry. Which is *true?*
   a Care label directions are followed.
   b Clothes are washed in hot water.
   c Clothes are ironed.
   d All white fabrics are washed together.

13 Usually ALR staff are allowed to
   a Give drugs
   b Give medication reminders
   c Refill drugs
   d Prepare pill organizers

14 Drugs are kept
   a In the person's closet
   b In the person's drawer
   c In a locked container, cabinet, or area
   d By the family

15 The ALR cannot provide a person with all needed services. Which is *true?*
   a The ALR must hire more staff.
   b The family must provide the needed care.
   c The ALR can ask the person to transfer.
   d The person's service plan needs to change.

Answers to these questions are on p. 720.

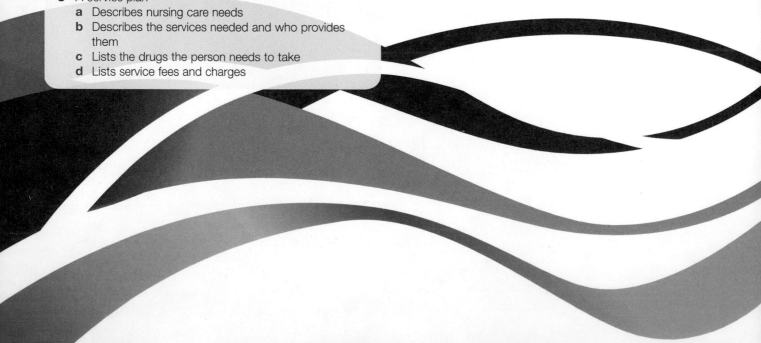

Measuring Vital Signs

- Define the key terms and key abbreviations listed in this chapter.
- Explain why vital signs are measured.
- List the factors affecting vital signs.
- Identify the normal ranges for each temperature site.
- Explain when to use each temperature site.
- Identify the pulse sites.

- Describe a normal pulse and normal respirations.
- Describe the practices to follow when measuring blood pressure.
- Perform the procedures described in this chapter.
- Explain how to promote quality of life.

KEY TERMS

apical-radial pulse Taking the apical and radial pulses at the same time

blood pressure (BP) The amount of force exerted against the walls of an artery by the blood

body temperature The amount of heat in the body that is a balance between the amount of heat produced and the amount lost by the body

bradycardia A slow *(brady)* heart rate *(cardia)*; less than 60 beats per minute

diastole The period of heart muscle relaxation; the heart is at rest

diastolic pressure The pressure in the arteries when the heart is at rest

fever Elevated body temperature

hypertension Blood pressure measurements remaining above *(hyper)* a systolic pressure of 140 mm Hg or a diastolic pressure of 90 mm Hg

hypotension When the systolic blood pressure is below *(hypo)* 90 mm Hg and the diastolic pressure is below 60 mm Hg

pulse The beat of the heart felt at an artery as a wave of blood passes through the artery

pulse deficit The difference between the apical and radial pulse rates

pulse rate The number of heartbeats or pulses felt in 1 minute

respiration Breathing air into *(inhalation)* and out of *(exhalation)* the lungs

sphygmomanometer A cuff and measuring device used to measure blood pressure

stethoscope An instrument used to listen to sounds produced by the heart, lungs, and other body organs

systole The period of heart muscle contraction; the heart is pumping blood

systolic pressure The pressure in the arteries when the heart contracts

tachycardia A rapid *(tachy)* heart rate *(cardia)*; more than 100 beats per minute

vital signs Temperature, pulse, respirations, and blood pressure

Copyright © 2011, 2007, 2003, 1999, 1994, 1988 by Mosby, Inc., an affiliate of Elsevier Inc.   473

KEY ABBREVIATIONS

BP	Blood pressure	**ID**	Identification
C	Centigrade	**IV**	Intravenous
F	Fahrenheit	**mm**	Millimeter
Hg	Mercury	**mm Hg**	Millimeters of mercury

Vital signs reflect the function of three body processes essential for life: regulation of body temperature, breathing, and heart function. The four vital signs of body function are:

- Temperature
- Pulse
- Respirations
- Blood pressure

Vital signs are often called TPR (temperature, pulse, and respiration) and BP (blood pressure). Some centers include "pain" as a vital sign (Chapter 27).

MEASURING AND REPORTING VITAL SIGNS

A person's vital signs vary within certain limits. They are affected by sleep, activity, eating, weather, noise, exercise, drugs, anger, fear, anxiety, pain, and illness.

Vital signs are measured to detect changes in normal body function. They tell about treatment response. They often signal life-threatening events. Vital signs are part of the assessment step in the nursing process. Vital signs are measured:

- During physical exams
- When the person is admitted to the center
- As often as the person's condition requires
- Before and after surgery, complex procedures, and diagnostic tests
- After some care measures, such as ambulation
- After a fall or other injury
- When drugs affect the respiratory or circulatory system
- When the person complains of pain, dizziness, light-headedness, feeling faint, shortness of breath, a rapid heart rate, or not feeling well
- As stated on the care plan (usually daily, twice a day, or weekly in nursing centers)

Vital signs show even minor changes in the person's condition. Accuracy is essential when you measure, record, and report vital signs. If unsure of your measurements, promptly ask the nurse to take them again. Unless otherwise ordered, take vital signs with the person at rest—lying or sitting. Report the following at once:

- Any vital sign that is changed from a prior measurement
- Vital signs above the normal range
- Vital signs below the normal range

Vital signs are recorded in the person's medical record. If measured often, a flow sheet is used. The doctor or nurse compares current and previous measurements.

See *Residents With Dementia: Measuring and Reporting Vital Signs.*

See *Focus on Communication: Measuring and Reporting Vital Signs.*

RESIDENTS WITH DEMENTIA
Measuring and Reporting Vital Signs

Measuring vital signs on persons with dementia may be difficult. The person may move about, hit at you, and grab equipment. This is not safe for the person or for you. Two workers may be needed. One uses touch and a soothing voice to calm and distract the person. The other measures the vital signs.

You may need to try the procedure when the person is calmer. Or take the pulse and respirations at one time. Then take the temperature and blood pressure at another time.

Always approach the person calmly. Use a soothing voice. Tell the person what you are going to do. Do not rush the person. Follow the care plan. If you cannot measure vital signs, tell the nurse right away.

FOCUS ON COMMUNICATION
Measuring and Reporting Vital Signs

Residents like to know their measurements. If center policy allows, tell the person the measurements. Remember, this information is private and confidential. Roommates and visitors must not hear what you are saying.

A measurement may be abnormal. Or you may not be able to feel a pulse or hear a blood pressure. Do not alarm the person. You can say:

* "I'm not sure that I counted your pulse correctly. I'll ask the nurse to take it."
* "I'm not sure that I heard your blood pressure correctly. I'll ask the nurse to take it again."
* "Your pulse is a little slow (or fast). I'll ask the nurse to check it."
* "Your temperature is higher than normal. I'm going to use another thermometer. I'll also ask the nurse to check you."

BODY TEMPERATURE

Body temperature is the amount of heat in the body. It is a balance between the amount of heat produced and the amount lost by the body. Heat is produced as cells use food for energy. It is lost through the skin, breathing, urine, and feces. Body temperature stays fairly stable. It is lower in the morning and higher in the afternoon and evening. See p. 474 for the factors affecting vital signs. Pregnancy and the menstrual cycle are other factors affecting body temperature.

You use thermometers to measure temperature. It is measured using the Fahrenheit (F) and centigrade (C) scales.

Temperature Sites

Temperature sites are the mouth, rectum, axilla (underarm), tympanic membrane (ear), and temporal artery (forehead) (Box 31-1). Each site has a normal range (Table 31-1). **Fever** means an elevated body temperature.

Older persons have lower body temperatures than younger persons. An oral temperature of 98.6° F may signal fever in an older person. Always report temperatures that are above or below the normal range.

See *Promoting Safety and Comfort: Temperature Sites.*

PROMOTING SAFETY AND COMFORT
Temperature Sites

Safety
Rectal temperatures are dangerous for persons with heart disease. The thermometer can stimulate the vagus nerve in the rectum. This nerve also affects the heart. Stimulation of the vagus nerve slows the heart rate. The heart rate can slow to dangerous levels in some persons.

Box 31-1 | Temperature Sites

Oral Site

Oral temperatures are *not* taken if the person:

* Is under 4 or 5 years of age
* Is unconscious
* Has had surgery or an injury to the face, neck, nose, or mouth
* Is receiving oxygen
* Breathes through the mouth
* Has a naso-gastric tube
* Is delirious, restless, confused, or disoriented
* Is paralyzed on one side of the body
* Has a sore mouth
* Has a convulsive (seizure) disorder

Rectal Site

Rectal temperatures are taken when the oral site cannot be used. Rectal temperatures are *not* taken if the person:

* Has diarrhea
* Has a rectal disorder or injury
* Has heart disease
* Had rectal surgery
* Is confused or agitated

Tympanic Membrane Site

The site has fewer microbes than the mouth or rectum. The risk of spreading infection is reduced. This site is *not* used if the person has:

* An ear disorder
* Ear drainage

Temporal Artery Site

Measures body temperature at the temporal artery in the forehead. The site is non-invasive.

Axillary Site

Less reliable than the other sites. It is used when the other sites cannot be used.

Table 31-1 | Normal Body Temperatures

Site	Baseline	Normal Range
Oral	98.6° F (37° C)	97.6° to 99.6° F (36.5° to 37.5° C)
Rectal	99.6° F (37.5° C)	98.6° to 100.6° F (37.0° to 38.1° C)
Axillary	97.6° F (36.5° C)	96.6° to 98.6° F (35.9° to 37.0° C)
Tympanic membrane	98.6° F (37° C)	98.6° F (37° C)
Temporal artery	99.6° F (37.5° C)	99.6° F (37.5° C)

Fig. 31-1 A, A Fahrenheit thermometer with a long or slender tip. The temperature measurement is 98.6° F. **B,** Centigrade thermometer with a stubby tip (rectal thermometer). The temperature measurement is 37.0° C. **C,** Fahrenheit thermometer with a pear-shaped tip. The temperature measurement is 99.2° F.

PROMOTING SAFETY AND COMFORT
Glass Thermometers

Safety
Mercury-glass thermometers are rarely used today. However, do not assume that a glass thermometer contains a mercury-free mixture. If a thermometer breaks, tell the nurse at once. Mercury is a hazardous substance. Do not touch the substance. Do not let the person do so. The center follows special procedures for handling all hazardous materials. See Chapter 12.

Fig. 31-2 The thermometer is held at the stem. It is read at eye level.

Glass Thermometers

The glass thermometer is a hollow glass tube (Fig. 31-1) with a bulb (tip) at the end. The device is filled with a substance. When heated, the substance expands and rises in the tube. When cooled, the substance contracts and moves down the tube.

Long- or slender-tip thermometers are used for oral and axillary temperatures. So are thermometers with stubby and pear-shaped tips. Rectal thermometers have stubby tips. Thermometers are color-coded:
* Blue—oral and axillary thermometers
* Red—rectal thermometers

Glass thermometers are re-usable. However, the following are problems:
* They take a long time to register—3 to 10 minutes, depending on the site.
* They break easily. Broken thermometers can injure the rectum and colon.
* The person may bite down and break an oral thermometer. Cuts in the mouth are risks. If the thermometer contains mercury, swallowed mercury can cause mercury poisoning.

See *Promoting Safety and Comfort: Glass Thermometers.*

Reading a Glass Thermometer Fahrenheit thermometers have long and short lines. Every other long line is an even degree from 94° to 108° F. The short lines mean 0.2 (two-tenths) of a degree (see Fig. 31-1, *A* and *C*).

On a centigrade thermometer, each long line means 1 degree. Degrees range from 34° to 42° C. Each short line means 0.1 (one-tenth) of a degree (see Fig. 31-1, *B*).

To read a glass thermometer:
* Hold it at the stem (Fig. 31-2). Bring it to eye level.
* Turn it until you can see the numbers and the long and short lines.
* Turn it back and forth slowly until you can see the silver or red line.
* Read the nearest degree (long line).
* Read the nearest tenth of a degree (short line)—an even number on a Fahrenheit thermometer.

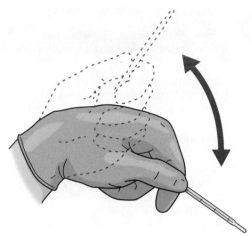

Fig. 31-3 The wrist is snapped to shake down the thermometer.

Fig. 31-4 The thermometer is inserted into a plastic cover.

Using a Glass Thermometer Do the following to prevent infection, promote safety, and obtain an accurate measurement:

- Follow Standard Precautions and the Bloodborne Pathogen Standard.
- Use the person's thermometer.
- Use a rectal thermometer only for rectal temperatures.
- Rinse the thermometer under cold, running water if it was soaking in a disinfectant. Dry it from the stem to the bulb end with tissues.
- Check the thermometer for breaks, cracks, and chips. Discard it following center policy if it is broken, cracked, or chipped.
- Shake down the thermometer to move the substance down in the tube. Hold it at the stem; stand away from walls, tables, or other hard surfaces. Flex and snap your wrist until the substance is below 94° F or 34° C. See Figure 31-3.
- Insert the thermometer into a plastic cover (Fig. 31-4). Remove the cover to read the thermometer. Discard the cover after use.
- Clean and store the thermometer following center policy. Wipe it with tissues first to remove mucus, feces, or sweat. Do not use hot water. It causes the substance in the thermometer to expand so much that the thermometer could break. After cleaning, rinse the thermometer under cold, running water. Then store it in a container with a disinfectant solution.

Taking Temperatures

Glass thermometers are used for oral, rectal, and axillary temperatures.

- *The oral site.* The glass thermometer remains in place 2 to 3 minutes or as required by center policy.
- *The rectal site.* Lubricate the bulb end of the rectal thermometer for easy insertion and to prevent injury. Hold the device in place so it is not lost into the rectum or broken. The glass thermometer remains in the rectum for 2 minutes or as required by center policy. Provide for privacy. The buttocks and anus are exposed. The procedure embarrasses many people.
- *The axillary site.* The axilla (underarm) must be dry. Do not use this site right after bathing. The glass thermometer stays in place for 5 to 10 minutes or as required by center policy.

See *Focus on Communication: Taking Temperatures.*
See *Delegation Guidelines: Taking Temperatures, p. 478.*
See *Promoting Safety and Comfort: Taking Temperatures,* p. 478.

FOCUS ON COMMUNICATION
Taking Temperatures

Checking a rectal temperature can be embarrassing and uncomfortable. Be professional. Tell the person what you are going to do. Explain why you must check the person's temperature using the rectal route. You can say: "Mr. Presney, I need to check your temperature. I must check a rectal temperature because your oxygen changes the temperature in your mouth. The thermometer has to stay in place for 2 minutes. Please tell me if you feel pain."

When using a glass thermometer, the thermometer remains in the rectum for at least 2 minutes. This can cause discomfort. To promote comfort, talk the person through the procedure. You can say: "I'm almost done. There's about 1 minute left. Are you doing okay?"

DELEGATION GUIDELINES
Taking Temperatures

Before taking temperatures, you need this information from the nurse and the care plan:

- What site to use for each person—oral, rectal, axillary, tympanic membrane, or temporal artery
- What thermometer to use for each person—glass, electronic (p. 480), or other type (p. 482)
- How long to leave a glass thermometer in place
- When to take temperatures
- Which persons are at risk for elevated temperatures
- What observations to report and record:
  - A temperature that is changed from a prior measurement
  - A temperature above or below the normal range for the site used
- When to report observations
- What specific resident concerns to report at once

PROMOTING SAFETY AND COMFORT
Taking Temperatures

Safety

Thermometers are inserted into the mouth, rectum, axilla, and ear. Each area has many microbes. The area may contain blood. Therefore each person has his or her own glass or digital (p. 482) thermometer. This prevents the spread of microbes and infection. Follow Standard Precautions and the Bloodborne Pathogen Standard when taking temperatures.

With rectal temperatures, your gloved hands may have contact with feces. If so, remove gloves and practice hand hygiene. Then note the temperature on your notepad or assignment sheet. Put on clean gloves to complete the procedure.

Comfort

Remove the thermometer in a timely manner. Do not leave it in place longer than needed. This affects the person's comfort. For example, an oral thermometer is left in place for 2 to 3 minutes. Do not leave it in place longer than that.

 ## TAKING A TEMPERATURE WITH A GLASS THERMOMETER

QUALITY OF LIFE

Remember to:
- Knock before entering the person's room.
- Address the person by name.
- Introduce yourself by name and title.

- Explain the procedure to the person before beginning and during the procedure.
- Protect the person's rights during the procedure.
- Handle the person gently during the procedure.

PRE-PROCEDURE

1 Follow *Delegation Guidelines: Taking Temperatures.* See *Promoting Safety and Comfort:*
   a *Glass Thermometers,* p. 476
   b *Taking Temperatures*
2 For an *oral temperature,* ask the person not to eat, drink, smoke, or chew gum for at least 15 to 20 minutes before the measurement or as required by center policy.
3 Practice hand hygiene.
4 Collect the following:
   - Oral or rectal thermometer and holder
   - Tissues

- Plastic covers if used
- Gloves
- Toilet tissue (rectal temperature)
- Water-soluble lubricant (rectal temperature)
- Towel (axillary temperature)

5 Decontaminate your hands.
6 Identify the person. Check the ID (identification) bracelet against the assignment sheet. Also call the person by name.
7 Provide for privacy.

PROCEDURE

8 Put on the gloves.
9 Rinse the thermometer in cold water if it was soaking in a disinfectant. Dry it with tissues.
10 Check for breaks, cracks, or chips.
11 Shake down the thermometer below the lowest number. Hold the device by the stem.
12 Insert it into a plastic cover if used.

13 For an *oral temperature:*
   a Ask the person to moisten his or her lips.
   b Place the bulb end of the thermometer under the tongue and to one side (Fig. 31-5).
   c Ask the person to close the lips around the thermometer to hold it in place.
   d Ask the person not to talk. Remind the person not to bite down on the thermometer.
   e Leave it in place for 2 to 3 minutes or as required by center policy.

TAKING A TEMPERATURE WITH A GLASS THERMOMETER—cont'd

PROCEDURE—cont'd

14 For a *rectal temperature:*
   a Position the person in Sims' position.
   b Put a small amount of lubricant on a tissue.
   c Lubricate the bulb end of the thermometer.
   d Fold back top linens to expose the anal area.
   e Raise the upper buttock to expose the anus (Fig. 31-6).
   f Insert the thermometer 1 inch into the rectum. Do not force the thermometer.
   g Hold the thermometer in place for 2 minutes or as required by center policy. Do not let go of it while it is in the rectum.
15 For an *axillary temperature:*
   a Help the person remove an arm from the gown. Do not expose the person.
   b Dry the axilla with the towel.
   c Place the bulb end of the thermometer in the center of the axilla.
   d Ask the person to place the arm over the chest to hold the thermometer in place (Fig. 31-7, p. 480). Hold it and the arm in place if he or she cannot help.
   e Leave the thermometer in place for 5 to 10 minutes or as required by center policy.
16 Remove the thermometer.

17 Use tissues to remove the plastic cover. Discard the cover and tissues. Wipe the thermometer with a tissue if no cover was used. Wipe from the stem to the bulb end. Discard the tissue.
18 Read the thermometer.
19 Note the person's name and temperature on your notepad or assignment sheet. Write *R* for a rectal temperature. Write *A* for an axillary temperature.
20 For a *rectal temperature:*
   a Place used toilet tissue on several thicknesses of clean toilet tissue.
   b Place the thermometer on clean toilet tissue.
   c Wipe the anal area to remove excess lubricant and any feces.
   d Cover the person.
21 For an *axillary temperature:* Help the person put the gown back on.
22 Shake down the thermometer.
23 Clean the thermometer according to center policy. Return it to the holder.
24 Discard tissues and dispose of toilet tissue.
25 Remove the gloves. Decontaminate your hands.

POST-PROCEDURE

26 Provide for comfort. (See the inside of the front book cover.)
27 Place the signal light within reach.
28 Unscreen the person.
29 Complete a safety check of the room. (See the inside of the front book cover.)

30 Decontaminate your hands.
31 Report and record the temperature. Note the temperature site when reporting and recording. Report an abnormal temperature at once.

Fig. 31-5 The thermometer is placed at the base of the tongue and to one side.

Frenulum of tongue
Tip of thermometer

Fig. 31-6 The rectal temperature is taken with the person in Sims' position. The buttock is raised to expose the anus.

Fig. 31-7 The thermometer is held in place in the axilla by bringing the person's arm over the chest.

Fig. 31-8 Electronic thermometer.

Fig. 31-9 Tympanic membrane thermometer.

Fig. 31-10 Temporal artery thermometer.

🔖 Electronic Thermometers

Electronic thermometers are battery-operated (Fig. 31-8). They measure temperature in a few seconds. The temperature is shown on the front of the device. Some have batteries. Others are kept in battery chargers when not in use.

Electronic thermometers have oral and rectal probes. A disposable cover (sheath) protects the probe. You discard the probe cover after use. This helps prevent the spread of infection.

Tympanic Membrane Thermometers Tympanic membrane thermometers measure temperature at the tympanic membrane in the ear (Fig. 31-9). The covered probe is gently inserted into the ear. The temperature is measured in 1 to 3 seconds.

Tympanic membrane thermometers are comfortable. They are not invasive like rectal thermometers and probes. There are fewer microbes in the ear than in the mouth or rectum. The risk of spreading infection is reduced. These devices are not used if there is ear drainage.

Temporal Artery Thermometers Body temperature is measured at the temporal artery in the forehead (Fig. 31-10). You gently stroke the device across the forehead and across the temporal artery. It measures the temperature of the blood in the temporal artery—the same temperature of the blood coming from the heart.

These non-invasive devices measure body temperature in 3 to 4 seconds. Follow the manufacturer's instructions to use, clean, and store the device. Some devices have probe covers. To measure temperature:

- Use the side of the head that is exposed. Do not use the side covered by hair, a dressing, a hat, or other covering. Do not use the side that was on a pillow.
- Place the device at the side of the forehead between the hairline and eyebrows.
- Slide the device across the forehead.
- Read the temperature display.

See *Residents With Dementia: Electronic Thermometers*, p. 482.

See *Teamwork and Time Management: Electronic Thermometers*, p. 482.

TAKING A TEMPERATURE WITH AN ELECTRONIC THERMOMETER

QUALITY OF LIFE

Remember to:
- Knock before entering the person's room.
- Address the person by name.
- Introduce yourself by name and title.

- Explain the procedure to the person before beginning and during the procedure.
- Protect the person's rights during the procedure.
- Handle the person gently during the procedure.

PRE-PROCEDURE

1 Follow *Delegation Guidelines: Taking Temperatures,* p. 478. See *Promoting Safety and Comfort: Taking Temperatures,* p. 478.
2 For an oral temperature, ask the person not to eat, drink, smoke, or chew gum for at least 15 to 20 minutes before the measurement or as required by center policy.
3 Practice hand hygiene.
4 Collect the following:
   - Thermometer—electronic or tympanic membrane
   - Probe (Blue for an oral or axillary temperature. Red for a rectal temperature.)

   - Probe covers
   - Toilet tissue (rectal temperature)
   - Water-soluble lubricant (rectal temperature)
   - Gloves
   - Towel (axillary temperature)
5 Plug the probe into the thermometer, if using an electronic thermometer.
6 Decontaminate your hands.
7 Identify the person. Check the ID bracelet against the assignment sheet. Also call the person by name.

PROCEDURE

8 Provide for privacy. Position the person for an oral, rectal, axillary, or tympanic membrane temperature.
9 Put on gloves if contact with blood, body fluids, secretions, or excretions is likely.
10 Insert the probe into a probe cover.
11 For an *oral temperature:*
   a Ask the person to open the mouth and raise the tongue.
   b Place the covered probe at the base of the tongue and to one side (see Fig. 31-5).
   c Ask the person to lower the tongue and close the mouth.
12 For a *rectal temperature:*
   a Place some lubricant on toilet tissue.
   b Lubricate the end of the covered probe.
   c Expose the anal area.
   d Raise the upper buttock.
   e Insert the probe ½ inch into the rectum.
   f Hold the probe in place.
13 For an *axillary temperature:*
   a Help the person remove an arm from the gown. Do not expose the person.
   b Dry the axilla with the towel.
   c Place the covered probe in the center of the axilla.
   d Place the person's arm over the chest.
   e Hold the probe in place.

14 For a *tympanic membrane temperature:*
   a Ask the person to turn his or her head so the ear is in front of you.
   b Pull up and back on the adult's ear to straighten the ear canal (Fig. 31-11, p. 482).
   c Insert the covered probe gently.
15 Start the thermometer.
16 Hold the probe in place until you hear a tone or see a flashing or steady light.
17 Read the temperature on the display.
18 Remove the probe. Press the eject button to discard the cover.
19 Note the person's name and temperature on your notepad or assignment sheet. Note the temperature site.
20 Return the probe to the holder.
21 Help the person put the gown back on (axillary temperature). For a rectal temperature:
   a Wipe the anal area with toilet tissue to remove lubricant.
   b Cover the person.
   c Dispose of used toilet tissue.
   d Remove the gloves. Practice hand hygiene.

POST-PROCEDURE

22 Provide for comfort. (See the inside of the front book cover.)
23 Place the signal light within reach.
24 Unscreen the person.
25 Complete a safety check of the room. (See the inside of the front book cover.)

26 Return the thermometer to the charging unit.
27 Decontaminate your hands.
28 Report and record the temperature. Note the temperature site when reporting and recording. Report an abnormal temperature at once.

RESIDENTS WITH DEMENTIA
Electronic Thermometers

Tympanic membrane and temporal artery thermometers are used for persons who are confused and resist care. They are fast and comfortable. Oral and rectal thermometers are unsafe because:

- A glass thermometer can easily break if the person moves, resists care, or bites down on it. Serious injury can occur.
- An electronic thermometer can injure the mouth and teeth if the person bites down on it. It also can cause injury if the person moves quickly and without warning.

TEAMWORK AND TIME MANAGEMENT
Electronic Thermometers

Electronic, tympanic membrane, and temporal artery thermometers are shared with your co-workers. When using these devices, tell your co-workers what thermometer you have. Work quickly, but carefully. Return the device to the charging unit in a timely manner.

Fig. 31-11 Using a tympanic membrane thermometer. **A,** The ear is pulled up and back. **B,** The probe is inserted into the ear canal.

Other Thermometers

Other thermometers are used. Follow the manufacturer's instructions.

- *Digital thermometers*—show the temperature on the front of the thermometer (Fig. 31-12). Depending on the type, the temperature is measured in 6 to 60 seconds.
- *Disposable oral thermometers*—have small chemical dots (Fig. 31-13). The dots change color when heated. Each dot is heated to a certain temperature before it changes color. These thermometers are used once. They measure temperatures in 45 to 60 seconds.
- *Temperature-sensitive tape*—changes color in response to body heat (Fig. 31-14). The tape is applied to the forehead. The measurement takes about 15 seconds.

Fig. 31-12 Digital thermometer.

Fig. 31-13 Disposable oral thermometer with chemical dots. The dots change color when heated by the body.

Fig. 31-14 Temperature-sensitive tape.

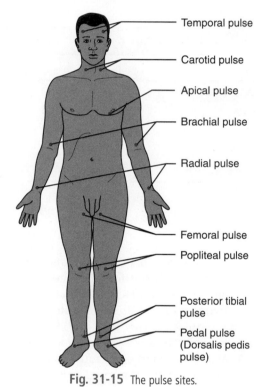

- Temporal pulse
- Carotid pulse
- Apical pulse
- Brachial pulse
- Radial pulse
- Femoral pulse
- Popliteal pulse
- Posterior tibial pulse
- Pedal pulse (Dorsalis pedis pulse)

Fig. 31-15 The pulse sites.

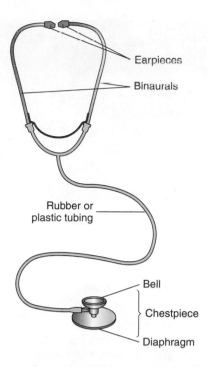

- Earpieces
- Binaurals
- Rubber or plastic tubing
- Bell
- Chestpiece
- Diaphragm

Fig. 31-16 Parts of a stethoscope.

PULSE

The **pulse** is the beat of the heart felt at an artery as a wave of blood passes through the artery. A pulse is felt every time the heart beats.

Pulse Sites

The temporal, carotid, brachial, radial, femoral, popliteal, posterior tibial, and dorsalis pedis (pedal) pulses are on each side of the body (Fig. 31-15). The arteries are close to the body surface and lie over a bone. Therefore they are easy to feel.

The radial pulse is used most often. It is easy to reach and find. You can take a radial pulse without disturbing or exposing the person. The carotid pulse is

taken during cardiopulmonary resuscitation (CPR) and other emergencies (Chapter 47).

The apical pulse is felt over the heart. The apex (*apical*) of the heart is at the tip of the heart, just below the left nipple (p. 487). This pulse is taken with a stethoscope.

Using a Stethoscope

A **stethoscope** is an instrument used to listen to the sounds produced by the heart, lungs, and other body organs (Fig. 31-16). It is used to take apical pulses and blood pressures. The device makes sounds louder for easy hearing.

To use a stethoscope:
- Wipe the earpieces and diaphragm with antiseptic wipes before and after use.
- Place the earpiece tips in your ears. The bend of the tips points forward. Earpieces should fit snugly to block out noises. They should not cause pain or ear discomfort.
- Tap the diaphragm gently. You should hear the tapping. If not, turn the chest piece at the tubing. Gently tap the diaphragm again. Proceed if you hear the tapping sound. Check with the nurse if you do not hear the tapping.
- Place the diaphragm over the artery. Hold it in place as in Figure 31-17, p. 484.
- Prevent noise. Do not let anything touch the tubing. Ask the person to be silent.

See *Focus on Communication: Using a Stethoscope,* p. 484.

See *Promoting Safety and Comfort: Using a Stethoscope* p. 484.

Fig. 31-17 The stethoscope is held in place with the fingertips of the index and middle fingers.

Fig. 31-18 The diaphragm of the stethoscope is warmed in the palm of the hand.

FOCUS ON COMMUNICATION
Using a Stethoscope

Hearing through the stethoscope is hard if the person is talking. Politely ask the person to be silent. Explain the procedure. Tell the person when and for how long he or she must remain silent. You can say:

> "Mr. Bradley, I am going to check your pulse with a stethoscope. It is hard for me to hear your heart beat when you talk. Please do not talk when my stethoscope is on your chest. It will take about 1 minute."

The person may forget and begin talking. You can politely say: "I am almost finished. Please stay quiet for just a little longer." Thank the person when you are done.

PROMOTING SAFETY AND COMFORT
Using a Stethoscope

Safety
Stethoscopes are in contact with many persons and staff. You must prevent infection. Wipe the earpieces and diaphragm with antiseptic wipes before and after use.

Comfort
Stethoscope diaphragms tend to be cold. Warm the diaphragm in your hand before applying it to the person (Fig. 31-18). Cold diaphragms can startle the person.

Table 31-2	Pulse Ranges by Age

Age	Pulse Rate per Minute
Birth to 1 year	80-190
2 years	80-160
6 years	75-120
10 years	70-110
12 years and older	60-100

Pulse Rate

The **pulse rate** is the number of heartbeats or pulses felt in 1 minute. The rate varies for each age-group (Table 31-2). The pulse rate is affected by many factors (p. 474). Some drugs increase the pulse rate. Other drugs slow down the pulse.

The adult pulse rate is between 60 and 100 beats per minute. A rate of less than 60 or more than 100 is considered abnormal. Report abnormal pulses to the nurse at once.

- **Tachycardia** is a rapid *(tachy)* heart rate *(cardia)*. The heart rate is more than 100 beats per minute.
- **Bradycardia** is a slow *(brady)* heart rate *(cardia)*. The heart rate is less than 60 beats per minute.

Fig. 31-19 A, The electrocardiogram shows a regular pulse. The beats occur at regular intervals. **B,** These beats are at irregular intervals.

Rhythm and Force of the Pulse

The pulse *rhythm* should be regular. That is, pulses are felt in a pattern. The same interval occurs between beats. An irregular pulse occurs when the beats are not evenly spaced or beats are skipped (Fig. 31-19).

Force relates to pulse strength. A forceful pulse is easy to feel. It is described as *strong, full,* or *bounding.* Hard-to-feel pulses are described as *weak, thready,* or *feeble.*

Electronic blood pressure equipment (p. 491) can also count pulses. The pulse rate and blood pressures are shown. Some show if the pulse is regular or irregular. However, you need to feel the pulse to determine its force.

Taking Pulses

You will take radial, apical, and apical-radial pulses. You must count, report, and record accurately.

See *Delegation Guidelines: Taking Pulses.*
See *Promoting Safety and Comfort: Taking Pulses.*

Taking a Radial Pulse The radial pulse is used for routine vital signs. Place the first 2 or 3 fingertips of one hand against the radial artery. The radial artery is on the thumb side of the wrist (Fig. 31-20). Count the pulse for 30 seconds. Then multiply the number by 2. This gives the number of beats per minute. If the pulse is irregular, count it for 1 minute.

In some centers, all radial pulses are taken for 1 minute. Follow center policy.

Fig. 31-20 The middle three fingertips are used to take the radial pulse.

TAKING A RADIAL PULSE

`VIDEO CLIP` `VIDEO` ◉ `NNAAP™ Skill`

QUALITY OF LIFE

Remember to:
- Knock before entering the person's room.
- Address the person by name.
- Introduce yourself by name and title.

- Explain the procedure to the person before beginning and during the procedure.
- Protect the person's rights during the procedure.
- Handle the person gently during the procedure.

PRE-PROCEDURE

1 Follow *Delegation Guidelines: Taking Pulses,* p. 485. See *Promoting Safety and Comfort: Taking Pulses,* p. 485.
2 Practice hand hygiene.

3 Identify the person. Check the ID bracelet against the assignment sheet. Also call the person by name.
4 Provide for privacy.

PROCEDURE

5 Have the person sit or lie down.
6 Locate the radial pulse on the thumb side of the person's wrist. Use your first 2 or 3 middle fingertips (see Fig. 31-20).
7 Note if the pulse is strong or weak, and regular or irregular.

8 Count the pulse for 30 seconds. Multiply the number of beats by 2. Or count the pulse for 1 minute if:
  a Directed by the nurse and care plan.
  b Required by center policy.
  c The pulse was irregular.
  d Required for your state competency test.
9 Note the person's name and pulse on your notepad or assignment sheet. Note the strength of the pulse. Note if it was regular or irregular.

POST-PROCEDURE

10 Provide for comfort. (See the inside of the front book cover.)
11 Place the signal light within reach.
12 Unscreen the person.
13 Complete a safety check of the room. (See the inside of the front book cover.)

14 Decontaminate your hands.
15 Report and record the pulse rate and your observations. Report an abnormal pulse at once.

Taking an Apical Pulse The apical pulse is on the left side of the chest slightly below the nipple (Fig. 31-21). It is taken with a stethoscope. Apical pulses are taken on persons who:

- Have heart disease
- Have irregular heart rhythms
- Take drugs that affect the heart

Count the apical pulse for 1 minute. The heartbeat normally sounds like a *lub-dub.* Count each *lub-dub* as one beat. Do not count the *lub* as one beat and the *dub* as another.

Fig. 31-21 The apical pulse is located 2 to 3 inches to the left of the sternum (breastbone) and below the left nipple.

TAKING AN APICAL PULSE   `VIDEO`

QUALITY OF LIFE

Remember to:
- Knock before entering the person's room.
- Address the person by name.
- Introduce yourself by name and title.

- Explain the procedure to the person before beginning and during the procedure.
- Protect the person's rights during the procedure.
- Handle the person gently during the procedure.

PRE-PROCEDURE

1 Follow *Delegation Guidelines: Taking Pulses,* p. 485. See *Promoting Safety and Comfort: Using a Stethoscope,* p. 484.
2 Practice hand hygiene.
3 Collect a stethoscope and antiseptic wipes.

4 Decontaminate your hands.
5 Identify the person. Check the ID bracelet against the assignment sheet. Also call the person by name.
6 Provide for privacy.

PROCEDURE

7 Clean the earpieces and diaphragm with the wipes.
8 Have the person sit or lie down.
9 Expose the nipple area of the left chest. Expose a woman's breasts to the extent necessary.
10 Warm the diaphragm in your palm.
11 Place the earpieces in your ears.
12 Find the apical pulse. Place the diaphragm 2 to 3 inches to the left of the breastbone and below the left nipple (see Fig. 31-21).

13 Count the pulse for 1 minute. Note if it was regular or irregular.
14 Cover the person. Remove the earpieces.
15 Note the person's name and pulse on your notepad or assignment sheet. Note if the pulse was regular or irregular.

POST-PROCEDURE

16 Provide for comfort. (See the inside of the front book cover.)
17 Place the signal light within reach.
18 Unscreen the person.
19 Complete a safety check of the room. (See the inside of the front book cover.)

20 Clean the earpieces and diaphragm with the wipes.
21 Return the stethoscope to its proper place.
22 Decontaminate your hands.
23 Report and record your observations. Record the pulse rate with *Ap* for apical. Report an abnormal pulse rate at once.

Taking an Apical-Radial Pulse The apical and radial pulse rates should be the same. Sometimes heart contractions are not strong enough to create pulses in the radial artery. Then the radial rate is less than the apical rate. Heart disease is a common cause.

To see if the apical and radial pulses are equal, two staff members are needed. One takes the radial pulse; the other takes the apical pulse. Taking the apical and radial pulses at the same time is called the **apical-radial pulse.**

The **pulse deficit** is the difference between the apical and radial pulse rates. That is, you subtract the radial rate from the apical rate. (The radial rate is never greater than the apical rate.) For example:

- The apical rate is 84 beats per minute. The radial rate is 84 beats per minute. The pulse deficit is zero (0).
- The apical rate is 90 beats per minute. The radial rate is 86 beats per minute. The pulse deficit is 4.

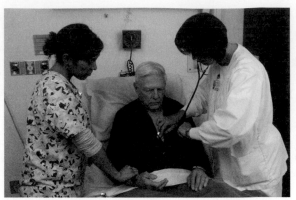

Fig. 31-22 Taking an apical-radial pulse. One worker takes the apical pulse. The other takes the radial pulse.

TAKING AN APICAL-RADIAL PULSE

QUALITY OF LIFE

Remember to:
- Knock before entering the person's room.
- Address the person by name.
- Introduce yourself by name and title.

- Explain the procedure to the person before beginning and during the procedure.
- Protect the person's rights during the procedure.
- Handle the person gently during the procedure.

PRE-PROCEDURE

1 Follow *Delegation Guidelines: Taking Pulses*, p. 485. See *Promoting Safety and Comfort:*
  a *Using a Stethoscope*, p. 484
  b *Taking Pulses*, p. 485
2 Ask a co-worker to help you.
3 Practice hand hygiene.

4 Collect a stethoscope and antiseptic wipes.
5 Decontaminate your hands.
6 Identify the person. Check the ID bracelet against the assignment sheet. Also call the person by name.
7 Provide for privacy.

PROCEDURE

8 Clean the earpieces and diaphragm with the wipes.
9 Have the person sit or lie down.
10 Expose the nipple area of the left chest. Expose a woman's breasts to the extent necessary.
11 Warm the diaphragm in your palm.
12 Place the earpieces in your ears.
13 Find the apical pulse. Your helper finds the radial pulse (Fig. 31-22).

14 Give the signal to begin counting.
15 Count the pulse for 1 minute.
16 Give the signal to stop counting.
17 Cover the person. Remove the stethoscope earpieces.
18 Note the person's name and the apical and radial pulses on your notepad or assignment sheet. Subtract the radial pulse from the apical pulse for the pulse deficit. Note whether the pulse was regular or irregular.

POST-PROCEDURE

19 Provide for comfort. (See the inside of the front book cover.)
20 Place the signal light within reach.
21 Unscreen the person.
22 Complete a safety check of the room. (See the inside of the front book cover.)
23 Clean the earpieces and diaphragm with the wipes.

24 Return the stethoscope to its proper place.
25 Decontaminate your hands.
26 Report and record your observations. (Report an abnormal pulse at once.) Include:
  a The apical and radial pulse rates
  b The pulse deficit

RESPIRATIONS

Respiration means breathing air into (*inhalation*) and out of (*exhalation*) the lungs. Oxygen enters the lungs during inhalation. Carbon dioxide leaves the lungs during exhalation. Each respiration involves one inhalation and one exhalation. The chest rises during inhalation. It falls during exhalation.

The healthy adult has 12 to 20 respirations per minute. See p. 474 for the factors affecting vital signs. Heart and respiratory diseases often increase the respiratory rate.

Respirations are normally quiet, effortless, and regular. Both sides of the chest rise and fall equally. See Chapter 28 for abnormal respiratory patterns.

Count respirations when the person is at rest. Position the person so you can see the chest rise and fall. To some extent, a person can control the rate and depth of breathing. People tend to change their breathing patterns when they know their respirations are being counted. Therefore do not tell the person that you are counting them.

Count respirations right after taking a pulse. Keep your fingers or stethoscope over the pulse site. (The person assumes you are taking the pulse). To count respirations, watch the chest rise and fall. Count them for 30 seconds. Multiply the number by 2 for the number of respirations in 1 minute. If you note an abnormal pattern, count the respirations for 1 minute.

In nursing centers, respirations may be counted for 1 minute. Follow center policy.

See *Delegation Guidelines: Respirations.*

DELEGATION GUIDELINES
Respirations

Before counting respirations, you need this information from the nurse and the care plan:
- How long to count respirations for each person— 30 seconds or 1 minute
- When to count respirations
- If the nurse has concerns about certain residents
- What other vital signs to measure
- What observations to report and record:
  - The respiratory rate
  - Equality and depth of respirations
  - If the respirations were regular or irregular
  - If the person has pain or difficulty breathing
  - Any respiratory noises
  - An abnormal respiratory pattern (Chapter 28)
- When to report observations
- What specific resident concerns to report at once

COUNTING RESPIRATIONS

PROCEDURE

1 Follow *Delegation Guidelines: Respirations.*
2 Keep your fingers or stethoscope over the pulse site.
3 Do not tell the person you are counting respirations.
4 Begin counting when the chest rises. Count each rise and fall of the chest as 1 respiration.
5 Note the following:
  a If respirations are regular
  b If both sides of the chest rise equally
  c The depth of respirations
  d If the person has any pain or difficulty breathing
  e An abnormal respiratory pattern

6 Count respirations for 30 seconds. Multiply the number by 2. Count respirations for 1 minute if:
  a Directed by the nurse and care plan.
  b Required by center policy.
  c They are abnormal or irregular.
  d Required for your state competency test.
7 Note the person's name, respiratory rate, and other observations on your notepad or assignment sheet.

POST-PROCEDURE

8 Provide for comfort. (See the inside of the front book cover.)
9 Place the signal light within reach.
10 Unscreen the person.
11 Complete a safety check of the room. (See the inside of the front book cover.)
12 Decontaminate your hands.
13 Report and record the respiratory rate and your observations. Report abnormal respirations at once.

BLOOD PRESSURE

Blood pressure (BP) is the amount of force exerted against the walls of an artery by the blood. Blood pressure is controlled by:

- The force of heart contractions
- The amount of blood pumped with each heartbeat
- How easily the blood flows through the blood vessels

Systole is the period of heart muscle contraction. The heart is pumping blood. Diastole is the period of heart muscle relaxation. The heart is at rest.

You measure systolic and diastolic pressures. The systolic pressure is the pressure in the arteries when the heart contracts. It is the higher pressure. The diastolic pressure is the pressure in the arteries when the heart is at rest. It is the lower pressure.

Blood pressure is measured in millimeters (mm) of mercury (Hg). The systolic pressure is recorded over the diastolic pressure. A systolic pressure of 120 mm Hg (millimeters of mercury) and a diastolic pressure of 80 mm Hg is written as 120/80 mm Hg.

Normal and Abnormal Blood Pressures

Blood pressure can change from minute to minute. Factors affecting blood pressure are listed in Box 31-2.

Blood pressure has normal ranges:

- *Systolic pressure*—less than 120 mm Hg
- *Diastolic pressure*—less than 80 mm Hg

Treatment is indicated for:

- Hypertension—BP measurements remaining above *(hyper)* a systolic pressure of 140 mm Hg or a diastolic pressure of 90 mm Hg. Report any systolic measurement at or above 120 mm Hg. Also report a diastolic pressure at or above 80 mm Hg.
- Hypotension—when the systolic blood pressure is below *(hypo)* 90 mm Hg and the diastolic pressure is below 60 mm Hg. Report a systolic pressure below 90 mm Hg. Also report a diastolic pressure below 60 mm Hg. Some people normally have low blood pressures. Older persons are at risk for orthostatic hypotension (Chapter 26). However, hypotension can signal a life-threatening problem.

Box 31-2   Factors Affecting Blood Pressure

- *Age.* BP increases with age. It is lowest in infancy and childhood. It is highest in adulthood.
- *Gender (male or female).* Women usually have lower blood pressures than men do. Blood pressures rise in women after menopause.
- *Blood volume.* This is the amount of blood in the system. Severe bleeding lowers the blood volume. Therefore BP lowers. Giving IV (intravenous) fluids rapidly increases the blood volume. The BP rises.
- *Stress.* Stress includes anxiety, fear, and emotions. BP increases as the body responds to stress.
- *Pain.* Pain generally increases BP. However, severe pain can cause *shock.* BP is seriously low in the state of shock (Chapter 47).
- *Exercise.* BP increases. Do not measure BP right after exercise.
- *Weight.* BP is higher in over-weight persons. It lowers with weight loss.

- *Race.* Black persons generally have higher blood pressures than white persons do.
- *Diet.* A high-sodium diet increases the amount of water in the body. The extra fluid volume increases BP.
- *Drugs.* Drugs can be given to raise or lower BP. Other drugs have the side effects of high or low BP.
- *Position.* BP is higher when lying down. It is lower in the standing position. Sudden changes in position can cause a sudden drop in BP (orthostatic hypotension). When standing suddenly, the person may have a sudden drop in BP. Dizziness and fainting can occur.
- *Smoking.* BP increases. Nicotine in cigarettes causes blood vessels to narrow. The heart must work harder to pump blood through narrowed vessels.
- *Alcohol.* Excessive alcohol intake can raise BP.

Equipment

You use a stethoscope and a sphygmomanometer to measure blood pressure. The **sphygmomanometer** has a cuff and a measuring device.

- The *aneroid type* has a round dial and a needle that points to the numbers (Fig. 31-23, *A*).
- The *mercury type* has a column of mercury within a calibrated tube (Fig. 31-23, *B*).
- The *electronic type* shows the systolic and diastolic blood pressures on the front of the device (Fig. 31-23, *C*). It also shows the pulse rate. To use the device, follow the manufacturer's instructions.

You wrap the blood pressure cuff around the upper arm. Tubing connects the cuff to the manometer. Another tube connects the cuff to a small, hand-held bulb. To inflate the cuff, turn the valve on the bulb clockwise to close the valve and then squeeze the bulb. The inflated cuff causes pressure over the brachial artery. Turn the valve counter-clockwise to open the valve to deflate the cuff. Measure BP as the cuff deflates.

Blood flowing through the arteries produces sounds. Use the stethoscope to listen to the sounds in the brachial artery as you deflate the cuff. You do not need a stethoscope for an electronic manometer.

See *Promoting Safety and Comfort: Equipment.*

PROMOTING SAFETY AND COMFORT
Equipment

Safety

Mercury is a hazardous substance. Mercury manometers are being phased out of health care. Some centers may still use them. Handle mercury manometers carefully. If one breaks, call for the nurse at once. Do not touch the mercury. Do not let the person touch it. The center follows special procedures for handling all hazardous substances. See Chapter 12.

Comfort

Inflate the cuff only to the extent necessary (see procedure: *Measuring Blood Pressure*, p. 493). The inflated cuff causes discomfort. The higher the inflation, the greater the discomfort.

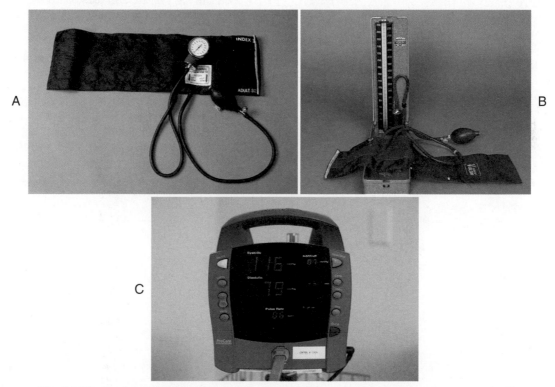

Fig. 31-23 Blood pressure equipment. **A,** Aneroid manometer and cuff. **B,** Mercury manometer and cuff. **C,** Electronic sphygmomanometer.

Measuring Blood Pressure

You measure blood pressure in the brachial artery. Box 31-3 lists the guidelines for measuring blood pressure.

See *Delegation Guidelines: Measuring Blood Pressure.*

DELEGATION GUIDELINES
Measuring Blood Pressure

Before measuring BP, you need this information from the nurse and the care plan:

- When to measure BP
- What arm to use
- The person's normal blood pressure range
- If the nurse has concerns about certain residents
- If the person needs to be lying down, sitting, or standing
- What size cuff to use—regular, child-size, or extra large
- What observations to report and record
- When to report the BP measurement
- What specific resident concerns to report at once

Box 31-3   Guidelines for Measuring Blood Pressure

- Do not take BP on an arm with an IV infusion, a cast, or a dialysis access site. If a person had breast surgery, do not take BP on that side. Avoid taking BP on an injured arm.
- Let the person rest for 10 to 20 minutes before measuring BP.
- Measure BP with the person sitting or lying. Sometimes the doctor orders BP measured in the standing position.
- Apply the cuff to the bare upper arm. Clothing can affect the measurement.
- Make sure the cuff is snug. Loose cuffs can cause inaccurate readings.
- Use a larger cuff if the person is obese or has a large arm. Use a small cuff if the person has a very small arm. Ask the nurse what size to use. Also check the care plan.
- Place the diaphragm of the stethoscope firmly over the brachial artery. The entire diaphragm must have contact with the skin.
- Make sure the room is quiet. Talking, TV, radio, and sounds from the hallway can affect an accurate measurement.
- Have the sphygmomanometer where you can clearly see it.
- Measure the systolic and diastolic pressures.
  - Expect to hear the first BP sound at the point where you last felt the radial or brachial pulse. The first sound is the systolic pressure.
  - The point where the sound disappears is the diastolic pressure.
- Take the BP again if you are not sure of an accurate measurement. Wait 30 to 60 seconds before repeating the measurement. Ask the nurse to take the BP if you are unsure of the measurement.
- Tell the nurse at once if you cannot hear the blood pressure.

MEASURING BLOOD PRESSURE

QUALITY OF LIFE

Remember to:
- Knock before entering the person's room.
- Address the person by name.
- Introduce yourself by name and title.

- Explain the procedure to the person before beginning and during the procedure.
- Protect the person's rights during the procedure.
- Handle the person gently during the procedure.

PRE-PROCEDURE

1 Follow *Delegation Guidelines: Measuring Blood Pressure.* See *Promoting Safety and Comfort:*
   a *Using a Stethoscope,* p. 484
   b *Equipment,* p. 491
2 Practice hand hygiene.
3 Collect the following:
   - Sphygmomanometer
   - Stethoscope
   - Antiseptic wipes

4 Decontaminate your hands.
5 Identify the person. Check the ID bracelet against the assignment sheet. Also call the person by name.
6 Provide for privacy.

PROCEDURE

7 Wipe the stethoscope earpieces and diaphragm with the wipes. Warm the diaphragm in your palm.
8 Have the person sit or lie down.
9 Position the person's arm level with the heart. The palm is up.
10 Stand no more than 3 feet away from the manometer. The mercury type is vertical, on a flat surface, and at eye level. The aneroid type is directly in front of you.
11 Expose the upper arm.
12 Squeeze the cuff to expel any remaining air. Close the valve on the bulb.
13 Find the brachial artery at the inner aspect of the elbow. (The brachial artery is on the little finger side of the arm.) Use your fingertips.
14 Locate the arrow on the cuff (Fig. 31-24, *A,* p. 494). Place the arrow on the cuff over the brachial artery (Fig. 31-24, *B,* p. 494). Wrap the cuff around the upper arm at least 1 inch above the elbow. It is even and snug.
15 Place the stethoscope earpieces in your ears.
16 Find the radial or brachial pulse.
17 *Method one:*
   a Inflate the cuff until you can no longer feel the pulse. Note this point.
   b Inflate the cuff 30 mm Hg beyond the point where you last felt the pulse.

18 *Method two:*
   a Inflate the cuff until you can no longer feel the pulse. Note this point.
   b Inflate the cuff 30 mm Hg beyond the point where you last felt the pulse.
   c Deflate the cuff slowly. Note the point when you feel the pulse.
   d Wait 30 seconds.
   e Inflate the cuff again, 30 mm Hg beyond the point where you felt the pulse return.
19 Place the diaphragm of the stethoscope over the brachial artery (Fig. 31-24, *C,* p. 494). Do not place it under the cuff.
20 Deflate the cuff at an even rate of 2 to 4 millimeters per second. Turn the valve counter-clockwise to deflate the cuff.
21 Note the point where you hear the first sound. This is the systolic reading. It is near the point where the radial pulse disappeared.
22 Continue to deflate the cuff. Note the point where the sound disappears. This is the diastolic reading.
23 Deflate the cuff completely. Remove it from the person's arm. Remove the stethoscope earpieces from your ears.
24 Note the person's name and blood pressure on your notepad or assignment sheet.
25 Return the cuff to the case or wall holder.

POST-PROCEDURE

26 Provide for comfort. (See the inside of the front book cover.)
27 Place the signal light within reach.
28 Unscreen the person.
29 Complete a safety check of the room. (See the inside of the front book cover.)

30 Clean the earpieces and diaphragm with the wipes.
31 Return the equipment to its proper place.
32 Decontaminate your hands.
33 Report and record the BP (Fig. 31-25, p. 494). Note which arm was used. Report an abnormal blood pressure at once.

Brachial
pulse

Fig. 31-24 Measuring blood pressure. **A,** The arrow is used for correct cuff alignment. **B,** The cuff is placed so the arrow is aligned with the brachial artery. **C,** The diaphragm of the stethoscope is over the brachial artery.

Date	Time	Weight	T	P	R	BP				Signatures
10/19	0700	126	98.4	72	20	142/84				Mary Smith CNA
10/26	0715	125	98.6	72	18	140/84				Jane Doe CNA
11/2	0715	126	98.6	70	18	144/82				Mary Smith CNA

Fig. 31-25 Charting sample.

QUALITY OF LIFE

Protect the right to privacy when measuring vital signs. This is very important when taking axillary or rectal temperatures and apical and apical-radial pulses. Expose the person only to the extent needed.

Always keep resident information confidential. Vital signs are just as private as other information. Do not share the information with family, visitors, and roommates.

The right to personal choice is important. Unless directed otherwise, vital signs are measured with the person sitting or lying down. Let the person choose the position. The person may also prefer that you use the right or left arm for pulses and blood pressure. If safe to do so, use the arm the person prefers.

REVIEW QUESTIONS

Circle the BEST answer.

1 Which statement is *false*?
a The vital signs are temperature, pulse, respirations, and blood pressure.
b Vital signs detect changes in body function.
c Vital signs change only during illness.
d Sleep, exercise, drugs, emotions, and noise affect vital signs.

2 Which should you report at once?
a An oral temperature of 98.4° F
b A rectal temperature of 101.6° F
c An axillary temperature of 97.6° F
d An oral temperature of 99.0° F

3 A rectal temperature is taken when the person
a Is unconscious
b Has heart disease
c Is confused
d Has diarrhea

4 Which gives the *least* accurate measurement of body temperature?
a Oral site
b Rectal site
c Axillary site
d Tympanic membrane site

5 Which is usually used to take an adult's pulse?
a The radial pulse
b The apical pulse
c The apical-radial pulse
d The brachial pulse

6 Which is reported to the nurse at once?
a An adult has a pulse of 124 beats per minute.
b An adult has a pulse of 90 beats per minute.
c An adult has a pulse of 86 beats per minute.
d An adult has a pulse of 64 beats per minute.

7 Which statement about the apical-radial pulse is *true*?
a The radial pulse can be greater than the apical pulse.
b The apical pulse can be greater than the radial pulse.
c The apical and radial pulses are always equal.
d The pulse deficit is 0.

8 In an adult, normal respirations are
a 10 to 18 per minute
b 12 to 20 per minute
c Less than 20 per minute
d More than 20 per minute

9 Normal respirations
a Are heard as the person inhales
b Are heard as the person exhales
c Are quiet
d Sound like wheezing with inhalation and exhalation

10 Respirations are usually counted
a After taking the temperature
b After taking the pulse
c Before taking the pulse
d After taking the blood pressure

11 Which blood pressure is normal for an adult?
a 88/54 mm Hg
b 140/90 mm Hg
c 100/58 mm Hg
d 112/78 mm Hg

12 When measuring BP, you should do the following *except*
a Use the arm with an intravenous infusion
b Apply the cuff to a bare upper arm
c Turn off the TV
d Locate the brachial artery

13 The systolic pressure is the point
a Where the pulse is no longer felt
b Where the first sound is heard
c Where the last sound is heard
d 30 mm Hg above where the pulse was felt

14 You are not sure of hearing an accurate BP measurement. What should you do?
a Record what you think that you heard.
b Measure the BP again after 60 seconds.
c Use the bell part of the stethoscope.
d Ask another nursing assistant to take the BP.

Answers to these questions are on p. 720.

Assisting With the Physical Examination

KEY TERMS

dorsal recumbent position The supine position with the legs together; horizontal recumbent position

genupectoral position See "knee-chest" position

horizontal recumbent position See "dorsal recumbent position"

knee-chest position The person kneels and rests the body on the knees and chest; the head is turned to one side, the arms are above the head or flexed at the elbows, the back is straight, and the body is flexed about 90 degrees at the hips; genupectoral position

laryngeal mirror An instrument used to examine the mouth, teeth, and throat

lithotomy position The woman lies on her back with her hips at the edge of the exam table, her knees are flexed, her hips are externally rotated, and her feet are in stirrups

nasal speculum An instrument used to examine the inside of the nose

ophthalmoscope A lighted instrument used to examine the internal eye structures

otoscope A lighted instrument used to examine the external ear and the eardrum (tympanic membrane)

percussion hammer An instrument used to tap body parts to test reflexes; reflex hammer

tuning fork An instrument vibrated to test hearing

vaginal speculum An instrument used to open the vagina for examining it and the cervix

Doctors and many RNs perform physical exams. Exams are done to:
- Promote health
- Determine fitness for work
- Diagnose disease

YOUR ROLE

Your role depends on center policies and procedures. It also depends on what the examiner prefers. You may do some or all of the following:
- Collect needed linens.
- Collect equipment and supplies.
- Prepare the room for the exam.
- Provide lighting.
- Transport the person to and from the exam room.
- Measure vital signs, weight, and height.
- Position and drape the person.
- Hand equipment and supplies to the examiner.
- Label specimen containers.
- Discard used supplies.
- Clean equipment.
- Help the person dress or to a comfortable position after the exam.
- Follow center policy for soiled linens.

EQUIPMENT

The instruments in Figure 32-1 are used in the exam:
- **Laryngeal mirror**—used to examine the mouth, teeth, and throat.
- **Nasal speculum**—used to examine the inside of the nose.
- **Ophthalmoscope**—a lighted instrument used to examine the internal eye structures.
- **Otoscope**—a lighted instrument used to examine the external ear and the eardrum (tympanic membrane). Some scopes can be changed into an ophthalmoscope.
- **Percussion hammer** *(reflex hammer)*—used to tap body parts to test reflexes.
- **Tuning fork**—vibrated to test hearing.
- **Vaginal speculum**—used to open the vagina to examine it and the cervix.

Some centers have exam trays in the supply department. If not, collect the items listed in the procedure: *Preparing the Person for an Examination*, p. 498. Arrange them on a tray or table.

🐦 PREPARING THE PERSON

The physical exam concerns many people. They worry about the findings. Some are confused or fearful about the procedure. Discomfort, embarrassment, fearing exposure, and not knowing the procedure cause anxiety. You must respect the person's feelings and concerns. To prepare the person physically and mentally, the nurse

Fig. 32-1 Instruments used for a physical exam.

explains the exam's purpose and what to expect. The person must give informed consent for the exam.

Privacy is protected. The person is screened and the room door closed. All clothes are removed for a complete exam. A patient gown is worn. It reduces the naked feeling and the fear of exposure. So does covering the person with a drape—paper drape, bath blanket, sheet, or drawsheet. Explain that only the part being examined is exposed.

The person voids before the exam to empty the bladder. This lets the examiner feel the abdominal organs. A full bladder can change the normal position and shape of organs. It also causes discomfort, especially when feeling the abdominal organs. If a urine specimen is needed, obtain it at this time. Explain how to collect the specimen (Chapter 33). Label the container.

Measure weight, height, and vital signs before the exam (Chapters 31 and 34). Record the measurements on the exam form. Then drape and position the person for the exam.

Nursing center residents have an exam at least once a year. The person is told who will do the exam and when it will be done. The person may want a different examiner. Or the person may want a family member present during the exam and when the results are explained.

See *Delegation Guidelines: Preparing the Person*, p. 498.
See *Promoting Safety and Comfort: Preparing the Person*, p. 498.

DELEGATION GUIDELINES
Preparing the Person

To prepare a person for an exam, you need this information from the nurse and the care plan:
- When to prepare the person
- Where it will be done—an exam room or the person's room
- How to position the person
- What equipment and supplies are needed
- If a urine specimen is needed
- What specific resident concerns to report at once

PROMOTING SAFETY AND COMFORT
Preparing the Person

Safety
Protect the person from falls and injury. Do not leave the person unattended.

Comfort
Warmth is a major concern during an exam. Protect the person from chilling. Have an extra bath blanket nearby. Also, take measures to prevent drafts.

PREPARING THE PERSON FOR AN EXAMINATION

QUALITY OF LIFE

Remember to:
- Knock before entering the person's room.
- Address the person by name.
- Introduce yourself by name and title.

- Explain the procedure to the person before beginning and during the procedure.
- Protect the person's rights during the procedure.
- Handle the person gently during the procedure.

PRE-PROCEDURE

1 Follow *Delegation Guidelines: Preparing the Person.* See *Promoting Safety and Comfort: Preparing the Person.*
2 Practice hand hygiene.
3 Collect the following:
- Flashlight
- Sphygmomanometer
- Stethoscope
- Thermometer
- Tongue depressors (blades)
- Laryngeal mirror
- Ophthalmoscope
- Otoscope
- Nasal speculum
- Percussion (reflex) hammer
- Tuning fork
- Tape measure
- Gloves
- Water-soluble lubricant
- Vaginal speculum
- Cotton-tipped applicators
- Specimen containers and labels
- Disposable bag

- Kidney basin
- Towel
- Bath blanket
- Tissues
- Drape (sheet, bath blanket, drawsheet, or paper drape)
- Paper towels
- Cotton balls
- Waterproof pad
- Eye chart (Snellen chart)
- Slides
- Gown
- Alcohol wipes
- Wastebasket
- Container for soiled instruments
- Marking pencils or pens

4 Decontaminate your hands.
5 Identify the person. Check the ID (identification) bracelet against the assignment sheet. Also call the person by name.
6 Provide for privacy.

PROCEDURE

7 Have the person put on the gown. Tell him or her to remove all clothes. Assist as needed.
8 Ask the person to void. Collect a urine specimen if needed. Provide for privacy.
9 Transport the person to the exam room. (This is not done for an exam in the person's room.)
10 Measure weight and height (Chapter 34). Record the measurements on the exam form.
11 Help the person onto the exam table. Provide a step stool if necessary. (Omit this step for an exam in the person's room.)

12 Raise the far bed rail (if used). Raise the bed to its highest level. (This step is not done if an exam table is used.)
13 Measure vital signs. Record them on the exam form.
14 Position the person as directed.
15 Drape the person.
16 Place a waterproof pad under the buttocks.
17 Raise the bed rail near you (if used).
18 Provide adequate lighting.
19 Put the signal light on for the examiner. Do not leave the person alone.

POSITIONING AND DRAPING

The examiner tells you how to position the person. Some positions are uncomfortable and embarrassing. Before helping the person assume and maintain the position, explain:

- Why the position is needed
- How to assume the position
- How the body is draped for warmth and privacy
- How long to expect to stay in the position

The **dorsal recumbent position (horizontal recumbent position)** is used to examine the abdomen, chest, and breasts. The person is supine with the legs together. To examine the perineal area, the knees are flexed and hips externally rotated. Drape the person as in Figure 32-2, *A.*

The **lithotomy position** (Fig. 32-2, *B*) is used to examine the vagina and cervix. The woman lies on her back. Hips are at the edge of the exam table. Knees are flexed and her hips externally rotated. Feet are in stirrups. Drape her as for perineal care (Chapter 20). Some centers provide socks for the feet and calves. Some women cannot assume this position. If so, the examiner tells you how to position the woman.

The **knee-chest position** (Fig. 32-2, *C*) is used to examine the rectum. It also is called the **genupectoral position.** (*Genu* means *knee. Pectoral* relates to the *breast.*) The person kneels and rests the body on the knees and chest. The head is turned to one side. The arms are above the head or flexed at the elbows. The back is straight. The body is flexed about 90 degrees at the hips. Apply the drape in a diamond shape to cover the back, buttocks, and thighs. This position is rarely used for older persons. For them, the side-lying position is used to examine the rectum.

The *Sims' position* (Fig. 32-2, *D*) is sometimes used to examine the rectum or vagina (Chapter 16). Apply the drape in a diamond shape. The examiner folds back the near corner to expose the rectum or vagina.

Fig. 32-2 Positioning and draping for the physical exam. **A,** Dorsal recumbent position. **B,** Lithotomy position. **C,** Knee-chest position. **D,** Sims' position.

Box 32-1 **Rules for Assisting With the Physical Exam**

- Practice hand hygiene before and after the exam.
- Provide for privacy.
  - Close doors and window coverings.
  - Screen and drape the person.
  - Expose only the body part being examined.
- Position the person as directed by the examiner.
- Place instruments and equipment near the examiner.
- Stay in the room when a female is examined (unless you are a male). When a man examines a female, another female is in the room. This is for the legal protection of the female and the male examiner. A female attendant also adds to the woman's mental comfort. A female examiner may want a male attendant present when examining a male. This also is for their legal protection.
- Protect the person from falling.
- Re-assure the person throughout the exam.
- Anticipate the examiner's need for equipment and supplies.
- Place paper or paper towels on the floor if the person is asked to stand.
- Follow Standard Precautions and the Bloodborne Pathogen Standard.

RESIDENTS WITH DEMENTIA

Assisting With the Exam

Persons with dementia may resist the examiner's efforts. The person may be agitated and aggressive because of confusion and fear. Do not restrain or force the person to have the exam. The exam is tried another time. Sometimes a family member can calm the person. The doctor may order drugs to help the person relax. The person's rights are always respected.

FOCUS ON COMMUNICATION

Assisting With the Exam

Each examiner has a routine. He or she does things in a certain order. To better assist, ask the examiner to explain the routine to you. Also ask him or her to tell you what equipment and supplies are needed. For example:

- "Dr. Weaver, I want to help in the best way that I can. Please tell me how you will start the exam and how you will proceed."
- "Ms. Carrigan, please ask for equipment and supplies as you need them. That way I can hand you the correct item."

ASSISTING WITH THE EXAM

You may be asked to prepare, position, and drape the person. If assisting with the exam, follow the rules in Box 32-1.

See *Residents With Dementia: Assisting With the Exam.*

See *Focus on Communication: Assisting With the Exam.*

After the Exam

After the exam, the person dresses or returns to bed. Lubricant is used to examine the vagina or rectum. The area is wiped or cleaned before the person dresses or returns to the room. Assist as needed. You also need to:

- Discard disposable items.
- Replace supplies so the tray is ready for the next exam.
- Clean re-usable items according to center policy. Return them to the tray or storage area. This includes the otoscope and ophthalmoscope tips and stethoscope.
- Send a re-usable speculum to the supply area. It needs to be sterilized.
- Cover the exam table with a clean drawsheet or paper.
- Label specimens. Take them to the designated area with a requisition slip.
- Clean and straighten the person's unit or exam room.
- Follow center policy for soiled linens.

See *Teamwork and Time Management: After the Exam.*

TEAMWORK AND TIME MANAGEMENT

After the Exam

Make sure that the exam room is clean and that supplies and equipment are ready for the next exam. Otherwise you delay the resident, examiner, and the staff member assisting.

You may find an exam room that is not clean. Or you may find that equipment and supplies are not ready for an exam. Call for the nurse before you start to prepare the room and ready supplies and equipment. The nurse needs to see the problem. The nurse can find out who last used the room or tray. The nurse can then talk to the staff members involved.

QUALITY OF LIFE

Resident care is given in a way that promotes dignity, self-esteem, and physical, mental, and social well-being. Often only a gown is worn for an exam. Sometimes an uncomfortable position is required. Often private body parts (breasts, vagina, penis, and rectum) are examined.

Fears about the exam affect the person's dignity, self-esteem, and well-being. These fears are common:

- Who will perform the exam?
- How will the exam be done?
- Why is the exam needed?
- Is the person dying?
- Will cancer be found?
- Will surgery be needed?
- Will more drugs be needed?
- Will an illness be found?

The person has the right to personal choice. The person also has the right to privacy and confidentiality. Protect the person from exposure. Only the examiner and the person assisting have the right to see the person's body. The person must consent for others to be present. Proper draping and screening are needed. Expose only the body part being examined. Remember to keep the person covered.

Only staff involved in the person's care need to know the reason for the exam and its results. If the person consents, the doctor tells the family. The person can share the information with others if he or she wants to.

The person needs to feel safe and secure. Protect the person from falls and other injuries. Keep the person covered to provide warmth and protect from chills and drafts. The person must feel covered and protected from exposure.

Safety and security affect mental well-being. The person should know the reasons for the exam and how it will be done. The person should feel comfortable with the examiner and the person assisting. Touch and comforting words also help the person feel safe and secure.

REVIEW QUESTIONS

Circle the BEST answer.

1   The otoscope is used to examine
   a   Internal eye structures
   b   The external ear and the eardrum
   c   Reflexes
   d   The vagina

2   Your are preparing a person for an exam. You should do the following *except*
   a   Ask the person to void
   b   Ask the person to undress
   c   Drape the person
   d   Go tell the nurse when the person is ready

3   Which part of an exam can you do?
   a   Test reflexes.
   b   Inspect the mouth, teeth, and throat.
   c   Measure weight, height, and vital signs.
   d   Observe the perineum and rectum.

4   A person is supine. The hips are flexed and externally rotated. The feet are supported in stirrups. The person is in the
   a   Dorsal recumbent position
   b   Lithotomy position
   c   Knee-chest position
   d   Sims' position

5   You will assist with Mrs. Janz's exam. Which is *false*?
   a   Hand hygiene is practiced before and after the exam.
   b   Instruments are placed near the examiner.
   c   A male nursing team member stays in the room.
   d   Provide for privacy by screening, closing the door, and proper draping.

Answers to these questions are on p. 720.

Collecting and Testing Specimens

OBJECTIVES

- Define the key terms and key abbreviations listed in this chapter.
- Explain why urine, stool, sputum, and blood specimens are collected.
- Explain the rules for collecting specimens.
- Describe the different types of urine specimens.
- Describe the equipment used for blood glucose testing.
- Identify the sites used for skin punctures.
- Explain how to promote quality of life.
- Perform the procedures described in this chapter.

KEY TERMS

acetone See "ketone"

glucosuria Sugar (*glucos*) in the urine (*uria*); glycosuria

glycosuria Sugar (*glycos*) in the urine (*uria*); glucosuria

hematoma A swelling (*oma*) that contains blood (*hemat*)

hematuria Blood (*hemat*) in the urine (*uria*)

hemoptysis Bloody (*hemo*) sputum (*ptysis* means to spit)

ketone A substance that appears in urine from the rapid breakdown of fat for energy; acetone, ketone body

ketone body See "ketone"

melena A black, tarry stool

sputum Mucus from the respiratory system that is expectorated (*expelled*) through the mouth

KEY ABBREVIATIONS

BM	Bowel movement	**mL**	Milliliter
ID	Identification	**oz**	Ounce
I&O	Intake and output		

Ordered by doctors, specimens *(samples)* are collected and tested to prevent, detect, and treat disease. Most specimens are tested in the laboratory. All specimens sent to the laboratory require requisition slips. The slip has the person's identifying information and the test ordered. And the specimen container is labeled according to center policy. Some tests are done at the bedside. When collecting specimens, follow the rules in Box 33-1.

See *Teamwork and Time Management: Collecting and Testing Specimens.*

Box 33-1   Rules for Collecting Specimens

- Follow the rules of medical asepsis.
- Follow Standard Precautions and the Bloodborne Pathogen Standard.
- Use a clean container for each specimen.
- Use the correct container.
- Do not touch the inside of the container or lid.
- Identify the person. Check the ID (identification) bracelet against the laboratory requisition slip or assignment sheet. Compare *all* information.
- Label the container in the person's presence. Provide accurate information.
- Collect the specimen at the correct time.
- Ask the person not to have a bowel movement (BM) when collecting a urine specimen. The specimen must not contain stools.
- Ask the person to void before collecting a stool specimen. The specimen must not contain urine.
- Ask the person to put toilet tissue in the toilet or wastebasket. Urine and stool specimens must not contain tissue.
- Place the specimen container in a labeled BIOHAZARD plastic bag. Do not let the container touch the outside of the bag. Seal the bag.
- Take the specimen and requisition slip to the storage area.

TEAMWORK AND TIME MANAGEMENT
Collecting and Testing Specimens

Nursing centers send specimens to a laboratory for study or analysis. The center has a storage area for specimens. A driver picks up specimens at a certain time and transports them to the laboratory.

Have ordered specimens collected and in the storage area by the pick-up time. If the specimen is not collected, the results are delayed at least one day. This can cause the person harm. If the specimen was not collected in time, it may need to be discarded. If discarded, another is collected the next day. This also causes a delay in the results and can harm the person. Using more supplies and equipment costs more money.

URINE SPECIMENS

Urine specimens are collected for urine tests. Follow the rules in Box 33-1.

See *Delegation Guidelines: Urine Specimens.*
See *Promoting Safety and Comfort: Urine Specimens.*

DELEGATION GUIDELINES
Urine Specimens

Before collecting a urine specimen, you need this information from the nurse and the care plan:

- If the person uses the toilet, bedpan, urinal, or commode for voiding
- The type of specimen needed
- What time to collect the specimen
- What special measures are needed
- If you need to test the specimen (p. 508)
- If measuring intake and output (I&O) is ordered
- What observations to report and record:
  - Problems obtaining the specimen
  - Color, clarity, and odor of urine
  - Blood in the urine
  - Particles in the urine
  - Complaints of pain, burning, urgency, difficulty voiding, or other problems
- When to report observations
- What specific resident concerns to report at once

PROMOTING SAFETY AND COMFORT
Urine Specimens

Safety
Microbes can grow in urine. Urine also may contain blood. Follow Standard Precautions and the Bloodborne Pathogen Standard.

Comfort
Urine specimens may embarrass some people. They do not like clear specimen containers that show urine. Placing the urine specimen container in a paper bag is often helpful.

The Random Urine Specimen

The random urine specimen is collected for a routine urinalysis. No special measures are needed. It is collected any time during a 24-hour period. Many people can collect the specimen themselves. Weak and very ill persons need help.

COLLECTING A RANDOM URINE SPECIMEN

QUALITY OF LIFE

Remember to:
- Knock before entering the person's room.
- Address the person by name.
- Introduce yourself by name and title.

- Explain the procedure to the person before beginning and during the procedure.
- Protect the person's rights during the procedure.
- Handle the person gently during the procedure.

PRE-PROCEDURE

1 Follow *Delegation Guidelines: Urine Specimens*, p. 503. See *Promoting Safety and Comfort: Urine Specimens*, p. 503.
2 Practice hand hygiene.
3 Collect the following before going to the person's room:
- Laboratory requisition slip
- Specimen container and lid
- Specimen label
- Plastic bag
- *BIOHAZARD* label (if needed)
- Gloves

4 Arrange collected items in the person's bathroom.
5 Decontaminate your hands.
6 Identify the person. Check the ID bracelet against the requisition slip. Also call the person by name.
7 Label the container in the person's presence.
8 Put on gloves.
9 Collect the following:
- Voiding receptacle—bedpan and cover, urinal, commode, or specimen pan (Fig. 33-1)
- Graduate to measure output
10 Provide for privacy.

PROCEDURE

11 Ask the person to void into the receptacle. Remind him or her to put toilet tissue into the wastebasket or toilet. Toilet tissue is not put in the bedpan or specimen pan.
12 Take the receptacle to the bathroom.
13 Pour about 120 mL (milliliters) (4 oz [ounces]) into the specimen container.
14 Place the lid on the specimen container. Put the container in the plastic bag. Do not let the container touch the outside of the bag. Apply a *BIOHAZARD* label according to center policy.

15 Measure urine if I&O are ordered. Include the amount in the specimen container.
16 Empty, clean, and disinfect equipment. Return equipment to its proper place.
17 Remove the gloves, and practice hand hygiene. Put on clean gloves.
18 Assist with hand washing.
19 Remove the gloves. Practice hand hygiene.

POST-PROCEDURE

20 Provide for comfort. (See the inside of the front book cover.)
21 Place the signal light within reach.
22 Raise or lower bed rails. Follow the care plan.
23 Unscreen the person.
24 Complete a safety check of the room. (See the inside of the front book cover.)

25 Decontaminate your hands.
26 Take specimen and requisition slip to the storage area. Follow center policy. Wear gloves.
27 Report and record your observations.

Fig. 33-1 The specimen pan is placed at the front of the toilet on the toilet rim. This pan has a color chart for urine. *(Courtesy Welcon, Inc., Forth Worth, Tex.)*

✉ The Midstream Specimen

The midstream specimen is also called a *clean-voided specimen* or *clean-catch specimen*. The perineal area is cleaned before collecting the specimen. This reduces the number of microbes in the urethral area. The person starts to void into a receptacle. Then the person stops the stream of urine, and a sterile specimen container is positioned. The person voids into the container until the specimen is obtained.

Stopping the stream of urine is hard for many people. You may need to position and hold the specimen container in place after the person starts to void (Fig. 33-2).

See *Focus on Communication: The Midstream Specimen.*

Fig. 33-2 The labia are separated to collect a midstream specimen.

Gloved hand is contaminated.

FOCUS ON COMMUNICATION
The Midstream Specimen

Some persons can collect the midstream specimen on their own. You may need to explain the procedure. Use words the person understands. Show what supplies to use. Also, ask if the person has any questions. For example:

"Ms. Jacobs, I need to collect a clean-catch urine specimen from you. This means I need urine that comes from the middle of your urine stream. First, wipe well with this towelette (show the towelette). Wipe from front to back. The specimen will go in this cup (show the specimen cup). Please do not touch the inside of the cup. Start your urine stream and then stop. Position the cup to catch urine and begin your stream again. If you cannot stop your stream, just position the cup during the middle of the stream. I need at least this much urine in the cup if possible (point to the 30 mL measure on the cup). Remove the cup when it is about that full. Finish urinating. Secure the lid on top of the cup. I will take the specimen when you are done. Do you have any questions?"

 COLLECTING A MIDSTREAM SPECIMEN   VIDEO

QUALITY OF LIFE

Remember to:
- Knock before entering the person's room.
- Address the person by name.
- Introduce yourself by name and title.

- Explain the procedure to the person before beginning and during the procedure.
- Protect the person's rights during the procedure.
- Handle the person gently during the procedure.

PRE-PROCEDURE

1 Follow *Delegation Guidelines: Urine Specimens*, p. 503. See *Promoting Safety and Comfort: Urine Specimens*, p. 503.
2 Practice hand hygiene.
3 Collect the following before going to the person's room:
   - Laboratory requisition slip
   - Midstream specimen kit—includes specimen container, label, and towelettes; may include sterile gloves
   - Plastic bag
   - Sterile gloves (if not part of the kit)
   - Disposable gloves
   - BIOHAZARD label (if needed)

4 Arrange your work area.
5 Decontaminate your hands.
6 Identify the person. Check the ID bracelet against the requisition slip. Also call the person by name.
7 Put on disposable gloves.
8 Collect the following:
   - Voiding receptacle—bedpan and cover, urinal, commode, or specimen pan if needed
   - Supplies for perineal care
   - Graduate to measure output
   - Paper towel
9 Provide for privacy.

Continued

COLLECTING A MIDSTREAM SPECIMEN—cont'd

VIDEO

PROCEDURE

10 Provide perineal care. (Wear gloves for this step. Decontaminate your hands after removing them.)
11 Open the sterile kit.
12 Put on the sterile gloves.
13 Open the packet of towelettes inside the kit.
14 Open the sterile specimen container. Do not touch the inside of the container or lid. Set the lid down so the inside is up.
15 *For a female*—clean the perineal area with the towelettes.
   a Spread the labia with your thumb and index finger. Use your non-dominant hand. (This hand is now contaminated. It must not touch anything sterile.)
   b Clean down the urethral area from front to back. Use a clean towelette for each stroke.
   c Keep the labia separated to collect the urine specimen (steps 17 through 20).
16 *For a male*—clean the penis with the towelettes.
   a Hold the penis with your non-dominant hand. (This hand is now contaminated. It must not touch anything sterile.)
   b Clean the penis starting at the meatus. Clean in a circular motion. Start at the center and work outward.
   c Keep holding the penis until the specimen is collected (steps 17 through 20).

17 Ask the person to void into a receptacle.
18 Pass the specimen container into the stream of urine. Keep the labia separated (see Fig. 33-2).
19 Collect about 30 to 60 mL (1 to 2 oz) of urine.
20 Remove the specimen container before the person stops voiding.
21 Release the labia or penis. Let the person finish voiding into the receptacle.
22 Put the lid on the specimen container. Touch only the outside of the container and lid. Wipe the outside of the container. Set the container on a paper towel.
23 Provide toilet tissue after the person is done voiding.
24 Take the receptacle to the bathroom.
25 Measure urine if I&O are ordered. Include the amount in the specimen container.
26 Empty, clean, and disinfect equipment. Return equipment to its proper place.
27 Remove the gloves, and practice hand hygiene. Put on clean disposable gloves.
28 Label the specimen container in the person's presence. Place the container in the plastic bag. Do not let the container touch the outside of the bag. Apply a *BIOHAZARD* label according to center policy.
29 Assist with hand washing.
30 Remove the gloves. Practice hand hygiene.

POST-PROCEDURE

31 Provide for comfort. (See the inside of the front book cover.)
32 Place the signal light within reach.
33 Raise or lower bed rails. Follow the care plan.
34 Unscreen the person.
35 Complete a safety check of the room. (See the inside of the front book cover.)

36 Decontaminate your hands.
37 Take the specimen and requisition slip to the storage area. Follow center policy. Wear gloves.
38 Report and record your observations.

 The 24-Hour Urine Specimen

All urine voided during a 24-hour period is collected for a 24-hour urine specimen. Urine is chilled on ice or refrigerated during this time. This prevents the growth of microbes. A preservative is added to the collection container for some tests.

The person voids to begin the test with an empty bladder. Discard this voiding. Save *all voidings* for the next 24 hours. The person and nursing staff must clearly understand the procedure and the test period. The test is re-started if:

• A voiding was not saved.
• Toilet tissue was discarded into the specimen.
• The specimen contains feces.

See *Promoting Safety and Comfort: The 24-Hour Urine Specimen.*

PROMOTING SAFETY AND COMFORT
The 24-Hour Urine Specimen

Safety

The collection container or preservative may contain an acid. Do not get the preservative or urine from the container on your skin or in your eyes. If you do, flush your skin or eyes with a large amount of water. Tell the nurse what happened and check the material safety data sheet (MSDS) (Chapter 12). Also complete an incident report.

Keep the specimen chilled to prevent the growth of microbes. If not refrigerated, place the urine collection container in a bucket with ice. Add ice to the bucket as needed.

Assist the person with hand washing after every voiding. This prevents the spread of microbes that may be in the urine.

COLLECTING A 24-HOUR URINE SPECIMEN

QUALITY OF LIFE

Remember to:
- Knock before entering the person's room.
- Address the person by name.
- Introduce yourself by name and title.

- Explain the procedure to the person before beginning and during the procedure.
- Protect the person's rights during the procedure.
- Handle the person gently during the procedure.

PRE-PROCEDURE

1 Follow *Delegation Guidelines: Urine Specimens*, p. 503. See *Promoting Safety and Comfort*:
   a *Urine Specimens*, p. 503
   b *The 24-Hour Urine Specimen*
2 Practice hand hygiene.
3 Collect the following before going to the person's room:
   - Laboratory requisition slip
   - Urine container for a 24-hour collection
   - Specimen label
   - Preservative if needed
   - Bucket with ice if needed
   - Two 24-HOUR URINE labels
   - Funnel
   - *BIOHAZARD* label
4 Arrange collected items in the person's bathroom.

5 Place one 24-HOUR URINE label in the bathroom. Place the other near the bed.
6 Decontaminate your hands.
7 Identify the person. Check the ID bracelet against the requisition slip. Also call the person by name.
8 Label the urine container in the person's presence. Apply the *BIOHAZARD* label.
9 Put on gloves.
10 Collect the following:
   - Voiding receptacle—bedpan and cover, urinal, commode, or specimen pan
   - Gloves
   - Graduate to measure output
11 Provide for privacy.

PROCEDURE

12 Ask the person to void. Provide a voiding receptacle.
13 Measure and discard the urine. Note the time. This starts the 24-hour collection period.
14 Mark the time on the collection container.
15 Empty, clean, and disinfect equipment. Return equipment to its proper place.
16 Remove the gloves, and practice hand hygiene. Put on clean gloves.
17 Assist with hand washing.
18 Remove the gloves. Practice hand hygiene.
19 Mark the time the test began and the time it ends on the room and bathroom labels.
20 Remind the person to:
   a Use the voiding receptacle when voiding during the next 24 hours.
   b Not have a BM when voiding.
   c Put toilet tissue in the toilet or wastebasket.
   d Put on the signal light after voiding.

21 Return to the room when the person signals for you. Knock before entering the room.
22 Do the following after every voiding:
   a Decontaminate your hands. Put on gloves.
   b Measure urine if I&O are ordered.
   c Pour urine into the container using the funnel. Do not spill any urine. Re-start the test if you spill or discard the urine.
   d Empty, clean, and disinfect equipment. Return equipment to its proper place.
   e Remove the gloves, and practice hand hygiene. Put on clean gloves.
   f Assist with hand washing.
   g Remove the gloves. Practice hand hygiene.
   h Follow "Post-Procedure" steps *except* for steps 28 and 33.
23 Ask the person to void at the end of the 24-hour period. Follow step 22a-g.

POST-PROCEDURE

24 Provide for comfort. (See the inside of the front book cover.)
25 Place the signal light within reach.
26 Raise or lower bed rails. Follow the care plan.
27 Put on gloves.
28 Remove the labels from the room and bathroom.
29 Clean and return equipment to its proper place. Discard disposable items.

30 Remove the gloves. Practice hand hygiene.
31 Unscreen the person.
32 Complete a safety check of the room. (See the inside of the front book cover.)
33 Take the specimen and requisition slip to the storage area. Wear gloves.
34 Report and record your observations.

Testing Urine

The nurse may ask you to do simple urine tests. You can test for pH, glucose, and blood using reagent strips (dipsticks). The doctor orders the type and frequency of urine tests. Random urine specimens are needed.

- *Testing for pH*—Urine pH measures if urine is acidic or alkaline. Changes in normal pH (4.6 to 8.0) occur from illness, food, and drugs.
- *Testing for glucose and ketones*—In diabetes, the pancreas does not secrete enough insulin (Chapter 41). The body needs insulin to use sugar for energy. If not used, sugar builds up in the blood. Some sugar appears in the urine. Glucosuria or glycosuria means sugar (*glucos, glycos*) in the urine (*uria*). The diabetic person may also have ketones (ketone bodies, acetone) in the urine. These substances appear in urine from the rapid breakdown of fat for energy. The body uses fat for energy if it cannot use sugar. Urine is also tested for ketones. These tests are usually done four times a day—30 minutes before each meal and at bedtime. The doctor uses the test to make drug and diet decisions.
- *Testing for blood*—Injury and disease can cause hematuria. It means blood (*hemat*) in the urine (*uria*). Sometimes blood is seen in the urine. At other times it is unseen (*occult*).

  See *Teamwork and Time Management: Testing Urine.*
  See *Delegation Guidelines: Testing Urine.*
  See *Promoting Safety and Comfort: Testing Urine.*

TEAMWORK AND TIME MANAGEMENT
Testing Urine

Blood glucose testing is usually used for persons with diabetes (p. 516). However, the nurse may want urine tested for glucose and ketones. Perform the tests when directed by the nurse and care plan. The nurse uses the test results to decide about giving the person diabetic drugs. The drugs are given at a certain time. The nurse needs the results before giving the drugs.

DELEGATION GUIDELINES
Testing Urine

When testing urine is delegated to you, you need this information from the nurse and the care plan:
- What test is needed
- What equipment to use
- When to test urine
- Instructions for the test ordered
- If the nurse wants to observe the results of each test
- What observations to report and record:
  - The time you collected and tested the specimen
  - Test results
  - Problems obtaining the specimen
  - Color, clarity, and odor of urine
  - Blood in the urine
  - Particles in the urine
  - Complaints of pain, burning, urgency, difficulty voiding, or other problems
- When to report test results and observations
- What specific resident concerns to report at once

PROMOTING SAFETY AND COMFORT
Testing Urine

Safety
You must be accurate when testing urine. Promptly report the results to the nurse. Ordered drugs may depend on the results.

Urine may contain microbes and blood. Follow Standard Precautions and the Bloodborne Pathogen Standard.

Comfort
The person may want to know the test results. If allowed by center policy, you can tell the person the results. Remember, this information is private and confidential. Make sure only the person hears what you are saying.

Using Reagent Strips Reagent strips (dipsticks) have sections that change color when they react with urine. To use a reagent strip:
- Do not touch the test area on the strip.
- Dip the strip into urine.
- Compare the strip with the color chart on the bottle (Fig. 33-3).

  See *Promoting Safety and Comfort: Using Reagent Strips.*

Fig. 33-3 Reagent strip for sugar and ketones.

TESTING URINE WITH REAGENT STRIPS

QUALITY OF LIFE

Remember to:
- Knock before entering the person's room.
- Address the person by name.
- Introduce yourself by name and title.

- Explain the procedure to the person before beginning and during the procedure.
- Protect the person's rights during the procedure.
- Handle the person gently during the procedure.

PRE-PROCEDURE

1 Follow *Delegation Guidelines: Testing Urine.* See *Promoting Safety and Comfort:*
   a *Testing Urine*
   b *Using Reagent Strips*
2 Practice hand hygiene.
3 Collect gloves and the reagent strips ordered.
4 Decontaminate your hands.

5 Identify the person. Check the ID bracelet against the assignment sheet. Also call the person by name.
6 Put on gloves.
7 Collect equipment for the urine specimen. (See procedure: *Collecting a Random Urine Specimen,* p. 504.)
8 Provide for privacy.

PROCEDURE

9 Collect the urine specimen. (See procedure: *Collecting a Random Urine Specimen,* p. 504.)
10 Remove the strip from the bottle. Put the cap on the bottle at once. It must be on tight.
11 Dip the strip test areas into the urine.
12 Remove the strip after the correct amount of time. See the manufacturer's instructions.
13 Tap the strip gently against the container. This removes excess urine.

14 Wait the required amount of time. See the manufacturer's instructions.
15 Compare the strip with the color chart on the bottle (see Fig. 33-3). Read the results.
16 Discard disposable items and the specimen.
17 Empty, clean, and disinfect equipment. Return equipment to its proper place.
18 Remove the gloves. Practice hand hygiene.

POST-PROCEDURE

19 Provide for comfort. (See the inside of the front book cover.)
20 Place the signal light within reach.
21 Raise or lower bed rails. Follow the care plan.
22 Unscreen the person.

23 Complete a safety check of the room. (See the inside of the front book cover.)
24 Decontaminate your hands.
25 Report and record the test results and other observations.

Straining Urine A stone *(calculus)* can develop in the kidney, ureter, or bladder. Stones *(calculi)* vary in size (Chapter 42). They can be as small as grains of sand, pearl-size, or larger. Stones causing severe pain and urinary system damage may require surgical removal. Some stones pass through urine. Therefore all urine is strained. Passed stones are sent to the laboratory.

The person drinks 8 to 12 glasses of water a day to help pass the stone. Expect the person to void in large amounts.

STRAINING URINE

QUALITY OF LIFE

Remember to:
- Knock before entering the person's room.
- Address the person by name.
- Introduce yourself by name and title.

- Explain the procedure to the person before beginning and during the procedure.
- Protect the person's rights during the procedure.
- Handle the person gently during the procedure.

PRE-PROCEDURE

1 Follow *Delegation Guidelines: Testing Urine*, p. 508. See *Promoting Safety and Comfort: Testing Urine*, p. 508.
2 Practice hand hygiene.
3 Collect the following before going to the person's room:
   - Laboratory requisition slip
   - Gauze or strainer
   - Specimen container
   - Specimen label
   - Two STRAIN ALL URINE labels
   - Plastic bag
   - BIOHAZARD label (if needed)
   - Gloves
4 Arrange collected items in the person's bathroom.

5 Place one STRAIN ALL URINE label in the bathroom. Place the other near the bed.
6 Decontaminate your hands.
7 Identify the person. Check the ID bracelet against the assignment sheet. Call the person by name.
8 Label the specimen container in the person's presence.
9 Put on gloves.
10 Collect the following:
   - Voiding receptacle—bedpan and cover, urinal, commode, or specimen pan
   - Graduate
   - Gloves
11 Provide for privacy.

PROCEDURE

12 Ask the person to use the voiding receptacle for urinating. Ask the person to put on the signal light after voiding.
13 Remove the gloves. Practice hand hygiene.
14 Return to the room when the person signals for you. Knock before entering the room.
15 Decontaminate your hands. Put on clean gloves.
16 Place the gauze or strainer into the graduate.
17 Pour urine into the graduate. Urine passes through the gauze or strainer (Fig. 33-4).
18 Place the gauze or strainer in the specimen container if any crystals, stones, or particles appear.

19 Place the specimen container in the plastic bag. Do not let the container touch the outside of the bag. Apply a BIOHAZARD label according to center policy.
20 Measure urine if I&O were ordered.
21 Empty, clean, and disinfect equipment. Return equipment to its proper place.
22 Remove the gloves, and practice hand hygiene. Put on clean gloves.
23 Assist with hand washing.
24 Remove the gloves. Practice hand hygiene.

POST-PROCEDURE

25 Provide for comfort. (See the inside of the front book cover.)
26 Place the signal light within reach.
27 Raise or lower bed rails. Follow the care plan.
28 Unscreen the person.
29 Complete a safety check of the room. (See the inside of the front book cover.)

30 Decontaminate your hands.
31 Take the specimen container and requisition slip to the laboratory or storage area. Wear gloves.
32 Report and record your observations.

Fig. 33-4 A strainer is placed in the graduate. Urine is poured through the strainer into the graduate.

STOOL SPECIMENS

When internal bleeding is suspected, stools are checked for blood. Stools also are studied for fat, microbes, worms, and other abnormal contents.

Urine must not contaminate the stool specimen. The person uses one receptacle for voiding and another for a BM. Some tests require a warm stool. The specimen is taken at once to the storage area for transport to the laboratory. Follow the rules in Box 33-1.

See *Focus on Communication: Stool Specimens.*
See *Delegation Guidelines: Stool Specimens.*
See *Promoting Safety and Comfort: Stool Specimens.*

DELEGATION GUIDELINES
Stool Specimens

Before collecting a stool specimen, you need this information from the nurse:
- What time to collect the specimen
- What special measures are needed
- What observations to report and record:
  - Problems obtaining the specimen
  - Color, amount, consistency, and odor of stools
  - Blood in the stool
  - Complaints of pain or discomfort
  - The time when the specimen was collected
- When to report observations
- What specific resident concerns to report at once

PROMOTING SAFETY AND COMFORT
Stool Specimens

Safety
Stools contain microbes. And they may contain blood. Follow Standard Precautions and the Bloodborne Pathogen Standard.

Comfort
Stools normally have an odor. A person may be embarrassed that you need to collect a specimen. Complete the task quickly and carefully. Also act in a professional manner.

FOCUS ON COMMUNICATION
Stool Specimens

Always explain the procedure before you begin. Explain what the person needs to do and what you will do. Also show what equipment and supplies you will use. For example:

"The doctor wants your stools tested. Meaning, we need a specimen from a bowel movement. I'm going to place this specimen pan (show the specimen pan) at the back of the toilet seat. You will urinate into the toilet. Your bowel movement will collect in the specimen pan rather than in the toilet. Please put toilet tissue in the toilet, not in the specimen pan. After you have a bowel movement, put your signal light on right away. I'll use a tongue blade (show the tongue blade) to take some stool from the specimen pan to put in this specimen container (show the specimen container)."

After explaining the procedure, ask the person if he or she has any questions. If you do not know the answer, refer questions to the nurse.

Also make sure the person understands what to do. You can say: "Mrs. Clark, please help me make sure that you understand what I said. To collect a stool specimen, please tell me what you're going to do."

COLLECTING A STOOL SPECIMEN

QUALITY OF LIFE

Remember to:
- Knock before entering the person's room.
- Address the person by name.
- Introduce yourself by name and title.

- Explain the procedure to the person before beginning and during the procedure.
- Protect the person's rights during the procedure.
- Handle the person gently during the procedure.

PRE-PROCEDURE

1 Follow *Delegation Guidelines: Stool Specimens*, p. 511. See *Promoting Safety and Comfort: Stool Specimens*, p. 511.
2 Practice hand hygiene.
3 Collect the following before going to the person's room:
   - Laboratory requisition slip
   - Specimen pan for the toilet
   - Specimen container and lid
   - Specimen label
   - Tongue blade
   - Disposable bag
   - Plastic bag
   - *BIOHAZARD* label (if needed)
   - Gloves

4 Arrange collected items in the person's bathroom.
5 Decontaminate your hands.
6 Identify the person. Check the ID bracelet against the requisition slip. Also call the person by name.
7 Label the specimen container in the person's presence.
8 Put on gloves.
9 Collect the following:
   - Receptacle for voiding—bedpan and cover, urinal, commode, or specimen pan
   - Toilet tissue
10 Provide for privacy.

PROCEDURE

11 Ask the person to void. Provide the receptacle for voiding if the person does not use the bathroom. Empty, clean, and disinfect the device. Return it to its proper place.
12 Put the specimen pan on the toilet if the person will use the bathroom. Place it at the back of the toilet (Fig. 33-5). Or provide a bedpan or commode.
13 Ask the person not to put toilet tissue into the bedpan, commode, or specimen pan. Provide a bag for toilet tissue.
14 Place the signal light and toilet tissue within reach. Raise or lower bed rails. Follow the care plan.
15 Remove the gloves. Decontaminate your hands. Leave the room.
16 Return when the person signals. Or check on the person every 5 minutes. Knock before entering.
17 Decontaminate your hands. Put on clean gloves.
18 Lower the bed rail near you if up.
19 Remove the bedpan (if used). Note the color, amount, consistency, and odor of stools.
20 Provide perineal care if needed.

21 Collect the specimen:
   a Use a tongue blade to take about 2 tablespoons of stool to the specimen container (Fig. 33-6). Take the sample from the middle of a formed stool.
   b Include pus, mucus, or blood present in the stool.
   c Take stool from 2 different places in the BM if required by center policy.
   d Put the lid on the specimen container.
   e Place the container in the plastic bag. Do not let the container touch the outside of the bag. Apply a *BIOHAZARD* label according to center policy.
22 Wrap the tongue blade in toilet tissue. Discard it into the disposable bag.
23 Empty, clean, and disinfect equipment. Return equipment to its proper place.
24 Remove the gloves, and practice hand hygiene. Put on clean gloves.
25 Assist with hand washing.
26 Remove the gloves. Practice hand hygiene.

POST-PROCEDURE

27 Provide for comfort. (See the inside of the front book cover.)
28 Place the signal light within reach.
29 Raise or lower bed rails. Follow the care plan.
30 Unscreen the person.

31 Complete a safety check of the room. (See the inside of the front book cover.)
32 Deliver the specimen and requisition slip to the storage area. Follow center policy. Wear gloves.
33 Report and record your observations.

Fig. 33-5 The specimen pan is placed at the back of the toilet for a stool specimen.

Fig. 33-6 A tongue blade is used to transfer a small amount of stool from the bedpan to the specimen container.

Testing Stools for Blood

Stools may contain blood. Ulcers, colon cancer, and hemorrhoids are common causes. Often blood is seen if bleeding is low in the bowels. Stools are black and tarry from bleeding in the stomach or upper gastro-intestinal tract. Melena is a black, tarry stool.

Sometimes bleeding occurs in very small amounts. Then stools are tested for *occult blood. Occult* means "hidden" or "not seen." The test is done to screen for colon cancer and other digestive disorders.

Occult blood test kits vary. Follow the manufacturer's instructions. The following procedure is presented as a guide.

See *Delegation Guidelines: Testing Stools for Blood.*

See *Promoting Safety and Comfort: Testing Stools for Blood.*

DELEGATION GUIDELINES
Testing Stools for Blood

Before testing a stool specimen for blood, you need this information from the nurse:
- What test is needed
- What equipment to use
- When to test the stool
- Instructions for the test ordered
- If the nurse wants to observe the results of each test
- What observations to report and record:
  - The time you collected and tested the specimen
  - Test results
  - Problems obtaining the specimen
  - Color, amount, consistency, and odor of feces
  - Blood in the stool
  - Complaints of pain or discomfort
- When to report observations
- What specific resident concerns to report at once

PROMOTING SAFETY AND COMFORT
Testing Stools for Blood

Safety
You must be accurate when testing stools. Follow the manufacturer's instructions for the test used. Promptly report the results to the nurse.

Stools contain microbes and may contain blood. Follow Standard Precautions and the Bloodborne Pathogen Standard.

QUALITY OF LIFE

Remember to:
- Knock before entering the person's room.
- Address the person by name.
- Introduce yourself by name and title.

- Explain the procedure to the person before beginning and during the procedure.
- Protect the person's rights during the procedure.
- Handle the person gently during the procedure.

PRE-PROCEDURE

1 Follow *Delegation Guidelines: Testing Stools for Blood,* p. 513. See *Promoting Safety and Comfort:*
  a *Stool Specimens,* p. 511
  b *Testing Stools for Blood,* p. 513
2 Practice hand hygiene.
3 Collect the following before going to the person's room:
  - Occult blood test kit
  - Tongue blades (if needed)
  - Gloves
4 Arrange collected items in the person's bathroom.

5 Decontaminate your hands.
6 Identify the person. Check the ID bracelet against the assignment sheet. Also call the person by name.
7 Put on gloves.
8 Collect the following:
  - Equipment for a stool specimen (see procedure: *Collecting a Stool Specimen,* p. 512)
  - Paper towels
9 Provide for privacy.

PROCEDURE

10 Collect a stool specimen. See procedure: *Collecting a Stool Specimen,* p. 512.
11 Practice hand hygiene. Put on clean gloves.
12 Open the test kit.
13 Use a tongue blade to obtain a small amount of stool.
14 Apply a thin smear of stool on *box A* on the test paper (Fig. 33-7, *A*).
15 Use another tongue blade to obtain stool from another part of the specimen.
16 Apply a thin smear of stool on *box B* on the test paper (Fig. 33-7, *B*).
17 Close the packet.

18 Turn the test packet to the other side. Open the flap. Apply developer (from the kit) to *boxes A* and *B.* Follow the manufacturer's instructions (Fig. 33-7, *C*).
19 Wait 10 to 60 seconds as required by the manufacturer.
20 Note the color changes on your assignment sheet (Fig. 33-7, *D*).
21 Dispose of the test packet.
22 Wrap the tongue blades with toilet tissue. Then discard them.
23 Empty, clean, and disinfect equipment. Return equipment to its proper place.
24 Remove the gloves. Practice hand hygiene.

POST-PROCEDURE

25 Provide for comfort. (See the inside of the front book cover.)
26 Place the signal light within reach.
27 Raise or lower bed rails. Follow the care plan.
28 Complete a safety check of the room. (See the inside of the front book cover.)

29 Decontaminate your hands.
30 Report and record the test results and your observations.

Fig. 33-7 Testing for occult blood. **A,** Stool is smeared on *box A.* **B,** Stool is smeared on *box B* and then the flap is closed. **C,** Developer is applied to *boxes A* and *B* on the back side of the test packet. **D,** Color changes are noted.

SPUTUM SPECIMENS

Respiratory disorders cause the lungs, bronchi, and trachea to secrete mucus. Mucus from the respiratory system is called sputum when expectorated (*expelled*) through the mouth. Sputum is not saliva. Saliva ("spit") is a thin, clear liquid produced by the salivary glands in the mouth.

Sputum specimens are studied for blood, microbes, and abnormal cells. The person coughs up sputum from the bronchi and trachea. This is often painful and hard to do. It is easier to collect a specimen in the morning. Secretions collect in the trachea and bronchi during sleep. They are coughed up on awakening.

To collect a specimen, follow the rules in Box 33-1. Also have the person rinse the mouth with water. Rinsing decreases saliva and removes food particles. Mouthwash is not used. It destroys some of the microbes in the mouth.

Older persons may lack the strength to cough up sputum. Coughing is easier after postural drainage. It drains secretions by gravity. Gravity causes fluids to flow down. The person is positioned so a lung part is higher than the airway (Fig. 33-8). The nurse or respiratory therapist does postural drainage.

See *Delegation Guidelines: Sputum Specimens*.
See *Promoting Safety and Comfort: Sputum Specimens*.

Fig. 33-8 Some positions for postural drainage. *(From Potter PA, Perry AG: Fundamentals of nursing, ed 7, 2009, Mosby.)*

DELEGATION GUIDELINES
Sputum Specimens

Before collecting a sputum specimen, you need this information from the nurse:
- When to collect the specimen
- How much sputum is needed—usually 1 to 2 teaspoons
- If the person uses the bathroom
- If the person can hold the specimen container
- What observations to report and record:
  - The time the specimen was collected
  - The amount of sputum collected
  - How easily the person raised the sputum
  - Sputum color—clear, white, yellow, green, brown, or red
  - Sputum odor—none or foul odor
  - Sputum consistency—thick, watery, or frothy (with bubbles or foam)
  - **Hemoptysis**—bloody *(hemo)* sputum (*ptysis*, meaning *to spit*)
  - If the person was not able to produce sputum
  - Any other observations
- When to report observations
- What specific resident concerns to report at once

PROMOTING SAFETY AND COMFORT
Sputum Specimens

Safety
Follow Standard Precautions and the Bloodborne Pathogen Standard to prevent contact with mucus. It may contain blood or microbes.

The person may have tuberculosis (TB) (Chapter 40). Follow isolation precautions and protect yourself by wearing a TB respirator (Chapter 15).

Comfort
The procedure can embarrass the person. Coughing and expectorating sounds can disturb others. Also, sputum is not pleasant to look at. For these reasons, privacy is important. Cover the specimen container and place it in a bag. Some sputum specimen containers are cloudy in color to hide the contents.

COLLECTING A SPUTUM SPECIMEN

QUALITY OF LIFE

Remember to:
- Knock before entering the person's room.
- Address the person by name.
- Introduce yourself by name and title.

- Explain the procedure to the person before beginning and during the procedure.
- Protect the person's rights during the procedure.
- Handle the person gently during the procedure.

PRE-PROCEDURE

1 Follow *Delegation Guidelines: Sputum Specimens,* p. 515. See *Promoting Safety and Comfort: Sputum Specimens,* p. 515.
2 Practice hand hygiene.
3 Collect the following before going to the person's room:
- Laboratory requisition slip
- Sputum specimen container and lid
- Specimen label
- Plastic bag
- *BIOHAZARD* label (if needed)

4 Arrange collected items in the person's bathroom.
5 Decontaminate your hands.
6 Identify the person. Check the ID bracelet against the requisition slip. Also call the person by name.
7 Label the specimen container in the person's presence.
8 Collect gloves and tissues.
9 Provide for privacy. If able, the person uses the bathroom for the procedure.

PROCEDURE

10 Put on gloves.
11 Ask the person to rinse the mouth out with clear water.
12 Have the person hold the container. Only the outside is touched.
13 Ask the person to cover the mouth and nose with tissues when coughing. Follow center policy for used tissues.
14 Ask him or her to take 2 or 3 deep breaths and cough up the sputum.
15 Have the person expectorate directly into the container (Fig. 33-9). Sputum should not touch the outside of the container.

16 Collect 1 to 2 teaspoons of sputum unless told to collect more.
17 Put the lid on the container.
18 Place the container in the plastic bag. Do not let the container touch the outside of the bag. Apply a *BIOHAZARD* label according to center policy.
19 Remove the gloves, and decontaminate your hands. Put on clean gloves.
20 Assist with hand washing.
21 Remove the gloves. Decontaminate your hands.

POST-PROCEDURE

22 Provide for comfort. (See the inside of the front book cover.)
23 Place the signal light within reach.
24 Raise or lower bed rails. Follow the care plan.
25 Unscreen the person.
26 Complete a safety check of the room. (See the inside of the front book cover.)

27 Decontaminate your hands.
28 Deliver the specimen and the requisition slip to the storage area. Follow center policy. Wear gloves.
29 Report and record your observations.

Fig. 33-9 The person expectorates into the center of the specimen container.

☒ BLOOD GLUCOSE TESTING

Blood glucose testing is used for persons with diabetes. The doctor uses the results to regulate the person's drugs and diet.

Capillary blood is obtained through a skin puncture. A drop of blood is collected. A fingertip is the most common site for skin punctures. This provides easy access and clothing is not removed.

Fig. 33-10 Site for skin punctures. *(From Bonewit-West K: Clinical procedures for medical assistants, ed 7, St Louis, 2008, Saunders.)*

Fig. 33-11 A lancet. *(From Bonewit-West K: Clinical procedures for medical assistants, ed 5, Philadelphia, 2000, Saunders.)*

Inspect the puncture site for signs of trauma and skin breaks. Do not use swollen, bruised, cyanotic (bluish color), scarred, or calloused sites. Such areas have poor blood flow. A *callus* is a thick, hardened area on the skin. Calluses often form over frequently used areas, such as the tips of the thumbs and index fingers. Therefore thumbs and index fingers are not good skin puncture sites.

Use the side toward the tip of the middle or ring finger (Fig. 33-10). Do not use the center, fleshy part of the fingertip. This site has many nerve endings, making punctures painful.

You use a sterile, disposable lancet to puncture the skin (Fig. 33-11). The person feels a brief, sharp pinch. A *lancet* is a short, pointed blade. It punctures but does not cut the skin. The lancet is inside a protective cover. You do not touch the blade. Discard it into the sharps container after use.

A *glucose meter (glucometer)* measures blood glucose. You apply a drop of blood to a reagent strip. Then you insert the strip into the glucose meter. The blood glucose level appears on the screen. Many types of glucose

---

meters are available. How fast results are displayed varies. Some take 5 seconds.

You will learn to use your center's device. Always follow the manufacturer's instructions.

See *Teamwork and Time Management: Blood Glucose Testing.*

See *Delegation Guidelines: Blood Glucose Testing.*

See *Promoting Safety and Comfort: Blood Glucose Testing,* p. 518.

PROMOTING SAFETY AND COMFORT
Blood Glucose Testing

Safety

Accurate results are important. Inaccurate results can harm the person. Follow the rules in Box 33-2.

You must know how to use the equipment. Use only the type of reagent strip specified by the manufacturer. Otherwise you will get inaccurate results.

Contact with blood is likely. Follow Standard Precautions and the Bloodborne Pathogen Standard.

Comfort

Older persons often have poor circulation in their fingers. To increase blood flow, apply a warm washcloth or wash the hands in warm water.

Fig. 33-12 The bar code on the bottle of reagent strips is scanned.

Box 33-2   Rules for Blood Glucose Testing

- Follow the manufacturer's instructions for the glucose meter.
- Know how to use the equipment. Request any necessary training.
- Make sure the glucose meter was tested for accuracy. Check the testing log.
- Enter a code or user-ID if required by the glucose meter. This is provided by the center. Do not share your user-ID with others.
- Make sure you have the correct reagent strips for the glucose meter you are using. Compare the code number on
- the strip with the code number on the glucose meter. The code numbers should be the same.
- Scan the bar code on the bottle of reagent strips if needed (Fig. 33-12).
- Check the color of reagent strips. Do not use discolored strips.
- Check the expiration date of the reagent strips. Do not use them if the date has passed.
- Report the result to the nurse at once.
- Record the result following center policy.

 ## MEASURING BLOOD GLUCOSE

QUALITY OF LIFE

Remember to:
- Knock before entering the person's room.
- Address the person by name.
- Introduce yourself by name and title.

- Explain the procedure to the person before beginning and during the procedure.
- Protect the person's rights during the procedure.
- Handle the person gently during the procedure.

PRE-PROCEDURE

1 Follow *Delegation Guidelines: Blood Glucose Testing,* p. 517. See *Promoting Safety and Comfort: Blood Glucose Testing.*
2 Practice hand hygiene.
3 Collect the following:
   - Sterile lancet
   - Antiseptic wipes
   - Gloves
   - Cotton balls
   - Glucose meter
   - Reagent strips (Use the correct ones for the meter. Check the expiration date.)

   - Paper towels
   - Warm washcloth
4 Read the manufacturer's instructions for the lancet and glucose meter.
5 Arrange your work area.
6 Identify the person. Check the ID bracelet against the assignment sheet. Also call the person by name.
7 Provide for privacy.
8 Raise the bed for body mechanics. The far bed rail is up if used.

MEASURING BLOOD GLUCOSE—cont'd

PROCEDURE

9 Help the person to a comfortable position.
10 Put on the gloves.
11 Prepare the supplies:
   a Open the antiseptic wipes.
   b Remove a reagent strip from the bottle. Place it on the paper towel. Place the cap securely on the bottle.
   c Prepare the lancet.
   d Turn on the glucose meter.
   e Follow the prompts. You may need to enter a user-ID and the person's ID number. Scan the bar code on the bottle of reagent strips if needed.
   f Insert a reagent strip into the glucose meter (Fig. 33-13).
12 Perform a skin puncture to obtain a drop of blood:
   a Inspect the person's fingers. Select a puncture site.
   b Warm the finger. Rub it gently or apply a warm washcloth.
   c Massage the hand and finger toward the puncture site. And lower the finger below the person's waist. These actions increase blood flow to the site.
   d Hold the finger with your thumb and forefinger. Use your non-dominant hand. Hold the finger until step 13, c.
   e Clean the site with an antiseptic wipe. *Do not touch the site after cleaning.*
   f Let the site dry.

   g Pick up the sterile lancet.
   h Place the lancet against the puncture site.
   i Push the button on the lancet to puncture the skin. (Follow the manufacturer's instructions.)
   j Wipe away the first blood drop. Use a cotton ball.
   k Apply gentle pressure below the puncture site.
   l Let a large drop of blood form.
13 Collect and test the specimen. Follow the manufacturer's instructions and center procedures for the glucose meter used.
   a Hold the test area of the reagent strip close to the drop of blood.
   b Lightly touch the reagent strip to the blood drop (Fig. 33-14). Do not smear the blood. The meter will test the sample when enough blood is applied.
   c Apply pressure to the puncture site until bleeding stops. Use a cotton ball. If able, let the person apply pressure to the site.
   d Read the result on the display (Fig. 33-15). Note the result on your notepad or assignment sheet. Tell the person the result.
   e Turn off the glucose meter.
14 Discard the lancet into the sharps container.
15 Discard the cotton balls and reagent strip following center policy.
16 Remove and discard the gloves. Decontaminate your hands.

POST-PROCEDURE

17 Provide for comfort. (See the inside of the front book cover.)
18 Place the signal light within reach.
19 Lower the bed to its lowest position.
20 Raise or lower bed rails. Follow the care plan.
21 Unscreen the person.

22 Discard used supplies.
23 Complete a safety check of the room. (See the inside of the front book cover.)
24 Follow center policy for soiled linen.
25 Decontaminate your hands.
26 Report and record the test result and your observations.

Fig. 33-13 A reagent strip is in the glucose meter.

Fig. 33-14 A drop of blood is applied to the reagent strip.

Fig. 33-15 The result is displayed on the glucose meter.

QUALITY OF LIFE

You must collect and test specimens on the right person. Otherwise one or more persons could suffer harm. Before collecting or testing a specimen, carefully identify the person. Check the ID bracelet against the laboratory requisition slip or assignment sheet. Compare all information, not just the person's name.

Some centers require placing the collection date, collection time, and the collector's name or initials on the container. This promotes safety. Follow center policy for labeling specimens.

Specimen collection embarrasses many people. To promote comfort and privacy:

- Politely ask visitors to leave the room.
- Close doors, the privacy curtain, and window coverings.
- Leave the room if it is safe to do so. If you cannot leave, explain this to the person.
- Place the specimen container in a paper bag or wrap it in a paper towel or washcloth so others do not see the specimen.
- Always act professionally. Do not say things that may embarrass the person.

Some people can collect their own urine and sputum specimens. Doing so promotes independence. It also helps reduce embarrassment. Explain the procedure to the person. This helps the person know how to correctly collect the specimen. Show the person the specimen container and how it is used. Also, ask the person where to place the container. When ready to collect the specimen, the person knows where to find the container.

REVIEW QUESTIONS

Circle the BEST answer.

1 A random urine specimen is collected
  a After sleep
  b Before meals
  c After meals
  d Any time

2 Perineal care is given before collecting a
  a Random specimen
  b Midstream specimen
  c 24-hour urine specimen
  d Stool specimen

3 A 24-hour urine specimen involves
  a Collecting all urine voided during a 24-hour period
  b Collecting a random specimen every hour for 24 hours
  c Testing urine for ketones every day
  d Measuring output every hour for 24 hours

4 Urine is tested for ketones
  a At bedtime
  b 30 minutes after meals and at bedtime
  c 30 minutes before meals and at bedtime
  d Before breakfast

5 You need to strain a person's urine. Straining is done to find
  a Blood
  b Stones
  c Ketones
  d Acetone

6 You note a black, tarry stool. This is called
  a Melena
  b Feces
  c Hemostool
  d Occult blood

7 A stool specimen must be kept warm. After collecting the specimen
  a Put it in an oven
  b Put it in a paper bag
  c Cover it with a towel
  d Take it to the storage area

8 The best time to collect a sputum specimen is
  a On awakening
  b After meals
  c At bedtime
  d After oral hygiene

9 A sputum specimen is needed. You should ask the person to
  a Use mouthwash
  b Rinse the mouth with clear water
  c Brush the teeth
  d Remove dentures

10 Which is the best site for a skin puncture?
  a The thumb
  b The index finger
  c The ring finger
  d The little finger

11 Which is used to measure blood glucose?
  a Glucose meter
  b Lancet
  c Reagent strip
  d Sphygmomanometer

12 Before using reagent strips for blood glucose testing, you need to
  a Check the expiration date
  b Make sure they are discolored
  c Label each strip with the person's name
  d Check the size of the test area

Answers to these questions are on p. 720.

Admissions, Transfers, and Discharges

OBJECTIVES

- Define the key terms listed in this chapter.
- Describe your role during admissions, transfers, discharges, and when moving the person to a new room.
- Explain how you can help the resident and family feel comfortable in the nursing center.
- Identify the rules for measuring weight and height.

- Explain the reasons for moving a resident to a new room.
- Perform the procedures described in this chapter.
- Explain how to promote quality of life.

KEY TERMS

admission Official entry of a person into a nursing center

discharge Official departure of a person from a nursing center

transfer Moving the person to another health care setting; moving the person to a new room within the center

KEY ABBREVIATIONS

CMS Centers for Medicare & Medicaid Services

OBRA Omnibus Budget Reconciliation Act of 1987

Admission is the official entry of a person into a nursing center. It causes anxiety and fear in residents and families. They are in a new, strange setting. They may have concerns and fears about:

- Where to go, what to do, and what to expect
- Never returning home
- Who gives care, how care is given, and if the correct care is given
- Getting meals
- Finding the bathroom
- How to get help
- Being abused
- Strange sights and sounds
- Being apart from family and friends
- Making new friends
- Leaving homes and possessions behind

Moving to another room may cause similar concerns. So may transfer to another health care setting—hospital or nursing center. Discharge to a home setting is usually a happy time. However, the person may need home care. Discharge and transfer are defined as follows:

- **Discharge** is the official departure of a person from a nursing center.
- **Transfer** is moving the person to another health care setting. In some centers it also means moving the person to a new room within the center.

Admission, transfer, and discharge are critical events. So is moving the person to a new room. Sometimes the new room is on another nursing unit. These events involve:

- Privacy and confidentiality
- Reporting and recording
- Understanding and communicating with the person
- Communicating with the health team
- Respect for the person and the person's property
- Being kind, courteous, and respectful

See *Teamwork and Time Management: Admissions, Transfers, and Discharges.*

See *Delegation Guidelines: Admissions, Transfers, and Discharges.*

See *Promoting Safety and Comfort: Admissions, Transfers, and Discharges.*

TEAMWORK AND TIME MANAGEMENT
Admissions, Transfers, and Discharges

Transfers and discharges are easier if a co-worker helps you. So is moving the person to a new room. When asking for help, politely tell your co-worker:

- The procedure you need help with
- When you plan to do the procedure
- What you need the person to do
- How much time it will take

Remember to thank the person for helping you.

DELEGATION GUIDELINES
Admissions, Transfers, and Discharges

When admitting, transferring, or discharging a person, you need this information from the nurse. You also need the same information when moving a person to a new room.

- If you need to admit, transfer, or discharge the person or move the person to a new room
- If moving to a new room, the person's new room and bed number
- The person's method of transportation to or from the center—car, ambulance, or wheelchair van
- How the person will move about within the center—walking, wheelchair, stretcher, or bed
- The person's room and bed number
- What equipment and supplies are needed
- If the person stays dressed or needs to wear a gown or sleepwear
- If the person stays in bed or can be in a chair
- When to report observations
- What specific resident concerns to report at once

PROMOTING SAFETY AND COMFORT
Admissions, Transfers, and Discharges

Safety

The person may develop pain or become distressed during admission, transfer, discharge, or when moving to a new room. If so, call for the nurse at once. Stay with the person. When the nurse arrives, assist as needed.

Comfort

Admission, transfer, or discharge may be stressful for the person. So may moving to a new room. Some persons are happy. Others are sad and fearful. Some anxiety is normal. To provide for the person's mental comfort:

- Explain what you are doing and why.
- Do not rush the person.
- Be sensitive to the person's needs and feelings.

ADMISSIONS

An admission coordinator starts the process. The goal is to make it simple and easy. Often the process starts 2 or 3 days before the person enters the center.

The person's identifying information is obtained. This includes the person's:

- Full name
- Age and birth date
- Doctor's name
- Medicare number
- Religion

A nurse or social worker explains the resident's rights to the person and family. They also receive the rights in writing.

Admitting papers and a consent for treatment are signed. The person signs them or the person's legal representative does so. The nurse or admission coordinator obtains needed signatures.

The person's photo is taken. Then the person may receive an ID (identification) bracelet. The photo or ID bracelet are used to identify the person (Chapter 12).

Admission is often a hard time for the person and family. They do not part until ready to do so. Remember, the center is now the person's home.

See *Residents With Dementia: Admissions.*

See *Focus on Rehabilitation: Admissions.*

Preparing the Room

You prepare the room before the person arrives. Figure 34-1 shows a room ready for a new resident.

Text continued on p. 526

RESIDENTS WITH DEMENTIA

Admissions

Persons with dementia and their families may need extra help during the admission process. Often confusion increases in a new setting. Fear, agitation, and wanting to leave are common. The family also is fearful. Many feel guilty about the need for nursing center care. The health team helps the person and family feel safe and welcome.

FOCUS ON REHABILITATION

Admissions

Patients are admitted to rehabilitation units from hospitals. Often they arrive with special equipment and supplies.

A nurse usually greets the person and starts the admission process. Assist as needed. The nurse may ask you to complete parts of the admission process if:

• The person's condition is stable
• The person has no serious discomfort or distress

Fig. 34-1 The room is ready for a new resident.

 PREPARING THE PERSON'S ROOM

PROCEDURE

1 Follow *Delegation Guidelines: Admissions, Transfers, and Discharges*
2 Practice hand hygiene.
3 Collect the following:
  • Admission kit—wash basin, soap, toothpaste, toothbrush, water pitcher and cup, and so on
  • Bedpan and urinal (for a man)
  • Admission form (Fig. 34-2, pp. 524-525)
  • Thermometer
  • Sphygmomanometer
  • Stethoscope
  • Gown or pajamas (if needed)
  • Towels and washcloth
  • IV (intravenous) pole (if needed)
  • Other items requested by the nurse
4 Place the following on the overbed table:
  • Thermometer
  • Sphygmomanometer
  • Stethoscope
  • Admission form
5 Place the water pitcher and cup on the bedside stand or overbed table.
6 Place the following in the bedside stand:
  • Admission kit
  • Bedpan and urinal
  • Gown or pajamas
  • Towels and washcloth
7 *If the person arrives by stretcher:*
  a Make a surgical bed (Chapter 19).
  b Raise the bed to its highest level.
8 *If the person is ambulatory or arrives by wheelchair:*
  a Leave the bed closed.
  b Lower the bed to its lowest position.
9 Attach the signal light to the bed linens.
10 Decontaminate your hands.

ADMISSION NURSING ASSESSMENT

STATUS UPON ADMISSION

Admission Notes

Date of admission _____/____/____   Time _____ a.m. / p.m.

Transported by _____

Accompanied by _____

Age _____ Sex _____ Weight _____ Height: _____ Ft. _____ In.

Vitals: T _____ P _____ (□ Reg □ Irreg) R _____ B/P _____/____

Attending physician notified? □ No □ Yes, date/time _____/____/____ _____ a.m. / p.m.

Diagnosis: _____ Date last chest x-ray or PPD _____/____/____

Allergies

Meds _____

Food _____

Other _____

Skin Condition

Using the diagrams provided, indicate all body marks such as old/recent scars (surgical and other), bruises, discolorations, abrasions, pressure ulcers, or questionable markings. Indicate size, depth (in cms), color and drainage.

COMMENTS: _____

_____

SPECIAL TREATMENTS & PROCEDURES:

_____

PAIN

(As described by resident/representative)

Frequency:
□ No pain   □ Daily, but not
□ Less than daily   constant
                   □ Constant

Location: _____

Intensity:
□ No pain   □ Severe pain
□ Mild pain   □ Horrible pain
□ Distressing pain □ Excruciating
                      pain

Pain on admission:
□ No □ Yes, describe _____

RIGHT   LEFT

CURRENT STATUS

General Skin Condition

Check all that apply.

□ Reddened □ Pale □ Jaundiced
  □ Cyanotic □ Ashen
□ Dry □ Moist □ Oily □ Warm □ Cold
□ Edema, site _____

Physical Status (describe if applicable otherwise indicate NA)

Paralysis/paresis-site, degree _____

Contracture(s)-site, degree _____

Congenital anomalies _____

Prosthesis: _____

Other _____

Functional Status

TRANSFERS-ABLE TO TRANSFER
□ Independently
□ 1 person assist
□ 2 person assist
□ Total assist

WEIGHT BEARING-ABLE TO BEAR
□ Full weight
□ Partial weight
□ Non-weight bearing

AMBULATION-ABLE TO AMBULATE
□ Independently
□ 1 person assist
□ 2 person assist
□ With device
   Type _____
□ Wheelchair only
□ Wheelchair/propels self
□ Bedrest

SUPPORTIVE DEVICES USED:
□ Elastic hose   □ Footboard
□ Bed cradle   □ Air mattress
□ Sheepskin   □ Eggcrate
□ Hand rolls □ Sling □ Trapeze
□ Other _____
_____
□ Other _____
_____

Drug Therapy

	DRUG	DOSE/FREQUENCY		DRUG	DOSE/FREQUENCY
1			6		
2			7		
3			8		
4			9		
5			10		

NAME-Last	First	Middle	Attending Physician	Record No.	Room/Bed

CFS 5-3HH   © 1992 Briggs Corporation, Des Moines, IA 50306 (800) 247-2343
R1001   PRINTED IN U.S.A.

ADMISSION NURSING ASSESSMENT
□ Continued on Reverse

Fig. 34-2 Admission form. *(Courtesy Briggs Corp., Des Moines, Iowa.)*

CURRENT STATUS - CONTINUED

Hearing	Right	Left	R & L	Vision	Right	Left	R & L	Communication
Adequate				Adequate				❏ Clear
Adequate w/aid				Adequate w/glasses				❏ Aphasic ❏ Dysphasic
Poor				Poor				Language(s) Spoken:
Deaf				Blind				

Oral Assessment / Eating/Nutrition

Oral Assessment	Eating/Nutrition	

Complete oral cavity exam: ❏ Yes ❏ No
  If yes, condition _____
 	
Own teeth: ❏ Yes ❏ No
  If yes, condition _____
 	
Dentures: Upper ❏ Comp ❏ Part
         Lower ❏ Comp ❏ Part
Do dentures fit? ❏ Yes ❏ No
	❏ Dependent ❏ Independent ❏ Needs assist
	❏ Dysphagic; reason _____
	❏ Adaptive equipment (specify) _____
	_____
	Type/consistency of diet _____
	_____
		Food likes _____
		_____
		Food dislikes _____
		_____
		Bev. preference _____
		HS snack preferred: ❏ Yes ❏ No

Sleep Patterns

Sleep Patterns	Bathing/Oral Hyg.	Indep.	Assist	Dep.	General Grooming	Indep.	Assist	Dep.
Usual bed time _____ a.m./p.m.	Tub				Shave			
Usual arising time _____ a.m./p.m.	Shower				Grooming			
Usual nap time _____ a.m./p.m.	Bed bath				Dressing			
Other _____	Oral hygiene				Shampoo			

Psychosocial Functioning

FAMILY RELATIONSHIPS:

Members visit (frequency) _____

_____

Closest relationship with _____

_____

ORIENTED: ❏ Yes ❏ No, if No _____
DISORIENTED TO: ❏ Time ❏ Place
❏ Person
RESIDENT GIVEN EXPLANATION OF/OR INVOLVED IN PLAN OF CARE? ❏ Yes ❏ No
RESIDENT ORIENTED TO FACILITY? ❏ Call light ❏ Bathroom ❏ Mealtime ❏ Activities

WHICH WORDS BEST DESCRIBE RESIDENT? ❏ Alert ❏ Angry ❏ Fearful
❏ Noisy ❏ Friendly ❏ Cooperative ❏ Lethargic ❏ _____
❏ Non-questioning ❏ Combative
ANSWERS QUESTIONS: ❏ Readily ❏ Reluctantly ❏ Inappropriately
MOOD: ❏ Passive ❏ Depressed ❏ Elated ❏ Quiet ❏ Secure
❏ Questioning ❏ Talkative ❏ Homesick ❏ Wanders mentally
❏ Hyperactive ❏ _____
COMPREHENSION: ❏ Slow ❏ Quick ❏ Unable to understand
MOTIVATION: ❏ Good ❏ Fair ❏ Poor
PERSONAL HABITS: Smokes? ❏ Yes ❏ No Uses alcohol? ❏ Yes ❏ No

Bowel and Bladder Evaluation

Uses: ❏ Toilet ❏ Urinal ❏ Bedpan ❏ Bedside commode
BOWEL HABITS: Continent? ❏ Yes ❏ No Constipated? ❏ Yes ❏ No Laxative used? ❏ Yes ❏ No
Enemas used? ❏ Yes ❏ No Last bowel movement _____ a.m./p.m.
BLADDER HABITS: Continent? ❏ Yes ❏ No Dribbles? ❏ Yes ❏ No Catheter? ❏ Yes, type _____ ❏ No
Urine color _____ Consistency _____ Time last voiding _____ a.m./p.m.

Restorative Programs Indicated / Therapy Indicated

Restorative Programs Indicated		Therapy Indicated
Based on the foregoing assessment, check all that apply. ❏ ROM ❏ Splint or brace assistance ❏ Bed mobility training & skill practice ❏ Transfer training & skill practice ❏ Walking training & skill practice	❏ Dressing/grooming training & skill practice ❏ Eating/swallowing training & skill practice ❏ Appliance/prosthesis training & skill practice ❏ Communication training & skill practice ❏ Scheduled toileting ❏ Bladder retraining	❏ Physical ❏ Occupational ❏ Speech Comments: _____ _____ _____ _____ _____

Comments: _____

_____

Completed by:
Signature/Title _____ Date _____

NAME–Last	First	Middle	Attending Physician	Record No.	Room/Bed

ADMISSION NURSING ASSESSMENT

Fig. 34-2—cont'd

Admitting the Person

The room assignment is made before the person arrives. Some residents arrive by ambulance or wheelchair van. Attendants take them to their rooms. Some arrive by car. A nurse usually greets and escorts the person to the room. The nurse may ask you to do so if the person has no discomfort or distress.

Admission is your first chance to make a good impression. You must:

- Greet the person by name and title. Use the admission form to find out the person's name.
- Introduce yourself by name and title to the person, family, and friends (Fig. 34-3).
- Make roommate introductions.
- Act in a professional manner.
- Treat the person with dignity and respect.

Fig. 34-3 The nursing assistant introduces herself to the person and family member.

Safety and Security Physical and mental comfort are important. So is feeling safe and secure. Do not rush the admission procedures. Rather, treat the person and family as guests in your home. Offer them a beverage. Visit with them. Tell them some of the good things about the center.

Introduce residents in nearby rooms. This way the person knows other residents. They can provide comfort and support. They understand, better than anyone else, what a nursing center is like.

The center is the person's home. Help make the room as home-like as possible. Also help the person unpack. Perhaps the person needs help putting clothes away. The person may want to hang pictures or display photos. Show care and compassion. Help the person feel safe, comfortable, and secure.

The Admission Procedure During the admission procedure the nurse may ask you to:

- Collect some information for the admission form.
- Measure the person's weight and height.
- Measure the person's vital signs.
- Complete a clothing and personal belongings list.
- Orient the person to the room, the nursing unit, and the center.

ADMITTING THE PERSON

QUALITY OF LIFE

Remember to:
- Knock before entering the person's room.
- Address the person by name.
- Introduce yourself by name and title.

- Explain the procedure to the person before beginning and during the procedure.
- Protect the person's rights during the procedure.
- Handle the person gently during the procedure.

PRE-PROCEDURE

1 Follow *Delegation Guidelines: Admissions, Transfers, and Discharges,* p. 522. See *Promoting Safety and Comfort: Admissions, Transfers, and Discharges,* p. 522.

2 Practice hand hygiene.
3 Prepare the room. See procedure: *Preparing the Person's Room,* p. 523.

PROCEDURE

4 Check the person's name on the admission form.
5 Greet the person by name. Ask if he or she prefers a certain name.
6 Introduce yourself to the person and others present. Give your name and title. Explain that you assist the nurses in giving care.

7 Introduce the roommate.
8 Provide for privacy. Ask family or friends to leave the room. Tell them how much time you need, and direct them to the waiting area. Let a family member or friend stay if the person prefers.

ADMITTING THE PERSON—cont'd

PROCEDURE—cont'd

9 Let the person stay dressed if his or her condition permits. Or help the person change into a gown or pajamas.

10 Provide for comfort. The person is in bed or in a chair as directed by the nurse.

11 Assist the nurse with assessment:
   a Measure vital signs (Chapter 31).
   b Measure weight and height.
   c Collect information for the admission form as requested by the nurse.

12 Complete a clothing and personal belongings list (Chapter 12).

13 Help the person put away clothes and personal items. Put them in the closet, drawers, and bedside stand. (The family may wish to help with this step.)

14 Explain ordered activity limits.

15 Orient the person and family to the area:
   a Give names of the nurses and nursing assistants.
   b Identify items in the bedside stand. Explain the purpose of each.
   c Explain how to use the overbed table.
   d Show how to use the signal light.
   e Show how to use the bed, TV, and light controls.
   f Explain how to make phone calls. Place the phone within reach.
   g Show the person the bathroom. Also show how to use the signal light in the bathroom.
   h Explain visiting hours and policies.
   i Explain where to find the nurses' station, lounge, chapel, dining room, and other areas.
   j Identify staff—housekeeping, dietary, physical therapy, and others. Also identify students who are in the center.
   k Explain when meals and snacks are served.

16 Fill the water pitcher and cup if oral fluids are allowed.

17 Place the signal light within reach.

18 Place other controls and needed items within reach.

19 Provide a denture container if needed. Label it with the person's name and room and bed number.

20 Label the person's property and personal care items with his or her name (if not done so by the family).

POST-PROCEDURE

21 Provide for comfort. (See the inside of the front book cover.)

22 Lower the bed to its lowest position.

23 Raise or lower bed rails. Follow the care plan.

24 Complete a safety check of the room. (See the inside of the front book cover.)

25 Decontaminate your hands.

26 Report and record your observations.

🔖 Weight and Height

Weight and height are measured on admission to the center. Then the person is weighed daily, weekly, or monthly. This is done to measure weight gain or loss.

Standing, chair, bed, and lift scales are used (Fig. 34-4, p. 528). Chair, bed, and lift scales are used for persons who cannot stand. Follow the manufacturer's instructions and center procedures.

When measuring weight and height, follow these guidelines:

- The person only wears a gown or pajamas. Clothes add weight. No footwear is worn. Footwear adds to the weight and height measurements.
- The person voids before being weighed. A full bladder adds weight.
- Weigh the person at the same time of day. Before breakfast is the best time. Food and fluids add weight.
- Use the same scale for daily, weekly, and monthly weights. Scales weigh differently.
- Balance the scale at zero (0) before weighing the person. For balance scales, move the weights to zero. A digital scale should read at zero.

See *Teamwork and Time Management: Weight and Height,* p. 528.

See *Delegation Guidelines: Weight and Height,* p. 528.

See *Promoting Safety and Comfort: Weight and Height,* p. 529.

Fig. 34-4 Types of scales. **A,** Standing scale. **B,** Chair scale. **C,** Lift scale. (**C,** *Courtesy ARJO, Morton Grove, Ill.*)

TEAMWORK AND TIME MANAGEMENT
Weight and Height

Nursing units usually have just one standing scale. In some centers, chair and lift scales are shared with other nursing units. Return the device to the storage area as quickly as possible. Do not have your co-workers wait or look for the scale.

DELEGATION GUIDELINES
Weight and Height

Before measuring weight and height, you need this information from the nurse and the care plan:
* When to measure weight and height
* What scale to use
* If height is measured with the person in bed
* When to report the measurements
* What specific resident concerns to report at once

PROMOTING SAFETY AND COMFORT
Weight and Height

Safety
Follow the manufacturer's instructions when using chair, bed, or lift scales. Also follow the center's procedures. Practice safety measures to prevent falls.

Comfort
The person wears only a gown or pajamas for the weight measurement. Prevent chilling and drafts (Chapter 18).

 MEASURING WEIGHT AND HEIGHT

QUALITY OF LIFE

Remember to:
- Knock before entering the person's room.
- Address the person by name.
- Introduce yourself by name and title.

- Explain the procedure to the person before beginning and during the procedure.
- Protect the person's rights during the procedure.
- Handle the person gently during the procedure.

PRE-PROCEDURE

1 Follow *Delegation Guidelines: Weight and Height.* See *Promoting Safety and Comfort: Weight and Height.*
2 Ask the person to void.
3 Practice hand hygiene.
4 Bring the scale and paper towels (for a standing scale) to the person's room.
5 Decontaminate your hands.

6 Identify the person. Check the ID bracelet against the assignment sheet. Also call the person by name.
7 Provide for privacy.

PROCEDURE

8 Place the paper towels on the scale platform.
9 Raise the height rod.
10 Move the weights to zero (0). The pointer is in the middle.
11 Have the person remove the robe and footwear. Assist as needed.
12 Help the person stand on the scale. The person stands in the center of the scale. Arms are at the sides.
13 Move the weights until the balance pointer is in the middle (Fig. 34-5, p. 530).
14 Note the weight on your notepad or assignment sheet.

15 Ask the person to stand very straight.
16 Lower the height rod until it rests on the person's head (Fig. 34-6, p. 530).
17 Note the height on your notepad or assignment sheet.
18 Raise the height rod. Help the person step off of the scale.
19 Help the person put on a robe and non-skid footwear if he or she will be up. Or help the person back to bed.
20 Lower the height rod. Adjust the weights to zero (0) if this is your center's policy.

POST-PROCEDURE

21 Provide for comfort. (See the inside of the front book cover.)
22 Place the signal light within reach.
23 Raise or lower bed rails. Follow the care plan.
24 Unscreen the person.
25 Complete a safety check of the room. (See the inside of the front book cover.)

26 Discard the paper towels.
27 Return the scale to its proper place.
28 Decontaminate your hands.
29 Report and record the measurements.

Fig. 34-5 A, The person is weighed. **B,** The weight is read when the balance pointer is in the middle.

Fig. 34-6 Height is measured.

MEASURING HEIGHT—THE PERSON IS IN BED

QUALITY OF LIFE

Remember to:
- Knock before entering the person's room.
- Address the person by name.
- Introduce yourself by name and title.

- Explain the procedure to the person before beginning and during the procedure.
- Protect the person's rights during the procedure.
- Handle the person gently during the procedure.

PRE-PROCEDURE

1 Follow *Delegation Guidelines: Weight and Height*, p. 528. See *Promoting Safety and Comfort: Weight and Height*, p. 529.
2 Practice hand hygiene.
3 Ask a co-worker to help you.
4 Collect a measuring tape and ruler.

5 Decontaminate your hands.
6 Identify the person. Check the ID bracelet against the assignment sheet. Also call the person by name.
7 Provide for privacy.
8 Raise the bed for body mechanics. Bed rails are up if used.

PROCEDURE

9 Lower the bed rails (if up).
10 Position the person supine if the position is allowed.
11 Have your co-worker hold the end of the measuring tape so it extends to the person's heel.
12 Pull the measuring tape along the person's body. Pull until it extends past the head (Fig. 34-7).

13 Place the ruler flat across the top of the person's head. It extends from the person's head to the measuring tape. Make sure the ruler is level.
14 Note the height on your notepad or assignment sheet.

POST-PROCEDURE

15 Provide for comfort. (See the inside of the front book cover.)
16 Place the signal light within reach.
17 Lower the bed to its lowest position.
18 Raise or lower bed rails. Follow the care plan.

19 Complete a safety check of the room. (See the inside of the front book cover.)
20 Return equipment to its proper place.
21 Decontaminate your hands.
22 Report and record the height.

Fig. 34-7 The person's height is measured in bed. The tape measure extends from the top of the head to the heel. The ruler is flat across the top of the person's head.

MOVING THE PERSON TO A NEW ROOM

Sometimes a person is moved to a new room. Reasons include:
- A change in condition.
- The person requests a room change.
- Roommates do not get along.
- Changes in care needs.

The doctor, nurse, or social worker explains the reasons for the move. The family and business office are told. You assist with the move or perform the entire procedure. The person is transported by wheelchair, stretcher, or the bed.

Support and reassure the person. If the new room is on another nursing unit, the person does not know the staff. Use good communication skills.
- Avoid pat answers. "It will be OK" is an example.
- Use touch to provide comfort.
- Introduce the person to the staff and roommate.
- Wish the person well as you leave him or her.

MOVING THE PERSON TO A NEW ROOM

QUALITY OF LIFE

Remember to:
- Knock before entering the person's room.
- Address the person by name.
- Introduce yourself by name and title.

- Explain the procedure to the person before beginning and during the procedure.
- Protect the person's rights during the procedure.
- Handle the person gently during the procedure.

PRE-PROCEDURE

1 Follow *Delegation Guidelines: Admissions, Transfers, and Discharges,* p. 522. See *Promoting Safety and Comfort: Admissions, Transfers, and Discharges,* p. 522.
2 Ask a co-worker to help you.
3 Practice hand hygiene.
4 Collect the following:
- Wheelchair or stretcher
- Utility cart
- Bath blanket

5 Decontaminate your hands.
6 Identify the person. Check the ID bracelet against the assignment sheet. Call the person by name.
7 Provide for privacy.

PROCEDURE

8 Collect the person's belongings and care equipment. Place them on the cart.
9 Transfer the person to a wheelchair or stretcher (Chapter 17). Cover him or her with the bath blanket.
10 Transport the person to the new room. Your co-worker brings the cart.
11 Help transfer the person to the bed or chair. Help position the person (Chapter 16).

12 Help arrange the person's belongings and equipment.
13 Report the following to the receiving nurse:
   a How the person tolerated the transfer
   b Any observations made during the transfer
   c That the nurse will bring the medical record, care plan, Kardex, and drugs

POST-PROCEDURE

14 Return the wheelchair or stretcher and the cart to the storage area.
15 Decontaminate your hands.
16 Report and record the following:
- The time of the transfer
- Who helped you with the transfer
- Where the person was taken
- How the person was transferred (bed, wheelchair, or stretcher)
- How the person tolerated the transfer

- Who received the person
- Any other observations

17 Strip the bed, and clean the unit. Decontaminate your hands, and put on gloves for this step. (The housekeeping staff may do this step.)
18 Remove the gloves. Decontaminate your hands.
19 Follow center policy for dirty linen.
20 Make a closed bed.
21 Decontaminate your hands.

✎ TRANSFERS AND DISCHARGES

When transferred or discharged, the person leaves the center. He or she goes home or to another health care setting. The Omnibus Budget and Reconciliation Act of 1987 (OBRA) and the Centers for Medicare & Medicaid Services (CMS) have standards for transfers and discharges. The person's rights are protected. Reasons for the transfer or discharge are part of the person's medical record. The person and family are informed in advance of the transfer or discharge plans. A procedure is followed if the person objects. An ombudsman protects the person's interests.

OBRA-CMS

According to OBRA and the CMS, reasons for a transfer or discharge are:
- The measure is necessary to meet the person's welfare. The person's welfare cannot be met in the center.
- The person's health has improved to the extent that he or she no longer needs the center's services.
- The health or safety of other people in the nursing center is in danger.
- The person has failed to pay for his or her stay in the nursing center.
- The nursing center closes.

OBRA-CMS

The person and family are told of the date and time of the transfer or discharge. And they are given the name and location of the hospital or nursing center where the person will be going.

Transfers and discharges are usually planned in advance. When transferred, the person goes to a hospital or another nursing center. Discharge is a happy time if the person is going home.

The health team plans the transfer or discharge. If being discharged, they teach the person and family about diet, exercise, and drugs. They also teach them about procedures and treatments. They arrange for home care, equipment, and therapies as needed. A doctor's appointment is given.

The nurse tells you when to start the transfer or discharge procedure. The doctor must give the order before the person can leave. The nurse tells you when the person is ready to leave. Usually a wheelchair is used. If leaving by ambulance, a stretcher is used.

Use good communication skills when assisting with a transfer or discharge. Wish the person and family well as they leave the center.

A person may want to leave the center without the doctor's permission. Tell the nurse at once. The nurse or social worker handles the matter.

Use the procedure that follows for discharges and transfers.

TRANSFERRING OR DISCHARGING THE PERSON

QUALITY OF LIFE

Remember to:
- Knock before entering the person's room.
- Address the person by name.
- Introduce yourself by name and title.

- Explain the procedure to the person before beginning and during the procedure.
- Protect the person's rights during the procedure.
- Handle the person gently during the procedure.

PRE-PROCEDURE

1 Follow *Delegation Guidelines: Admissions, Transfers, and Discharges*, p. 522. See *Promoting Safety and Comfort: Admissions, Transfers, and Discharges*, p. 522.
2 Ask a co-worker to help you.

3 Practice hand hygiene.
4 Identify the person. Check the ID bracelet against the assignment sheet. Also call the person by name.
5 Provide for privacy.

PROCEDURE

6 Help the person dress as needed.
7 Help the person pack. Check all drawers and closets. Make sure all items are collected.
8 Check off the clothing list and personal belongings list. Give the lists to the nurse.
9 Tell the nurse that the person is ready for the final visit. The nurse:
  a Gives prescriptions written by the doctor
  b Provides discharge instructions
  c Gets valuables from the safe
  d Has the person sign the clothing and personal belongings lists

10 If the person will leave by wheelchair:
  a Get a wheelchair and a utility cart for the person's items. Ask a co-worker to help you.
  b Help the person into the wheelchair.
  c Take the person to the exit area.
  d Lock the wheelchair wheels.
  e Help the person out of the wheelchair and into the car (Fig. 34-8, p. 534).
  f Help put the person's items into the car.
11 If the person will leave by ambulance:
  a Raise the bed rails.
  b Raise the bed to its highest level.
  c Place the signal light within reach.
  d Wait for the ambulance attendants.

POST-PROCEDURE

12 Return the wheelchair and cart to the storage area.
13 Decontaminate your hands.
14 Report and record the following:
- The time of the discharge
- Who helped you with the procedure
- How the person was transported
- Who was with the person
- The person's destination
- Any other observations

15 Strip the bed, and clean the unit. Decontaminate your hands, and put on gloves for this step. (The housekeeping staff may do this step.)
16 Remove the gloves. Decontaminate your hands.
17 Follow center policy for dirty linen.
18 Make a closed bed.
19 Decontaminate your hands.

Fig. 34-8 This resident is going home with her husband.

QUALITY OF LIFE

Admission to a nursing center usually is a hard time for the person and family. Transfers and discharges also can cause fear and worry. Discharge often is a happy and pleasant event. However, it may cause worries and concerns if more care and treatment are needed. To help the person and family:

- Be courteous, caring, efficient, and competent.
- Be sensitive to fears and concerns.
- Handle the person's property and valuables carefully and with respect. Protect them from loss or damage.
- Treat the person and family like you want your loved ones treated.

The first hours and days in the center are often very lonely. Visit new residents often. Introduce them to other residents. Encourage them to take part in activities.

Explain all procedures and what the various sounds mean. Repeat information as needed. The new resident is in a new place. There is much new information. It may take time to remember things. Knowing what is happening and why helps the person feel safer and more secure. Remember to always protect the person's rights and to promote quality of life.

REVIEW QUESTIONS

Circle T if the statement is TRUE. Circle F if the statement is FALSE.

1 T F Identifying information is obtained when the person arrives in the room.
2 T F You are admitting a new resident. You must introduce yourself by name and title.
3 T F A person arrives at the center by ambulance. You transport the person to his or her room.
4 T F The person is greeted by name and title during the admission process.
5 T F Vital signs are measured during the admission procedure.
6 T F You explain the resident's rights to the person and family.
7 T F A person complains of pain. Report the complaint after completing the admission form.
8 T F The person arrives by stretcher. You make an occupied bed.
9 T F You help orient the person to the new setting.
10 T F A robe and footwear are worn when measuring weight.
11 T F A robe and footwear are worn when measuring height.
12 T F Clothing and personal belongings lists are made during the admission process.
13 T F A person's condition may require a transfer to another nursing unit.
14 T F A doctor's order is required for transfer or discharge from the center.
15 T F You teach the person about diet and drugs.
16 T F Starting with admission, the person's rights are protected.
17 T F A person with dementia may become more confused in a new setting.
18 T F A person objects to a transfer. An ombudsman makes sure the person's rights are protected.

Answers to these questions are on p. 721.

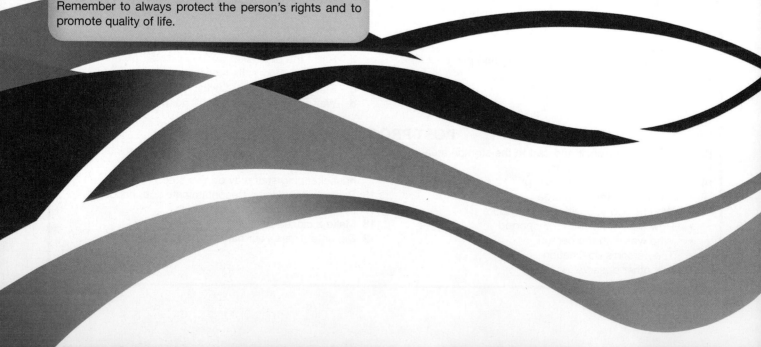

Wound Care

OBJECTIVES

- Define the key terms and key abbreviations listed in this chapter.
- Describe skin tears, circulatory ulcers, and diabetic foot ulcers; the persons at risk; and how to prevent them.
- Describe the process and complications of wound healing.
- Describe what to observe about wounds.
- Explain how to secure dressings.
- Explain the rules for applying dressings.

- Explain the purpose of binders and how to apply them.
- Explain the purpose, effects, and complications of heat and cold applications.
- Describe the rules for applying heat and cold.
- Describe how to meet the basic needs of persons with wounds.
- Perform the procedures described in this chapter.
- Explain how to promote quality of life.

KEY TERMS

abrasion A partial-thickness wound caused by the scraping away or rubbing of the skin

arterial ulcer An open wound on the lower legs or feet caused by poor arterial blood flow

chronic wound A wound that does not heal easily

circulatory ulcer An open sore on the lower legs or feet caused by decreased blood flow through the arteries or veins; vascular ulcer

clean-contaminated wound Occurs from the surgical entry of the reproductive, urinary, respiratory, or gastro-intestinal system

clean wound A wound that is not infected

closed wound Tissues are injured but the skin is not broken

compress A soft pad applied over a body area

constrict To narrow

contaminated wound A wound with a high risk of infection

contusion A closed wound caused by a blow to the body; a bruise

dehiscence The separation of wound layers

diabetic foot ulcer An open wound on the foot caused by complications from diabetes

dilate To expand or open wider

dirty wound See "infected wound"

edema Swelling caused by fluid collecting in tissues

embolus A blood clot that travels through the vascular system until it lodges in a vessel

evisceration The separation of the wound along with the protrusion of abdominal organs

full-thickness wound The dermis, epidermis, and subcutaneous tissue are penetrated; muscle and bone may be involved

gangrene A condition in which there is death of tissue

hyperthermia A body temperature *(thermia)* that is much higher *(hyper)* than the person's normal range

Continued

KEY TERMS—cont'd

hypothermia A very low *(hypo)* body temperature *(thermia)*

incision A cut produced surgically by a sharp instrument; it creates an opening into an organ or body space

infected wound A wound containing large amounts of microbes that shows signs of infection; a dirty wound

intentional wound A wound created for therapy

laceration An open wound with torn tissues and jagged edges

open wound The skin or mucous membrane is broken

pack Wrapping a body part with a wet or dry application

partial-thickness wound The dermis and epidermis of the skin are broken

penetrating wound An open wound that breaks the skin and enters a body area, organ, or cavity

phlebitis Inflammation *(itis)* of a vein *(phleb)*

puncture wound An open wound made by a sharp object

purulent drainage Thick green, yellow, or brown drainage

sanguineous drainage Bloody *(sanguis)* drainage

serosanguineous drainage Thin, watery drainage *(sero)* that is blood-tinged *(sanguineous)*

serous drainage Clear, watery fluid *(serum)*

skin tear A break or rip in the outer layers of the skin; the epidermis (top skin layer) separates from the underlying tissues

stasis ulcer See "venous ulcer"

thrombus A blood clot

trauma An accident or violent act that injures the skin, mucous membranes, bones, and organs

ulcer A shallow or deep crater-like sore of the skin or a mucous membrane

unintentional wound A wound resulting from trauma

vascular ulcer See "circulatory ulcer"

venous ulcer An open sore on the lower legs or feet caused by poor venous blood flow; stasis ulcer

wound A break in the skin or mucous membrane

KEY ABBREVIATIONS

C	Centigrade	ID	Identification
F	Fahrenheit	PPE	Personal protective equipment
GI	Gastro-intestinal		

A wound is a break in the skin or mucous membrane. Common causes are:
- Surgery
- Trauma—an accident or violent act that injures the skin, mucous membranes, bones, and organs. Falls, vehicle crashes, gun shots, stabbings, human and animal bites, burns, and frostbite are examples.
- Pressure ulcers from unrelieved pressure (Chapter 36).
- Decreased blood flow through the arteries or veins.
- Nerve damage.

Infection is a major threat. Wound care involves preventing infection and further injury to the wound and nearby tissues. Blood loss and pain also are prevented.

The nurse uses the nursing process to keep the person's skin healthy. Some centers have a skin care team to manage all skin problems. The team includes an RN, physical therapist, and a dietitian.

See *Focus on Rehabilitation: Wound Care.*

FOCUS ON REHABILITATION
Wound Care

Some persons have poor or delayed wound healing. Others have complications from wound healing. Rehabilitation and subacute care units often provide special wound care.

Box 35-1   Types of Wounds

Intentional and Unintentional Wounds
- Intentional wound—is created for therapy. Surgical incisions are examples. So are venipunctures for starting intravenous therapy and for drawing blood specimens.
- Unintentional wound—results from trauma.

Open and Closed Wounds
- Open wound—when the skin or mucous membrane is broken. Intentional and most unintentional wounds are open.
- Closed wound—tissues are injured but the skin is not broken. Bruises, twists, and sprains are examples.

Clean and Dirty Wounds
- Clean wound—is not infected. Microbes have not entered the wound. Closed wounds are usually clean. So are intentional wounds created under surgical asepsis. The reproductive, urinary, respiratory, and gastrointestinal (GI) systems are not entered.
- Clean-contaminated wound—occurs from the surgical entry of the reproductive, urinary, respiratory, or GI system. Some or all parts of these systems are not sterile and contain normal flora.

Clean and Dirty Wounds—cont'd
- Contaminated wound—has a high risk of infection. Unintentional wounds are generally contaminated. Wound contamination occurs from breaks in surgical asepsis and spillage of intestinal contents. Tissues may show signs of inflammation.
- Infected wound (dirty wound)—contains large amounts of microbes and shows signs of infection. Examples include old wounds, surgical incisions into infected areas, and traumatic injuries that rupture the bowel.
- Chronic wound—does not heal easily. Pressure ulcers and circulatory ulcers are examples.

Partial- and Full-Thickness Wounds (Describe Wound Depth)
- Partial-thickness wound—the dermis and epidermis of the skin are broken.
- Full-thickness wound—the dermis, epidermis, and subcutaneous tissue are penetrated. Muscle and bone may be involved.

TYPES OF WOUNDS

Types of wounds are described in Box 35-1. Wounds also are described by their cause:

- Abrasion—a partial-thickness wound caused by the scraping away or rubbing of the skin (Fig. 35-1).
- Contusion—a closed wound caused by a blow to the body (a bruise) (Fig. 35-2).
- Incision—a cut produced surgically by a sharp instrument. It creates an opening into an organ or body space (Fig. 35-3, p. 538).
- Laceration—an open wound with torn tissues and jagged edges (Fig. 35-4, p. 538).
- Penetrating wound—an open wound that breaks the skin and enters a body area, organ, or cavity (Fig. 35-5, p. 538).
- Puncture wound—an open wound made by a sharp object (knife, nail, metal, wood, glass). Entry of the skin and underlying tissues may be intentional or unintentional. See Figure 35-6, p. 538.
- Ulcer—a shallow or deep crater-like sore of the skin or a mucous membrane (p. 539).

Fig. 35-1 An abrasion. *(From Kumar V, Abbas AK, Fausto N:* Robbins and Cotran pathologic basis of disease, *ed 7, Philadelphia, 2005, Saunders.)*

Fig. 35-2 Contusion. *(From Finkbeiner W, Ursell P, Davis R:* Autopsy pathology: a manual and atlas, *London, 2004, Churchill Livingstone.)*

Fig. 35-3 A surgical incision closed with staples. *(From Elkin MK, Perry AG, Potter PA: Nursing interventions and clinical skills, ed 4, St Louis, 2007, Mosby.)*

Fig. 35-4 Laceration. *(From Roberts JR, Hedges JR: Clinical Procedures in Emergency Medicine, ed. 5, St. Louis, 2009, Saunders.)*

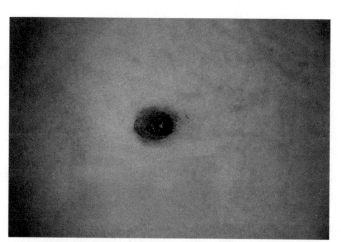

Fig. 35-5 Penetrating wound. *(From McCance KL, Huether SE: Pathophysiology: The biologic basis for disease in adults and children, ed 6, St. Louis, 2010, Mosby.)*

Fig. 35-6 Puncture wound. *(From McCance KL, Huether SE: Pathophysiology: The biologic basis for disease in adults and children, ed 6, St. Louis, 2010, Mosby.)*

SKIN TEARS

A **skin tear** is a break or rip in the outer layers of the skin (Fig. 35-7). The epidermis (top skin layer) separates from the underlying tissues (Chapter 9). The skin is "peeled back." The hands, arms, and lower legs are common sites for skin tears. Very thin and fragile skin is common in older persons. Slight pressure can cause a skin tear.

Causes

Skin tears are caused by:
* Friction, shearing (Chapter 17), pulling, or pressure on the skin.
* Falls or bumping a hand, arm, or leg on any hard surface. Beds, bed rails, chairs, wheelchair footplates, and tables are dangers.
* Holding the person's arm or leg too tight.
* Removing tape or adhesives.
* Bathing, dressing, and other tasks.
* Pulling buttons and zippers across fragile skin.
* Jewelry—yours or the person's. Rings, watches, and bracelets are examples.

Skin tears are painful. They are portals of entry for microbes. Infection is a risk. Tell the nurse at once if you cause or find a skin tear.

Fig. 35-7 Skin tear. *(Used with permission from Dr. Rosemary Kohr, RN, PhD, ACNP (cert), www.lhsc.on.ca/wound)*

Persons at Risk

Persons at risk for skin tears:

- Need some to total help in moving
- Have poor nutrition
- Have poor hydration
- Have altered mental awareness
- Are very thin

See *Residents With Dementia: Persons at Risk (Skin Tears).*

Prevention and Treatment

Careful and safe care helps prevent skin tears and further injury. Follow the measures in Box 35-2. Also follow the care plan and the nurse's directions. They may include dressings (p. 550) and elastic bandages (p. 543) to protect the skin and promote healing.

RESIDENTS WITH DEMENTIA

Persons at Risk (Skin Tears)

Some persons are confused and may resist care. They often move quickly and without warning. Or they pull away from you during care. Some try to hit or kick. These sudden movements can cause skin tears.

Never force care on a person. Chapter 44 describes how to care for persons who are confused and resist care. Always follow the care plan.

CIRCULATORY ULCERS

Some diseases affect blood flow to and from the legs and feet. Such poor circulation can lead to pain, open wounds, and edema. Edema is swelling caused by fluid collecting in tissues. Infection and gangrene can result from the open wound and poor circulation. Gangrene is a condition in which there is death of tissue.

Circulatory ulcers (vascular ulcers) are open sores on the lower legs or feet. They are caused by decreased blood flow through the arteries or veins. Persons with diseases affecting the blood vessels are at risk. These wounds are painful and hard to heal.

The doctor orders drugs and treatments as needed. The nurse uses the nursing process to meet the person's needs (Box 35-3, p. 540). You must help prevent skin breakdown on the legs and feet.

Venous Ulcers

Venous ulcers (stasis ulcers) are open sores on the lower legs or feet. *Stasis* means stopped or slowed fluid flow. These ulcers are caused by poor venous blood flow (Fig. 35-8, p. 540).

Venous ulcers can develop when valves in the leg's veins do not close well. The veins do not pump blood back to the heart in a normal way. Blood and fluid collect in the legs and feet. Small skin veins rupture. This allows hemoglobin to enter the tissue, causing the skin to turn brown. (Hemoglobin gives blood its red color.) The skin is dry, leathery, and hard. Itching is common.

Box 35-2 Measures to Prevent Skin Tears

- Keep your fingernails short and smoothly filed.
- Keep the person's fingernails short and smoothly filed. Report long and tough toenails.
- Do not wear rings with large or raised stones. Do not wear bracelets.
- Be patient and calm when the person is confused or agitated or resists care.
- Follow the care plan and safety rules to handle, move, turn, position, or transfer the person.
  - Prevent shearing and friction.
  - Use an assist device to move and turn the person in bed.
  - Use pillows to support arms and legs. Follow the care plan.
- Pad bed rails and wheelchair arms, footplates, and leg supports. Follow the care plan.

- Follow the care plan and safety rules to bathe the person.
- Dress and undress the person carefully.
- Dress the person in soft clothes with long sleeves and long pants.
- Provide good lighting so the person can see. The person needs to avoid bumping into furniture, walls, and equipment.
- Provide a safe area for wandering (Chapter 44).
- Keep the skin moisturized. Apply lotion according to the care plan.
- Offer fluids. Follow the care plan.
- Remove tape carefully (p. 551).
- Do not apply adhesive tape (p. 551).

Box 35-3 Measures to Prevent Circulatory Ulcers

- Remind the person not to sit with the legs crossed.
- Re-position the person according to the care plan—at least every 2 hours.
- Do not use elastic or rubber band–type garters to hold socks or hose in place.
- Do not dress the person in tight clothes.
- Provide good skin care daily. Keep the feet clean and dry. Clean and dry between the toes.
- Do not scrub or rub the skin during bathing and drying.
- Keep linens clean, dry, and wrinkle-free.
- Avoid injury to the legs and feet.
- Make sure shoes fit well.
- Keep pressure off the heels and other bony areas. Use pillows or other devices as the nurse and care plan direct.
- Check the person's legs and feet. Report skin breaks or changes in skin color.
- Do not massage over pressure points (Chapter 36). *Never rub or massage reddened areas.*
- Use protective devices as the nurse directs. Follow the care plan.
- Follow the care plan for walking and exercise.

The heels and inner part of the ankles are common sites for venous ulcers. They can occur from skin injury. Scratching is an example. Or they can occur without trauma.

Venous ulcers are painful and walking is difficult. Fluid may seep from the wound. Infection is a risk. Healing is slow.

Risk Factors Risk factors for venous ulcers include:
- History of blood clots
- History of varicose veins (Fig. 35-9)
- Decreased mobility
- Obesity
- Leg or foot surgery
- Advanced age
- Surgery on the bones and joints
- Phlebitis (inflammation [*itis*] of a vein [*phleb*])

Prevention and Treatment To prevent venous ulcers:
- Follow the care plan to prevent skin breakdown. See the measures in Box 35-3.
- Prevent injury. Do not bump the legs and feet.
- Handle, move, and transfer the person carefully and gently.

Persons at risk need professional foot care. Attention is given to toenails, corns, calluses, and other toe and foot problems. *You do not cut the toenails of persons with diseases affecting the circulation.*

Venous ulcers are hard to heal. The doctor may order drugs for infection and to decrease swelling. Medicated bandages and other wound care products are often ordered. So are devices used for pressure ulcers. The doctor may order elastic stockings or elastic bandages to:
- Promote comfort
- Promote circulation by providing support and pressure to the veins
- Promote healing
- Prevent injury

Fig. 35-8 Venous ulcer.

Fig. 35-9 Varicose veins. Veins under the skin are dilated (wide) and bulging. *(From Belch J and others: Color atlas of peripheral vascular diseases, ed 2, London, 1996, Wolfe Medical Publishers.)*

Elastic Stockings. Elastic stockings exert pressure on the veins. The pressure promotes venous blood return to the heart. The stockings help prevent venous ulcers and blood clots in leg veins.

A blood clot is called a **thrombus**. If blood flow is sluggish, blood clots may form. They can form in the deep leg veins in the lower leg or thigh (Fig. 35-10, *A*). A thrombus can break loose and travel through the bloodstream. It then becomes an embolus. An **embolus** is a blood clot that travels through the vascular system until it lodges in a vessel (Fig. 35-10, *B*). An embolus from a vein lodges in the lungs *(pulmonary embolism)*. A pulmonary embolus can cause severe respiratory problems and death. Report chest pain or shortness of breath at once.

Elastic stockings also are called AE stockings (AE means *anti-embolism* or *anti-embolic*). They also are called TED hose (TED means *thrombo-embolic disease*). Persons at risk for thrombi include those who:
- Have heart and circulatory disorders
- Are on bedrest
- Have had surgery
- Are older
- Are pregnant

The person usually has two pairs of stockings. Wash one pair while the other pair is worn. Wash them by hand with a mild soap. Hang them to dry.

See *Delegation Guidelines: Elastic Stockings.*
See *Promoting Safety and Comfort: Elastic Stockings.*

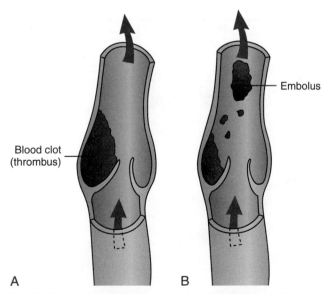

A   B

Fig. 35-10 A, A blood clot is attached to the wall of a vein. The arrow shows the direction of blood flow. **B,** Part of the thrombus breaks off and becomes an embolus. The embolus travels in the bloodstream until it lodges in a distant vessel.

Blood clot (thrombus)

Embolus

DELEGATION GUIDELINES
Elastic Stockings

Before applying elastic stockings, you need this information from the nurse and the care plan:
- What size to use—small, medium, or large
- What length to use—thigh-high or knee-high
- When to remove them and for how long—usually every 8 hours for 30 minutes
- What observations to report and record:
  - The size and length of stockings applied
  - When you applied the stockings
  - Skin color and temperature
  - Leg and foot swelling
  - Skin tears, wounds, or signs of skin breakdown
  - Complaints of pain, tingling, or numbness
  - When you removed the stockings and for how long
  - When you re-applied the stockings
  - When you washed the stockings
- When to report observations
- What specific resident concerns to report at once

PROMOTING SAFETY AND COMFORT
Elastic Stockings

Safety
Apply the stocking so the opening in the toe area is over the top of the toes. Use the opening to check circulation, skin color, and skin temperature in the toes.

Stockings should not have twists, creases, or wrinkles after you apply them. Twists can affect circulation. Creases and wrinkles can cause skin breakdown.

Loose stockings do not promote venous blood return to the heart. Stockings that are too tight can affect circulation. Tell the nurse if the stockings are too loose or too tight.

Comfort
Apply stockings before the person gets out of bed. Otherwise the person's legs can swell from sitting or standing. Stockings are hard to put on when the legs are swollen. The person lies in bed while they are off. This prevents the legs from swelling.

Gently handle and move the person's foot and leg. Do not force the joints (toes, foot, ankle, knee, and hip) beyond their range of motion or to the point of pain.

APPLYING ELASTIC STOCKINGS

QUALITY OF LIFE

Remember to:
- Knock before entering the person's room.
- Address the person by name.
- Introduce yourself by name and title.

- Explain the procedure to the person before beginning and during the procedure.
- Protect the person's rights during the procedure.
- Handle the person gently during the procedure.

PRE-PROCEDURE

1. Follow *Delegation Guidelines: Elastic Stockings*, p. 541. See *Promoting Safety and Comfort: Elastic Stockings*, p. 541.
2. Practice hand hygiene.
3. Obtain elastic stockings in the correct size and length.

4. Identify the person. Check the ID (identification) bracelet against the assignment sheet. Also call the person by name.
5. Provide for privacy.
6. Raise the bed for body mechanics. Bed rails are up if used.

PROCEDURE

7. Lower the bed rail near you if up.
8. Position the person supine.
9. Expose the legs. Fan-fold top linens toward the thighs.
10. Turn the stocking inside out down to the heel.
11. Slip the foot of the stocking over the toes, foot, and heel (Fig. 35-11, *A*). Make sure the stocking heel is properly positioned on the person's heel.

12. Grasp the stocking top. Pull the stocking up the leg. It turns right side out as it is pulled up. The stocking is even and snug (Fig. 35-11, *B*).
13. Remove twists, creases, or wrinkles.
14. Repeat steps 10 through 13 for the other leg.

POST-PROCEDURE

15. Cover the person.
16. Provide for comfort. (See the inside of the front book cover.)
17. Place the signal light within reach.
18. Lower the bed to its lowest position.
19. Raise or lower bed rails. Follow the care plan.

20. Unscreen the person.
21. Complete a safety check of the room. (See the inside of the front book cover.)
22. Decontaminate your hands.
23. Report and record your observations.

Fig. 35-11 Applying elastic stockings. **A,** The stocking is slipped over the toes, foot, and heel. **B,** The stocking turns right side out as it is pulled up over the leg.

Elastic Bandages. Elastic bandages have the same purposes as elastic stockings. They provide support and reduce swelling from injuries. Sometimes they are used to hold dressings in place. They are applied to arms and legs. When applying bandages:

- Use the correct size—length and width—to bandage the extremity.
- Position the person in good alignment.
- Face the person during the procedure.
- Start at the lower (distal) part of the extremity. Work upward to the top (proximal) part.
- Expose fingers or toes if possible. This allows circulation checks.
- Apply the bandage with firm, even pressure.
- Check the color and temperature of the extremity every hour.
- Re-apply a loose or wrinkled bandage.
- Replace a moist or soiled bandage.
  See *Focus on Communication: Elastic Bandages.*
  See *Delegation Guidelines: Elastic Bandages.*
  See *Promoting Safety and Comfort: Elastic Bandages.*

DELEGATION GUIDELINES
Elastic Bandages

Before applying elastic bandages, you need this information from the nurse and the care plan:
- Where to apply the bandage
- What width and length to use
- When to remove the bandage and for how long—usually every 8 hours for 30 minutes
- What to do if the bandage is wet or soiled
- What observations to report and record:
  - The width and length applied
  - When you applied the bandage
  - Skin color and temperature
  - Swelling of the part
  - Skin tears, wounds, or signs of skin breakdown
  - Complaints of pain, itching, tingling, or numbness
  - When you removed the bandage and for how long
  - When you re-applied the bandage
- When to report observations
- What specific resident concerns to report at once

FOCUS ON COMMUNICATION
Elastic Bandages

Elastic bandages should promote comfort. To check for comfort, you can ask:
- "Does the bandage feel too tight?"
- "Do you feel pain, itching, tingling, or numbness?" If yes: "What do you feel?" "Where do you feel it?"

PROMOTING SAFETY AND COMFORT
Elastic Bandages

Safety
Elastic bandages must be firm and snug, but not tight. A tight bandage can affect circulation.

Bandages are secured in place with clips, tape, or Velcro. Clips are made of metal or plastic. Clips can injure the skin if they become loose, fall off, or cause pressure. Use clips only if the nurse tells you to. Check the bandage often to make sure the clips are correctly in place.

Some centers do not allow you to apply elastic bandages. Know your center's policy.

Comfort
A tight bandage can cause pain and discomfort. Apply it with firm, even pressure. If the person complains of pain, tingling, or numbness, remove the bandage. Tell the nurse at once.

APPLYING ELASTIC BANDAGES

QUALITY OF LIFE

Remember to:
- Knock before entering the person's room.
- Address the person by name.
- Introduce yourself by name and title.

- Explain the procedure to the person before beginning and during the procedure.
- Protect the person's rights during the procedure.
- Handle the person gently during the procedure.

PRE-PROCEDURE

1 Follow *Delegation Guidelines: Elastic Bandages*, p. 543. See *Promoting Safety and Comfort: Elastic Bandages*, p. 543.
2 Practice hand hygiene.
3 Collect the following:
- Elastic bandage as directed by the nurse
- Tape or clips (unless the bandage has Velcro)

4 Identify the person. Check the ID bracelet against the assignment sheet. Also call the person by name.
5 Provide for privacy.
6 Raise the bed for body mechanics. Bed rails are up if used.

PROCEDURE

7 Lower the bed rail near you if up.
8 Help the person to a comfortable position. Expose the part you will bandage.
9 Make sure the area is clean and dry.
10 Hold the bandage so the roll is up. The loose end is on the bottom (Fig. 35-12, *A*).
11 Apply the bandage to the smallest part of the wrist, foot, ankle, or knee.
12 Make two circular turns around the part (Fig. 35-12, *B*).
13 Make overlapping spiral turns in an upward direction. Each turn overlaps about ½ to ⅔ of the previous turn (Fig. 35-12, *C*). Each overlap is equal.

14 Apply the bandage smoothly with firm, even pressure. It is not tight.
15 End the bandage with two circular turns.
16 Secure the bandage in place with Velcro, tape, or clips. Clips are not under the body part.
17 Check the fingers or toes for coldness or cyanosis (bluish color). Ask about pain, itching, numbness, or tingling. Remove the bandage if any are noted. Report your observations.

POST-PROCEDURE

18 Provide for comfort. (See the inside of the front book cover.)
19 Place the signal light within reach.
20 Lower the bed to its lowest position.
21 Raise or lower bed rails. Follow the care plan.

22 Unscreen the person.
23 Complete a safety check of the room. (See the inside of the front book cover.)
24 Decontaminate your hands.
25 Report and record your observations.

Fig. 35-12 Applying an elastic bandage. **A,** The roll of the bandage is up. The loose end is at the bottom. **B,** The bandage is applied to the smallest part with two circular turns. **C,** The bandage is applied with spiral turns in an upward direction.

Arterial Ulcers

Arterial ulcers are open wounds on the lower legs or feet caused by poor arterial blood flow. They are found between the toes, on top of the toes, and on the outer side of the ankle (Fig. 35-13). The leg and foot may feel cold and look blue or shiny. The ulcer is very painful.

These ulcers are caused by diseases or injuries that decrease arterial blood flow to the legs and feet. High blood pressure and diabetes are common causes. So are narrowed arteries from aging. Smoking is a risk factor.

The doctor treats the disease causing the ulcer. Drugs, wound care, and a walking and exercise program are ordered. Professional foot care is important. Follow the care plan (see Box 35-3) and prevent further injury.

Fig. 35-13 Arterial ulcer. *(From Black JM, Hawks JH: Medical-surgical nursing: clinical management for positive outcomes, ed 7, St Louis, 2005, WB Saunders.)*

Diabetic Foot Ulcers

A diabetic foot ulcer is an open wound on the foot caused by complications from diabetes. Diabetes (Chapter 41) can affect the nerves and blood vessels.
* *Nerves.* The person can lose sensation in a foot or leg. Loss of sensation can be complete or partial. The person may not feel pain, heat, or cold. Therefore the person may not feel a cut, blister, burn, or other trauma to the foot. Infection and a large sore can develop.
* *Blood vessels.* Blood flow decreases. Tissues and cells do not get needed oxygen and nutrients. Sores heal poorly. Tissue death (gangrene) can occur.

Some persons have both nerve and blood vessel damage. Both problems can lead to diabetic foot ulcers. Infection and gangrene are risks. Sometimes the affected part is amputated to prevent the spread of gangrene.

Check the person's feet every day. Look for the foot problems described in Box 35-4. Report any sign of a foot problem to the nurse at once. Follow the care plan to prevent and treat diabetic foot ulcers.

Box 35-4 Foot Problems Common in Persons With Diabetes

* *Corns and calluses* (Fig. 35-14, *A*, p. 546). These are thick layers of the skin caused by too much rubbing or pressure on the same spot. They occur over bony areas or the soles of the feet. Infection is a risk.
* *Blisters* (Fig. 35-14, *B*, p. 546). These form when shoes rub on the same spot. Shoes that do not fit well and wearing shoes without socks are causes. Infection is a risk.
* *In-grown toenails* (Fig. 35-14, *C*, p. 546). An edge of a toenail grows into the skin. This occurs when the skin is cut while trimming toenails or from tight shoes. The skin becomes red and infected.
* *Bunions* (Fig. 35-14, *D*, p. 546). The big toe slants toward the small toes. The space between the bones near the base of the big toe grows larger. Bunions can occur on one or both feet. Heredity is a factor. Shoes that fit poorly and pointy shoes are causes. Bunions are removed by surgery.
* *Plantar warts* (Fig. 35-14, *E*, p. 546). *Plantar* means sole. Plantar warts occur on the soles (bottoms) of the feet. Caused by a virus, plantar warts are painful.

* *Hammer toes* (Fig. 35-14, *F*, p. 546). One or more toes are permanently flexed. They form when a foot muscle weakens. Diabetic nerve damage can weaken foot muscles. The second toe is commonly affected. Because of deformed toes, the person has problems walking. Shoes do not fit well. Sores can develop on the tops of the toes and on the bottoms of the feet.
* *Dry and cracked skin* (Fig. 35-14, *G*, p. 546). Dry skin can occur from nerve damage in the legs and feet. These areas do not receive messages from the brain to keep the skin soft and moist. The dry skin can crack, causing portals of entry for microbes. Infection can occur.
* *Athlete's foot* (Fig. 35-14, *H*, p. 546). This is a fungus causing redness and cracked skin between the toes and on the bottoms of the feet. The cracks are portals of entry for microbes. The fungus can spread to the toenails. The toenails become thick, yellow, and hard to cut.

Fig. 35-14 Diabetic foot problems. **A,** Corns. **B,** A blister. **C,** An in-grown toenail. **D,** A bunion. **E,** Plantar warts. **F,** Hammer toe. **G,** Dry and cracked skin. **H,** Athlete's foot. *(Redrawn from* Prevent diabetes problems: keep your feet and skin healthy, *National Diabetes Information Clearinghouse [NDIC], NIH Publication No. 08-4282, May 2008, Bethesda, Md.)*

WOUND HEALING

The healing process has three phases:

- *Inflammatory phase* (3 days). Bleeding stops. A scab forms over the wound. The scab protects against microbes entering the wound. Blood supply to the wound increases. The blood brings nutrients and healing substances. Because blood supply increases, signs and symptoms of inflammation appear— redness, swelling, heat or warmth, and pain. Loss of function may occur.
- *Proliferative phase* (day 3 to day 21). Proliferate means to multiply rapidly. Tissue cells multiply to repair the wound.
- *Maturation phase* (day 21 to 2 years). The scar gains strength. The red, raised scar becomes thin and pale.

Types of Wound Healing

Healing occurs in three ways:

- *First intention (primary intention, primary closure).* Wound edges are brought together to close the wound. Sutures (stitches), staples, clips, special glue, or adhesive strips hold the wound edges together. See Figure 35-15, *A.*
- *Second intention (secondary intention).* This is for contaminated and infected wounds. Wounds are cleaned and dead tissue removed. Wound edges are not brought together. The wound gaps. Healing takes longer and leaves a larger scar. Infection is a great risk. See Figure 35-15, *B.*
- *Third intention (delayed intention, tertiary intention).* The wound is left open and closed later. It combines first and second intention. Infection and poor circulation are common reasons for third intention. See Figure 35-15, *C.*

► Healing by First Intention

A

Clean incision

Early suture

"Hairline" scar

► Healing by Second Intention (Granulation and Contraction)

B

Gaping, irregular wound

Healing

Growth of epithelium over scar

► Healing by Third Intention (Delayed Closure)

C

Infected wound

Healing

Closure with wide scar

Fig. 35-15 Wound healing. **A,** First intention. **B,** Second intention. **C,** Third intention. *(Modified from Ignatavicius DD, Workman ML: Medical-surgical nursing: critical thinking for collaborative care, ed 5, St Louis, 2006, Saunders.)*

Complications of Wound Healing

Many factors affect healing and increase the risk of complications. They include wound type and the person's age, general health, nutrition, and life-style.

Good circulation is needed. Age, smoking, circulatory disease, and diabetes all affect circulation. Certain drugs (Coumadin and heparin) prolong bleeding.

Good nutrition is needed. Protein is needed for tissue growth and repair.

Infection is a risk for persons with immune system changes and for those taking antibiotics. Antibiotics kill pathogens. Specific antibiotics kill specific pathogens. In doing so, other pathogens may be allowed to grow and multiply.

See *Focus on Rehabilitation: Complications of Wound Healing.*

FOCUS ON REHABILITATION
Complications of Wound Healing

Some persons need rehabilitation or subacute care because of:
- *Infection.* Contamination can occur during or after the injury. Trauma is a common cause. Surgical wounds can be contaminated during or after surgery. An infected wound appears inflamed (reddened) and has drainage. The wound is painful and tender. The person has a fever.
- *Dehiscence.* **Dehiscence** is the separation of wound layers (Fig. 35-16). It may involve the skin layer or underlying tissues. Abdominal wounds are commonly affected. Coughing, vomiting, and abdominal distention place stress on the wound. The person often describes the sensation of the wound "popping open."
- *Evisceration.* **Evisceration** is the separation of the wound along with the protrusion of abdominal organs (Fig. 35-17). Causes are the same as for dehiscence.

Dehiscence and evisceration are surgical emergencies. Tell the nurse at once. The nurse covers the wound with large sterile dressings saturated with saline. Help prepare the person for surgery as directed.

Wound Appearance

Doctors and nurses observe the wound and its drainage. They observe for healing and complications. See Box 35-5 for the observations to make when assisting with wound care. Report and record your observations according to center policy.

Wound Drainage

During injury and the inflammatory phase of wound healing, fluid and cells escape from the tissues. Drainage amounts may be large or small. This depends on wound size and site. Bleeding and infection also affect the amount and kind of drainage. Wound drainage is observed and measured.
- **Serous drainage**—clear, watery fluid (Fig. 35-19, *A*). Serous comes from the word *serum.* The fluid in a blister is serous. Serum is the clear, thin, fluid portion of blood. Serum does not contain blood cells or platelets.
- **Sanguineous drainage**—bloody drainage (Fig. 35-19, *B*). The Latin word *sanguis* means blood. The amount and color of sanguineous drainage is important. Hemorrhage is suspected when large amounts are present. Bright drainage means fresh bleeding. Older bleeding is darker.
- **Serosanguineous drainage**—thin, watery drainage *(sero)* that is blood-tinged *(sanguineous)* (Fig. 35-19, *C*).
- **Purulent drainage**—thick green, yellow, or brown drainage (Fig. 35-19, *D*).

Drainage must leave the wound for healing. Trapped drainage causes swelling of underlying tissues. The wound may heal at the skin level, but underlying tissues do not close. Infection and complications can occur.

When large amounts of drainage are expected, the doctor inserts a drain. A *Penrose drain* is a rubber tube that drains onto a dressing (Fig. 35-20, p. 550). It opens onto the dressing. Therefore it is an open drain. Microbes can enter the drain and wound.

Closed drainage systems prevent microbes from entering the wound. A drain is attached to suction. The *Hemovac* (Fig. 35-21, p. 550) and *Jackson-Pratt* systems are examples (Fig. 35-22, p. 550). Other systems are used depending on wound type, size, and site.

Drainage is measured in three ways:
- Weighing dressings before applying them to the wound. The weight of each new dressing is noted. Dressings are weighed after removal. The dry dressing weight is subtracted from the wet dressing weight. (Wet dressings weigh more.)
- Noting the number and size of dressings with drainage. What is the amount and kind of drainage? Are dressings saturated? Is drainage on just part of the dressing? If so, which part? Is drainage through some or all layers?
- Measuring the amount of drainage in the collection container. This is done for closed drainage.

Fig. 35-16 Wound dehiscence. *(Courtesy KCI Licensing, Inc., San Antonio, Tex.)*

Fig. 35-17 Wound evisceration. *(From Ignatavicius DD, Workman ML: Medical-surgical nursing: critical thinking for collaborative care, ed 5, St Louis, 2006, Saunders.)*

Fig. 35-18 The size and depth of the wound are measured. *(From Potter PA, Perry AG: Fundamentals of nursing, ed 7, St Louis, 2009, Mosby.)*

Fig. 35-19 Wound drainage. **A,** Serous drainage. **B,** Sanguineous drainage. **C,** Serosanguineous drainage. **D,** Purulent drainage. *(From Potter PA, Perry AG: Fundamentals of nursing, ed 7, St Louis, 2009, Mosby.)*

Box 35-5   Wound Observations

- Wound site
  - The person may have multiple wounds from surgery or trauma.
- Wound size and depth (measure in centimeters)
  - Size: Measure from top to bottom and side to side (Fig. 35-18).
  - Depth. To measure depth, the nurse:
    - Inserts a swab inside the deepest part of the wound
    - Removes the swab
    - Measures the distance on the swab
  - Use a disposable ruler.
- Wound appearance
  - Is the wound red and swollen?
  - Is the area around the wound warm to touch?
  - Are sutures, staples, or clips intact or broken?
  - Are wound edges closed or separated?
  - Did the wound break open?
- Drainage
  - Is the drainage serous, sanguineous, serosanguineous, or purulent?
  - What is the amount of drainage?
- Odor
  - Does the wound or drainage have an odor?
- Surrounding skin
  - Is surrounding skin intact?
  - What is the color of surrounding skin?
  - Are surrounding tissues swollen?

Fig. 35-20 Penrose drain. *(From Potter PA, Perry AG: Fundamentals of nursing, ed 7, St Louis, 2009, Mosby.)*

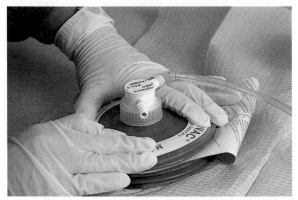

Fig. 35-21 Hemovac. Drains are sutured to the wound and connected to a reservoir. *(From Potter PA, Perry AG: Fundamentals of nursing, ed 7, St Louis, 2009, Mosby.)*

Fig. 35-22 Jackson-Pratt drainage system. *(From Potter PA, Perry AG: Fundamentals of nursing, ed 7, St Louis, 2009, Mosby.)*

DRESSINGS

Wound dressings have many functions. They:
- Protect wounds from injury and microbes.
- Absorb drainage.
- Remove dead tissue.
- Promote comfort.
- Cover unsightly wounds.
- Provide a moist environment for wound healing.
- Apply pressure (pressure dressings) to help control bleeding.

Dressing type and size depend on many factors. These include the type of wound, its size and site, and amount of drainage. Infection is a factor. The dressing's function and the frequency of dressing changes are other factors. The doctor and nurse choose the dressing for each wound.

Types of Dressings

Dressings are described by the material used and how applied. There are many dressing products (Fig. 35-23). The following are common:
- *Gauze.* It comes in squares, rectangles, pads, and rolls. Gauze dressings absorb drainage and moisture.
- *Non-adherent gauze.* It is a gauze dressing with a nonstick surface. It does not stick to the wound. It removes easily without injuring tissue.
- *Transparent adhesive film.* Air can reach the wound but fluids and microbes cannot. The wound is kept moist. Drainage is not absorbed. The transparent film allows wound observation.

Fig. 35-23 Types of dressings. *(From deWit SC: Fundamental concepts and skills for nursing, ed 3, St Louis, 2009, Saunders.)*

Some dressings contain special agents to promote wound healing. If you assist with a dressing change, the nurse explains its use to you.

Dressings are wet or dry:

- *Dry dressing.* A dry gauze dressing is placed over the wound. More dressings are placed on top of the first dressing as needed. The dressings absorb drainage. The drainage is removed with the dressing. A dry dressing can stick to the wound. The dressing is removed carefully to prevent tissue injury and discomfort.
- *Wet-to-dry dressing.* This is used to remove dead tissue from the wound. Gauze dressings are saturated with a solution. These "wet" dressings are applied to the wound. The solution softens dead tissue. The dressing absorbs the dead tissue, which is removed when the dressings are dry.
- *Wet-to-wet dressing.* Gauze dressings saturated with solution are placed in the wound. The dressing is kept moist. It is not allowed to dry.

Securing Dressings

Dressings must be secured over wounds. Microbes can enter the wound, and drainage can escape if the dressing is dislodged. Tape and Montgomery ties are used to secure dressings. Binders hold dressings in place.

Tape Adhesive, paper, plastic, cloth, and elastic tapes are common. Adhesive tape sticks well to the skin. However, adhesive remaining on the skin is hard to remove. It can irritate the skin. An abrasion occurs if skin is removed with tape. Many people are allergic to adhesive tape. Paper, plastic, and cloth tapes usually do not cause allergic reactions. Elastic tape allows movement of the body part.

Tape comes in different sizes—½, ¾, 1, 2, and 3 inch widths. Tape is applied to the top, middle, and bottom parts of the dressing. The tape extends several inches beyond each side of the dressing (Fig. 35-24). *Do not apply tape to circle the entire body part. If swelling occurs, circulation to the part is impaired.*

See *Focus on Communication: Tape.*

Fig. 35-24 Tape is applied at the top, middle, and bottom of the dressing. The tape extends several inches beyond both sides of the dressing.

Fig. 35-25 Montgomery ties.

Montgomery Ties Montgomery ties (Fig. 35-25) are used for large dressings and frequent dressing changes. A Montgomery tie has an adhesive strip and a cloth tie. When the dressing is in place, the adhesive strips are placed on both sides of the dressing. Then the cloth ties are secured over the dressing. A wound may need 2 or 3 Montgomery ties on each side. The ties are undone for the dressing change. The adhesive strips stay in place. They are not removed unless soiled. Montgomery ties protect the skin from frequent tape application and removal.

Applying Dressings

The nurse may ask you to assist with dressing changes. Some centers let you apply simple, dry, non-sterile dressings to simple wounds. Follow the rules in Box 35-6, p. 552.

See *Focus on Communication: Applying Dressings,* p. 552.

See *Teamwork and Time Management: Applying Dressings,* p. 552.

See *Delegation Guidelines: Applying Dressings,* p. 552.

See *Promoting Safety and Comfort: Applying Dressings,* p. 552.

Text continued on p. 554

Box 35-6 Rules for Applying Dressings

- Let pain drugs take effect, usually 30 minutes. The dressing change may cause discomfort. The nurse gives the drug and tells you how long to wait.
- Meet the person's fluid and elimination needs before you begin.
- Collect equipment and supplies before you begin.
- Do not bend or reach over your work area.
- Control your non-verbal communication. Wound odors, appearance, and drainage may be unpleasant. Do not communicate your thoughts or reactions to the person.
- Remove soiled dressings so the person cannot see the soiled side. The drainage and its odor may upset the person.

- Do not force the person to look at the wound. A wound can affect body image and self-esteem. The nurse helps the person deal with the wound.
- Remove tape by pulling it toward the wound.
- Remove dressings gently. They may stick to the wound, drain, or surrounding skin. If the dry dressing sticks, the nurse may have you wet the dressing with a saline solution. A wet dressing is easier to remove.
- Touch only the outer edges of old and new dressings (Chapter 15).
- Report and record your observations. See *Delegation Guidelines: Applying Dressings.*

FOCUS ON COMMUNICATION
Applying Dressings

The person may not report discomfort from a dressing. You should ask:
- "Is the dressing comfortable?"
- "Does the tape cause pain or itching?"

TEAMWORK AND TIME MANAGEMENT
Applying Dressings

Collect all needed items before starting the procedure. Have extra dressings, tape, and other supplies on-hand. Leave unused items in the room for the next dressing change. Wound contamination can occur if you need to leave the room during the procedure.

PROMOTING SAFETY AND COMFORT
Applying Dressings

Safety
Contact with blood, body fluids, secretions, or excretions is likely. Follow Standard Precautions and the Bloodborne Pathogen Standard. Wear personal protective equipment (PPE) as needed.

Do not apply tape to irritated, injured, or non-intact skin. Tape can further damage the skin.

Older persons have thin, fragile skin. Prevent skin tears. Use extreme care when removing tape.

Comfort
Wounds and dressing changes can cause discomfort or pain. If so, the nurse gives a pain-relief drug before the dressing change. Allow time for the drug to take effect. Be gentle when applying and removing tape and dressings.

DELEGATION GUIDELINES
Applying Dressings

When applying a dressing is delegated to you, make sure that:
- Your state allows you to perform the procedure.
- The procedure is in your job description.
- You have the necessary training.
- You know how to use the equipment.
- You review the procedure with the nurse.
- A nurse is available to answer questions and to supervise you.

If the above conditions are met, you need this information from the nurse:
- When to change the dressing
- When the person received a pain-relief drug; when it will take effect
- What to do if the dressing sticks to the wound
- How to clean the wound
- What dressings to use
- How to secure the dressing—tape or Montgomery ties
- What kind of tape to use—adhesive, paper, plastic, cloth, or elastic
- What size tape to use—½, ¾, 1, 2, or 3 inch width

- What observations to report and record:
  - What you used to dress the wound and secure the dressing
  - A red or swollen wound
  - An area around the wound that is warm to touch
  - If wound edges are closed or separated
  - A wound that has broken open
  - Drainage appearance—clear, bloody, or watery and blood-tinged; thick and green, yellow, or brown
  - The amount of drainage
  - Wound or drainage odor
  - Intactness and color of surrounding tissues
  - Swelling of surrounding tissues
  - Possible dressing contamination—urine, feces; other body fluids, secretions, or excretions; dislodged dressing
  - Pain
  - Fever
- When to report observations
- What specific resident concerns to report at once

APPLYING A DRY, NON-STERILE DRESSING   VIDEO

QUALITY OF LIFE

Remember to:
- Knock before entering the person's room.
- Address the person by name.
- Introduce yourself by name and title.

- Explain the procedure to the person before beginning and during the procedure.
- Protect the person's rights during the procedure.
- Handle the person gently during the procedure.

PRE-PROCEDURE

1 Follow *Delegation Guidelines: Applying Dressings.* See *Promoting Safety and Comfort: Applying Dressings.*
2 Practice hand hygiene.
3 Collect the following:
  - Gloves
  - PPE as needed
  - Tape or Montgomery ties
  - Dressings as directed by the nurse
  - Saline solution as directed by the nurse
  - Cleansing solution as directed by the nurse
  - Adhesive remover

  - Dressing set with scissors and forceps
  - Plastic bag
  - Bath blanket
4 Decontaminate your hands.
5 Identify the person. Check the ID bracelet against the assignment sheet. Also call the person by name.
6 Provide for privacy.
7 Arrange your work area. You should not have to reach over or turn your back on your work area.
8 Raise the bed for body mechanics. Bed rails are up if used.

PROCEDURE

9 Lower the bed rail near you if up.
10 Help the person to a comfortable position.
11 Cover the person with a bath blanket. Fan-fold top linens to the foot of the bed.
12 Expose the affected body part.
13 Make a cuff on the plastic bag. Place it within reach.
14 Decontaminate your hands.
15 Put on needed PPE. Put on gloves.
16 Remove tape or undo Montgomery ties.
  a *Tape:* hold the skin down. Gently pull the tape toward the wound.
  b *Montgomery ties:* fold ties away from the wound.
17 Remove any adhesive from the skin. Wet a 4×4 gauze dressing with adhesive remover. Clean away from the wound.
18 Remove gauze dressings. Start with the top dressing, and remove each layer. Keep the soiled side away from the person's sight. Put dressings in the plastic bag. They must not touch the outside of the bag.

19 Remove the dressing over the wound very gently. It may stick to the wound or drain site. Moisten the dressing with saline if it sticks to the wound.
20 Observe the wound, drain site, and wound drainage.
21 Remove the gloves, and discard into the plastic bag. Decontaminate your hands.
22 Open the new dressings.
23 Cut the length of tape needed.
24 Put on clean gloves.
25 Clean the wound with saline as directed by the nurse. See Figure 35-26, p. 554.
26 Apply dressings as directed by the nurse.
27 Secure the dressings in place. Use tape or Montgomery ties.
28 Remove the gloves. Put them in the bag.
29 Remove and discard PPE.
30 Decontaminate your hands.
31 Cover the person. Remove the bath blanket.

POST-PROCEDURE

32 Provide for comfort. (See the inside of the front book cover.)
33 Place the signal light within reach.
34 Lower the bed to its lowest position.
35 Raise or lower bed rails. Follow the care plan.
36 Return equipment and supplies to the proper place. Leave extra dressings and tape in the room.
37 Discard used supplies into the bag. Tie the bag closed. Discard the bag following center policy. (Wear gloves for this step.)

38 Clean your work area. Follow the Bloodborne Pathogen Standard.
39 Unscreen the person.
40 Complete a safety check of the room. (See the inside of the front book cover.)
41 Decontaminate your hands.
42 Report and record your observations.

Fig. 35-26 Cleaning a wound. **A,** Clean starting at the wound and stroking out to the surrounding skin. Use new gauze for each stroke. **B,** Clean the wound from the top to the bottom. Start at the wound. Then clean the surrounding areas. Use new gauze for each stroke. *(Redrawn from Potter PA, Perry AG:* Fundamentals of nursing, *ed 7, St Louis, 2009, Mosby.)*

Box 35-7   Rules for Applying Binders

- Follow the manufacturer's instructions.
- Apply the binder so there is firm, even pressure over the area.
- Apply the binder so it is snug. It must not interfere with breathing or circulation.
- Position the person in good alignment.
- Re-apply the binder if it is loose or wrinkled.
- Re-apply the binder if it is out of position or causes discomfort.
- Secure safety pins so they point away from the wound (if used).
- Change binders that are moist or soiled. This prevents the growth of microbes.
- Tell the nurse at once if there is a change in the person's breathing.
- Check the person's skin under and around the binder. Tell the nurse at once if there is redness, irritation, or other signs of a skin problem.

Fig. 35-27 Abdominal binder.

BINDERS

Binders are wide bands of elastic fabric. They are applied to the abdomen, chest, or perineal areas. Binders promote healing because they support wounds and hold dressings in place. They also prevent or reduce swelling, promote comfort, and prevent injury.

Box 35-7 lists the rules for applying these binders:

- *Abdominal binder*—provides abdominal support and holds dressings in place (Fig. 35-27). The top part is at the person's waist. The lower part is over the hips. Binders are secured in place with Velcro or with hook and loop closures.
- *Breast binder*—supports the breasts after surgery (Fig. 35-28). They are secured in place with Velcro or padded zippers.

See *Focus on Communication: Binders.*
See *Promoting Safety and Comfort: Binders.*

Fig. 35-28 Breast binder.

The person may not tell you about pain or discomfort. Therefore, you need to ask these questions:
- "Is the binder too tight or too loose?"
- "Does the binder cause pain?"
- "Do you feel pressure from the binder?" If yes: "Where? Please show me."

Safety
Apply binders properly. Otherwise, severe discomfort, skin irritation, and circulatory and respiratory problems can occur. Correct application is needed for safety and for the binder to work effectively.

Comfort
A binder should promote comfort. Re-apply the binder if it causes pain or discomfort.

HEAT AND COLD APPLICATIONS

Heat and cold applications promote healing and comfort. They also reduce tissue swelling. Heat and cold have opposite effects on body function. Severe injuries and changes in body function can occur. The risks are great.

Heat Applications

Heat applications are often used for musculo-skeletal injuries or problems (arthritis). Heat:
- Relieves pain
- Relaxes muscles
- Decreases joint stiffness
- Promotes healing
- Reduces tissue swelling

When heat is applied to the skin, blood vessels in the area dilate. **Dilate** means to expand or open wider (Fig. 35-29, p. 556). Blood flow increases. Tissues have more oxygen and nutrients for healing. Excess fluid is removed from the area faster. The skin is red and warm.

Complications High temperatures can cause burns. Report pain, excessive redness, and blisters at once.

Also observe for pale skin. When heat is applied too long, blood vessels **constrict** (narrow) (see Fig. 35-29, p. 556). Blood flow decreases. Tissues receive less blood. Tissue damage occurs, and the skin is pale.

Confused persons and those with dementia may not recognize pain. Look for changes in the person's behavior. Behavior changes can signal pain.

Older and fair-skinned persons have fragile skin that is easily burned. Persons with problems sensing heat and pain are also at risk. Nervous system damage, loss of consciousness, and circulatory disorders affect sensation. So do confusion and some drugs.

Metal implants pose risks. Metal conducts heat. Deep tissues can be burned. Pacemakers (cardiac devices) and joint replacements are made of metal. Do not apply heat to an implant area.

See *Residents With Dementia: Complications.*

Moist and Dry Heat Applications With a *moist heat application,* water is in contact with the skin. Water conducts heat. Moist heat has greater and faster effects than dry heat. Heat penetrates deeper with a moist application. To prevent injury, moist heat applications have lower (cooler) temperatures than dry heat applications. Moist heat applications include:
- *Hot compresses* (Fig. 35-30, *A*, p. 556)—a **compress** is a soft pad applied over a body area. It is usually made of cloth. Sometimes an aquathermia pad (p. 556) is applied over the compress. It maintains the temperature of the compress.
- *Hot soaks* (Fig. 35-30, *B*, p. 556)—a body part is put into water. This is usually used for small parts—a hand, lower arm, foot, or lower leg. A tub is used for larger areas.
- *Sitz baths* (Fig. 35-30, *C*, p. 556)—the perineal and rectal areas are immersed in warm or hot water. (*Sitz* means *seat* in German.) Sitz baths are common for hemorrhoids and after rectal or pelvic surgeries. They are used to:
  - Clean perineal and anal wounds
  - Promote healing
  - Relieve pain and soreness
  - Increase circulation
  - Stimulate voiding
- *Hot packs* (Fig. 35-30, *D*, p. 556)—a **pack** involves wrapping a body part with a wet or dry application. There are single-use and re-usable packs. Some can be used for heat or cold. Follow the manufacturer's instructions to activate the heat or cold. Clean re-usable packs after use. To clean them, follow center policy and the manufacturer's instructions.

Fig. 35-29 A, Blood vessel under normal conditions. **B,** Dilated blood vessel. **C,** Constricted blood vessel.

Fig. 35-30 Wet heat applications. **A,** Compress. **B,** Hot soak. **C,** Disposable sitz bath. **D,** Hot pack.

With *dry heat applications,* water is not in contact with the skin. A dry heat application stays at the desired temperature longer. Dry heat does not penetrate as deeply as moist heat. Because water is not used, dry heat needs higher (hotter) temperatures to achieve the desired effect. Therefore burns are still a risk.

Some *hot packs* and the *aquathermia pad* are dry heat applications. The aquathermia pad is an electrical device (Fig. 35-31). Tubes inside the pad are filled with distilled water. Heated water flows to the pad through a hose. Another hose returns water to the heating unit. The water is reheated and returned back into the pad.

Fig. 35-31 The aquathermia pad.

Cold Applications

Cold applications reduce pain, prevent swelling, and decrease circulation and bleeding. Cold cools the body when fever is present.

Cold has the opposite effect of heat. When cold is applied to the skin, blood vessels constrict (see Fig. 35-29). Blood flow decreases. Tissues receive less oxygen and nutrients.

Cold applications are useful right after an injury. Decreased blood flow reduces the amount of bleeding. Less fluid collects in the tissues. Cold has a numbing effect on the skin. This helps reduce or relieve pain in the part.

Complications Complications include pain, burns, blisters, and poor circulation. Burns and blisters occur from intense cold. They also occur when dry cold is in direct contact with the skin.

When cold is applied for a long time, blood vessels dilate. Blood flow increases. The prolonged application of cold has the same effect as heat applications.

Older and fair-skinned persons have fragile skin. They are at great risk for complications. So are persons with sensory impairments.

See *Residents With Dementia: Complications,* p. 555.

Moist and Dry Cold Applications Moist cold applications penetrate deeper than dry ones. Therefore moist applications are not as cold as dry applications.

The cold compress is a moist cold application (see Fig. 35-30, *A*). Dry cold applications include ice bags, ice collars, and ice gloves. Cold packs can be moist or dry applications.

Applying Heat and Cold

Protect the person from injury during heat and cold applications. Follow the rules listed in Box 35-8. Temperature ranges for heat and cold are listed in Table 35-1.

See *Focus on Communication: Applying Heat and Cold,* p. 558.

See *Teamwork and Time Management: Applying Heat and Cold,* p. 558.

See *Delegation Guidelines: Applying Heat and Cold,* p. 558.

See *Promoting Safety and Comfort: Applying Heat and Cold,* p. 558.

Box 35-8 Rules for Applying Heat and Cold

- Know how to use the equipment. Follow the manufacturer's instructions for commercial devices.
- Measure the temperature of moist applications. Use a bath thermometer. Or follow center policy for measuring temperature.
- Follow center policies for safe temperature ranges. See Table 35-1.
- Do not apply *very hot* (above 106° F [Fahrenheit] or 46.1° C [centigrade]) applications. Tissue damage can occur. A nurse applies *very hot* applications.
- Ask the nurse what the temperature should be.
  - Heat—cooler temperatures are needed for persons at risk.
  - Cold—warmer temperatures are needed for persons at risk.
- Know the exact site of the application. Ask the nurse to show you the site.
- Cover dry heat or cold applications before applying them. Use a flannel cover, towel, or other cover as directed by the nurse.
- Provide for privacy. Properly screen and drape the person. Expose only the body part involved. Avoid unnecessary exposure.
- Maintain comfort and body alignment during the procedure.
- Observe the skin every 5 minutes for signs of complications. See *Delegation Guidelines: Applying Heat and Cold,* p. 558.
- Do not let the person change the temperature of the application.
- Know how long to leave the application in place. See *Delegation Guidelines: Applying Heat and Cold,* p. 558. Carefully watch the time. Heat and cold are applied no longer than 15 to 20 minutes.
- Follow the rules of electrical safety when using electrical appliances to apply heat.
- Place the signal light within the person's reach.
- Complete a safety check before leaving the room. (See the inside of the front book cover.)

Table 35-1 Heat and Cold Temperature Ranges

Temperature	Fahrenheit Range	Centigrade Range
Hot	98° to 106° F	36.6° to 41.1° C
Warm	93° to 98° F	33.8° to 36.6° C
Tepid	80° to 93° F	26.6° to 33.8° C
Cool	65° to 80° F	18.3° to 26.6° C
Cold	50° to 65° F	10.0° to 18.3° C

Modified from Perry AG, Potter PA: Clinical nursing skills and techniques, ed 7, St Louis, 2010, Mosby.

FOCUS ON COMMUNICATION
Applying Heat and Cold

The person may not tell you about pain or discomfort. The person may not know what symptoms to report. For heat and cold applications, you need to ask:

- "Does the application feel too hot or too cold?"
- "Do you feel any pain, numbness, or burning?"
- "Are you warm enough?"
- "Do you feel weak, faint, or drowsy?" If yes: "Tell me how you feel."

TEAMWORK AND TIME MANAGEMENT
Applying Heat and Cold

After applying heat or cold, check the person and the application every 5 minutes. Plan your work so that you can stay in or near the person's room. For example, during the application:

- Make the bed and straighten the person's unit.
- Provide care to the roommate if you are assigned to him or her.
- Help the person complete his or her daily or weekly menu.
- Read cards and letters to the person, with his or her consent.
- Address envelopes and other correspondence for the person.
- Take time to visit with the person.

DELEGATION GUIDELINES
Applying Heat and Cold

Before applying heat or cold, you need this information from the nurse and the care plan:

- The type of application—hot compress or pack, commercial compress, hot soak, sitz bath, aquathermia pad; ice bag, ice collar, ice glove, cold pack, or cold compress
- How to cover the application
- What temperature to use (see Table 35-1)
- The application site
- How long to leave the application in place
- What observations to report and record:
  - Complaints of pain or discomfort, numbness, or burning
  - Excessive redness
  - Blisters
  - Pale, white, or gray skin
  - *Cyanosis* (bluish color)
  - Shivering
  - Rapid pulse, weakness, faintness, and drowsiness (sitz bath)
  - Time, site, and length of application
- When to report observations
- What specific resident concerns to report at once

PROMOTING SAFETY AND COMFORT
Applying Heat and Cold

Safety

Check the person every 5 minutes. Also follow these safety measures:

- *Sitz bath.* Blood flow increases to the perineum and rectum. Therefore less blood flows to other body parts. The person may become weak or feel faint. Drowsiness can occur from the bath's relaxing effect. Observe for signs of weakness, fainting, or fatigue. Also protect the person from injury. Keep the signal light within reach, and prevent chills and burns.
- *Commercial hot and cold packs.* Read warning labels and follow the manufacturer's instructions.
- *Aquathermia pad:*
  - Follow electrical safety precautions (Chapter 12).
  - Check the device for damage or flaws.
  - Follow the manufacturer's instructions.
  - Place the heating unit on an even, uncluttered surface. This prevents it from being knocked over or knocked off of the surface.
  - Make sure the hoses do not have kinks or bubbles.
  - Use a flannel cover to insulate the pad. It absorbs perspiration at the application site. (Some centers use towels or pillowcases.)
  - Secure the pad in place with ties, tape, or rolled gauze. Do not use pins. They can puncture the pad and cause leaks.
  - Do not place the pad under the person or under a body part. This prevents the escape of heat. Burns can result if heat cannot escape.
  - Give the key used to set the temperature to the nurse. This prevents anyone from changing the temperature.

Some persons have medicated patches or ointments applied to the skin. Do not apply heat over such areas.

Comfort

Cold applications can cause chills and shivering. Provide for warmth. Use bath blankets or other blankets as needed.

APPLYING HEAT AND COLD APPLICATIONS `VIDEO`

QUALITY OF LIFE

Remember to:
- Knock before entering the person's room.
- Address the person by name.
- Introduce yourself by name and title.

- Explain the procedure to the person before beginning and during the procedure.
- Protect the person's rights during the procedure.
- Handle the person gently during the procedure.

PRE-PROCEDURE

1 Follow *Delegation Guidelines: Applying Heat and Cold.* See *Promoting Safety and Comfort: Applying Heat and Cold.*
2 Practice hand hygiene.
3 Collect needed equipment.
   a For a *hot compress:*
   - Basin
   - Bath thermometer
   - Small towel, washcloth, or gauze squares
   - Plastic wrap or aquathermia pad
   - Ties, tape, or rolled gauze
   - Bath towel
   - Waterproof pad
   b For a *hot soak:*
   - Water basin or arm or foot bath
   - Bath thermometer
   - Waterproof pad
   - Bath blanket
   - Towel
   c For a *sitz bath:*
   - Disposable sitz bath
   - Bath thermometer
   - Two bath blankets, bath towels, and a clean gown

   d For a *hot or cold pack:*
   - Commercial pack
   - Pack cover
   - Ties, tape, or rolled gauze (if needed)
   - Waterproof pad
   e For an *aquathermia pad:*
   - Aquathermia pad and heating unit
   - Distilled water
   - Flannel cover or other cover as directed by the nurse
   - Ties, tape, or rolled gauze
   f For an *ice bag, ice collar, ice glove, or dry cold pack:*
   - Ice bag, collar, or glove or cold pack
   - Crushed ice (except for a cold pack)
   - Flannel cover or other cover as directed by the nurse
   - Paper towels
   g For a *cold compress:*
   - Large basin with ice
   - Small basin with cold water
   - Gauze squares, washcloths, or small towels
   - Waterproof pad
4 Identify the person. Check the ID bracelet against the assignment sheet. Also call the person by name.
5 Provide for privacy.

PROCEDURE

6 Position the person for the procedure.
7 Place the waterproof pad (if needed) under the body part.
8 For a *hot compress:*
   a Fill the basin ½ to ⅔ full with hot water as directed by the nurse. Measure water temperature.
   b Place the compress in the water.
   c Wring out the compress.
   d Apply the compress over the area. Note the time.
   e Cover the compress quickly. Use one of the following as directed by the nurse:
      (1) Apply plastic wrap and then a bath towel. Secure the towel in place with ties, tape, or rolled gauze.
      (2) Apply an aquathermia pad.
9 For a *hot soak:*
   a Fill the container ½ full with hot water as directed by the nurse. Measure water temperature.
   b Place the part into the water. Pad the edge of the container with a towel. Note the time.
   c Cover the person with a bath blanket for warmth.

10 For a *sitz bath:*
   a Place the disposable sitz bath on the toilet seat.
   b Fill the sitz bath ⅔ full with water as directed by the nurse. Measure water temperature.
   c Secure the gown above the waist.
   d Help the person sit on the sitz bath. Note the time.
   e Provide for warmth. Place a bath blanket around the shoulders. Place another over the legs.
   f Stay with the person if or she is weak or unsteady.
11 For a *hot or cold pack:*
   a Squeeze, knead, or strike the pack as directed by the manufacturer.
   b Place the pack in the cover.
   c Apply the pack. Note the time.
   d Secure the pack in place with ties, tape, or rolled gauze. Some packs are secured with Velcro straps.

Continued

APPLYING HEAT AND COLD APPLICATIONS—cont'd   `VIDEO`

PROCEDURE—cont'd

12 For an *aquathermia pad:*

  a Fill the heating unit to the fill line with distilled water.

  b Remove the bubbles. Place the pad and tubing below the heating unit. Tilt the heating unit from side to side.

  c Set the temperature as the nurse directs (usually 105° F [40.5° C]). Remove the key.

  d Place the pad in the cover.

  e Plug in the unit. Let water warm to the desired temperature.

  f Set the heating unit on the bedside stand. Keep the pad and connecting hoses level with the unit. Hoses must not have kinks.

  g Apply the pad to the part. Note the time.

  h Secure the pad in place with ties, tape, or rolled gauze. Do not use pins.

13 For an *ice bag, collar, or glove:*

  a Fill the device with water. Put in the stopper. Turn the device upside down to check for leaks.

  b Empty the device.

  c Fill the device ½ to ⅔ full with crushed ice or ice chips (Fig. 35-32).

  d Remove excess air. Bend, twist, or squeeze the device. Or press it against a firm surface.

  e Place the cap or stopper on securely.

  f Dry the device with paper towels.

  g Place the device in the cover.

  h Apply the device. Note the time.

  i Secure the device in place with ties, tape, or rolled gauze.

14 For a *cold compress:*

  a Place the small basin with cold water into the large basin with ice.

  b Place the compresses into the cold water.

  c Wring out a compress.

  d Apply the compress to the part. Note the time.

15 Place the signal light within reach. Unscreen the person.

16 Raise or lower bed rails. Follow the care plan.

17 Check the person every 5 minutes. Check for signs and symptoms of complications (see *Delegation Guidelines: Applying Heat and Cold,* p. 558). Remove the application if any occur. Tell the nurse at once.

18 Check the application every 5 minutes. Change the application if cooling (hot applications) or warming (cold applications) occurs.

19 Remove the application at the specified time. Heat and cold applications are left on for 15 to 20 minutes. (If bed rails are up, lower the near one for this step.)

POST-PROCEDURE

20 Provide for comfort. (See the inside of the front book cover.)

21 Place the signal light within reach.

22 Raise or lower bed rails. Follow the care plan.

23 Unscreen the person.

24 Clean and return re-usable items to their proper place. Follow center policy for soiled linen. Wear gloves for this step.

25 Complete a safety check of the room. (See the inside of the front book cover.)

26 Remove and discard the gloves. Decontaminate your hands.

27 Report and record your observations (Fig. 35-33).

Fig. 35-32 Ice bags.

Date	Time	Nursing Margin	Other Depts Margin
3/6	1000	Aquathermia heating unit set at 105° F. The pad was placed in a flannel cover and applied to the anterior R thigh. Secured in place with tape. Resident positioned in semi-Fowler's position. States she is comfortable. States the pad does not feel too hot. Overbed table with water pitcher and water glass within reach. Bed in the low position. Signal light within reach. Adam Aims, CNA	
3/6	1005	Aquathermia pad checked. Resident states she feels comfortable. States the pad is not too hot. Denies pain or discomfort. There is no redness, swelling, or blistering of the skin under the pad. Pad re-secured with tape. Overbed table with water pitcher and glass within reach. Bed in the low position. Signal light within reach. Adam Aims, CNA	

Fig. 35-33 Charting sample.

Cooling and Warming Blanket

Hyperthermia is a body temperature *(thermia)* that is much higher *(hyper)* than the person's normal range. Body temperature is usually greater than 103° F (39.4° C). It is often called *heat stroke* when caused by hot weather. Other causes include illness, dehydration, and not being able to perspire. Lowering the body temperature is necessary. Otherwise death can occur. The doctor orders ice packs applied to the head, neck, underarms, and groin. Sometimes cooling blankets are used alone or with ice packs.

A cooling blanket is an electrical device. Made of rubber or plastic, the device has tubes filled with fluid. The fluid flows through the tubes. The blanket is placed on the bed and covered with a sheet. The blanket is turned on the cool setting and allowed to cool. The person lies on the blanket.

Hypothermia is a very low *(hypo)* body temperature *(thermia)*. Body temperature is less than 95° F (35° C). Cold weather is a common cause. The person is warmed to prevent death. Treatment may include a warming blanket. A warming blanket is like a cooling blanket except warm settings are used.

When used for cooling, the device is called a *hypothermia blanket.* When used for warming, it is called a *hyperthermia blanket.* The device has warm and cool settings. Vital signs are measured often. Rapid and excess cooling or warming are prevented.

MEETING BASIC NEEDS

The wound can affect basic needs. However, it is only one part of the person's care. Remember, the *person* has the wound.

The person is recovering from surgery or trauma. The wound causes pain and discomfort. These may affect breathing and moving. Turning, re-positioning, and walking may be painful. Handle the person gently. Allow pain drugs to take effect before giving care.

Good nutrition is needed for healing. However, pain and discomfort can affect appetite. So can odors from wound drainage. Promptly remove soiled dressings from the room. Use room deodorizers as directed. Also keep drainage containers out of the person's sight. Tell the nurse if the person wants certain foods or drinks.

Infection is always a threat. Follow Standard Precautions and the Bloodborne Pathogen Standard. Carefully observe the wound for signs and symptoms of infection.

Delayed healing is a risk for persons who are older, obese, or have poor nutrition. Protein is needed for tissue growth and repair. Poor circulation and diabetes also affect healing. These conditions are risk factors for infection.

Many factors affect safety and security needs. The person fears scarring, disfigurement, delayed healing, and infection. Fears about the wound "popping open" are common. Medical bills are other concerns. The person may need care for a long time.

Victims of violence have many other concerns. Future attacks, finding and convicting the attacker, and fear for family members are common concerns. Victims of domestic, child, and elder abuse often hide the source of their injuries.

Wounds may be large or small. Others can see wounds on the face, arms, or legs. Clothing can hide some wounds. Wound drainage may have odors. Some wounds are disfiguring. They can affect sexual performance or feelings of sexual attraction. Amputation of a finger, hand, arm, toe, foot, or leg can affect function, everyday activities, and jobs. Eye injuries can affect vision. Abdominal trauma and surgery can affect eating and elimination.

Whatever the wound site or size, it affects function and body image. Love and belonging and self-esteem needs are affected. The person may be sad and tearful or angry and hostile. Adjustment may be hard and rehabilitation necessary. Be gentle and kind, give thoughtful care, and practice good communication. Other health team members—therapists, social workers, psychiatrists, and the clergy—may be involved in the person's care.

QUALITY OF LIFE

Wounds result from surgery, trauma, pressure (Chapter 36), and circulatory problems. Many factors affect wound healing. They include wound type and site. The person's age, general health, nutrition, and life-style are other factors. Wounds cause pain and discomfort. Basic needs are affected. Treat the person with dignity and respect.

Many persons have poor arterial or venous circulation. They are at risk for open wounds on the lower legs and feet. Persons with diabetes are at risk for foot ulcers. Follow the person's care plan. Be very careful not to injure the skin during care.

Heat and cold applications promote healing and comfort. They also reduce tissue swelling. A person may worry about the need for a heat or cold application. Be kind, caring, and patient. Refer questions to the nurse. Remember the right to personal choice. The person has the right to be involved in planning care. To do so, the person must know the reason for the application.

Remember to explain procedures to residents. They can plan if they know what will happen. A person may want to make a phone call or finish an activity first. Or a person may want the procedure done by a certain time—before visitors arrive, before a TV program, or before an activity. You protect the right to personal choice when the person helps plan procedure times.

Protect the right to privacy. It shows respect and protects the person's dignity. Expose only the body part involved in the procedure. Unnecessary exposure violates the person's right to privacy. It also affects comfort and chilling.

Heat and cold are usually applied for 15 to 20 minutes. The person cannot move about during this time. To promote comfort and safety:

- Meet elimination needs before the procedure.
- Keep the room free of unpleasant equipment and odors.
- Place needed items within the person's reach. These include the signal light, water pitcher and cup, reading material, needlework, phone, and other items requested by the person.
- Check the person often.

REVIEW QUESTIONS

Circle the BEST answer.

1 A person has a laceration on the right leg from a fall. The wound is
  a Open, unintentional, and contaminated
  b Open, unintentional, and infected
  c Closed, intentional, and clean
  d Closed, intentional, and chronic

2 A person had rectal surgery. The person has a
  a Clean wound
  b Dirty wound
  c Clean-contaminated wound
  d Contaminated wound

3 The skin and underlying tissues are pierced. This is
  a A penetrating wound   **c** A contusion
  b An incision   **d** An abrasion

4 Which can cause skin tears?
  a Keeping your nails trimmed and smooth
  b Dressing the person in soft clothing
  c Wearing rings
  d Padding wheelchair footplates

5 A person has a circulatory ulcer. Which measure should you question?
  a Hold socks in place with elastic garters.
  b Do not cut or trim toenails.
  c Apply elastic stockings.
  d Re-position the person every hour.

6 Elastic stockings
  a Hold dressings in place
  b Prevent blood clots
  c Reduce swelling after injury
  d Prevent venous blood flow

7 Elastic stockings are applied
  a Before the person gets out of bed
  b When the person is standing
  c After the person's shower or bath
  d For 30 minutes and then removed

8 When applying an elastic bandage
  a Position the part in good alignment
  b Cover the fingers or toes if possible
  c Apply it from the largest to smallest part of the extremity
  d Apply it from the upper to lower part of the extremity

9 Persons with diabetes are at risk for diabetic foot ulcers because of
   a Gangrene
   b Amputation
   c Infection
   d Nerve and blood vessel damage

10 A person has diabetes. You should check the person's feet every
   a 2 hours
   b Day
   c Week
   d Month

11 A person with diabetes needs to wear socks with shoes to prevent
   a Corns
   b Bunions
   c Plantar warts
   d Blisters

12 A wound is separating. This is called
   a Primary intention
   b Third intention
   c Dehiscence
   d Evisceration

13 Clear, watery drainage from a wound is called
   a Purulent drainage
   b Serous drainage
   c Sero-purulent drainage
   d Serosanguineous drainage

14 A dressing does the following except
   a Protect the wound from injury
   b Absorb drainage
   c Provide moisture for wound healing
   d Support the wound and reduce swelling

15 To secure a dressing, apply tape
   a Around the entire part
   b Along the sides of the dressing
   c To the top, middle, and bottom of the dressing
   d As the person prefers

16 A person has frequent dressing changes. The nurse will likely have the dressings secured with
   a A binder
   b Montgomery ties
   c Paper or cloth tape
   d An elastic bandage

17 A person receives a pain-relief drug before a dressing change. How long should you wait for the drug to take effect?
   a 5 minutes
   b 10 minutes
   c 15 minutes
   d 30 minutes

18 To remove tape
   a Pull it toward the wound
   b Pull it away from the wound
   c Use an adhesive remover
   d Use a saline solution

19 An abdominal binder is used to
   a Prevent blood clots
   b Prevent wound infection
   c Provide support and hold dressings in place
   d Decrease swelling and circulation

20 Heat applications have these effects except
   a Pain relief
   b Muscle relaxation
   c Healing
   d Decreased blood flow

21 The greatest threat from heat applications is
   a Infection
   b Burns
   c Chilling
   d Venous ulcers

22 These statements are about moist heat applications. Which is false?
   a Water is in contact with the skin.
   b The effects from moist heat are less than from a dry heat application.
   c Moist heat penetrates deeper than dry heat.
   d A moist heat application has a lower temperature than a dry heat application.

23 A hot application is usually
   a 80° to 93° F
   b 93° to 98° F
   c 98° to 106° F
   d Above 106° F

24 These statements are about sitz baths. Which is false?
   a The perineal and rectal areas are immersed in warm or hot water.
   b Sitz baths last 25 to 30 minutes.
   c They clean the perineum, relieve pain, increase circulation, or stimulate voiding.
   d Weakness and fainting can occur.

25 A person uses an aquathermia pad. Which is false?
   a It is a dry heat application.
   b A flannel cover is used.
   c Electrical safety precautions are practiced.
   d Pins secure the pad in place.

26 Cold applications
   a Reduce pain, prevent swelling, and decrease circulation
   b Dilate blood vessels
   c Prevent the spread of microbes
   d Prevent infection

27 Which is not a complication of cold applications?
   a Pain
   b Burns
   c Blisters
   d Infection

28 Before applying an ice bag
   a Place the bag in the freezer
   b Measure the temperature of the bag
   c Place the bag in a cover
   d Provide perineal care

Answers to these questions are on p. 721.

Pressure Ulcers

OBJECTIVES

- Define the key terms and key abbreviations listed in this chapter.
- Describe the causes and risk factors for pressure ulcers.
- Identify the persons at risk for pressure ulcers.
- Describe the stages of pressure ulcers.
- Identify the sites for pressure ulcers.
- Explain how to prevent pressure ulcers.
- Identify the complications from pressure ulcers.
- Explain how to promote quality of life.

KEY TERMS

avoidable pressure ulcer A pressure ulcer that develops from the improper use of the nursing process

bedfast Confined to bed

bony prominence An area where the bone sticks out or projects from the flat surface of the body

chairfast Confined to a chair

colonized The presence of bacteria on the wound surface or in wound tissue; the person does not have signs and symptoms of an infection

eschar Thick, leathery dead tissue that may be loose or adhered to the skin; it is often black or brown

friction The rubbing of one surface against another

pressure ulcer A localized injury to the skin and/or underlying tissue usually over a bony prominence; results from pressure or pressure in combination with shear; any lesion caused by unrelieved pressure that results in damage to underlying tissues

shear When layers of the skin rub against each other; when the skin remains in place and underlying tissues move and stretch and tear underlying capillaries and blood vessels, causing tissue damage

slough Dead tissue that is shed from the skin; it is usually light colored, soft, and moist; may be stringy at times

unavoidable pressure ulcer A pressure ulcer that occurs despite efforts to prevent one through proper use of the nursing process

KEY ABBREVIATIONS

CMS	Centers for Medicare & Medicaid Services	**TJC**	The Joint Commission

Fig. 36-1 A pressure ulcer. *(From Proceedings from the November National V.A.C.®,* Ostomy Wound Management, *Feb 2005, 51[2A, Suppl]:7S, HMP Communications.)*

The National Pressure Ulcer Advisory Panel (NPUAP) defines a **pressure ulcer** as a localized injury to the skin and/or underlying tissue usually over a bony prominence (Fig. 36-1). It is the result of pressure or pressure in combination with shear. *Prominence* means to stick out. A **bony prominence** is an area where the bone sticks out or projects from the flat surface of the body. The back of the head, shoulder blades, elbows, hips, spine, sacrum, knees, ankles, heels, and toes are bony prominences (Fig. 36-2). *Decubitus ulcer, bed sore,* or *pressure sore* are other terms for pressure ulcer.

Fig. 36-2 Bony prominences (pressure points). **A,** The supine position. **B,** The lateral position. **C,** The prone position. **D,** Fowler's position. **E,** Sitting position.

The Centers for Medicare & Medicaid Services (CMS) defines a pressure ulcer as any lesion caused by unrelieved pressure that results in damage to underlying tissues. According to the CMS, friction and shear are not the main causes of pressure ulcers. However, friction and shear are important contributing factors. Shear is when layers of the skin rub against each other. Or shear is when the skin remains in place and underlying tissues move and stretch and tear underlying capillaries and blood vessels. Tissue damage occurs. Friction is the rubbing of one surface against another. The skin is dragged across a surface. Friction is always present with shearing.

The CMS has standards focusing on pressure ulcers. Some persons are admitted to the center with pressure ulcers. They come from hospitals or from home. According to the CMS, nursing centers must ensure that:

- A person does not develop a pressure ulcer after entering the center. However, for some persons, developing a pressure ulcer cannot be avoided. A pressure ulcer occurs despite efforts to prevent one through proper use of the nursing process. This is called an unavoidable pressure ulcer. An avoidable pressure ulcer is one that develops from the improper use of the nursing process. The center must:
  - Evaluate the person's condition and pressure ulcer risk factors.
  - Identify and implement measures that meet the resident's needs and goals.
  - Monitor and evaluate the effect of such measures.
  - Revise the measures as needed.
- A person with a pressure ulcer must receive the necessary treatment and services to promote healing, prevent infection, and prevent new sores.

Centers must identify persons at risk for developing pressure ulcers. Some persons are at greater risk than others. And the person's risk may increase during an illness (cold, flu) or when his or her condition changes. Many pressure ulcers occur within the first 4 weeks of admission to a nursing center. A person at risk can develop a pressure ulcer within 2 to 6 hours after the onset of pressure. The center must develop a comprehensive care plan to meet the person's needs. The care plan must include measures to reduce or remove the person's risk factors.

RISK FACTORS

Pressure is the major cause of pressure ulcers. Shearing and friction are important factors. They also cause skin breakdown (Box 36-1) that can lead to a pressure ulcer. Risk factors include breaks in the skin, poor circulation to an area, moisture, dry skin, and irritation by urine and feces. Older and disabled persons are at great risk for pressure ulcers. Their skin is easily injured. Causes include age-related skin changes, chronic disease, and general debility.

Box 36-1   Skin Breakdown—Common Causes

- Age-related changes in the skin
- Dryness
- Fragile and weak capillaries
- General thinning of the skin
- Loss of the fatty layer under the skin
- Decreased sensation to touch, heat, and cold
- Decreased mobility
- Sitting in a chair or lying in bed most or all of the day
- Chronic diseases (diabetes, high blood pressure)
- Diseases that decrease circulation
- Poor nutrition
- Poor hydration
- Incontinence (urinary, fecal)
- Moisture in dark body areas (skin folds, under breasts, perineal area)
- Pressure on bony parts
- Poor fingernail and toenail care
- Friction and shearing
- Edema

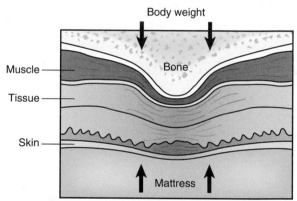

Fig. 36-3 Tissue under pressure. The skin is squeezed between two hard surfaces: the bone and the mattress. *(Redrawn from* Understanding your body: what are pressure ulcers? *U.S. Department of Health & Human Services, Agency for Healthcare Research and Quality, Sept 2009.)*

Unrelieved pressure squeezes tiny blood vessels. The skin does not receive oxygen and nutrients. Tissues die and a pressure ulcer forms when the skin is starved of oxygen and nutrients for too long. For example, pressure occurs when the skin over a bony area is squeezed between hard surfaces (Fig. 36-3). The bone is one hard surface. The other is usually the mattress or chair seat. Squeezing or pressure prevents blood flow to the skin and underlying tissues. Oxygen and nutrients cannot get to the cells. Involved skin and tissues die.

Friction scrapes the skin, causing an open area. The open area needs to heal. A good blood supply is needed. A poor blood supply or an infection can lead to a pressure ulcer.

Shear occurs when the person slides down in the bed or chair. Blood vessels and tissues are damaged. Blood flow to the area is reduced.

PERSONS AT RISK

Persons at risk for pressure ulcers are those who:

- Are bedfast (confined to a bed) or chairfast (confined to a chair). Pressure occurs from lying or sitting in the same position for too long.
- Need some or total help in moving. Coma, paralysis, or a hip fracture increases the risk for pressure ulcers.
- Are agitated or have involuntary muscle movements. The person's movements cause rubbing (friction) against linens and other surfaces.
- Have urinary or fecal incontinence. Urine and feces contain substances that irritate the skin and lead to skin breakdown. They are also sources of moisture.
- Are exposed to moisture. Urine, feces, wound drainage, sweat, and saliva expose the person to moisture. Moisture irritates the skin. It also increases the risk of damage from friction and shearing during repositioning.
- Have poor nutrition. A balanced diet is needed to properly nourish the skin. The risk for pressure ulcers increases when the skin is not healthy.
- Have poor fluid balance. Fluid balance is needed for healthy skin.
- Have lowered mental awareness. The person cannot act (move, change positions) to prevent pressure ulcers. Drugs and health problems affect mental awareness.
- Have problems sensing pain or pressure. These are symptoms of tissue damage. If the person cannot sense pain or pressure, he or she does not know to alert the staff to the symptoms.
- Have circulatory problems. Good blood flow is needed to bring oxygen and nutrients to the cells. Cells and tissues die when starved of oxygen and nutrients.
- Are older. Older persons have thin and fragile skin. Such skin is easily injured. They may have chronic diseases that affect mobility, nutrition, circulation, and mental awareness.
- Are obese or very thin. Friction can damage the skin.
- Refuse care. The person needs proper care to prevent pressure ulcers. The CMS requires that the person make informed choices. The center and resident must discuss the person's condition, treatment options, expected outcomes, and problems from refusing treatment. The center must address the person's concerns and offer options if a certain treatment is refused. The presence of a "Do Not Resuscitate" order (Chapter 48) does not mean the person is refusing measures to prevent or treat a pressure ulcer. It only means that the person will not be resuscitated in the event of a cardiac or respiratory arrest.
- Have a healed pressure ulcer. According to the CMS, areas of healed Stage 3 or 4 pressure ulcers are more likely to recur. See "Pressure Ulcer Stages."

PRESSURE ULCER STAGES

In persons with light skin, a reddened bony area is the first sign of a pressure ulcer. In persons with dark skin, skin color may differ from surrounding areas. The color change remains after the pressure is relieved. The area may feel warm or cool. The person may complain of pain, burning, tingling, or itching in the area. Some persons do not feel anything unusual. Box 36-2 describes pressure ulcer stages.

See *Focus on Communication: Pressure Ulcer Stages.*

Text continued on p. 570

Box 36-2 Pressure Ulcer Stages

Stage 1 The skin is intact. There is usually redness over a bony prominence. The color does not return to normal when the skin is relieved of pressure. In persons with dark skin, skin color may differ from surrounding areas. It may appear to be a persistent red, blue, or purple. See Figures 36-4, *A*, p. 568, and 36-5, *A*, p. 569.

Stage 2 Partial-thickness skin loss (Figs. 36-4, *B*, p. 568, and 36-5, *B*, p. 569). The wound may involve a blister or shallow ulcer. An ulcer may appear to be reddish-pink. A blister may be intact or open.

Stage 3 Full-thickness tissue loss (Figs. 36-4, *C*, p. 568, and 36-5, *C*, p. 569). The skin is gone. Subcutaneous fat may be exposed. Slough may be present. Slough is dead tissue that is shed from the skin. Usually light colored, soft, and moist. It may be stringy at times.

Stage 4 Full-thickness tissue loss with muscle, tendon, and bone exposure (Figs. 36-4, *D*, p. 568 and 36-5, *D*, p. 569). Slough and eschar may be present. Eschar is thick, leathery dead tissue that may be loose or adhered to the skin. It is often black or brown.

Unstageable Full-thickness tissue loss with the ulcer covered by slough and/or eschar (Figs. 36-4, *E*, p. 568 and 36-6, p. 570). Slough is yellow, tan, gray, green, or brown. Eschar is tan, brown, or black.

FOCUS ON COMMUNICATION
Pressure Ulcer Stages

Tell the nurse if you see areas of redness, skin color changes, blisters, or skin or tissue loss. Describe what you observed as best as you can. Tell the nurse the site. The nurse needs to assess the area. For example, you can say:

- "I saw a reddened area on Mr. Drake's left heel. It was about the size of a quarter. The skin looked intact. Would you please take a look at it?"
- "I just gave Ms. Richards a bath. I noticed a reddened area with a blister on her left buttock. I didn't see any drainage. Would you please take a look at it? I can help you turn her."

Fig. 36-4 Stages of pressure ulcers. **A,** Stage 1—the skin is intact. There is usually redness over a bony prominence. The color does not return to normal when the skin is relieved of pressure. In persons with dark skin, skin color may differ from surrounding areas. **B,** Stage 2—partial-thickness skin loss. The wound may involve a blister or shallow ulcer. An ulcer may appear to be reddish-pink. A blister may be intact or open. **C,** Stage 3—full-thickness tissue loss. The skin is gone. Subcutaneous fat may be exposed. Tissue shedding *(slough)* may be present. **D,** Stage 4—full-thickness tissue loss with muscle, tendon, and bone exposure. Slough (tissue shedding) or *eschar* (a scab or dry crust) may be present. **E,** Unstageable—full-thickness tissue loss with the ulcer covered by slough and/or eschar. Slough is yellow, tan, gray, green, or brown. Eschar is tan, brown, or black. *(Redrawn from National Pressure Ulcer Advisory Panel, 2007.)*

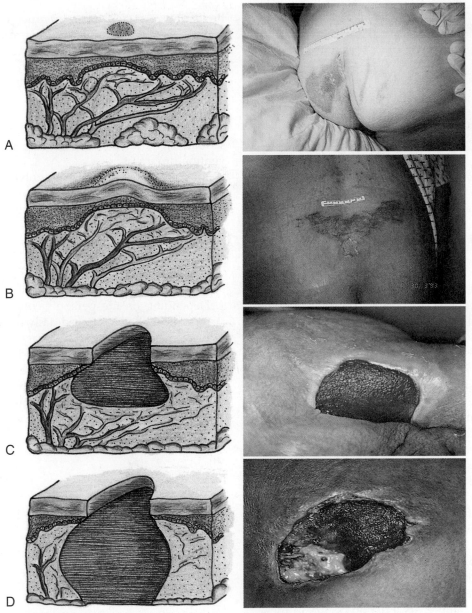

Fig. 36-5 Stages of pressure ulcers. **A,** Stage 1. **B,** Stage 2. **C,** Stage 3. **D,** Stage 4. *(Courtesy Laurel Wiersema-Bryant, RN, MSN, Clinical Nurse Specialist, Barnes-Jewish Hospital, St Louis, Mo.)*

Fig. 36-6 Unstageable pressure ulcer. *(From Bryant RA, Nix DP:* Acute & Chronic Wounds: Current Management Concepts, *ed. 3, St. Louis, 2007, Mosby.)*

SITES

Pressure ulcers usually occur over bony areas. The bony areas are called *pressure points*. This is because they bear the weight of the body in a certain position (see Fig. 36-2). Pressure from body weight can reduce the blood supply to the area. According to the CMS, the sacrum is the most common site for a pressure ulcer. However, pressure ulcers on the heels often occur.

The ears also are sites for pressure ulcers. This is from pressure of the ear on the mattress when in the side-lying position. Eyeglasses and oxygen tubing also can cause pressure on the ears. A urinary catheter can cause pressure and friction on the meatus. Tubes, casts, braces, and other devices can cause pressure on arms, hands, legs, and feet. A pressure ulcer can develop where medical equipment is attached to the skin for a prolonged time.

In obese people, pressure ulcers can occur in areas where skin has contact with skin. Common sites are between abdominal folds, the legs, the buttocks, the thighs, and under the breasts. Friction occurs in these areas.

PREVENTION AND TREATMENT

Preventing pressure ulcers is much easier than trying to heal them. The Joint Commission (TJC) estimates that it costs $1119 to $70,000 to treat a hospital-acquired pressure ulcer. Pressure ulcers also occur in long-term care and home settings. TJC estimates that it costs $11 billion a year to treat pressure ulcers in the United States.

Good nursing care, cleanliness, and skin care are essential. TJC and the CMS require pressure ulcer prevention programs.

Pressure ulcer prevention involves:

- Identifying persons at risk. The nurse assesses the person when he or she is admitted to the center. The person's risk factors and skin condition are assessed. The CMS requires that the nurse use the Minimum Data Set (MDS). See Appendix B. The Braden Scale for Predicting Pressure Sore Risk is a popular tool (Fig. 36-7). Existing pressure ulcers are identified. Depending on the person's condition and risk factors, he or she is assessed daily or weekly.
- Implementing prevention measures for those at risk. Managing moisture, good nutrition and fluid balance, and relieving pressure are key measures. The measures in Box 36-3, p. 572 help prevent skin breakdown and pressure ulcers. Follow the person's care plan.

BRADEN SCALE FOR PREDICTING PRESSURE SORE RISK

Patient's name _____ Evaluator's name _____ Date of assessment _____

SENSORY PERCEPTION Ability to respond meaningfully to pressure-related discomfort	**1. Completely Limited** Unresponsive (does not moan, flinch, or grasp) to painful stimuli, due to diminished level of consciousness or sedation OR limited ability to feel pain over most of body	**2. Very Limited** Responds only to painful stimuli. Cannot communicate discomfort except by moaning or restlessness OR has a sensory impairment which limits the ability to feel pain or discomfort over 1/2 of body.	**3. Slighty Limited** Responds to verbal commands, but cannot always communicate discomfort or the need to be turned OR has some sensory impairment which limits ability to feel pain or discomfort in 1 or 2 extremities.	**4. No Impairment** Responds to verbal commands. Has no sensory deficit which would limit ability to feel or voice pain or discomfort.				
MOISTURE Degree to which skin is exposed to moisture	**1. Constantly Moist** Skin is kept moist almost constantly by perspiration, urine, etc. Dampness is detected every time patient is moved or turned.	**2. Very Moist** Skin is often, but not always moist. Linen must be changed at least once a shift.	**3. Occasionally Moist** Skin is occasionally moist, requiring an extra linen change approximately once a day.	**4. Rarely Moist** Skin is usually dry, linen only requires changing at routine intervals.				
ACTIVITY Degree of physical activity	**1. Bedfast** Confined to bed.	**2. Chairfast** Ability to walk severly limited or non-existent. Cannot bear own weight and/or must be assisted into chair or wheelchair.	**3. Walks Occasionally** Walks occasionally during day, but for very short distances, with or without assistance. Spends majority of each shift in bed or chair.	**4. Walks Frequently** Walks outside room at least twice a day and inside room at least once every two hours during waking hours.				
MOBILITY Ability to change and control body position	**1. Completely Immobile** Does not make even slight changes in body or extremity position without assistance.	**2. Very Limited** Makes occasional slight changes in body or extremity position but unable to make frequent or significant changes independently.	**3. Slightly Limited** Makes frequent though slight changes in body or extremity position independently.	**4. No Limitation** Makes major and frequent changes in position without assistance.				
NUTRITION Usual food intake pattern	**1. Very Poor** Never eats a complete meal. Rarely eats more than 1/3 of any food offered. Eats 2 servings or less of protein (meat or dairy products) per day. Takes fluids poorly. Does not take a liquid dietary supplement OR is NPO and/or maintained on clear liquids or IV's for more than 5 days.	**2. Probably Inadequate** Rarely eats a complete meal and generally eats only about 1/2 of any food offered. Protein intake includes only 3 servings of meat or dairy products per day. Occasionally will take a dietary supplement OR receives less than optimum amount of liquid diet or tube feeding.	**3. Adequate** Eats over half of most meals. Eats a total of 4 servings of protein (meat, dairy products) per day. Occasionally will refuse a meal, but will usually take a supplement when offered OR is on a tube feeding or TPN regimen which probably meets most of nutritional needs.	**4. Excellent** Eats most of every meal. Never refuses a meal. Usually eats a total of 4 or more servings of meat and dairy products. Occasionally eats between meals. Does not require supplementation.				
FRICTION & SHEAR	**1. Problem** Requires moderate to maximum assistance in moving. Complete lifting without sliding against sheets is impossible. Frequently slides down in bed or chair, requiring frequent repositioning with maximum assistance. Spasticity, contractures or agitation leads to almost constant friction.	**2. Potential Problem** Moves feebly or requires minimum assitance. During a move skin probably slides to some extent against sheets, chair, restraints or other devices. Maintains relatively good position in chair or bed most of the time, but occasionally slides down.	**3. No Apparent Problem** Moves in bed and in chair independently and has sufficient muscle strength to lift up completely during move. Maintains good position in bed or chair.					
				Total score				

Fig. 36-7 Braden Scale for Predicting Pressure Sore Risk. *(Copyright 1988. Used with permission of Barbara Braden, PhD, RN, Professor, Creighton University School of Nursing, Omaha, Neb, and Nancy Bergstrom, Professor, University of Texas-Houston, School of Nursing, Houston, Tex.)*

Box 36-3   Measures to Prevent Pressure Ulcers

Handling, Moving, and Positioning

- Follow the re-positioning schedule in the person's care plan (Fig. 36-8). Re-position bedfast persons at least every 1 to 2 hours. Re-position chairfast persons every hour. Some persons are re-positioned every 15 minutes. Some persons are allowed to sit in a chair 3 times a day for 60 minutes or less.
- Use assist devices (Chapter 17) according to the care plan.
- Position the person according to the care plan. Use pillows for support as instructed by the nurse. The 30-degree lateral position is recommended (Fig. 36-9).
- Do not position the person on a pressure ulcer.
- Do not position the person on a reddened area.
- Do not position the person on tubes or other medical devices.
- Do not leave a person on a bedpan longer than necessary.
- Prevent shearing and friction during handling, moving, and transfer procedures. Use assist devices as directed by the nurse and the care plan.
- Prevent friction in bed. Powder sheets lightly to prevent friction. Follow the care plan.
- Prevent shearing. Do not raise the head of the bed more than 30 degrees. Follow the care plan. The care plan tells you:
  - When to raise the head of the bed
  - How far to raise the head of the bed
  - How long (in minutes) to raise the head of the bed
- Use pillows, foam wedges, or other devices to prevent bony areas from contact with bony areas. The ankles, knees, hips, and sacrum are examples. Follow the care plan.
- Keep the heels and ankles off the bed. Use pillows or other devices as the nurse directs. Place the pillows or devices under the lower legs from mid-calf to the ankles.
- Use protective devices as the nurse and care plan direct.
- Remind persons sitting in chairs to shift their positions every 15 minutes. This decreases pressure on bony points.
- Support the person's feet properly. Use a footrest if the person's feet do not touch the floor when he or she is sitting in a chair. The body slides forward when the person's feet do not touch the floor. If the person is in a wheelchair, position the feet on the footplates.

Skin Care

- Inspect the person's skin every time you provide care. This includes during or after transfers, re-positioning, bathing, and elimination procedures. Report any concern at once.
- Follow the care plan for the person's bathing schedule. Some persons do not need a bath every day.
- Do not use hot water to bathe or clean the skin. Hot water can irritate the skin.
- Use a cleansing agent as directed by the nurse and the care plan. Soap can dry and irritate the skin.
- Provide good skin care. The skin is clean and dry after bathing. The skin is free of moisture from a bath, urine, stools, perspiration, wound drainage, and other secretions.
- Follow the care plan to prevent incontinence.
- Prevent skin exposure to moisture. Check persons who are incontinent of urine or feces often. Provide good skin care and change linens and garments at the time of soiling. Use incontinence products as directed by the nurse and the care plan.
- Apply an ointment or moisture barrier if the person is incontinent of urine or feces. Follow the care plan.
- Check persons often who perspire heavily or have wound drainage. Change linens and garments as needed. Provide good skin care.
- Apply moisturizer to dry areas—hands, elbows, legs, ankles, heels, and so on. The nurse tells you what to use and what areas need attention.
- Give a back massage when re-positioning the person. *Do not massage bony areas.*
- Do not massage over pressure points. *Never rub or massage reddened areas.*
- Keep linens clean, dry, and wrinkle-free.
- Do not irritate the skin. Avoid scrubbing or vigorous rubbing when bathing or drying the person.
- Use pillows and blankets to prevent skin from being in contact with skin. They also reduce moisture and friction.
- Make sure socks and shoes are in good repair. Socks should not have wrinkles or creases. Make sure there is nothing in the shoes before the person puts them on.
- Do not apply heat (Chapter 35) directly on a pressure ulcer.

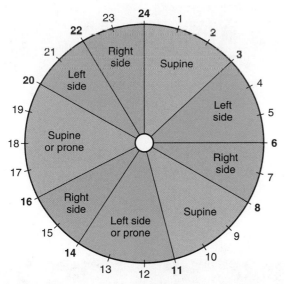

Fig. 36-8 Turn clock in 24-hour time. The clock shows the times to turn the person and to what position.

30-degree side-lying position, using pillows and foam wedge.

Hipbone

30 degrees

Hipbone

Tailbone

Fleshy part of buttocks

Fig. 36-9 The 30-degree lateral position. Pillows are placed under the head, shoulder, and leg. This position inclines (lifts up) the hip to avoid pressure on the hip. The person does not lie on the hip as in the side-lying position.

Some centers use symbols or colored stickers as pressure ulcer alerts. They are placed on the person's door or chart. They remind the staff that the person is at risk for a pressure ulcer.

Support surfaces are used to relieve or reduce pressure. Such surfaces include foam, air, alternating air, gel, or water mattresses. The best surface for the person is used.

Protective Devices

The doctor orders wound care products, drugs, treatments, and special equipment to promote healing. The nurse and care plan tell you what to do. Protective devices are often used to prevent and treat pressure ulcers and skin breakdown. These devices are common:

- *Bed cradle*—A bed cradle is a metal frame placed on the bed and over the person (Chapter 26). Top linens are brought over the cradle to prevent pressure on the legs, feet, and toes. Protect the person from drafts and chilling. To do so, tuck and miter linens at the bottom of the mattress. Also tuck them in under the mattress sides.
- *Heel and elbow protectors*—These devices are made of foam padding, pressure-relieving gel, sheepskin, and other cushion materials. They fit the shape of heels and elbows (Fig. 36-10, p. 574). Some are inserted inside sleeves or mesh. Others are secured in place with straps. These devices promote comfort. And they reduce shear and friction.
- *Heel and foot elevators*—These raise the heels and feet off of the bed (Fig. 36-11, p. 574). They prevent pressure. Some also prevent footdrop (Chapter 26).
- *Gel or fluid-filled pads and cushions*—These devices involve a pressure-relieving gel or fluid (Fig. 36-12, p. 574). They are used for chairs and wheelchairs to prevent pressure. The outer case is vinyl. The pad or cushion is placed in a fabric cover to protect the person's skin. Some covers are two colors (Fig. 36-13, p. 574). The colors remind the staff to re-position the person.
- *Eggcrate-type pads*—If used, these devices are placed on beds or in chairs or wheelchairs (Fig. 36-14, p. 575). The foam pad looks like an egg carton. Peaks in the pad distribute the person's weight more evenly. The pad is put in a special cover. The cover protects against heat, moisture, and soiling. Only a bottom sheet is used over the eggcrate-type pad and cover. No other bottom linens are used.
- *Special beds*—Some beds have air flowing through the mattresses (Fig. 36-15, p. 575). The person *floats* on the mattress. Body weight is distributed evenly. There is little pressure on body parts. Some beds allow re-positioning without moving the person. The person is turned to the prone or supine position or the bed is tilted various degrees. Alignment does not change. Pressure points change as the position changes. There is little friction. Some beds constantly rotate from side to side. They are useful for persons with spinal cord injuries.
- *Other equipment*—Pillows, trochanter rolls, footboards, and other positioning devices are used (Chapter 26). They help keep the person in good alignment.

See *Teamwork and Time Management: Prevention and Treatment*, p. 575.

Fig. 36-10 Elbow and heel protectors. *(Images courtesy J. T. Posey Co., Arcadia, Calif.)*

Fig. 36-11 Heel elevator.

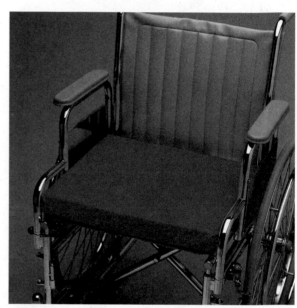

Fig. 36-12 Gel and foam cushion. *(Image courtesy Posey Company, Arcadia, Calif.)*

Fig. 36-13 Gel and foam cushion with a two-color cover. *(Image courtesy Posey Company, Arcadia, Calif.)*

Fig. 36-14 Eggcrate-type pad on the bed.

Fig. 36-15 Air flotation bed.

TEAMWORK AND TIME MANAGEMENT
Prevention and Treatment

The entire nursing team must prevent pressure ulcers. As you walk down hallways, look into rooms to see if a person has slid down in bed or in a chair. Do the same when people are in dining and lounge areas. Help re-position the person. Ask a co-worker to help you as needed. Report the re-positioning to the nurse.

Dressings

The nurse decides what dressing to use (Chapter 35). Sometimes wet dressings are used. The wound must be moist enough to promote healing. However, it must not be too moist. If too moist, the dressing can interfere with healing.

A pressure ulcer may have drainage. A dressing that absorbs drainage is used.

Wet-to-dry gauze dressings are sometimes used. The dressing absorbs slough. The slough is removed when the dressing is removed.

COMPLICATIONS

TJC estimates that about 60,000 people die each year from pressure ulcer complications. Infection is the most common complication. According to the CMS, all Stage 2, 3, and 4 pressure ulcers are colonized with bacteria. *Colonized* refers to the presence of bacteria on the wound surface or in wound tissue. The person does not have signs and symptoms of an infection.

Wounds are infected if the person has signs and symptoms of infection (Chapter 15). For some persons, pain and delayed healing signal an infection. For the pressure ulcer to heal, infection must be diagnosed and treated.

Osteomyelitis is a risk if the pressure ulcer is over a bony prominence. The risk is great if the ulcer is not healing. *Osteomyelitis* means inflammation *(itis)* of the bone *(osteo)* and bone marrow *(myel)*. The person has severe pain. The person is treated with bedrest and antibiotics. Careful and gentle positioning is needed. Surgery may be needed to remove dead bone and tissue.

Pressure ulcers can cause pain. Pain management is important (Chapter 27). Pain may interfere with movement and activity. The immobility is a risk factor for pressure ulcers. And it may delay healing of an existing pressure ulcer.

REPORTING AND RECORDING

Report and record any signs of skin breakdown or pressure ulcers at once. See Figure 36-16, p. 576. See "Wound Appearance" in Chapter 35.

See *Focus on Communication: Reporting and Recording,* p. 576.

OBRA-CMS

Date	Time	Nursing Margin	Other Depts Margin
8-27	0830	While assisting resident with a tub bath, a blister the size of a quarter was noted on the outer aspect of the L heel. There is a 1/4 inch reddened area around the blister. No drainage noted. Resident states "It hurts a little." She said she thinks her shoes are rubbing Asked Barbara Lane, RN to observe the area. Jean Hein, CNA	

Fig. 36-16 Charting sample.

FOCUS ON COMMUNICATION
Reporting and Recording

During a site survey, CMS staff may interview you. They might ask questions about:

- How you are involved in the person's care.
- What measures the center uses to prevent and treat pressure ulcers.
- What skin changes you should report and when.
- To whom you should report skin changes.
- Your knowledge of measures in a person's care plan.

Respond to the surveyor in a professional manner. Answer questions honestly and completely.

QUALITY OF LIFE

Residents have the right to care that promotes healthy skin and prevents skin breakdown and pressure ulcers. The Omnibus Budget Reconciliation Act of 1987 (OBRA), the CMS, and TJC require a care plan for each person. It must address correct skin care. Use skin care products and protective devices as directed by the nurse and the care plan. Everyone must keep the person's skin healthy.

The skin is the body's first line of defense against changes in the environment. Keep the skin clean and intact. This promotes comfort and prevents infection. Giving good skin care is an important part of your job. Older persons require special skin care. Their skin is thin and fragile.

Preventing pressure ulcers is easier than trying to heal them. Prolonged infection, pain, amputation, and longer hospital or nursing center stays are complications. The person's quality of life is reduced. Depression and death are risks.

REVIEW QUESTIONS

Circle the BEST answer.

1 A pressure ulcer is
- **a** An open wound
- **b** A localized injury to the skin and/or underlying tissue
- **c** A bony prominence
- **d** Dead tissue

2 Pressure ulcers are the result of
- **a** Unrelieved pressure
- **b** Moisture
- **c** Medical devices
- **d** Aging

3 Which of the following contribute to the development of pressure ulcers?
- **a** Shear and friction
- **b** Slough and eschar
- **c** Bony prominences
- **d** CMS and TJC

4 A pressure ulcer can develop within
- **a** 2 to 6 hours
- **b** 6 to 10 hours
- **c** 10 to 14 hours
- **d** 14 to 18 hours

5 The following are risk factors for pressure ulcers *except*
- **a** Urinary and fecal incontinence
- **b** Lowered mental awareness
- **c** Moisture
- **d** Balanced diet

6 Which is the most common site for a pressure ulcer?
- **a** Back of the head
- **b** Hip
- **c** Sacrum
- **d** Heel

7 In a light-skinned person, the first sign of a pressure ulcer is
- **a** A blister
- **b** A reddened area
- **c** Drainage
- **d** Gangrene

8 A person's care plan includes the following. Which should you question?
- **a** Re-position the person every 2 hours.
- **b** Scrub and rub the skin during bathing.
- **c** Apply lotion to dry areas.
- **d** Keep linens clean, dry, and wrinkle-free.

9 When positioning a person, you should position the person
   a On an existing pressure ulcer
   b On a reddened area
   c On tubes or other medical devices
   d Using assist devices

10 What is the preferred position for preventing pressure ulcers?
   a 30-degree lateral position
   b Semi-Fowler's position
   c Prone position
   d Supine position

11 Besides heel and foot elevators, which are used to keep the heels and ankles off of the bed?
   a Bed cradles   c Heel protectors
   b Pillows   d Eggcrate-type pads

12 Persons sitting in chairs should shift their positions every
   a 15 minutes   c Hour
   b 30 minutes   d Two hours

13 A person is sitting in a chair. The feet do not touch the floor. What should you do?
   a Have the person slide forward until the feet touch the floor.
   b Let the feet dangle.
   c Stack pillows under the person's feet.
   d Position the feet on a footrest.

14 Which are *not* used to treat pressure ulcers?
   a Special beds
   b Gel or fluid-filled pads and cushions
   c Plastic drawsheets and waterproof pads
   d Heel and elbow protectors

15 The following are sources of moisture *except*
   a Urine and feces   c Perspiration
   b Wound drainage   d Barrier ointment

16 You see a reddened area on the person's skin. What should you do?
   a Rub or massage the area.
   b Apply a moisturizer.
   c Apply a moisture barrier.
   d Tell the nurse.

17 The nurse tells you that the person's pressure ulcer is colonized. This means that
   a The wound is infected
   b Bacteria are present
   c The person has osteomyelitis
   d The person has a wet-to-dry gauze dressing

Circle T if the statement is TRUE. Circle F if the statement is FALSE.

18 T F   All pressure ulcers are avoidable.
19 T F   Skin breakdown can lead to a pressure ulcer.
20 T F   Unrelieved pressure squeezes tiny blood vessels. Tissues do not receive needed oxygen and nutrients.
21 T F   Persons who are bedfast or chairfast are at risk for pressure ulcers.
22 T F   Pressure ulcers can develop on the ears.
23 T F   Pressure ulcers can develop where medical devices are attached to the skin.
24 T F   You are responsible for identifying persons at risk for pressure ulcers.
25 T F   A person has a "Do Not Resuscitate" order. This means that the person is refusing treatment for a pressure ulcer.
26 T F   You use the Resident Assessment Instrument to assess a person's risk factors and skin condition.
27 T F   Pressure ulcers can involve muscles, tendons, and bones.
28 T F   To prevent pressure ulcers, the head of the bed is raised higher than 30 degrees.
29 T F   You should inspect the person's skin every time you provide care.
30 T F   A person is at risk for pressure ulcers. A bath is needed every day.
31 T F   You are giving a back massage. You should massage bony areas.
32 T F   You can use pillows and blankets to prevent skin from being in contact with skin.

Answers to these questions are on p. 721.

Hearing, Speech, and Vision Problems

OBJECTIVES

- Define the key terms and key abbreviations listed in this chapter.
- Describe the common ear disorders.
- Describe how to communicate with persons who have hearing loss.
- Explain the purpose of a hearing aid.
- Describe how to care for hearing aids.
- Describe the common speech disorders.
- Explain how to communicate with speech-impaired persons.

- Describe the common eye disorders.
- Explain how to assist persons who are visually impaired or blind.
- Explain how to protect an ocular prosthesis from loss or damage.
- Perform the procedure described in this chapter.
- Explain how to promote quality of life.

KEY TERMS

aphasia The total or partial loss *(a)* of the ability to use or understand language *(phasia);* a language disorder resulting from damage to parts of the brain responsible for language

blindness The absence of sight

braille A touch reading and writing system that uses raised dots for each letter of the alphabet; the first 10 letters also represent the numbers 0 through 9

Broca's aphasia See "expressive aphasia"

cerumen Earwax

deafness Hearing loss in which it is impossible for the person to understand speech through hearing alone

expressive aphasia Difficulty expressing or sending out thoughts; motor aphasia, Broca's aphasia

expressive-receptive aphasia Difficulty expressing or sending out thoughts and difficulty understanding language; global aphasia, mixed aphasia

global aphasia See "expressive-receptive aphasia"

hearing loss Not being able to hear the normal range of sounds associated with normal hearing

low vision Eyesight that cannot be corrected with eyeglasses, contact lenses, drugs, or surgery

mixed aphasia See "expressive-receptive aphasia"

motor aphasia See "expressive aphasia"

receptive aphasia Difficulty understanding language; Wernicke's aphasia

tinnitus A ringing, roaring, hissing, or buzzing sound in the ears or head

vertigo Dizziness

Wernicke's aphasia See "receptive aphasia"

Hearing, speech, and vision allow communication, learning, and moving about. They are important for self-care, work, and most activities. They also are important for safety and security needs. For example, you see dark clouds and hear tornado warning sirens. You know to seek shelter. With speech, you can alert others.

Many people have some degree of hearing or vision loss. Common causes are birth defects, accidents, infections, diseases, and aging.

EAR DISORDERS

The ear functions in hearing and balance. To review the structures and functions of the ear, see Chapter 9.

Otitis Media

Otitis media is infection (*itis*) of the middle (*media*) ear (*ot*). It often begins with infections that cause sore throats, colds, or other respiratory infections that spread to the middle ear. Viruses and bacteria are causes.

Otitis media is acute or chronic. Chronic otitis media can damage the tympanic membrane (eardrum) or the ossicles (Chapter 9). These structures are needed for hearing. Permanent hearing loss can occur.

Fluid builds up in the ear. Pain (earache) and hearing loss occur. So do fever and tinnitus. Tinnitus is a ringing, roaring, hissing, or buzzing sound in the ears or head. An untreated infection can travel to the brain and other structures in the head. The doctor orders antibiotics, drugs for pain relief, or drugs to relieve congestion.

See *Residents With Dementia: Otitis Media.*

> **RESIDENTS WITH DEMENTIA**
> ### Otitis Media
>
> Some persons with dementia cannot tell you about pain or when something is wrong. Be alert for behavior changes. Report the following to the nurse. They may signal otitis media:
> - Unusual irritability
> - Problems sleeping
> - Tugging or pulling at one or both ears
> - Fever
> - Fluid draining from the ear
> - Balance problems
> - Signs of hearing problems (p. 580)

Meniere's Disease

Meniere's disease involves the inner ear. It is a common cause of hearing loss. Usually one ear is affected. Symptoms include:
- Vertigo (dizziness)
- Tinnitus
- Hearing loss
- Pain or pressure in the affected ear

With Meniere's disease, there is increased fluid in the inner ear. The increased fluid causes swelling and pressure in the inner ear. Symptoms occur suddenly. They can occur daily or just once a year. An attack can last several hours.

An attack usually involves vertigo, tinnitus, and hearing loss. Vertigo causes whirling and spinning sensations. The dizziness causes severe nausea and vomiting.

Drugs, fluid restriction, a low-salt diet, and no alcohol or caffeine decrease fluid in the inner ear. Safety is needed during vertigo. The person must lie down. Falls are prevented. Bed rails are used according to the care plan. The person's head is kept still. The person avoids turning the head. To talk to the person, stand directly in front of him or her. When movement is necessary, move the person slowly. Sudden movements are avoided. So are bright or glaring lights. Assist with walking. The person should not walk alone in case vertigo occurs.

Hearing Loss

Hearing loss is not being able to hear the normal range of sounds associated with normal hearing. Losses are mild to severe. Deafness is the most severe form. Deafness is hearing loss in which it is impossible for the person to understand speech through hearing alone.

Hearing loss occurs in all age-groups. According to the National Institute on Deafness and Other Communication Disorders (NIDCD), about one third (33%) of Americans between ages 65 and 74 have hearing problems. About half (50%) of persons age 75 years and older have hearing loss. Hearing loss is more common in men than in women.

Common causes of hearing loss are:
- Damage to the outer, middle, or inner ear
- Damage to the auditory nerve

Risk factors that can damage ear structures include:
- Aging
- Exposure to very loud sounds and noises—job-related noises, loud music, loud engines from vehicles, shooting firearms
- Drugs—antibiotics, too much aspirin
- Infections
- Reduced blood flow to the ear caused by high blood pressure, heart and vascular diseases, and diabetes
- Stroke
- Head injuries
- Tumors
- Heredity
- Birth defects

Temporary hearing loss can occur from earwax (cerumen). Hearing improves after the earwax is removed.

Clear speech, responding to others, safety, and awareness of surroundings require hearing. Many people deny hearing problems. They relate hearing loss to aging.

See *Focus on Communication: Hearing Loss.*
See *Promoting Safety and Comfort: Hearing Loss.*

FOCUS ON COMMUNICATION
Hearing Loss

The National Association of the Deaf (NAD) uses the terms *deaf* and *hard-of-hearing* to describe persons with hearing loss. Do not use the terms "deaf and dumb," "deaf-mute," or "hearing-impaired." Such terms offend persons who are deaf or hard-of-hearing.

PROMOTING SAFETY AND COMFORT
Hearing Loss

Safety
Do not try to remove earwax. This is done by a doctor or a nurse. Do not insert anything, including cotton swabs, into the ear.

Effects on the Person A person may not notice gradual hearing loss. Others may see changes in the person's behavior or attitude. They may not relate the changes to hearing loss. Obvious signs and symptoms of hearing loss include:
- Speaking too loudly
- Leaning forward to hear
- Turning and cupping the better ear toward the speaker
- Answering questions or responding inappropriately
- Asking for words to be repeated
- Asking others to speak louder or to speak more slowly and clearly
- Having trouble hearing over the phone
- Finding it hard to follow conversations when two or more people are talking
- Turning up the TV, radio, or music volume so loud that others complain
- Thinking that others are mumbling or slurring words
- Having problems understanding women and children

Psychological and social changes are less obvious. People may give wrong answers or responses. Therefore they tend to shun social events to avoid embarrassment. Often they feel lonely, bored, and left out. Only parts of conversations are heard. They may become suspicious. They think others are talking about them or are talking softly on purpose. Some control conversations to avoid responding or being labeled "senile" because of poor answers. Straining and working hard to hear can cause fatigue, frustration, and irritability.

Hearing is needed for speech. How you pronounce words and voice volume depend on how you hear yourself. Hearing loss may result in slurred speech. Words may be pronounced wrong. Some have monotone speech or drop word endings. It may be hard to understand what the person says. Do not assume or pretend that you understand what the person says. Otherwise, serious problems can result. See "Speech Disorders" on p. 583.

Communication Persons with hearing loss may wear hearing aids or lip-read (speech-read). They watch facial expressions, gestures, and body language. Some people learn American Sign Language (ASL) (Figs. 37-1 and 37-2). ASL uses signs made with the hands and other movements such as facial expressions, gestures, and postures. To promote communication, practice the measures in Box 37-1, p. 582. (Different sign languages are used in different countries and regions. For example, British Sign Language is different from ASL.)

Some people have *hearing assistance dogs* (hearing dogs). The dog alerts the person to sounds. Phones, doorbells, smoke detectors, alarm clocks, sirens, and on-coming cars are examples.

Fig. 37-1 Manual alphabet. *(Courtesy National Association of the Deaf, Silver Spring, Md.)*

Wash

Eat, Food

Begin, Start

Help, Aid, Assist

Bath, Bathe

Good

Lie (lie down)

Sit, Seat, Chair

Hot

Thank you

Stand (arise)

Dress, Clothing

Cold, Winter

Tired

Walk

Permission, Privilege

Shower

Invite, Welcome

Thirsty

Better

Fig. 37-2 American Sign Language examples.

Box 37-1   Measures to Promote Hearing

The Environment
- Reduce or eliminate background noises. Turn off radios, stereos, music players, TVs, air conditioners, fans, and so on.
- Provide a quiet place to talk.
- Have the person sit in small groups or where he or she can hear best.

The Person
- Have the person wear his or her hearing aid. It must be turned on and working.
- Have the person wear needed eyeglasses or contact lenses. The person needs to see your face for lip-reading (speech-reading).

You
- Gain attention. Alert the person to your presence. Raise an arm or hand, or lightly touch the person's arm. Do not startle or approach the person from behind.
- Position yourself at the person's level. If the person is sitting, you sit. If the person is standing, you stand.
- Face the person when speaking. Do not turn or walk away while you are talking. Do not talk to the person from the doorway or another room.
- Stand or sit in good light. Shadows and glares affect the person's ability to see your face clearly.
- Speak clearly, distinctly, and slowly.
- Speak in a normal tone of voice. Do not shout.

You—cont'd
- Adjust the pitch of your voice as needed. Ask the person if he or she can hear you better:
  - If the person does not wear a hearing aid, lower the pitch if you are a female. Women's voices are higher-pitched and harder to hear than lower-pitched male voices.
  - If the person wears a hearing aid, raise the pitch slightly.
- Do not cover your mouth, smoke, eat, or chew gum while talking. Mouth movements are affected.
- Keep your hands away from your face. The person must be able to clearly see your face.
- Stand or sit on the side of the better ear.
- State the topic of conversation first.
- Tell the person when you are changing the subject. State the new subject of conversation.
- Use short sentences and simple words.
- Use gestures and facial expressions to give useful clues.
- Write out important names and words.
- Say things in another way if the person does not seem to understand.
- Keep conversations and discussions short. This avoids tiring the person.
- Repeat and rephrase statements as needed.
- Be alert to messages sent by your facial expressions, gestures, and body language.

Hearing Aids *Hearing aids* are electronic devices that fit inside or behind the ear (Fig. 37-3). They make sounds louder. They do not correct, restore, or cure hearing problems. Hearing ability does not improve. The person hears better because the device makes sounds louder. Background noise and speech are louder. The measures in Box 37-1 apply.

Hearing aids are battery-operated. Sometimes they do not seem to work properly. Try these simple measures:

- Check if the hearing aid is *on.* It has an *on* and *off* switch.
- Check the battery position.
- Insert a new battery if needed.
- Clean the hearing aid. *Follow the nurse's directions and the manufacturer's instructions.*

Hearing aids are turned off when not in use. And the battery is removed. These measures help prolong battery life. The person should not use hair spray or other hair care products while wearing a hearing aid. They can damage the device.

Hearing aids are costly. Handle and care for them properly. When not in the person's ear, store a hearing aid in its case. Place the case in the top drawer of the bedside stand. Report lost or damaged hearing aids to the nurse at once.

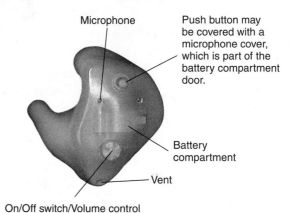

Fig. 37-3 A hearing aid. *(Courtesy Siemens Hearing Instruments, Inc., Piscataway, NJ.)*

Other Hearing Devices Other devices can help the person with hearing loss. They include:

- *Telephone amplifying devices.* Special telephone receivers make sounds louder. Some phones work with hearing aids.
- *TV and radio listening systems.* These can be used with or without hearing aids. The person does not have to turn the TV or radio volume up high.

SPEECH DISORDERS

Speech is used to communicate with others. Speech disorders result in impaired or ineffective oral communication. Hearing loss, developmental disabilities (Chapter 45), and brain injury are common causes. The following are common problems.

- Aphasia. See "Aphasia."
- *Apraxia* means not *(a)* to act, do, or perform *(praxia)*. The person with *apraxia of speech* cannot use the speech muscles to produce understandable speech. The person understands speech and knows what to say. However, the brain cannot coordinate the speech muscles to make the words. Apraxia is caused by damage to the motor speech area in the brain.
- *Dysarthria* means difficult or poor *(dys)* speech *(arthria)*. It is caused by damage to the nervous system. Mouth and face muscles are affected. Slurred speech, speaking slowly or softly, hoarseness, and drooling are other problems that can occur.

To communicate with the speech-impaired person, practice the measures in Box 37-2.

See *Focus on Rehabilitation: Speech Disorders.*

Box 37-2   Measures to Communicate With the Speech-Impaired Person

The Person
- Ask the person to repeat or rephrase statements if necessary.
- Repeat what the person has said. Ask if your understanding is correct.
- Ask the person to write down key words or the message.
- Ask the person to point, gesture, or draw to communicate key words.

You
- Follow the care plan. A consistent approach is needed.
- Provide a calm, quiet setting. Turn off the TV, radio, music, and other distractions.
- Include the person in conversations.
- Listen, and give the person your full attention.
- Use short, simple sentences.
- Repeat what you are saying as needed.
- Write down key words as needed.
- Speak to the person in a normal, adult tone. Do not treat or talk to the adult in a babyish or child-like way.
- Ask the person questions to which you know the answers. This helps you learn how the person speaks.
- Allow the person plenty of time to talk.
- Determine the topic being discussed. This helps you understand main points. Watch the person's lip movements.
- Watch facial expressions, gestures, and body language. They give clues about what is being said.
- Do not correct the person's speech.

FOCUS ON REHABILITATION
Speech Disorders

Some persons need speech rehabilitation. The goal is to improve the person's ability to communicate. A speech-language pathologist and other health team members help the person:
- Improve affected language skills
- Use remaining abilities
- Restore language abilities to the extent possible
- Learn other methods of communicating
- Strengthen the muscles of speech

The amount of improvement possible depends on many factors. They include the cause, amount, and area of brain damage and the person's age and health. The person's willingness and ability to learn are other factors.

Aphasia

Aphasia is the total or partial loss *(a)* of the ability to use or understand language *(phasia)*. Aphasia is a language disorder. It results from damage to parts of the brain responsible for language. Stroke, head injury, brain infections, and cancer are common causes. Most people who have aphasia are middle-aged adults and older.

Expressive aphasia (motor aphasia, Broca's aphasia) relates to difficulty expressing or sending out thoughts. Thinking is clear. The person knows what to say but has difficulty or cannot speak the words. There are problems speaking, spelling, counting, gesturing, or writing. The person may:
- Omit small words such as "is," "and," "of," and "the."
- Speak in single words or short sentences. For example, "Walk dog" can mean "I will take the dog for a walk" or "You take the dog for a walk."
- Put words in the wrong order. Instead of "bathroom," the person may say "room bath."
- Think one thing but say another. The person may want food but asks for a book.
- Call people by the wrong names.
- Make up words.
- Produce sounds and no words.
- Cry or swear for no reason.

Receptive aphasia (Wernicke's aphasia) is difficulty understanding language. The person has trouble understanding what is said or read. The person may speak in long sentences that have no meaning. Because of difficulty understanding speech, the person may not be aware of his or her mistakes. People and common objects are not recognized. The person may not know how to use a fork, toilet, cup, TV, phone, or other items.

With *expressive aphasia,* the person has difficulty expressing or sending out thoughts. With *receptive aphasia,* the person has difficulty understanding language. Some people have both types. This is called expressive-receptive aphasia (global aphasia, mixed aphasia). The person has problems speaking and understanding language.

The person has many emotional needs. Frustration, depression, and anger are common. Communication is needed to function and relate to others. The person wants to communicate but cannot. Be patient and kind.

EYE DISORDERS

Vision loss occurs at all ages. Problems range from mild loss to complete blindness. Blindness is the absence of sight. Vision loss is sudden or gradual. One or both eyes are affected.

Glaucoma

Glaucoma causes damage to the optic nerve. The eye produces a fluid that nourishes certain eye structures. The fluid normally drains from the eye. When the fluid cannot drain properly, it builds up in the eye, causing pressure on the optic nerve. The optic nerve is damaged. Vision loss with eventual blindness occurs.

Glaucoma can develop in one or both eyes. Onset is sudden or gradual. Peripheral vision (side vision) is lost. The person sees through a tunnel (Fig. 37-4), has blurred vision, and sees halos around lights. Severe eye pain, nausea, and vomiting occur with sudden onset.

Risk Factors Glaucoma is a leading cause of vision loss in the United States. Persons at risk include:
- African Americans over 40 years of age
- Everyone over 60 years of age
- Those with a family history of the disease
- Those who have diabetes, high blood pressure, or heart disease
- Those who have eye diseases or eye injuries
- Those who have had eye surgery

Treatment Glaucoma has no cure. Prior damage cannot be reversed. Drugs and surgery can control glaucoma and prevent further damage to the optic nerve.

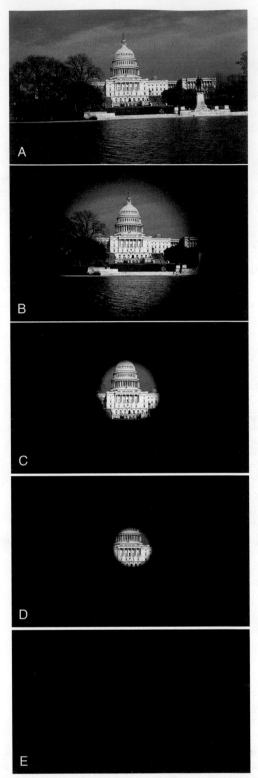

Fig. 37-4 Vision loss from glaucoma. **A,** Normal vision. **B,** Loss of peripheral vision begins. **C, D,** and **E,** Vision loss continues, with eventual blindness.

Fig. 37-5 One eye is normal. The other has a cataract. *(From Swartz MH: Textbook of physical diagnosis, ed 5, Philadelphia, 2006, Saunders.)*

Cataracts

Cataract is a clouding of the lens (Fig. 37-5). The normal lens is clear. *Cataract* comes from the Greek word that means *waterfall*. Trying to see is like looking through a waterfall. A cataract can occur in one or both eyes. Signs and symptoms include:

- Cloudy, blurry, or dimmed vision (Fig. 37-6).
- Colors seem faded. Blues and purples are hard to see.
- Sensitivity to light and glares.
- Poor vision at night.
- Halos around lights.
- Double vision in the affected eye.

Risk Factors Most cataracts are caused by aging. By age 80, more than 50% of all Americans have a cataract or have had cataract surgery. Diabetes, smoking, alcohol use, and prolonged exposure to sunlight are risk factors. So is a family history of cataracts.

Treatment Surgery is the only treatment. The lens is removed, and a plastic lens implanted. Surgery is done when the cataract starts to interfere with daily activities. Driving, reading, and watching TV are examples. Vision improves after surgery.

Post-operative care includes the following:

- Keep the eye shield in place as directed. The shield is worn for sleep, including naps.
- Follow measures for persons who are visually impaired or blind (p. 587) when an eye shield is worn. The person may have vision loss in the other eye.
- Remind the person not to rub or press the affected eye.
- Do not bump the eye.
- Place the overbed table and the bedside stand on the un-operative side.
- Place the signal light within reach.
- Report eye drainage or complaints of pain at once.

Fig. 37-6 Vision loss from a cataract. **A,** Normal vision. **B,** Scene viewed with a cataract. *(From National Eye Institute:* Cataract: what you should know, *National Institutes of Health, Bethesda, Md.)*

Age-Related Macular Degeneration

Age-related macular degeneration (AMD) blurs central vision. *Central vision* is what you see "straight-ahead." AMD causes a blind spot in the center of vision (Fig. 37-7, p. 586). Central vision is needed for reading, sewing, driving, and seeing faces and fine detail.

The disease damages the macula in the center of the retina. The retina receives light and sends messages to the brain through the optic nerve. Normal signals are not sent to the brain. Onset is gradual and painless. AMD is the leading cause of blindness in persons 60 years of age and older.

The two types of AMD are:

- *Wet AMD*—Blood vessels behind the retina start to grow under the macula. The blood vessels leak blood and fluid. Loss of central vision occurs quickly. An early symptom is that straight lines appear wavy. Wet AMD is considered advanced. It is more severe than dry AMD.
- *Dry AMD*—Light-sensitive cells in the macula slowly break down. Central vision gradually blurs. As dry AMD gets worse, a blurred spot is seen in the center of the eye. Usually both eyes are affected.

Dry AMD is more common than wet AMD. People who have wet AMD had dry AMD first. Dry AMD can suddenly turn into wet AMD.

Fig. 37-7 Vision loss from macular degeneration. **A,** Normal vision. **B,** Central vision is blurred. *(From National Eye Institute:* Age-related macular degeneration: what you should know, *National Institutes of Health, Bethesda, Md.)*

Fig. 37-8 Vision loss from diabetic retinopathy. **A,** Normal vision. **B,** Vision with diabetic retinopathy. *(From National Eye Institute:* Diabetic retinopathy: what you should know, *National Institutes of Health, Bethesda, Md.)*

Risk Factors AMD can occur during middle age. However, the risk increases with aging. Besides age, risk factors include:

- Smoking.
- Obesity.
- Race. Whites are at greater risk than any other group.
- Family history.
- Gender. Women are at greater risk than men.
- Light-colored eyes.
- Exposure to sunlight.
- Cardiovascular disease. This includes high blood pressure, coronary artery disease, and stroke.

Treatment For advanced dry AMD, no treatment can prevent vision loss. For wet AMD, some treatments may stop or slow the disease progress. They may save what is left of central vision. Laser surgery is an example.

The following can reduce the risk of AMD:

- Eating a healthy diet high in green leafy vegetables and fish
- Not smoking
- Maintaining a normal blood pressure
- Managing cardiovascular diseases
- Maintaining a normal weight
- Exercising
- Wearing sunglasses
- Having regular eye exams

Diabetic Retinopathy

In diabetic retinopathy, the tiny blood vessels in the retina are damaged. A complication of diabetes, it is a leading cause of blindness. Usually both eyes are affected.

Vision blurs (Fig. 37-8). The person may see spots "floating." Often there are no early warning signs.

Risk Factors Everyone with diabetes (Chapter 41) is at risk for diabetic retinopathy.

Treatment The person needs to control diabetes, blood pressure, and blood cholesterol. Laser surgery may help. In another surgery, blood is removed from the center of the eye. The person may need low vision services.

Low Vision

Low vision is eyesight that cannot be corrected with eyeglasses, contact lenses, drugs, or surgery. Reading, shopping, cooking, watching TV, writing, and other tasks are hard to do.

While wearing eyeglasses or contact lenses, the person has problems:

- Recognizing the faces of family and friends
- Doing tasks that require close vision—reading, cooking, sewing, and so on
- Picking out and matching the color of clothing
- Reading signs
- Doing things because lighting seems dimmer

Risk Factors Persons at risk for low vision have:

- Eye diseases
- Glaucoma
- Cataracts
- Age-related macular degeneration
- Diabetes
- Eye injuries
- Birth defects

Treatment The person learns to use one or more visual and adaptive devices. The devices used depend on the person's needs. Examples include:

- Prescription reading glasses
- Large-print reading materials
- Magnifying aids for close vision
- Telescopic aids for far vision
- A black felt tip marker for writing
- Paper with bold lines for writing
- Audio tapes
- Electronic reading machines
- Computer systems using large print
- Computer systems that talk
- Closed-circuit TV
- Phones, clocks, and watches with large numbers
- Phones designed for people who have low vision, are visually impaired, or blind
- Lighting that can be adjusted
- Dark-colored light switches and electrical outlets against light-colored walls
- Motion lights that turn on when the person enters a room

Impaired Vision and Blindness

Birth defects, accidents, and eye diseases are among the causes of impaired vision and blindness. They also are complications of some diseases. Some people are totally blind. Others sense some light but have no usable vision. Others have some usable vision but cannot read newsprint. The legally blind person sees at 20 feet what a person with normal vision sees at 200 feet. See Box 37-3 for the signs and symptoms of vision problems.

Box 37-3 Signs and Symptoms of Vision Problems

The Person Complains of:

- Halos or rings around lights
- Headaches with blurry vision
- Not being able to see at night
- Spots in front of the eyes
- Eyes hurting
- Seeing flashes of light
- Seeing double
- Things looking distorted
- Needing more light

You Observe the Person:

- Bumping into things
- Hesitating when moving
- Walking close to the wall
- Groping for objects
- Touching things in an uncertain way
- Squinting to see
- Tilting the head to see
- Asking for more or different lighting
- Holding books, newspapers, and so on close to the face
- Dropping food when eating
- Having trouble making out faces
- Having trouble reading signs
- Not seeing stains on clothing
- Wearing clothes that do not match
- Acting disoriented or confused in strange settings
- Tripping on rugs

Information from the American Foundation for the Blind, Understanding Vision Loss, 2010.

According to the American Foundation for the Blind (AFB), about 1.3 million Americans are legally blind. According to AFB reports, about 6.2 million older persons (65 and older) are blind or visually impaired.

Loss of sight is serious. Adjustments can be hard and long. Special education and training are needed. Moving about, performing daily tasks, reading and writing, communicating with others, and using a guide dog are among the tasks the person needs to learn. All are needed for quality of life. The person may need some of the devices used for low vision. When caring for blind or visually impaired persons, follow the practices in Box 37-4, p. 588.

See *Focus on Rehabilitation: Impaired Vision and Blindness*, p. 589.

Box 37-4   Caring for Blind and Visually Impaired Persons

The Environment

- Report worn carpeting and other flooring.
- Keep furniture, equipment, and electrical cords out of areas where the person will walk.
- Keep table and desk chairs pushed in under the table or desk.
- Keep doors fully open or fully closed. This includes room, closet, and cabinet doors.
- Keep drawers fully closed.
- Report burnt out bulbs in rooms, lounges, dining areas, hallways, stairways, and other areas.
- Provide lighting as the person prefers. Tell the person when the lights are on or off.
- Adjust window coverings to prevent glares. Sunny days and bright, snowy days cause glares.
- Provide a consistent meal time setting:
  - Avoid plates, napkins, placemats, and tablecloths with patterns and designs. Use solid colors and provide contrast. For example, place a white plate on a dark placemat or tablecloth.
  - Have the person sit in good light above the table where he or she will eat.
  - Keep place settings the same. The knife and spoon are to the right of the plate. The fork and napkin are to the left of the plate. The glass or cup is to the right of the plate if the person is right-handed. It is to the left of the plate if the person is left-handed.
  - Arrange main dishes, side dishes, seasonings, and condiments in a straight line or in a semi-circle just beyond the person's place setting. Arrange things in the same way for each meal.
  - Explain the location of food and beverages. Use the face of a clock (Chapter 24). Or guide the person's hand to each item on the tray or place setting.
  - Cut meat, open containers, butter bread, and perform other tasks as needed.
- Keep the signal light and TV, light, and other controls within the person's reach.
- Turn on night-lights in the person's room, bathroom, and in hallways.
- Practice safety measures to prevent falls (Chapter 13).
- Orient the person to the room. Describe the layout. Also describe the location and purpose of furniture and equipment.
- Let the person move about. Let him or her touch and find furniture and equipment.
- Do not rearrange furniture and equipment.
- Complete a safety check before leaving the room. (See the inside of the front book cover.)

The Person

- Have the person use railings when climbing stairs.
- Make sure the person wears comfortable shoes that fit correctly.
- Assist with walking as needed. Offer to guide the person. Ask if he or she would like help. Respect the person's answers. If your help is accepted:
  - Offer your arm. Tell the person which arm is offered. Tap the back of your hand against the person's hand.
  - Have the person hold on to your arm just above the elbow (Fig. 37-9). Do not grab the person's arm.
  - Walk at a normal pace. Walk one step ahead of the person. Stand next to the person at the top and bottom of stairs and when crossing streets.
  - Never push, pull, or guide the person in front of you.
  - Pause when changing direction, stepping up, and stepping down.
  - Tell the person about stairs, elevators, escalators, doors, turns, furniture, and other obstructions. State if steps are up or down.
  - Have the person hold onto a railing, the wall, or other strong surface if you need to leave his or her side. Tell the person that you are leaving and what to hold on to.
- Guide the person to a seat by placing your guiding arm on the seat. The person will move his or her hand down your arm to the seat.
- Let the person do as much for himself or herself as possible. Do not do things that the person can do. Cutting meat, seasoning food, getting dressed, and putting on shoes are examples.
- Provide visual and adaptive devices. Follow the care plan.

You

- Identify yourself when you enter the room. Give your name, title, and reason for being there. Do not touch the person until you have indicated your presence.
- Ask the person how much he or she can see. Do not assume the person is totally blind or that the person has some vision.
- Identify others. Explain where each person is located and what the person is doing.
- Offer to help. Simply say "May I help you?" Respect the person's answer.
- Leave the person's belongings in the same place that you found them. Do not move or rearrange things. If you have to move things, tell the person what you moved and where.

Information from the American Foundation for the Blind, Understanding Vision Loss, 2010.

Box 37-4 Caring for Blind and Visually Impaired Persons—cont'd

Communication

- Face the person when speaking. Speak slowly and clearly.
- Use a normal tone of voice. Do not shout or speak loudly. Vision loss does not mean the person has hearing loss.
- Address the person by name. This tells the person that you are directing a comment or question to him or her.
- Speak directly to the person. Do not just talk to family and friends who are present.
- Feel free to use words such as "see," "look," "read," or "watch TV." You also can use "blind" and "visually impaired."
- Feel free to refer to colors, sizes, shapes, patterns, designs, and so on.
- Describe people, places, and things thoroughly. Do not leave out a detail because you do not think it is important.
- Warn the person of dangers. Provide a calm and clear warning. You can say "wait" first. Then describe the danger. For example, "Wait, there is ice on the walk."
- Greet the person by name when he or she enters a room. This alerts the person to your presence in the room. Tell the person who you are. Also identify others in the room.

Communication—cont'd

- Listen to the person. Give the person verbal cues that you are listening. Say "yes," "ok," "I see," "tell me more," "I don't understand," and so on.
- Answer the person's questions. Provide specific and descriptive responses.
- Give step-by-step explanations of procedures as you perform them. Say when the procedure is over.
- Give specific directions:
  - Say "right behind you," "on your left," or "in front of you." Avoid phrases like "over here" or "over there."
  - Tell the distance. For example, "Three steps in front of you" or "At the end of the hallway by the nurses' station."
  - Give landmarks if possible. Sounds and scents can serve as "landmarks." "By the kitchen" is an example.
- Tell the person when you are leaving the room or the area. If appropriate, tell the person where you are going. For example, "I'm going to go into your bathroom now."
- Tell the person when you are ending a conversation. For example, "I enjoyed hearing about your children. Thank you for sharing stories with me."

Fig. 37-9 The blind person walks slightly behind the nursing assistant. She touches the nursing assistant's arm lightly.

FOCUS ON REHABILITATION
Impaired Vision and Blindness

Rehabilitation programs help the person adjust to the vision loss and to learn to be independent. The goal is for the person to be as active as possible and to have quality of life. The AFB describes these rehabilitation services:

- Counseling to help with adjusting to the vision loss.
- Support groups. Members talk about their problems and how to cope.
- Training in home and personal skills. Preparing meals, personal care, managing money, and labeling drugs are examples.
- Communication skills. This includes using large print, special computers, tape recorders, braille, talking watches and clocks, phones with large buttons, and so on.
- Movement and travel skills. How to orient oneself in new settings, asking for help, using a long cane, and using a guide dog are examples.

Braille Braille is a touch reading and writing system using raised dots for each letter of the alphabet (Fig. 37-10, p. 590). The first 10 letters also represent the numbers 0 through 9. Braille is read by moving the hands from left to right along each line of braille (Fig. 37-11, p. 590).

Special devices allow computer access. A "braille display" sits on a desk. Using braille, the person reads information on the computer display. Braille printers allow printing computer information in braille. Braille keyboards also are available.

	a	b	c	d	e	f	g	h	i	j
	1	2	3	4	5	6	7	8	9	0

k	l	m	n	o	p	q	r	s	t

u	v	w	x	y	z	Capital sign	Numeral sign

Fig. 37-10 Braille.

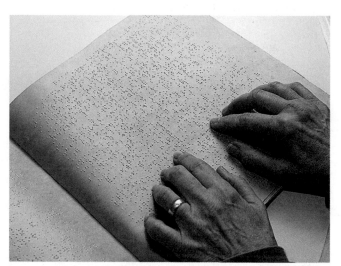

Fig. 37-11 Braille is read by moving the fingers left to right across the braille lines.

Mobility Blind and visually impaired persons learn to move about using a long cane with a red tip or using a guide dog. Both are used worldwide. The AFB describes them and measures to help as follows:

- Long canes are white or silver-gray. Some are one piece. Others fold or collapse for storage. To assist a person, announce your presence first. Ask if you can assist before trying to help. Do not interfere with the arm holding the cane. The person stores the cane. If you store it, tell the person where to find the cane.
- The guide dog sees for the person. The dog moves in response to the master's commands. Commands are disobeyed to avoid danger. For example, the master wants to cross the street. The guide dog disobeys the command if a car is approaching. Do not pet, feed, or distract a guide dog. Such actions can place the person in danger.

Corrective Lenses

Eyeglasses and contact lenses can correct many vision problems. Some people wear eyeglasses for reading or seeing at a distance. Others wear them for all activities. Contact lenses are usually worn while awake. Some contacts can be worn day and night for up to 30 days.

Eyeglasses

Lenses are hardened glass or plastic. Clean them daily and as needed. Wash glass lenses with warm water. Dry them with a lens cloth or cotton cloth. Plastic lenses scratch easily. Use special cleaning solutions and cloths.

See *Delegation Guidelines: Eyeglasses.*
See *Promoting Safety and Comfort: Eyeglasses.*

DELEGATION GUIDELINES
Eyeglasses

Cleaning eyeglasses is a routine care measure. Do not wait until the nurse tells you to clean them. Clean them daily and as needed.

To clean eyeglasses, find out if you need a special cleaning solution. Then follow the manufacturer's instructions.

PROMOTING SAFETY AND COMFORT
Eyeglasses

Safety
Eyeglasses are costly. Protect them from loss or damage. When not worn, put them in their case. Place the case in the top drawer of the bedside stand.

CARING FOR EYEGLASSES

QUALITY OF LIFE

Remember to:
- Knock before entering the person's room.
- Address the person by name.
- Introduce yourself by name and title.

- Explain the procedure to the person before beginning and during the procedure.
- Protect the person's rights during the procedure.
- Handle the person gently during the procedure.

PRE-PROCEDURE

1 Follow *Delegation Guidelines: Eyeglasses.* See *Promoting Safety and Comfort: Eyeglasses.*
2 Practice hand hygiene.

3 Collect the following:
   - Eyeglass case
   - Cleaning solution or warm water
   - Disposable lens cloth or cotton cloth

PROCEDURE

4 Remove the eyeglasses.
   a Hold the frames in front of the ears (Fig. 37-12, *A*).
   b Lift the frames from the ears. Bring the eyeglasses down away from the face (Fig. 37-12, *B*).
5 Clean the lenses with cleaning solution or warm water. Clean in a circular motion. Dry the lenses with the cloth.
6 If the person will not wear the eyeglasses:
   a Open the eyeglass case.
   b Fold the glasses. Put them in the case. Do not touch the clean lenses.
   c Place the case in the top drawer of the bedside stand.

7 If the person wears the eyeglasses:
   a Unfold the eyeglasses.
   b Hold the frames at each side. Place them over the ears.
   c Adjust the eyeglasses so the nosepiece rests on the nose.
   d Return the case to the top drawer in the bedside stand.

POST-PROCEDURE

8 Provide for comfort. (See the inside of the front book cover.)
9 Place the signal light within reach.
10 Return the cleaning solution to its proper place.
11 Discard the disposable cloth.

12 Complete a safety check of the room. (See the inside of the front book cover.)
13 Decontaminate your hands.
14 Report and record your observations.

A   B

Fig. 37-12 Removing eyeglasses. **A,** Hold the frames in the front of the ears. **B,** Lift the frames from the ears. Bring the glasses down away from the face.

Contact Lenses

Contact lenses fit on the eye. There are hard and soft contacts. Disposable ones are discarded daily, weekly, or monthly. Contacts are cleaned, removed, and stored according to the manufacturer's instructions.

Report and record the following:
- Eye redness or irritation
- Eye drainage
- Complaints of eye pain, blurred or fuzzy vision, uncomfortable lenses

See *Promoting Safety and Comfort: Contact Lenses.*

Ocular Prosthesis

Removal of an eyeball is sometimes done because of injury or disease. The person is fitted with an ocular (eye) prosthesis. See Figure 37-13. This artificial eye does not provide vision. It matches the other eye in color and shape. The other eye may have normal, some, or no vision.

Some prostheses are permanent implants. Others are removable. If removable, the person is taught to remove, clean, and insert it.

Follow these measures if the prosthesis is not inserted after removal:
- Wash it with mild soap and warm water. Rinse well.
- Line a container with a soft cloth or 4 × 4 gauze. This prevents scratches and damage.
- Fill the container with sterile water or saline (salt) solution.
- Place the eye in the container. Close the container.
- Label the container with the person's name and room and bed number.
- Place the labeled container in the top drawer of the bedside stand.
- Wash the eye socket with warm water or saline. Use a washcloth or gauze square. Remove excess moisture with a gauze square.
- Wash the eyelid and eyelashes with warm water. Clean from the inner to the outer aspect of the eye (Chapter 20). Dry the eyelid.
- Rinse the prosthesis with sterile water before the person inserts the eye.

See *Promoting Safety and Comfort: Ocular Prosthesis.*

PROMOTING SAFETY AND COMFORT
Contact Lenses

Safety
Some centers let nursing assistants remove and insert contact lenses. Others do not. Know your center's policy. If allowed to insert and remove contacts, follow the center's procedures.

PROMOTING SAFETY AND COMFORT
Ocular Prosthesis

Safety
When an ocular prosthesis is removed, you must prevent chips and scratches. It must not fall on the floor or other hard surface. Always hold the eye over a towel or other soft surface.

The prosthesis is the person's property. Protect it from loss or damage.

Fig. 37-13 An ocular prosthesis is inserted. *(From Lewis SM, Heitkemper MM, Dirksen SR: Medical-surgical nursing: assessment and management of clinical problems, ed 5, St Louis, 2000, Mosby.)*

QUALITY OF LIFE

Hearing, speech, and vision problems can interfere with quality of life. Adjustment is often long and hard. The focus is on the person's abilities. The health team promotes independence to improve quality of life. The person is allowed to control his or her life to the extent possible. He or she is encouraged to take part in the care planning process.

Provide a safe and secure setting. See Boxes 37-1, 37-2, and 37-4. And follow the person's care plan for specific safety measures. Always protect communication, hearing, and vision devices from loss or damage. This includes hearing aids, eyeglasses, and contact lenses.

Always treat the person with dignity and respect. Refer to the person first, then the disability. Say "The person who is blind" rather than "the blind person." Do not pity the person. Treat the person like an adult, not like a child. Be patient, understanding, and sensitive to the person's needs and feelings.

REVIEW QUESTIONS

Circle the BEST answer.

1 A person with Meniere's disease has
   a A middle ear infection
   b Vertigo
   c A hearing aid to correct the problem
   d A speech problem

2 Care of the person with Meniere's disease includes preventing
   a Infection   c Pain
   b Falls   d Deafness

3 Which is *not* an obvious sign of hearing loss?
   a Loneliness and boredom
   b Speaking too loudly
   c Asking to repeat things
   d Answering questions poorly

4 You are talking to a person with hearing loss. You should do the following *except*
   a Speak clearly, distinctly, and slowly
   b Sit or stand in good light
   c Shout
   d Stand or sit on the side of the better ear

5 You are talking to a person with hearing loss. You can do the following *except*
   a State the topic
   b Change the subject if the person does not seem to understand
   c Use short sentences and simple words
   d Write out key words and names

6 A hearing aid
   a Corrects a hearing problem   c Makes speech clearer
   b Makes sounds louder   d Lowers background noise

7 A hearing aid does not seem to be working. Your *first* action is to
   a See if it is turned on
   b Wash it with soap and water
   c Have it repaired
   d Remove the batteries

8 A person has aphasia. You know that
   a The person cannot use the muscles of speech
   b Mouth and face muscles are affected
   c The person has a language disorder
   d The person cannot speak

9 A person with receptive aphasia has trouble
   a Talking   c Understanding messages
   b Writing   d Using gestures

10 A person has a speech disorder. You should do the following *except*
   a Correct the person's speech
   b Have the person write key words
   c Ask the person to repeat or rephrase when necessary
   d Watch lip movements

11 A person has a cataract. Which is *false*?
   a Vision is cloudy, blurry, or dimmed.
   b Colors seem faded.
   c Central vision is lost.
   d The person is sensitive to light and glares.

12 A person had cataract surgery. You should do the following *except*
   a Follow measures for blind or visually impaired persons if an eye shield is worn
   b Let the person rub the eye
   c Place the overbed table on the un-operative side
   d Have the person wear an eye shield during naps

13 A person has age-related macular degeneration. Which is *true*?
   a There is a blind spot in the center of the eye.
   b Lost vision can be restored with surgery.
   c Peripheral (side) vision is lost.
   d Vision is blurry with spots.

14 These statements are about low vision. Which is *false*?
   a The person has usable vision.
   b Eyesight can be corrected.
   c The person needs visual or adaptive devices.
   d The person has problems doing things that require close vision.

15 Who is at risk for low vision?
   a The person with diabetic retinopathy
   b The person with global aphasia
   c The person with Meniere's disease
   d The person who is blind

16 Braille involves
   a A long cane for walking
   b Raised dots arranged for letters of the alphabet
   c A guide dog
   d Special computers and printers

17 Which are dangers to persons who are blind or visually impaired?
   a Drawers that are fully closed   c Burnt out bulbs
   b Doors that are fully open   d Night-lights

18 A person is blind. The meal time setting should
   a Be the same for every meal
   b Provide variety for mental stimulation
   c Include plates, napkins, and placemats with designs
   d Be arranged like the face of a clock

19 A person is blind. You should do the following *except*
   a Identify yourself
   b Move furniture to provide variety
   c Explain procedures step-by-step
   d Have the person walk behind you

20 You are talking to a person who is visually impaired. You should
   a Face the person when talking to him or her
   b Avoid words such as "see" and "look"
   c Avoid using colors when describing things
   d Assume that the person has no sight

21 A person is blind. To give directions you can say
   a "Over there."   c "Across the room."
   b "Right here."   d "On your left."

22 When eyeglasses are not worn they should be
   a Soaked in a cleansing solution
   b Kept within the person's reach
   c Put in the eyeglass case
   d Placed on the overbed table

Answers to these questions are on p. 721.

Cancer, Immune System, and Skin Disorders

OBJECTIVES

- Define the key terms and key abbreviations listed in this chapter.
- Explain the difference between benign tumors and cancer.
- Identify cancer risk factors.
- Identify the signs and symptoms of cancer.
- Explain the common cancer treatments.
- Describe the needs of a person with cancer.
- Explain how immune system disorders occur.
- Describe the common immune system disorders.

- Explain how the human immunodeficiency virus is spread.
- Identify the signs and symptoms of acquired immunodeficiency syndrome.
- Explain how to assist in the care of persons with acquired immunodeficiency syndrome.
- Describe the causes, signs and symptoms, and treatment of shingles.
- Explain how to promote quality of life.

KEY TERMS

benign tumor A tumor that does not spread to other body parts; it can grow to a large size

cancer See "malignant tumor"

malignant tumor A tumor that invades and destroys nearby tissue and can spread to other body parts; cancer

metastasis The spread of cancer to other body parts

stomatitis Inflammation *(itis)* of the mouth *(stomat)*

tumor A new growth of abnormal cells; tumors are benign or malignant

KEY ABBREVIATIONS

AIDS	Acquired immunodeficiency syndrome	**IV**	Intravenous
HIV	Human immunodeficiency virus		

Understanding cancer, immune system, and skin disorders gives meaning to the required care. Refer to Chapter 9 while you study this chapter.

CANCER

Cells reproduce for tissue growth and repair. Cells divide in an orderly way. Sometimes cell division and growth are out of control. A mass or clump of cells develops. This new growth of abnormal cells is called a **tumor**. Tumors are benign or malignant (Fig. 38-1):

- **Benign tumors** do not spread to other body parts. They can grow to a large size, but rarely threaten life. They usually do not grow back when removed.
- **Malignant tumors (cancer)** invade and destroy nearby tissue (Fig. 38-2). They can spread to other body parts. They may be life-threatening. Sometimes they grow back after removal.

Metastasis is the spread of cancer to other body parts (Fig. 38-3). Cancer cells break off the tumor and travel to other body parts. New tumors grow in other body parts. This occurs if cancer is not treated and controlled.

Cancer can occur almost anywhere. Common sites are the skin, lung and bronchus, colon and rectum, breast, prostate, uterus, ovary, urinary bladder, kidney, mouth and pharynx, pancreas, and thyroid gland. Cancer is the second leading cause of death in the United States.

Fig. 38-2 Malignant tumor on the skin. *(From Belcher AE: Cancer nursing, St Louis, 1992, Mosby.)*

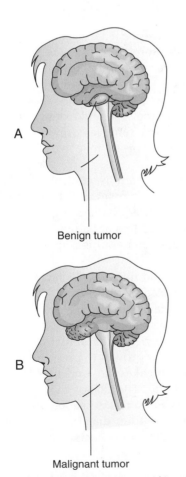

Benign tumor

Malignant tumor

Fig. 38-1 Tumors. **A,** A benign tumor grows within a local area. **B,** A malignant tumor invades other tissues.

A
Primary tumor

B
Metastases

Fig. 38-3 **A,** Tumor in the lung. **B,** Tumor has metastasized to the other lung. *(Modified from Belcher AE: Cancer nursing, St Louis, 1992, Mosby.)*

Risk Factors

Certain factors increase the risk of cancer. The National Cancer Institute describes these risk factors:

- *Growing older.* Cancer occurs in all age-groups. However, most cancers occur in persons over 65 years of age.
- *Tobacco.* This includes using tobacco (smoking, snuff, and chewing tobacco) and being around tobacco (second-hand smoke). This risk can be avoided.
- *Sunlight.* Sun, sunlamps, and tanning booths cause early aging of the skin and skin damage. These can lead to skin cancer. Limit time in the sun. Avoid sunlamps and tanning booths.
- *Ionizing radiation.* This can cause cell damage that leads to cancer. Sources are x-rays and radon gas that forms in the soil and some rocks. Miners are at risk for radon exposure. Radon is found in some homes. Radioactive fallout is another source. It can come from nuclear power plant accidents and from the production, testing, or use of atomic weapons.
- *Certain chemicals and other substances.* Painters, construction workers, and those in the chemical industry are at risk. Household substances also carry risks—paint, pesticides, used engine oil, and other chemicals.
- *Some viruses and bacteria.* Certain viruses increase the risk of these cancers—cervical, liver, lymphoma, leukemia, Kaposi's sarcoma (a cancer associated with AIDS, p. 598), stomach.
- *Certain hormones.* Hormone replacement therapy for menopause may increase the risk of breast cancer. Some pregnant women received diethylstilbestrol (DES), a form of estrogen, between the early 1940s and 1971. They are at risk for breast cancer. Their daughters are at risk for a certain type of cervical cancer.
- *Family history of cancer.* Certain cancers tend to occur in families. They include melanoma and cancers of the breast, ovary, prostate, and colon.
- *Alcohol.* More than 2 drinks a day increases the risk of certain cancers. Such cancers are of the mouth, throat, esophagus, larynx, liver, and breast. Women should have only 1 drink a day. Men should have only 2 drinks a day.
- *Poor diet, lack of physical activity, and being over-weight.* A high-fat diet increases the risk of cancers of the colon, uterus, and prostate. Lack of physical activity and being over-weight increase the risk for cancers of the breast, colon, esophagus, kidney, and uterus.

Box 38-1   Some Signs and Symptoms of Cancer

- Thickening or lump in the breast or any other part of the body
- New mole or an obvious change in an existing mole
- A sore that does not heal
- Hoarseness or cough that does not go away
- Changes in bowel or bladder habits
- Discomfort after eating
- A hard time swallowing
- Weight gain or loss with no known reason
- Unusual bleeding or discharge
- Feeling weak or very tired

From National Cancer Institute: What you need to know about™ cancer, *NIH Publication No. 06-1566, Bethesda, Md, August 2006.*

Treatment

If detected early, cancer can be treated and controlled (Box 38-1). Treatment depends on the tumor type, its site and size, and if it has spread. The treatment goal may be to:

- Cure the cancer
- Control the disease
- Reduce symptoms for as long as possible

Some cancers respond to one type of treatment. Others respond best to two or more types. Cancer treatments also damage healthy cells and tissues. Side effects depend on the type and extent of the treatment.

Surgery Surgery removes tumors. It is done to cure or control cancer or to relieve pain from advanced cancer.

Post-operative pain is controlled with pain-relief drugs. The person may feel weak or tired for a while.

Radiation Therapy Radiation therapy (*radiotherapy*) kills cells. X-ray beams are aimed at the tumor. Sometimes radioactive material is implanted in or near the tumor.

Cancer cells and normal cells receive radiation. Both are destroyed. Radiation therapy:

- Destroys certain tumors
- Shrinks a tumor before surgery
- Destroys cancer cells that remain after surgery
- Controls tumor growth to prevent or relieve pain

Burns, skin breakdown, and hair loss can occur at the treatment site. The doctor may order special skin care measures. Extra rest is needed for fatigue. Discomfort, nausea, vomiting, diarrhea, and loss of appetite (*anorexia*) are other side effects.

Chemotherapy Chemotherapy involves drugs that kill cells. It is used to:

- Shrink a tumor before surgery.
- Kill cells that break off the tumor. The goal is to prevent metastasis.
- Relieve symptoms caused by the cancer.

Cancer cells and normal cells are affected. Side effects depend on the drug used:

- Hair loss (*alopecia*).
- Gastro-intestinal irritation. Poor appetite, nausea, vomiting, and diarrhea can occur. Stomatitis, an inflammation (*itis*) of the mouth (*stomat*), may occur.
- Decreased blood cell production. Bleeding and infection are risks. The person may feel weak and tired.

Hormone Therapy Hormone therapy prevents cancer cells from getting or using hormones needed for their growth. Drugs are given that prevent the production of certain hormones. Organs or glands that produce a certain hormone are removed. For example, the ovaries are removed if a breast cancer needs estrogen for growth. A prostate cancer may need testosterone for growth. The testicles may be removed.

Side effects include fatigue, fluid retention, weight gain, hot flashes, nausea, vomiting, appetite changes, and blood clots. Fertility is affected in men and women. Men may experience impotence (Chapter 11) and loss of sexual desire.

Biological Therapy Biological therapy (*immunotherapy*) helps the immune system fight the cancer. It also protects the body from the side effects of cancer treatments.

Side effects include flu-like symptoms—chills, fever, muscle aches, weakness, loss of appetite, nausea, vomiting, and diarrhea. Bleeding, bruising, swelling, and skin rashes may occur.

The Person's Needs

Persons with cancer have many needs. They include:

- Pain relief or control
- Rest and exercise
- Fluids and nutrition
- Preventing skin breakdown
- Preventing bowel problems (constipation from pain-relief drugs; diarrhea from some cancer treatments)
- Dealing with treatment side effects
- Psychological and social needs
- Spiritual needs
- Sexual needs

Psychological and social needs are great. Anger, fear, and depression are common. Some surgeries are disfiguring. The person may feel unwhole, unattractive, or unclean. The person and family need support.

Talk to the person. Do not avoid the person because you are uncomfortable. Cancer is not contagious. Listen and use touch to show that you care. Often the person needs to talk and have someone listen. Being there when needed is important. You may not have to say anything. Just listen.

Spiritual needs are important. A spiritual leader may provide comfort. To many people, spiritual needs are just as important as physical needs.

Persons dying of cancer often receive hospice care (Chapters 1 and 48). Support is given to the person and family.

IMMUNE SYSTEM DISORDERS

The immune system protects the body from microbes, cancer cells, and other harmful substances. It defends against threats inside and outside the body.

Immune system disorders occur from problems with the immune response. The response may be inappropriate, too strong, or lacking. *Autoimmune disorders* can occur. The immune system can attack the body's own (*auto*) normal cells, tissues, or organs. One of the following may occur:

- One or more types of body tissues are destroyed.
- An organ grows abnormally.
- There is a change in how an organ functions.

The organs and tissues commonly affected are:

- Red blood cells
- Blood vessels
- Connective tissue
- The endocrine glands (thyroid gland, pancreas)
- Muscles
- Joints
- Skin

Common autoimmune disorders include:

- Graves' disease—the most common form of hyperthyroidism. The immune system attacks the thyroid gland. The thyroid gland produces excess (*hyper*) amounts of the hormone thyroxine. Signs and symptoms include anxiety, problems sleeping, rapid heart rate, weight loss, and bulging of the eyeballs (Fig. 38-4, p. 598).
- Lupus—an inflammatory disease affecting the blood cells, joints, skin, kidneys, lungs, heart, or brain. Lupus comes from the Latin word for *wolf*. It was thought that the lupus rash looked like a wolf bite (Fig. 38-5, p. 598).
- Multiple sclerosis (Chapter 39)
- Rheumatoid arthritis (Chapter 39)
- Type 1 diabetes (Chapter 41)

Signs and symptoms depend on the type of disease. Fatigue, dizziness, not feeling well, and fever are common.

Fig. 38-4 Bulging of the eyes occurs in Graves' disease. *(From Belchetz PE, Hammond P: Diabetes and endocrinology, London, 2003, Mosby.)*

Fig. 38-5 The rash from lupus is across the nose and cheeks. *(Redrawn from National Institute of Arthritis and Musculoskeletal and Skin Diseases: Do I have lupus? Bethesda, Md, National Institutes of Health. April, 2009)*

Most autoimmune disorders are chronic. Treatment depends on the disorder and the tissues and organs affected. Treatment is aimed at:
- Reducing symptoms
- Controlling the autoimmune response
- Maintaining the body's ability to fight disease

Acquired Immunodeficiency Syndrome

Acquired immunodeficiency syndrome (AIDS) is caused by a virus. The virus is called the *human immunodeficiency virus (HIV)*. It attacks the immune system. Therefore it destroys the body's ability to fight infections and certain cancers. Some infections are life-threatening.

The virus is spread through body fluids—blood, semen, vaginal secretions, and breast milk. HIV is not spread by saliva, tears, sweat, sneezing, coughing, insects, or casual contact. The virus is transmitted mainly by:
- Unprotected anal, vaginal, or oral sex with an infected person. "Unprotected" is without a new latex or polyurethane condom.
- Needle and syringe sharing among IV (intravenous) drug users.
- HIV-infected mothers before or during childbirth.
- HIV-infected mothers through breast-feeding.

The virus enters the bloodstream through the rectum, vagina, penis, mouth, or skin breaks. Small breaks in the vagina or rectum may occur when the penis, finger, or other objects are inserted. Gum disease can cause breaks in the gums. The virus can enter the bloodstream through these mucous membrane breaks (mouth, vagina, rectum). Breaks in the skin pose a risk. The virus can enter the bloodstream when infected body fluids come in contact with open skin areas. Babies can become infected during pregnancy, shortly after birth, or from breast-feeding.

The virus is carried in contaminated blood left in needles or syringes. When the devices are shared, contaminated blood enters the bloodstream. Needle-sticks are a threat to the health team.

The virus is very fragile. It cannot live outside the body. HIV is not spread by casual, everyday contact. Such contact includes using public telephones, restrooms, swimming pools, hot tubs, or water fountains. Other forms of casual contact include talking to, hugging, or dancing with an infected person. HIV is not transmitted by food prepared by the infected person.

Box 38-2 lists the signs and symptoms of AIDS. Some HIV-infected persons have symptoms within a few months. Others are symptom-free for more than 10 years. However, they carry the virus. They can spread it to others.

The person with AIDS can develop other health problems. The immune system is damaged. Pneumonia, tuberculosis, Kaposi's sarcoma (a cancer), and nervous system damage are risks. Memory loss, loss of coordination, paralysis, mental health disorders, and dementia signal nervous system damage.

Many new drugs help slow the spread of HIV in the body. They also reduce complications and prolong life. AIDS has no vaccine and no cure at present. It is a life-threatening disease.

Box 38-2   Signs and Symptoms of AIDS

- Appetite: loss of
- Cough
- Depression
- Diarrhea lasting more than a week
- Energy: lack of
- Fever
- Headache
- Memory loss, confusion, and forgetfulness
- Mouth or tongue:
  - Brown, red, pink, or purple spots or blotches
  - Sores or white patches
- Night sweats
- Pneumonia
- Shortness of breath
- Skin:
  - Rashes or flaky skin
  - Brown, red, pink, or purple spots or blotches on the skin, eyelids, or nose
- Swallowing: painful or difficult
- Swollen glands: neck, underarms, and groin
- Tiredness: may be extreme
- Vision loss
- Weight loss

Box 38-3   Caring for the Person With AIDS

- Practice Standard Precautions.
- Follow the Bloodborne Pathogen Standard.
- Provide daily hygiene. Avoid irritating soaps.
- Provide oral hygiene according to the care plan. A toothbrush with soft bristles is best.
- Provide oral fluids as ordered.
- Measure and record intake and output.
- Measure weight daily.
- Encourage deep-breathing and coughing exercises as ordered.
- Prevent pressure ulcers.
- Assist with range-of-motion exercises and ambulation as ordered.
- Encourage self-care as able. The person may need assistive devices (walker, commode, eating devices).
- Encourage the person to be as active as possible.
- Change linens and garments as often as needed when fever or night sweats are present.
- Be a good listener. Provide emotional support.

You may care for persons with AIDS or persons who are HIV carriers (Box 38-3). You may have contact with the person's blood or body fluids. Protect yourself and others from the virus. Follow Standard Precautions and the Bloodborne Pathogen Standard. A person may have the HIV virus but no symptoms. In some persons, HIV or AIDS is not yet diagnosed.

Persons age 45 years and older are at risk. The Centers for Disease Control and Prevention (CDC) reported that through 2007, there were over 244,566 cases of AIDS in persons age 45 years and older.

- Ages 45 to 54—over 176,300 cases
- Ages 55 to 64—over 52,400 cases
- Ages 65 and older—15,800 cases

Older persons get and spread HIV through sexual contact and IV drug use. Many do not consider themselves to be at risk. Older persons tend to be less informed about the disease. They tend not to practice safe sex. A blood transfusion between 1978 and 1985 increases the HIV risk.

Aging and some diseases can mask the signs and symptoms of AIDS. Older persons are less likely to be tested for HIV/AIDS. Often the person dies without the disease being diagnosed. You must follow Standard Precautions and the Bloodborne Pathogen Standard.

SKIN DISORDERS

There are many types of skin disorders. Alopecia, hirsutism, dandruff, lice, and scabies are discussed in Chapter 21. Skin tears and pressure ulcers are discussed in Chapters 35 and 36. Burns are discussed in Chapter 47. Shingles is discussed here.

Shingles

Shingles (herpes zoster) is caused by the same virus that causes chicken pox. The virus lies dormant in nerve tissue. (*Dormant* means to be *inactive*.) The virus can become active years later.

A rash or blisters occur on the skin. At first there is burning or tingling pain, numbness, or itching. This occurs in an area on one side of the body or one side of the face. After a few days or a week, a rash with fluid-filled blisters appears (Fig. 38-6, p. 600). Pain is mild to intense. Itching is a common complaint.

Shingles is most common in persons over 50 years of age. Persons who have had chicken pox are at risk. So are persons with weakened immune systems from HIV infection, cancer treatments, transplant surgeries, and stress.

The doctor orders anti-viral drugs and drugs for pain relief. For many healthy people, blisters heal and pain is gone in 3 to 5 weeks. A vaccine is now available to prevent shingles.

Fig. 38-6 Shingles. *(Courtesy Department of Dermatology, School of Medicine, University of Utah, Salt Lake City, Utah. In McCance KL, Huether SE: Pathophysiology: The biologic basis for disease in adults and children, ed. 6, St Louis, 2010, Mosby.)*

QUALITY OF LIFE

Any illness changes and affects the family. This is especially true of cancer. Unlike a cold or the flu, the person with cancer may have health problems for a long time. Cancer treatments require hospital stays and medical and clinical appointments. The same is true for AIDS and some immune system disorders. Nursing center care may be needed short- or long-term.

The person and family have many reactions. Fear, anger, worry, and guilt are common. Good communication skills are important. Sometimes all you have to do is just listen.

Remember to protect the person's rights. Privacy, confidentiality, and personal choice are very important. Also meet the person's basic needs to the best of your ability.

REVIEW QUESTIONS

Circle the BEST answer.

1 A person has cancer. You know that
   a The tumor will not threaten life
   b The tumor can spread to other body parts
   c The tumor is benign
   d The person's mouth is inflamed

2 Who has the greatest risk for cancer?
   a The person who smokes
   b The person who is physically active
   c The person who limits time in the sun
   d The person who is 40 years old

3 Which is *not* a warning sign of cancer?
   a Painful, swollen joints
   b A sore that does not heal
   c Unusual bleeding or discharge
   d Discomfort after eating

4 A person had surgery for cancer. The person's care will likely include
   a Pain-relief measures
   b Mouth care for stomatitis
   c Skin care for burns at the treatment site
   d Measures to prevent hair loss

5 A person receiving chemotherapy will likely experience
   a Diarrhea
   b Burns
   c Skin breakdown
   d Weight gain

6 Mrs. Jones has cancer. She is telling you about her treatments and how she feels. What should you do?
   a Listen.
   b Change the subject.
   c Call for the nurse.
   d Ask about her feelings.

7 HIV is spread through
   a Body fluids
   b Coughing and sneezing
   c Using public telephones and restrooms
   d Hugging or dancing with an infected person

8 HIV can enter the bloodstream in the following ways *except*
   a Through gum disease
   b Through the rectum, vagina, penis, mouth, or skin breaks
   c Through needle-sharing
   d Through swimming pools and hot tubs used by infected persons

9 Which of the following is used to prevent the spread of HIV and AIDS?
   a Isolation precautions
   b Radiation therapy
   c Chemotherapy
   d Standard Precautions

10 A person has shingles. You will likely assist the nurse with measures to
   a Prevent diarrhea
   b Relieve pain
   c Prevent skin breakdown
   d Prevent weight loss

Circle T if the statement is TRUE. Circle F if the statement is FALSE.

11 T   F   Cancer treatments damage healthy cells and tissues.

12 T   F   A person has an autoimmune disorder. The person's body has attacked its own cells, tissues, or organs.

13 T   F   Autoimmune disorders commonly affect the heart.

14 T   F   Autoimmune disorders are usually chronic.

15 T   F   A person infected with HIV does not have signs and symptoms. The person can spread the virus to others.

Answers to these questions are on p. 721.

Nervous System and Musculo-Skeletal Disorders

OBJECTIVES

- Define the key terms and key abbreviations listed in this chapter.
- Describe stroke and the care required.
- Describe Parkinson's disease and the care required.
- Describe multiple sclerosis and the care required.
- Describe amyotrophic lateral sclerosis and the care required.
- Describe traumatic brain injury and spinal cord injury and the care required.

- Describe autonomic dysreflexia and the care required.
- Describe arthritis and the care required.
- Explain how to assist in the care of persons after total joint replacement surgery.
- Describe the care required for osteoporosis.
- Explain how to assist in the care of persons in casts, in traction, and with hip pinnings.
- Describe the effects of amputation.
- Explain how to promote quality of life.

KEY TERMS

amputation The removal of all or part of an extremity

arthritis Joint (*arthr*) inflammation (*itis*)

arthroplasty The surgical replacement (*plasty*) of a joint (*arthr*)

closed fracture The bone is broken but the skin is intact; simple fracture

compound fracture See "open fracture"

fracture A broken bone

gangrene A condition in which there is death of tissue

hemiplegia Paralysis (*plegia*) on one side (*hemi*) of the body

open fracture The broken bone has come through the skin; compound fracture

paralysis Loss of motor function, loss of sensation, or both

paraplegia Paralysis in the legs and trunk

quadriplegia Paralysis in the arms, legs, and trunk; tetraplegia

simple fracture See "closed fracture"

tetraplegia See "quadriplegia"

KEY ABBREVIATIONS

ADL	Activities of daily living	**RA**	Rheumatoid arthritis
ALS	Amyotrophic lateral sclerosis	**ROM**	Range-of-motion
CVA	Cerebrovascular accident	**TBI**	Traumatic brain injury
MS	Multiple sclerosis	**TIA**	Transient ischemic attack

Understanding disorders of the nervous and musculo-skeletal systems gives meaning to the required care. Refer to Chapter 9 while you study this chapter.

NERVOUS SYSTEM DISORDERS

Nervous system disorders can affect mental and physical function. They can affect the ability to speak, understand, feel, see, hear, touch, think, control bowels and bladder, and move.

Stroke

Stroke is a disease affecting the arteries that supply blood to the brain. It also is called a *brain attack* or *cerebrovascular accident (CVA)*. It occurs when one of the following happens:

- A blood vessel in the brain bursts. Bleeding occurs in the brain (cerebral hemorrhage).
- A blood clot blocks blood flow to the brain.

Brain cells in the affected area do not get enough oxygen and nutrients. Brain cells die. Brain damage occurs. Functions controlled by that part of the brain are lost (Fig. 39-1).

Stroke is the third leading cause of death in the United States. It is a leading cause of disability in adults. See Box 39-1 for warning signs. The person needs emergency care. Blood flow to the brain must be restored as soon as possible.

Sometimes warning signs last a few minutes. This is called a *transient ischemic attack (TIA)*. (*Transient* means temporary or short term. *Ischemic* means to hold back [*ischein*] blood [*hemic*].) Blood supply to the brain is interrupted for a short time. Sometimes a TIA occurs before a stroke. All stroke-like symptoms signal the need for emergency care.

Box 39-1   Warning Signs of Stroke

- Sudden numbness or weakness of the face, arm, or leg, especially on one side of the body
- Sudden confusion, trouble speaking, or understanding speech
- Sudden trouble seeing in one or both eyes
- Sudden trouble walking, dizziness, loss of balance or coordination
- Sudden severe headache with no known cause

From National Institute for Neurological Disorders and Stroke: What you need to know about stroke, National Institutes of Health, NIH Publication No. 04-5517, Bethesda, Md, updated September 11, 2007.

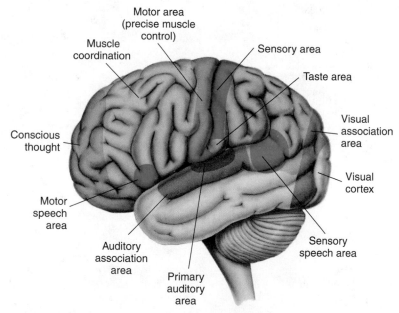

Fig. 39-1 Functions lost from a stroke depend on the area of brain damage. *(Modified from Thibodeau GA, Patton KT: The human body in health & disease, ed 5, St Louis, 2010, Mosby.)*

Risk Factors There are several risk factors for stroke. Some can be controlled, others cannot.

- *Age.* Older persons are at greater risk than younger persons.
- *Family history.* The risk increases if a parent, sister, or brother had a stroke.
- *Gender.* Both men and women are affected.
- *Race.* Blacks are at greater risk than other groups. This is because they have high rates of hypertension and diabetes.
- *Hypertension (high blood pressure).* This damages and weakens blood vessels. Clots can form. Or arteries can burst.
- *Heart disease.* Heart diseases can increase the risk of stroke. They include heart failure, heart attack, valve diseases, abnormal heart rhythm, and atherosclerosis (Chapter 40).
- *Smoking.* Blood vessels are damaged. The nicotine in cigarettes makes the heart work harder, increases the heart rate, and raises blood pressure. The amount of oxygen in the blood decreases.
- *Diabetes.* Blood vessels are damaged. The person is at risk for high blood pressure and blood clots.
- *High blood cholesterol.* Fatty materials build up on the walls of the artery and block blood flow.
- *Obesity.* The over-weight person is at risk for high blood pressure, heart disease, diabetes, and high blood cholesterol.
- *Previous stroke or TIA.* Persons who had a stroke or a TIA are at great risk.

Signs and Symptoms Stroke can occur suddenly. The person may have warning signs (see Box 39-1). The person also may have nausea, vomiting, and memory loss. Unconsciousness, noisy breathing, high blood pressure, slow pulse, redness of the face, and seizures may occur. So can hemiplegia—paralysis *(plegia)* on one side *(hemi)* of the body. The person may lose bowel and bladder control and the ability to speak. (See "Aphasia" in Chapter 37.)

Effects on the Person If the person survives, some brain damage is likely. Functions lost depend on the area of brain damage (see Fig. 39-1). The effects of stroke include:

- Loss of face, hand, arm, leg, or body control
- Hemiplegia
- Changing emotions (crying easily or mood swings, sometimes for no reason)
- Difficulty swallowing (dysphagia)
- Aphasia or slowed or slurred speech (Chapter 37)
- Changes in sight, touch, movement, and thought
- Impaired memory
- Urinary frequency, urgency, or incontinence
- Loss of bowel control or constipation
- Depression and frustration

Behavior changes occur. The person may forget about or ignore the weaker side. This is called neglect. It is from the loss of vision or movement and feeling on that side. Sometimes thinking is affected. The person may not recognize or know how to use common items. Activities of daily living (ADL) and other tasks are hard to do. The person may forget what to do and how to do it. If the person does know, the body may not respond.

Rehabilitation starts at once. The person may depend in part or totally on others for care. The health team helps the person regain the highest possible level of function (Box 39-2).

Box 39-2   Care of the Person With a Stroke

- Position the person in the lateral (side-lying) position to prevent aspiration.
- Keep the bed in semi-Fowler's position.
- Approach the person from the strong (unaffected) side. Place objects on the strong (unaffected) side. The person may have loss of vision on the affected side.
- Turn and re-position the person at least every 2 hours.
- Use assist devices to move, turn, re-position, and transfer the person.
- Encourage incentive spirometry and deep breathing and coughing.
- Prevent contractures.
- Meet food and fluids needs. The person may need a dysphagia diet (Chapter 24).
- Apply elastic stockings to prevent thrombi (blood clots) in the legs.
- Assist with range-of-motion (ROM) exercises to prevent contractures. They also strengthen affected extremities.
- Meet elimination needs:
  - The person has a catheter or bladder training program.
  - A bowel training program is started if needed.
- Practice safety precautions:
  - Keep the signal light within reach. It is on the person's strong (unaffected) side.
  - Check the person often if he or she cannot use the signal light. Follow the care plan.
  - Use bed rails according to the care plan.
  - Prevent falls.
- Have the person do as much self-care as possible. This includes turning, positioning, and transferring. The person uses assistive, self-help, and ambulation aids as needed.
- Follow established communication methods (Chapters 8 and 37).
- Give support, encouragement, and praise.
- Complete a safety check before leaving the room. (See the inside of the front book cover.)

Fig. 39-2 Signs of Parkinson's disease. *(From Thibodeau GA, Patton KT: The human body in health & disease, ed 5, St Louis, 2010, Mosby.)*

Parkinson's Disease

Parkinson's disease is a slow, progressive disorder with no cure. The area of the brain controlling muscle movement is affected. Persons over the age of 50 are at risk. Signs and symptoms become worse over time (Fig. 39-2). They include:

- *Tremors*—often start in one finger and spread to the whole arm. Pill-rolling movements—rubbing the thumb and index finger—may occur. The person may have trembling in the hands, arms, legs, jaw, and face.
- *Rigid, stiff muscles*—in the arms, legs, neck, and trunk.
- *Slow movements*—the person has a slow, shuffling gait.
- *Stooped posture and impaired balance*—it is hard to walk. Falls are a risk.
- *Mask-like expression*—the person cannot blink and smile. A fixed stare is common.

Other signs and symptoms develop over time. They include swallowing and chewing problems, constipation, and bladder problems. Sleep problems, depression, and emotional changes (fear, insecurity) can occur. So can memory loss and slow thinking. The person may have slurred, monotone, and soft speech. Some people talk too fast or repeat what they say.

Medications are ordered to treat and control the disease. Exercise and physical therapy are ordered to improve strength, posture, balance, and mobility. Therapy is needed for speech and swallowing problems. The person may need help with eating and self-care. Normal elimination is a goal. Safety measures are needed to prevent falls and injury.

Multiple Sclerosis

Multiple sclerosis (MS) is a chronic disease. *Multiple* means many. *Sclerosis* means hardening or scarring. The myelin (which covers nerve fibers) in the brain and spinal cord is destroyed. Nerve impulses are not sent to and from the brain in the normal way. Functions are impaired or lost. There is no cure.

Symptoms often start between the ages of 20 and 40. More women are affected than men. Whites are at greater risk than other groups. A person's risk increases if a family member has MS.

Signs and symptoms depend on the damaged area. They may include:

- Vision problems—blurred or double vision, blindness in one eye
- Numbness or weakness in the arms and legs
- Balance problems that affect standing and walking
- Tingling, prickling, or numb sensations
- Partial or complete paralysis
- Pain
- Speech problems
- Tremors
- Dizziness
- Problems with concentration, attention, memory, and judgment
- Depression
- Bowel and bladder problems
- Problems with sexual function
- Hearing loss
- Fatigue
- Coordination problems and clumsiness

MS can present as follows:

- *Relapsing-remitting.* Symptoms last for a few weeks or a few months. They gradually disappear with partial or total recovery. That is, symptoms *remit* or the person is in *remission*. Later, symptoms flare-up again *(relapse).*
- *Primary-progressive.* The person's condition gradually declines with more and more symptoms. There are no remissions.
- *Secondary-progressive.* Symptoms relapse and remit. More symptoms occur with each flare-up. The person's condition declines.
- *Progressive relapsing.* The person's condition gradually declines. Flare-ups occur. They leave new symptoms and more damage.

The person is kept active and independent as long as possible. The care plan reflects the person's changing needs. Skin care, hygiene, and ROM exercises are important. So are turning, positioning, and deep breathing and coughing. Bowel and bladder elimination is promoted. Injuries and complications from bedrest are prevented.

Amyotrophic Lateral Sclerosis

Amyotrophic lateral sclerosis (ALS) attacks the nerve cells that control voluntary muscles. Commonly called *Lou Gehrig's disease*, it is rapidly progressive and fatal. (Lou Gehrig was a New York Yankees baseball player. He died of the disease in 1941.)

ALS usually strikes between 40 and 60 years of age. The person usually dies 3 to 5 years after onset. Some survive for 10 or more years.

Motor nerve cells in the brain, brainstem, and spinal cord degenerate or die. They stop sending messages to the muscles. Muscles weaken, waste away (atrophy), and twitch. Over time, the brain cannot start voluntary movements or control them. The person cannot move the arms, legs, and body. Muscles for speaking, chewing, swallowing, and breathing also are affected. Eventually muscles in the chest wall fail. The person needs a ventilator for breathing (Chapter 29). The disease usually does not affect the mind or memory. Sight, smell, taste, hearing, and touch are not affected. Usually bowel and bladder functions remain intact.

ALS has no cure. Medications may slow disease progression. Damage cannot be reversed. The person is kept active and independent as long as possible. The care plan reflects the person's changing needs. The care plan may include:

*   Physical, occupational, and speech/language therapies
*   ROM exercises
*   Braces, a walker, or a wheelchair for mobility
*   Measures to relieve pain and promote comfort
*   Communication methods
*   Dysphagia diet or feeding tube
*   Suctioning to remove excess fluids and saliva
*   Mechanical ventilation
*   Safety measures to prevent falls and injuries
*   Psychological and social support
*   Hospice care

Traumatic Brain Injury

Head injuries result from trauma to the scalp, skull, or brain. Some injuries are minor and do not need health care. Or the person only needs emergency care.

Traumatic brain injury (TBI) occurs when a sudden trauma damages the brain. Brain tissue is bruised or torn. Bleeding is in the brain or in nearby tissues. Spinal cord injuries are likely. Motor vehicle crashes, falls, and firearms are common causes. So are assaults and sports and recreation injuries.

Death can occur at the time of injury or later. If the person survives TBI, some permanent damage is likely. Disabilities depend on the severity and site of the injury. They include:

*   Cognitive problems—thinking, memory, reasoning
*   Sensory problems—sight, hearing, touch, taste, smell
*   Communication problems—expressing or understanding language
*   Behavior or mental health problems—depression, anxiety, personality changes, aggressive behavior, socially inappropriate behavior
*   Stupor—an unresponsive state; the person can be briefly aroused
*   Coma—the person is unconscious, does not respond, is unaware, and cannot be aroused
*   Vegetative state—the person is unconscious and unaware of surroundings; he or she has sleep-wake cycles and alert periods
*   Persistent vegetative state (PVS)—being in a vegetative state for more than one month

Rehabilitation is required. Physical, occupational, speech/language, and mental health therapies are ordered depending on the person's needs. Nursing care depends on the person's needs and remaining abilities.

Spinal Cord Injury

Spinal cord injuries can permanently damage the nervous system. Paralysis (loss of motor function, loss of sensation, or both) can result. Young adult men have the highest risk. Common causes are stab or gunshot wounds, motor vehicle crashes, falls, and sports injuries.

Problems depend on the amount of damage to the spinal cord and the level of injury. Damage may be:

*   *Incomplete*—the spinal cord can send messages to and from the brain. The person has some sensory (feeling) and motor (movement) function below the level of the injury.
*   *Complete*—the spinal cord cannot send messages to and from the brain. The person has no sensory or motor function below the level of the injury.

The higher the level of injury, the more functions lost (Fig. 39-3, p. 606):

*   *Lumbar injuries*—sensory and muscle function in the legs is lost. Paraplegia is paralysis in the legs and trunk. (*Para* means beside or beyond; *plegia* means paralysis.)
*   *Thoracic injuries*—sensory and muscle function below the chest is lost. The person has paraplegia.
*   *Cervical injuries*—sensory and muscle function of the arms, legs, and trunk is lost. Paralysis in the arms, legs, and trunk is called quadriplegia or tetraplegia. (*Quad* and *tetra* mean four.)

Fig. 39-3 The *shaded areas* show the area of paralysis. **A,** Quadriplegia (tetraplegia). **B,** Paraplegia.

Cervical traction may be needed (p. 613). Cervical traction requires a special bed to keep the spine straight at all times. See Box 39-3 for care measures. Emotional needs require attention. Reactions to paralysis and loss of function are often severe.

If the person survives, rehabilitation is necessary. See *Focus on Rehabilitation: Spinal Cord Injury.*

Autonomic Dysreflexia This syndrome affects persons with spinal cord injuries above the mid-thoracic level. There is uncontrolled stimulation of the sympathetic nervous system (Chapter 9). If untreated, stroke, heart attack, and death are risks. Report any of these signs and symptoms to the nurse at once:
- High blood pressure
- Throbbing or pounding headache
- Bradycardia—heart rate less than 60 beats per minute
- Blurred vision
- Sweating above the level of injury
- Flushing, reddening of the skin above the level of injury
- Cold, clammy skin below the level of injury
- "Goose bumps" (*piloerection*) below the level of injury
- Nasal congestion or stuffiness
- Nausea
- Anxiety

The head of the bed is raised 45 degrees or the person sits upright if allowed. The identified cause is removed. The most common causes are a full bladder, constipation or fecal impaction, and skin disorders. The measures in Box 39-4 are part of the person's care plan.

See *Promoting Safety and Comfort: Autonomic Dysreflexia.*

Box 39-3   Care of Persons With Paralysis

- Prevent falls. Follow the care plan for safety measures and bed rail use.
- Keep the bed in the low position.
- Keep the signal light within reach. If unable to use the signal light, check the person often.
- Prevent burns. Check bath water, heat applications, and food for proper temperature.
- Turn and re-position the person at least every 2 hours. Follow the care plan.
- Prevent pressure ulcers. Follow the care plan.
- Maintain good alignment at all times. Use supportive devices according to the care plan.
- Follow bowel and bladder training programs.
- Keep intake and output records.
- Maintain muscle function and prevent contractures. Assist with ROM exercises.
- Assist with food and fluids as needed. Provide self-help devices as ordered.
- Give emotional and psychological support.
- Follow the person's rehabilitation plan.
- Complete a safety check of the room. (See the inside of the front book cover.)

FOCUS ON REHABILITATION
Spinal Cord Injury

Some rehabilitation centers focus on spinal cord injuries. The person learns to function at the highest possible level. He or she learns to use self-help, assistive, and other devices.

Some persons return home and live independently. Others need nursing center care, home care, or assisted-living settings.

Box 39-4   Preventing Autonomic Dysreflexia

- Monitor urinary output.
- Follow measures for the person with an indwelling catheter. See Box 22-3 in Chapter 22. Do not let the drainage bag get too full.
- Prevent urinary tract infections.
- Promote bowel elimination. Prevent constipation and fecal impaction.
- Prevent pressure ulcers.
- Prevent skin injuries—skin tears, cuts, bruises, blisters, and so on.
- Check the person's feet for ingrown toenails, blisters, pressure ulcers, and so on. Report any problems to the nurse.
- Prevent burns. This includes burns from hot water.
- Have the person wear clothing that is loose and comfortable. Avoid tight clothing.
- Make sure the person does not sit or lie on wrinkled clothing or linens.
- Re-position the person at least every 2 hours. Avoid prolonged pressure from the bed or chair.
- Report menstrual cramps to the nurse.

Fig. 39-4 Bony growths called *Heberden nodes* occur in the finger joints. *(From Swartz MH: Textbook of physical diagnosis, ed 5, Philadelphia, 2006, Saunders.)*

MUSCULO-SKELETAL DISORDERS

Musculo-skeletal disorders affect movement. ADL, social activities, and quality of life are affected. Injury and age-related changes are common causes.

Arthritis

Arthritis means joint *(arthr)* inflammation *(itis)*. It is the most common joint disease. Pain, swelling, and stiffness occur in the affected joints. Joints are hard to move.

Osteoarthritis (Degenerative Joint Disease) This is the most common type of arthritis. Aging, being overweight, and joint injury are causes. Stress, muscle weakness, and heredity are other causes. The fingers, spine (neck and lower back), and weight-bearing joints (hips, knees, and feet) are often affected (Fig. 39-4).

Signs and symptoms include joint stiffness, pain, swelling, and tenderness. Joint stiffness occurs with rest and lack of motion. Pain occurs with weight-bearing and joint motion. Or pain can be constant or occur from lack of motion. Pain can affect rest, sleep, and mobility. Swelling is common after using the joint. Cold weather and dampness seem to increase symptoms.

There is no cure. Treatment involves:

- *Pain relief.* Medications to decrease swelling and inflammation and relieve pain.
- *Heat and cold applications.* Heat relieves pain, increases blood flow to the part, and reduces swelling. Heat applications and warm baths or showers are helpful. So is water therapy in a heated pool. Sometimes cold applications are used after joint use.
- *Exercise.* Exercise decreases pain, increases flexibility, and improves blood flow. It helps with weight control and promotes fitness. Mental well-being improves. The person is taught what exercises to do.
- *Rest and joint care.* Good body mechanics, posture, and regular rest protect the joints. Relaxation methods are helpful. Canes and walkers provide support. Splints support weak joints and keep them in alignment. Adaptive and self-help devices for hands and wrists are useful for ADL. See Chapters 24 and 46.
- *Weight control.* Weight loss reduces stress and injury on weight-bearing joints.
- *Healthy life-style.* Arthritis support programs can help the person develop a healthy outlook. Abilities and strengths are stressed. The focus is on fitness, exercise, rest, managing stress, and good nutrition.

Falls are prevented. Help is given with ADL as needed. Toilet seat risers are helpful when hips and knees are affected. So are chairs with higher seats and armrests. Some people need joint replacement surgery (p. 608).

Rheumatoid Arthritis Rheumatoid arthritis (RA) is a chronic inflammatory disease. It causes joint pain, swelling, stiffness, and loss of function. More common in women than in men, it generally develops between the ages of 20 and 50.

RA occurs on both sides of the body. For example, if the right wrist is involved, so is the left wrist. The wrist and finger joints closest to the hand are often affected (Fig. 39-5). Other joints affected are the neck, shoulders,

Fig. 39-5 Deformities caused by rheumatoid arthritis. *(From Swartz MH: Textbook of physical diagnosis, ed 5, Philadelphia, 2006, Saunders.)*

elbows, hips, knees, ankles, and feet. Joints are tender, warm, and swollen. Fatigue and fever are common. The person does not feel well. Symptoms may last for several years.

Other body parts may be affected. Decreased red blood cell production and dry eyes and mouth are common. Inflammation of the linings of the heart, blood vessels, and lungs can occur but is rare.

RA varies from person to person. Some people have flare-ups and then feel better. In others, the disease is active most of the time.

Treatment goals are to:
• Relieve pain
• Reduce inflammation
• Slow down or stop joint damage
• Improve well-being and function
The person's care plan may include:
• *Rest balanced with exercise.* More rest is needed when RA is active. More exercise is needed when it is not. Short rest periods during the day are better than long times in bed. The doctor and physical therapist prescribe an exercise program. ROM exercises are included. Exercise helps maintain healthy and strong muscles, joint mobility, and flexibility. Exercise also promotes sleep, reduces pain, and helps weight control.
• *Proper positioning.* Prevent contractures and deformities. Bed-boards, a bed cradle, trochanter rolls, and pillows are used.
• *Joint care.* Good body mechanics and body alignment, wrist and hand splints, and self-help devices for ADL reduce stress on the joints. Walking aids may be needed.
• *Weight control.* Excess weight places stress on the weight-bearing joints. Exercise and a healthy diet help control weight.
• *Measures to reduce stress.* Relaxation, distraction, and regular rest help reduce stress. So does exercise.
• *Measures to prevent falls.* See Chapter 13.

Medications are given for pain relief and to reduce inflammation. Heat and cold applications may be ordered. Some persons need joint replacement surgery.

Emotional support is needed. A good outlook is important. Persons with RA need to stay as active as possible. The more they can do for themselves, the better off they are. Give encouragement and praise. Listen when the person needs to talk.

Total Joint Replacement Surgery   Arthroplasty is the surgical replacement (*plasty*) of a joint (*arthro*). The damaged joint is removed and replaced with an artificial joint—a prosthesis (Fig. 39-6).

Hip and knee replacements are the most common (Box 39-5). Ankle, foot, shoulder, elbow, and finger joints also can be replaced. The surgery can relieve pain, restore or preserve joint function, or correct a deformed joint.

Fig. 39-6 A, Hip replacement prosthesis. Hip replacement prosthesis stems. **B,** Knee replacement prosthesis. *(Courtesy Zimmer, Inc., a Bristol-Meyers Squibb Co., Warsaw, Ind.)*

Box 39-5 Care of the Person After Total Joint Replacement Surgery—Hip and Knee

- Incentive spirometry and deep-breathing and coughing exercises to prevent respiratory complications.
- Elastic stockings to prevent thrombi (blood clots) in the legs.
- Exercises to strengthen the hip or knee. These are taught by a physical therapist.
- Measures to protect the hip as shown in Figure 39-7.
- Food and fluids for tissue healing and to restore strength.

- Safety measures to prevent falls.
- Measures to prevent infection. Wound, urinary tract, and skin infections must be prevented.
- Measures to prevent pressure ulcers.
- Assist devices for moving, turning, re-positioning, and transfers.
- Assistance with walking and a walking aid. The person may need a cane, walker, or crutches.

Do

Do Not

Do not cross your operated leg past the midline of the body or turn your kneecap in toward your body.

Do not sit in low chairs or cross your legs.

To sit: Use a high chair with arms or add pillows to elevate the seat.

Avoid flexing your hips past 90 degrees.

To bend: Keep the operative leg behind you or as instructed by your therapist.

To reach: Use long-handled grabbers or as therapist advises.

Use an elevated toilet.

Sleep with a pillow between the legs.

Fig. 39-7 Measures to protect the hip after total hip replacement surgery. *(Modified from Monahan FD and others:* Phipps' medical-surgical nursing: health and illness perspectives, *ed 8, St Louis, 2007, Mosby.)*

Osteoporosis With osteoporosis, the bone (*osteo*) becomes porous and brittle (*porosis*). Bones are fragile and break easily. Spine, hip, wrist, and rib fractures are common. Older men and women are at risk. The risk for women increases after menopause. The ovaries do not produce estrogen after menopause. The lack of estrogen causes bone changes. So do low levels of dietary calcium.

All ethnic groups are at risk. A family history of the disease, being thin or having a small frame, eating disorders (Chapter 43), tobacco use, alcoholism, lack of exercise, bedrest, and immobility are risk factors. Exercise and activity are needed for bone strength. To form properly, bone must bear weight. If not, calcium leaves the bone. The bone becomes porous and brittle.

Back pain, gradual loss of height, and stooped posture occur. Fractures are a major threat. Even slight activity can cause fractures. They can occur from turning in bed, getting up from a chair, or coughing. Fractures are great risks from falls and accidents.

Prevention is important. Doctors often order calcium and vitamin supplements. Estrogen is ordered for some women. Other preventive measures include:

- Exercising weight-bearing joints—walking, jogging, stair climbing
- Strength-training (lifting weights)
- No smoking
- Limiting alcohol and caffeine
- Back supports or corsets if needed for good posture
- Walking aids if needed
- Safety measures to prevent falls and accidents
- Good body mechanics
- Safe handling, moving, transfer, and turning and positioning procedures

Fractures

A fracture is a broken bone. Tissues around the fracture muscles, blood vessels, nerves, and tendons—are injured. Fractures are open or closed (Fig. 39-8):

- **Closed fracture (simple fracture).** The bone is broken but the skin is intact.
- **Open fracture (compound fracture).** The broken bone has come through the skin.

Falls and accidents are causes. Bone tumors, metastatic cancer, and osteoporosis are other causes. Signs and symptoms of a fracture are:

- Pain
- Swelling
- Loss of function
- Limited or no movement of the part
- Movement where motion should not occur
- Deformity (the part is in an abnormal position)
- Bruising and skin color changes at the fracture site
- Bleeding (internal or external)

For healing, bone ends are brought into and held in normal position. This is called *reduction* and *fixation*:

- *Closed reduction and external fixation.* The bone is moved back into place. The bone is not exposed.
- *Open reduction and internal fixation.* This requires surgery. The bone is exposed and moved into alignment. Nails, rods, pins, screws, plates, or wires keep the bone in place (Fig. 39-9).

After reduction, movement of the bone ends is prevented. This is done with a cast or traction. Other devices—splints, walking boots, external fixators—also are used (Fig. 39-10).

Fig. 39-8 A, Open fracture. **B,** Closed fracture. *(From Thibodeau GA, Patton KT: The human body in health & disease, ed 5, St Louis, 2010, Mosby.)*

Fig. 39-9 Devices used for open reduction of a fracture. *(From Beare PG, Meyers JL:* Adult health nursing, *ed 3, St Louis, 1998, Mosby.)*

Fig. 39-10 External fixator. *(From Lewis SM, Heitkemper MM, Dirksen SR:* Medical-surgical nursing: assessment and management of clinical problems, *ed 7, St Louis, 2007, Mosby.)*

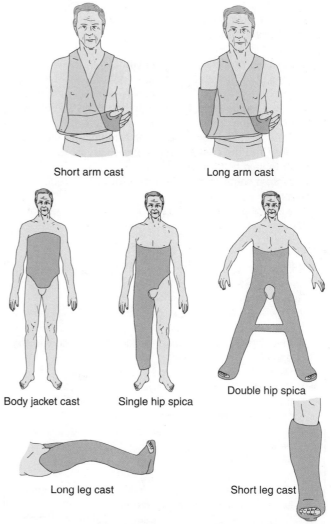

Short arm cast   Long arm cast

Body jacket cast   Single hip spica   Double hip spica

Long leg cast   Short leg cast

Fig. 39-11 Common casts.

Casts Casts are made of plaster of paris, plastic, or fiberglass (Fig. 39-11). Before casting, the skin is protected with stockinette or cotton padding. Moistened cast rolls are wrapped around the part. Plastic and fiberglass casts dry quickly. A plaster of paris cast dries in 24 to 48 hours. It is odorless, white, and shiny when dry. A wet cast is gray and cool and has a musty smell. Assist with care as directed (Box 39-6, p. 612).

Box 39-6 Rules for Cast Care

- Do not cover the cast with blankets, plastic, or other material. A cast gives off heat as it dries. Covers prevent the escape of heat. Burns can occur if heat cannot escape.
- Turn the person every 2 hours or as directed by the nurse and the care plan. All cast surfaces need exposure to air. Turning promotes even drying.
- Do not place a wet cast on a hard surface. It flattens the cast. The cast must keep its shape. Use pillows to support the entire length of the cast (Fig. 39-12).
- Support the wet cast with your palms when turning and positioning the person (Fig. 39-13). Fingertips can dent the cast. The dents can cause pressure areas that lead to skin breakdown.
- Report rough cast edges. The nurse needs to cover the cast edges with tape.
- Keep the cast dry. A wet cast loses its shape. Some casts are near the perineal area. The nurse may apply a waterproof material around the perineal area after the cast dries.
- Do not let the person insert anything into the cast. Itching under the cast causes an intense desire to scratch. Items used for scratching (pencils, coat hangers, knitting needles, back scratchers, and so on) can open the skin. Infection is a risk. Scratching items can wrinkle the stockinette or cotton padding. Or they can be lost into the cast. Both can cause pressure and lead to skin breakdown.
- Elevate a casted arm or leg on pillows. This reduces swelling.
- Have enough help to turn and re-position the person. Plaster casts are heavy and awkward. Balance is lost easily.
- Position the person as directed.
- Follow the care plan for elimination needs. Some persons use a fracture pan.
- Report these signs and symptoms at once:
  - *Pain*—pressure ulcer, poor circulation, nerve damage
  - *Swelling and a tight cast*—reduced blood flow to the part
  - *Pale skin*— reduced blood flow to the part
  - *Cyanosis (bluish skin color)*—reduced blood flow to the part
  - *Odor*—infection
  - *Inability to move the fingers or toes*—pressure on a nerve
  - *Numbness*—pressure on a nerve, reduced blood flow to the part
  - *Temperature changes*—cool skin means poor circulation; hot skin means inflammation
  - *Drainage on or under the cast*—infection or bleeding
  - *Chills, fever, nausea, and vomiting*—infection
- Complete a safety check before leaving the room. (See the inside of the front book cover.)

Fig. 39-12 Pillows support the entire length of the wet cast. *(From Harkness GA, Dincher JR: Medical-surgical nursing: total patient care, ed 10, St Louis, 1999, Mosby.)*

Fig. 39-13 The cast is supported with the palms.

Traction Traction reduces and immobilizes fractures. A steady pull from two directions keeps the bone in place. Traction also is used for muscle spasms and to correct deformities or contractures. Weights, ropes, and pulleys are used (Fig. 39-14). Traction is applied to the neck, arms, legs, or pelvis.

Skin traction is applied to the skin. Boots, wraps, tape, or splints are used. Weights are attached to the device (see Fig. 39-14). *Skeletal traction* is applied to the bone. Wires or pins are inserted through the bone (Fig. 39-15). For cervical traction, tongs are applied to the skull (Fig. 39-16). Weights are attached to the device.

Assist with the person's care as directed (Box 39-7).

Fig. 39-14 Traction set-up. Note the weights, pulleys, and ropes. *(From Monahan FD and others:* Phipps' medical-surgical nursing: health and illness perspectives, *ed 8, St Louis, 2007, Mosby.)*

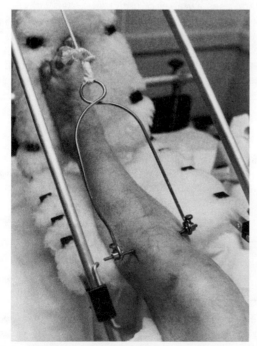

Fig. 39-15 Skeletal traction is attached to the bone. *(From Christensen BL, Kockrow EO:* Adult health nursing, *ed 6, St Louis, 2011, Mosby.)*

Fig. 39-16 Tongs are inserted into the skull for cervical spine traction. *(From Monahan FD and others:* Phipps' medical-surgical nursing: health and illness perspectives, *ed 8, St Louis, 2007, Mosby.)*

Box 39-7   Caring for Persons in Traction

- Keep the person in good alignment.
- Do not remove the traction.
- Keep the weights off the floor. Weights must hang freely from the traction set-up (see Fig. 39-14).
- Do not add or remove weights from the traction set-up.
- Check for frayed ropes. Report fraying at once.
- Perform ROM exercises for the uninvolved joints as directed.
- Position the person as directed. Usually only the back-lying position is allowed. Sometimes slight turning is allowed.
- Provide the fracture pan for elimination.
- Give skin care as directed.
- Put bottom linens on the bed from the top down. The person uses a trapeze to raise the body off the bed.
- Check pin, nail, wire, or tong sites for redness, drainage, and odors. Report observations at once.
- Observe for the signs and symptoms listed under cast care (see Box 39-6). Report them at once.
- Complete a safety check before leaving the room. (See the inside of the front book cover.)

Fractures
in head
and neck
of femur

Fig. 39-17 Hip fracture repaired with a prosthesis. *(Modified from Christensen BL, Kockrow EO:* Adult health nursing, *ed 6, St Louis, 2011, Mosby.)*

Hip Fractures Fractured hips are common in older persons (Fig. 39-17). Older women are at risk. Slow healing and other health problems affect the older person's condition and care.

Post-operative problems present life-threatening risks. They include pneumonia, atelectasis (collapse of a part of a lung), urinary tract infections, and thrombi (blood clots) in the leg veins. Pressure ulcers, constipation, and confusion are other risks.

The fracture requires internal fixation (p. 610). Some hip fractures require partial or total hip replacement. Adduction, internal rotation, external rotation, and severe hip flexion are avoided after surgery. Rehabilitation is usually needed. If home care is not possible, the person needs subacute or long-term care. Recovery can take 6 months. Some persons return home after successful rehabilitation. Others stay in nursing centers. See Box 39-8 for the care required after surgery for a hip fracture.

Box 39-8 Care of the Person With a Hip Fracture

- Give good skin care. Skin breakdown can occur rapidly.
- Follow the care plan to prevent pressure ulcers.
- Follow the care plan to prevent wound, skin, and urinary tract infections.
- Encourage incentive spirometry and deep-breathing and coughing exercises as directed.
- Turn and position the person as directed. Turning and positioning depend on the type of fracture and the surgery. Usually the person is not positioned on the operative side.
- Prevent external rotation of the hip. Use trochanter rolls, pillows, and sandbags as directed.
- Keep the leg abducted at all times. The leg is abducted when the person is supine, being turned, or in a side-lying position. Use pillows (Fig. 39-18) or a hip abduction wedge (abductor splint) as directed. Do not exercise the affected leg.
- Provide a straight-back chair with armrests. The person needs a high, firm seat. A low, soft chair is not used.
- Place the chair on the unaffected side.
- Use assist devices to move, turn, re-position, and transfer the person.
- Do not let the person stand on the operated leg unless allowed by the doctor.
- Elevate the leg according to the care plan. With an internal fixation device, the leg is not elevated when the person sits in a chair. Elevating the leg puts strain on the device.
- Apply elastic stockings to prevent thrombi (blood clots) in the legs.
- Remind the person not to cross his or her legs.
- Assist with ambulation according to the care plan. The person uses a walker or crutches.
- Follow measures to protect the hip. See Box 39-5 and Figure 39-7, p. 609.
- Practice safety measures to prevent falls.
- Complete a safety check before leaving the room. (See the inside of the front book cover.)

Fig. 39-18 Pillows are used to keep the hip in abduction. *(From Monahan FD and others:* Phipps' medical-surgical nursing: health and illness perspectives, *ed 8, St Louis, 2007, Mosby.)*

Loss of Limb

An amputation is the removal of all or part of an extremity. Most amputations involve a lower extremity. Severe injuries, tumors, severe infection, gangrene, and vascular disorders are common causes. Diabetes is a common cause of vascular changes leading to amputation.

Gangrene is a condition in which there is death of tissue. It can cause death. Causes include infection, injuries, and vascular disorders. Blood flow is affected. Tissues do not get enough oxygen and nutrients. Poisonous substances and wastes build up in the tissues. Tissues die and become black, cold, and shriveled (Fig. 39-19). Surgery is needed to remove dead tissue. If untreated, gangrene spreads throughout the body. For example, in diabetes the toes are usually affected first. If affected toes are not removed, gangrene spreads up the foot and to the knee.

The amputation affects the person's life. Body image, appearance, daily activities, movement, and work are some areas affected. Fear, shock, anger, denial, and depression are common emotions. Much support is needed.

The person is fitted with a prosthesis—an artificial replacement for a missing body part (Fig. 39-20). First the stump is conditioned so the prosthesis fits. This involves shrinking and shaping the stump into a cone shape with bandages (Fig. 39-21). The person learns exercises to strengthen other limbs. Occupational and physical therapists help the person use the prosthesis.

The person may feel that the limb is still there. Aching, tingling, and itching are common sensations. Or the person may complain of pain in the amputated part. Called *phantom limb pain,* this is a normal reaction. It may occur for a short time or for many years.

Lower limb amputations are common in older persons. Because of other health problems, many cannot use a prosthesis. They need to use wheelchairs. After amputation, most older persons need temporary or permanent nursing center care.

Fig. 39-20 Leg prostheses. **A,** Above-the-knee prosthesis. **B,** Below-the-knee prosthesis. *(Courtesy Otto Bock Health Care, Minneapolis, Minn.)*

Fig. 39-21 A mid-thigh amputation is bandaged to shrink and shape the stump. *(From Monahan FD and others: Phipps' medical-surgical nursing: health and illness perspectives, ed 8, St Louis, 2007, Mosby.)*

QUALITY OF LIFE

A person may have one or many problems affecting the nervous and musculo-skeletal systems. For example, a person with a stroke may fall and fracture a hip. He or she may also have arthritis and osteoporosis. The care plan depends on the person's problems and needs.

The care you give affects the person's quality of life. Safety, good alignment, and turning and re-positioning are important. So is skin care. Quality-of-life issues discussed for such care apply.

Always protect the person's rights. Privacy, confidentiality, and personal choice are examples. Also guard against abuse, mistreatment, and neglect.

Fig. 39-19 Gangrene. *(Courtesy Cameron Bangs, MD. From Auerbach PS: Wilderness medicine, management of wilderness and environmental emergencies, ed 3, St Louis, 1995, Mosby.)*

REVIEW QUESTIONS

Circle the BEST answer.

1 A stroke also is called
   a A cerebrovascular accident
   b Aphasia
   c Hemiplegia
   d A transient ischemic attack

2 Warning signs of stroke occur
   a With exertion
   b Suddenly
   c Between the ages of 20 and 40
   d At rest

3 A person had a stroke. Which measure should you question?
   a Semi-Fowler's position
   b Range-of-motion exercises every 2 hours
   c Turn, re-position, and give skin care every 2 hours
   d Bed in the highest horizontal position

4 A person has Parkinson's disease. Which is *false*?
   a The part of the brain controlling muscle movements is affected.
   b Mental function is affected first.
   c Tremors, slow movements, and a shuffling gait occur.
   d The person needs protection from injury.

5 Parkinson's disease
   a Can be cured with medications
   b Can be cured with surgery
   c Is a slow, progressive disorder
   d Progresses rapidly

6 A person has multiple sclerosis. Which is *false*?
   a There is no cure.
   b Only voluntary muscles are affected.
   c Symptoms begin in young adulthood.
   d Over time, the person depends on others for care.

7 A person has multiple sclerosis. Signs, symptoms, and the care required depend on the area of damage.
   a True
   b False

8 Amyotrophic lateral sclerosis affects nerve cells that control
   a Involuntary muscles   **c** The brain
   b Voluntary muscles   **d** The lungs

9 A person has amyotrophic lateral sclerosis. Which measure should you question?
   a ROM exercises
   b Dysphagia diet
   c Walker for mobility
   d Measures to prevent confusion

10 Persons with brain or spinal cord injuries require
   a Rehabilitation   **c** Long-term care
   b Speech therapy   **d** Chemotherapy

11 A person has quadriplegia from a spinal cord injury. Which measure should you question?
   a Keep the bed in the low position.
   b Assist with active ROM exercises.
   c Follow the bowel training program.
   d Turn and re-position every hour.

12 Autonomic dysreflexia occurs
   a After spinal cord injuries
   b In Parkinson's disease
   c With Lou Gehrig's disease
   d Following stroke

13 Autonomic dysreflexia is usually triggered by
   a High blood sugar
   b High blood pressure
   c A full bladder
   d A virus

14 Arthritis affects
   a The joints
   b The bones
   c The muscles
   d The hips and knees

15 A person has arthritis. Care includes the following *except*
   a Preventing contractures
   b ROM exercises
   c A cast or traction
   d Assisting with ADL

16 A person had hip replacement surgery. Which measure should you question?
   a Provide a chair with a low seat.
   b Do not cross the legs.
   c Keep a hip abduction wedge between the legs.
   d Provide a long-handled brush for bathing.

17 A person with osteoporosis is at risk for
   a Fractures
   b An amputation
   c Phantom limb pain
   d Paralysis

18 A cast needs to dry. Which is *false*?
   a The cast is covered with blankets and plastic.
   b The person is turned so the cast dries evenly.
   c The entire cast is supported with pillows.
   d The cast is supported by the palm when lifted.

19 A person has a cast. You report the following at once *except*
   a Pain, numbness, or inability to move the fingers
   b Chills, fever, nausea, or vomiting
   c Odor, cyanosis, or temperature changes of the skin
   d Pulse rate of 75 beats per minute

20 A person is in traction. Care includes the following *except*
   a Performing ROM exercises as directed
   b Keeping weights off the floor
   c Removing weights if the person is uncomfortable
   d Giving skin care at frequent intervals

21 After a hip pinning, the operated leg is
   a Abducted at all times
   b Adducted at all times
   c Externally rotated at all times
   d Flexed at all times

22 After an amputation, the person
   a Is fitted with a prosthesis
   b Needs a wheelchair
   c Has quadriplegia
   d Needs arthroplasty

Answers to these questions are on p. 721.

Cardiovascular and Respiratory Disorders

OBJECTIVES

- Define the key terms and key abbreviations listed in this chapter.
- Describe hypertension, its risk factors, signs and symptoms, complications, and treatment.
- Describe coronary artery disease, its risk factors, and complications.
- Describe cardiac rehabilitation.
- Describe angina, its signs and symptoms, and treatment.
- Describe myocardial infarction, its signs and symptoms, and treatment.
- Describe heart failure, its signs and symptoms, and treatment.

- Describe chronic obstructive pulmonary disease, its signs and symptoms, and treatment.
- Describe asthma, its signs and symptoms, and treatment.
- Explain the difference between a cold and influenza.
- Explain how influenza is treated.
- Describe pneumonia, its signs and symptoms, and treatment.
- Describe tuberculosis, its signs and symptoms, and treatment.
- Explain how to promote quality of life.

KEY TERMS

high blood pressure See "hypertension"

hypertension The systolic pressure is 140 mm Hg or higher *(hyper)*, or the diastolic pressure is 90 mm Hg or higher; high blood pressure

pre-hypertension When the systolic pressure is between 120 and 139 mm Hg or the diastolic pressure is between 80 and 89 mm Hg

KEY ABBREVIATIONS

CAD	Coronary artery disease	**MI**	Myocardial infarction
CDC	Centers for Disease Control and Prevention	**mm Hg**	Millimeters of mercury
CO$_2$	Carbon dioxide	**O$_2$**	Oxygen
COPD	Chronic obstructive pulmonary disease	**TB**	Tuberculosis

Cardiovascular and respiratory system disorders are leading causes of death in the United States. Many people have these disorders. Refer to Chapter 9 while you study this chapter.

CARDIOVASCULAR DISORDERS

Problems occur in the heart or blood vessels. See Chapter 35 for circulatory ulcers. Risk factors for cardiovascular disorders are listed in Box 40-1.

Hypertension

With **hypertension (high blood pressure)**, the resting blood pressure is too high. The systolic pressure is 140 mm Hg (millimeters of mercury) or higher (*hyper*). Or the diastolic pressure is 90 mm Hg or higher. Such measurements must occur several times. **Pre-hypertension** is when the systolic pressure is between 120 and 139 mm Hg or the diastolic pressure is between 80 and 89 mm Hg.

The person with pre-hypertension will likely develop hypertension in the future. Most people have hypertension some time during their lives. See Box 40-1 for risk factors.

Narrowed blood vessels are a common cause. The heart pumps with more force to move blood through narrowed vessels. Kidney disorders, head injuries, some pregnancy problems, and adrenal gland tumors are causes.

A person can be unaware of hypertension for many years. That is why hypertension is called "the silent killer." Hypertension is found when blood pressure is measured. Signs and symptoms develop over time. Headache, blurred vision, dizziness, and nose bleeds occur. Hypertension can lead to stroke, hardening of the arteries, heart attack, heart failure, kidney failure, and blindness.

Life-style changes can lower blood pressure. A diet low in fat and salt, a healthy weight, and regular exercise are needed. No smoking is allowed. Alcohol and caffeine are limited. Managing stress and sleeping well also lower blood pressure. Certain medications lower blood pressure.

Coronary Artery Disease

The coronary arteries are in the heart. They supply the heart with blood. In coronary artery disease (CAD), the coronary arteries become hardened and narrow. One or all are affected. The heart muscle gets less blood and oxygen (O_2). CAD also is called *coronary heart disease* and *heart disease*.

The most common cause is *atherosclerosis* (Fig. 40-1). Plaque—made up of cholesterol, fat, and other substances—collects on artery walls. The narrowed arteries block blood flow. Blockage may be total or partial. Blood clots can form along the plaque and block blood flow.

Box 40-1   Risk Factors for Cardiovascular Disorders

Hypertension

Factors You Cannot Change
- Age—45 years or older for men; 55 years or older for women
- Gender—younger men are at greater risk than younger women; the risk increases for women after menopause
- Race—African-Americans are at greater risk than whites
- Family history—tends to run in families

Factors You Can Change
- Being over-weight
- Stress
- Tobacco use
- High-salt diet
- Excessive alcohol
- Lack of exercise
- Atherosclerosis
- Pre-hypertension

Coronary Artery Disease

Factors You Cannot Change
- Gender—men are at greater risk than women
- Age—in men, the risk increases after age 45; in women, the risk increases after age 55
- Family history
- Race—African-Americans are at greater risk than other groups

Factors You Can Change
- Being over-weight
- Lack of exercise
- High blood cholesterol
- Hypertension
- Smoking
- Diabetes

Fig. 40-1 **A,** Normal artery. **B,** Plaque on the artery wall in atherosclerosis.

The major complications of CAD are angina, myocardial infarction (heart attack), irregular heartbeats, and sudden death. The more risk factors, the greater the chance of CAD and its complications. See Box 40-1 for risk factors.

CAD can be treated. Treatment goals are to:
- Relieve symptoms (see "Angina")
- Slow or stop atherosclerosis
- Lower the risk of blood clots
- Widen or bypass clogged arteries
- Reduce cardiac events (see "Angina" and "Myocardial Infarction," p. 620)

Persons with CAD need to make life-style changes. The person must quit smoking, exercise, and reduce stress. A healthy diet is needed to reduce high blood pressure, lower blood cholesterol, and maintain a healthy weight. If over-weight, the person must lose weight.

Some persons need medications to decrease the heart's workload and relieve symptoms. Other medications are given to prevent a heart attack or sudden death. Medications can delay the need for medical and surgical procedures that open or bypass diseased arteries (Fig. 40-2).

See *Focus on Rehabilitation: Coronary Artery Disease.*

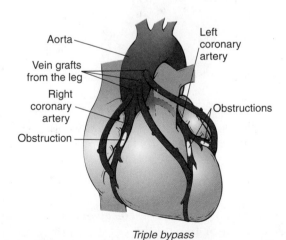

Fig. 40-2 Triple coronary artery bypass surgery. *(Modified from Thibodeau GA, Patton KT: The human body in health & disease, ed 5, St Louis, 2010, Mosby.)*

Labels in figure: Aorta; Left coronary artery; Vein grafts from the leg; Right coronary artery; Obstructions; Obstruction; *Triple bypass*

FOCUS ON REHABILITATION
Coronary Artery Disease

Persons with complications from CAD may need cardiac rehabilitation (cardiac rehab). The cardiac rehab team includes doctors (the person's doctor, a heart specialist, a heart surgeon), nurses, exercise specialists, physical and occupational therapists, dietitians, and mental health professionals.

Cardiac rehab has two parts:
- Exercise training. The person learns to exercise safely. Exercises are done to strengthen muscles and improve stamina (staying power, endurance). The exercise plan is based on the person's abilities, needs, and interests.
- Education, counseling, and training. The person learns about:
  - His or her heart condition
  - How to reduce the risk of future problems
  - How to adjust to a new life-style
  - How to deal with fears about the future

Angina

Angina *(pain)* is chest pain from reduced blood flow to part of the heart muscle (myocardium). It occurs when the heart needs more O_2. Normally blood flow to the heart increases when O_2 needs increase. Exertion, a heavy meal, stress, and excitement increase the heart's need for O_2. So does smoking and very hot or cold temperatures. In CAD, narrowed vessels prevent increased blood flow.

Chest pain is described as a tightness, pressure, squeezing, or burning in the chest (Fig. 40-3, p. 620). Pain can occur in the shoulders, arms, neck, jaw, or back. Pain in the jaw, neck, and down one or both arms is common. The person may be pale, feel faint, and perspire. Dyspnea is common. Nausea, fatigue, and weakness may occur. Some persons complain of "gas" or indigestion. Rest often relieves symptoms in 3 to 15 minutes. Rest reduces the heart's need for O_2. Therefore normal blood flow is achieved. Heart damage is prevented.

Besides rest, a nitroglycerin tablet is taken when angina occurs. It is placed under the tongue. There it dissolves and is rapidly absorbed into the bloodstream. Tablets are kept within the person's reach at all times. The person takes a tablet and then tells the nurse. Some persons have nitroglycerin patches. The nurse applies and removes them.

Things that cause angina are avoided. These include over-exertion, heavy meals and over-eating, and emotional stress. The person needs to stay indoors during cold weather or during hot, humid weather. Doctor-supervised programs are helpful.

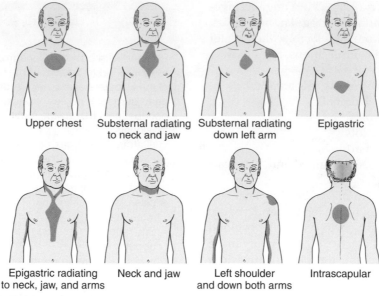

Fig. 40-3 *Shaded areas* show where the pain of angina is located. *(From Lewis SM, Heitkemper MM, Dirksen SR: Medical-surgical nursing: assessment and management of clinical problems, ed 7, St Louis, 2007, Mosby.)*

See "Coronary Artery Disease" for the treatment of angina. The goal is to increase blood flow to the heart. Doing so may prevent or lower the risk of heart attack and death. Chest pain lasting longer than a few minutes and not relieved by rest and nitroglycerin may signal heart attack. The person needs emergency care.

Myocardial Infarction

Myocardial refers to the heart muscle. *Infarction* means tissue death. With myocardial infarction (MI), part of the heart muscle dies. Sudden cardiac death *(sudden cardiac arrest)* can occur (Chapter 47).

MI also is called:
- Heart attack
- Acute myocardial infarction (AMI)
- Acute coronary syndrome (ACS)
- Coronary
- Coronary thrombosis
- Coronary occlusion

In MI, blood flow to the heart muscle is suddenly blocked. A thrombus (blood clot) blocks blood flow in an artery with atherosclerosis. The damaged area may be small or large (Fig. 40-4).

CAD, angina, and previous MI are risk factors. See Box 40-2 for signs and symptoms. MI is an emergency. Efforts are made to:
- Relieve pain
- Restore blood flow to the heart
- Stabilize vital signs
- Give oxygen
- Calm the person
- Prevent death and life-threatening problems

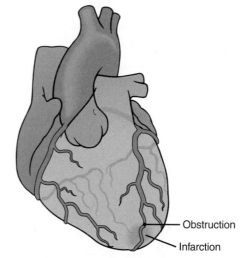

Fig. 40-4 Myocardial infarction. *(Modified from Lewis SM, Heitkemper MM, Dirksen SR: Medical-surgical nursing: assessment and management of clinical problems, ed 7, St Louis, 2007, Mosby.)*

The person may need medical or surgical procedures to open or bypass the diseased artery. Cardiac rehabilitation is needed. The goals are to:
- Recover and resume normal activities
- Prevent another MI
- Prevent complications such as heart failure or sudden cardiac arrest

Box 40-2	Signs and Symptoms of Myocardial Infarction

- Chest pain
  - Sudden, severe; usually on the left side
  - Described as crushing, stabbing, or squeezing; some describe it as someone sitting on the chest
  - More severe and lasts longer than angina
  - Not relieved by rest and nitroglycerin
- Pain or numbness in one or both arms, the back, neck, jaw, or stomach
- Indigestion or "heartburn"
- Dyspnea
- Nausea
- Dizziness
- Perspiration and cold, clammy skin
- Pallor or cyanosis
- Blood pressure: low
- Pulse: weak and irregular
- Fear, apprehension, and a feeling of doom

Heart Failure

Heart failure or congestive heart failure (CHF) occurs when the weakened heart cannot pump normally. Blood backs up. Tissue congestion occurs.

When the left side of the heart cannot pump blood normally, blood backs up into the lungs. Respiratory congestion occurs. The person has dyspnea, increased sputum, cough, and gurgling sounds in the lungs. The body does not get enough blood. Signs and symptoms occur from the effects on other organs. Poor blood flow to the brain causes confusion, dizziness, and fainting. The kidneys produce less urine. The skin is pale. Blood pressure falls.

When the right side of the heart cannot pump blood normally, blood backs up into the venous system. Feet and ankles swell. Neck veins bulge. Liver congestion affects liver function. The abdomen is congested with fluid. Less blood is pumped to the lungs. The left side of the heart receives less blood from the lungs. The left side has less blood to pump to the body. As with left-sided heart failure, organs receive less blood. The signs and symptoms of left-sided failure occur.

Pulmonary edema (fluid in the lungs) is a very severe form of heart failure. It is an emergency. The person can die.

A damaged or weak heart usually causes heart failure. CAD, MI, hypertension, diabetes, age, and irregular heart rhythms are common causes. So are damaged heart valves and kidney disease.

Drugs strengthen the heart. They also reduce the amount of fluid in the body. A sodium-controlled diet is ordered. Oxygen is given. Semi-Fowler's position is preferred for breathing. The person must reduce CAD risk factors. If acutely ill, the person needs hospital care.

You assist with these aspects of the person's care:
- Promoting rest and activity as ordered
- Measuring intake and output
- Measuring weight daily
- Assisting with pulse oximetry
- Restricting fluids as ordered
- Promoting a diet that is low in sodium, fat, and cholesterol
- Preventing skin breakdown and pressure ulcers
- Assisting with range-of-motion and other exercises
- Assisting with transfers and ambulation
- Assisting with self-care activities
- Maintaining good alignment
- Applying elastic stockings

Many older persons have heart failure. Skin breakdown is a risk. Tissue swelling, poor circulation, and fragile skin combine to increase the risk of pressure ulcers. Good skin care and regular position changes are needed.

RESPIRATORY DISORDERS

The respiratory system brings oxygen (O_2) into the lungs and removes carbon dioxide (CO_2) from the body. Respiratory disorders interfere with this function and threaten life.

Chronic Obstructive Pulmonary Disease

Chronic obstructive pulmonary disease (COPD) involves two disorders—chronic bronchitis and emphysema. These disorders interfere with O_2 and CO_2 exchange in the lungs. They obstruct airflow. Lung function is gradually lost.

Cigarette smoking is the most important risk. Pipe, cigar, and other smoking tobaccos are also risk factors. So is exposure to second-hand smoke. Not smoking is the best way to prevent COPD. COPD has no cure.

COPD affects the airways and alveoli (Chapter 9). Less air gets into the lungs; less air leaves the lungs. These changes occur:
- The airways and alveoli (air sacs) become less elastic. They are like old rubber bands.
- The walls between many alveoli are destroyed.
- Airway walls become thick, inflamed, and swollen.
- The airways secrete more mucus than usual. Excess mucus clogs the airways.

Chronic Bronchitis Chronic bronchitis occurs after repeated episodes of bronchitis. Bronchitis means inflammation (*itis*) of the bronchi (*bronch*). Smoking is the major cause. Infection, air pollution, and industrial dusts are risk factors.

Smoker's cough in the morning is often the first symptom. At first the cough is dry. Over time, the person coughs up mucus. Mucus may contain pus. The cough becomes more frequent. The person has difficulty breathing and tires easily. Mucus and inflamed breathing passages obstruct airflow into the lungs. The body cannot get normal amounts of O_2.

The person must stop smoking. Oxygen therapy and breathing exercises are often ordered. Respiratory tract infections are prevented. If one occurs, the person needs prompt treatment.

Emphysema In emphysema, the alveoli enlarge. They become less elastic. They do not expand and shrink normally with breathing in and out. As a result, some air is trapped in the alveoli when exhaling. Trapped air is not exhaled. Over time, more alveoli are involved. O_2 and CO_2 exchange cannot occur in affected alveoli. As more air is trapped in the lungs, the person develops a *barrel chest* (Fig. 40-5).

Smoking is the most common cause. Air pollution and industrial dusts are risk factors.

The person has shortness of breath and a cough. At first, shortness of breath occurs with exertion. Over time, it occurs at rest. Sputum may contain pus. Fatigue is common. The person works hard to breathe in and out. And the body does not get enough O_2. Breathing is easier when the person sits upright and slightly forward (Chapter 28).

The person must stop smoking. Respiratory therapy, breathing exercises, oxygen, and medications are ordered.

Fig. 40-5 Barrel chest from emphysema.

Asthma

Asthma comes from the Greek word that means *panting*. With asthma, the airway becomes inflamed and narrow. Extra mucus is produced. Dyspnea results. Wheezing and coughing are common. So are pain and tightening in the chest. Symptoms are mild to severe.

Asthma usually is triggered by allergies. Other triggers include air pollutants and irritants, smoking and second-hand smoke, respiratory infections, exertion, and cold air.

Sudden attacks *(asthma attacks)* can occur. There is shortness of breath, wheezing, coughing, rapid pulse, sweating, and cyanosis. The person gasps for air and is very frightened. Fear makes the attack worse.

Asthma is treated with medications. Severe attacks may require emergency care. The person and family learn how to prevent asthma attacks. Repeated attacks can damage the respiratory system.

Influenza

Influenza *(flu)* is a respiratory infection. Table 40-1 contrasts *cold* and the *flu*. Caused by viruses, November through March is the usual flu season. According to the Centers for Disease Control and Prevention (CDC), about 36,000 people die every year from flu-related causes. Older persons are at great risk.

Older persons may not have the signs and symptoms listed in Table 40-1. The following may signal flu in older persons:

* Changes in mental status
* Worsening of other health problems
* A body temperature below the normal range
* Fatigue
* Decreased appetite and fluid intake

Treatment involves fluids and rest. The doctor orders medications for symptom relief and to shorten the flu episode. Most people are better in about one week.

Coughing and sneezing spread flu viruses. Follow Standard Precautions. The flu vaccine is the best way to prevent the disease. The CDC recommends the flu vaccine for persons who:

* Are 50 years of age and older
* Have chronic heart, lung, liver, or kidney diseases
* Have diabetes
* Have immune system problems
* Have nervous system disorders
* Have a severe form of anemia (a decrease in hemoglobin in the blood)
* Are pregnant
* Are nursing center or other long-term care residents
* Are in close contact with children under 5 years of age
* Are health care workers
* Have contact with persons at high risk for flu-related complications

Pneumonia is a common complication.

Table 40-1	Cold vs the Flu	
Symptoms	Cold	Flu
Fever	Rare	Usually high (100° to 102° F); lasts 3 to 4 days
Headache	Rare	Common
General aches and pains	Slight	Usual; often severe
Fatigue; weakness	Sometimes	Usual; can last 2 to 3 weeks
Extreme exhaustion	Never	Usual; at the beginning of the illness
Stuffy nose	Common	Sometimes
Sneezing	Usual	Sometimes
Sore throat	Common	Sometimes
Chest discomfort; cough	Mild to moderate; hacking cough	Common; can be severe
Complications	Sinus congestion; middle ear infection (otitis media); asthma	Bronchitis, pneumonia; can worsen chronic conditions; can be life-threatening

Modified from National Institute of Allergy and Infectious Disease: Is it a cold or the flu? National Institutes of Health, November 2008, Bethesda, Md.

Pneumonia

Pneumonia is an inflammation and infection of lung tissue. (*Pneumo* means lungs.) Affected tissues fill with fluid. O_2 and CO_2 exchange is affected.

Bacteria, viruses, and other microbes are causes. Microbes reach the lungs by being inhaled, aspirated, or carried in the blood to the lungs from an infection elsewhere in the body. Children under 2 years of age and adults over 65 years of age are at risk. Smoking, aging, stroke, bedrest, immobility, chronic diseases, and tube feedings are some factors that increase the pneumonia risk.

Onset may be sudden. The person is very ill. Signs and symptoms are listed in Box 40-3.

Older adults are at great risk of dying from the disease. Changes from aging, diseases, and decreased mobility increase the risk of pneumonia in older persons. Decreased mobility after surgery also is a risk factor. Aspiration pneumonia is common in older persons. Dysphagia, decreased cough and gag reflexes, and nervous system disorders are risk factors. So are substances that depress the brain—narcotics, sedatives, alcohol, and medications for anesthesia.

Older persons may not have the signs and symptoms listed in Box 40-3. Medications and other diseases can mask signs and symptoms. Older persons may show signs of confusion, dehydration, and rapid respirations.

Medications are ordered for infection and pain. Fluid intake is increased because of fever and to thin secretions. Thin secretions are easier to cough up. Intravenous therapy and oxygen may be needed. Semi-Fowler's position eases breathing. Rest is important. Standard Precautions are followed. Isolation precautions are used depending on the cause. Mouth care is important. Frequent linen changes are needed because of fever.

Box 40-3 Signs and Symptoms of Pneumonia

- High fever
- Chills
- Painful cough
- Chest pain on breathing
- Pulse: rapid
- Shortness of breath
- Breathing: rapid
- Cyanosis
- Sputum: thick and white, green, yellow, or rust-colored
- Nausea
- Vomiting
- Headache
- Tiredness
- Muscle aches

Tuberculosis

Tuberculosis (TB) is a bacterial infection in the lungs. It also can occur in the kidneys, bones, joints, nervous system (including the spine), muscles, and other parts of the body. If TB is not treated, the person can die.

TB is spread by airborne droplets with coughing, sneezing, speaking, singing, or laughing (Chapter 15). Nearby persons can inhale the bacteria. Those who have close, frequent contact with an infected person are at risk. TB is more likely to occur in close, crowded areas. Age, poor nutrition, and HIV (human immunodeficiency virus) infection are other risk factors.

TB can be present in the body but not cause signs and symptoms. An active infection may not occur for many years. Only persons with an active infection can spread the disease to others. Increased numbers of nursing center residents have active TB. Infected long ago, the TB becomes active because general health declines with aging. Other older people become newly infected from lengthy, extended contact with those already infected.

Chest x-rays and TB testing can detect the disease. Signs and symptoms are tiredness, loss of appetite, weight loss, fever, and night sweats. Cough and sputum increase over time. Sputum may contain blood. Chest pain occurs.

Medications for TB are given. Standard Precautions and isolation precautions are needed (Chapter 15). The person must cover the mouth and nose with tissues when sneezing, coughing, or producing sputum. Tissues are flushed down the toilet, placed in a BIOHAZARD bag, or placed in a paper bag and burned. Hand washing after contact with sputum is essential.

QUALITY OF LIFE

A person's condition can change very quickly. A person with angina may have an MI. A person with hypertension may have a stroke. Sudden changes in a person's condition require the nurse's attention. Assist the nurse as directed. You may need to help other residents while the nurse readies the person for transport to a hospital. Always help willingly. The entire nursing team may need to make that "extra effort" to meet resident needs.

To promote quality of life, follow the care plan to meet the person's basic needs. This includes the person's emotional needs. Heart and lung function are essential for life. Fears of death are common.

Also protect the person's rights. Privacy, confidentiality, and personal choice are important to the person. So is the right to be free of abuse, mistreatment, or neglect. This is very important for persons with TB, a cold, or the flu. Do not avoid the person out of fear of getting the disease. Treat the person with dignity and respect. Follow Standard Precautions and the Bloodborne Pathogen Standard. They protect you and others from contamination.

REVIEW QUESTIONS

Circle the BEST answer.

1 In hypertension, the systolic blood pressure is
   a Over 140 mm Hg
   b Over 120 mm Hg
   c Over 90 mm Hg
   d Over 80 mm Hg

2 Which is *not* a complication of hypertension?
   a Stroke
   b Heart attack
   c Renal failure
   d Diabetes

3 Treatment of hypertension may include the following *except*
   a No smoking and regular exercise
   b A high-sodium diet
   c A low-calorie diet if the person is obese
   d Medications to lower blood pressure

4 A person has angina. Which is *true*?
   a There is heart muscle damage.
   b Pain is described as crushing, stabbing, or squeezing.
   c Pain is relieved with rest and nitroglycerin.
   d Pain is always on the left side of the chest.

5 Cardiac rehabilitation involves
   a Exercise   c Catheter procedures
   b Surgery   d Receiving a vaccine

6 A person is having an MI. Which is *false*?
   a The person is having a heart attack.
   b This is an emergency.
   c The person may have a cardiac arrest.
   d The person does not have enough blood.

7 The pain of MI is usually
   a On the left side of the chest
   b On the right side of the chest
   c In the upper abdomen
   d In the mid-back region

8 A person has heart failure. Which should you question?
   a Encourage fluids.
   b Measure intake and output.
   c Measure weight daily.
   d Perform range-of-motion exercises.

9 The most common cause of COPD is
   a Smoking   c Being over-weight
   b Allergies   d A high-sodium diet

10 A person has emphysema. Which is *false*?
   a The person has dyspnea.
   b The person has an infection.
   c Breathing is usually easier sitting upright.
   d Sputum may contain pus.

11 The flu virus is spread by
   a Coughing and sneezing c Blood
   b The fecal-oral route   d Needle sharing

12 A person has pneumonia. You know that this is
   a An inflammation of the airway
   b A narrowing of the airway
   c An inflammation and infection of lung tissue
   d A bacterial infection in the lungs

13 Which position eases breathing in the person with pneumonia?
   a Supine   c Semi-Fowler's
   b Prone   d Trendelenburg's

14 Tuberculosis is spread by
   a Coughing and sneezing
   b Contaminated drinking water
   c Contact with wound drainage
   d The fecal-oral route

15 A person has TB. You had contact with the person's sputum. What should you do?
   a Wash your hands.
   b Put on gloves.
   c Use an alcohol-based hand rub.
   d Tell the nurse.

Answers to these questions are on p. 721.

Digestive and Endocrine Disorders

OBJECTIVES

- Define the key terms and key abbreviations listed in this chapter.
- Describe gastro-esophageal reflux disease and the care required.
- Describe the care required for vomiting.
- Describe diverticular disease and the care required.
- Describe gallstones and the care required.
- Describe hepatitis and the care required.
- Describe cirrhosis and the care required.
- Describe diabetes and the care required.
- Explain how to promote quality of life.

KEY TERMS

emesis See "vomitus"

heartburn A burning sensation in the chest and sometimes the throat

hyperglycemia High *(hyper)* sugar *(glyc)* in the blood *(emia)*

hypoglycemia Low *(hypo)* sugar *(glyc)* in the blood *(emia)*

jaundice Yellowish color of the skin or whites of the eyes

vomitus Food and fluids expelled from the stomach through the mouth; emesis

KEY ABBREVIATIONS

GERD	Gastro-esophageal reflux disease	**I&O**	Intake and output
HBV	Hepatitis B virus	**IV**	Intravenous

Problems can develop in any part of the digestive system. This includes the liver, gallbladder, and pancreas—the accessory organs of digestion. The pancreas also is part of the endocrine system. Refer to Chapter 9 while you study this chapter.

DIGESTIVE DISORDERS

The digestive system breaks down food for the body to absorb. Solid wastes are eliminated. Diarrhea, constipation, flatulence, and fecal incontinence are discussed in Chapter 23. So is ostomy care.

Gastro-Esophageal Reflux Disease

In gastro-esophageal reflux disease (GERD) stomach contents flow back (*reflux*) from the stomach (*gastro*) into the esophagus (*esophageal*). Stomach contents contain acid. The acid can irritate and inflame the esophagus lining. This is called *esophagitis*—inflammation (*itis*) of the esophagus.

Heartburn is the most common symptom of GERD. Heartburn is a burning sensation in the chest and sometimes the throat. The person may have a sour taste in the back of the mouth. Occasional heartburn is not a problem. If it occurs more than twice a week, the person may have GERD. Besides heartburn, other signs and symptoms of GERD include:

- Chest pain, often when lying down
- Hoarseness in the morning
- Dysphagia
- Choking sensation
- Feeling like food is stuck in the throat
- Feeling like the throat is tight
- Dry cough
- Sore throat
- Bad breath

GERD risk factors include being over-weight, alcohol use, pregnancy, and smoking. Hiatal hernia is a risk. With hiatal hernia, the upper part of the stomach is above the diaphragm. Large meals and lying down after eating can cause gastric reflux. So can certain foods—citrus fruits, chocolate, caffeine drinks, fried and fatty foods, garlic, onions, spicy foods, tomato-based foods (pasta sauce, chili, pizza).

The doctor may order medications to prevent stomach acid production or to promote stomach emptying. Surgery may be needed if medications and life-style changes do not work. Life-style changes include:

- No smoking
- Not drinking alcohol
- Losing weight
- Eating small meals
- Wearing loose belts and loose-fitting clothes
- Not lying down for 3 hours after meals
- Raising the head of the bed 6 to 8 inches. See "reverse Trendelenburg's position" in Chapter 18.

Vomiting

Vomiting means expelling stomach contents through the mouth. It signals illness or injury. Vomitus (emesis) is the food and fluids expelled from the stomach through the mouth. Aspirated vomitus can obstruct the airway. Vomiting large amounts of blood can lead to shock. These measures are needed:

- Follow Standard Precautions and the Bloodborne Pathogen Standard.
- Turn the person's head well to one side. This prevents aspiration.
- Place a kidney basin under the person's chin.
- Move vomitus away from the person.
- Provide oral hygiene. This helps remove the bitter taste of vomitus.
- Observe vomitus for color, odor, and undigested food. If it looks like coffee grounds, it contains undigested blood. This signals bleeding. Report your observations.
- Measure, report, and record the amount of vomitus. Also record the amount on the I&O (intake and output) record.
- Save a specimen for laboratory study.
- Dispose of vomitus after the nurse observes it.
- Eliminate odors.
- Provide for comfort. (See the inside of the front book cover.)

Diverticular Disease

Small pouches can develop in the colon. The pouches bulge outward through weak spots in the colon (Fig. 41-1). Each pouch is called a *diverticulum*. (*Diverticulare* means *to turn inside out*.) *Diverticulosis* is the condition of having these pouches. (*Osis* means *condition of*.) The pouches can become infected or inflamed—*diverticulitis*. (*Itis* means *inflammation*.)

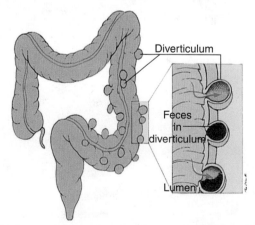

Fig. 41-1 Diverticulosis. *(From Christensen BL, Kockrow EO:* Adult health nursing, *ed 6, St Louis, 2011, Mosby.)*

About half of all people over 60 years of age have diverticulosis. Age, a low-fiber diet, and constipation are risk factors.

When feces enter the pouches, they can become inflamed and infected. The person has abdominal pain and tenderness in the lower left abdomen. Fever, nausea and vomiting, chills, cramping, and constipation are likely. Bloating, rectal bleeding, frequent urination, and pain while voiding can occur.

A ruptured pouch is a rare complication. Feces spill out into the abdomen. This leads to a severe, life-threatening infection. A pouch also can cause a blockage in the intestine (intestinal obstruction). Feces and gas cannot move past the blocked part.

Dietary changes are ordered. Sometimes antibiotics are ordered. Surgery is needed for severe disease, obstruction, and ruptured pouches. The diseased part of the bowel is removed. Sometimes a colostomy is necessary (Chapter 23).

Gallstones

Bile is a greenish liquid made in the liver. It is stored in the gallbladder until needed to digest fat. Gallstones form when the bile hardens into stone-like pieces (Fig. 41-2).

Bile is carried from the liver to the gallbladder through ducts (tubes). The gallbladder contracts and pushes bile through the common bile duct to the small intestine. Gallstones can lodge in any of the ducts (Fig. 41-3). Bile flow is blocked. The trapped bile can cause inflammation of the gallbladder and the ducts. Liver and pancreas involvement are possible. Death can result from severe infections or damage.

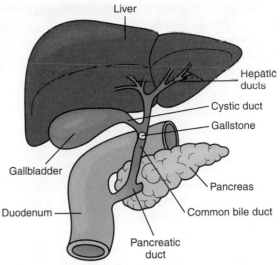

Fig. 41-3 The gallbladder and ducts that carry bile from the liver, gallbladder, and pancreas to the small intestine. *(Modified from National Digestive Diseases Information Clearinghouse [NDDIC]: Gallstones, National Institutes of Health, NIH Publication No. 07-2897, Bethesda, Md, July 2007.)*

Gallstones vary in size. They can be as small as a grain of sand or as large as a golf ball. A person may have one large stone. Some people have large and small stones. Risk factors include:

- Gender. Women are at greater risk than men.
- Family history. A genetic link is possible.
- Diet. A diet high in fat and cholesterol increases the risk. So does a low-fiber diet.
- Age. People over age 60 are at greater risk than younger people.
- American Indians. They have genetic factors that increase the risk of gallstones. High levels of cholesterol are secreted into the bile.
- Mexican Americans. Men and women of all ages are at risk.
- Being over-weight. Increased cholesterol reduces gallbladder emptying.
- Rapid weight loss and fasting. To burn fat, the liver secretes more cholesterol into the bile. Cholesterol can cause gallstones. And the gallbladder does not empty properly.
- Cholesterol-lowering medications. They increase the amount of cholesterol secreted into bile.
- Diabetes. Persons with diabetes have high levels of fatty acids. The fatty acids may increase the risk of gallstones.

Signs and symptoms of a "gallbladder attack" or "gallstone attack" occur suddenly (Box 41-1, p. 628). They often follow a fatty meal. The most common treatment is surgical removal of the gallbladder.

Fig. 41-2 Inflamed gallbladder filled with gallstones. *(From Thompson JM, Wilson SF: Health assessments for nursing practice, St Louis, 1996, Mosby.)*

Box 41-1   Signs and Symptoms of Gallstones

- Steady pain in the upper abdomen
  - Increases rapidly
  - Lasts 30 minutes to several hours
- Pain
  - In the back between the shoulder blades
  - Under the right shoulder
- Prolonged pain—lasting more than 5 hours
- Nausea and vomiting
- Chills
- Fever
- Jaundice—yellowish color of the skin or whites of the eyes (Fig. 41-4) (Jaundice comes from the French word *jaune* meaning *yellow*.)
- Clay-colored stools

Modified from National Digestive Diseases Information Clearinghouse (NDDIC): Gallstones, National Institutes of Health, NIH Publication No. 07-2897, Bethesda, Md, July 2007.

Box 41-2   Signs and Symptoms of Hepatitis

- Jaundice (yellowish color of the skin or whites of the eyes)
- Fatigue, weakness
- Pain and discomfort: abdominal, joint, muscles
- Appetite: loss of
- Nausea and vomiting
- Diarrhea
- Bowel movements: light, clay-colored
- Urine: dark
- Fever
- Chills
- Headache
- Itching
- Weight loss
- Skin rash

Fig. 41-4 Jaundice. *(From Emond RT, Welsby PD, Rowland HA: Color atlas of infectious diseases, ed 4, London, 2004, Mosby.)*

Hepatitis

Hepatitis is an inflammation *(itis)* of the liver *(hepat)*. It can be mild or cause death. Signs and symptoms are listed in Box 41-2. Some people do not have symptoms.

Protect yourself and others. Follow Standard Precautions and the Bloodborne Pathogen Standard. Isolation precautions are ordered as necessary (Chapter 15). Assist the person with hygiene and hand washing as needed.

There are five major types of hepatitis. See Box 41-3 for persons at risk.

Hepatitis A This type is spread by food or water contaminated with feces from an infected person. Spread through the fecal-oral route, the hepatitis A virus is ingested when:
- Eating or drinking food or water contaminated with feces
- Eating or drinking from a contaminated vessel

Treatment involves rest, a healthy diet, fluids, and no alcohol. Recovery takes 1 to 2 months.

Persons with fecal incontinence, confusion, and dementia can cause contamination. Carefully look for contaminated items and areas.

Handle bedpans, feces, and rectal thermometers carefully. Good hand washing is needed by everyone, including the person. Assist with hand washing after bowel movements. The hepatitis A vaccine provides protection against the disease.

Hepatitis B This is caused by the hepatitis B virus (HBV). It is spread through infected blood or blood products and body fluids (saliva, semen, vaginal secretions) of infected persons. It is spread by:
- IV (intravenous) drug use and sharing needles and syringes
- Accidental needle-sticks
- Sex without a condom, especially anal sex
- Contaminated tools used for tattoos or body piercings
- Sharing a toothbrush, razor, or nail clippers with an infected person

For the HBV vaccine, see Chapter 15. Medications are ordered to treat chronic hepatitis B.

Modified from National Digestive Diseases Information Clearinghouse (NDDIC): Viral hepatitis: A through E and beyond, National Institutes of Health, NIH Publication No. 08-4762, Bethesda, Md, February 2008.

Box 41-3 Persons at Risk for Hepatitis

Hepatitis A
- International travelers (especially to developing countries)
- People who live with an infected person
- People who have sex with an infected person
- People living in areas where children are not routinely vaccinated against hepatitis A
- Children in day care (during outbreaks)
- Day-care workers (during outbreaks)
- Men who have sex with men
- Users of illegal drugs

Hepatitis B
- People who live with an infected person
- People who have sex with an infected person
- People who have multiple sex partners
- Injection drug users
- Immigrants from areas with high rates of hepatitis B
- Children of immigrants from areas with high rates of hepatitis B
- Infants born to infected mothers
- Health care workers
- Hemodialysis patients (Chapter 42)
- People who received blood or blood products before 1987
- International travelers (especially to developing countries)

Hepatitis C
- Injection drug users
- People who have sex with an infected person
- People who have multiple sex partners
- Health care workers
- Infants born to infected mothers
- Hemodialysis patients
- People who received blood or blood products before 1992
- People who received blood clotting factors made before 1987

Hepatitis D
- People who have sex with an infected person
- People who received blood or blood products before 1987

Hepatitis E
- International travelers (especially to developing countries)
- People living in areas where hepatitis E outbreaks are common
- People who live with an infected person
- People who have sex with an infected person

Hepatitis C This type is spread by blood contaminated with the hepatitis C virus. A person may have the virus but no symptoms. Serious liver disease and damage may show up years later. Even without symptoms, the person can transmit the disease. Hepatitis C is treated with medications. The virus is spread by:
- Blood contaminated with the virus
- IV drug use and sharing needles
- Inhaling cocaine through contaminated straws
- Contaminated tools used for tattoos or body piercings
- High-risk sexual activity—sex with an infected person, multiple sex partners
- Sharing a toothbrush, razor, or nail clippers with an infected person

Hepatitis D and Hepatitis E Hepatitis D occurs only in people infected with hepatitis B. It is spread the same way as HBV.

Hepatitis E is spread through food or water contaminated by feces from an infected person. It is spread by the fecal-oral route. This disease is not common in the United States.

Cirrhosis

Cirrhosis is a liver condition caused by chronic damage to the liver (Fig. 41-5, p. 630). (*Cirrho* comes from the Greek word meaning *yellow-orange. Osis* means *condition.*) Healthy tissue is replaced by scar tissue. Blood flow through the liver is blocked. Normal liver functions are affected:
- Controlling infection
- Removing bacteria and toxins from the blood
- Processing nutrients, hormones, and drugs
- Making proteins for blood clotting
- Producing bile for fat digestion

Cirrhosis has many causes. Chronic alcohol abuse and chronic hepatitis B and C are common causes. Obesity is becoming a common cause.

Signs and symptoms do not appear early in the disease. The following may occur as the disease progresses:
- Weakness
- Fatigue
- Loss of appetite
- Nausea
- Vomiting
- Weight loss
- Abdominal pain and bloating when fluid collects in the membrane lining the abdominal cavity (Fig. 41-6, p. 630)
- Itching
- Spider-like blood vessels on the skin

Fig. 41-5 Liver damage from alcohol. (*A from Thibodeau GA, Patton KT:* The human body in health & disease, *ed 5, St Louis, 2010, Mosby. **B** from Kumar V and others:* Robbins basic pathology, *ed 8, Philadelphia, 2007, Saunders.)*

Fig. 41-6 Fluid in the membrane lining the abdominal cavity (ascites). (*From Swartz MH:* Textbook of physical diagnosis, *ed 5, Philadelphia, 2006, Saunders.)*

Cirrhosis has many serious complications. Fluid collects in the legs *(edema)* and abdomen *(ascites)*. Infection, jaundice, and bruising and bleeding occur. Blood vessels in the esophagus and stomach may enlarge and can burst. Gallstones may develop. Toxins build up in the brain causing confusion, personality changes, and memory loss. The person is at risk for diabetes and liver cancer.

Treatment is aimed at preventing the progress of scar tissue. Complications also are treated. The person must have a healthy diet limited in protein. A low-sodium diet is needed for edema and ascites. Diuretic medications (water pills) are ordered to remove fluid from the body. Antibiotics are ordered for infection. Medications and enemas are ordered to remove toxins. The person must avoid alcohol. The person may need a liver transplant.

Assist with the person's care as directed. The measures listed in Box 41-4 may be part of the person's care plan.

Box 41-4   Care of the Person With Cirrhosis

- Use bed rails according to the care plan.
- Keep the signal light within reach.
- Observe vomitus and stools for blood.
- Observe for signs of decreased mental function—confusion, memory loss, behavior changes, and so on.
- Measure vital signs every 2 to 4 hours. Follow the care plan.
- Measure I&O.
- Follow fluid restriction orders.
- Weigh the person daily.
- Provide good skin care.
- Apply lotion to the skin.
- Turn the person at least every 2 hours or as noted on the care plan.
- Provide mouth care every 2 hours.
- Use warm water with baking soda for bathing. This decreases itching.
- Assist with activities of daily living (ADL) as needed.
- Complete a safety check before leaving the room. (See the inside of the front book cover.)

ENDOCRINE DISORDERS

The endocrine system is made up of glands. The endocrine glands secrete hormones that affect other organs and glands. Diabetes is the most common endocrine disorder.

Diabetes

In this disorder, the body cannot produce or use insulin properly. Insulin is needed for glucose to move from the blood into the cells. The cells need glucose for energy. The pancreas secretes insulin. Without enough insulin, sugar builds up in the blood. Blood glucose (sugar) is high. Cells do not have enough sugar for energy and cannot function.

Types of Diabetes A family history of the disease is a common risk factor for the three types of diabetes:

- *Type 1 diabetes.* Occurs most often in children, teens, and young adults. It is more common in whites than in non-whites. The pancreas produces little or no insulin. Onset is rapid.
- *Type 2 diabetes.* This type is more common after age 45. However, it is becoming more common in children, teens, and young adults. Being over-weight, lack of exercise, and hypertension are risk factors. The pancreas secretes insulin. However, the body cannot use it well. Onset is slow. Infections are frequent. Wounds heal slowly. Gum disease (Chapter 20) is common. These ethnic groups are at risk:
  - Alaskan Natives
  - American Indians
  - African-Americans
  - Hispanics and Latinos
  - Asian Americans
  - Pacific Islanders
- *Gestational diabetes*—develops during pregnancy. (Gestation comes from *gestare*. It means to *bear*.) It usually goes away after the baby is born. However, the mother is at risk for type 2 diabetes later in life.

Signs and Symptoms Signs and symptoms of diabetes are:

- Being very thirsty
- Urinating often
- Feeling very hungry or tired
- Losing weight without trying
- Having sores that heal slowly
- Having dry, itchy skin
- Tingling or loss of feeling in the feet
- Blurred vision

Complications Diabetes must be controlled to prevent complications. They include blindness, renal failure, nerve damage, and damage to the gums and teeth. Heart and blood vessel diseases are very serious problems. They can lead to stroke, heart attack, and slow healing. Foot and leg wounds and ulcers are very serious (Chapter 35). Infection and gangrene can occur. Sometimes amputation is necessary.

Treatment Type 1 diabetes is treated with daily insulin therapy, healthy eating (Chapter 24), and exercise. Type 2 diabetes is treated with healthy eating and exercise. Many persons with type 2 take oral medications. Some need insulin. Over-weight persons need to lose weight. Types 1 and 2 involve controlling blood pressure, cholesterol, and the risk factors for coronary artery disease.

Good foot care is needed. Corns, blisters, calluses, and other foot problems can lead to an infection and amputation. See Chapters 21 and 35.

The person's blood sugar level can fall too low or go too high. Blood glucose (Chapter 33) is monitored daily or 3 or 4 times a day for:

- **Hypoglycemia** means low *(hypo)* sugar *(glyc)* in the blood *(emia)*.
- **Hyperglycemia** means high *(hyper)* sugar *(glyc)* in the blood *(emia)*.

See Table 41-1, p. 632 for the causes, signs, and symptoms of hypoglycemia and hyperglycemia. Both can lead to death if not corrected. You must call for the nurse at once.

Assist with the person's care as directed by the nurse. Also follow the person's care plan.

Table 41-1   Hypoglycemia and Hyperglycemia

	Causes	Signs and Symptoms
Hypoglycemia (low blood sugar)	Too much insulin or diabetic drugs Omitting or missing a meal Delayed meal Eating too little food Increased exercise Vomiting Drinking alcohol	Hunger Fatigue; weakness Trembling; shakiness Sweating Headache Dizziness Faintness Pulse: rapid Blood pressure: low Respirations: rapid and shallow Motions: clumsy and jerky Tingling around the mouth Confusion Vision: changes in Skin: cold and clammy Convulsions Unconsciousness
Hyperglycemia (high blood sugar)	Undiagnosed diabetes Not enough insulin or diabetic drugs Eating too much food Too little exercise Emotional stress Infection or sickness	Weakness Drowsiness Thirst Dry mouth (very) Hunger Urination: frequent Leg cramps Face: flushed Breath odor: sweet Respirations: rapid, deep, and labored Pulse: rapid, weak Blood pressure: low Skin: dry Vision: blurred Headache Nausea and vomiting Convulsions Coma

QUALITY OF LIFE

For some health problems, family history is a risk factor. Others result from life-style choices. Poor diet, drug abuse, and alcohol abuse are examples. So is lack of exercise. Do not judge the person or his or her actions. Always treat the person with dignity and respect.

Also protect the person's rights. Privacy, confidentiality, and personal choice are important to the person. So is the right to be free of abuse, mistreatment, or neglect. Always provide a safe setting to protect the person from harm and injury.

REVIEW QUESTIONS

Circle the BEST answer.

1 A person has gastro-esophageal reflux disease. Which nursing measure should you question?
   a Person to wear loose clothing
   b Supine position after meals
   c Person to have small meals
   d No smoking or alcohol

2 A person with gastro-esophageal reflux disease has the following food choices. Which is best for the person?
   a Baked chicken
   b Pasta with tomato sauce
   c Pizza
   d Salad with orange slices

3 A person is vomiting. How should you position the person?
   a Supine
   b Prone
   c Semi-Fowler's
   d With the head turned to the side

4 Vomiting is dangerous because of
   a Aspiration
   b Diverticular disease
   c Fluid loss
   d Jaundice

5 Vomitus looks like coffee grounds. You need to report this at once because it signals
   a Bleeding
   b Gastro-esophageal reflux disease
   c Gallstones
   d A ruptured pouch

6 A person has diverticular disease. You will likely assist the nurse with
   a Preventing diarrhea
   b Giving antibiotics
   c Giving enemas
   d Preventing constipation

7 Gallbladder attacks usually occur
   a On awakening
   b During a fast
   c After a fatty meal
   d When the person is lying down

8 Which is *not* a sign of gallstones?
   a Jaundice
   b Pain under the right shoulder
   c Clay-colored stools
   d Hoarseness and choking sensation

9 Hepatitis is an inflammation of the
   a Liver
   b Gallbladder
   c Pancreas
   d Stomach

10 Hepatitis A is spread by
   a Needle sharing
   b IV drug use
   c Contaminated blood
   d The fecal-oral route

11 Hepatitis requires
   a Sterile gloves
   b Double-bagging
   c Standard Precautions
   d Masks, gowns, and goggles

12 Which is a common cause of cirrhosis?
   a Alcohol abuse
   b Diabetes
   c Gallstones
   d GERD

13 A person has cirrhosis. Which measure should you question?
   a Measure I&O.
   b Weigh the person daily.
   c Use warm water with baking soda for bathing.
   d Encourage fluids.

14 A person has cirrhosis. You should observe stools and vomitus for blood.
   a True
   b False

15 Which is *not* a sign of diabetes?
   a Increased urine production
   b Weight gain
   c Hunger
   d Increased thirst

16 A person with diabetes needs the following *except*
   a Exercise
   b Good foot care
   c A sodium-controlled diet
   d Healthy eating

17 A person with diabetes is vomiting after a meal. The person is at risk for
   a Hypoglycemia
   b Hyperglycemia
   c Jaundice
   d Bleeding

18 A person has diabetes. Blood glucose is monitored daily or
   a 2 or 3 times a day
   b 3 or 4 times a day
   c 4 or 5 times a day
   d 5 or 6 times a day

Answers to these questions are on p. 721.

Urinary and Reproductive Disorders

OBJECTIVES

- Define the key terms and key abbreviations listed in this chapter.
- Describe urinary tract infections and the care required.
- Describe prostate enlargement and the care required.
- Describe urinary diversions and the care required.

- Describe renal calculi and the care required.
- Describe acute and chronic kidney failure and the care required.
- Describe sexually transmitted diseases and the care required.
- Explain how to promote quality of life.

KEY TERMS

dialysis The process of removing waste products from the blood

diuresis The process *(esis)* of passing *(di)* urine *(ur)*; large amounts of urine are produced—1000 to 5000 mL (milliliters) a day

dysuria Difficult or painful *(dys)* urination *(uria)*

hematuria Blood *(hemat)* in the urine *(uria)*

oliguria Scant *(olig)* urine *(uria)*

pyuria Pus *(py)* in the urine *(uria)*

urinary diversion A new pathway for urine to exit the body

urostomy A surgically created opening *(stomy)* between a ureter *(uro)* and the abdomen

KEY ABBREVIATIONS

AIDS	Acquired immunodeficiency syndrome	**mL**	Milliliter
BPH	Benign prostatic hyperplasia	**STD**	Sexually transmitted disease
HIV	Human immunodeficiency virus	**UTI**	Urinary tract infection

Understanding urinary and reproductive disorders gives meaning to the required care. Refer to Chapter 9 while you study this chapter.

URINARY SYSTEM DISORDERS

The kidneys, ureters, bladder, and urethra are the major urinary system structures. Disorders can occur in these structures. Men can develop prostate problems.

Urinary Tract Infections

Urinary tract infections (UTIs) are common. Infection in one area can progress through the entire system. Microbes can enter the system through the urethra. Catheterization, urological exams, intercourse, poor perineal hygiene, immobility, and poor fluid intake are common causes. UTI is a common healthcare-associated infection (Chapter 15).

Women are at high risk. Microbes can easily enter the short female urethra. Prostate gland secretions help protect men from UTIs. However, an enlarged prostate increases the risk of UTI.

Older persons are at high risk for UTIs. Incomplete bladder emptying, perineal soiling from fecal incontinence, poor fluid intake, and poor nutrition increase the risk of UTI in older men and women.

Cystitis Cystitis is a bladder *(cyst)* infection *(itis)* caused by bacteria. These signs and symptoms are common:
- Urinary frequency
- **Oliguria**—scant *(olig)* urine *(uria)*
- Urgency
- **Dysuria**—difficult or painful *(dys)* urination *(uria)*
- Pain or burning on urination
- Foul-smelling urine
- **Hematuria**—blood *(hemat)* in the urine *(uria)*
- **Pyuria**—pus *(py)* in the urine *(uria)*
- Fever

Antibiotics are ordered. Fluids are encouraged—usually 2000 mL (milliliters) per day. If untreated, cystitis can lead to pyelonephritis.

Pyelonephritis Pyelonephritis is inflammation *(itis)* of the kidney *(nephr)* pelvis *(pyelo)*. Infection is the most common cause. Cloudy urine may contain pus, mucus, and blood. Chills, fever, back pain, and nausea and vomiting occur. So do the signs and symptoms of cystitis. Treatment involves antibiotics and fluids.

Prostate Enlargement

The prostate is a gland in men. It lies in front of the rectum and just below the bladder (Chapter 9). The prostate also surrounds the urethra. In young men, the prostate is about the size of a walnut. The prostate grows larger (enlarges) as the man grows older. This is called benign prostatic hyperplasia (BPH). See Figure 42-1. (*Benign* means non-malignant. *Hyper* means excessive. *Plasia* means formation or development.) Benign prostatic hypertrophy is another name for enlarged prostate. (*Trophy* means growth.)

Most men age 60 and older have some symptoms of BPH. The enlarged prostate presses against the urethra, obstructing urine flow. Bladder function is gradually lost. These problems are common:
- A weak urine stream
- Frequent voidings of small amounts of urine
- Urgency and leaking or dribbling of urine
- Frequent voiding at night
- Urinary retention (The man cannot void. Urine remains in the bladder.)

Treatment depends on the extent of the problem. For mild BPH, medications can shrink the prostate or stop its growth. Some microwave and laser treatments destroy excess prostate tissue.

Fig. 42-1 A, Normal prostate size. **B,** Enlarged prostate. The prostate presses against the urethra. Urine flow is obstructed. *(Redrawn from National Kidney and Urologic Diseases Information Clearinghouse:* Prostate enlargement: benign prostatic hyperplasia, *National Institutes of Health, NIH Publication No. 07-3012, Bethesda, Md, June 2006, National Institutes of Health.)*

Transurethral resection of the prostate (TURP) is a common surgical procedure. The doctor inserts a lighted scope through the penis. The scope has a wire loop. The loop is used to cut tissue and seal blood vessels. The removed tissue is flushed out of the bladder. A special catheter is inserted and left in place for a few days. Flushing fluid enters the bladder through the catheter. Urine and the flushing fluid flow out of the bladder through the same catheter. Some bleeding and blood clots are normal. After surgery, the person's care plan may include the following:

- No straining or sudden movements
- Drinking at least 8 cups of water daily to flush the bladder
- No straining to have a bowel movement
- A balanced diet to prevent constipation
- No heavy lifting

Urinary Diversions

Sometimes the urinary bladder is surgically removed. Cancer and bladder injuries are common reasons. When the bladder is removed, urine must still leave the body. A new pathway—**urinary diversion**—is needed for urine to exit the body.

Often an ostomy is involved. A **urostomy** is a surgically created opening *(stomy)* between a ureter *(uro)* and the abdomen (Fig. 42-2). The nurse provides care after surgery. You may care for persons with long-standing urostomies. The person assists with care as able.

Fig. 42-2 Urostomies. **A,** Both ureters are brought through the skin onto the abdomen. The person has two stomas. **B,** The ileal conduit. A small section of the small intestine is removed. One end is sutured closed. The other end is brought through the skin onto the abdomen to form a stoma. The ureters are attached to this part of the small intestine. *(From Beare PA, Myers JL: Principles and practices of adult health nursing, ed 3, St Louis, 1998, Mosby.)*

A pouch is applied over the stoma (Fig. 42-3). Urine drains through the stoma into the pouch. Pouches are changed every 5 to 7 days. A pouch is replaced anytime it leaks. Skin irritation, breakdown, and infection can occur if urine leaks onto the skin.

Urine drains constantly into the pouch. Empty pouches every 3 to 4 hours. Or empty them when they are becoming ⅓ (one-third) full. Pouches become heavy as they fill with urine. A heavy pouch can loosen the seal between the pouch and the skin. Urine can leak onto the skin.

The person needs good skin care. You must help prevent skin breakdown. Observe the skin for changes around the stoma. Report changes to the nurse. See "The Person With an Ostomy" in Chapter 23.

See *Promoting Safety and Comfort: Urinary Diversions.*

Fig. 42-3 Urostomy pouch.

PROMOTING SAFETY AND COMFORT
Urinary Diversions

Safety
Microbes can grow in urine. And urine may contain blood. Also, you have contact with mucous membranes. Follow Standard Precautions and the Bloodborne Pathogen Standard.

Comfort
The best time to change a pouch is after sleep and before eating or drinking fluids. Urine flow is less when the person has not had anything to eat or drink for 2 to 3 hours.

The stoma does not have sensation. Touching the stoma does not cause pain or discomfort.

| Smooth | Golf-ball–sized and brown | Staghorn | Jagged and yellow |

Fig. 42-4 Kidney stones.

Fig. 42-5 *Shaded areas* show where the pain from kidney stones is located.

Kidney Stones

Kidney stones (calculi) are the most common in white men between the ages of 20 and 40 years. Bedrest, immobility, and poor fluid intake are risk factors. Stones vary in size from as small as grains of sand to as big as golf balls (Fig. 42-4). Signs and symptoms include:

- Severe, cramping pain in the back and side just below the ribs (Fig. 42-5)
- Pain in the abdomen, thigh, and urethra
- Nausea and vomiting
- Fever and chills
- Dysuria—difficult or painful *(dys)* urination *(uria)*
- Urinary frequency
- Urinary urgency
- Burning on urination
- Oliguria—scant *(olig)* urine *(uria)*
- Hematuria—blood *(hemat)* in the urine *(uria)*
- Cloudy urine
- Foul-smelling urine

Medications are given for pain relief. The person needs to drink 2000 to 3000 mL of fluid a day. The fluids help stones pass from the body through the urine. All urine is strained (Chapter 33). Surgical removal of the stone may be necessary. Some dietary changes can prevent stones.

Kidney Failure

In kidney failure (renal failure), the kidneys do not function or are severely impaired. Waste products are not removed from the blood. Fluid is retained. Heart failure and hypertension easily result. Kidney failure may be acute or chronic. The person is very ill.

Acute Kidney Failure Acute kidney failure is sudden. Blood flow to the kidneys is severely decreased. Causes include severe injury or bleeding, heart attack, heart failure, burns, infection, and severe allergic reactions. Hospital care is needed.

At first, *oliguria* (scant amount of urine) occurs. Urine output is less than 400 mL in 24 hours. This phase lasts a few days to 2 weeks. Then **diuresis** occurs—the process *(esis)* of passing *(di)* urine *(ur)*. Large amounts of urine are produced—1000 to 5000 mL a day. Kidney function improves and returns to normal during the recovery phase. This can take from 1 month to 1 year. Some persons develop chronic kidney failure.

Every system is affected when waste products build up in the blood. Death can occur.

Treatment involves medications, restricted fluids, and diet therapy. The diet is high in carbohydrates and low in protein and potassium. The care plan may include:

- Measuring and recording urine output every hour. Report an output of less than 30 mL per hour to the nurse at once.
- Measuring and recording intake and output.
- Restricting fluid intake.
- Measuring weight daily.
- Turning and re-positioning at least every 2 hours.
- Measures to prevent pressure ulcers.
- Frequent oral hygiene.
- Measures to prevent infection.
- Deep-breathing and coughing exercises.
- Measures to meet emotional needs.

Box 42-1	Signs and Symptoms of Chronic Kidney Failure

- Skin
  - Color: yellow, tan, or dusky
  - Dry, itchy
  - Thin, brittle
- Bruises
- Breath: bad breath *(halitosis)*
- Mouth: inflammation of *(stomatitis)*
- Nausea
- Vomiting
- Appetite: loss of
- Weight loss
- Diarrhea or constipation
- Urine output: decreased
- Bleeding tendencies
- Infection: susceptible to
- Hypertension
- Heart failure
- Gastric ulcers
- Gastro-intestinal bleeding
- Pulse: irregular
- Breathing: abnormal patterns
- Legs and ankles: swelling
- Legs and feet: burning sensation in
- Muscles: twitching and cramps
- Fatigue
- Sleep disorders
- Headache
- Convulsions
- Confusion
- Coma

Fig. 42-6 Dialysis machine. *(Courtesy Baxter Healthcare Corp., Deerfield, Ill.)*

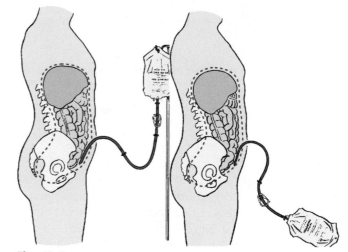

Fig. 42-7 Peritoneal dialysis system. *(From Tucker S et al: Patient care standards: collaborative practice planning guides, ed 6, St Louis, 1996, Mosby.)*

Chronic Kidney Failure The kidneys cannot meet the body's needs. Nephrons in the kidney are destroyed over many years. Hypertension and diabetes are common causes. Infections, urinary tract obstructions, and tumors are other causes.

Signs and symptoms appear when 75% of kidney function is lost (Box 42-1). Every system is affected as waste products build up in the blood.

Treatment includes fluid restriction, diet therapy, medications, and dialysis. Dialysis is the process of removing waste products from the blood.

- *Hemodialysis* removes waste and fluid by filtering the blood *(hemo)* through an artificial kidney (Fig. 42-6).
- *Peritoneal dialysis* uses the lining of the abdominal cavity *(peritoneal membrane)* to remove waste and fluid from the blood (Fig. 42-7).

You will assist the nurse in the care of persons with chronic kidney failure. See Box 42-2.

Box 42-2 Care of the Person in Chronic Kidney Failure

- A diet low in protein, potassium, and sodium
- Fluid restriction
- Measuring blood pressure in the supine, sitting, and standing positions
- Measuring daily weight
- Measuring and recording intake and output
- Turning and re-positioning
- Measures to prevent pressure ulcers
- Range-of-motion exercises
- Measures to prevent itching (bath oils, lotions, creams)
- Measures to prevent injury and bleeding
- Frequent oral hygiene
- Measures to prevent infection
- Measures to prevent diarrhea or constipation
- Measures to meet emotional needs
- Measures to promote rest

REPRODUCTIVE DISORDERS

Sexual activities involve the structures and functions of the reproductive system. The male reproductive system:

- Produces and transports sperm
- Deposits sperm in the female reproductive tract
- Secretes hormones
  The female reproductive system:
- Produces eggs (ova)
- Secretes hormones
- Protects and nourishes the fetus during pregnancy
  Aging affects the reproductive system (Chapter 10). Many injuries, diseases, and surgeries can affect reproductive structures and functions.

Sexually Transmitted Diseases

A sexually transmitted disease (STD) is spread by oral, vaginal, or anal sex (Table 42-1). Some people do not have signs and symptoms or are not aware of an infection. Others know but do not seek treatment because of embarrassment.

STDs often occur in the genital and rectal areas. They also occur in the ears, mouth, nipples, throat, tongue, eyes, and nose. Condom use helps prevent the spread of STDs, especially the human immunodeficiency virus (HIV) and acquired immunodeficiency syndrome (AIDS). (HIV and AIDS are discussed in Chapter 38.) Some STDs are also spread through skin breaks, by contact with infected body fluids (blood, semen, saliva), or by contaminated blood or needles.

Standard Precautions and the Bloodborne Pathogen Standard are followed.

Table 42-1 Sexually Transmitted Diseases

Disease	Signs and Symptoms	Treatment
Herpes	Painful, blister-like sores on or near the genitals, mouth, or anus (Fig. 42-8, p. 640) Sores may have a watery discharge Pain, itching, burning, and tingling in the affected area Vaginal discharge Pain during urination or intercourse Fever Swollen glands	No known cure Anti-viral medications
Genital warts	*Male*—Warts in or on the penis, anus, genitalia, mouth, or throat *Female*—Warts in or on the vagina, cervix, labia, anus, mouth, or throat	Application of special ointment that causes the warts to dry up and fall off Surgical removal may be necessary if the ointment is not effective
HIV/AIDS	See Chapter 38	See Chapter 38
Gonorrhea	Burning and pain on urination Urinary frequency and urgency Genital discharge (vagina, urethra, rectum)	Antibiotic medications

Continued

Table 42-1	Sexually Transmitted Diseases—cont'd	
Disease	**Signs and Symptoms**	**Treatment**
Chlamydia	May not show symptoms Discharge from the penis or vagina Burning or pain on urination Testicular pain or swelling Vaginal bleeding Rectal inflammation and/or discharge Pain during intercourse Diarrhea Nausea Abdominal pain Fever	Antibiotic medications
Pubic lice (Chapter 21)	Intense itching	Over-the-counter or prescription lice treatment Washing or dry-cleaning all exposed clothing, bedding, and towels
Trichomoniasis (occurs in women; men are carriers)	No symptoms in men Frothy, thick, foul-smelling, yellow vaginal discharge Genital itching and irritation Burning and pain on urination Genital swelling	Metronidazole
Syphilis	*Stage 1*—10 to 90 days after exposure • Painless sores (chancres) on the penis, in the vagina, or on the genitalia; the chancre may also be on the lips or inside the mouth, or anywhere on the body *Stage 2*—About 3 to 6 weeks after the sores • General fatigue, loss of appetite, nausea, fever, headache, rash, swollen glands, sore throat, bone and joint pain, hair loss, lesions on the lips and genitalia • Symptoms may come and go for many years *Stage 3*—3 to 15 years after infection • Central nervous system damage (including paralysis), heart damage, blindness, liver damage, mental health problems, death	Penicillin and other antibiotic medications

Fig. 42-8 Herpes. **A,** Sores on the penis. **B,** Sores on the female perineum. *(Courtesy United States Public Health Service, Washington, DC.)*

QUALITY OF LIFE

Urinary and reproductive disorders can vary from mild, to severely uncomfortable, to life-threatening. Follow the care plan and the nurse's directions carefully. Report your observations promptly. They can make a difference in the person's life.

Many older people are sexually active. They get and can spread STDs in the same ways that younger persons do. However, many do not think they are at risk. Always practice Standard Precautions and the Bloodborne Pathogen Standard. Do not assume that older people are too old to have sex.

REVIEW QUESTIONS

Circle the BEST answer.

1   A person has cystitis. This is a
   a   Kidney infection
   b   Kidney stone
   c   Urinary diversion
   d   Bladder infection

2   The person with cystitis needs to drink about
   a   500 mL daily
   b   1000 mL daily
   c   1500 mL daily
   d   2000 mL daily

3   BPH causes urinary problems because
   a   The person has a weak urine stream
   b   The person voids frequently at night
   c   The enlarged prostate presses against the urethra
   d   Voidings are in small amounts

4   Mr. Jones had a TURP. Which measure should you question?
   a   No sudden movements
   b   No heavy lifting
   c   No straining to have a bowel movement
   d   No oral fluids

5   A person with a urostomy
   a   Has a new pathway for urine to exit the body
   b   Needs dialysis
   c   Had surgery for an enlarged prostate
   d   Has pyuria

6   A person has kidney stones. You need to
   a   Strain all urine
   b   Empty the pouch
   c   Collect a urine specimen
   d   Change the urinary drainage bag

7   A person has kidney failure. Which statement is *false*?
   a   The kidneys remove waste products from the blood.
   b   The body retains fluid.
   c   Every body system is affected.
   d   Diuresis follows oliguria.

8   For chronic kidney failure, care includes the following *except*
   a   A diet low in protein, potassium, and sodium
   b   Measuring urine output every hour
   c   Measures to prevent pressure ulcers
   d   Measuring weight daily

9   These statements are about STDs. Which is *false*?
   a   They are usually spread by sexual contact.
   b   They can affect the genital area and other body parts.
   c   Signs and symptoms are obvious.
   d   Some result in death.

10   STDs require
   a   Masks and protective eyewear
   b   Gowns
   c   Double-bagging
   d   Standard Precautions

Answers to these questions are on p. 721.

Mental Health Problems

OBJECTIVES

- Define the key terms and key abbreviations listed in this chapter.
- Explain the difference between mental health and mental illness.
- List the causes of mental illness.
- Describe four anxiety disorders.
- Explain the defense mechanisms used to relieve anxiety.
- Describe common phobias.

- Explain schizophrenia.
- Describe bipolar disorder and depression.
- Describe personality disorders.
- Describe substance abuse and addiction.
- Describe suicide and the persons at risk.
- Describe the care required by persons with mental health disorders.
- Explain how to promote quality of life.

KEY TERMS

affect Feelings and emotions

anxiety A vague, uneasy feeling in response to stress

compulsion Repeating an act over and over again

defense mechanism An unconscious reaction that blocks unpleasant or threatening feelings

delusion A false belief

delusion of grandeur An exaggerated belief about one's importance, wealth, power, or talents

delusion of persecution A false belief that one is being mistreated, abused, or harassed

emotional illness See "mental disorder"

flashback Reliving the trauma in thoughts during the day and in nightmares during sleep

hallucination Seeing, hearing, smelling, or feeling something that is not real

mental Relating to the mind; something that exists in the mind or is done by the mind

mental disorder A disturbance in the ability to cope with or adjust to stress; behavior and function are impaired; mental illness, emotional illness, psychiatric disorder

mental health The person copes with and adjusts to everyday stresses in ways accepted by society

mental illness See "mental disorder"

obsession A recurrent, unwanted thought, idea, or image

panic An intense and sudden feeling of fear, anxiety, terror, or dread

paranoia A disorder (*para*) of the mind (*noia*); false beliefs (delusions) and suspicion about a person or situation

phobia An intense fear

psychiatric disorder See "mental disorder"

psychosis A state of severe mental impairment

stress The response or change in the body caused by any emotional, physical, social, or economic factor

stressor The event or factor that causes stress

suicide To kill oneself

KEY TERMS—cont'd

suicide contagion Exposure to suicide or suicidal behaviors within one's family, one's peer group, or media reports of suicide

withdrawal syndrome The person's physical and mental response after stopping or severely reducing the use of a substance that was used regularly

KEY ABBREVIATIONS

BPD	Borderline personality disorder
GI	Gastro-intestinal
NIAAA	National Institute on Alcohol Abuse and Alcoholism

NIMH	National Institute of Mental Health
OCD	Obsessive-compulsive disorder
PTSD	Post-traumatic stress disorder

The whole person has physical, social, psychological, and spiritual parts. Each part affects the other.

- A physical problem has social, mental, and spiritual effects.
- A mental health problem can affect the person physically, socially, and spiritually.
- A social problem can have physical, mental health, and spiritual effects.

BASIC CONCEPTS

Mental relates to the mind. It is something that exists in the mind or is done by the mind. Therefore mental health involves the mind. Mental health and mental disorders involve stress:

- Stress—is the response or change in the body caused by any emotional, physical, social, or economic factor.
- Mental health—means that the person copes with and adjusts to everyday stresses in ways accepted by society.
- Mental disorder—is a disturbance in the ability to cope with or adjust to stress. Behavior and function are impaired. Mental illness, emotional illness, and psychiatric disorder are other names.

Causes of mental health disorders include:

- Not being able to cope or adjust to stress
- Chemical imbalances
- Genetics
- Physical or biologic factors
- Psychological factors
- Drug or substance abuse
- Social and cultural factors

ANXIETY DISORDERS

Anxiety is a vague, uneasy feeling in response to stress. The person may not know why or the cause. Danger or harm—real or imagined—is sensed. The person acts to relieve the unpleasant feeling. Often anxiety occurs when needs are not met.

Some anxiety is normal. Persons with mental health problems have higher levels of anxiety. Signs and symptoms depend on the degree of anxiety (Box 43-1).

Anxiety level depends on the stressor. A stressor is the event or factor that causes stress. It can be physical, emotional, social, or economic. Past experiences affect how a person reacts. So does the number of stressors. A stressor may produce mild anxiety. The same stressor can cause higher anxiety at another time.

Box 43-1 Signs and Symptoms of Anxiety

- A "lump" in the throat
- "Butterflies" in the stomach
- Pulse: rapid
- Respirations: rapid
- Blood pressure: increased
- Speech: rapid, voice changes
- Mouth: dry
- Sweating
- Nausea
- Diarrhea
- Urinary frequency and urgency
- Attention span: poor
- Directions: difficulty following
- Sleep: difficulty
- Appetite: loss of

Box 43-2 Defense Mechanisms

Compensation. *Compensate* means to make up for, replace, or substitute. The person makes up for or substitutes a strength for a weakness.
EXAMPLE: Not good in sports, a child develops another talent.

Conversion. *Convert* means to change. An emotion is shown as a physical symptom or changed into a physical symptom.
EXAMPLE: Not wanting to read out loud in school, a child complains of a headache.

Denial. *Deny* means refusing to accept or believe something that is true. The person refuses to face or accept unpleasant or threatening things.
EXAMPLE: After a heart attack, a person continues to smoke.

Displacement. *Displace* means to move or take the place of. An individual moves behaviors or emotions from one person, place, or thing to a safe person, place, or thing.
EXAMPLE: Angry at your boss, you yell at a friend.

Identification. *Identify* means to relate or recognize. A person assumes the ideas, behaviors, and traits of another person.
EXAMPLE: A neighbor is a high school cheerleader. A little girl practices cheerleading in her backyard.

Projection. *Project* means to blame another. An individual blames another person or object for unacceptable behaviors, emotions, ideas, or wishes.
EXAMPLE: Sleeping too long, a worker blames the traffic when late for work.

Rationalization. *Rational* means sensible, reasonable, or logical. An acceptable reason or excuse is given for behaviors or actions. The real reason is not given.
EXAMPLE: Often late for work, an employee does not get a raise. The employee thinks "My boss doesn't like me."

Reaction formation. A person acts in a way opposite to what he or she truly feels.
EXAMPLE: A worker does not like his boss. He buys the boss an expensive gift.

Regression. *Regress* means to move back or to retreat. The person retreats or moves back to an earlier time or condition.
EXAMPLE: A 3-year-old wants a baby bottle when a new baby comes into the family.

Repression. *Repress* means to hold down or keep back. The person keeps unpleasant or painful thoughts or experiences from the conscious mind. They cannot be recalled or remembered.
EXAMPLE: A child was sexually abused. Now 33 years old, there is no memory of the event.

Coping and defense mechanisms are used to relieve anxiety. Some are healthy. Others are not—eating, drinking, smoking, fighting are examples. Healthy ways to cope include discussing the problem, exercising, playing music, taking a hot bath, wanting to be alone.

Defense mechanisms are unconscious reactions that block unpleasant or threatening feelings (Box 43-2). Some use of defense mechanisms is normal. In mental disorders, they are used poorly.

Panic Disorder

Panic is the highest level of anxiety. Panic is an intense and sudden feeling of fear, anxiety, terror, or dread. Onset is sudden with no obvious reason. The person cannot function. Signs and symptoms of anxiety are severe (see Box 43-1). The person may also have:

- Chest pain
- Shortness of breath
- Rapid heart rate ("heart pounding")
- Numbness and tingling in the hands
- Dizziness
- A smothering sensation
- Feeling of impending doom or loss of control

The person may feel that he or she is having a heart attack, losing his or her mind, or on the verge of death. Attacks can occur at any time, even during sleep.

Panic attacks can last for 10 minutes or longer. They can occur often. Panic disorder can last for a few months or for many years.

Many people avoid places where panic attacks occurred. For example, a person had a panic attack in a shopping mall. Malls are avoided.

Phobias

Phobia means an intense fear. The person has an intense fear of an object, situation, or activity that has little or no actual danger. Common phobias are fear of:

- Being in an open, crowded, or public place (agoraphobia—*agora* means marketplace)
- Being in pain or seeing others in pain (algophobia—*algo* means pain)
- Water (aquaphobia—*aqua* means water)
- Being in or being trapped in an enclosed or narrow space (claustrophobia—*claustro* means closing)
- The slightest uncleanliness (mysophobia—*myso* means anything that is disgusting)
- Night or darkness (nyctophobia—*nycto* means night or darkness)
- Fire (pyrophobia—*pyro* means fire)
- Strangers (xenophobia—*xeno* means strange)

The person avoids what is feared. When faced with the fear, the person has high anxiety and cannot function.

Obsessive-Compulsive Disorder

The person with obsessive-compulsive disorder (OCD) has obsessions and compulsions. An **obsession** is a recurrent, unwanted thought, idea, or image. Some people are obsessed with microbes, dirt, violent thoughts, or things forbidden by religious beliefs. **Compulsion** is repeating an act over and over again (a ritual). The act may not make sense. However, the person has much anxiety if the act is not done.

Common rituals are hand washing, constant checking to make sure the stove is off, cleaning, counting things to a certain number, or touching things in a certain order. Such rituals can take over an hour every day. They are very distressing and affect daily life. Some persons with OCD also have depression, eating disorders, substance abuse, and other anxiety disorders.

Post-Traumatic Stress Disorder

Post-traumatic stress disorder (PTSD) occurs after a terrifying ordeal. The ordeal involved physical harm or the threat of physical harm. Signs and symptoms of PTSD are listed in Box 43-3. PTSD can develop:

- After being harmed
- After a loved one was harmed
- After seeing a harmful event happen to loved ones or strangers

PTSD can result from many traumatic events. They include:

- War
- A terrorist attack
- Mugging
- Rape
- Torture
- Kidnapping
- Being held captive
- Child abuse
- A crash—vehicle, train, plane
- Bombing
- A natural disaster—flood, tornado, hurricane

Most people with PTSD have flashbacks. A **flashback** is reliving the trauma in thoughts during the day and in nightmares during sleep. Flashbacks may involve images, sounds, smells, or feelings. Everyday things can trigger them. A door slamming is an example. During a flashback, the person may lose touch with reality. He or she may believe that the trauma is happening all over again.

Signs and symptoms usually develop about 3 months after the harmful event. However, they may not emerge until years later. Some people recover within 6 months. PTSD lasts longer in other people. The condition may become chronic.

PTSD can develop at any age including during childhood. The person may also suffer from depression, substance abuse, and other anxiety disorders.

Box 43-3 Signs and Symptoms of Post-Traumatic Stress Disorder

- Startles easily
- Emotionally numb—especially to those with whom the person used to be close
- Difficulty trusting people
- Difficulty feeling close to people
- Loss of interest in things he or she used to enjoy
- Problems being affectionate
- Feelings of intense guilt
- Irritability
- Avoiding situations that remind of the harmful event
- Difficulty around the anniversary of the harmful event
- Gets mad easily
- Outbursts of anger
- Problems sleeping
- Increasingly aggressive
- Becoming more violent
- Physical symptoms:
  - Headache
  - Gastro-intestinal (GI) distress
  - Immune system problems
  - Dizziness
  - Chest pain
  - Discomfort in other body parts

SCHIZOPHRENIA

Schizophrenia means split *(schizo)* mind *(phrenia)*. It is a severe, chronic, disabling brain disorder. It involves:

- **Psychosis**—a state of severe mental impairment. The person does not view the real or unreal correctly.
- **Delusion**—a false belief. For example, the person believes that a radio station is broadcasting the person's thoughts.
- **Hallucination**—seeing, hearing, smelling, or feeling something that is not real. A person may see animals, insects, or people that are not real. "Voices" are the most common type of hallucination in schizophrenia. "Voices" may comment on behavior, order the person to do things, warn of danger, or talk to other voices.
- **Paranoia**—a disorder *(para)* of the mind *(noia)*. The person has false beliefs (delusions). He or she is suspicious about a person or situation. For example, a person may believe that others are cheating, harassing, poisoning, spying upon, or plotting against him or her.
- **Delusion of grandeur**—an exaggerated belief about one's importance, wealth, power, or talents. For example, a man believes he is Superman. Or a woman believes she is the Queen of England.
- **Delusion of persecution**—the false belief that one is being mistreated, abused, or harassed. For example, a person believes that someone is "out to get" him or her.

FOCUS ON COMMUNICATION
Schizophrenia

Delusions, hallucinations, and paranoia can frighten a person. Good communication is important. Remember to:
- Speak slowly and calmly.
- Do not pretend you experience what the person does. Help the person focus on reality.
- Do not try to convince the person that the experience is not real. To the person, it is real.
  For example, a person is hearing voices. You can say: "I don't hear the voices, but I believe that you do. Try to listen to my voice and not the other voices."

The person with schizophrenia has severe mental impairment *(psychosis)*. Thinking and behavior are disturbed. The person has false beliefs *(delusions).* He or she also has *hallucinations.* That is, the person sees, hears, smells, or feels things that are not real. The person has problems relating to others. He or she may be *paranoid.* That is, the person is suspicious about a person or situation. The person may have difficulty organizing thoughts. Responses are not appropriate. Communication is disturbed. The person may ramble or repeat what another says. Sometimes speech cannot be understood. He or she may make up words. The person may withdraw. That is, the person lacks interest in others. He or she is not involved with people or society.

Disorders of movement occur. These include:
- Being clumsy and uncoordinated
- Involuntary movements
- Grimacing
- Unusual mannerisms
- Sitting for hours without moving, speaking, or responding

Some persons regress. To *regress* means to retreat or move back to an earlier time or condition. For example, a 5-year-old wets the bed when there is a new baby. This is normal. Healthy adults do not act like infants or children.

In men, the symptoms usually begin in the late teens or early 20s. In women, symptoms usually begin in their 20s and 30s. In rare cases, it can appear in childhood. People with schizophrenia do not tend to be violent. However, if a person with paranoid schizophrenia becomes violent, it is often directed at family members. The violence usually occurs at home. Some persons with schizophrenia attempt suicide (p. 652).

See *Focus on Communication: Schizophrenia.*

MOOD DISORDERS

Mood or **affect** relates to feelings and emotions. Mood (or affective) disorders involve feelings, emotions, and moods.

Bipolar Disorder

Bipolar means two *(bi)* poles or ends *(polar.)* The person with bipolar disorder has severe extremes in mood, energy, and ability to function. There are emotional lows *(depression)* and emotional highs *(mania).* The disorder also is called manic-depressive illness. The person may:
- Be more depressed than manic
- Be more manic than depressed
- Alternate between depression and mania

The disorder tends to run in families. It usually develops in the late teens or in early adulthood. Life-long management is required.

Signs and symptoms can range from mild to severe (Box 43-4). Mood changes are called "episodes." Bipolar disorder can damage relationships and affect school or work performance. Some people are suicidal.

Box 43-4   Signs and Symptoms of Bipolar Disorder

Mania (Manic Episode)
- Increased energy, activity, and restlessness
- Excessively "high," overly good mood
- Extreme irritability
- Racing thoughts and talking very fast
- Jumping from one idea to another
- Easily distracted; problems concentrating
- Little sleep needed
- Unrealistic beliefs in one's abilities and powers
- Poor judgment
- Spending sprees
- A lasting period of behavior that is different from usual
- Increased sexual drive
- Drug abuse (particularly cocaine, alcohol, and sleeping pills)
- Aggressive behavior
- Denial that anything is wrong

Depression (Depressive Episode)
- Lasting sad, anxious, or empty mood
- Feelings of hopelessness
- Feelings of guilt, worthlessness, or helplessness
- Loss of interest or pleasure in activities once enjoyed
- Loss of interest in sex
- Decreased energy; a feeling of fatigue or being "slowed down"
- Problems concentrating, remembering, or making decisions
- Restlessness or irritability
- Sleeping too much, or unable to sleep
- Change in appetite
- Unintended weight loss or gain
- Chronic pain or other symptoms not caused by physical illness or injury
- Thoughts of death or suicide
- Suicide attempts

Major Depression

Depression involves the body, mood, and thoughts. Symptoms (see Box 43-4) affect work, study, sleep, eating, and other activities. The person is very sad. He or she loses interest in daily activities.

Depression may occur because of a stressful event such as the death of a partner, parent, or child. Divorce and job loss are other stressful events. Some physical disorders can cause depression. Stroke, heart attack, cancer, and Parkinson's disease are examples. Hormonal factors may cause depression in women—menstrual cycle changes, pregnancy, miscarriage, after childbirth (post-partum depression), and before and during menopause.

Depression in Older Persons Depression is common in older persons. They have many losses—death of family and friends, loss of health, loss of body functions, loss of independence. Loneliness and the side effects of some medications also are causes. See Box 43-5 for the signs and symptoms of depression in older persons.

Depression in older persons is often overlooked or a wrong diagnosis is made. Often the person is thought to have a cognitive disorder (Chapter 44). Therefore depression is often not treated.

PERSONALITY DISORDERS

Personality disorders involve rigid and maladaptive behaviors. To *adapt* means to change or adjust. *Mal* means bad, wrong, or ill. *Maladaptive* means to change or adjust in the wrong way. Because of their behaviors, those with personality disorders cannot function well in society.

Antisocial Personality Disorder

This is a chronic disorder in which the person's thinking and behaviors show no regard for right and wrong. The person has poor judgment, lacks responsibility, and is hostile. The person is not loyal to any person or group. Morals and ethics are lacking. The rights of others do not matter. The person lies, charms, or cons others for personal gain or pleasure. The person has no guilt. He or she does not learn from experiences or punishment. The person is often in trouble with the police.

Signs and symptoms may include:
- Lying or cheating
- Child abuse or neglect
- Aggressive or violent behaviors
- Poor or abusive relationships
- Blaming others for actions and behaviors
- Problems functioning in work or school

Symptoms tend to peak during the 20s and then decrease. Risk factors include:
- A conduct disorder in childhood
- A family history of antisocial personality disorder
- A family history of mental disorders
- Childhood abuse—verbal, physical, sexual
- Unstable family life during childhood
- Loss of parents during childhood—death, divorce

Borderline Personality Disorder (BPD)

The person has problems with moods, relationships, self-image, and behavior. The person has problems controlling emotions. He or she may have intense bouts of anger, depression, and anxiety that last hours or most of the day. Aggression, self-injury, and drug or alcohol abuse may occur. The person may engage in risky behaviors—unsafe driving, unsafe sex, gambling sprees. The person may greatly admire and love family and friends and then suddenly shift to intense anger and dislike. The person may have thoughts of suicide and other mental health disorders.

BPD is more common in women than in men. Risk factors may include:
- A family history of BPD
- Childhood abuse—sexual, physical
- Childhood neglect or being abandoned
- Changes in the brain
- Brain chemicals that do not function properly

Box 43-5 Signs and Symptoms of Depression in Older Persons

- Fatigue and lack of interest
- Inability to experience pleasure
- Feelings of uselessness, hopelessness, and helplessness
- Decreased sexual interest
- Increased dependency
- Anxiety
- Slow or unreliable memory
- Paranoia
- Agitation
- Focus on the past
- Thoughts of death and suicide
- Difficulty completing activities of daily living
- Changes in sleep patterns
- Poor grooming
- Withdrawal from people and interests
- Muscle aches, abdominal pain, and headaches
- Nausea and vomiting
- Dry mouth
- Loss of appetite
- Weight loss

SUBSTANCE ABUSE AND ADDICTION

Substance abuse or addiction occurs when a person over-uses or depends on alcohol or drugs. Physical and mental health are affected. So is the welfare of others.

Substances involved in abuse and addiction affect the nervous system. Some depress the nervous system. Others stimulate it. All affect the mind and thinking.

Alcoholism and Alcohol Abuse

Alcohol slows down brain activity. It affects alertness, judgment, coordination, and reaction time. Over time, heavy drinking damages the brain, central nervous system, liver, heart, kidneys, blood vessels, and stomach. It also can cause forgetfulness and confusion.

According to the National Institute on Alcohol Abuse and Alcoholism (NIAAA), *alcoholism* (alcohol dependence) includes these symptoms:
- *Craving.* The person has a strong need or urge to drink.
- *Loss of control.* The person cannot stop drinking once drinking has begun.
- *Physical dependence.* The person has withdrawal symptoms when he or she stops drinking. They include nausea, sweating, shakiness, and anxiety.
- *Tolerance.* The person needs to drink greater amounts of alcohol to get "high."

Alcoholism is a chronic disease. It lasts throughout life. Life-style and genetics are risk factors. Some people drink alcohol for relief from life stresses—retirement, lowered income, job loss, failing health, loneliness, or the deaths of loved ones or friends. The alcohol craving can be as strong as the need for food or water. An alcoholic will continue to drink despite serious family, health, or legal problems.

Alcoholism can be treated but not cured. Counseling and medications are used to help the person stop drinking. The person must avoid all alcohol to avoid a relapse.

Alcohol abuse is just as harmful as alcoholism. A person who abuses alcohol drinks too much but is not dependent on alcohol.

Problems linked to alcoholism and alcohol abuse include:
- Not being able to meet work, school, or family responsibilities
- Motor vehicle crashes
- Drunk-driving arrests
- Drinking-related medical conditions

Drinking occasionally or regularly does not mean a drinking problem. According to the NIAAA, a person needs help if he or she:
- Drinks to calm nerves, forget worries, or reduce depression
- Has lost interest in food
- Gulps drinks down fast
- Lies or tries to hide drinking habits
- Drinks alone more often

- Has hurt oneself or someone else while drinking
- Was drunk more than 3 or 4 times in one year
- Needs more alcohol to get "high"
- Feels irritable, resentful, or unreasonable when not drinking
- Has medical, social, or money problems caused by drinking

Alcohol and Older Persons Alcohol effects vary with age. Even small amounts can make older persons feel "high." Older persons are at risk for falls, vehicle crashes, and other injuries from drinking. They have:
- Slower reaction times
- Hearing and vision problems
- A lower tolerance for alcohol

Older people tend to take more medications than younger persons. Mixing alcohol with some medications can be harmful, even fatal. Alcohol also makes some health problems worse. High blood pressure is an example.

Drug Abuse and Addiction

Drugs interfere with normal brain function. While they create powerful feelings of pleasure, they have long-term effects on the brain. At some point, changes in the brain can turn drug abuse into addiction.
- *Drug abuse*—is the over-use of a drug for non-medical or non-therapy effects.
- *Drug addiction*—is a chronic, relapsing brain disease. The person has an overwhelming desire to take a drug. The person repeatedly takes the drug because of its effect. Usually the effect is altered mental awareness. The person has to have the drug. Often higher doses are needed. The person cannot stop taking the drug without treatment.

A diagnosis of drug abuse or addiction is based on 3 or more of the following. They must have occurred any time during a 12-month period.
- The substance is often taken in larger amounts. Or it is taken longer than intended.
- There is a constant desire for the substance. Or the person cannot cut down or control substance use.
- A lot of time is spent using the substance or recovering from its effects. Or a great deal of time is spent trying to obtain the substance. For example, the person visits many doctors to obtain the substance. Or he or she drives long distances to get the substance.
- The person gave up or reduced important social, occupational, or recreational activities because of substance abuse.
- The person continues to use the substance. The person does so despite knowing that a constant or recurring problem is caused by or made worse by using the substance. The problem may be physical or psychological.

- The person has tolerance to the substance:
  - Increased amounts are needed to achieve intoxication or the desired effect.
  - Continued use of the same amount has a greatly reduced effect on the person.
- Withdrawal from the substance (*withdraw* means to stop, remove, or take away):
  - The withdrawal syndrome is that expected for the drug. **Withdrawal syndrome** is the person's physical and mental response after stopping or severely reducing the use of a substance that was used regularly. The body responds with anxiety, restlessness, insomnia, irritability, impaired attention, and physical illness.
  - The same (or similar) substance is taken to relieve or avoid withdrawal symptoms.

Drug abuse and addiction affect social and mental function. Drug abuse and addiction are linked to crimes, violence, and motor vehicle crashes. Physical effects can occur from one use, high doses, or prolonged use:

- HIV and AIDS (Chapter 38)
- Cardiovascular disease
- Stroke
- Sudden death
- Hepatitis
- Lung disease
- Cancer

Legal and illegal drugs are abused (Table 43-1). Legal drugs are approved for use in the United States. Doctors prescribe them. Illegal drugs are not approved for use. They are obtained through illegal means. Often legal drugs also are obtained through illegal means.

Treatment depends on the drug and the person. A drug treatment program combines various therapies and services to meet the person's needs. The person's age, race, culture, sexual orientation, and gender are considered. So are issues such as pregnancy, parenting, housing, employment, and physical and sexual abuse.

Drug abuse and addiction are chronic problems. Relapses can occur. A short-term, one-time treatment is often not enough. Treatment is a long-term process.

Text continued on p. 652

Table 43-1 Commonly Abused Drugs

Substance (How Administered)	Commercial and Street Names	Effects and Potential Health Problems
Cannabinoids		
		Euphoria; slowed thinking and reaction time; confusion; impaired balance and coordination; frequent respiratory infections; impaired memory and learning; increased heart rate; anxiety; panic attacks; tolerance; addiction
hashish *(swallowed; smoked)*	boom, chronic gangster, hash, hash oil, hemp	See "Cannabinoids"
marijuana *(swallowed; smoked)*	blunt, dope, ganja, grass, herb, joints, Mary Jane, pot, reefer, sinsemilla, skunk, weed	See "Cannabinoids"
Depressants		
		Reduced anxiety; feeling of well-being; lowered inhibitions; slowed pulse and breathing; lowered blood pressure; poor concentration; fatigue; confusion; impaired coordination, memory, and judgment; addiction; respiratory depression and arrest; death
barbiturates *(injected; swallowed)*	*Amytal, Nembutal, Seconal, Phenobarbital*; barbs, reds, red birds, phennies, tooies, yellows, yellow jackets	See "Depressants;" sedation; drowsiness; depression; unusual excitement; fever, irritability; poor judgment; slurred speech; dizziness; life-threatening withdrawal
benzodiazepines *(swallowed; injected)* NOTE: Other than flunitrazepam	*Ativan, Halcion, Librium, Valium, Xanax*; candy, downers, sleeping pills, tranks	See "Depressants;" sedation; drowsiness; dizziness

Modified from National Institute on Drug Abuse: Commonly abused drugs, *National Institutes of Health, Bethesda, Md, updated May 19, 2010.*

Continued

Table 43-1	Commonly Abused Drugs—cont'd	

Substance (How Administered)	Commercial and Street Names	Effects and Potential Health Problems
Depressants—cont'd		
flunitrazepam *(swallowed; snorted)* NOTE: Drug is associated with sexual assaults.	*Rohypnol;* forget-me pill, Mexican Valium, R2, Roche, roofies, roofinol, rope, rophies	See "Depressants;" visual and GI disturbances, urinary retention, memory loss for the time under the drug's effects
GHB *(swallowed)* NOTE: Drug is associated with sexual assaults.	*gamma-hydroxybutyrate;* G, Georgia home boy, grievous bodily harm, liquid ecstasy	See "Depressants;" drowsiness; nausea and vomiting; headache; loss of consciousness; loss of reflexes; seizures; coma; death
methaqualone *(injected; swallowed)*	*Quaalude, Sopor, Parest;* ludes, mandrex, quad, quay	See "Depressants;" euphoria and depression; poor reflexes; slurred speech; coma
Dissociative Anesthetics		
		Increased heart rate and blood pressure; impaired motor function and memory loss; numbness; nausea and vomiting
ketamine *(injected; snorted; smoked)*	*Ketalar SV;* cat Valiums, K, Special K, vitamin K	See "Dissociative Anesthetics;" delirium; depression; respiratory depression and arrest
PCP and analogs *(injected; swallowed; smoked)*	*phencyclidine;* angel dust, boat, hog, love boat, peace pill	See "Dissociative Anesthetics;" possible decrease in blood pressure and heart rate; panic; aggression; violence; loss of appetite; depression
Hallucinogens		
		Altered states of perception and feeling; nausea; flashbacks
LSD *(swallowed; absorbed through mouth tissues)*	*lysergic acid diethylamide;* acid, blotter, boomers, cubes, microdot, yellow sunshines	See "Hallucinogens;" increased body temperature, pulse, and blood pressure; loss of appetite; sleeplessness; numbness; weakness; tremors; persistent mental disorders
mescaline *(smoked; swallowed)*	buttons, cactus, mesc, peyote	See "Dissociative Anesthetics;" see "LSD"
psilocybin *(swallowed)*	magic mushroom, purple passion, shrooms	See "Dissociative Anesthetics;" nervousness; paranoia
Opioids and Morphine Derivatives		
		Pain relief; euphoria; drowsiness; nausea; constipation; confusion; sedation; respiratory depression and arrest; tolerance; addiction; unconsciousness; coma; death
codeine *(injected; swallowed)*	*Empirin with Codeine, Fiorinal with Codeine, Robitussin A-C, Tylenol with Codeine;* Captain Cody, schoolboy, doors & fours, loads, pancakes and syrup	See "Opioids and Morphine Derivatives;" less analgesia, sedation, and respiratory depression than from morphine
fentanyl and fentanyl analogs *(injected; smoked; snorted)*	*Actiq, Duragesic, Sublimaze;* Apache, China girl, China white, dance fever, friend, goodfella, jackpot, murder 8, TNT, Tango and Cash	See "Opioids and Morphine Derivatives"
heroin *(injected; smoked; snorted)*	*diacetyl-morphine;* brown sugar, dope, H, horse, junk, skag, skunk, smack, white horse	See "Opioids and Morphine Derivatives"

Table 43-1 Commonly Abused Drugs—cont'd

Substance (How Administered)	Commercial and Street Names	Effects and Potential Health Problems
Opioids and Morphine Derivatives—cont'd		
morphine *(injected; smoked; snorted)*	*Roxanol, Duramorph;* M, Miss Emma, monkey, white stuff	See "Opioids and Morphine Derivatives"
opium *(swallowed; smoked)*	*laudanum, paregoric;* big O, black stuff, block, gum, hop	See "Opioids and Morphine Derivatives"
oxycodone HCl *(swallowed; snorted; injected)*	*OxyContin;* Oxy, O.C., killer	See "Opioids and Morphine Derivatives"
hydrocodone bitartrate, ac- etaminophen *(swallowed)*	*Vicodin;* vike, Watson-387	See "Opioids and Morphine Derivatives"
Stimulants		
		Increased pulse, blood pressure, and metabolism; feelings of exhilaration; energy; increased mental awareness; rapid or irregular heartbeat; reduced appetite; weight loss; heart failure; nervousness; insomnia
amphetamine *(injected; swal- lowed; smoked; snorted)*	*Biphetamine, Dexedrine;* bennies, black beauties, crosses, hearts, LA turnaround, speed, truck drivers, uppers	See "Stimulants;" rapid breathing; tremor; loss of co- ordination; irritability; anxiousness; restlessness; delirium; panic, paranoia; impulsive behavior; ag- gressiveness; tolerance; addiction; psychosis
cocaine *(injected; smoked; snorted)*	*Cocaine hydrochloride;* blow, bump, C, candy, Charlie, coke, crack, flake, rock, snow, toot	See "Stimulants;" increased temperature; chest pain; respiratory failure; nausea; abdominal pain; strokes; seizures; headaches; malnutrition; panic attacks
MDMA *(swallowed)*	*methylenedioxymethamphet- amine;* Adam, clarity, ecstasy, Eve, lover's speed, peace, STP, X, XTC	See "Stimulants;" mild hallucinogenic effects; in- creased sensitivity to touch; empathic feelings; im- paired memory and learning; hyperthermia; cardiac toxicity; kidney failure; liver toxicity
methamphetamine *(injected; swallowed; smoked; snorted)*	*Desoxyn;* chalk, crank, crystal, fire, glass, go fast, ice, meth, speed	See "Stimulants;" aggression, violence; psychotic be- havior; memory loss; cardiac and nervous system damage; impaired memory and learning; tolerance; addiction
methylphenidate *(injected; swallowed; snorted)*	*Ritalin;* JIF, MPH, R-ball, Skippy, the smart drug, vitamin R	See "Stimulants"
nicotine *(smoked; snorted; taken in snuff and spit tobacco)*	cigarettes, cigars, smokeless to- bacco, snuff, spit tobacco, bidis, chew	See "Stimulants;" adverse pregnancy outcomes; chronic lung disease; cardiovascular disease; stroke; cancer; tolerance; addiction
Other Compounds		
anabolic steroids *(injected; swallowed; applied to the skin)*	*Anadrol, Oxandrin, Durabolin, Depo-Testosterone, Equipoise;* roids, juice	Hypertension; blood clotting and cholesterol changes; liver cysts and cancer; kidney cancer; hostility and aggression; acne; premature growth stoppage in adolescents; prostate cancer; reduced sperm pro- duction; shrunken testicles; breast enlargement (males); menstrual irregularities; beard and other male characteristics (females)
Inhalants *(inhaled through the nose or mouth)*	*Solvents (paint thinners, gasoline, glues), gases (butane, propane, aerosol propellants, nitrous ox- ide), nitrites (isoamyl, isobutyl, cyclohexyl);* laughing gas, pop- pers, snappers, whippets	Stimulation; loss of inhibition; headache; nausea or vomiting; slurred speech; loss of motor coordina- tion; wheezing; unconsciousness; cramps; weight loss; muscle weakness; depression; memory im- pairment; damage to cardiovascular and nervous systems; sudden death

SUICIDE

Suicide means to kill oneself. According to a 2009 National Institute of Mental Health (NIMH) report and a 2009 report from the Centers for Disease Control and Prevention (CDC):

- Suicide was the 11th leading cause of death in the United States. In 2006, there were 33,000 deaths from suicide.
- Risk factors for attempted suicide include:
  - Depression and other mental health disorders
  - Alcohol or other substance abuse
  - Separation or divorce
- Firearms, suffocation, and poison are the most common methods of suicide. Firearms are the most common method for men. For women, poison is the most common method.
- More men than women die by suicide.
- American Indians and Alaskan Natives have high rates of suicide.
- Youth, the elderly, and veterans are at risk for suicide.
- The highest rate of suicide was among white men aged 85 years and older.
- Suicide was the third leading cause of death among persons aged 15 to 24. More males than females in this age-group died by suicide. Risk factors for attempted suicide are:
  - Depression
  - Alcohol or other substance abuse
  - Physical or sexual abuse
  - Disruptive behavior

Risk factors for suicide are listed in Box 43-6. *If a person mentions or talks about suicide, take the person seriously. Call for the nurse at once. Do not leave the person alone.*

Box 43-6　Risk Factors for Suicide

- Depression and other mental disorders
- History of alcohol or drug abuse
- Stressful life event or loss (Divorce is an example.)
- Prior suicide attempt
- Family history of a mental disorder or substance abuse
- Family history of suicide
- Family violence (including physical or sexual abuse)
- Firearms in the home
- Easy access to lethal methods
- Incarceration
- Exposure to suicidal behavior of others (family, peers, media figures)

Modified from National Institute of Mental Health: Suicide in the U.S.: statistics and prevention, *National Institutes of Health, NIH Publication No. 06-4594, reviewed July 27, 2009.*

FOCUS ON COMMUNICATION
Suicide

Persons thinking of suicide may talk about their thoughts. A person may say:
- "I just don't want to live anymore."
- "I wish I was dead."
- "I wish I had never been born."
- "Everyone would be better off without me."

Call for the nurse at once if a person mentions thoughts of suicide.

A person may ask you not to tell anyone about his or her suicidal thoughts. Protecting personal information is important. But the person's safety is the priority. Never promise the person that you will not tell anyone. Report the statements to the nurse at once. It is the right thing to do.

Centers that treat persons with mental health problems must identify persons at risk for suicide. They must:
- Identify specific factors or features that increase or decrease the risk for suicide.
- Meet the person's immediate safety needs.
- Provide the most appropriate setting for treating the person.
- Provide crisis information to the person and family. A crisis "hotline" phone number is an example.

See *Focus on Communication: Suicide.*

Suicide and Older Persons

According to NIMH, older persons have higher suicide rates than younger persons. Older white males have the highest rates. Among white males 65 and older, the risk goes up with age. White men 85 and older have the highest suicide rates. Some older persons are less likely to recover from a suicide attempt.

Many older persons suffer from depression (p. 647). Depression often occurs with other serious illnesses. Heart disease, stroke, diabetes, cancer, and Parkinson's disease are examples. The person also may have social and financial problems.

Most older victims did not report depression to their doctors. Or depression was not detected by the doctors.

Suicide Contagion

The NIMH defines suicide contagion as exposure to suicide or suicidal behaviors within the family, peer group, or media reports of suicide. The exposure has led to an increase in suicide and suicidal behaviors in persons at risk for suicide. Adolescents and young adults are at risk for suicide contagion.

Following suicide exposure, those close to the victim should be evaluated by a mental health professional. They include family, friends, peers, and co-workers. Persons at risk for suicide need mental health services.

CARE AND TREATMENT

Treatment of mental health problems involves having the person explore his or her thoughts and feelings. This is done through psychotherapy and behavior, group, occupational, art, and family therapies. Often medications are ordered.

The care plan reflects the person's needs. The needs of the total person must be met. This includes physical, safety and security, and emotional needs.

Communication is important. Be alert to nonverbal communication. This includes the person's nonverbal communication and your own.

Persons with mental health problems may respond to stress with anxiety, panic, or anger. Some may become violent. You must take responsibility for your safety. Your first priority is to protect yourself. Once you are safe, the health team can work together to protect the person and others. To protect yourself:

- Call for help. Do not try to handle the situation on your own.
- Keep a safe distance between you and the person.
- Be aware of your surroundings. Do not let the person between you and the exit.

See *Focus on Communication: Care and Treatment.*

FOCUS ON COMMUNICATION
Care and Treatment

Nonverbal communication involves eye contact, tone of voice, facial expressions, body movements, and posture. Persons with major depression often have little eye contact, poor posture, and speak softly. Some do not speak much at all. Facial expressions may not change. Some persons cry.

Persons with anxiety feel uneasy. They may be restless and unable to sit still. Anxious persons often speak quickly. Eye contact may be prolonged and intense. Others have poor eye contact. The eyes may move quickly from one place to another. Be alert to nonverbal cues. Tell the nurse what you observe.

Your nonverbal communication also is important. When interacting with persons with mental disorders:

- Face the person.
- Maintain eye contact.
- Position yourself near the person but not too close. Do not invade the person's space.
- Crouch, sit, or stand at the person's level if it is safe to do so.
- Show interest and concern through your posture and facial expressions.
- Speak calmly.

QUALITY OF LIFE

Persons with mental health problems have the right to quality of life. They have the same rights as other residents. Some are very ill. They cannot exercise their rights. Legal representatives do so for them.

People do not choose to have physical or mental health problems. Just as a person does not choose to have diabetes, a person does not choose to have anxiety or depression. How you view the person's illness affects the way you treat the person. Persons with mental health problems deserve the same dignity and respect given to persons with physical illnesses.

Persons with mental health problems may respond to stress in different ways. They may say or do things that seem strange or odd to you. Do not laugh at or insult the person. Do not joke with others about the person. Treat the person with kindness and respect. Also protect the right to privacy and confidentiality. Share what the person said or did only with the nurse. The nurse shares it with the health team as needed. No one else needs to know what the person said or did.

Protect the right to personal choice. The person may have problems making choices. Follow the care plan. Sometimes choices are limited. This helps the person make simple choices. It helps the person feel in control.

Protect the person from abuse, mistreatment, and neglect. Some persons cannot protect themselves. They do not know that they are being mistreated. Report signs of abuse, mistreatment, or neglect to the nurse.

Provide a safe setting. Some persons with mental disorders are dangerous to themselves or others. The care plan includes safety measures. If suicide is a threat, all harmful items are removed from the person's setting. The nurse tells you what to do.

REVIEW QUESTIONS

Circle the BEST answer.

1 Stress is
  a The way a person copes with and adjusts to everyday living
  b A response or change in the body caused by some factor
  c A mental disorder
  d A thought or idea
2 Defense mechanisms are used to
  a Blame others
  b Make excuses for behavior
  c Return to an earlier time
  d Block unpleasant feelings
3 These statements are about defense mechanisms. Which is *false*?
  a Mentally healthy persons use them.
  b They relieve anxiety.
  c They prevent mental disorders.
  d Persons with mental disorders use them.

4 A phobia is
   a The event that causes stress
   b A false belief
   c An intense fear of something
   d Feelings and emotions

5 A person cleans and cleans. This behavior is
   a A delusion
   b A hallucination
   c A compulsion
   d An obsession

6 A person has nightmares about a trauma. The person is having
   a Phobias
   b Panic attacks
   c Flashbacks
   d Anxiety

7 A woman believes she is married to a rock singer. This is called a
   a Fantasy
   b Delusion of grandeur
   c Delusion of persecution
   d Hallucination

8 A man believes that someone is trying to kill him. This belief is called a
   a Fantasy
   b Delusion of grandeur
   c Delusion of persecution
   d Hallucination

9 These statements are about schizophrenia. Which is *false*?
   a It is a brain disorder.
   b It can be cured with medications and therapy.
   c Thinking and behavior are disturbed.
   d Suicide is a risk.

10 Bipolar disorder means that the person
   a Is very suspicious
   b Has anxiety
   c Is very unhappy and feels unwanted
   d Has severe mood swings

11 In bipolar disorder, an "emotional high" is called
   a Depression
   b Psychosis
   c An obsession
   d Mania

12 These statements are about antisocial personality disorder. Which is *false*?
   a The person has regard for right and wrong.
   b The person blames others.
   c The person lies or cons others for pleasure.
   d The person is hostile and lacks morals.

13 Substances involved in abuse and addiction affect the
   a Circulatory system
   b Respiratory system
   c Nervous system
   d Immune system

14 These statements are about alcoholism. Which is *false*?
   a The person has a strong craving for alcohol.
   b The disease lasts throughout life.
   c After treatment, the person can have a social drink.
   d The person physically depends on alcohol.

15 These statements are about drug addiction. Which is *false*?
   a It is a chronic brain disease.
   b Higher doses of the drug may be needed.
   c The person has to have the drug.
   d The person can stop taking the drug without treatment.

16 A person has withdrawal syndrome. This means that
   a The person has a physical and mental response when the drug is not taken
   b The person needs higher doses of the drug
   c The effect is reduced with the same amount of drug
   d The person has a relapse after treatment

17 Which group has the highest suicide rate?
   a White men over 85 years of age
   b Persons between the ages of 15 and 24
   c Men
   d Women

18 For men, the most common method of suicide involves
   a Firearms
   b Suffocation
   c Self-poisoning
   d Drug overdose

19 Most persons who commit suicide have
   a A mental disorder
   b Schizophrenia
   c A phobia
   d Suicide contagion

20 A person talks about suicide. What should you do?
   a Call for the nurse.
   b Identify factors that increase the risk of suicide.
   c Ask what method the person intends to use.
   d Restrain the person.

Circle T if the statement is TRUE. Circle F if the statement is FALSE.

21 T F   Some anxiety is normal.
22 T F   Anxiety is an intense and sudden feeling of fear or dread.
23 T F   Panic is the highest level of anxiety.
24 T F   Depression is common in older persons.
25 T F   Sudden death can occur from one use of a substance.
26 T F   A person is talking about suicide. You can leave the person alone to get the nurse.

Answers to these questions are on p. 721

Confusion and Dementia

OBJECTIVES

- Define the key terms and key abbreviations listed in this chapter.
- Describe confusion and its causes.
- List the measures that help confused persons.
- Explain the differences between delirium, depression, and dementia.
- Describe Alzheimer's disease (AD).

- Describe the signs, symptoms, and behaviors of AD.
- Explain the care required by persons with AD and other dementias.
- Describe the effects of AD on the family.
- Explain validation therapy.
- Explain how to promote quality of life.

KEY TERMS

cognitive function Involves memory, thinking, reasoning, ability to understand, judgment, and behavior

delirium A state of sudden, severe confusion and rapid brain changes

delusion A false belief

dementia The loss of cognitive function that interferes with routine personal, social, and occupational activities

elopement When a person leaves the center without staff knowledge

hallucination Seeing, hearing, smelling, or feeling something that is not real

paranoia A disorder *(para)* of the mind *(noia)*; the person has false beliefs (delusions) and suspicion about a person or situation

pseudodementia False *(pseudo)* dementia

sundowning Signs, symptoms, and behaviors of AD increase during hours of darkness

KEY ABBREVIATIONS

AD	Alzheimer's disease	**OBRA**	Omnibus Budget Reconciliation Act of 1987
ADL	Activities of daily living		
NIA	National Institute on Aging		

Box 44-1 Changes in the Nervous System From Aging

- Nerve cells are lost.
- Nerve conduction slows.
- Responses and reaction times are slower.
- Reflexes are slower.
- Vision and hearing decrease.
- Taste and smell decrease.
- Touch and sensitivity to pain decrease.
- Blood flow to the brain is reduced.
- Sleep patterns change.
- Memory is shorter.
- Forgetfulness occurs.
- Dizziness can occur.

Changes in the brain and nervous system occur with aging (Box 44-1). Certain diseases affect the brain. Changes in the brain can affect cognitive function. (*Cognitive* relates to knowledge.) Quality of life is affected. **Cognitive function** involves:

- Memory
- Thinking
- Reasoning
- Ability to understand
- Judgment
- Behavior

CONFUSION

Confusion has many causes. Diseases, infections, hearing and vision loss, and medication side effects are some causes. So is brain injury. With aging, blood supply to the brain is reduced. Personality and mental changes can result. Memory and the ability to make good judgments are lost. A person may not know people, the time, or the place. Some people gradually lose the ability to perform daily activities. Behavior changes are common. The person may be angry, restless, depressed, and irritable.

Acute confusion (delirium) occurs suddenly. It is usually temporary. Causes include infection, illness, injury, medications, and surgery. Treatment is aimed at the cause.

Confusion caused by physical changes cannot be cured. Some measures help to improve function (Box 44-2). You must meet the person's basic needs.

Box 44-2 Caring for the Person With Confusion

- Follow the person's care plan.
- Provide for safety.
- Face the person. Speak clearly.
- Call the person by name every time you are in contact with him or her.
- State your name. Show your name tag.
- Give the date and time each morning. Repeat as needed during the day or evening.
- Explain what you are going to do and why.
- Give clear, simple directions and answers to questions.
- Ask clear and simple questions. Give the person time to respond.
- Keep calendars and clocks with large numbers in the person's room and in nursing areas (Fig. 44-1). Remind the person of holidays, birthdays, and special events.
- Have the person wear eyeglasses and hearing aids as needed.
- Use touch to communicate (Chapter 8).
- Place familiar objects and pictures within the person's view.
- Provide newspapers, magazines, TV, and radio. Read to the person if appropriate.
- Discuss current events with the person.
- Maintain the day-night cycle.
  - Open window coverings during the day. Close them at night.
  - Use night-lights at night. Use them in rooms, bathrooms, hallways, and other areas.
  - Have the person wear regular clothes during the day—not sleepwear.
- Provide a calm, relaxed, and peaceful setting. Prevent loud noises, rushing, and congested hallways and dining rooms.
- Follow the person's routine. Meals, bathing, exercise, TV, bedtime, and other activities have a schedule. This promotes a sense of order and what to expect.
- Break tasks into small steps when helping the person.
- Do not re-arrange furniture or the person's belongings.
- Encourage the person to take part in self-care.
- Be consistent.

Fig. 44-1 A large calendar can help persons who are confused.

DEMENTIA

Dementia is the loss of cognitive function that interferes with routine personal, social, and occupational activities. (*De* means from. *Mentia* means mind.) The person may have changes in personality, mood, or behavior. Dementia is a group of symptoms that may occur with certain diseases or conditions.

Dementia is not a normal part of aging. Most older people do not have dementia. Early warning signs include:

- Recent memory loss that affects job skills
- Problems with common tasks (for example, dressing, cooking, driving)
- Problems with language; forgetting simple words
- Getting lost in familiar places
- Misplacing things and putting things in odd places (for example, putting a watch in the oven)
- Personality changes
- Poor or decreased judgment (for example, going outdoors in the snow without shoes)
- Loss of interest in life

If changes in the brain have not occurred, some dementias can be reversed. When the cause is removed, so are the signs and symptoms. Treatable causes include:

- Drugs and alcohol
- Delirium and depression
- Tumors
- Heart, lung, and blood vessel problems
- Head injuries
- Infection
- Vision and hearing problems

Permanent dementias result from changes in the brain. They have no cure. Function declines over time. Causes of permanent dementia are listed in Box 44-3. Alzheimer's disease is the most common type of permanent dementia.

Box 44-3 **Causes of Permanent Dementia**

- Alcohol-related dementia and Korsakoff's syndrome
- Alzheimer's disease
- AIDS-related dementia
- Brain tumors
- Cerebrovascular disease
- Huntington's disease (a nervous system disease)
- Multi-infarct dementia (MID) (many *[multi]* strokes leave areas of damage *[infarct]*)
- Multiple sclerosis
- Parkinson's disease
- Stroke
- Syphilis
- Trauma and head injury

Pseudodementia means false (*pseudo*) dementia. The person has signs and symptoms of dementia. However, there are no changes in the brain. This can occur with delirium and depression. Both can be mistaken for dementia.

Delirium

Delirium is a state of sudden, severe confusion and rapid brain changes. It occurs with physical or mental illness. Usually temporary and reversible, it is common in older persons with acute or chronic illnesses. Infections, heart and lung diseases, and poor nutrition are common causes. So are hormone disorders. Hypoglycemia is also a cause (Chapter 41). Alcohol and many drugs (including prescription medications) can cause delirium. Delirium often lasts for about 1 week. However, it may take several weeks for normal mental function to return.

Delirium signals physical illness in older persons and in persons with dementia. It is an emergency. The cause must be found and treated. Signs and symptoms are listed in Box 44-4.

Box 44-4 **Signs and Symptoms of Delirium**

- Alertness: changes in. The person is usually more alert in the morning and less alert at night.
- Sensation: changes in.
- Awareness: changes in.
- Movement: inactive or slow moving.
- Drowsiness.
- Confusion about time or place.
- Memory:
  - Decreased short-term memory and recall. Cannot remember events since the delirium began.
  - Cannot remember past events.
- Thinking and behavior are without purpose.
- Problems concentrating.
- Speech does not make sense.
- Emotional changes:
  - Anger
  - Anxiety
  - Apathy
  - Depression
  - Euphoria
  - Irritability
- Incontinence.
- Restlessness.

Modified from Medline Plus: Delirium, U.S. National Library of Medicine, National Institutes of Health, Bethesda, Md, updated February 6, 2010.

Depression

Depression is the most common mental health problem in older persons. It is often overlooked. Depression, aging, and some medication side effects have similar signs and symptoms. See Chapter 43 for signs and symptoms of depression in older persons.

Mild Cognitive Impairment

Mild cognitive impairment (MCI) is a type of memory change. The person has problems with memory, language, and other mental functions (attention, judgment, reading, writing). The person or others may notice the problems. However, the problems do not interfere with daily life. The person is at risk for Alzheimer's disease.

ALZHEIMER'S DISEASE

Alzheimer's disease (AD) is a brain disease. Many nerve cells that control intellectual and social function are damaged and die (Fig. 44-2). These functions are affected:

- Memory
- Thinking
- Reasoning
- Judgment
- Language
- Behavior
- Mood
- Personality

The person has problems with work and everyday functions. Problems with family and social relationships occur. There is a steady decline in memory and mental function.

The disease is gradual in onset. It gets worse and worse over time. Persons with AD usually live 8 to 10 years after diagnosis. Some persons live as few as 3 years. Others live as long as 20 years. Some people in their 40s and 50s have AD. However, usually symptoms first appear after the age of 60. The risk increases with age. It is often diagnosed around the age of 80. Nearly half of the persons age 85 and older have AD.

The cause is unknown. A family history of AD increases a person's risk of developing the disease. More women than men have AD. Women live longer than men.

Signs of AD

The classic sign of AD is *gradual loss of short-term memory.* At first, the only symptom may be forgetfulness. Box 44-5 lists the warning signs and other signs of AD. See Box 44-6 for the difference between AD and normal age-related changes.

Fig. 44-2 A, Normal brain. **B,** Dark patches show damage to brain tissue. *(From Thibodeau GA, Patton KT: The human body in health & disease, ed 5, St Louis, 2010, Mosby.)*

Box 44-5 Signs of Alzheimer's Disease

Warning Signs

- Gradual loss of short-term memory.
- Asking the same question over and over again.
- Repeating the same story—word for word, again and again.
- Forgetting how to cook, how to make repairs, or how to play cards. The person forgets activities that were once done regularly and with ease.
- Losing the ability to pay bills or balance a checkbook.
- Getting lost in familiar places.
- Misplacing household items.
- Neglecting to bathe. Or wearing the same clothes over and over again. Meanwhile, the person insists that a bath was taken or that clothes are clean.
- Relying on someone else to make decisions or answer questions that he or she would have handled.

Other Signs

- Forgets recent events, conversations, and appointments.
- Forgets simple directions.
- Forgets names (including family members).
- Forgets the names of everyday things (clock, radio, TV, and so on).
- Forgets words, loses train of thought.
- Substitutes unusual words and names for what is forgotten.

Other Signs—cont'd

- Speaks in a native language.
- Curses or swears.
- Misplaces things. Puts things in odd places.
- Has problems writing checks.
- Gives away large amounts of money.
- Does not recognize or understand numbers.
- Has problems following conversations.
- Has problems reading and writing.
- Becomes lost in familiar settings.
- Forgets where he or she is.
- Does not know how to get back home.
- Wanders from home.
- Cannot tell or understand time or dates.
- Cannot solve everyday problems (iron is left on, stove burners left on, food burning on the stove, and so on).
- Cannot perform everyday tasks (dressing, bathing, brushing teeth, and so on).
- Distrusts others.
- Is stubborn.
- Withdraws socially.
- Is restless.
- Becomes suspicious.
- Becomes fearful.
- Does not want to do things.
- Sleeps more than usual.

Warning signs written by Eric Pfeiffer, MD, the director of the University of South Florida Suncoast Alzheimer's and Gerontology Center. Reprinted with permission.

Box 44-6 Alzheimer's Disease and Normal Age-Related Changes

Signs of AD

Poor judgment and decision making.
Cannot manage a budget.
Loses track of the date or season.
Problems having a conversation.
Misplaces things. Cannot retrace steps to find them.

Normal Age-Related Changes

Makes a bad decision once in a while.
Misses a monthly payment.
Forgets which day it is but remembers later.
Sometimes forgets which word to use.
Loses things from time to time.

Modified from Alzheimer's Association: 10 signs of Alzheimer's, Chicago, April 6, 2010.

Stages of AD

Signs and symptoms become more severe as the disease progresses. The disease ends in death. AD is often described in terms of 3 stages (Box 44-7). See Figure 44-3. The Alzheimer's Association describes seven stages:

- *No impairment.* The person does not show signs of memory problems.
- *Very mild cognitive decline.* The person thinks that he or she has memory loss or lapses. Familiar words or names are forgotten. The person does not know where to find keys, eyeglasses, or other objects. These problems are not apparent to family, friends, or the health team.
- *Mild cognitive decline.* Family, friends, and others notice problems. The person has problems with memory or concentration and with words or names. The person loses or misplaces something valuable. Functioning in social or work settings declines.
- *Moderate cognitive decline (mild or early stage).* Memory of recent or current events declines. There are problems with shopping, paying bills, and managing money. The person may withdraw or be quiet in social situations.

- *Moderately severe cognitive decline (moderate or mid-stage).* The person has major memory problems. There may be confusion about the date or day of the week. He or she may need help choosing the correct clothing to wear. The person knows his or her own name, a partner's name, and children's names. Usually help is not needed with eating or elimination.
- *Severe cognitive decline (moderately severe or mid-stage).* Memory problems are worse. Personality and behavior changes develop—delusions, hallucinations, repetitive behavior. The person needs much help with daily activities, including dressing and elimination. Names may be forgotten, but faces may be recognized. Sleep problems, incontinence (urinary and fecal), and wandering are common.
- *Very severe cognitive decline (severe or late stage).* The person cannot respond to his or her setting, speak, or control movement. The person cannot walk without help. Over time, he or she cannot sit up without support or hold the head up. Muscles become rigid. Swallowing is impaired.

Box 44-7 Stages of Alzheimer's Disease

Stage 1: Mild AD
- Memory loss—forgetfulness; forgets recent events
- Problems finding words, finishing thoughts, following directions, and remembering names
- Poor judgment; bad decisions (including when driving)
- Disoriented to time and place
- Lack of spontaneity—less outgoing or interested in things
- Blames others for mistakes, forgetfulness, and other problems
- Moodiness
- Problems performing everyday tasks

Stage 2: Moderate AD
- Restlessness—increases during the evening hours
- Sleep problems
- Memory loss increases:
  - May not know family and friends
  - May not know where he or she is
  - May not know the day or year
- May wander
- Dulled senses—cannot tell the difference between hot and cold; cannot recognize dangers
- Fecal and urinary incontinence
- Needs help with activities of daily living (ADL)—bathing, feeding, and dressing self; afraid of bathing; will not change clothes
- Loses impulse control—foul language, poor table manners, sexual aggression, rudeness

Stage 2: Moderate AD—cont'd
- Movement and gait problems—walks slowly, has a shuffling gait
- Communication problems—cannot follow directions; problems with reading, writing, and math; speaks in short sentences or single words; statements may not make sense
- Repeats motions and statements—moves things back and forth constantly; says the same thing over and over again
- Agitation—behavior may be violent
- May make threats, accuse others of stealing, curse, kick, hit, bite, scream, or grab things

Stage 3: Severe AD
- Seizures (Chapter 47)
- Cannot speak—may groan, grunt, or scream
- Does not recognize self or family members
- Depends totally on others for all ADL
- Disoriented to person, time, and place
- Totally incontinent of urine and feces
- Cannot swallow—choking and aspiration are risks
- Sleep problems increase
- Becomes bed bound—cannot sit or walk
- Coma
- Death

memory, language skills perception, or cognitive skills such as reasoning & judgement

Fig. 44-3 A, Very early AD. **B,** Mild to moderate AD. **C,** Severe AD. *(From Alzheimer's Disease Education & Referral [ADEAR] Center:* Alzheimer's disease fact sheet, *National Institutes of Health, NIH Publication No. 08-6423, updated February 19, 2010.*

Behaviors and Problems

AD changes how a person behaves and acts. These changes are common:

- Getting upset, worried, or angry more easily
- Acting depressed
- Losing interest in things
- Hiding things (p. 666)
- Believing other people are hiding things
- Pacing a lot of the time
- Wandering (p. 662)
- Sundowning (p. 662)
- Hallucinations (p. 663)
- Delusions (p. 663)
- Catastrophic reactions (p. 663)
- Agitation and restlessness (p. 663)
- Aggression and combativeness (p. 664)
- Screaming (p. 666)
- Problems with intimacy and sexuality (p. 664)
- Repetitive behaviors (p. 664)
- Communication problems (p. 665)

Health-related issues can make the problems worse. Examples include illness, infection, medications, lack of sleep, constipation, hunger, thirst, poor vision or hearing, alcohol, and caffeine. So can problems in the person's setting. According to the National Institute on Aging (NIA), they include:

- A strange setting. The person does not know the setting well.
- Too much noise. TV, radio, people talking at once, and other noises can cause confusion and frustration.
- Stepping from one type of flooring to another. With changes in floor color or texture, the person may want to step down.
- Not understanding signs. The person may think that a "Wet Floor" sign means to urinate on the floor.
- Mirrors. The person may think that a mirror image is another person in the room.

See *Promoting Safety and Comfort: Behaviors and Problems* (p. 662).

drs. diagnose dementia only if 2 or more (brain functions) are significantly impaired w/o loss of consciousness.

Safety

Some behaviors and problems are not caused by AD. They may be caused by an illness, injury, or medication. If the cause is not treated, it may threaten the person's life. Always report changes in behaviors to the nurse.

TEAMWORK AND TIME MANAGEMENT
Wandering

Every staff member must be alert to persons who wander. Such persons are allowed to wander in safe areas (Fig. 44-4). However, the person may wander into an unsafe area. Kitchens, shower rooms, and utility rooms are examples.

Tell your team members when you are caring for a person who wanders. You cannot be with the person all the time. The team can assist and monitor the person. Help your team members in the same way. If you see a person wandering into an unsafe area, gently guide the person to a safe place (Fig. 44-5). Report the problem to the nurse.

Fig. 44-4 An enclosed garden allows persons with AD to wander in a safe setting.

Fig. 44-5 Guide the person who wanders to a safe area.

Wandering Persons with AD are not oriented to person, time, and place. They may wander away and not find their way back. Wandering may be by foot, car, bike, or other means. They may be with you one moment and gone the next.

Judgment is poor. They cannot tell what is safe or dangerous. Life-threatening accidents are great risks. They can walk into traffic or into a nearby river, lake, ocean, or forest. If not properly dressed, heat or cold exposure is a risk.

Residents may try to wander to another nursing unit or out of the center. Leaving the center without staff knowledge is called **elopement**. Serious injury and death have resulted from elopement. Centers must follow state and federal guidelines to prevent elopement.

Wandering may have no cause. Or the person may be looking for something or someone—the bathroom, the bedroom, a child, or a partner. Pain, medication side effects, stress, restlessness, and anxiety are possible causes. Sometimes finding the cause prevents wandering.

See *Teamwork and Time Management: Wandering.*

MedicAlert + Safe Return. *MedicAlert + Safe Return* is a 24-hour emergency service for persons who wander or have a medical emergency. It was formed by the MedicAlert Foundation International and the Alzheimer's Association. The program is nationwide.

The purpose is to identify and safely return persons who wander and become lost. A small fee is charged. A family member completes a form and provides a photo. These are entered into a national database. The person receives an ID (wallet card, bracelet, or necklace).

When reported missing, the person's information is sent to the police. When the person is found, someone calls the toll-free number on the ID. *MedicAlert + Safe Return* then calls the family member or caregiver. The person is returned home safely.

Sundowning With **sundowning,** signs, symptoms, and behaviors of AD increase during hours of darkness. It occurs in the late afternoon and evening hours. As daylight ends and darkness starts, confusion and restlessness increase. So do anxiety, agitation, and other symptoms. Behavior is worse after the sun goes down. It may continue throughout the night.

Sundowning may relate to being tired or hungry. Poor light and shadows may cause the person to see things that are not there. Persons with AD may be afraid of the dark.

Hallucinations and Delusions A *hallucination* is seeing, hearing, smelling, or feeling something that is not real. Senses are dulled. Affected persons see animals, insects, or people that are not present. Some hear voices. They may feel bugs crawling or feel that they are being touched.

Sometimes the problem is caused by poor vision or hearing. The person needs to wear eyeglasses and hearing aids as prescribed.

Delusions are false beliefs. People with AD may think they are some other person. Some believe they are in jail, are being killed, or are being attacked. A person may believe that the caregiver is someone else. Many other false beliefs can occur.

Paranoia *Paranoia* is a disorder (*para*) of the mind (*noia*). The person has false beliefs (delusions) and suspicion about a person or situation. Paranoia is a type of delusion. The person believes that others are mean, lying, not fair, or "out to get" him or her. The person may be suspicious, fearful, or jealous.

According to the NIA, paranoia may worsen as memory loss gets worse. The NIA uses these examples:

* The person forgets where he or she put something. The person may believe that someone is taking his or her things.
* The person forgets that you are a caregiver. The person may think that you are a stranger and not trust you.
* The person forgets people to whom he or she was introduced. The person may believe that strangers are harmful.
* The person forgets directions that you gave. The person may think that you are trying to trick him or her.

The person may express loss through paranoia. Reasons for the loss do not make sense. Therefore the person blames or accuses others. The NIA offers these helpful measures:

* Do not react if the person blames you for something.
* Do not argue with the person.
* Let the person know that he or she is safe.
* Use touch or gently hug the person. This shows that you care.
* Search for missing things. This helps distract the person. Talk about what you found. For example, you find a photo. Talk about the photo.

See *Promoting Safety and Comfort: Paranoia.*

PROMOTING SAFETY AND COMFORT
Paranoia

Safety

The person's behaviors may not mean paranoia. Fears of harm, strangers, stealing, mistreatment, and so on may be real. Some people do take advantage of vulnerable adults (Chapter 4). This includes sexual abuse and financial abuse.

The abuse may be by phone, mail, e-mail, or in person. The abuser may be a friend or family member. The NIA describes financial abuse as including:

* "Scams" such as identity theft, phony prizes, and threats
* Borrowing money and not paying it back
* Giving away or selling the person's property without permission
* Signing or cashing the person's check without permission
* Mis-using bank cards or credit cards
* Forcing the person to sign over property
* Stealing prescription medications

You must protect the person from harm, abuse, and mistreatment. Report the following at once:

* What the person is saying
* The person seems afraid or worried about money
* Some of the person's items are missing
* The person's behaviors
* Signs and symptoms of problems
* Visitors or family members acting strangely

Catastrophic Reactions These are extreme responses. The person reacts as if there is a disaster or tragedy. The person may scream, cry, or be agitated or combative. These reactions are common from too many stimuli. Eating, music or TV playing, and being asked questions all at once can overwhelm the person.

Agitation and Restlessness The person may pace, hit, or yell. Common causes are pain or discomfort, anxiety, lack of sleep, and too many or too few stimuli. Hunger, the need to eliminate, and incontinence also are causes. A calm, quiet setting helps calm the person. So does meeting basic needs.

Caregivers can cause these behaviors. A caregiver may rush the person or be impatient. Or mixed verbal and nonverbal messages are sent. For example, a caregiver may talk too fast or too loud. Caregivers always need to look at how their behaviors affect other persons.

The NIA suggests these measures to help with agitation and restlessness:

- Observe for early signs of agitation and restlessness. Such signs may help you remove the cause before the behaviors worsen.
- Do not ignore the problem. Try to find the cause.
- Allow personal choice. Let the person decide things to the extent possible.
- Try to distract the person. A snack, safe object, or an activity may help.
- Reassure the person:
  - Speak calmly.
  - Listen to the person's concerns.
  - Try to show that you understand the person's anger or fears.
- Keep personal items within the person's sight. Photos and treasures are examples.
- Reduce noise and clutter.
- Limit the number of people in the room.
- Use gentle touch.
- Provide soothing music.
- Read to the person using a gentle voice.
- Provide quiet times.
- Follow a set routine for bathing, dressing, eating, and so on.

Aggression and Combativeness These behaviors include hitting, pinching, grabbing, biting, or swearing. They may result from agitation and restlessness. They frighten others.

Sometimes these behaviors are personality traits. Or pain, fatigue, too much stimulation, caregiver stress, and feeling lost or abandoned are causes. The behaviors can occur during care measures (bathing, dressing) that upset or frighten the person. See Chapter 8 for dealing with the angry person. See Chapter 12 for workplace violence. Also follow the person's care plan. The measures listed for agitation and restlessness may be helpful.

Intimacy and Sexuality *Intimacy* is a special bond between people who love and respect each other. It involves the way people talk and act toward each other. *Sexuality* is a type of intimacy. It is the way partners physically express their feelings for each other. AD can affect intimacy and sexuality. The person with AD may:

- Depend on and cling to his or her partner
- Not remember life with his or her partner
- Not remember feelings for his or her partner
- Fall in love with another person
- Have side effects from medications that affect sexual interest
- Have memory loss, changes in the brain, or depression that affect sexual interest
- Have abnormal sexual behaviors

Sexual behaviors are labeled abnormal because of how and when they occur. Persons with AD are not oriented to person, time, and place. Sexual behaviors may involve the wrong person, the wrong place, and the wrong time. Also, persons with AD cannot control behavior.

Healthy persons do not undress or expose themselves in front of others. They do not masturbate or engage in sexual pleasures in public. They know their sexual partners. Persons with AD often mistake someone else for a sexual partner. The person kisses and hugs the other person.

Being overly *(hyper)* interested in sex is called *hypersexuality*. The person may try to seduce others. Or the person may masturbate often. These behaviors are symptoms of AD. They may not mean that the person wants to have sex. When a person masturbates in public, lead the person to his or her room. Provide for privacy and safety.

Some behaviors are not sexual. Touching, scratching, and rubbing the genitals can signal infection, pain, or discomfort in the urinary or reproductive systems. Poor hygiene is another cause. So is being wet or soiled from urine or feces. Good hygiene prevents itching. Clean the person quickly and thoroughly after elimination. Do not let the person stay wet or soiled. The nurse assesses the person for urinary or reproductive system problems. The doctor is contacted as necessary.

The nurse encourages the person's partner to show affection. Their normal practices are encouraged. Examples include hand holding, hugging, kissing, touching, and dancing.

Repetitive Behaviors *Repetitive* means to repeat over and over again. Persons with AD repeat the same motions over and over again. For example, the person folds the same napkin over and over. Or the person says the same words over and over. Or the same question is asked. Such behaviors do not harm the person. However, they can annoy caregivers and the family.

Harmless acts are allowed. Music, picture books, exercise, and movies are distracting. Taking the person for a walk can help. Such measures help when words or questions are repeated.

CARING ABOUT CULTURE
Communication Problems

Some persons with AD learned English as a second language. For example, the first language learned may be Spanish, Italian, French, Russian, Chinese, Japanese, and so on. With AD the person may forget or no longer understand English. He or she may only use and understand the first language learned.

Communication Problems People with AD have trouble remembering things. Communication problems include:

- Struggling to find the right word
- Forgetting what he or she wants to say
- Problems understanding the meaning of words
- Attention problems during conversations
- Losing one's train of thought when talking
- Problems blocking background noises—radio, TV, phones, and so on
- Frustration with problems communicating
- Being sensitive to touch, tone, and voice volume
  See *Caring About Culture: Communication Problems.*
  See *Focus on Communication: Communication Problems.*

FOCUS ON COMMUNICATION
Communication Problems

Impaired communication is a common problem among persons with AD and other dementias. Communication abilities decline over time. Some persons can have brief conversations. To promote communication, practice the measures in Box 44-8. Avoid the following:

- *Giving orders.* For example: "Sit down and eat." The statement is bossy. It does not show respect for the person. Instead you can say: "Let me help you sit down."
- *Wanting the truth.* For example, do not say: "Don't you remember?" "What's my name?" "What day is it?" Instead you can say, "Today is Friday."
- *Correcting the person's errors.* For example, do not say: "No, that is your daughter Rose. That's not Mary." Or, "I just told you that it's time to get dressed. You already had breakfast." Instead you can say, "Let me help you get dressed."
- *Pointing out errors.* Instead of saying "You missed a button," say "Let's try it this way."
- *Giving many choices.* For example, "What would you like for dinner?" involves many choices. Instead, limit choices. You can say: "Do you want potatoes or rice?"
- *Asking open-ended questions.* For example, do not say "How did you sleep last night?" Instead, ask "yes" or "no" questions. You can say: "Did you sleep OK last night?"

Box 44-8 Communicating With Persons With AD and Other Dementias

- Approach the person in a calm, quiet manner.
- Approach the person from the front—not from the side or the back. This avoids startling the person.
- Make eye contact to get the person's attention.
- Have the person's attention before you start speaking.
- Call the person by name.
- Identify other people by their names. Avoid pronouns (he, she, them, and so on).
- Follow the rules of communication (Chapters 6 and 8).
- Practice measures to promote communication (Chapter 8).
- Use gestures or cues. Point to objects.
- Speak in a calm, gentle voice.
- Hold the person's hand while you talk.
- Speak slowly. Use simple words and short sentences.
- Ask or say one thing at a time. Present one idea, question, or instruction at a time.
- Do not "baby talk" or use a "baby voice."
- Let the person speak. Do not interrupt or rush the person.
- Give the person time to respond.
- Try different words if the person does not seem to understand.
- Do not criticize, correct, interrupt, argue, or try to reason with the person.
- Give simple, step-by-step instructions.
- Repeat instructions as needed. Give the person time to respond or react.
- Ask simple questions having simple answers. Do not ask complex questions.
- Do not present the person with many questions.
- Provide simple explanations of all procedures and activities.
- Give consistent responses.
- Practice measures to promote hearing (Chapter 37).
- Practice measures to communicate with speech-impaired persons (Chapter 37).
- Practice measures for blind and visually impaired persons (Chapter 37).

Screaming Persons with AD have communication problems. At first, it is hard to find the right words. As AD progresses, the person speaks in short sentences or just in words. Often speech is not understandable.

The person screams to communicate. This is common in persons who are very confused and have poor communication skills. The person may scream a word or a name. Or the person just makes screaming sounds.

Possible causes include hearing and vision problems, pain or discomfort, fear, and fatigue. Too much or not enough stimulation is another cause. The person may react to a caregiver or family member by screaming.

Sometimes these measures are helpful:

* Providing a calm, quiet setting
* Playing soft music
* Having the person wear hearing aids and eyeglasses
* Having a family member or favorite caregiver comfort and calm the person
* Using touch to calm the person

Rummaging and Hiding Things To *rummage* means to search for things by moving things around, turning things over, or looking through something such as a drawer or closet. The behavior may not have meaning. Or the person may be looking for a certain item but cannot tell you what or why.

The person may hide things, throw things away, or lose something. Some things need to stay with the person. Eyeglasses, hearing aids, and dentures are examples. Always make sure these items are safe. Look for them before discarding linens, returning food trays, or emptying wastebaskets. Money, jewelry, and other important items usually are sent home with the family.

These measures may help with rummaging and hiding behaviors:

* Keep harmful items and products out of the person's sight and reach.
* Remove spoiled items from refrigerators and cabinets. The person may go into a kitchen looking for food and snacks. He or she may not know or be able to taste spoiled food.
* Do not let the person go into another resident's room.
* Keep wastebaskets covered or out of sight. The person may rummage through a wastebasket or throw things away.
* Check wastebaskets before you empty them. Look for items thrown away or hidden.
* Keep bathroom doors closed and toilet seats down. This helps prevent the person from flushing things down the toilet.
* Allow the person to rummage in a safe place. The center may have a drawer, closet, bag, box, basket, or chest with safe items.

CARE OF PERSONS WITH AD AND OTHER DEMENTIAS

Usually the person is cared for at home until symptoms are severe. Adult day care may help. Often assisted living or nursing center care is required. Sometimes hospital care is needed for other illnesses. You may care for persons with AD or other dementias in such settings. The person and family need your support and understanding.

People with AD do not choose to be forgetful, incontinent, agitated, or rude. Nor do they choose to have other behaviors, signs, and symptoms of the disease. They cannot control what is happening to them. The disease causes the behaviors. *The disease is responsible, not the person.*

Currently AD has no cure. Symptoms worsen over many years. The rate varies from person to person. Over time, persons with AD depend on others for care. Safety, hygiene, nutrition and fluids, elimination, and activity needs must be met. So must comfort and sleep needs. The person's care plan will include many of the measures listed in Box 44-9.

Comfort and safety are important. Good skin care and alignment prevent skin breakdown and contractures. You must treat these persons with dignity and respect. They have the same rights as persons who are alert and active. Talk to them in a calm voice. Always explain what you are going to do. Massage, soothing touch, music, and aromatherapy are comforting and relaxing. Range-of-motion exercises and touch are also important therapies. The person may need hospice care as death nears (Chapter 48).

The person can have other health problems and injuries. However, the person may not be aware of pain, fever, constipation, incontinence, or other signs and symptoms. Carefully observe the person. Report any change in the person's usual behavior to the nurse.

Infection is a risk. The person cannot fully tend to self-care. Infection can occur from poor hygiene. This includes poor skin care, oral hygiene, and perineal care after bowel and bladder elimination. Inactivity and immobility can cause pneumonia and pressure ulcers.

The person needs to feel useful, worthwhile, and active. This promotes self-esteem. Therapists work with one person, a small group, or a large group. Therapies and activities focus on the person's strengths and past successes. For example:

* A woman used to cook. She helps clean fruit.
* A man was a good dancer. Activities are planned so he can dance.
* A man likes to clean. He helps with dusting.

Supervised activities meet the person's needs and cognitive abilities. The person's interests are considered. Activities are based on what the person enjoys and can do. Some people like crafts, exercise, gardening, and listening and moving to music. Others like sing-alongs, reminiscing, and board games. Some like to string beads, fold towels, or roll dough.

See *Teamwork and Time Management: Care of Persons With AD and Other Dementias.*

TEAMWORK AND TIME MANAGEMENT
Care of Persons With AD and Other Dementias

The entire staff must protect the person from harm. Always look for dangers in the person's room and in hallways, lounges, dining areas, and other areas on the nursing unit. Remove the danger if you can, and tell the nurse at once. If you cannot remove the danger, also tell the nurse at once.

Box 44-9 Care of Persons With AD and Other Dementias

Environment
- Follow set routines.
- Avoid changing rooms or roommates.
- Place picture signs by room doors, bathrooms, dining rooms, and other areas (Fig. 44-6, p. 668).
- Keep personal items where the person can see them.
- Stay within the person's sight to the extent possible.
- Place memory aids (large clocks and calendars) where the person can see them.
- Keep noise levels low.
- Play music and show movies from the person's past.
- Select tasks and activities that fit the person's abilities and interests.

Safety
- Reassure the person that you are there to help.
- Remove harmful, sharp, and breakable items from the area. This includes knives, scissors, glass, dishes, razors, and tools.
- Provide plastic eating and drinking utensils. This helps prevent breakage and cuts.
- Place safety plugs in electrical outlets or cover outlets with safety plates.
- Keep cords and electrical items out of reach.
- Remove electrical appliances from the bathroom. Hair dryers, curling irons, make-up mirrors, and electric shavers are examples.
- Store personal care items (shampoo, deodorant, lotion, and so on) in a safe place.
- Keep childproof caps on medication containers and household cleaners.
- Store household cleaners and medications in locked storage areas.
- Store dangerous equipment and tools in a safe place.
- Remove knobs from stoves or place safety covers on the knobs (Fig. 44-7).
- Remove dangerous appliances and power tools from the home.
- Remove firearms from the home.
- Store car keys in a safe place.
- Supervise the person who smokes.
- Store cigarettes, cigars, pipes, matches, and other smoking materials in a safe place.
- Practice safety measures to prevent falls (Chapter 13).
- Practice safety measures to prevent fires (Chapter 12).
- Practice safety measures to prevent burns (Chapter 12).
- Practice safety measures to prevent poisoning (Chapter 12).
- Lock all doors to kitchens, utility rooms, and housekeeping closets. Keep them locked.

Wandering
- Follow center policy for locking doors and windows. Locks are often placed at the top and bottom of doors (Fig. 44-8, p. 669). The person is not likely to look for a lock in such places.
- Keep door alarms and electronic doors turned on. The alarm goes off when the door is opened. Respond to door alarms at once.
- Follow center policy for fire exits. Everyone must be able to leave the building if there is a fire.
- Make sure the person wears an ID bracelet or *MedicAlert + Safe Return* at all times.
- Exercise the person as ordered. Adequate exercise may reduce wandering.
- Involve the person in activities—folding napkins, dusting a table, sorting socks, rolling yarn, sweeping, sanding blocks of wood, or watering plants.
- Do not use restraints. Restraints require a doctor's order. They also tend to increase confusion and disorientation.
- Do not argue with the person who wants to leave. The person does not understand what you are saying.
- Go with the person who insists on going outside. Make sure he or she is properly dressed. Guide the person inside after a few minutes.
- Let the person wander in enclosed areas. The center may have enclosed areas for walking about. They provide a safe place for the person to wander.

Sundowning
- Complete treatments and activities early in the day.
- Provide a calm, quiet setting late in the day.
- Do not restrain the person.
- Encourage exercise and activity early in the day.
- Meet nutrition needs. Hunger can increase restlessness.
- Promote elimination. The need to eliminate can increase restlessness.
- Do not try to reason with the person. He or she cannot understand what you are saying.
- Do not ask the person to tell you what is bothering him or her. Communication is impaired. The person does not understand what you are asking. He or she cannot think or speak clearly.

Continued

Box 44-9 Care of Persons With AD and Other Dementias—cont'd

Hallucinations and Delusions

- Have the person wear eyeglasses and hearing aids as needed. Follow the care plan.
- Do not argue with the person. He or she does not understand what you are saying.
- Reassure the person. Tell him or her that you will provide protection from harm.
- Try to comfort the person if he or she is afraid.
- Distract the person with some item or activity. Go to another room. Taking the person for a walk may be helpful.
- Turn off TV or movies when violent and disturbing programs are on. The person may believe that the story is real.
- Use touch to calm and reassure the person (Fig. 44-9).
- Eliminate noises that the person could misinterpret. TV, radio, stereos, furnaces, air conditioners, and other things could affect the person.
- Check lighting. Make sure there are no glares, shadows, or reflections.
- Cover or remove mirrors. The person could misinterpret his or her reflection.
- Make sure the person cannot reach anything that could be used to hurt self or others.

Sleep

- Develop a regular bedtime. Keep the bedtime at the same time each evening.
- Provide a quiet, peaceful mood in the evening—dim lights, low noise level, and soothing music.
- Follow bedtime rituals.
- Use night-lights so the person can see. Use them in rooms, hallways, bathrooms, and other areas. They help prevent accidents and disorientation.
- Limit caffeine during the day.
- Discourage naps during the day.
- Follow the person's exercise plan. Play music to the exercise.
- Reduce noises.

Basic Needs

- Follow a daily routine. This helps the person know when certain things will happen.
- Meet food and fluid needs (Chapter 24). Provide finger foods. Cut food and pour liquids as needed.

Basic Needs—cont'd

- Provide good skin care (Chapters 20, 35, and 36). Keep the person's skin free of urine and feces.
- Promote urinary and bowel elimination (Chapters 22 and 23).
- Provide incontinence care as needed (Chapters 22 and 23).
- Promote exercise and activity during the day (Chapter 26). This helps reduce wandering and sundowning behaviors. The person may also sleep better.
- Reduce intake of coffee, tea, and cola drinks. These contain caffeine. Caffeine is a stimulant. It can increase restlessness, confusion, and agitation.
- Provide a quiet, restful setting. Soft music is better than loud TV programs.
- Play music during care activities such as bathing and during meals.
- Promote personal hygiene (Chapter 20). Do not force the person into a shower or tub. People with AD are often afraid of bathing. Try bathing the person when he or she is calm. Use the person's preferred bathing method (tub bath, shower). Provide privacy and keep the person warm. Do not rush the person.
- Provide oral hygiene (Chapter 20).
- Choose clothing that is comfortable and simple to put on. Front-opening garments are easy to put on. Pullover tops are harder to put on. And the person may become frightened when his or her head is inside the pullover top.
- Select clothing that closes with Velcro. Such items are easy to put on and take off. Buttons, zippers, snaps, and other closures can frustrate the person.
- Offer simple clothing choices (Fig. 44-10). Let the person choose between two shirts or two blouses, two pants or two slacks, and so on.
- Lay clothing out in the order it will be put on. Hand the person one clothing item at a time. Tell or show the person what to do. Do not rush him or her.
- Have equipment ready for any procedure. This reduces the amount of time the person is involved in care measures.
- Observe for signs and symptoms of health problems (Chapter 7).
- Prevent infection (Chapter 15).

Fig. 44-6 Signs give cues to persons with dementia.

Fig. 44-7 Safety covers are on stove knobs.

Fig. 44-8 A slide lock is at the top of the door.

Fig. 44-9 Use touch to calm the person.

Fig. 44-10 The person with AD is offered simple clothing choices.

Special Care Units

Many nursing centers have special units for persons with AD and other dementias. Some units are secured. This means that entrances and exits are locked. Persons in these units have a safe setting for moving about. They cannot wander away. Some persons have aggressive behaviors that disrupt or threaten others. They may need a secured unit.

According to the Omnibus Budget Reconciliation Act of 1987 (OBRA), secured units are physical restraints. The center must follow OBRA rules. They must use the least restrictive approach. A dementia diagnosis and a doctor's order are needed to place a person on a secured unit. At least every 90 days, the health team reviews the person's need for a secured unit. The person's rights are always protected.

At some point, the secured unit is no longer needed for safe care. For example, the person's condition progresses from stage 2 to stage 3. The person cannot sit or walk. Wandering is not a concern. The person is transferred to another unit.

Licensing and accrediting agencies have standards of care for special care units. Staff must have special training in the care of persons with dementia. The unit must have programs that promote dignity, personal freedom, and safety.

The Family

The person may live at home or with a partner, children, or other family members. The family gives care. Or someone stays with the person. Health care is sought when the family cannot deal with the situation or meet the person's needs. Home health care may help for a while. Adult day care is an option. Long-term care is needed when:

- Family members cannot meet the person's needs.
- The person no longer knows the caregiver.
- Family members have health problems.
- Money problems occur.
- The person's behavior presents dangers to self and others.

Diagnostic tests, doctor's visits, medications, and home care are costly. So is long-term care. The person's medical care can drain family finances.

The family has special needs. Home care and nursing center care are stressful. There are physical, emotional, social, and financial stresses. Adult children are in the *sandwich generation.* They are caught between their own children needing attention and an ill parent needing care. Caring for two families is stressful. Often adult children have jobs too.

Caregivers can suffer from anger, anxiety, guilt, depression, and sleeplessness. Some cannot concentrate or are irritable. Health problems can develop. They need to focus on their own health. They need a healthy diet, exercise, and plenty of rest. Asking family and friends for help is important. However, asking for help is hard for some people. According to the NIA, they may feel that:

- They should do everything themselves.
- It is wrong to leave the person with someone else.
- No one will help if they ask.
- They do not have money to pay someone to help or watch the person for 1 or 2 hours.

Caregivers need much support and encouragement. AD support groups are helpful. They are sponsored by hospitals, nursing centers, and the Alzheimer's Association. The Alzheimer's Association has chapters in cities across the country. Support groups offer encouragement and advice. Members share their feelings, anger, frustration, guilt, and other emotions. They also share coping and caregiving ideas.

The family often feels hopeless. No matter what is done, the person gets worse. Much time, money, energy, and emotion are needed to care for the person. Anger and resentment may result. Guilt feelings are common. The family knows that the person did not

OBRA-CMS

choose the disease. They know that the person does not choose to have its signs, symptoms, and behaviors. Sometimes behaviors are embarrassing. The family may be upset and angry that the loved one cannot show love or affection.

The family is an important part of the health team. They help plan care whenever possible. They need to learn how to bathe, feed, dress, and give oral hygiene to the person. They also need to learn how to provide a safe setting. The nurse and support group help the family learn how to give necessary care.

Some family members take part in unit activities. For many persons, family members provide comfort. They also need support and understanding from the health team.

The NIA suggests ways that family members can take care of themselves. See Box 44-10.

Validation Therapy

Validation therapy may be part of the person's care plan. The therapy is based on these principles:

- All behavior has meaning.
- Development occurs in a sequence, order, and pattern (Chapter 10). Certain tasks must be completed during a stage of development. A stage cannot be skipped. Each stage is the basis of the next stage.
- If a person does not successfully complete a stage of development, unresolved issues and emotions may surface later in life.
- A person may return to the past to resolve such issues and emotions.
- Caregivers need to listen and provide empathy.
- Attempts are not made to correct the person's thoughts or bring the person back to reality. For example:
  - While going from room to room, Mrs. Bell calls for her daughter. In reality, her daughter died 20 years ago. The caregiver does not tell Mrs. Bell that her daughter died. Instead, the caregiver says: "Tell me about your daughter."
  - Mrs. Brown sits all day on a bench by the window. She says that she is at the train station waiting to meet her husband. In reality, her husband was killed during World War II. Buried in England, he never returned home. The caregiver does not remind Mrs. Brown of what happened. Instead, the caregiver encourages Mrs. Brown to talk about her husband.
  - Mr. Garcia was 3 years old when his father died. He holds a ball constantly. He is very upset when anyone tries to remove it from his hand. He calls for his father and repeats "play ball, play ball." The caregiver does not remind Mr. Garcia that he is 80 years old and that his father died many years ago. Instead, the caregiver says, "Tell me about playing ball."

Box 44-10 Family Caregivers—Taking Care of Yourself

- Ask for help when you need it. Asking for something specific may be useful. For example:
  - "Can you make Mom's dinner Sunday night?"
  - "Can you stay with Dad from 2 to 4 Monday afternoon?"
  - "Can Mom stay at your house Saturday afternoon?"
- Join a support group.
- Take breaks every day.
- Spend time with friends.
- Maintain hobbies and interests.
- Eat healthy foods.
- Exercise often.
- See a doctor regularly.
- Keep health, legal, and financial information current.
- Remember that these feelings are normal—being sad, lonely, frustrated, confused, angry. Say the following to yourself:
  - "I'm doing the best I can."
  - "What I'm doing would be hard for anyone."
  - "I'm not perfect, and that's okay."
  - "I can't control some things."
  - "I need to do what works for right now."
  - "Even when I do everything that I can, the person with AD will still have problem behaviors. They are caused by the illness, not what I do."
  - "I will enjoy the times when we can be together in peace."
  - "I will get counseling if caregiving becomes too much for me."
- Meet spiritual needs—attending religious services, believing that larger forces or a higher power is at work.
  - Understand that you may feel powerless and hopeless about what is happening.
  - Understand that you feel a sense of loss and sadness.
  - Understand why you are caring for a person with AD. Was the choice made out of love, loyalty, duty, religious obligation, money concerns, fear, habit, or self-punishment?
  - Let yourself feel "uplifts." Examples include good feelings about the person, support from caring people, time for your own interests.
  - Keep connected to something "higher than yourself." This may be believing in a higher power, religion, or that something good comes from every experience.

Modified from National Institute on Aging: Caring for a person with Alzheimer's disease: your easy-to-use guide, *NIH Publication No. 09-6173, May 2009.*

The health team decides if validation therapy might help a person. If so, it will be part of the person's care plan. Proper use of validation therapy requires special training. If the therapy is used in your center, you will receive the training needed to use it correctly.

QUALITY OF LIFE

Quality of life is important for all persons with confusion and dementia. Nursing center residents have rights under OBRA. They may not know or be able to exercise their rights. However, the family knows the person's rights. They want those rights protected. They want respect and dignity for the loved one.

The person has the right to privacy and confidentiality. Protect the person from exposure. Only those involved in the person's care are present for care and procedures. The person is allowed to visit in private. Protect confidentiality. Do not share information about the person's care and condition with others.

Personal choice is important. Encourage simple choices. For example, a person chooses to wear a shirt or sweater. Watching or not watching TV may be a simple choice. The family makes choices if the person cannot. They choose bath times, menus, clothing, activities, and other care.

The person has the right to keep and use personal items. Some items provide comfort. A pillow, blanket, afghan, or sweater may have meaning to the person. The person may not know why or even recognize the item. Still, it is important. Keep personal items safe. Protect the person's property from loss or damage.

These persons must be kept free from abuse, mistreatment, and neglect. Caring for persons with confusion and dementia is often very frustrating. Some behaviors are hard to deal with. Family and staff can become short-tempered and angry. Protect the person from abuse. Report any signs and symptoms of abuse to the nurse at once. Be patient and calm when caring for these persons. Talk with the nurse if you are becoming upset. Sometimes an assignment change is needed for a while.

All persons have the right to be free from restraints. Restraints require a doctor's order. They are used only if it is the best way to protect the person. They are not used for staff convenience. Restraints can make confusion and demented behaviors worse. The nurse tells you when to use restraints.

Activity and a safe setting promote quality of life. Safe, calm, and quiet activities are needed. The recreational therapist and other health team members will find activities that are best for each person. These are part of the person's care plan.

REVIEW QUESTIONS

Circle the BEST answer.

1 Cognitive function relates to the following *except*
   a Memory loss and personality
   b Thinking and reasoning
   c Ability to understand
   d Judgment and behavior

2 A person is confused after surgery. The confusion is likely to be
   a Permanent
   b Temporary
   c Caused by an infection
   d Caused by a brain injury

3 A person is confused. The care plan includes the following. Which should you question?
   a Restrain in bed at night.
   b Give clear, simple directions.
   c Use touch to communicate.
   d Open drapes during the day.

4 A person has delusions. A delusion is
   a A false belief
   b An illness caused by changes in the brain
   c Seeing, hearing, or feeling something that is not real
   d Alzheimer's disease

5 A person has AD. Which is *true*?
   a AD occurs only in older persons.
   b Diet and medications can cure the disease.
   c AD and delirium are the same.
   d AD ends in death.

6 The following are common in persons with AD *except*
   a Memory loss, poor judgment, and sleep disturbances
   b Loss of impulse control and loss of the ability to communicate
   c Wandering, delusions, and hallucinations
   d Paralysis, dyspnea, and pain

7 A person leaves the center without staff knowledge. This is called
   a Elopement
   b Wandering
   c Bad behavior
   d Poor judgment

8 Sundowning means that
   a The person becomes sleepy when the sun sets
   b Behaviors become worse in the late afternoon and evening hours
   c Behavior improves at night
   d The person goes to bed when the sun sets

9 A person with AD keeps telling you that someone is stealing things. What should you do?
   a Nothing. You know that the person suffers from paranoia.
   b Tell the nurse. Someone could be abusing the person.
   c Replace missing items.
   d Send other items home with the family.

10 A person has AD. To communicate with him or her, you should
   a Give orders
   b Correct the person's mistakes
   c Ask open-ended questions
   d Limit the person's choices

Continued

11 A person with AD is screaming. You know that this is
  a An agitated reaction
  b A way to communicate
  c Caused by a delusion
  d A repetitive behavior

12 A person with AD is rummaging through a drawer. Which is *false?*
  a The person may be looking for something.
  b The behavior may have no meaning.
  c The behavior is allowed if items in the drawer are safe.
  d You must distract the person with another activity.

13 Which is the best way to approach a person with AD?
  a From the front
  b From the back
  c From the right side
  d From the left side

14 A person with AD tends to wander. You should do the following *except*
  a Make sure door alarms are turned on
  b Make sure an ID bracelet is worn
  c Assist with exercise as ordered
  d Tell the person where to wander safely

15 Safety is important for the person with AD. Which is *false?*
  a Safety plugs are placed in electrical outlets.
  b Cleaners and medications are kept locked up.
  c The person can keep smoking materials.
  d Sharp and breakable objects are removed from the person's setting.

16 Which of these can cause delusions in persons with AD?
  a Eyeglasses
  b Hearing aids
  c Mirrors
  d Night-lights

17 You are caring for a person with AD. Which is *false?*
  a You can reason with the person.
  b Touch can calm and reassure the person.
  c A calm, quiet setting is important.
  d Help is needed with ADL.

18 Which helps prevent many of the behaviors and problems of AD?
  a Soothing music
  b Support groups
  c Caffeine
  d Validation therapy

19 AD support groups do the following *except*
  a Provide care
  b Offer encouragement and care ideas
  c Provide support for the family
  d Promote the sharing of feelings and frustrations

Circle T if the statement is TRUE. Circle F if the statement is FALSE.

20 T F   A person with AD is agitated and restless. You or other caregivers may have caused the behaviors.

21 T F   A person with AD may mistake you for a sexual partner. This is called hypersexuality.

22 T F   A person with AD keeps moving an empty cup back and forth across the table. The behavior is not harming the person or others. The behavior is allowed to continue.

23 T F   A person with AD tends to hide things. You should check wastebaskets before emptying them.

24 T F   The person with AD can control his or her behaviors.

25 T F   The person with AD can tell you about pain, constipation, and other discomforts.

26 T F   The person with AD is at risk for infection from poor hygiene after elimination.

27 T F   A set routine is important for the person with AD.

28 T F   You can use gestures or point to things to communicate with persons who have AD.

29 T F   Restraints can help improve the behaviors of AD.

30 T F   Family members continue their hobbies and holiday events. They are abusing the person with AD.

Answers to these questions are on p. 721.

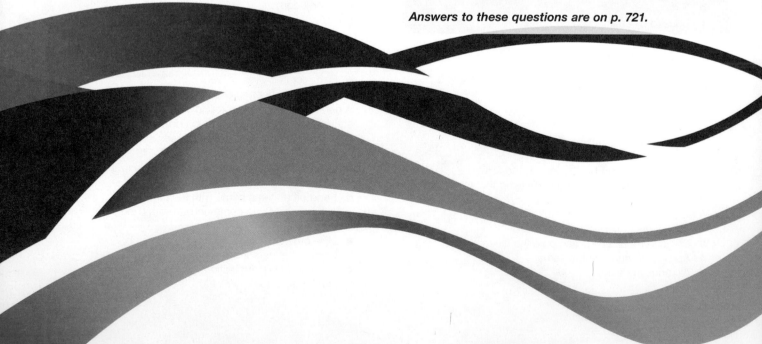

Box 45-1 Causes of Intellectual Disabilities

Genetic Conditions
- Abnormal genes from parents
- Errors when genes combine
- Gene disorders during pregnancy caused by infections, over-exposure to x-rays, and other factors
- Down syndrome (p. 676)
- Fragile X syndrome (p. 677)

Problems During Pregnancy
- Alcohol use (fetal alcohol syndrome)
- Drug use
- Smoking
- Malnutrition (*mal* means *bad*)
- Rubella (German measles)
- Diabetes
- Lack of oxygen to the brain
- Syphilis
- Rh blood disease

Problems at Birth
- Prematurity
- Low birth weight
- Head injury
- Lack of oxygen to the brain

Problems After Birth
- Childhood diseases (whooping cough, chicken pox, measles, Hib disease, meningitis, encephalitis)
- Head injuries
- Near drowning
- Lead poisoning
- Poisoning (alcohol, ammonia, bleaches, detergent, household cleaners and polishes, gasoline, kerosene, lighter fluid, drugs, lye, paint thinners and removers, pesticides, turpentine, weed killers, mercury, and so on)
- Shaken baby syndrome
- Malnutrition
- Dehydration
- Reye's syndrome (a disease caused by medications that contain aspirin)
- Poor health care

Modified from Causes and prevention of intellectual disabilities, *The Arc of the United States, revised August 2009, Silver Spring, Md.*

The Arc describes an intellectual disability as:
- An IQ score of about 70 or below. (IQ means intelligence quotient.) The person learns at a slower rate than normal. Learning ability is less than normal.
- A significant limit in at least one adaptive behavior. Adaptive behaviors are skills needed to function in everyday life—to live, work, and play. They involve communication, reading and writing, and money concepts.
  - Social skills involve interpersonal skills, responsibility, not being tricked by others, following rules, and obeying laws.
  - Practical skills involve personal activities of daily living: eating, dressing, mobility, and elimination.
  - Other personal skills include preparing meals, taking medications, using the phone, managing money, using transportation, housekeeping, job skills, and maintaining a safe setting.

Brain development is impaired. It can occur before birth, during birth, or before age 18. Causes are listed in Box 45-1. According to the Arc, alcohol is the leading preventable cause of intellectual disabilities.

Intellectual disabilities range from mild to severe. Persons mildly affected are slow to learn in school. As adults, they can function in society with some support. For example, they need help finding a job. Support is not needed every day. Some people need much support every day at home and at work. Still others need constant support in all areas.

The Arc believes that persons with intellectual disabilities must be able to enjoy and maintain a good quality of life. A good quality of life involves friendships, health and safety, and the right to make choices and take risks.

The Arc believes that children should live in a family. They should learn and play with children without disabilities. As adults, they should control their lives to the greatest extent possible. They should speak, make choices, and act for themselves. They should live in a home and have friends. They should do meaningful work and enjoy adult activities.

Sexuality

Persons with intellectual and developmental disabilities have physical, emotional, and social needs and desires. Reproductive organs develop. Some have life partners. Others marry and have children. Some persons can control their sexual urges. Others cannot. The type and location of sexual responses may be inappropriate. Also, sometimes persons with intellectual disabilities are sexually abused.

The Arc's beliefs about sexuality include the right to:

- Develop friendships and emotional and sexual relationships. This involves the right to:
  - Love and be loved
  - End a relationship as he or she chooses
- Dignity and respect.
- Privacy and confidentiality.
- Freely choose associations.
- Sexual expression.
- Learn about sex, marriage and family, abstinence, safe sex, sexual orientation, sexual abuse, and emotional abuse.
- Be protected from sexual harassment and abuses—physical, sexual, emotional.
- Decide about having and raising children.
- Make birth control decisions.
- Have control over their own bodies.
- Protection from sterilization because of the disability. *Sterilization* means to remove or block sex organs so the person cannot have children.

DOWN SYNDROME

Down syndrome (DS) is named for the doctor who identified the syndrome. DS is a common genetic cause of mild to moderate intellectual disabilities. It is caused by an error in cell division. At fertilization, a male sex cell (sperm) unites with a female sex cell (ovum). Each cell has 23 chromosomes. When they unite, the cell has 46 chromosomes. In DS, an extra 21st chromosome is present. The fertilized cell has 47 chromosomes. Thus DS occurs at fertilization.

The DS child has certain features caused by the extra chromosome (Fig. 45-1):

- Small head
- Eyes that slant upward
- Flat face
- Short, wide neck
- Large tongue
- Wide, flat nose
- Abnormally shaped ears
- Short stature
- Short, wide hands with stubby fingers
- Poor muscle tone

Many children with DS have heart defects and thyroid gland problems. They tend to have hearing and vision problems and to be over-weight. They are at risk for ear and respiratory infections. Leukemia is a risk. (*Leukemia* is a malignant disease in which there is an abnormal increase in the number of white blood cells.) Dementia may appear in adults with DS.

Fig. 45-1 A, An infant with Down syndrome. **B,** A child with Down syndrome. (**A** *from Hockenberry MJ, Wilson D:* Wong's nursing care of infants and children, *ed 9, St Louis, 2011, Mosby.* **B** *from Zitelli BJ, Davis HW:* Atlas of pediatric physical diagnosis, *ed 5, Philadelphia, 2007, Mosby.*)

Persons with DS need speech, language, physical, and occupational therapies. Most learn self-care skills. They also need health and sex education. Weight gain and constipation are problems. They need a healthy diet and regular exercise.

FRAGILE X SYNDROME

Fragile X syndrome (FXS) is inherited from one's parents. Inherited means to be passed down from parents to children. FXS is the most common form of inherited intellectual disabilities. With FXS there is a change in the gene that makes a protein needed for brain development. The body makes only a little or none of the protein.

Signs and symptoms vary from person to person. Girls often have milder symptoms than boys. FXS has no cure. The person needs help to reduce or eliminate these common signs and symptoms:

- *Learning.* The person may have mild learning disabilities or severe intellectual disabilities.
- *Physical.* Teenagers and adults may have long ears, faces, and jaws. Joints may be loose and flexible. They may be able to extend the elbow, thumb, and knee further than normal.
- *Social and emotional.* Behavior problems are common:
  - Fear and anxiety in new situations
  - Boys: attention problems, aggression
  - Girls: shy around new people
- *Speech and language.* Girls usually do not have severe problems. Most boys may have these problems:
  - Speaking clearly
  - Stuttering
  - Leaving out parts of words
  - Understanding "clues" when talking to people (voice tone, body language)
- *Sensory.* Bright lights, loud noises, and how something feels may bother many children. Some do not like being touched. They may have trouble making eye contact with others.

CEREBRAL PALSY

Cerebral palsy (CP) is a term applied to a group of disorders involving muscle weakness or poor muscle control (*palsy*). The defect is in the motor region of the brain (*cerebral*). CP permanently affects the ability to move and to maintain balance and posture. Abnormal movements, posture, and coordination result. Problems walking are likely.

The defects result from brain damage. It occurs before, during, or within a few years after birth. Lack of oxygen to the brain is the usual cause. Brain defects (from faulty brain development) are other causes. There is no cure.

Infants at risk include those who:
- Are premature
- Have low birth weight
- Do not cry within the first 5 minutes after birth
- Need mechanical ventilation
- Have bleeding in the brain
- Have heart, kidney, or spinal cord defects
- Have blood problems
- Have seizures
- Have fetal alcohol syndrome

Brain damage in infancy and early childhood also can result in CP. Lack of oxygen to the brain can occur from:
- Poisoning
- Traumatic brain injuries from accidents, falls, or child abuse (including shaken baby syndrome)
- Encephalitis and meningitis
- Rubella (German measles)

Body movements and body parts are affected. These types are the most common:

- *Spastic.* Spastic comes from *spastikos.* It means to *draw in.* Spastic means uncontrolled contractions of skeletal muscles. Muscles contract or shorten. They are stiff and cannot relax. One or both sides of the body may be involved. Posture, balance, and movement are affected. The arms may be affected. If so, there are problems with eating, writing, dressing, and other activities of daily living.
- *Athetoid.* The person cannot control movements. *Athetoid* comes from *athetos.* It means *not fixed.* The person has constant, slow, weaving, or writhing motions. These occur in the trunk, arms, hands, legs, and feet. Sometimes the tongue, face, and neck muscles are involved. Drooling and grimacing result.

Certain terms describe the body parts involved:
- *Hemiplegia.* The arm and leg on one side are paralyzed.
- *Diplegia. Di* means *twice.* Diplegia means that similar body parts are affected on both sides of the body. Both arms or both legs are paralyzed. The legs are commonly involved.
- *Quadriplegia.* Both arms and both legs are paralyzed. So are the trunk and neck muscles.

The person with CP can have many other impairments. They include:

- Intellectual disabilities
- Learning disabilities
- Hearing, vision, and speech impairments
- Drooling
- Bladder and bowel control problems
- Seizures
- Difficulty swallowing
- Attention deficit hyperactivity disorder (short attention span, poor concentration, increased activity)
- Breathing problems from poor posture
- Pressure ulcers from immobility

Care needs depend on the degree of brain damage. Disabilities range from mild to severe. Some persons are very smart. Others have severe intellectual disabilities. The goal is independence to the extent possible. Physical, occupational, and speech therapies can help. Some persons need braces and use walkers or crutches. Others need wheelchairs. Some need vision and hearing aids. Medications can control seizures. Surgery and medications can help some muscle problems.

AUTISM

Autism begins in early childhood. Some signs of delayed development are seen at about 18 months of age. (*Autos* means *self.*) It is a brain disorder with no cure. The child has:

- Problems with social skills
- Verbal and nonverbal communication problems
- Repetitive behaviors and routines and narrow interests (*Repetitive* means to repeat or repeated.)

Early signs of autism are:

- No babbling or pointing by the age of 1
- No single words by 16 months
- No 2-word phrases by age 2
- No response to his or her name
- Loss of language or social skills
- Poor eye contact
- Excessive lining up of toys or objects
- No smiling or social responses

Autism is more common in boys than in girls. The cause is unknown. Genetics and environmental factors may be involved.

The disorder can range from mild to severe. Signs of autism are listed in Box 45-2. With therapy, the person can learn to change or control behaviors. The therapies used include:

- Behavior modification
- Speech and language therapy
- Music therapy

Box 45-2	Signs of Autism

- Shows no interest in other people
- Poor eye contact
- Wants to be alone
- Has trouble understanding the feelings of others
- Has trouble talking about his or her own feelings
- Does not like to be held or cuddled; screams to be put down
- Over-reacts to touch
- Shows little reaction to pain
- Has frequent tantrums for no apparent reason
- Does not notice when others try to talk to him or her
- May not know how to talk, play, or relate to others
- May not talk
- Has slow language development
- Talks later than other children
- Repeats what others say at the moment or later
- Repeats words or phrases
- May not understand gestures (such as waving good-bye)
- Has a voice that sounds flat
- Cannot control voice volume (loudness or softness)
- Does not start or maintain conversations
- Stands too close to people when talking to them
- Stays with one topic of conversation for too long
- Has problems listening to what others say
- May act deaf
- Does not respond to his or her name
- Repeats actions over and over again
- Has routines where things stay the same
- Does not like change
- Repeats body movements (hand flapping, hand twisting, rocking)
- Has strong attachment to one item, idea, activity, or person
- Is very active or very quiet

- Auditory therapy
- Sensory therapies
- Physical and occupational therapies
- Drug therapy
- Diet therapy
- Communication therapy
- Recreation therapy

The person needs to develop social and work skills. Children with autism become adults. Some adults work and live independently. Others need support from family and community services. Some live in group homes or residential facilities.

Persons with autism may have other disorders. They include fragile X syndrome and seizures.

SPINA BIFIDA

Spina bifida (SB) is a defect of the spinal column. (*Spina* means *backbone*. *Bifid* means *split in two parts*.) The defect occurs during the first month of pregnancy. Hydrocephalus often occurs with SB (p. 680).

Spinal column bones (*vertebrae*) protect the spinal cord. In SB, vertebrae do not form properly. This leaves a split in the vertebrae. The split leaves the spinal cord unprotected. Only a membrane covers the spinal cord, which contains nerves. The nerves send messages to and from the brain. If the spinal cord is not protected, nerve damage occurs. Affected body parts do not function properly. Paralysis may occur. Bowel and bladder problems are common. Infection is a threat.

SB can occur anywhere in the spine. The lower back is the most common site. Types of SB include:

- *Spina bifida occulta*. *Occult* means *hidden*. Vertebrae are closed. A defect occurs in the vertebrae closure. In other words, the defect is hidden. The spinal cord and nerves are normal. The person has a dimple or tuft of hair on the back (Fig. 45-2). Often there are no symptoms. Foot weakness and bowel and bladder problems can occur.

- *Spina bifida cystica*. *Cystica* means *pouch* or *sac*. Part of the spinal column is in the pouch or sac. A membrane or a thin layer of skin covers the sac. It looks like a large blister. The pouch is easily injured. Infection is a threat. The two types of spina bifida cystica are (Fig. 45-3):
  - *Meningocele*. *Meningo* comes from *meninx*. It means *membrane*. *Cele* means *hernia* or *swelling*. Meninges are the connective tissue that covers and protects the brain and spinal cord. Cerebrospinal fluid also protects the brain and spinal cord. The sac contains meninges and cerebrospinal fluid (see Fig. 45-3, *A*, and Fig. 45-4, p. 680). The sac does not contain nerve tissue. The spinal cord and nerves are usually normal. Nerve damage usually does not occur. Surgery corrects the defect.
  - *Myelomeningocele* (or *meningomyelocele*). *Myelo* means *spinal cord*. The pouch contains nerves, spinal cord, meninges, and cerebrospinal fluid (see Fig. 45-3, *B*). Nerve damage occurs. Loss of function occurs below the level of damage. Leg paralysis and lack of sensation are common problems. So is the lack of bowel and bladder control. The defect is closed with surgery. Some children walk with braces or crutches. Others use wheelchairs.

Some children have learning problems. They may have problems with attention, language, reading, and math. They are at high risk for gastro-intestinal disorders and mobility problems. Skin breakdown, depression, and social and sexual issues are other risks.

Fig. 45-2 Spina bifida occulta.

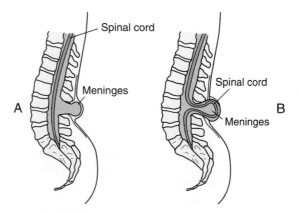

Fig. 45-3 **A,** Meningocele. **B,** Meningomyelocele.

Fig. 45-4 Meningocele. *(From Zitelli BJ, Davis HW: Atlas of pediatric physical diagnosis, St Louis, 1987, Gower Medical Publishing.)*

Fig. 45-5 Hydrocephalus. *(From Hart CA, Broadhead RL: Color atlas of pediatric infectious diseases, London, 1992, Mosby-Wolfe.)*

HYDROCEPHALUS

With hydrocephalus, cerebrospinal fluid collects in and around the brain. (*Hydro* means *water*. *Cephalo* means *head*.) The head enlarges (Fig. 45-5). Pressure inside the head increases. Intellectual disabilities and neurological damage occur without treatment.

A shunt is placed in the brain. It allows cerebrospinal fluid to drain from the brain. The shunt is a long flexible tube. It goes from the brain into a body cavity (Fig. 45-6). Usually it drains into the abdomen or a heart chamber. The shunt must remain open (*patent*). If blocked, the cerebrospinal fluid cannot drain from the brain.

The person can have many problems. Vision problems, seizures, and learning disabilities can occur.

Fig. 45-6 A shunt drains fluid from the brain. *(From Hockenberry MJ, Wilson D: Wong's nursing care of infants and children, ed 8, St Louis, 2007, Mosby.)*

QUALITY OF LIFE

Persons with DD have the same rights as every citizen. They have the right to live, learn, work, and enjoy life. The Americans With Disabilities Act of 1990 (ADA) further protects their rights. So does the Developmental Disabilities Assistance and Bill of Rights Act of 2000. Some persons with DD need nursing center care. They are further protected by OBRA.

Independence to the extent possible is the goal for these persons. This includes having a job and living in the community. The many resources to assist the person and family include:

- Assistive and self-help devices
- Education
- Job training
- Personal assistive services
- Home and vehicle changes
- Financial help
- Physical and occupational therapies
- Speech and language therapy
- Respiratory therapy
- Recreation therapy
- Assistance with hearing and vision

REVIEW QUESTIONS

Circle the BEST answer.

1 All developmental disabilities occur
   a At birth
   b From trauma
   c During pregnancy
   d Before 22 years of age

2 These statements are about developmental disabilities. Which is *true*?
   a Self-care, learning, and mobility are always affected.
   b The disability is severe and permanent.
   c Physical and intellectual impairment occur together.
   d The person cannot hold a job.

3 The person with intellectual disabilities
   a Has delayed development of sexual organs
   b Does not have the skills to live, work, and play
   c Needs care in a special setting
   d Learns at a slower rate than normal

4 Intellectual disabilities
   a Are always severe
   b Can occur before, during, or after birth
   c Are caused by an extra chromosome
   d Affect the motor region of the brain

5 Down syndrome occurs
   a At fertilization
   b During the first month of pregnancy
   c Any time before, during, or after birth
   d From trauma

6 The person with Down syndrome always has some degree of
   a Cerebral palsy
   b Autism
   c Impaired mobility
   d Intellectual disability

7 Fragile X syndrome is
   a The result of brain injury
   b Inherited from parents
   c Caused by drug and alcohol use
   d Caused by an infection

8 Cerebral palsy is usually caused by
   a An extra chromosome
   b High fever
   c Lack of oxygen to the brain
   d Infection during pregnancy

9 The person with the spastic type of cerebral palsy has problems with
   a Learning
   b Drooling
   c Posture, balance, and movement
   d Weaving motions of the trunk, arms, and legs

10 Autism begins
   a At fertilization
   b During pregnancy
   c At birth
   d In early childhood

11 The person with autism has
   a Impaired movement
   b Social and communication problems
   c Diplegia and brain damage
   d Intellectual disabilities

12 Spina bifida involves
   a Nerve damage
   b A defect in the spinal column
   c Seizures
   d Intellectual disabilities

13 Which is common in spina bifida?
   a Short attention span
   b Hearing and vision problems
   c Seizures
   d Bowel and bladder problems

14 Hydrocephalus often occurs with
   a Down syndrome   c Spina bifida
   b Cerebral palsy   d Autism

15 Hydrocephalus is treated with
   a Braces and crutches   c Medications
   b A shunt   d Social services

Answers to these questions are on p. 721.

CHAPTER 46

Rehabilitation and Restorative Nursing Care

OBJECTIVES

- Define the key terms and key abbreviations listed in this chapter.
- Describe how rehabilitation and restorative care involve the whole person.
- Identify the complications to prevent.
- Identify the common reactions to rehabilitation.

- List the common rehabilitation programs and services.
- Explain your role in rehabilitation and restorative care.
- Explain how to promote quality of life.

KEY TERMS

activities of daily living (ADL) The activities usually done during a normal day in a person's life

disability Any lost, absent, or impaired physical or mental function

prosthesis An artificial replacement for a missing body part

rehabilitation The process of restoring the person to his or her highest possible level of physical, psychological, social, and economic function

restorative aide A nursing assistant with special training in restorative nursing and rehabilitation skills

restorative nursing care Care that helps persons regain health, strength, and independence

KEY ABBREVIATIONS

ADL	Activities of daily living	**ROM**	Range-of-motion

Disease, injury, and surgery can affect body function. So can birth injuries and birth defects (Chapter 45). Often more than one function is lost. Losses are temporary or permanent. Eating, bathing, dressing, and walking are hard or seem impossible. Some persons cannot work. Others cannot care for children or family.

A disability is any lost, absent, or impaired physical or mental function. Causes are acute or chronic (Box 46-1).

- An *acute problem* has a short course. Recovery is complete. A fracture is an acute problem.
- A *chronic problem* has a long course. The problem is controlled—not cured—with treatment. Diabetes and arthritis are chronic health problems.

Disabilities are short-term or long-term. A leg fracture is short-term. The person has a cast. Crutches are used until the bone heals. A spinal cord injury is long-term if paralysis results.

The person may depend totally or in part on others for basic needs. The degree of disability affects how much function is possible.

A goal of health care is to prevent and reduce the degree of disability. Helping the person adjust is another goal. Rehabilitation is the process of restoring the person to his or her highest possible level of physical, psychological, social, and economic function. The focus is on improving abilities. This promotes function at the highest level of independence. For some persons the goal is to return to a job. For others, self-care is the goal. Sometimes improved function is not possible. Then the goal is to prevent further loss of function. This helps the person maintain the best possible quality of life.

Some nursing center residents have physical disabilities. Causes include strokes, fractures, amputations, and injuries. They need to regain function or adjust to a long-term disability. Often these residents return home. The rehabilitation may continue in home or community settings.

Box 46-1 Common Health Problems Requiring Rehabilitation

- Amputation
- Birth defects
- Brain tumor
- Burns
- Cerebral palsy
- Chronic obstructive pulmonary disease
- Fractures
- Head injury
- Myocardial infarction (heart attack)
- Spinal cord injury
- Spinal cord tumor
- Stroke
- Substance abuse—drug, alcohol

RESTORATIVE NURSING

Some persons are weak. Many cannot perform daily functions. They need restorative nursing care. Restorative nursing care is care that helps persons regain health, strength, and independence. With progressive illnesses, the person becomes more and more disabled. Restorative nursing programs:

- Help maintain the highest level of function
- Prevent unnecessary decline in function

Restorative nursing may involve measures that promote:

- Self-care
- Elimination
- Positioning
- Mobility
- Communication
- Cognitive function

Many persons need restorative nursing and rehabilitation. Often it is hard to separate them. In many centers, they mean the same thing. Both focus on the whole person.

Restorative Aides

Some centers have restorative aides. A restorative aide is a nursing assistant with special training in restorative nursing and rehabilitation skills. These aides assist the nursing and health teams as needed.

Usually nursing assistants are promoted to restorative aide positions. Professional behaviors are highly valued when considering staff to promote. Restorative aides need patience, kindness, and good communication skills. Those chosen have a positive attitude and excellent work ethics, job performance, and skills. Required training varies among states. If there are no state requirements, the center provides needed training.

REHABILITATION AND THE WHOLE PERSON

A health problem has physical, psychological, and social effects. So does a disability. Suppose an illness left you paralyzed from the waist down.

- Would you be angry, afraid, or depressed?
- How would you move about?
- How would you care for yourself?
- How would you care for your family?
- How would you worship, shop, or visit friends?
- What job could you do?
- How would you support yourself?

The person needs to adjust physically, psychologically, socially, and economically. Abilities—what the person can do—are stressed. Complications are prevented. They can cause further disability.

Rehabilitation takes longer in older persons than in other age-groups. Changes from aging affect healing, mobility, vision, hearing, and other functions. Chronic health problems can slow recovery. Older persons also are at risk for injuries. Fast-paced rehabilitation programs are hard for them. Their programs usually are slower-paced.

Physical Aspects

Rehabilitation starts when the person first seeks health care. Complications are prevented. They can occur from bedrest, a long illness, or recovery from surgery or injury. Bowel and bladder problems are prevented. So are contractures and pressure ulcers. Good alignment, turning and re-positioning, range-of-motion (ROM) exercises, and supportive devices are needed (Chapters 16, 17, and 26). Good skin care also prevents pressure ulcers (Chapters 20 and 36).

Elimination Some persons need bladder training (Chapter 22). The method depends on the person's problems, abilities, and needs. Some need bowel training (Chapter 23). Control of bowel movements and regular elimination are goals. Fecal impaction, constipation, and fecal incontinence are prevented. Follow the care plan and the nurse's instructions.

Self-Care Self-care is a major goal. **Activities of daily living (ADL)** are the activities usually done during a normal day in a person's life. ADL include bathing, oral hygiene, dressing, eating, elimination, and moving about. The health team evaluates the person's ability to perform ADL. The need for self-help devices is considered.

Sometimes the hands, wrists, and arms are affected. Self-help devices are often needed. Equipment is changed, made, or bought to meet the person's needs.

- Eating devices include glass holders, plate guards, and silverware with curved handles or cuffs (Chapter 24). Some devices attach to splints (Fig. 46-1).
- Electric toothbrushes are helpful. They have back-and-forth brushing motions for oral hygiene.
- Longer handles attach to combs, brushes, and sponges. Or the devices have long handles. See Chapters 20 and 21.
- Self-help devices are useful for cooking, dressing, writing, phone calls, and other tasks. Some are shown in Figure 46-2.

Mobility The person may need crutches or a walker, cane, or brace. Physical and occupational therapies are common for musculo-skeletal and nervous system problems (Fig. 46-3). Some people need wheelchairs. If possible, they learn wheelchair transfers. Such transfers include to and from the bed, toilet, bathtub, sofa, and chair and in and out of vehicles (Fig. 46-4 and Figs. 46-5 and 46-6, p. 686).

A **prosthesis** is an artificial replacement for a missing body part. The person learns how to use the artificial arm or leg (Chapter 39). The goal is for the device to be like the missing body part in function and appearance.

Fig. 46-1 Eating device attached to a splint.

Fig. 46-2 A, Light switch extender. **B,** Power gripper. **C,** Cutting board. **D,** Pot stabilizer. *(**A, C, D,** Courtesy Parsons ADL, Inc., Tottenham, Ontario. **B,** Courtesy OXO International, Inc., New York, NY.)*

Fig. 46-3 The person is assisted with walking in physical therapy.

Transfer board

Fig. 46-4 The person uses a transfer board to transfer from the wheelchair to bed.

Fig. 46-5 The person transfers from the wheelchair to the bathtub. A transfer board is used.

Fig. 46-6 The person transfers from the wheelchair to the car.

Nutrition Difficulty swallowing *(dysphagia)* may occur after a stroke. The person may need a dysphagia diet (Chapter 24). When possible, the person learns exercises to improve swallowing. Some persons cannot swallow. They need enteral nutrition (Chapter 25).

Communication *Aphasia* may occur from a stroke (Chapter 37). Aphasia is the total or partial loss *(a)* of the ability to use or understand language *(phasia)*. It is a language disorder resulting from damage to parts of the brain responsible for language. The person does not have normal speech. Speech therapy and communication devices are helpful (Chapter 8).

See *Focus on Communication: Communication.*

Mechanical Ventilation Some persons need mechanical ventilation (Chapter 29). Some are weaned from the ventilator. That is, the person learns to breathe without the machine. The process may take many weeks. Other persons must learn to live with life-long mechanical ventilation.

Psychological and Social Aspects

A disability can affect function and appearance. Self-esteem and relationships may suffer. Some persons may feel unwhole, useless, unattractive, unclean, or undesirable. They may deny the disability and expect therapy to correct the problem. Some persons are depressed, angry, and hostile.

Successful rehabilitation depends on the person's attitude. The person must accept his or her limits and be motivated. The focus is on abilities and strengths. Despair and frustration are common. Progress may be slow. Learning a new task is a reminder of the disability. Old fears and emotions may recur.

Remind persons of their *progress.* They need help accepting disabilities and limits. Give support, reassurance, and encouragement. Psychological and social needs are part of the care plan. Spiritual support helps some persons.

See *Focus on Communication: Psychological and Social Aspects.*

Economic Aspects

Some persons return to their jobs. Others cannot do so. They are assessed for work skills, work history, interests, and talents. A job skill may be restored or a new one learned. The goal is for the person to become gainfully employed. Help is given finding a job.

FOCUS ON COMMUNICATION
Communication

Speaking is difficult or impossible for some persons. Persons with speech disorders may need other communication methods. Pictures, reading, writing, facial expressions, and gestures are examples. The person and health team decide on the best method. All health team members and the family use the same method with the person. Changing methods can cause confusion and delay progress.

FOCUS ON COMMUNICATION
Psychological and Social Aspects

Denial, anger, depression, fear, and frustration are common during rehabilitation. Good communication and support provide encouragement. To deal with such emotions:
- Listen to the person.
- Show concern, not pity.
- Focus on what the person can do. Point out even slight progress.
- Be polite but firm. Do not let the person control you.
- Do not shout at or insult the person. Such behaviors are abuse and mistreatment.
- Do not argue with the person.
- Tell the nurse. The person may need other support measures.

THE REHABILITATION TEAM

Rehabilitation is a team effort. The person is the key team member. The family, doctor, nursing team, and other health team members help the person set goals and plan care. The focus is on regaining function and independence.

The team meets often to discuss the person's progress. The rehabilitation plan is changed as needed. The person and family attend the meetings when possible. Families are important. They provide support and encouragement. Often they help with care when the person returns home.

Your Role

Every part of your job focuses on promoting the person's independence. Preventing decline in function also is a goal. The many procedures, care measures, and rules in this book apply. Safety, communication, legal, and ethical aspects apply. So do the measures in Box 46-2.

See *Focus on Communication: Your Role.*
See *Teamwork and Time Management: Your Role.*

FOCUS ON COMMUNICATION
Your Role

You may need to guide and direct the person during care measures. First, listen to how the nurse or therapist guides and directs the person. Use those words. Hearing the same thing helps the person learn and remember what to do.

TEAMWORK AND TIME MANAGEMENT
Your Role

Rehabilitation can frustrate the person, you, and other team members. Teamwork is about helping with care. But it is also about giving each other emotional support. Talking about your feelings may help. The team can help you control or express your feelings. You may need to assist with other residents for a while.

Box 46-2 Assisting With Rehabilitation and Restorative Care

- Follow the nurse's instructions carefully.
- Follow the person's care plan.
- Follow the person's daily routine.
- Provide for safety.
- Protect the person's rights. Privacy and personal choice are very important.
- Report early signs and symptoms of complications. They include pressure ulcers, contractures, and bowel and bladder problems.
- Keep the person in good alignment at all times.
- Turn and re-position the person as directed.
- Use safe transfer methods.
- Practice measures to prevent pressure ulcers.
- Perform ROM exercises as instructed.
- Apply assistive devices as ordered.
- Do not pity the person or give sympathy.
- Encourage the person to perform ADL to the extent possible.
- Give the person time to complete tasks. Do not rush the person.
- Give praise when even a little progress is made.
- Provide emotional support and reassurance.
- Try to understand and appreciate the person's situation, feelings, and concerns.
- Provide for spiritual needs.
- Practice the methods developed by the rehabilitation team. This helps you better assist the person.
- Practice the task that the person must do. This helps you guide and direct the person.
- Know how to apply the person's self-help devices.
- Know how to use the person's equipment.
- Stress what the person can do. Focus on abilities and strengths. Do not focus on disabilities and weaknesses.
- Remember that muscles will atrophy if not used. And contractures can develop.
- Have a hopeful outlook.

REHABILITATION PROGRAMS AND SERVICES

Rehabilitation begins when the person first needs health care. Often this is in the hospital. Common rehabilitation programs include:

- *Cardiac rehabilitation*—for heart disorders (Chapter 40)
- *Brain injury rehabilitation*—for nervous system disorders including traumatic brain injury (Chapter 39)
- *Spinal cord rehabilitation*—for spinal cord injuries (Chapter 39)
- *Stroke rehabilitation*—after a stroke (Chapter 39)
- *Respiratory rehabilitation*—for respiratory system disorders such as chronic obstructive pulmonary disease, after lung surgery, for respiratory complications from other health problems (Chapter 40), and for mechanical ventilation (Chapter 29)
- *Musculo-skeletal rehabilitation*—for fractures, joint replacement surgery, and so on (Chapter 39)
- *Rehabilitation for complex medical and surgical conditions*—for wound care (Chapters 35 and 36), diabetes (Chapter 41), burns (Chapter 47), and so on

Depending on the person's needs and problems, the process may continue after the person leaves the hospital. The person may need nursing center care. Some persons transfer to rehabilitation agencies. There are agencies for persons who are blind or deaf, have intellectual disabilities (formerly called mental retardation), are physically disabled, or have speech problems. Some agencies are for persons who are mentally ill. Many substance abuse programs are available.

Home care agencies also provide rehabilitation services. So do some assisted living residences (Chapter 30) and adult day-care centers.

OBRA Requirements

The Omnibus Budget Reconciliation Act of 1987 (OBRA) requires that nursing centers provide rehabilitation services. If not provided by center staff, the service is obtained from another source. For example, a center does not have a speech therapist. Instead, the service is obtained from a hospital or other agency.

The center must provide services required by a person's comprehensive care plan. If a person requires physical therapy, it must be provided. If a person requires occupational therapy, it must be provided. If a person requires speech therapy, it must be provided. Such services require a doctor's order.

QUALITY OF LIFE

Successful rehabilitation and restorative care improves the person's quality of life. The goal is independence to the greatest extent possible. A hopeful and winning outlook is needed. The more the person can do alone, the better his or her quality of life. To promote independence:

- Focus on what the person can do.
- Offer support and encouragement.
- Remain patient. Do not rush the person.
- Resist the urge to do things for the person that he or she can do. This hinders the person's ability to regain function. Remind the family to resist as well.
- Use self-help devices as needed.

Promoting quality of life helps the person's attitude. To promote quality of life:

- *Protect the right to privacy.* The person re-learns old skills or practices new skills in private. No one needs to watch. They do not need to see mistakes, falls, spills, or clumsiness. Nor do they need to see anger or tears. Privacy protects dignity and promotes self-respect.
- *Encourage personal choice.* This gives the person control. Not being able to control body movements or functions is very frustrating. Allow and encourage persons to control their lives to the extent possible. Persons who are sad and depressed may not want to make choices. Encourage them to do so. It can help them feel in control of those things that affect them. Personal choice is important in planning care.
- *Protect the right to be free from abuse and mistreatment.* Sometimes improvement is not seen for weeks. Learning to use a self-help device takes time. Learning to speak again can take a long time. So can learning how to dress when there is paralysis. What seems simple is often very hard to do. Repeated explanations and demonstrations may have no or little results. You may become upset and short-tempered. Other staff or the family may have such behaviors. Protect the person from abuse and mistreatment. No one can shout at, scream at, yell at, or call the person names. They cannot hit or strike the person. Unkind remarks are not allowed. Report signs of abuse or mistreatment to the nurse.
- *Learn to deal with your anger and frustration.* The person does not choose loss of function. If the process upsets you, think how the person must feel. Share your feelings with the nurse. The nurse can suggest ways to help you control or express your feelings. Perhaps you can assist other persons for a while.
- *Encourage activities.* Often a person worries about how others view the disability. Provide support and reassurance. Remind the person that others have disabilities. They can give support and understanding. Allow personal choice. Let the person do what interests him or her. The person usually chooses activities that he or she can do.

Continued

QUALITY OF LIFE—cont'd

- *Provide a safe setting.* It must meet the person's needs. Needed changes are made. The overbed table, bedside stand, signal light, and other needed items are moved to the person's strong side. If unable to use the signal light, another way is used to communicate with the staff. The person may need a special chair. The rehabilitation team suggests these and other changes. They explain the need and purpose to the person and family.

- *Show patience, understanding, and sensitivity.* Disability affects the whole person. Many emotions are felt. Anger and frustration are common. Some persons have trouble controlling such feelings. They may have outbursts. Progress may be slow and hard to see. The person may be upset and discouraged. You may feel short-tempered. You still must show respect. Control your words and actions. Give support, encouragement, and praise. Stress the person's abilities and strengths. Do not give pity or sympathy.

REVIEW QUESTIONS

Circle the BEST answer.

1 Rehabilitation and restorative nursing care focus on
   a What the person cannot do
   b Self-care
   c The whole person
   d The person's rights

2 Rehabilitation begins with preventing
   a Angry feelings
   b Contractures and pressure ulcers
   c Illness and injury
   d Loss of self-esteem

3 A person has weakness on the right side. ADL are
   a Done by the person to the extent possible
   b Done by you
   c Postponed until the right side can be used
   d Supervised by a therapist

4 Persons with disabilities are likely to feel the following *except*
   a Undesirable
   b Angry and hostile
   c Depressed
   d Relief

5 During a therapy, a person asks to have music played. You should
   a Explain that music is not allowed
   b Choose some music
   c Ask the person to choose some music
   d Ask a therapist to choose some music

6 A person's right side is weak. You move the signal light to the left side. You have promoted quality of life by
   a Protecting the person from abuse and mistreatment
   b Allowing personal choice
   c Providing for safety
   d Taking part in activities

Circle T if the statement is TRUE. Circle F if the statement is FALSE.

7 T F You should give praise even when slight progress is made.

8 T F A person's speech therapy should be done in private.

9 T F You tell a person that dessert is not allowed until exercises are done. This is abuse and mistreatment.

10 T F A person refuses to attend a concert at the nursing center. The person must attend. It is part of the rehabilitation plan.

11 T F Rehabilitation programs for older persons are usually slower-paced than those for younger persons.

12 T F You need to stress the person's abilities and strengths.

13 T F Sympathy and pity help the person adjust.

14 T F You should know how to apply self-help devices.

15 T F You should know how to use the person's care equipment.

16 T F You need to convey hopefulness to the person.

Answers to these questions are on p. 721.

Basic Emergency Care

OBJECTIVES

- Define the key terms and key abbreviations listed in this chapter.
- Describe the rules of emergency care.
- Identify the signs of sudden cardiac arrest and the emergency care required.
- Describe the signs, symptoms, and emergency care for hemorrhage.
- Identify the common causes and emergency care for fainting.
- Identify the signs, symptoms, and emergency care for shock.

- Describe the signs, symptoms, and emergency care for stroke.
- Explain the causes and types of seizures and how to care for a person during a seizure.
- Identify the causes, types, and emergency care for burns.
- Perform the procedures described in this chapter.
- Explain how to promote quality of life.

KEY TERMS

anaphylaxis A life-threatening sensitivity to an antigen

cardiac arrest See "sudden cardiac arrest"

convulsion See "seizure"

fainting The sudden loss of consciousness from an inadequate blood supply to the brain

first aid Emergency care given to an ill or injured person before medical help arrives

hemorrhage The excessive loss of blood in a short time

respiratory arrest Breathing stops but heart action continues for several minutes

seizure Violent and sudden contractions or tremors of muscle groups; convulsion

shock Results when organs and tissues do not get enough blood

sudden cardiac arrest (SCA) The heart stops suddenly and without warning; cardiac arrest

KEY ABBREVIATIONS

AED	Automated external defibrillator	**EMS**	Emergency Medical Services
AHA	American Heart Association	**SCA**	Sudden cardiac arrest
BLS	Basic Life Support	**VF**	Ventricular fibrillation
CPR	Cardiopulmonary resuscitation	**V-fib**	Ventricular fibrillation

Emergencies can occur anywhere. Sometimes you can save a life if you know what to do. You are encouraged to take a first aid course and a Basic Life Support (BLS) course. These courses prepare you to give emergency care.

The BLS procedures in this chapter are given as basic information. They do not replace certification training. You need a BLS course for health care providers.

EMERGENCY CARE

First aid is the emergency care given to an ill or injured person before medical help arrives. The goals of first aid are to:

- Prevent death
- Prevent injuries from becoming worse

In an emergency, the Emergency Medical Services (EMS) system is activated. Emergency personnel (paramedics, emergency medical technicians) rush to the scene. They treat, stabilize, and transport persons with life-threatening problems. Their ambulances have emergency medications, equipment, and supplies. They have guidelines for care and communicate with doctors in hospital emergency departments. The doctors can tell them what to do. To activate the EMS system, do one of the following:

- Dial 911.
- Call the local fire or police department.
- Call the phone operator.

In nursing centers, a nurse decides when to activate the EMS system. The nurse tells you how to help. If a person has stopped breathing or is in sudden cardiac arrest, the nurse may start cardiopulmonary resuscitation (CPR) (p. 694). Some centers allow nursing assistants to start CPR. Others do not. Know your center's policy about CPR.

Death is expected in persons with terminal illnesses. Usually these persons are not resuscitated (Chapter 48). This information is on the care plan.

Each emergency is different. The rules in Box 47-1 apply to any emergency.

See *Focus on Communication: Emergency Care.*
See *Promoting Safety and Comfort: Emergency Care.*
See *Teamwork and Time Management: Emergency Care.*

Box 47-1   Rules of Emergency Care

- Know your limits. Do not do more than you are able. Do not perform an unfamiliar procedure. Do what you can under the circumstances.
- Stay calm. This helps the person feel more secure.
- Know where to find emergency supplies.
- Follow Standard Precautions and the Bloodborne Pathogen Standard to the extent possible.
- Check for life-threatening problems. Check for breathing, a pulse, and bleeding.
- Keep the person lying down or as you found him or her. Moving the person could make an injury worse.
- Move the person only if the setting is unsafe. Examples include:
  - A burning building or car
  - A building that might collapse
  - Stormy conditions with lightning
  - In water
  - Near electrical wires
- Wait for help to arrive if the scene is not safe enough for you to approach.
- Perform necessary emergency measures.

- Call for help. Or have someone activate the EMS system. *Do not hang up until the operator has hung up.* Give the operator the following information:
  - Your location: street address and city, cross streets or roads, and landmarks.
  - Phone number you are calling from.
  - What seems to have happened (for example: heart attack, crash, fire)—police, fire equipment, and ambulances may be needed.
  - How many people need help.
  - Conditions of victims, obvious injuries, and life-threatening situations.
  - What aid is being given.
- Do not remove the person's clothes unless you have to. If you must remove clothing, tear or cut garments along the seams.
- Keep the person warm. Cover the person with a blanket, coats, or sweaters.
- Reassure the person. Explain what is happening and that help was called.
- Do not give the person food or fluids.
- Keep onlookers away. They invade privacy and tend to stare, give advice, and comment about the person's condition. The person may think the situation is worse than it really is.

BASIC LIFE SUPPORT FOR ADULTS

When the heart and breathing stop, the person is clinically dead. Blood is not circulated through the body. Heart, brain, and other organ damage occurs within minutes. The American Heart Association's (AHA) Basic Life Support (BLS) procedures support circulation and breathing.

AHA guidelines are updated every 5 years. Any changes to the material presented here are available on Evolve at http://evolve.elsevier.com/Sorrentino/longterm.

Chain of Survival for Adults

The AHA's BLS courses teach the adult *Chain of Survival.* These actions are taken for heart attack (Chapter 40), sud-

den cardiac arrest, respiratory arrest (p. 694), stroke (Chapter 39 and p. 705), and choking (Chapter 12). They also apply to other life-threatening problems. They are done as soon as possible. Any delay reduces the person's chance of surviving.

Chain of Survival actions for the adult are:
- *Recognizing cardiac arrest and activating the EMS system at once.*
- *Early cardiopulmonary resuscitation (CPR).*
- *Early defibrillation.* See p. 698.
- *Early advanced care.* This is given by EMS staff, doctors, and nurses. They give drugs and perform life-saving measures.
- *Organized post-cardiac arrest care.* This care is given to improve survival following cardiac arrest.

You will learn the Chain of Survival for children in the AHA's *BLS for Healthcare Providers* course.

See *Focus on Communication: Chain of Survival for Adults.*

Sudden Cardiac Arrest

Sudden cardiac arrest (SCA) or cardiac arrest is when the heart stops suddenly and without warning. Within moments, breathing stops as well. Permanent brain and other organ damage occurs unless circulation and breathing are restored. There are three major signs of SCA:
- No response.
- No breathing or no normal breathing. The person may have *agonal gasps* or *agonal respirations* early during SCA. (*Agonal* comes from the Greek word that means to *struggle.* Agonal is used in relation to death and dying.) Agonal gasps do not bring enough oxygen into the lungs. Gasps are not normal breathing.
- No pulse.

The person's skin is cool, pale, and gray. The person is not coughing or moving.

SCA is a sudden, unexpected, and dramatic event. It can occur anywhere and at any time—while driving, shoveling snow, playing golf or tennis, watching TV, eating, or sleeping. Common causes include heart disease, drowning, electric shock, severe injury, choking (Chapter 12), and drug over-dose. These causes lead to an abnormal heart rhythm called ventricular fibrillation (p. 698). The heart cannot pump blood. A normal rhythm must be restored. Otherwise the person will die.

Respiratory Arrest

Respiratory arrest is when breathing stops but heart action continues for several minutes. If breathing is not restored, cardiac arrest occurs. Causes of respiratory arrest include:

- Drowning
- Stroke
- Choking
- Drug over-dose
- Electric shock (including lightning strikes)
- Smoke inhalation
- Suffocation
- Heart attack
- Coma
- Other injuries

Rescue Breathing Rescue breaths are given when there is a pulse but no breathing or only gasping. To give rescue breaths:

- Open the airway (p. 695).
- Give 1 breath every 5 to 6 seconds for adults.
- Give each breath over 1 second. The chest should rise when breaths are given.
- Check the pulse every 2 minutes. If there is no pulse, begin CPR.

Cardiopulmonary Resuscitation for Adults

When the heart and breathing stop, blood and oxygen are not supplied to the body. Brain and other organ damage occurs within minutes.

Cardiopulmonary resuscitation (CPR) must be started at once when a person has SCA. CPR supports circulation and breathing. It provides blood and oxygen to the heart, brain, and other organs until advanced emergency care is given. CPR involves:

- Chest compressions
- Airway
- Breathing
- Defibrillation

CPR procedures require speed, skill, and efficiency. Chest compressions and airway and breathing procedures are done until a defibrillator arrives. The defibrillator is used as soon as possible.

See *Promoting Safety and Comfort: Cardiopulmonary Resuscitation for Adults.*

PROMOTING SAFETY AND COMFORT
Cardiopulmonary Resuscitation for Adults

Safety

The discussion and procedures that follow assume that the person does not have injuries from trauma (Chapter 35). If injuries are present, special measures are needed to position the person and open the airway. Such measures are learned during a BLS certification course.

You will learn CPR for infants and children in the AHA's *BLS for Healthcare Providers* course.

Chest Compressions The heart, brain, and other organs must receive blood. Otherwise, permanent damage results. In cardiac arrest, the heart has stopped beating. Blood must be pumped through the body in some other way. Chest compressions force blood through the circulatory system.

Before starting chest compressions, check for a pulse. Use the carotid artery on the side near you. To find the carotid pulse, place 2 or 3 fingertips on the trachea (windpipe). Then slide your fingertips down to the groove of the neck (Fig. 47-1). While checking for a pulse, look for signs of circulation. See if the person has started breathing or is coughing or moving.

The heart lies between the sternum (breastbone) and the spinal column. When pressure is applied to the sternum, the sternum is depressed. This compresses the heart between the sternum and spinal column (Fig. 47-2). For effective chest compressions, the person must

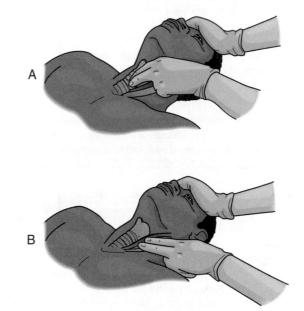

Fig. 47-1 Locating the carotid pulse. **A,** Two fingers are placed on the trachea. **B,** The fingertips are moved down into the groove of the neck to the carotid artery.

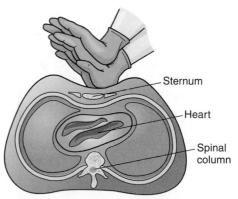

Fig. 47-2 The heart lies between the sternum and the spinal column. The heart is compressed when pressure is applied to the sternum.

be supine on a hard, flat surface—floor or back-board. You are positioned at the person's side.

Hand position is important for effective chest compressions (Fig. 47-3). You use the heels of your hands—one on top of the other—for chest compressions. For proper placement:

- Expose the person's chest. Remove clothing or move it out of the way. You need to be able to see the person's bare skin for proper hand position.
- Place the heel of one hand (usually your dominant hand) in the center of the bare chest. The heel of this hand is placed on the sternum between the nipples.
- Place the heel of your other hand on top of the heel of the first hand.

To give chest compressions, your arms are straight. Your shoulders are directly over your hands. And your fingers are interlocked (Fig. 47-4). Exert firm downward pressure to depress the adult sternum at least 2 inches. Then release pressure without removing your hands from the chest. Releasing pressure allows the chest to recoil—to return to its normal position. Recoil lets the heart fill with blood.

The AHA recommends that you:

- Give compressions at a rate of 100 per minute.
- Push hard, and push fast.
- Push deeply into the chest.
- Interrupt chest compressions only when necessary. Interruptions should be less than 10 seconds. When there are no chest compressions, blood does not flow to the heart, brain, and other organs.

Airway The respiratory passages (airway) must be open to restore breathing. The airway is often obstructed (blocked) during SCA. The person's tongue falls toward the back of the throat and blocks the airway. The head tilt–chin lift method opens the airway (Fig. 47-5):

- Place the palm of one hand on the forehead.
- Tilt the head back by pushing down on the forehead with your palm.
- Place the fingers of your other hand under the lower jaw. Use your index and middle fingers. Do not use your thumb.
- Lift the jaw. This brings the chin forward.
- Do not close the person's mouth. The mouth should

Fig. 47-3 Proper hand position for CPR. **A,** The heel of the dominant hand is placed in the center of the chest between the nipples. **B,** The heel of the non-dominant hand is placed on top of the dominant hand.

Fig. 47-4 Giving chest compressions. The arms are straight. The shoulders are over the hands. The fingers are interlocked.

Fig. 47-5 The head tilt-chin lift method opens the airway. One hand is on the person's forehead. Pressure is applied to tilt the head back. The chin is lifted with the fingers of the other hand.

be slightly open unless you need to do mouth-to-nose breathing (p. 697).

Breathing Air is not inhaled when breathing stops. The person must get oxygen. If not, permanent heart, brain, and other organ damage occurs. The person is given *breaths*. That is, a rescuer inflates the person's lungs.

Each breath should take 1 second. *You should see the chest rise with each breath.* Then two breaths are given after every 30 chest compressions.

Mouth-to-Mouth Breathing. Mouth-to-mouth breathing (Fig. 47-6) is one way to give breaths. You place your mouth over the person's mouth. Contact with the person's blood, body fluids, secretions, or excretions is likely. To give mouth-to-mouth breathing:

- Keep the airway open with the head tilt-chin lift method.
- Pinch the person's nostrils shut. Use your thumb and index finger. Use the hand on the forehead. Shutting the nostrils prevents air from escaping through the nose.
- Take a breath. A regular breath is needed, not a deep breath.
- Place your mouth tightly over the person's mouth. Seal the person's mouth with your lips.
- Blow air into the person's mouth. You should see the chest rise as the lungs fill with air. You should also hear air escape when the person exhales.
- Repeat the head tilt-chin lift method if the person's chest did not rise.
- Remove your mouth from the person's mouth. Then take in a quick breath.
- Give another breath. You should see the chest rise.

Barrier Device Breathing. A barrier device is used for giving breaths whenever possible. The device prevents contact with the person's mouth and blood, body fluids, secretions, or excretions. A face shield may be used (Fig. 47-7 and 47-8). A face shield is replaced with a face mask as soon as possible (Fig. 47-9, *A*). The mask is placed over the person's mouth and nose (Fig. 47-9, *B*, p. 697). When using a barrier device, seal the device against the person's face. The seal must be tight. Then open the airway with the head tilt-chin lift method.

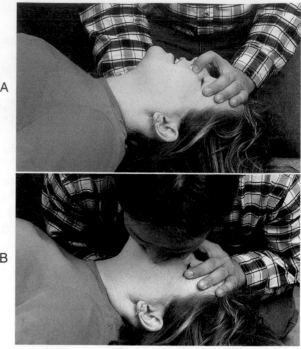

Fig. 47-6 Mouth-to-mouth breathing. **A,** The person's airway is opened. The nostrils are pinched shut. **B,** The person's mouth is sealed by the rescuer's mouth.

Fig. 47-7 Face shield.

Fig. 47-8 The face shield is in place.

Fig. 47-9 A, Mask for giving breaths. **B,** The mask is in place.

Fig. 47-10 A bag valve mask.

Fig. 47-11 Mouth-to-nose breathing.

A bag valve mask (Fig. 47-10) is another device used to give rescue breaths. The device consists of a hand-held bag attached to a mask. The mask is held securely to the person's face. And the bag is squeezed to give breaths. The bag can be connected to an oxygen source.

Mouth-to-Nose Breathing. Mouth-to-nose breathing is used when:
- You cannot breathe through the person's mouth.
- You cannot open the mouth.
- Your mouth is too small to make a tight seal for mouth-to-mouth breathing.
- The mouth or jaw is severely injured.
- The person is bleeding from the mouth.

The mouth is closed for mouth-to-nose breathing. The head tilt-chin lift method opens the airway. Pressure is placed on the chin to close the mouth. To give a

breath, place your mouth over the person's nose and blow air into the nose (Fig. 47-11). After giving a breath, remove your mouth from the person's nose.

Mouth-to-Stoma Breathing. Some people breathe through *stomas* (openings) in their necks (Fig. 47-12). To give mouth-to-stoma breathing:
- Keep the person's mouth closed.
- Do not tilt the person's head back.
- Seal your mouth around the stoma.
- Blow air into the stoma (Fig. 47-13).

If the person's chest does not rise, you may need to pinch the nostrils shut.

Before giving mouth-to-mouth or mouth-to-nose breathing, always check to see if the person has a stoma. Other rescue breathing methods are not effective if the person has a stoma.

Fig. 47-12 A stoma in the neck. The person breathes in and out of the stoma.

Fig. 47-13 Mouth-to-stoma breathing.

Defibrillation Ventricular fibrillation (VF, V-fib) is an abnormal heart rhythm (Fig. 47-14). It causes sudden cardiac arrest. Rather than beating in a regular rhythm, the heart shakes and quivers like a bowl of Jell-O. The heart does not pump blood. The heart, brain, and other organs do not receive blood and oxygen.

A *defibrillator* is used to deliver a shock to the heart. The shock stops the VF (V-fib). This allows the return of a regular heart rhythm. Defibrillation as soon as possible after the onset of VF (V-fib) increases the person's chance of survival.

For adults, the AHA recommends that rescuers:
- Attach and use the AED as soon as it is available.
- Minimize interruptions in chest compressions before and after a shock is delivered.
- Give one shock. Then resume CPR at once. Begin with compressions. Do 5 cycles of 30 compressions and 2 breaths.
- Check for a heart rhythm.

Fig. 47-14 **A,** Normal rhythm. **B,** Ventricular fibrillation.

Fig. 47-15 An automated external defibrillator (AED).

Automated external defibrillators (AEDs) are found in hospitals, nursing centers, dental offices, and other health care agencies (Fig. 47-15). They are on airplanes and in airports, health clubs, malls, and many other public places. Many people have them in their homes.

You will learn more about using an AED in the AHA's *BLS for Healthcare Providers* course.

Performing Adult CPR CPR is done only for cardiac arrest. You must determine if cardiac arrest or fainting (p. 000) has occurred. *CPR is done if the person does not respond, is not breathing (or has no normal breathing), and has no pulse.*

CPR is done alone or with another person. When done alone, chest compressions and rescue breathing are done by the one rescuer. With two rescuers, one person gives chest compressions, and the other does rescue breathing. Rescuers switch tasks about every 2 minutes to avoid fatigue and inadequate compressions. The second rescuer uses the AED if one is available.

See *Promoting Safety and Comfort: Performing Adult CPR.*

See *Focus On Communication: Performing Adult CPR.*

PROMOTING SAFETY AND COMFORT
Performing Adult CPR

Safety

Never practice CPR on another person. Serious damage can be done. Mannequins are used to learn and practice CPR.

Make sure you have a safe setting for CPR. Move the person only if the setting is unsafe (see Box 47-1). Do not approach the person if the scene is unsafe for you.

The person must be on a hard, flat surface for CPR. If the person is in bed, place a board under the person. Or move the person to the floor.

FOCUS ON COMMUNICATION
Performing Adult CPR

Good communication is needed when 2 rescuers perform CPR. The rescuer giving compressions must count out loud so the other rescuer is ready to give breaths. Clear communication prevents delays and minimizes interruptions in chest compressions.

Hands-Only CPR. When an adult has sudden cardiac arrest, the person's survival depends on others nearby. Outside of the health care setting, persons trained in BLS are often not available. Bystanders may worry that they will not do CPR correctly or they may injure the person.

The AHA developed "Hands-Only CPR" to improve the response of bystanders who witness an adult collapse suddenly in the out-of-hospital setting. In "Hands-Only CPR," CPR is simplified to 2 steps:

1 Call 911.
2 Push hard and fast in the center of the chest.

"Hands-Only CPR" is used to educate persons not trained in BLS. As a health care provider, use the CPR method presented in this chapter and in a BLS course.

 ADULT CPR—ONE RESCUER

PROCEDURE

1 Make sure the scene is safe.
2 Take 5 to 10 seconds to check for a response and breathing:
  a Check if the person is responding. Tap or gently shake the person. Call the person by name, if known. Shout, "Are you OK?"
  b Check for no breathing or no normal breathing (gasping).
3 Call for help. Activate the EMS system or the center's emergency response system if the person is not responding and not breathing or not breathing normally (gasping).
4 Get or ask someone to bring an AED if available.
5 Position the person supine on a hard, flat surface. Logroll the person so there is no twisting of the spine. Place the arms alongside the body.
6 Check for a carotid pulse. This should take 5 to 10 seconds. Start chest compressions if you do not feel a pulse.

7 Expose the person's chest.
8 Give chest compressions at a rate of 100 per minute. Push hard and fast. Establish a regular rhythm. Count out loud. Press down at least 2 inches. Allow the chest to recoil between compressions. Give 30 chest compressions.
9 Open the airway. Use the head tilt-chin lift method.
10 Give 2 breaths. Each breath should take only 1 second. Each breath must make the chest rise. (If the first breath does not make the chest rise, try opening the airway again. Use the head tilt-chin lift method.)
11 Continue the cycle of 30 compressions followed by 2 breaths. Limit interruptions in compressions to less than 10 seconds. Continue cycles until the AED arrives. See procedure *Adult CPR With AED—Two Rescuers* (p. 702). Or continue until help arrives or the person begins to move. If movement occurs, place the person in the recovery position (p. 703).

ADULT CPR—TWO RESCUERS

PROCEDURE

1 Make sure the scene is safe.
2 *Rescuer 1*—Take 5 to 10 seconds to check for a response and breathing:
   a Check if the person is responding. Tap or gently shake the person. Call the person by name, if known. Shout, "Are you OK?"
   b Check for no breathing or no normal breathing (gasping).
3 *Rescuer 2:*
   a Activate the EMS system or the center's emergency response system if the person is not responding and not breathing or not breathing normally (gasping).
   b Get a defibrillator (AED) if one is available. (See procedure: *Adult CPR With AED—Two Rescuers,* p. 702.)
4 *Rescuer 1:* Position the person supine on a hard, flat surface. Logroll the person so there is no twisting of the spine. Place the arms alongside the body. Begin 1-rescuer CPR until the second rescuer returns. (See procedure: *Adult CPR—One Rescuer,* steps 6 to 11.)
5 When the second rescuer returns, perform 2-person CPR (Fig. 47-16).
   a *Rescuer 1:* Give chest compressions at a rate of 100 per minute. Push hard and fast. Establish a regular rhythm. Count out loud. Press down at least 2 inches. Allow the chest to recoil between compressions. Give 30 chest compressions. Pause to allow the other rescuer to give 2 breaths.
   b *Rescuer 2:*
      (1) Open the airway. Use the head tilt-chin lift method.
      (2) Give 2 breaths after every 30 compressions. Each breath should take only 1 second and make the chest rise. (If the first breath does not make the chest rise, try opening the airway again. Use the head tilt-chin lift method.)
   c Continue cycles of 30 compressions and 2 breaths.
   d Change positions every 2 minutes (after about 5 cycles of 30 compressions and 2 breaths). The switch should take no more than 5 seconds.
   e Continue until the AED arrives. See procedure *Adult CPR With AED—Two Rescuers* (p. 702). Or continue until help takes over or the person begins to move. If movement occurs, place the person in the recovery position (p. 703).

Fig. 47-16 Two people perform CPR.

ADULT CPR WITH AED—TWO RESCUERS

PROCEDURE

1 Make sure the scene is safe.
2 *Rescuer 1*—Take 5 to 10 seconds to check for a response and breathing:
   a Check if the person is responding. Tap or gently shake the person. Call the person by name, if known. Shout, "Are you OK?"
3 *Rescuer 2:*
   a Activate the EMS system or the center's emergency response system if the person is not responding and not breathing or not breathing normally (gasping).
   b Get a defibrillator (AED) if one is available.
4 *Rescuer 1:*
   a Position the person supine on a hard, flat surface. Logroll the person so there is no twisting of the spine. Place the arms alongside the body.
   b Check for a carotid pulse. This should take 5 to 10 seconds. Start chest compressions if you do not feel a pulse.
   c Expose the person's chest.
   d Give chest compressions at a rate of 100 per minute. Push hard and fast. Establish a regular rhythm. Count out loud. Press down at least 2 inches. Allow the chest to recoil between compressions. Give 30 chest compressions.
   e Open the airway. Use the head tilt-chin lift method.
   f Give 2 breaths. Each breath should take only 1 second. Each breath must make the chest rise. (If the first breath does not make the chest rise, try opening the airway again. Use the head tilt-chin lift method.)
   g Continue the cycle of 30 chest compressions followed by 2 breaths. Limit interruptions in compressions to less than 10 seconds.

5 *Rescuer 2:*
   a Open the case with the AED.
   b Turn on the AED (Fig. 47-17, *A*).
   c Apply adult electrode pads to the person's chest (Fig. 47-17, *B*). Follow the instructions and diagram provided with the AED.
   d Attach the connecting cables to the AED (Fig. 47-17, *C*).
   e Clear away from the person. Make sure no one is touching the person (Fig. 47-17, *D*).
   f Let the AED check the person's heart rhythm.
   g Make sure everyone is clear of the person if the AED advises a "shock" (see Fig. 47-17, *D*). Loudly instruct others not to touch the person. Say: "I am clear, you are clear, everyone is clear!" Look to make sure no one is touching the person.
   h Press the "SHOCK" button if the AED advises a "shock" (Fig. 47-17, *E*).
6 *Rescuers 1 and 2:*
   a Perform 2-person CPR:
      (1) Begin with compressions. One rescuer gives chest compressions at a rate of at least 100 per minute. Push hard and fast. Establish a regular rhythm. Count out loud. Allow the chest to recoil between compressions. Give 30 chest compressions. Pause to allow the other rescuer to give 2 breaths.
      (2) The other rescuer gives 2 breaths after every 30 chest compressions.
7 Repeat steps 5 e, f, g, and h after 2 minutes of CPR (5 cycles of 30 compressions and 2 breaths). Change positions and continue CPR beginning with compressions.
8 Continue until help takes over or the person begins to move. If movement occurs, place the person in the recovery position (p. 703).

Fig. 47-17 **A,** The rescuer turns on the AED. **B,** Electrode pads are placed on the person's chest. **C,** The cables are connected to the AED. **D,** The rescuer "clears" the person. The rescuer makes sure no one is touching the person. **E,** The "SHOCK" button is pressed to deliver a shock.

A   B   C   D   E

Fig. 47-18 Recovery position.

Recovery Position

The recovery position is used when the person is breathing and has a pulse but is not responding (Fig. 47-18). The position helps keep the airway open and prevents aspiration.

Logroll the person into the recovery position. Keep the head, neck, and spine straight. A hand supports the head. *Do not use this position if the person might have neck injuries or other trauma.*

HEMORRHAGE

Life and body functions require an adequate blood supply. If a blood vessel is cut or torn, bleeding occurs. The larger the blood vessel, the greater the bleeding and blood loss. Hemorrhage is the excessive loss of blood in a short time. If bleeding is not stopped, the person will die.

Hemorrhage is internal or external. You cannot see internal hemorrhage. The bleeding is inside body tissues and body cavities. Pain, shock (p. 704), vomiting blood, coughing up blood, and loss of consciousness signal internal hemorrhage. There is little you can do for internal bleeding.

- Follow the rules in Box 47-1. This includes activating the EMS system.
- Keep the person warm, flat, and quiet until help arrives.
- Do not give fluids.

If not hidden by clothing, external bleeding is usually seen. Bleeding from an artery occurs in spurts. There is a steady flow of blood from a vein. To control external bleeding:

- Follow the rules in Box 47-1. This includes activating the EMS system.
- Do not remove any objects that have pierced or stabbed the person.
- Elevate the affected part—hand, arm, foot, or leg.
- Place a sterile dressing directly over the wound. Or use any clean material (handkerchief, towel, cloth, or sanitary napkin).
- Apply pressure with your hand directly over the bleeding site (Fig. 47-19). Do not release pressure until bleeding stops.

Fig. 47-19 Direct pressure is applied to the wound to stop bleeding.

Fig. 47-20 Pressure points to control bleeding.

- If direct pressure does not control bleeding, apply pressure over the artery above the bleeding site (Fig. 47-20). For example, if bleeding is from the lower arm, apply pressure over the brachial artery.
- Bind the wound when bleeding stops. Tape or tie the dressing in place. You can tie the dressing with such things as clothing, a scarf, a necktie, or a belt.
See *Promoting Safety and Comfort: Hemorrhage,* p. 704.

PROMOTING SAFETY AND COMFORT
Hemorrhage

Safety
Contact with blood is likely with hemorrhage. Follow Standard Precautions and the Bloodborne Pathogen Standard to the extent possible. Wear gloves if possible. Practice hand hygiene as soon as you can.

Fig. 47-21 The person bends forward and lowers her head between her knees to prevent fainting.

FAINTING

Fainting is the sudden loss of consciousness from an inadequate blood supply to the brain. Hunger, fatigue, fear, and pain are common causes. Some people faint at the sight of blood or injury. Standing in one position for a long time and being in a warm, crowded room are other causes. Dizziness, perspiration, and blackness before the eyes are warning signals. The person looks pale. The pulse is weak. Respirations are shallow if consciousness is lost. Emergency care for fainting includes the following:

- Have the person sit or lie down before fainting occurs.
- If sitting, the person bends forward and places the head between the knees (Fig. 47-21).
- If the person is lying down, raise the legs.
- Loosen tight clothing (belts, ties, scarves, collars, and so on).
- Keep the person lying down if fainting has occurred. Raise the legs.
- Do not let the person get up until symptoms have subsided for about 5 minutes.
- Help the person to a sitting position after recovery from fainting. Observe for fainting.

SHOCK

Shock results when organs and tissues do not get enough blood. Blood loss, heart attack (myocardial infarction), burns, and severe infection are causes. Signs and symptoms include:

- Low or falling blood pressure
- Rapid and weak pulse
- Rapid respirations
- Cold, moist, and pale skin
- Thirst
- Restlessness
- Confusion and loss of consciousness as shock worsens

Shock is possible in any person who is acutely ill or severely injured. Follow the rules in Box 47-1. Keep the person lying down, maintain an open airway, and control bleeding. Begin CPR if cardiac arrest occurs.

Anaphylactic Shock

Some people are allergic or sensitive to foods, insects, chemicals, and medications. For example, many people are allergic to *penicillin*—an antibiotic medication. An *antigen* is a substance that the body reacts to. The body releases chemicals to fight or attack the antigen. The person may react with an area of redness, swelling, or itching. Or the reaction can involve the entire body.

Anaphylaxis is a life-threatening sensitivity to an antigen. (*Ana* means without. *Phylaxis* means protection.) The reaction can occur within seconds. Signs and symptoms include:

- Sweating
- Shortness of breath
- Low blood pressure
- Irregular pulse
- Respiratory congestion
- Swelling of the larynx (laryngeal edema)
- Hoarseness
- Dyspnea

Anaphylactic shock is an emergency. The EMS system must be activated. The person needs special medications to reverse the allergic reaction. Keep the person lying down and the airway open. Start CPR if cardiac arrest occurs.

STROKE

Stroke (cerebrovascular accident) occurs when the brain is suddenly deprived of its blood supply (Chapter 39). Usually only part of the brain is affected. A stroke may be caused by a thrombus, an embolus, or hemorrhage if a blood vessel in the brain ruptures.

Signs of stroke vary (Chapter 39). They depend on the size and location of brain injury. Loss of consciousness or semi-consciousness, rapid pulse, labored respirations, high blood pressure, facial drooping, and hemiplegia (paralysis on one side of the body) are signs of a stroke. The person may have slurred speech or aphasia (the inability to have normal speech). Loss of vision in one eye, unsteadiness, and falling also are signs. Seizures may occur.

Emergency care includes the following:

- Follow the rules in Box 47-1. This includes activating the EMS system.
- Position the person in the recovery position on the affected side (see Fig. 47-18). The affected side is limp, and the cheek appears puffy.
- Raise the head without flexing the neck.
- Loosen tight clothing (belts, ties, scarves, collars, and so on).
- Keep the person quiet and warm.
- Reassure the person.
- Provide CPR if necessary.
- Provide emergency care for seizures (p. 706) if necessary.

SEIZURES

Seizures (convulsions) are violent and sudden contractions or tremors of muscle groups. Movements are uncontrolled. The person may lose consciousness. Seizures are caused by an abnormality in the brain. Causes include head injury during birth or from trauma, high fever, brain tumors, poisoning, and nervous system disorders or infections. Lack of blood flow to the brain, seizure disorders, and epilepsy are other causes.

Epilepsy

Epilepsy is a brain disorder in which clusters of nerve cells sometimes signal abnormally. There are brief changes in the brain's electrical function. The person can have strange sensations, emotions, and behavior. Sometimes there are seizures, muscle spasms, and loss of consciousness.

A single seizure does not mean epilepsy. In epilepsy, seizures recur. The person has a permanent brain injury or defect.

Children and young adults are commonly affected. However, epilepsy can develop at any time in a person's life. It can occur with any problem affecting the brain. Such causes include:

- Brain injury before, during, or after birth (Chapter 45)
- Problems with brain development before birth
- The mother having an injury or infection during pregnancy
- Head injury (accidents, gunshot wounds, sports injuries, falls, blows to the head)
- Poor nutrition
- Brain tumor
- Childhood fevers
- Poisoning—such as lead and alcohol
- Infection—such as meningitis and encephalitis
- Stroke

There is no cure at this time. Doctors order medications to prevent seizures. The medications control seizures in many people. For others, drug therapy does not work.

When controlled, epilepsy usually does not affect learning and activities of daily living. Activity and job limits occur in severe cases. For example, a person has seizures at any time. The person may not be allowed to drive. This may limit job choices. Also, the person is at risk for accidents and injuries. Safety measures are needed. They are needed for the home, workplace, transportation, and recreation.

Types of Seizures

The major types of seizures are:

- *Partial seizure.* Only one part of the brain is involved. A body part may jerk. Or the person has a hearing or vision problem or stomach discomfort. The person does not lose consciousness.
- *Generalized tonic-clonic seizure (grand mal seizure).* This type has two phases. In the *tonic phase,* the person loses consciousness. If standing or sitting, the person falls to the floor. The body is rigid because all muscles contract at once. The *clonic phase* follows. Muscle groups contract and relax. This causes jerking and twitching movements. Urinary and fecal incontinence may occur. A deep sleep is common after the seizure. Confusion and headache may occur on awakening.
- *Generalized absence (petit mal) seizure.* This type usually lasts a few seconds. There is loss of consciousness, twitching of the eyelids, and staring. No first aid is necessary. However, you should guide the person away from dangers—stairs, streets, a hot stove, fireplaces, and so on.

Emergency Care for Seizures

You cannot stop a seizure. However, you can protect the person from injury:

- Follow the rules in Box 47-1. This includes activating the EMS system.
- Do not leave the person alone.
- Lower the person to the floor. This protects the person from falling.
- Note the time the seizure started.
- Place something soft under the person's head (Fig. 47-22). It prevents the person's head from striking the floor. You can use a pillow, a cushion, or a folded blanket, towel, or jacket. Or cradle the person's head in your lap.
- Loosen tight jewelry and clothing around the person's neck. Ties, scarves, collars, and necklaces are examples.
- Turn the person onto his or her side. Make sure the head is turned to the side.
- Do not put any object or your fingers between the person's teeth. The person can bite down on your fingers during the seizure.
- Do not try to stop the seizure or control the person's movements.
- Move furniture, equipment, and sharp objects away from the person. He or she may strike these objects during the seizure.
- Note the time when the seizure ends.
- Make sure the mouth is clear of food, fluids, and saliva after the seizure.
- Provide BLS if the person is not breathing after the seizure.

Fig. 47-22 A pillow protects the person's head during a seizure.

BURNS

Burns can severely disable a person (Fig. 47-23). They can also cause death. Most burns occur in the home. Infants and children are at risk. So are older persons. Common causes of burns and fires are:

- Scalds from hot liquids
- Playing with matches and lighters
- Electrical injuries (Fig. 47-24)
- Cooking accidents (barbecues, microwaves, stoves, ovens)
- Falling asleep while smoking
- Fireplaces
- Space heaters
- No smoke detectors or non-functioning smoke detectors
- Sunburn
- Chemicals

Fig. 47-23 Full-thickness burn. *(From Ignatavicius DD, Workman ML: Medical-surgical nursing: critical thinking for collaborative care, ed 6, St Louis, 2010, Saunders.)*

Fig. 47-24 An electrical burn. **A,** The electrical current enters through the hand. **B,** The electrical current exits through the foot. *(From Sanders M: Mosby's paramedic textbook, ed 3, St Louis, 2007, Mosby.)*

The skin has two layers: the dermis and epidermis. Burns are described as superficial, partial-thickness, and full-thickness:

- *Superficial (first degree) burns*—involve the epidermis only. They are painful, but the burn is not severe.
- *Partial-thickness (second degree) burns*—involve the epidermis and part of the dermis. They are very painful. Nerve endings are exposed.
- *Full-thickness (third degree) burns*—involve the entire epidermis and dermis. Fat, muscle, and bone may be injured or destroyed. These burns are not painful. Nerve endings are destroyed.

Some burns are minor; others are severe. Severity depends on burn size and depth, the body part involved, and the person's age. Burns to the face, eyes, ears, hands, and feet are more serious than burns to an arm or leg. Infants, young children, and older persons are at high risk for death.

Emergency care for severe burns includes the following:

- Follow the rules in Box 47-1. This includes activating the EMS system.
- Do not touch the person if he or she is in contact with an electrical source. Have the power source turned off, or remove the electrical source. Use an object that does not conduct electricity (rope or wood) to remove the electrical source.
- Remove the person from the fire or burn source.
- Stop the burning process. Put out flames with water or roll the person in a blanket. Or smother flames with a coat, sheet, or towel.
- Do not remove burned clothing.
- Remove hot clothing that is not sticking to the skin. If you cannot remove hot clothing, cool the clothing with water.
- Remove jewelry and any tight clothing that is not sticking to the skin.
- Provide rescue breathing and CPR as needed.
- Cover burns with sterile, cool, moist coverings. Or use towels, sheets, or any other clean cloth. Keep the covering wet.
- Do not put oil, butter, salve, or ointments on the burns.
- Cover the person with a blanket or coat to prevent heat loss.

QUALITY OF LIFE

During emergencies, promoting quality of life is important. Remember the person's rights. And treat the person with dignity and respect.

Protect the right to privacy. Do not expose the person unnecessarily. You may be in a place where you cannot close doors or window coverings. The person may be in a lounge, dining area, or public place. Do what you can to provide privacy.

Protect the person from onlookers. (See *Teamwork and Time Management: Emergency Care* on p. 693.) People are curious. They want to know what happened, the extent of injuries or illness, and if the person will be okay. Do not discuss the situation or offer ideas of what is wrong with the person. Information about the person's care, treatment, and condition is confidential.

Protect the right to personal choice. Choices are few in emergencies. They are given when possible. Hospital care may be required. The person has the right to choose a hospital. Sometimes the person may choose to refuse care. The EMS has guidelines to follow for persons refusing care. For example, the person must be competent and able to legally make his or her own medical decisions. The person must also be informed of the risks, benefits, and alternatives to the care recommended.

Protect personal items from loss and damage. Dentures, eyeglasses, and hearing aids are often lost or broken in emergencies. Watches and jewelry are easily lost. Clothing may be torn or cut. Be very careful to protect the person's property. In public places, personal items are given to police or EMS personnel.

Physical and psychological safety is important. Protect the person from further injury. For example, protect the person from falls after a stroke. Protect the person's head during a seizure. The person needs to feel safe and secure. Reassurance, explanations about care, and a calm approach are helpful.

REVIEW QUESTIONS

Circle the BEST answer.

1 The goals of first aid are to
   a Call for help and keep the person warm
   b Prevent death and prevent injuries from becoming worse
   c Stay calm and give emergency care
   d Calm the person and keep bystanders away

2 When giving first aid, you should
   a Be aware of your own limits
   b Move the person
   c Give the person fluids
   d Remove clothing

Continued

3 Sudden cardiac arrest is
   a The same as stroke
   b The sudden stopping of heart action
   c The sudden loss of consciousness
   d When organs and tissues do not get enough blood

4 The signs of sudden cardiac arrest are
   a Confusion, hemiplegia, and slurred speech
   b Restlessness, rapid breathing, and a weak pulse
   c No response, no normal breathing, and no pulse
   d Dizziness, pale skin, and rapid breathing

5 Rescue breathing for an adult involves
   a Giving each breath over 2 seconds
   b Watching the abdomen rise with each breath
   c Giving a breath every 3 to 5 seconds
   d Giving a breath every 5 to 6 seconds

6 In adult CPR, the chest is compressed
   a 1½ inches with the index and middle fingers
   b 2 inches with the heel of one hand
   c At least 2 inches with two hands
   d At least 1 inch with two hands

7 When checking for breathing,
   a Use the head tilt–chin lift method to open the airway
   b Look for no breathing or gasping
   c Look, listen, and feel for air moving in and out of the lungs
   d Take 10 to 15 seconds to listen for breathing

8 Which pulse is used during adult CPR?
   a The apical pulse
   b The brachial pulse
   c The carotid pulse
   d The femoral pulse

9 Which compression rate is used for CPR?
   a At least 150 compressions per minute
   b At least 100 compressions per minute
   c At least 30 compressions per minute
   d At least 15 compressions per minute

10 When doing adult CPR alone,
   a Give 2 breaths after every 15 compressions
   b Give 2 breaths after every 30 compressions
   c Give 1 breath after every 5 compressions
   d Give 2 breaths when you are tired from giving compressions

11 After delivering a shock with an AED, you should
   a Deliver another shock
   b Place the person in the recovery position
   c Look, listen, and feel for breathing
   d Perform CPR beginning with compressions

12 Arterial bleeding
   a Cannot be seen
   b Occurs in spurts
   c Is dark red
   d Oozes from the wound

13 A person is hemorrhaging from the left forearm. Your first action is to
   a Lower the arm
   b Apply pressure to the brachial artery
   c Apply direct pressure to the wound
   d Tape a dressing in place

14 A person is about to faint. Which is *false*?
   a Take the person outside for fresh air.
   b Have the person sit or lie down.
   c Loosen tight clothing.
   d Raise the legs if the person is lying down.

15 Which is *not* a sign of shock?
   a High blood pressure
   b Rapid pulse
   c Rapid respirations
   d Cold, moist, and pale skin

16 A person in shock needs
   a Rescue breathing
   b To be kept lying down
   c Clothes removed
   d The recovery position

17 A person is having a stroke. Emergency care involves the following *except*
   a Positioning the person on the affected side
   b Giving the person sips of water
   c Loosening tight clothing
   d Keeping the person quiet and warm

18 These statements relate to tonic-clonic seizures. Which is *false*?
   a There is contraction of all muscles at once.
   b Incontinence may occur.
   c The seizure lasts 5 seconds.
   d There is loss of consciousness.

19 A person was burned. There are no complaints or signs of pain. You know that
   a The burn is minor
   b The burn is partial-thickness
   c The burn is full-thickness
   d The dermis was destroyed

20 Burns are covered with
   a A clean, moist cloth or dressing
   b Butter, oil, or salve
   c Water
   d Nothing

Answers to these questions are on p. 721.

End-of-Life Care

OBJECTIVES

- Define the key terms and key abbreviations listed in this chapter.
- Describe terminal illness.
- Describe the factors that affect attitudes about death.
- Describe how different age-groups view death.
- Describe the five stages of dying.
- Explain how to meet the needs of the dying person and family.
- Describe palliative care and hospice care.

- Explain the purpose of the Patient Self-Determination Act.
- Explain what is meant by a "Do Not Resuscitate" order.
- Identify the signs of approaching death and the signs of death.
- Explain how to assist with post-mortem care.
- Perform the procedure described in this chapter.
- Explain how to promote quality of life.

KEY TERMS

advance directive A document stating a person's wishes about health care when that person cannot make his or her own decisions

autopsy The examination of the body after death

end-of-life care The support and care given during the time surrounding death

palliative care Care that involves relieving or reducing the intensity of uncomfortable symptoms without producing a cure

post-mortem care Care of the body after *(post)* death *(mortem)*

reincarnation The belief that the spirit or soul is reborn in another human body or in another form of life

rigor mortis The stiffness or rigidity *(rigor)* of skeletal muscles that occurs after death *(mortis)*

terminal illness An illness or injury from which the person will not likely recover

KEY ABBREVIATIONS

DNR	Do not resuscitate	**OBRA**	Omnibus Budget Reconciliation Act of 1987
ID	Identification		

End-of-life care describes the support and care given during the time surrounding death. Sometimes death is sudden. Often it is expected. Some people gradually fail. End-of-life care may involve days, weeks, or months.

According to the National Institute on Aging, most people die in hospitals or nursing centers. Hospice care is becoming a common option. Therefore, the health team sees death often. Many team members are not sure of their feelings about death. Dying persons and the subject of death cause discomfort. Death and dying mean helplessness and failure to cure. They also remind us that our loved ones and we will die.

Your feelings about death affect the care you give. You will help meet the dying person's physical, psychological, social, and spiritual needs. Therefore you must understand the dying process. Then you can approach the dying person with caring, kindness, and respect.

See *Teamwork and Time Management: End-of-Life Care.*

TERMINAL ILLNESS

Many illnesses and diseases have no cure. Some injuries are so serious that the body cannot function. Recovery is not expected. The disease or injury ends in death. An illness or injury from which the person will not likely recover is a terminal illness.

Doctors cannot predict the time of death. A person may have days, months, weeks, or years to live. People expected to live for a short time have lived for years. Others have died sooner than expected.

Modern medicine has found cures or has prolonged life in many cases. Research will bring new cures. However, hope and the will to live strongly influence living and dying. Many people have died for no apparent reason when they have lost hope or the will to live.

TEAMWORK AND TIME MANAGEMENT
End-of-Life Care

The nurse may need to spend a lot of time with the dying person. Often it is a busy time before and after someone dies. Offer to take equipment and supplies to and from the room. Also offer to help with other residents.

Types of Care

Persons with terminal illnesses can choose palliative care or hospice care. The person may opt for palliative care and then change to hospice care.

- *Palliative care.* *Palliate* comes from the Latin word meaning *to cloak.* It means to soothe or relieve. Palliative care involves relieving or reducing the intensity of uncomfortable symptoms without producing a cure. The person receives care to relieve symptoms. His or her illness also is treated. The intent is to improve the person's quality of life and provide support for the family. This type of care is for anyone with a long-term illness that will cause death. Settings include hospitals, nursing centers, and the person's home.
- *Hospice care.* Hospice care focuses on the physical, emotional, social, and spiritual needs of dying persons and their families (Chapter 1). Often the person has less than 6 months to live. No attempts are made to cure the person. It is not concerned with cure or life-saving measures. Pain relief and comfort are stressed. The goal is to improve the dying person's quality of life. Hospitals, nursing centers, and home care agencies offer hospice care. Or a hospice may be a separate agency. Follow-up care and support groups for survivors are hospice services. Hospice also provides support for the health team to help deal with a person's death.

ATTITUDES ABOUT DEATH

Experiences, culture, religion, and age influence attitudes about death. Many people fear death. Others do not believe they will die. Some look forward to and accept death. Attitudes about death often change as a person grows older and with changing circumstances.

Dying people often need hospital, nursing center, hospice, or home care. The family is often involved in the person's care. They usually gather at the bedside to comfort the person and each other. When death occurs, the funeral director is called. He or she takes the body to the funeral home to prepare it for funeral practices.

Many adults and children never have had contact with a dying person. Nor have they been present at the time of death. Some have not attended a visitation (wake) or funeral. They have not seen the process of dying and death. Therefore it is frightening, morbid, and a mystery.

Culture and Spiritual Needs

Practices and attitudes about death differ among cultures. See *Caring About Culture: Death Rites.* In some cultures, dying people are cared for at home by the family. Some families prepare the body for burial.

Spiritual needs relate to the human spirit and to religion and religious beliefs. They do not involve material or physical things. Rather, they involve finding meaning in one's life. Some people need to resolve issues with family and friends. Many people strengthen their religious beliefs when dying. Religion provides comfort for the dying person and the family.

Attitudes about death are closely related to religion. Some believe that life after death is free of suffering and hardship. They also believe in reunion with loved ones. Many believe sins and misdeeds are punished in the afterlife. Others do not believe in the afterlife. To them, death is the end of life.

There also are religious beliefs about the body's form after death. Some believe the body keeps its physical form. Others believe that only the spirit or soul is present in the afterlife. Reincarnation is the belief that the spirit or soul is reborn in another human body or in another form of life.

Many religions practice rites and rituals during the dying process and at the time of death. Prayers, blessings, scripture readings, and religious music are common and sources of comfort. So are visits from a spiritual leader—minister, priest, rabbi, or other cleric.

See *Focus on Communication: Culture and Spiritual Needs.*

Age

Infants and toddlers do not understand the nature or meaning of death. They know or sense that something is different. They sense that a caregiver is absent or that there is a different caregiver. They also sense changes in when and how their needs are met. They may feel a sense of loss.

Between 2 and 6 years old, children think death is temporary. It can be reversed. The dead person continues to live and function in some ways and can come back to life. These ideas come from fairy tales, cartoons, movies, video games, and TV. For example, a cartoon character is injured and dies. Later the character comes back to life, whole and intact. Children this age often blame themselves when someone or something dies. To them, death is punishment for being bad. They know when family members or pets die. They notice dead birds or bugs. Answers to questions about death often cause fear and confusion. Children who are told "He is sleeping" may be afraid to go to sleep.

CARING ABOUT CULTURE
Death Rites

In *Vietnam*, dying persons are helped to recall past good deeds and to achieve a fitting mental state. Death at home is preferred over death in the hospital. In some areas, a coin or jewels (a wealthy family) and rice (a poor family) are put in the dead person's mouth. This is from the belief that they will help the soul go through encounters with gods and devils and the soul will be born rich in the next life.

The *Chinese* have an aversion to death and anything concerning death. Autopsy and disposal of the body are not prescribed by religion. Donating body parts is encouraged. The eldest son makes all arrangements. The body is buried in a coffin. After 7 years, the body is exhumed and cremated. The urn, containing the ashes, is buried in the family tomb. White, yellow, or black clothing is worn for mourning.

In *India*, Hindu persons are often accepting of God's will. The person's desire to be clear-headed as death nears must be assessed in planning treatment. A time and place for prayer are essential for the family and the person. Prayer helps them deal with anxiety and conflict. The Hindu priest reads from Holy Sanskrit books. Some priests tie strings (meaning a blessing) around the neck or wrist. After death, the son pours water into the mouth of the deceased. Blood transfusions, organ transplants, and autopsies are allowed. Cremation is preferred.

From D'Avanzo CE: Pocket guide to cultural health assessment, ed 4, St Louis, 2008, Mosby.

Between 6 and 11 years, children learn that death is final. They do not think that they will die. Death happens to others, especially adults. It can be avoided. Children relate death to punishment and body mutilation. It also involves witches, ghosts, goblins, and monsters.

By age 11, death is more fully understood. Death is still viewed as something that happens to other people. One's own death is an event in the distant future. Without correct information, they may have some wrong ideas. However, understanding increases as they grow older and have more experiences with death.

Adults fear pain and suffering, dying alone, and the invasion of privacy. They also fear loneliness and separation from loved ones. They worry about the care and support of those left behind. Adults often resent death because it affects plans, hopes, dreams, and ambitions.

Older persons usually have fewer fears than younger adults. They know death will occur. They have had more experiences with dying and death. Many have lost family and friends. Some welcome death as freedom from pain, suffering, and disability. Death also means reunion with those who have died. Like younger adults, many fear dying alone.

THE STAGES OF DYING

Dr. Elisabeth Kubler-Ross described five stages of dying. They also are known as the "stages of grief." *Grief* is the person's response to loss.

- *Stage 1: Denial.* The person refuses to believe that he or she is dying. "No, not me" is a common response. The person believes a mistake was made. Information about the illness or injury is not heard. The person cannot deal with any problem or decision about the matter. This stage can last for a few hours, days, or much longer. Some people are still in denial when they die.
- *Stage 2: Anger.* The person thinks "Why me?" There is anger and rage. Dying persons envy and resent those with life and health. Family, friends, and the health team are often targets of anger. The person blames others and finds fault with those who are loved and needed the most. It is hard to deal with the person during this stage. Anger is normal and healthy. Do not take the person's anger personally. Control any urge to attack back or avoid the person.
- *Stage 3: Bargaining.* Anger has passed. The person now says "Yes, me, but...." Often the person bargains with God or a higher power for more time. Promises are made in exchange for more time. The person may want to see a child marry, see a grandchild, have one more Christmas, or live for some other event. Usually more promises are made as the person makes "just one more" request. You may not see this stage. Bargaining is usually private and spiritual.

- *Stage 4: Depression.* The person thinks "Yes, me" and is very sad. The person mourns things that were lost and the future loss of life. The person may cry or say little. Sometimes the person talks about people and things that will be left behind.
- *Stage 5: Acceptance.* The person is calm and at peace. The person has said what needs to be said. Unfinished business is completed. The person accepts death. This stage may last for many months or years. Reaching the acceptance stage does not mean death is near.

Dying persons do not always pass through all five stages. A person may never get beyond a certain stage. Some move back and forth between stages. For example, Mr. Jones reached acceptance but moves back to bargaining. Then he moves forward to acceptance. Some people stay in one stage.

COMFORT NEEDS

Comfort is a basic part of end-of-life care. It involves physical, mental and emotional, and spiritual needs. For spiritual needs, see "Culture and Spiritual Needs" on p. 711. Comfort goals are to:
- Prevent or relieve suffering to the extent possible
- Respect and follow end-of-life wishes

They may want family and friends present. They may want to talk about their fears, worries, and anxieties. Some want to be alone. Often they need to talk during the night. Things are quiet, distractions are few, and there is more time to think. You need to listen and use touch.

- *Listening.* The person needs to talk and share worries and concerns. Let the person express feelings and emotions in his or her own way. Do not worry about saying the wrong thing or finding comforting words. You do not need to say anything. Being there for the person is what counts.
- *Touch.* Touch shows caring and concern when words cannot. Sometimes the person does not want to talk but needs you nearby. Do not feel that you need to talk. Silence, along with touch, is a powerful and meaningful way to communicate.

Some people may want to see a spiritual leader. Or they want to take part in religious practices. Provide privacy during prayer and spiritual moments. Be courteous to the spiritual leader. The person has the right to have religious objects nearby—medals, pictures, statues, writings, and so on. Handle these valuables with care and respect.

See *Focus on Communication: The Person's Needs.*
See *Residents With Dementia: The Person's Needs.*

> **PROMOTING SAFETY AND COMFORT**
> Care of the Body After Death
>
> **Safety**
> Standard Precautions and the Bloodborne Pathogen Standard are followed. You may have contact with blood, body fluids, secretions, or excretions.

ASSISTING WITH POST-MORTEM CARE

PRE-PROCEDURE

1 Follow *Delegation Guidelines: Care of the Body After Death*, p. 715. See *Promoting Safety and Comfort: Care of the Body After Death*.
2 Practice hand hygiene.
3 Collect the following:
- Post-mortem kit (shroud or body bag, gown, ID [identification] tags, gauze squares, safety pins)
- Bed protectors
- Wash basin
- Bath towel and washcloths
- Denture cup
- Tape
- Dressings
- Gloves
- Cotton balls
- Valuables envelope
4 Provide for privacy.
5 Raise the bed for body mechanics.
6 Make sure the bed is flat.

PROCEDURE

7 Put on the gloves.
8 Position the body supine. Arms and legs are straight. A pillow is under the head and shoulders. Or raise the head of the bed 15 to 20 degrees if this is center policy.
9 Close the eyes. Gently pull the eyelids over the eyes. Apply moist cotton balls gently over the eyelids if the eyes will not stay closed.
10 Insert dentures if it is center policy to do so. If not, put them in a labeled denture cup.
11 Close the mouth. If necessary, place a rolled towel under the chin to keep the mouth closed.
12 Follow center policy for jewelry. Remove all jewelry, except for wedding rings if this is center policy. List the jewelry that you removed. Place the jewelry and the list in a valuables envelope.
13 Place a cotton ball over the rings. Tape them in place.
14 Remove drainage containers.
15 Remove tubes and catheters. Use the gauze squares as needed.
16 Bathe soiled areas with plain water. Dry thoroughly.
17 Place a bed protector under the buttocks.
18 Remove soiled dressings. Replace them with clean ones.
19 Put a clean gown on the body. Position the body as in step 8.
20 Brush and comb the hair if necessary.
21 Cover the body to the shoulders with a sheet if the family will view the body.
22 Gather the person's belongings. Put them in a bag labeled with the person's name. Make sure you include eyeglasses, hearing aids, and other valuables.
23 Remove supplies, equipment, and linens. Straighten the room. Provide soft lighting.
24 Remove the gloves. Decontaminate your hands.
25 Let the family view the body. Provide for privacy. Return to the room after they leave.
26 Decontaminate your hands. Put on gloves.
27 Fill out the ID tags. Tie one to the ankle or to the right big toe.
28 Place the body in the body bag or cover it with a sheet. Or apply the shroud (Fig. 48-1).
   a Position the shroud under the body.
   b Bring the top down over the head.
   c Fold the bottom up over the feet.
   d Fold the sides over the body.
   e Pin or tape the shroud in place.
29 Attach the second ID tag to the shroud, sheet, or body bag.
30 Leave the denture cup with the body.
31 Pull the privacy curtain around the bed. Or close the door.

POST-PROCEDURE

32 Remove the gloves. Decontaminate your hands.
33 Strip the unit after the body has been removed. Wear gloves for this step.
34 Remove the gloves. Decontaminate your hands.
35 Report the following:
- The time the body was taken by the funeral director
- What was done with jewelry, other valuables, and personal items
- What was done with dentures

> **FOCUS ON COMMUNICATION**
> The Person's Needs
>
> You may not know what to say to the dying person. That is hard for many experienced health team members. Unless you have been near death yourself, do not say "I understand what you are going through." The statement is a communication barrier. Instead you can say:
> - "Would you like to talk? I have time to listen."
> - "You seem sad. How can I help?"
> - "Is it okay if I quietly sit with you for a while?"

> **RESIDENTS WITH DEMENTIA**
> The Person's Needs
>
> Persons with Alzheimer's disease (AD) become more and more disabled. Those with advanced AD cannot share their concerns, discomforts, or problems. And it is hard to provide emotional and spiritual comfort.
>
> Focusing on the person's senses—hearing, touch, sight—can promote comfort. Comforting touch or massage can be soothing. So can soft music or sounds from nature—birds chirping, gentle breezes, ocean waves, and so on.

Physical Needs

Dying may take a few minutes, hours, days, or weeks. Body processes slow. The person is weak. Changes occur in levels of consciousness. To the extent possible, independence is allowed. As the person weakens, basic needs are met. The person may depend on others for basic needs and activities of daily living. Every effort is made to promote physical and psychological comfort. The person is allowed to die in peace and with dignity.

Pain Some dying persons do not have pain. Others do, and it may be severe. Always report signs and symptoms of pain at once (Chapter 27). Pain management is important. The nurse can give pain-relief medications ordered by the doctor. Preventing and controlling pain is easier than relieving pain.

Skin care, personal and oral hygiene, back massages, and good alignment promote comfort. Frequent position changes and supportive devices promote comfort. Turn the person slowly and gently. The person's care plan will include other measures to prevent and control pain.

Breathing Problems Shortness of breath and difficulty breathing (dyspnea) are common end-of-life problems. Semi-Fowler's position is usually best for breathing problems. The doctor may order oxygen (Chapter 28). Opening a window for fresh air may help some people. For others, a fan circulating air is helpful.

Noisy breathing—called the *death rattle*—is common as death nears. This is due to mucus collecting in the airway. The following may help:
- The side-lying position
- Suctioning by the nurse
- Medications ordered by the doctor to reduce the amount of mucus

Vision, Hearing, and Speech Vision blurs and gradually fails. The person naturally turns toward light. A darkened room may frighten the person. The eyes may be half-open. Secretions may collect in the eye corners.

Because of failing vision, explain who you are and what you are doing to the person or in the room. The room should be well lit. However, avoid bright lights and glares.

Good eye care is essential (Chapter 20). If the eyes stay open, a nurse may apply a protective ointment. Then the eyes are covered with moist pads to prevent injury.

Hearing is one of the last functions lost. Many people hear until the moment of death. Even unconscious persons may hear. Always assume that the person can hear. Speak in a normal voice. Provide reassurance and explanations about care. Offer words of comfort. Avoid topics that could upset the person. Do not talk about the person.

Speech becomes harder. It may be hard to understand the person. Sometimes the person cannot speak. Anticipate the person's needs. Do not ask questions that need long answers. Ask "yes" or "no" questions. These should be few in number. Despite speech problems, you must talk to the person.

Mouth, Nose, and Skin Oral hygiene promotes comfort. Give routine mouth care if the person can eat and drink. Give frequent oral hygiene as death nears and when taking oral fluids is difficult. Oral hygiene is needed if mucus collects in the mouth and the person cannot swallow. A lip balm may help dry lips.

Crusting and irritation of the nostrils can occur. Nasal secretions, an oxygen cannula, and a naso-gastric tube are common causes. Carefully clean the nose. Apply lubricant as directed by the nurse and the care plan.

Circulation fails and body temperature rises as death nears. The skin feels cool, pale, and mottled (blotchy). Perspiration increases. Skin care, bathing, and preventing pressure ulcers are necessary. Linens and gowns are changed whenever needed. Although the skin feels cool, only light bed coverings are needed. Blankets may make the person feel warm and cause restlessness. However, observe for signs of cold. Shivering, hunching the shoulders, and pulling covers up may signal that the person is cold. Prevent drafts and provide more blankets.

Nutrition Nausea, vomiting, and loss of appetite are common at the end of life. The doctor can order medications for nausea and vomiting.

Some persons are too tired or too weak to eat. You may need to feed them. Providing the person's favorite foods may help loss of appetite. So may small, frequent meals.

As death nears, loss of appetite is common. The person may choose not to eat or drink. Do not force the person to eat or drink. Doing so may add to the person's discomfort. Report refusal to eat or drink to the nurse.

Elimination Urinary and fecal incontinence may occur. Use incontinence products or bed protectors as directed. Give perineal care as needed. Constipation and urinary retention are common. Enemas and catheters may be needed. Provide catheter care according to the care plan.

The Person's Room Provide a comfortable and pleasant room. It should be well lit and well ventilated. Remove unnecessary equipment. Some equipment is upsetting to look at (suction machines, drainage containers). If possible, keep these items out of the person's sight.

Mementos, pictures, cards, flowers, and religious items provide comfort. Arrange them within the person's view. The person and family arrange the room as they wish. This helps meet love, belonging, and esteem needs. The room should reflect the person's choices.

Mental and Emotional Needs

Mental and emotional needs are very personal. Some persons are anxious or depressed. Others have specific fears and concerns. Examples include:
- Severe pain
- When and how death will occur
- What will happen to loved ones
- Dying alone

The doctor may order medications for anxiety or depression. Simple measures may soothe the person—touch, holding a hand, back massage, soft lighting, music at a low volume.

THE FAMILY

This is a hard time for the family. You may find it hard to find comforting words. To show you care, be available, courteous, and considerate. Use touch to show your concern.

The family usually can stay as long as they wish. Sometimes family members keep a *vigil*. That is, someone is with the person at all times including during the night. They watch over or pray for the person. The health team makes them as comfortable as possible.

Respect the right to privacy. The person and family need time together. However, do not neglect care because the family is present. Most centers let family members help give care. Or you can suggest that they take a break for a beverage or meal.

The family may be very tired, sad, and tearful. Watching a loved one die is very painful. So is dealing with the eventual loss of that person. The family goes through stages like the dying person. They need support, understanding, courtesy, and respect. A spiritual leader may provide comfort. Communicate this request to the nurse at once.

LEGAL ISSUES

Much attention is given to the right to die. Many people do not want machines or other measures keeping them alive. Consent is needed for any treatment. When able, the person makes care decisions. Some people make end-of-life wishes known.

The Patient Self-Determination Act

OBRA-CMS The Patient Self-Determination Act and the Omnibus Budget Reconciliation Act of 1987 (OBRA) give persons the right to accept or refuse treatment. They also give the right to make advance directives. An **advance directive** is a document stating a person's wishes about health care when that person cannot make his or her own decisions. It lets others know the type of care he or she wants if seriously ill or dying. Advance directives usually forbid certain care if there is no hope of recovery. Living wills and durable power of attorney for health care are common advance directives.

These laws protect quality of care. Quality of care cannot be less because of the person's advance directives.

Nursing centers must inform all persons of the right to advance directives on admission. This information is in writing. The medical record must document whether or not the person has made them.

Living Wills A living will is a document about measures that support or maintain life when death is likely. Tube feedings, ventilators, and resuscitation are examples. A living will may instruct doctors:
- Not to start measures that prolong dying
- To remove measures that prolong dying

Durable Power of Attorney for Health Care This advance directive gives the power to make health care decisions to another person. That person is often called a *health care proxy*. Usually this is a family member, friend, or lawyer. When a person cannot make health care decisions, the health care proxy can do so. This advance directive does not cover property or financial matters.

"Do Not Resuscitate" Orders

When death is sudden and unexpected, efforts are made to save the person's life. See Chapter 47.

For terminally ill persons, doctors often write "Do Not Resuscitate" (DNR) or "No Code" orders. The person will not be resuscitated. The person is allowed to die with peace and dignity. The orders are written after consulting with the person and family. The family and doctor make the decision if the person is not mentally able to do so. Some advance directives address resuscitation.

You may not agree with care and resuscitation decisions. However, you must follow the person's or family's wishes and the doctor's orders. These may be against your personal, religious, and cultural values. If so, discuss the matter with the nurse. You may need an assignment change.

SIGNS OF DEATH

In the weeks before death, the following may occur:
- Restlessness and agitation
- Shortness of breath (dyspnea)
- Depression
- Anxiety
- Drowsiness
- Confusion
- Constipation or incontinence
- Nausea
- Loss of appetite
- Healing problems
- Swelling in the hands, feet, or other body areas
- Pauses in breathing
As death nears, these signs may occur fast or slowly:
- Movement, muscle tone, and sensation are lost. This usually starts in the feet and legs. When mouth muscles relax, the jaw drops. The mouth may stay open. The facial expression is often peaceful.
- Peristalsis and other gastro-intestinal functions slow down. Abdominal distention, fecal incontinence, nausea, and vomiting are common.
- Body temperature rises. The person feels cool or cold, looks pale, and perspires heavily.
- Circulation fails. The pulse is fast or slow, weak, and irregular. Blood pressure starts to fall.
- The respiratory system fails. Slow or rapid and shallow respirations are observed. Mucus collects in the airway. Breathing sounds are noisy and gurgling—commonly called the *death rattle*.
- Pain decreases as the person loses consciousness. However, some people are conscious until the moment of death.

The signs of death include no pulse, no respirations, and no blood pressure. The pupils are fixed and dilated. A doctor determines that death has occurred. He or she pronounces the person dead. The cause, time, and place are noted for the death certificate.

CARE OF THE BODY AFTER DEATH

Care of the body after (*post*) death (*mortem*) is called **post-mortem care**. A nurse gives post-mortem care. You may be asked to assist. Post-mortem care begins when the doctor pronounces the person dead.

Post-mortem care is done to maintain a good appearance of the body. Discoloration and skin damage are prevented. Valuables and personal items are gathered for the family. The right to privacy and the right to be treated with dignity and respect apply after death.

Within 2 to 4 hours after death, rigor mortis develops. **Rigor mortis** is the stiffness or rigidity (*rigor*) of skeletal muscles that occurs after death (*mortis*). The body is positioned in normal alignment before rigor mortis sets in. The family may want to see the body. The body should appear in a comfortable and natural position for this viewing.

In some centers, the body is prepared only for viewing by the family. The funeral director completes post-mortem care.

Sometimes an autopsy is done. An **autopsy** is the examination of the body after death. (*Autos* means *self. Opsis* means *view.*) Its purpose is to determine the cause of death. The coroner or medical examiner can order an autopsy. Or the family can request one. Follow center procedures when an autopsy is to be done. Post-mortem care is not done. Doing so could remove or destroy evidence.

Post-mortem care involves moving the body. For example, soiled areas are bathed and the body is placed in good alignment. Moving the body can cause remaining air in the lungs, stomach, and intestines to be expelled. When air is expelled, sounds are produced. Do not let these sounds alarm or frighten you. They are normal and expected.

See *Delegation Guidelines: Care of the Body After Death.*

See *Promoting Safety and Comfort: Care of the Body After Death,* p. 716.

> ### DELEGATION GUIDELINES
> #### Care of the Body After Death
>
> When assisting with post-mortem care, you need this information from the nurse:
> - If dentures are inserted or placed in a denture cup
> - If tubes and dressings are removed or left in place
> - If rings are removed or left in place
> - If the family wants to view the body
> - Special center policies and procedures

Fig. 48-1 Applying a shroud. **A,** Position the shroud under the body. **B,** Bring the top of the shroud down over the head. **C,** Fold the bottom up over the feet. **D,** Fold the sides over the body. Tape or pin the sides together. Attach the ID tag.

QUALITY OF LIFE

A person has the right to die in peace and with dignity. Box 48-1, p. 718 contains the dying person's bill of rights. The dying person also has these rights under OBRA:

- *The right to privacy before and after death.* Do not expose the person unnecessarily. The person has the right not to have his or her body seen by others. Properly drape and screen the person.
- *The right to visit others in private.* If the person is too weak to leave the room, the roommate may have to do so. The nurse and social worker develop a plan that satisfies everyone. Moving the dying person to a private room provides privacy. The family can also stay as long as they like.
- *The right to confidentiality before and after death.* Only those involved in care need to know the person's diagnosis and condition. The final moments and cause of death also are kept confidential. So are statements, conversations, and family reactions.
- *The right to be free from abuse, mistreatment, and neglect.* Some health team members avoid dying persons. They are uncomfortable with death and dying. Others have religious or cultural beliefs about being near dying people. Neglect is possible. So is abuse or mistreatment. Family, friends, or staff may be sources of such actions. The dying person may be too weak to report the abuse or mistreatment. Or the person may feel that the punishment is deserved for needing so much care. The person has the right to receive kind and respectful care before and after death. Always report signs of abuse, mistreatment, or neglect to the nurse at once.
- *Freedom from restraint.* Restraints are used only if ordered by the doctor. Dying persons are often too weak to pose dangers to themselves or others.
- *The right to have personal possessions.* You must protect the person's property. The person may want photos and religious items nearby. Protect the person's property from loss or damage before and after death. They may be family treasures or mementos.
- *The right to a safe and home-like setting.* Dying persons depend on others for safety. Everyone must keep the setting safe and home-like. The center is the person's home. Try to keep equipment and supplies out of view. The room also should be free from unpleasant odors and noises. Do your best to keep the room neat and clean.
- *The right to personal choice.* The person has the right to be involved in treatment and care. The dying person may refuse treatment. Advance directives are common. Some persons cannot make treatment decisions. The family or health care proxy does so. The decision may be to allow the person to die with peace and dignity. The health team must respect choices to refuse treatment or not prolong life.

Box 48-1 A Dying Patient's Bill of Last Rights

- *The Right to BE IN CONTROL.* Grant me the right to make as many decisions as possible regarding my care. Please do not take choices from me. Let me make my own decisions.
- *The Right to HAVE A SENSE OF PURPOSE.* I have lost my job. I can no longer fulfill my role in my family. Please help me find some sense of purpose in my last days.
- *The Right to REMINISCE.* There has been pleasure in my life, moments of pride, moments of love. Please give some time to recollect those moments. And please listen to my recollections.
- *The Right to TOUCH AND BE TOUCHED.* Sometimes I need distance. Yet sometimes I have a strong need to be close. When I want to reach out, please come to me and hold me as I hold you.
- *The Right to LAUGH.* People often—far too often—come to me wearing masks of seriousness. Although I am dying, I still need to laugh. Please laugh with me and help others to laugh as well.
- *The Right to BE ANGRY AND SAD.* It is difficult to leave behind all my attachments and all that I love. Please allow me the opportunity to be angry and sad.
- *The Right to HAVE A RESPECTED SPIRITUALITY.* Whether I am questioning or affirming, doubting or praising, I sometimes need your ear, a non-judging ear. Please let my spirit travel its own journey, without judging its direction.
- *The Right to HEAR THE TRUTH.* If you withhold the truth from me, you will treat me as if I am no longer living. I am still living, and I need to know the truth about my life. Please help me find that truth.
- *The Right to BE IN DENIAL.* If I hear the truth and choose not to accept it, that is my right.

  Honor these Rights. One day you too will want the same Rights.

Modified from The Hospice RN: Patient's bill of rights: a dying patient's bill of last rights.

REVIEW QUESTIONS

Circle the BEST answer.

1 Which is *true*?
  a Death from terminal illness is sudden and unexpected.
  b Doctors know when death will occur.
  c An illness is terminal when recovery is not likely.
  d All severe injuries end in death.

2 These statements relate to attitudes about death. Which is *false*?
  a Dying people are often cared for in health care agencies.
  b Religion influences attitudes about death.
  c Infants and toddlers understand death.
  d Young children often blame themselves when someone dies.

3 Reincarnation is the belief that
  a There is no afterlife
  b The spirit or soul is reborn into another human body or another form of life
  c The body keeps its physical form in the afterlife
  d Only the spirit or soul is present in the afterlife

4 A 6-year-old views death as
  a Temporary   c Adults do
  b Final   d Going to sleep

5 Adults and older persons usually fear
  a Dying alone   c The five stages of dying
  b Reincarnation   d Advance directives

6 Persons in the stage of denial
  a Are angry
  b Are calm and at peace
  c Are sad and quiet
  d Refuse to believe they are dying

7 A dying person tries to gain more time during the stage of
  a Anger   c Depression
  b Bargaining   d Acceptance

8 When caring for the dying person, you should
  a Use touch and listen
  b Do most of the talking
  c Keep the room darkened
  d Speak in a loud voice

9 As death nears, the last sense lost is
  a Sight   c Smell
  b Taste   d Hearing

10 The dying person's care includes the following *except*
  a Eye care
  b Mouth care
  c Active range-of-motion exercises
  d Position changes

11 The dying person is positioned in
  a The supine position
  b The Fowler's position
  c Good body alignment
  d The dorsal recumbent position

12 A "DNR" order was written. This means that
  a CPR will not be done
  b The person has a living will
  c Life-prolonging measures will be carried out
  d The person is kept alive as long as possible

13 Which are *not* signs of approaching death?
  a Increased body temperature and rapid pulse
  b Loss of movement and muscle tone
  c Increased pain and blood pressure
  d Slow or rapid and shallow respirations

14 The signs of death are
  a Convulsions and incontinence
  b No pulse, respirations, or blood pressure
  c Loss of consciousness and convulsions
  d The eyes stay open, no muscle movements, and the body is rigid

15 Post-mortem care is done
  a After rigor mortis sets in
  b After the doctor pronounces the person dead
  c When the funeral director arrives for the body
  d After the family has viewed the body

Answers to these questions are on p. 721.

REVIEW QUESTION ANSWERS

CHAPTER 1
1 d
2 c
3 b
4 b
5 a
6 a
7 c
8 a
9 b
10 a
11 a
12 d

CHAPTER 2
1 b
2 b
3 c
4 d
5 b
6 a
7 a
8 a
9 b
10 a
11 d
12 d
13 b
14 a
15 b
16 d
17 T
18 T
19 F
20 F
21 F
22 F
23 T
24 F
25 F

CHAPTER 3
1 b
2 c
3 c
4 d
5 c
6 b
7 c
8 c
9 c
10 b

11 a
12 a
13 b
14 c
15 b

CHAPTER 4
1 b
2 c
3 d
4 a
5 c
6 c
7 d
8 a
9 d
10 c
11 b
12 a
13 d
14 d
15 a
16 b
17 a
18 b
19 c
20 c

CHAPTER 5
1 T
2 T
3 F
4 T
5 T
6 T
7 F
8 F
9 T
10 F
11 c
12 d
13 a
14 d
15 b
16 d
17 c
18 b
19 c
20 d
21 c
22 b
23 a

24 a
25 b
26 c
27 d
28 c
29 b
30 a
31 d
32 d

CHAPTER 6
1 F
2 F
3 T
4 F
5 a
6 c
7 d
8 c
9 c
10 c
11 d
12 d
13 b
14 b
15 c
16 a
17 d
18 b

CHAPTER 7
1 a
2 d
3 b
4 c
5 d
6 b
7 a
8 c
9 c
10 b
11 c
12 d

CHAPTER 8
1 c
2 d
3 c
4 b
5 a
6 d

7 a
8 c
9 b
10 c
11 b
12 d
13 c
14 a
15 c
16 a
17 d
18 a
19 d
20 c
21 d
22 b

CHAPTER 9
1 a
2 b
3 d
4 c
5 c
6 a
7 b
8 c
9 d
10 d
11 b
12 a
13 b
14 b
15 b
16 c
17 d
18 a
19 d
20 a
21 b

CHAPTER 10
1 c
2 c
3 a
4 d
5 c
6 b
7 c
8 a
9 b
10 a
11 b

12 d
13 c
14 d
15 c
16 a
17 d
18 b
19 a
20 b
21 d
22 c
23 c
24 a

CHAPTER 11
1 a
2 d
3 c
4 a
5 b
6 b
7 d
8 b
9 b
10 b

CHAPTER 12
1 a
2 d
3 c
4 a
5 a
6 b
7 c
8 d
9 a
10 d
11 b
12 a
13 b
14 b
15 c
16 b
17 d
18 b
19 h
20 a
21 b
22 c
23 c
24 c

25 b
26 d

CHAPTER 13
1 a
2 d
3 c
4 a
5 a
6 c
7 d
8 c
9 a
10 b
11 a
12 c
13 c
14 a

CHAPTER 14
1 F
2 T
3 T
4 F
5 F
6 T
7 T
8 T
9 F
10 F
11 T
12 F
13 F
14 T
15 F
16 a
17 c
18 b
19 c
20 a
21 d
22 c
23 c
24 d

CHAPTER 15
1 F
2 T
3 T
4 F
5 F

6	F
7	F
8	T
9	T
10	b
11	d
12	d
13	b
14	a
15	b
16	a
17	d
18	c
19	a
20	d
21	c
22	a
23	d
24	b
25	d
26	c
27	b
28	a

CHAPTER 16

1	d
2	b
3	a
4	b
5	a
6	c
7	c
8	b
9	a
10	b
11	c
12	a

CHAPTER 17

1	b
2	a
3	a
4	b
5	a
6	b
7	a
8	a
9	a
10	a
11	b
12	a
13	d
14	b
15	c
16	c

CHAPTER 18

1	c
2	d
3	a
4	b
5	d
6	a
7	b
8	d
9	c
10	b
11	c
12	c
13	T
14	T
15	F
16	T
17	T
18	T
19	T
20	T
21	F
22	F

CHAPTER 19

1	F
2	T
3	F
4	T
5	T
6	F
7	T
8	b
9	d
10	b
11	a
12	b
13	a
14	d
15	c

CHAPTER 20

1	T
2	T
3	F
4	F
5	F
6	F
7	F
8	T
9	F
10	F
11	F
12	F
13	T

14	T
15	T
16	d
17	d
18	b
19	b
20	c
21	c
22	d

CHAPTER 21

1	d
2	b
3	c
4	a
5	d
6	d
7	b
8	d
9	b
10	F
11	T
12	T
13	F
14	F

CHAPTER 22

1	b
2	d
3	a
4	b
5	a
6	b
7	d
8	a
9	a
10	a
11	a
12	d
13	d
14	a

CHAPTER 23

1	a
2	b
3	d
4	a
5	c
6	a
7	a
8	c
9	d
10	d

CHAPTER 24

1	b
2	a
3	a
4	d
5	d
6	c
7	a
8	c
9	a
10	c
11	d
12	a
13	b
14	c
15	c
16	b
17	b
18	c
19	d
20	b
21	c
22	d

CHAPTER 25

1	c
2	a
3	a
4	b
5	d
6	a
7	a
8	a
9	a
10	c
11	a
12	b
13	a
14	d
15	b
16	b
17	b
18	a

CHAPTER 26

1	b
2	b
3	c
4	b
5	c
6	b
7	c
8	a
9	a
10	c

11	b
12	F
13	F
14	T
15	T

CHAPTER 27

1	a
2	c
3	d
4	c
5	a
6	b
7	c
8	d
9	b
10	c
11	d
12	a
13	b
14	T
15	F
16	T

CHAPTER 28

1	a
2	c
3	c
4	b
5	b
6	d
7	c
8	d
9	a
10	a
11	b
12	d

CHAPTER 29

1	a
2	d
3	d
4	b
5	b
6	a
7	d
8	c
9	d
10	b
11	c
12	d

CHAPTER 30

1	a
2	a
3	b
4	d
5	d
6	b
7	d
8	b
9	b
10	d
11	b
12	a
13	b
14	c
15	c

CHAPTER 31

1	c
2	b
3	a
4	c
5	a
6	a
7	b
8	b
9	c
10	b
11	d
12	a
13	b
14	b

CHAPTER 32

1	b
2	d
3	c
4	b
5	c

CHAPTER 33

1	d
2	b
3	a
4	c
5	b
6	a
7	d
8	b
9	b
10	c
11	a
12	a

CHAPTER 34

1 F
2 T
3 F
4 T
5 T
6 F
7 F
8 F
9 T
10 F
11 F
12 T
13 T
14 T
15 F
16 T
17 T
18 T

CHAPTER 35

1 a
2 c
3 a
4 c
5 a
6 b
7 a
8 a
9 d
10 b
11 d
12 c
13 b
14 d
15 c
16 b
17 d
18 a
19 c
20 d
21 b
22 b
23 c
24 b
25 d
26 a
27 d
28 c

CHAPTER 36

1 b
2 a
3 a
4 a
5 d

6 c
7 b
8 b
9 d
10 a
11 b
12 a
13 d
14 c
15 d
16 d
17 b
18 F
19 T
20 T
21 T
22 T
23 T
24 F
25 F
26 F
27 T
28 F
29 T
30 F
31 F
32 T

CHAPTER 37

1 b
2 b
3 a
4 c
5 b
6 b
7 a
8 c
9 c
10 a
11 c
12 b
13 a
14 b
15 a
16 b
17 c
18 a
19 b
20 a
21 d
22 c

CHAPTER 38

1 b
2 a

3 a
4 a
5 a
6 a
7 a
8 d
9 d
10 b
11 T
12 T
13 F
14 T
15 T

CHAPTER 39

1 a
2 b
3 d
4 b
5 c
6 b
7 a
8 b
9 d
10 a
11 b
12 a
13 c
14 a
15 c
16 a
17 a
18 a
19 d
20 c
21 a
22 a

CHAPTER 40

1 a
2 d
3 b
4 c
5 a
6 d
7 a
8 a
9 a
10 b
11 a
12 c
13 c
14 a
15 a

CHAPTER 41

1 b
2 a
3 d
4 a
5 a
6 d
7 c
8 d
9 a
10 d
11 c
12 a
13 d
14 a
15 b
16 c
17 a
18 b

CHAPTER 42

1 d
2 d
3 c
4 d
5 a
6 a
7 a
8 b
9 c
10 d

CHAPTER 43

1 b
2 d
3 c
4 c
5 c
6 c
7 b
8 c
9 b
10 d
11 d
12 a
13 c
14 c
15 d
16 a
17 a
18 a
19 a
20 a
21 T
22 F

23 T
24 T
25 T
26 F

CHAPTER 44

1 a
2 b
3 a
4 a
5 d
6 d
7 a
8 b
9 b
10 d
11 b
12 d
13 a
14 a
15 c
16 c
17 a
18 a
19 a
20 T
21 F
22 T
23 T
24 F
25 F
26 T
27 T
28 T
29 F
30 F

CHAPTER 45

1 d
2 b
3 d
4 b
5 a
6 d
7 b
8 c
9 c
10 d
11 b
12 b
13 d
14 c
15 b

CHAPTER 46

1 c
2 b
3 a
4 d
5 c
6 c
7 T
8 T
9 T
10 F
11 T
12 T
13 F
14 T
15 T
16 T

CHAPTER 47

1 b
2 a
3 b
4 c
5 d
6 c
7 b
8 c
9 b
10 b
11 d
12 b
13 c
14 a
15 a
16 b
17 b
18 c
19 c
20 a

CHAPTER 48

1 c
2 c
3 b
4 a
5 a
6 d
7 b
8 a
9 d
10 c
11 c
12 a
13 c
14 b
15 b

APPENDIX A

NATIONAL NURSE AIDE ASSESSMENT PROGRAM (NNAAP™) WRITTEN EXAMINATION CONTENT OUTLINE

The NNAAP Written Examination is comprised of seventy (70) multiple choice questions. Ten (10) of these questions are pre-test (non-scored) questions on which statistical information will be collected.

I. Physical Care Skills

A. Activities of Daily Living   14% of exam
1. Hygiene
2. Dressing and Grooming
3. Nutrition and Hydration
4. Elimination
5. Rest/Sleep/Comfort

B. Basic Nursing Skills   39% of exam
1. Infection Control
2. Safety/Emergency
3. Therapeutic/Technical Procedures
4. Data Collection and Reporting

C. Restorative Skills   7% of exam
1. Prevention
2. Self Care/Independence

II. Psychosocial Care Skills

A. Emotional and Mental Health Needs   11% of exam
B. Spiritual and Cultural Needs   2% of exam

III. Role of the Nurse Aide

A. Communication   8% of exam
B. Client Rights   7% of exam
C. Legal and Ethical Behavior   3% of exam
D. Member of the Health Care Team   9% of exam

NATIONAL NURSE AIDE ASSESSMENT PROGRAM (NNAAP™) SKILLS EVALUATION

List of Skills

1. Washes hands
2. Applies one knee high stocking
3. Assists to ambulate using transfer belt
4. Assists client with use of bedpan
5. Cleans upper or lower denture
6. Counts and records radial pulse
7. Counts and records respirations
8. Donning and removing PPE (gown and gloves)
9. Dresses client with affected (weak) right arm
10. Feeds client who cannot feed self
11. Gives modified bed bath (face and one arm, hand and underarm)
12. Makes an occupied bed (client does not need assistance to turn)
13. Measures and records blood pressure
14. Measures and records blood pressure (two-step procedure) (for use in PA only)
15. Measures and records urinary output
16. Measures and records weight of ambulatory client
17. Performs passive range of motion (ROM) for one knee and ankle
18. Performs passive range of motion (ROM) for one shoulder
19. Positions client on side
20. Provides catheter care
21. Provides fingernail care on one hand
22. Provides foot care on one foot
23. Provides mouth care
24. Provides perineal care (peri-care) for female
25. Transfers client from bed to wheelchair using transfer belt

Resident _____   Identifier _____   Date _____

MINIMUM DATA SET (MDS) - Version 3.0
RESIDENT ASSESSMENT AND CARE SCREENING
ALL ITEM LISTING

Section A	Identification Information

A0100. Facility Provider Numbers

A. National Provider Identifier (NPI):

☐☐☐☐☐☐☐☐☐☐

B. CMS Certification Number (CCN):

☐☐☐☐☐☐☐☐☐☐☐☐

C. State Provider Number:

☐☐☐☐☐☐☐☐☐☐☐☐☐☐

A0200. Type of Provider

Enter Code ☐

Type of provider
1. **Nursing home (SNF/NF)**
2. **Swing Bed**

A0310. Type of Assessment

Enter Code ☐☐

A. Federal OBRA Reason for Assessment
01. **Admission** assessment (required by day 14)
02. **Quarterly** review assessment
03. **Annual** assessment
04. **Significant change in status** assessment
05. **Significant correction** to **prior comprehensive** assessment
06. **Significant correction** to **prior quarterly** assessment
99. **Not OBRA required** assessment

Enter Code ☐☐

B. PPS Assessment
PPS Scheduled Assessments for a Medicare Part A Stay
01. **5-day** scheduled assessment
02. **14-day** scheduled assessment
03. **30-day** scheduled assessment
04. **60-day** scheduled assessment
05. **90-day** scheduled assessment
06. **Readmission/return** assessment
PPS Unscheduled Assessments for a Medicare Part A Stay
07. **Unscheduled assessment used for PPS** (OMRA, significant or clinical change, or significant correction assessment)
Not PPS Assessment
99. **Not PPS** assessment

Enter Code ☐

C. PPS Other Medicare Required Assessment - OMRA
0. **No**
1. **Start of therapy** assessment
2. **End of therapy** assessment
3. **Both Start and End of therapy** assessment

Enter Code ☐

D. Is this a Swing Bed clinical change assessment? Complete only if A0200 = 2
0. **No**
1. **Yes**

Enter Code ☐

E. Is this assessment the first assessment (OBRA, PPS, or Discharge) **since the most recent admission?**
0. **No**
1. **Yes**

Enter Code ☐☐

F. Entry/discharge reporting
01. **Entry** record
10. **Discharge** assessment-**return not anticipated**
11. **Discharge** assessment-**return anticipated**
12. **Death in facility** record
99. **Not entry/discharge** record

MDS 3.0 Item Listing-Version 1.00.2 10/01/2010

Resident _____   Identifier _____   Date _____

Section A	Identification Information

A0410. Submission Requirement

Enter Code [ ]
1. **Neither federal nor state required submission**
2. **State but not federal required submission** (FOR NURSING HOMES ONLY)
3. **Federal required submission**

A0500. Legal Name of Resident

A. First name:
[ ][ ][ ][ ][ ][ ][ ][ ][ ][ ][ ][ ]

B. Middle initial:
[ ]

C. Last name:
[ ][ ][ ][ ][ ][ ][ ][ ][ ][ ][ ][ ][ ][ ][ ][ ][ ][ ]

D. Suffix:
[ ][ ][ ]

A0600. Social Security and Medicare Numbers

A. Social Security Number:
[ ][ ][ ] - [ ][ ] - [ ][ ][ ][ ]

B. Medicare number (or comparable railroad insurance number):
[ ][ ][ ][ ][ ][ ][ ][ ][ ][ ][ ][ ]

A0700. Medicaid Number - Enter "+" if pending, "N" if not a Medicaid recipient

[ ][ ][ ][ ][ ][ ][ ][ ][ ][ ][ ][ ][ ][ ]

A0800. Gender

Enter Code [ ]
1. **Male**
2. **Female**

A0900. Birth Date

[ ][ ] - [ ][ ] - [ ][ ][ ][ ]
Month   Day   Year

A1000. Race/Ethnicity

↓ Check all that apply

[ ] A. **American Indian or Alaska Native**

[ ] B. **Asian**

[ ] C. **Black or African American**

[ ] D. **Hispanic or Latino**

[ ] E. **Native Hawaiian or Other Pacific Islander**

[ ] F. **White**

A1100. Language

Enter Code [ ]
A. **Does the resident need or want an interpreter to communicate with a doctor or health care staff?**
0. **No**
1. **Yes** → Specify in A1100B, Preferred language
9. **Unable to determine**

B. **Preferred language:**
[ ][ ][ ][ ][ ][ ][ ][ ][ ][ ][ ][ ][ ][ ][ ][ ][ ]

Resident _____   Identifier _____   Date _____

Section A	Identification Information

A1200. Marital Status

Enter Code ☐
1. **Never married**
2. **Married**
3. **Widowed**
4. **Separated**
5. **Divorced**

A1300. Optional Resident Items

A. **Medical record number:**

☐☐☐☐☐☐☐☐☐☐☐☐☐

B. **Room number:**

☐☐☐☐☐☐☐☐☐

C. **Name by which resident prefers to be addressed:**

☐☐☐☐☐☐☐☐☐☐☐☐☐☐☐☐☐☐☐☐☐☐☐☐☐

D. **Lifetime occupation(s)** - put "/" between two occupations:

☐☐☐☐☐☐☐☐☐☐☐☐☐☐☐☐☐☐☐☐☐☐☐☐☐

A1500. Preadmission Screening and Resident Review (PASRR)

Complete only if A0310A = 01

Enter Code ☐
Has the resident been evaluated by Level II PASRR and determined to have a serious mental illness and/or mental retardation or a related condition?
0. **No**
1. **Yes**
9. **Not a Medicaid certified unit**

A1550. Conditions Related to MR/DD Status

If the resident is 22 years of age or older, complete only if A0310A = 01
If the resident is 21 years of age or younger, complete only if A0310A = 01, 03, 04, or 05

↓ **Check all conditions that are related to MR/DD status** that were manifested before age 22, and are likely to continue indefinitely

	MR/DD With Organic Condition
☐	A. **Down syndrome**
☐	B. **Autism**
☐	C. **Epilepsy**
☐	D. **Other organic condition related to MR/DD**
	MR/DD Without Organic Condition
☐	E. **MR/DD with no organic condition**
	No MR/DD
☐	Z. **None of the above**

A1600. Entry Date (date of this admission/reentry into the facility)

☐☐ - ☐☐ - ☐☐☐☐
Month   Day   Year

A1700. Type of Entry

Enter Code ☐
1. **Admission**
2. **Reentry**

Resident _____ Identifier _____ Date _____

Section A — Identification Information

A1800. Entered From

Enter Code [ ][ ]

01. **Community** (private home/apt., board/care, assisted living, group home)
02. **Another nursing home or swing bed**
03. **Acute hospital**
04. **Psychiatric hospital**
05. **Inpatient rehabilitation facility**
06. **MR/DD facility**
07. **Hospice**
99. **Other**

A2000. Discharge Date

Complete only if A0310F = 10, 11, or 12

[ ][ ] – [ ][ ] – [ ][ ][ ][ ]
Month   Day   Year

A2100. Discharge Status

Complete only if A0310F = 10, 11, or 12

Enter Code [ ][ ]

01. **Community** (private home/apt., board/care, assisted living, group home)
02. **Another nursing home or swing bed**
03. **Acute hospital**
04. **Psychiatric hospital**
05. **Inpatient rehabilitation facility**
06. **MR/DD facility**
07. **Hospice**
08. **Deceased**
99. **Other**

A2200. Previous Assessment Reference Date for Significant Correction

Complete only if A0310A = 05 or 06

[ ][ ] – [ ][ ] – [ ][ ][ ][ ]
Month   Day   Year

A2300. Assessment Reference Date

Observation end date:

[ ][ ] – [ ][ ] – [ ][ ][ ][ ]
Month   Day   Year

A2400. Medicare Stay

Enter Code [ ]

A. Has the resident had a Medicare-covered stay since the most recent entry?

0. **No** → Skip to B0100, Comatose
1. **Yes** → Continue to A2400B, Start date of most recent Medicare stay

B. Start date of most recent Medicare stay:

[ ][ ] – [ ][ ] – [ ][ ][ ][ ]
Month   Day   Year

C. End date of most recent Medicare stay - Enter dashes if stay is ongoing:

[ ][ ] – [ ][ ] – [ ][ ][ ][ ]
Month   Day   Year

Resident _____ Identifier _____ Date _____

Look back period for all items is 7 days unless another time frame is indicated

Section B	Hearing, Speech, and Vision

B0100. Comatose

Enter Code ☐

Persistent vegetative state/no discernible consciousness
- 0. **No** → Continue to B0200, Hearing
- 1. **Yes** → Skip to G0110, Activities of Daily Living (ADL) Assistance

B0200. Hearing

Enter Code ☐

Ability to hear (with hearing aid or hearing appliances if normally used)
- 0. **Adequate** - no difficulty in normal conversation, social interaction, listening to TV
- 1. **Minimal difficulty** - difficulty in some environments (e.g., when person speaks softly or setting is noisy)
- 2. **Moderate difficulty** - speaker has to increase volume and speak distinctly
- 3. **Highly impaired** - absence of useful hearing

B0300. Hearing Aid

Enter Code ☐

Hearing aid or other hearing appliance used in completing B0200, Hearing
- 0. **No**
- 1. **Yes**

B0600. Speech Clarity

Enter Code ☐

Select best description of speech pattern
- 0. **Clear speech** - distinct intelligible words
- 1. **Unclear speech** - slurred or mumbled words
- 2. **No speech** - absence of spoken words

B0700. Makes Self Understood

Enter Code ☐

Ability to express ideas and wants, consider both verbal and non-verbal expression
- 0. **Understood**
- 1. **Usually understood** - difficulty communicating some words or finishing thoughts **but** is able if prompted or given time
- 2. **Sometimes understood** - ability is limited to making concrete requests
- 3. **Rarely/never understood**

B0800. Ability To Understand Others

Enter Code ☐

Understanding verbal content, however able (with hearing aid or device if used)
- 0. **Understands** - clear comprehension
- 1. **Usually understands** - misses some part/intent of message **but** comprehends most conversation
- 2. **Sometimes understands** - responds adequately to simple, direct communication only
- 3. **Rarely/never understands**

B1000. Vision

Enter Code ☐

Ability to see in adequate light (with glasses or other visual appliances)
- 0. **Adequate** - sees fine detail, including regular print in newspapers/books
- 1. **Impaired** - sees large print, but not regular print in newspapers/books
- 2. **Moderately impaired** - limited vision; not able to see newspaper headlines but can identify objects
- 3. **Highly impaired** - object identification in question, but eyes appear to follow objects
- 4. **Severely impaired** - no vision or sees only light, colors or shapes; eyes do not appear to follow objects

B1200. Corrective Lenses

Enter Code ☐

Corrective lenses (contacts, glasses, or magnifying glass) used in completing B1000, Vision
- 0. **No**
- 1. **Yes**

MDS 3.0 Item Listing-Version 1.00.2 10/01/2010

Resident _____   Identifier _____   Date _____

Section C   Cognitive Patterns

C0100. Should Brief Interview for Mental Status (C0200-C0500) be Conducted?

Attempt to conduct interview with all residents

Enter Code ☐

   0. **No** (resident is rarely/never understood) → Skip to and complete C0700-C1000, Staff Assessment for Mental Status

   1. **Yes** → Continue to C0200, Repetition of Three Words

Brief Interview for Mental Status (BIMS)

C0200. Repetition of Three Words

Enter Code ☐

Ask resident: *"I am going to say three words for you to remember. Please repeat the words after I have said all three. The words are: **sock, blue, and bed.** Now tell me the three words."*

Number of words repeated after first attempt

   0. **None**
   1. **One**
   2. **Two**
   3. **Three**

After the resident's first attempt, repeat the words using cues ("*sock, something to wear; blue, a color; bed, a piece of furniture*"). You may repeat the words up to two more times.

C0300. Temporal Orientation (orientation to year, month, and day)

Enter Code ☐

Ask resident: "*Please tell me what year it is right now.*"

A. Able to report correct year

   0. **Missed by > 5 years** or no answer
   1. **Missed by 2-5 years**
   2. **Missed by 1 year**
   3. **Correct**

Enter Code ☐

Ask resident: "*What month are we in right now?*"

B. Able to report correct month

   0. **Missed by > 1 month** or no answer
   1. **Missed by 6 days to 1 month**
   2. **Accurate within 5 days**

Enter Code ☐

Ask resident: "*What day of the week is today?*"

C. Able to report correct day of the week

   0. **Incorrect** or no answer
   1. **Correct**

C0400. Recall

Enter Code ☐

Ask resident: "*Let's go back to an earlier question. What were those three words that I asked you to repeat?*"

If unable to remember a word, give cue (something to wear; a color; a piece of furniture) for that word.

A. Able to recall "sock"

   0. **No** - could not recall
   1. **Yes, after cueing** ("something to wear")
   2. **Yes, no cue required**

Enter Code ☐

B. Able to recall "blue"

   0. **No** - could not recall
   1. **Yes, after cueing** ("a color")
   2. **Yes, no cue required**

Enter Code ☐

C. Able to recall "bed"

   0. **No** - could not recall
   1. **Yes, after cueing** ("a piece of furniture")
   2. **Yes, no cue required**

C0500. Summary Score

☐☐
Enter Score

Add scores for questions C0200-C0400 and fill in total score (00-15)
Enter 99 if the resident was unable to complete the interview

---

Resident _____ Identifier _____ Date _____

Section C   Cognitive Patterns

C0600. Should the Staff Assessment for Mental Status (C0700 - C1000) be Conducted?

Enter Code
☐
  0. **No** (resident was able to complete interview) → Skip to C1300, Signs and Symptoms of Delirium
  1. **Yes** (resident was unable to complete interview) → Continue to C0700, Short-term Memory OK

Staff Assessment for Mental Status

Do not conduct if Brief Interview for Mental Status (C0200-C0500) was completed

C0700. Short-term Memory OK

Enter Code
☐
Seems or appears to recall after 5 minutes
  0. **Memory OK**
  1. **Memory problem**

C0800. Long-term Memory OK

Enter Code
☐
Seems or appears to recall long past
  0. **Memory OK**
  1. **Memory problem**

C0900. Memory/Recall Ability

↓ Check all that the resident was normally able to recall

☐	**A. Current season**
☐	**B. Location of own room**
☐	**C. Staff names and faces**
☐	**D. That he or she is in a nursing home**
☐	**Z. None of the above** were recalled

C1000. Cognitive Skills for Daily Decision Making

Enter Code
☐
Made decisions regarding tasks of daily life
  0. **Independent** - decisions consistent/reasonable
  1. **Modified independence** - some difficulty in new situations only
  2. **Moderately impaired** - decisions poor; cues/supervision required
  3. **Severely impaired** - never/rarely made decisions

Resident _____   Identifier _____   Date _____

Section D — Mood

D0100. Should Resident Mood Interview be Conducted? - Attempt to conduct interview with all residents

Enter Code ☐

0. **No** (resident is rarely/never understood) → Skip to and complete D0500-D0600, Staff Assessment of Resident Mood (PHQ-9-OV)
1. **Yes** → Continue to D0200, Resident Mood Interview (PHQ-9©)

D0200. Resident Mood Interview (PHQ-9©)

Say to resident: "Over the last 2 weeks, have you been bothered by any of the following problems?"

If symptom is present, enter 1 (yes) in column 1, Symptom Presence.
If yes in column 1, then ask the resident: "About **how often** have you been bothered by this?"
Read and show the resident a card with the symptom frequency choices. Indicate response in column 2, Symptom Frequency.

1. Symptom Presence
0. **No** (enter 0 in column 2)
1. **Yes** (enter 0-3 in column 2)
9. **No response** (leave column 2 blank)

2. Symptom Frequency
0. **Never or 1 day**
1. **2-6 days** (several days)
2. **7-11 days** (half or more of the days)
3. **12-14 days** (nearly every day)

	1. Symptom Presence	2. Symptom Frequency
	↓ Enter Scores in Boxes ↓	
A. *Little interest or pleasure in doing things*	☐	☐
B. *Feeling down, depressed, or hopeless*	☐	☐
C. *Trouble falling or staying asleep, or sleeping too much*	☐	☐
D. *Feeling tired or having little energy*	☐	☐
E. *Poor appetite or overeating*	☐	☐
F. *Feeling bad about yourself - or that you are a failure or have let yourself or your family down*	☐	☐
G. *Trouble concentrating on things, such as reading the newspaper or watching television*	☐	☐
H. *Moving or speaking so slowly that other people could have noticed. Or the opposite - being so fidgety or restless that you have been moving around a lot more than usual*	☐	☐
I. *Thoughts that you would be better off dead, or of hurting yourself in some way*	☐	☐

D0300. Total Severity Score

Enter Score ☐☐

Add scores for all frequency responses in Column 2, Symptom Frequency. Total score must be between 00 and 27. Enter 99 if unable to complete interview (i.e., Symptom Frequency is blank for 3 or more items).

D0350. Safety Notification - Complete only if D0200I1 = 1 indicating possibility of resident self harm

Enter Code ☐

Was responsible staff or provider informed that there is a potential for resident self harm?
0. **No**
1. **Yes**

MDS 3.0 Item Listing-Version 1.00.2 10/01/2010

Resident _____   Identifier _____   Date _____

Section D   Mood

D0500. Staff Assessment of Resident Mood (PHQ-9-OV*)

Do not conduct if Resident Mood Interview (D0200-D0300) was completed

Over the last 2 weeks, did the resident have any of the following problems or behaviors?

If symptom is present, enter 1 (yes) in column 1, Symptom Presence.
Then move to column 2, Symptom Frequency, and indicate symptom frequency.

		1. Symptom Presence	2. Symptom Frequency
1. Symptom Presence 0. **No** (enter 0 in column 2) 1. **Yes** (enter 0-3 in column 2)	**2. Symptom Frequency** 0. **Never or 1 day** 1. **2-6 days** (several days) 2. **7-11 days** (half or more of the days) 3. **12-14 days** (nearly every day)	↓ Enter Scores in Boxes ↓	
A. Little interest or pleasure in doing things		☐	☐
B. Feeling or appearing down, depressed, or hopeless		☐	☐
C. Trouble falling or staying asleep, or sleeping too much		☐	☐
D. Feeling tired or having little energy		☐	☐
E. Poor appetite or overeating		☐	☐
F. Indicating that s/he feels bad about self, is a failure, or has let self or family down		☐	☐
G. Trouble concentrating on things, such as reading the newspaper or watching television		☐	☐
H. Moving or speaking so slowly that other people have noticed. Or the opposite - being so fidgety or restless that s/he has been moving around a lot more than usual		☐	☐
I. States that life isn't worth living, wishes for death, or attempts to harm self		☐	☐
J. Being short-tempered, easily annoyed		☐	☐

D0600. Total Severity Score

☐☐ **Add scores for all frequency responses in Column 2**, Symptom Frequency. Total score must be between 00 and 30.

Enter Score

D0650. Safety Notification - Complete only if D0500I1 = 1 indicating possibility of resident self harm

Enter Code	**Was responsible staff or provider informed that there is a potential for resident self harm?**
☐	0. **No** 1. **Yes**

MDS 3.0 Item Listing-Version 1.00.2 10/01/2010

Resident _____ Identifier _____ Date _____

Section E	Behavior

E0100. Psychosis

↓ Check all that apply

☐	**A. Hallucinations** (perceptual experiences in the absence of real external sensory stimuli)
☐	**B. Delusions** (misconceptions or beliefs that are firmly held, contrary to reality)
☐	**Z. None of the above**

Behavioral Symptoms

E0200. Behavioral Symptom - Presence & Frequency

Note presence of symptoms and their frequency

Coding:	↓ Enter Codes in Boxes
Coding: 0. **Behavior not exhibited** 1. **Behavior of this type occurred 1 to 3 days** 2. **Behavior of this type occurred 4 to 6 days,** but less than daily 3. **Behavior of this type occurred daily**	☐ **A. Physical behavioral symptoms directed toward others** (e.g., hitting, kicking, pushing, scratching, grabbing, abusing others sexually) ☐ **B. Verbal behavioral symptoms directed toward others** (e.g., threatening others, screaming at others, cursing at others) ☐ **C. Other behavioral symptoms not directed toward others** (e.g., physical symptoms such as hitting or scratching self, pacing, rummaging, public sexual acts, disrobing in public, throwing or smearing food or bodily wastes, or verbal/vocal symptoms like screaming, disruptive sounds)

E0300. Overall Presence of Behavioral Symptoms

Enter Code ☐	**Were any behavioral symptoms in questions E0200 coded 1, 2, or 3?** 0. **No** → Skip to E0800, Rejection of Care 1. **Yes** → Considering all of E0200, Behavioral Symptoms, answer E0500 and E0600 below

E0500. Impact on Resident

	Did any of the identified symptom(s):
Enter Code ☐	**A. Put the resident at significant risk for physical illness or injury?** 0. **No** 1. **Yes**
Enter Code ☐	**B. Significantly interfere with the resident's care?** 0. **No** 1. **Yes**
Enter Code ☐	**C. Significantly interfere with the resident's participation in activities or social interactions?** 0. **No** 1. **Yes**

E0600. Impact on Others

	Did any of the identified symptom(s):
Enter Code ☐	**A. Put others at significant risk for physical injury?** 0. **No** 1. **Yes**
Enter Code ☐	**B. Significantly intrude on the privacy or activity of others?** 0. **No** 1. **Yes**
Enter Code ☐	**C. Significantly disrupt care or living environment?** 0. **No** 1. **Yes**

E0800. Rejection of Care - Presence & Frequency

Enter Code ☐	**Did the resident reject evaluation or care** (e.g., bloodwork, taking medications, ADL assistance) **that is necessary to achieve the resident's goals for health and well-being?** Do not include behaviors that have already been addressed (e.g., by discussion or care planning with the resident or family), and/or determined to be consistent with resident values, preferences, or goals. 0. **Behavior not exhibited** 1. **Behavior of this type occurred 1 to 3 days** 2. **Behavior of this type occurred 4 to 6 days,** but less than daily 3. **Behavior of this type occurred daily**

Resident _____ Identifier _____ Date _____

Section E	Behavior

E0900. Wandering - Presence & Frequency

Enter Code	**Has the resident wandered?** 0. **Behavior not exhibited** → Skip to E1100, Change in Behavioral or Other Symptoms 1. **Behavior of this type occurred 1 to 3 days** 2. **Behavior of this type occurred 4 to 6 days,** but less than daily 3. **Behavior of this type occurred daily**

E1000. Wandering - Impact

Enter Code	**A. Does the wandering place the resident at significant risk of getting to a potentially dangerous place** (e.g., stairs, outside of the facility)? 0. **No** 1. **Yes**
Enter Code	**B. Does the wandering significantly intrude on the privacy or activities of others?** 0. **No** 1. **Yes**

E1100. Change in Behavior or Other Symptoms

Consider all of the symptoms assessed in items E0100 through E1000

Enter Code	How does resident's current behavior status, care rejection, or wandering **compare to prior assessment (OBRA or PPS)?** 0. **Same** 1. **Improved** 2. **Worse** 3. **N/A** because no prior MDS assessment

Resident _____   Identifier _____   Date _____

Section F	Preferences for Customary Routine and Activities

F0300. Should Interview for Daily and Activity Preferences be Conducted? - Attempt to interview all residents able to communicate. If resident is unable to complete, attempt to complete interview with family member or significant other

Enter Code [ ]
- 0. **No** (resident is rarely/never understood <u>and</u> family/significant other not available) → Skip to and complete F0800, Staff Assessment of Daily and Activity Preferences
- 1. **Yes** → Continue to F0400, Interview for Daily Preferences

---

F0400. Interview for Daily Preferences

Show resident the response options and say: **"While you are in this facility..."**

Coding:
1. **Very important**
2. **Somewhat important**
3. **Not very important**
4. **Not important at all**
5. **Important, but can't do or no choice**
9. **No response or non-responsive**

↓ Enter Codes in Boxes

[ ] A. how important is it to you to **choose what clothes to wear?**

[ ] B. how important is it to you to **take care of your personal belongings or things?**

[ ] C. how important is it to you to **choose between a tub bath, shower, bed bath, or sponge bath?**

[ ] D. how important is it to you to **have snacks available between meals?**

[ ] E. how important is it to you to **choose your own bedtime?**

[ ] F. how important is it to you to **have your family or a close friend involved in discussions about your care?**

[ ] G. how important is it to you to **be able to use the phone in private?**

[ ] H. how important is it to you to **have a place to lock your things to keep them safe?**

F0500. Interview for Activity Preferences

Show resident the response options and say: **"While you are in this facility..."**

Coding:
1. **Very important**
2. **Somewhat important**
3. **Not very important**
4. **Not important at all**
5. **Important, but can't do or no choice**
9. **No response or non-responsive**

↓ Enter Codes in Boxes

[ ] A. how important is it to you to **have books, newspapers, and magazines to read?**

[ ] B. how important is it to you to **listen to music you like?**

[ ] C. how important is it to you to **be around animals such as pets?**

[ ] D. how important is it to you to **keep up with the news?**

[ ] E. how important is it to you to **do things with groups of people?**

[ ] F. how important is it to you to **do your favorite activities?**

[ ] G. how important is it to you to **go outside to get fresh air when the weather is good?**

[ ] H. how important is it to you to **participate in religious services or practices?**

F0600. Daily and Activity Preferences Primary Respondent

Enter Code [ ]

Indicate primary respondent for Daily and Activity Preferences (F0400 and F0500)
1. **Resident**
2. **Family or significant other** (close friend or other representative)
9. **Interview could not be completed** by resident or family/significant other ("No response" to 3 or more items)

Resident _____   Identifier _____   Date _____

Section F — Preferences for Customary Routine and Activities

F0700. Should the Staff Assessment of Daily and Activity Preferences be Conducted?

Enter Code	
☐	0. **No** (because Interview for Daily and Activity Preferences (F0400 and F0500) was completed by resident or family/significant other) → Skip to and complete G0110, Activities of Daily Living (ADL) Assistance
	1. **Yes** (because 3 or more items in Interview for Daily and Activity Preferences (F0400 and F0500) were not completed by resident or family/significant other) → Continue to F0800, Staff Assessment of Daily and Activity Preferences

F0800. Staff Assessment of Daily and Activity Preferences

Do not conduct if Interview for Daily and Activity Preferences (F0400-F0500) was completed

Resident Prefers:

↓ **Check all that apply**

- ☐ **A.** Choosing clothes to wear
- ☐ **B.** Caring for personal belongings
- ☐ **C.** Receiving tub bath
- ☐ **D.** Receiving shower
- ☐ **E.** Receiving bed bath
- ☐ **F.** Receiving sponge bath
- ☐ **G.** Snacks between meals
- ☐ **H.** Staying up past 8:00 p.m.
- ☐ **I.** Family or significant other involvement in care discussions
- ☐ **J.** Use of phone in private
- ☐ **K.** Place to lock personal belongings
- ☐ **L.** Reading books, newspapers, or magazines
- ☐ **M.** Listening to music
- ☐ **N.** Being around animals such as pets
- ☐ **O.** Keeping up with the news
- ☐ **P.** Doing things with groups of people
- ☐ **Q.** Participating in favorite activities
- ☐ **R.** Spending time away from the nursing home
- ☐ **S.** Spending time outdoors
- ☐ **T.** Participating in religious activities or practices
- ☐ **Z.** None of the above

Resident _____   Identifier _____   Date _____

Section G	**Functional Status**

G0110. Activities of Daily Living (ADL) Assistance
Refer to the ADL flow chart in the RAI manual to facilitate accurate coding

Instructions for Rule of 3
- When an activity occurs three times at any one given level, code that level.
- When an activity occurs three times at multiple levels, code the most dependent, exceptions are total dependence (4), activity must require full assist every time, and activity did not occur (8), activity must not have occurred at all. Example, three times extensive assistance (3) and three times limited assistance (2), code extensive assistance (3).
- When an activity occurs at various levels, but not three times at any given level, apply the following:
  - When there is a combination of full staff performance, and extensive assistance, code extensive assistance.
  - When there is a combination of full staff performance, weight bearing assistance and/or non-weight bearing assistance code limited assistance (2).

If none of the above are met, code supervision.

1. ADL Self-Performance
Code for **resident's performance** over all shifts - not including setup. If the ADL activity occurred 3 or more times at various levels of assistance, code the most dependent - except for total dependence, which requires full staff performance every time

Coding:
  Activity Occurred 3 or More Times
  0. **Independent** - no help or staff oversight at any time
  1. **Supervision** - oversight, encouragement or cueing
  2. **Limited assistance** - resident highly involved in activity; staff provide guided maneuvering of limbs or other non-weight-bearing assistance
  3. **Extensive assistance** - resident involved in activity, staff provide weight-bearing support
  4. **Total dependence** - full staff performance every time during entire 7-day period
  Activity Occurred 2 or Fewer Times
  7. **Activity occurred only once or twice** - activity did occur but only once or twice
  8. **Activity did not occur** - activity (or any part of the ADL) was not performed by resident or staff at all over the entire 7-day period

2. ADL Support Provided
Code for **most support provided** over all shifts; code regardless of resident's self-performance classification

Coding:
  0. **No** setup or physical help from staff
  1. **Setup** help only
  2. **One** person physical assist
  3. **Two+** persons physical assist
  8. ADL activity itself **did not occur** during entire period

	1. Self-Performance	2. Support
	↓ Enter Codes in Boxes ↓	
A. Bed mobility - how resident moves to and from lying position, turns side to side, and positions body while in bed or alternate sleep furniture	☐	☐
B. Transfer - how resident moves between surfaces including to or from: bed, chair, wheelchair, standing position (**excludes** to/from bath/toilet)	☐	☐
C. Walk in room - how resident walks between locations in his/her room	☐	☐
D. Walk in corridor - how resident walks in corridor on unit	☐	☐
E. Locomotion on unit - how resident moves between locations in his/her room and adjacent corridor on same floor. If in wheelchair, self-sufficiency once in chair	☐	☐
F. Locomotion off unit - how resident moves to and returns from off-unit locations (e.g., areas set aside for dining, activities or treatments). **If facility has only one floor**, how resident moves to and from distant areas on the floor. If in wheelchair, self-sufficiency once in chair	☐	☐
G. Dressing - how resident puts on, fastens and takes off all items of clothing, including donning/removing a prosthesis or TED hose. Dressing includes putting on and changing pajamas and housedresses	☐	☐
H. Eating - how resident eats and drinks, regardless of skill. Do not include eating/drinking during medication pass. Includes intake of nourishment by other means (e.g., tube feeding, total parenteral nutrition, IV fluids administered for nutrition or hydration)	☐	☐
I. Toilet use - how resident uses the toilet room, commode, bedpan, or urinal; transfers on/off toilet; cleanses self after elimination; changes pad; manages ostomy or catheter; and adjusts clothes. Do not include emptying of bedpan, urinal, bedside commode, catheter bag or ostomy bag	☐	☐
J. Personal hygiene - how resident maintains personal hygiene, including combing hair, brushing teeth, shaving, applying makeup, washing/drying face and hands (**excludes** baths and showers)	☐	☐

Resident _____ Identifier _____ Date _____

Section G — Functional Status

G0120. Bathing

How resident takes full-body bath/shower, sponge bath, and transfers in/out of tub/shower (**excludes** washing of back and hair). Code for **most dependent** in self-performance and support

Enter Code	A. Self-performance
☐	0. **Independent** - no help provided
	1. **Supervision** - oversight help only
	2. **Physical help limited to transfer only**
	3. **Physical help in part of bathing activity**
	4. **Total dependence**
	8. **Activity itself did not occur** during the entire period

Enter Code	B. Support provided
☐	(Bathing support codes are as defined in item **G0110 column 2, ADL Support Provided**, above)

G0300. Balance During Transitions and Walking

After observing the resident, **code the following walking and transition items for most dependent**

Coding:
0. **Steady at all times**
1. **Not steady, but able to stabilize without human assistance**
2. **Not steady, only able to stabilize with human assistance**
8. **Activity did not occur**

↓ Enter Codes in Boxes

☐	A. **Moving from seated to standing position**
☐	B. **Walking** (with assistive device if used)
☐	C. **Turning around** and facing the opposite direction while walking
☐	D. **Moving on and off toilet**
☐	E. **Surface-to-surface transfer** (transfer between bed and chair or wheelchair)

G0400. Functional Limitation in Range of Motion

Code for limitation that interfered with daily functions or placed resident at risk of injury

Coding:
0. **No impairment**
1. **Impairment on one side**
2. **Impairment on both sides**

↓ Enter Codes in Boxes

☐	A. **Upper extremity** (shoulder, elbow, wrist, hand)
☐	B. **Lower extremity** (hip, knee, ankle, foot)

G0600. Mobility Devices

↓ Check all that were normally used

☐	A. **Cane/crutch**
☐	B. **Walker**
☐	C. **Wheelchair** (manual or electric)
☐	D. **Limb prosthesis**
☐	Z. **None of the above** were used

G0900. Functional Rehabilitation Potential
Complete only if A0310A = 01

Enter Code	A. **Resident believes he or she is capable of increased independence** in at least some ADLs
☐	0. **No**
	1. **Yes**
	9. **Unable to determine**

Enter Code	B. **Direct care staff believe resident is capable of increased independence** in at least some ADLs
☐	0. **No**
	1. **Yes**

Resident _____　Identifier _____　Date _____

Section H	**Bladder and Bowel**

H0100. Appliances

↓ Check all that apply

- [ ] **A. Indwelling catheter** (including suprapubic catheter and nephrostomy tube)
- [ ] **B. External catheter**
- [ ] **C. Ostomy** (including urostomy, ileostomy, and colostomy)
- [ ] **D. Intermittent catheterization**
- [ ] **Z. None of the above**

H0200. Urinary Toileting Program

Enter Code ☐　**A. Has a trial of a toileting program (e.g., scheduled toileting, prompted voiding, or bladder training)** been attempted on admission/reentry or since urinary incontinence was noted in this facility?
- 0. **No** → Skip to H0300, Urinary Continence
- 1. **Yes** → Continue to H0200B, Response
- 9. **Unable to determine** → Skip to H0200C, Current toileting program or trial

Enter Code ☐　**B. Response -** What was the resident's response to the trial program?
- 0. **No improvement**
- 1. **Decreased wetness**
- 2. **Completely dry** (continent)
- 9. **Unable to determine** or trial in progress

Enter Code ☐　**C. Current toileting program or trial -** Is a toileting program (e.g., scheduled toileting, prompted voiding, or bladder training) currently being used to manage the resident's urinary continence?
- 0. **No**
- 1. **Yes**

H0300. Urinary Continence

Enter Code ☐　**Urinary continence -** Select the one category that best describes the resident
- 0. **Always continent**
- 1. **Occasionally incontinent** (less than 7 episodes of incontinence)
- 2. **Frequently incontinent** (7 or more episodes of urinary incontinence, but at least one episode of continent voiding)
- 3. **Always incontinent** (no episodes of continent voiding)
- 9. **Not rated,** resident had a catheter (indwelling, condom), urinary ostomy, or no urine output for the entire 7 days

H0400. Bowel Continence

Enter Code ☐　**Bowel continence -** Select the one category that best describes the resident
- 0. **Always continent**
- 1. **Occasionally incontinent** (one episode of bowel incontinence)
- 2. **Frequently incontinent** (2 or more episodes of bowel incontinence, but at least one continent bowel movement)
- 3. **Always incontinent** (no episodes of continent bowel movements)
- 9. **Not rated,** resident had an ostomy or did not have a bowel movement for the entire 7 days

H0500. Bowel Toileting Program

Enter Code ☐　**Is a toileting program currently being used to manage the resident's bowel continence?**
- 0. **No**
- 1. **Yes**

H0600. Bowel Patterns

Enter Code ☐　**Constipation present?**
- 0. **No**
- 1. **Yes**

Resident _____ Identifier _____ Date _____

Section I	Active Diagnoses

Active Diagnoses in the last 7 days - Check all that apply

Diagnoses listed in parentheses are provided as examples and should not be considered as all-inclusive lists

Cancer
- ☐ I0100. **Cancer** (with or without metastasis)

Heart/Circulation
- ☐ I0200. **Anemia** (e.g., aplastic, iron deficiency, pernicious, and sickle cell)
- ☐ I0300. **Atrial Fibrillation or Other Dysrhythmias** (e.g., bradycardias and tachycardias)
- ☐ I0400. **Coronary Artery Disease (CAD)** (e.g., angina, myocardial infarction, and atherosclerotic heart disease (ASHD))
- ☐ I0500. **Deep Venous Thrombosis (DVT), Pulmonary Embolus (PE), or Pulmonary Thrombo-Embolism (PTE)**
- ☐ I0600. **Heart Failure** (e.g., congestive heart failure (CHF) and pulmonary edema)
- ☐ I0700. **Hypertension**
- ☐ I0800. **Orthostatic Hypotension**
- ☐ I0900. **Peripheral Vascular Disease (PVD) or Peripheral Arterial Disease (PAD)**

Gastrointestinal
- ☐ I1100. **Cirrhosis**
- ☐ I1200. **Gastroesophageal Reflux Disease (GERD) or Ulcer** (e.g., esophageal, gastric, and peptic ulcers)
- ☐ I1300. **Ulcerative Colitis, Crohn's Disease, or Inflammatory Bowel Disease**

Genitourinary
- ☐ I1400. **Benign Prostatic Hyperplasia (BPH)**
- ☐ I1500. **Renal Insufficiency, Renal Failure, or End-Stage Renal Disease (ESRD)**
- ☐ I1550. **Neurogenic Bladder**
- ☐ I1650. **Obstructive Uropathy**

Infections
- ☐ I1700. **Multidrug-Resistant Organism (MDRO)**
- ☐ I2000. **Pneumonia**
- ☐ I2100. **Septicemia**
- ☐ I2200. **Tuberculosis**
- ☐ I2300. **Urinary Tract Infection (UTI) (LAST 30 DAYS)**
- ☐ I2400. **Viral Hepatitis** (e.g., Hepatitis A, B, C, D, and E)
- ☐ I2500. **Wound Infection** (other than foot)

Metabolic
- ☐ I2900. **Diabetes Mellitus (DM)** (e.g., diabetic retinopathy, nephropathy, and neuropathy)
- ☐ I3100. **Hyponatremia**
- ☐ I3200. **Hyperkalemia**
- ☐ I3300. **Hyperlipidemia** (e.g., hypercholesterolemia)
- ☐ I3400. **Thyroid Disorder** (e.g., hypothyroidism, hyperthyroidism, and Hashimoto's thyroiditis)

Musculoskeletal
- ☐ I3700. **Arthritis** (e.g., degenerative joint disease (DJD), osteoarthritis, and rheumatoid arthritis (RA))
- ☐ I3800. **Osteoporosis**
- ☐ I3900. **Hip Fracture** - any hip fracture that has a relationship to current status, treatments, monitoring (e.g., sub-capital fractures, and fractures of the trochanter and femoral neck)
- ☐ I4000. **Other Fracture**

Neurological
- ☐ I4200. **Alzheimer's Disease**
- ☐ I4300. **Aphasia**
- ☐ I4400. **Cerebral Palsy**
- ☐ I4500. **Cerebrovascular Accident (CVA), Transient Ischemic Attack (TIA), or Stroke**
- ☐ I4800. **Dementia** (e.g. Non-Alzheimer's dementia such as vascular or multi-infarct dementia; mixed dementia; frontotemporal dementia such as Pick's disease; and dementia related to stroke, Parkinson's or Creutzfeldt-Jakob diseases)

Neurological Diagnoses continued on next page

MDS 3.0 Item Listing-Version 1.00.2 10/01/2010

Resident _____ Identifier _____ Date _____

Section I	Active Diagnoses

Active Diagnoses in the last 7 days - Check all that apply
Diagnoses listed in parentheses are provided as examples and should not be considered as all-inclusive lists

Neurological - Continued

☐ I4900. **Hemiplegia or Hemiparesis**

☐ I5000. **Paraplegia**

☐ I5100. **Quadriplegia**

☐ I5200. **Multiple Sclerosis (MS)**

☐ I5250. **Huntington's Disease**

☐ I5300. **Parkinson's Disease**

☐ I5350. **Tourette's Syndrome**

☐ I5400. **Seizure Disorder or Epilepsy**

☐ I5500. **Traumatic Brain Injury (TBI)**

Nutritional

☐ I5600. **Malnutrition** (protein or calorie) or at risk for malnutrition

Psychiatric/Mood Disorder

☐ I5700. **Anxiety Disorder**

☐ I5800. **Depression** (other than bipolar)

☐ I5900. **Manic Depression** (bipolar disease)

☐ I5950. **Psychotic Disorder** (other than schizophrenia)

☐ I6000. **Schizophrenia** (e.g., schizoaffective and schizophreniform disorders)

☐ I6100. **Post Traumatic Stress Disorder (PTSD)**

Pulmonary

☐ I6200. **Asthma, Chronic Obstructive Pulmonary Disease (COPD), or Chronic Lung Disease** (e.g., chronic bronchitis and restrictive lung diseases such as asbestosis)

☐ I6300. **Respiratory Failure**

Vision

☐ I6500. **Cataracts, Glaucoma, or Macular Degeneration**

None of Above

☐ I7900. **None of the above active diagnoses** within the last 7 days

Other

☐ I8000. **Additional active diagnoses**
Enter diagnosis on line and ICD code in boxes. Include the decimal for the code in the appropriate box.

A. _____ ☐☐☐☐☐☐☐☐

B. _____ ☐☐☐☐☐☐☐☐

C. _____ ☐☐☐☐☐☐☐☐

D. _____ ☐☐☐☐☐☐☐☐

E. _____ ☐☐☐☐☐☐☐☐

F. _____ ☐☐☐☐☐☐☐☐

G. _____ ☐☐☐☐☐☐☐☐

H. _____ ☐☐☐☐☐☐☐☐

I. _____ ☐☐☐☐☐☐☐☐

J. _____ ☐☐☐☐☐☐☐☐

MDS 3.0 Item Listing-Version 1.00.2 10/01/2010

Resident _____   Identifier _____   Date _____

Section J	Health Conditions

J0100. Pain Management - Complete for all residents, regardless of current pain level

At any time in the last **5** days, has the resident:

Enter Code	A. **Been on a scheduled pain medication regimen?**
☐	0. **No**
	1. **Yes**

Enter Code	B. **Received PRN pain medications?**
☐	0. **No**
	1. **Yes**

Enter Code	C. **Received non-medication intervention for pain?**
☐	0. **No**
	1. **Yes**

J0200. Should Pain Assessment Interview be Conducted?

Attempt to conduct interview with all residents. If resident is comatose, skip to J1100, Shortness of Breath (dyspnea)

Enter Code	0. **No** (resident is rarely/never understood) → Skip to and complete J0800, Indicators of Pain or Possible Pain
☐	1. **Yes** → Continue to J0300, Pain Presence

Pain Assessment Interview

J0300. Pain Presence

Enter Code	Ask resident: "***Have you had pain or hurting at any time*** in the last 5 days?"
☐	0. **No** → Skip to J1100, Shortness of Breath
	1. **Yes** → Continue to J0400, Pain Frequency
	9. **Unable to answer** → Skip to J0800, Indicators of Pain or Possible Pain

J0400. Pain Frequency

Enter Code	Ask resident: "***How much of the time have you experienced pain or hurting*** over the last 5 days?"
☐	1. **Almost constantly**
	2. **Frequently**
	3. **Occasionally**
	4. **Rarely**
	9. **Unable to answer**

J0500. Pain Effect on Function

Enter Code	A. Ask resident: "*Over the past 5 days, **has pain made it hard for you to sleep at night**?*"
☐	0. **No**
	1. **Yes**
	9. **Unable to answer**

Enter Code	B. Ask resident: "*Over the past 5 days, **have you limited your day-to-day activities because of pain**?*"
☐	0. **No**
	1. **Yes**
	9. **Unable to answer**

J0600. Pain Intensity - Administer **ONLY ONE** of the following pain intensity questions (A or B)

Enter Rating	A. **Numeric Rating Scale (00-10)**
☐☐	Ask resident: "*Please rate your worst pain over the last 5 days on a zero to ten scale, with zero being no pain and ten as the worst pain you can imagine.*" (Show resident 00 -10 pain scale)
	Enter two-digit response. Enter 99 if unable to answer.

Enter Code	B. **Verbal Descriptor Scale**
☐	Ask resident: "*Please rate the intensity of your worst pain over the last 5 days.*" (Show resident verbal scale)
	1. **Mild**
	2. **Moderate**
	3. **Severe**
	4. **Very severe, horrible**
	9. **Unable to answer**

MDS 3.0 Item Listing-Version 1.00.2 10/01/2010

Resident _____   Identifier _____   Date _____

Section J   Health Conditions

J0700. Should the Staff Assessment for Pain be Conducted?

Enter Code	0. **No** (J0400 = 1 thru 4) → Skip to J1100, Shortness of Breath (dyspnea)
☐	1. **Yes** (J0400 = 9) → Continue to J0800, Indicators of Pain or Possible Pain

Staff Assessment for Pain

J0800. Indicators of Pain or Possible Pain in the last 5 days

↓ **Check all that apply**

☐	A. **Non-verbal sounds** (e.g., crying, whining, gasping, moaning, or groaning)
☐	B. **Vocal complaints of pain** (e.g., that hurts, ouch, stop)
☐	C. **Facial expressions** (e.g., grimaces, winces, wrinkled forehead, furrowed brow, clenched teeth or jaw)
☐	D. **Protective body movements or postures** (e.g., bracing, guarding, rubbing or massaging a body part/area, clutching or holding a body part during movement)
☐	Z. **None of these signs observed or documented** → If checked, skip to J1100, Shortness of Breath (dyspnea)

J0850. Frequency of Indicator of Pain or Possible Pain in the last 5 days

Enter Code	Frequency with which resident complains or shows evidence of pain or possible pain
☐	1. **Indicators of pain** or possible pain observed **1 to 2 days**
	2. **Indicators of pain** or possible pain observed **3 to 4 days**
	3. **Indicators of pain** or possible pain observed **daily**

Other Health Conditions

J1100. Shortness of Breath (dyspnea)

↓ **Check all that apply**

☐	A. **Shortness of breath** or trouble breathing **with exertion** (e.g., walking, bathing, transferring)
☐	B. **Shortness of breath** or trouble breathing **when sitting at rest**
☐	C. **Shortness of breath** or trouble breathing **when lying flat**
☐	Z. **None of the above**

J1300. Current Tobacco Use

Enter Code	Tobacco use
☐	0. **No**
	1. **Yes**

J1400. Prognosis

Enter Code	Does the resident have a condition or chronic disease that may result in a **life expectancy of less than 6 months?** (Requires physician documentation)
☐	0. **No**
	1. **Yes**

J1550. Problem Conditions

↓ **Check all that apply**

☐	A. **Fever**
☐	B. **Vomiting**
☐	C. **Dehydrated**
☐	D. **Internal bleeding**
☐	Z. **None of the above**

Resident _____   Identifier _____   Date _____

Section J	Health Conditions

J1700. Fall History on Admission
Complete only if A0310A = 01 or A0310E = 1

Enter Code ☐	**A.** Did the resident have a fall any time in the **last month** prior to admission?
	   0. **No**
	   1. **Yes**
	   9. **Unable to determine**

Enter Code ☐	**B.** Did the resident have a fall any time in the **last 2-6 months** prior to admission?
	   0. **No**
	   1. **Yes**
	   9. **Unable to determine**

Enter Code ☐	**C.** Did the resident have any **fracture related to a fall in the 6 months** prior to admission?
	   0. **No**
	   1. **Yes**
	   9. **Unable to determine**

J1800. Any Falls Since Admission or Prior Assessment (OBRA, PPS, or Discharge), whichever is more recent

Enter Code ☐	Has the resident **had any falls since admission or the prior assessment** (OBRA, PPS, or Discharge), whichever is more recent?
	   0. **No** → Skip to K0100, Swallowing Disorder
	   1. **Yes** → Continue to J1900, Number of Falls Since Admission or Prior Assessment (OBRA, PPS, or Discharge)

J1900. Number of Falls Since Admission or Prior Assessment (OBRA, PPS, or Discharge), whichever is more recent

	↓ **Enter Codes in Boxes**	
Coding: 0. **None** 1. **One** 2. **Two or more**	☐	**A. No injury** - no evidence of any injury is noted on physical assessment by the nurse or primary care clinician; no complaints of pain or injury by the resident; no change in the resident's behavior is noted after the fall
	☐	**B. Injury (except major)** - skin tears, abrasions, lacerations, superficial bruises, hematomas and sprains; or any fall-related injury that causes the resident to complain of pain
	☐	**C. Major injury** - bone fractures, joint dislocations, closed head injuries with altered consciousness, subdural hematoma

Resident _____   Identifier _____   Date _____

Section K	**Swallowing/Nutritional Status**

K0100. Swallowing Disorder

Signs and symptoms of possible swallowing disorder

↓ **Check all that apply**

☐	A. Loss of liquids/solids from mouth when eating or drinking
☐	B. Holding food in mouth/cheeks or residual food in mouth after meals
☐	C. Coughing or choking during meals or when swallowing medications
☐	D. Complaints of difficulty or pain with swallowing
☐	Z. None of the above

K0200. Height and Weight - While measuring, if the number is X.1 - X.4 round down; X.5 or greater round up

☐☐ inches	A. **Height** (in inches). Record most recent height measure since admission
☐☐☐ pounds	B. **Weight** (in pounds). Base weight on most recent measure in last 30 days; measure weight consistently, according to standard facility practice (e.g., in a.m. after voiding, before meal, with shoes off, etc.)

K0300. Weight Loss

Enter Code ☐	Loss of 5% or more in the last month or loss of 10% or more in last 6 months 0. **No** or unknown 1. **Yes, on** physician-prescribed weight-loss regimen 2. **Yes, not on** physician-prescribed weight-loss regimen

K0500. Nutritional Approaches

↓ **Check all that apply**

☐	A. **Parenteral/IV feeding**
☐	B. **Feeding tube** - nasogastric or abdominal (PEG)
☐	C. **Mechanically altered diet** - require change in texture of food or liquids (e.g., pureed food, thickened liquids)
☐	D. **Therapeutic diet** (e.g., low salt, diabetic, low cholesterol)
☐	Z. **None of the above**

K0700. Percent Intake by Artificial Route - Complete K0700 only if K0500A or K0500B is checked

Enter Code ☐	A. **Proportion of total calories the resident received through parenteral or tube feeding** 1. **25% or less** 2. **26-50%** 3. **51% or more**
Enter Code ☐	B. **Average fluid intake per day by IV or tube feeding** 1. **500 cc/day or less** 2. **501 cc/day or more**

Section L	**Oral/Dental Status**

L0200. Dental

↓ **Check all that apply**

☐	A. **Broken or loosely fitting full or partial denture** (chipped, cracked, uncleanable, or loose)
☐	B. **No natural teeth or tooth fragment(s)** (edentulous)
☐	C. **Abnormal mouth tissue** (ulcers, masses, oral lesions, including under denture or partial if one is worn)
☐	D. **Obvious or likely cavity or broken natural teeth**
☐	E. **Inflamed or bleeding gums or loose natural teeth**
☐	F. **Mouth or facial pain, discomfort or difficulty with chewing**
☐	G. **Unable to examine**
☐	Z. **None of the above were present**

Resident _____ Identifier _____ Date _____

Section M Skin Conditions

Report based on highest stage of existing ulcer(s) at its worst; do not "reverse" stage

M0100. Determination of Pressure Ulcer Risk

↓ Check all that apply

- ☐ **A.** Resident has a stage 1 or greater, a scar over bony prominence, or a non-removable dressing/device
- ☐ **B.** Formal assessment instrument/tool (e.g., Braden, Norton, or other)
- ☐ **C.** Clinical assessment
- ☐ **Z.** None of the above

M0150. Risk of Pressure Ulcers

Enter Code ☐ Is this resident at risk of developing pressure ulcers?
- 0. **No**
- 1. **Yes**

M0210. Unhealed Pressure Ulcer(s)

Enter Code ☐ Does this resident have one or more unhealed pressure ulcer(s) at Stage 1 or higher?
- 0. **No** → Skip to M0900, Healed Pressure Ulcers
- 1. **Yes** → Continue to M0300, Current Number of Unhealed (non-epithelialized) Pressure Ulcers at Each Stage

M0300. Current Number of Unhealed (non-epithelialized) **Pressure Ulcers at Each Stage**

Enter Number ☐
A. Number of Stage 1 pressure ulcers
Stage 1: Intact skin with non-blanchable redness of a localized area usually over a bony prominence. Darkly pigmented skin may not have a visible blanching; in dark skin tones only it may appear with persistent blue or purple hues

B. Stage 2: Partial thickness loss of dermis presenting as a shallow open ulcer with a red or pink wound bed, without slough. May also present as an intact or open/ruptured blister

Enter Number ☐
1. Number of Stage 2 pressure ulcers - If 0 → Skip to M0300C, Stage 3

Enter Number ☐
2. Number of these Stage 2 pressure ulcers that were present upon admission/reentry - enter how many were noted at the time of admission

3. Date of oldest Stage 2 pressure ulcer - Enter dashes if date is unknown:

☐☐ – ☐☐ – ☐☐☐☐
Month   Day   Year

C. Stage 3: Full thickness tissue loss. Subcutaneous fat may be visible but bone, tendon or muscle is not exposed. Slough may be present but does not obscure the depth of tissue loss. May include undermining and tunneling

Enter Number ☐
1. Number of Stage 3 pressure ulcers - If 0 → Skip to M0300D, Stage 4

Enter Number ☐
2. Number of these Stage 3 pressure ulcers that were present upon admission/reentry - enter how many were noted at the time of admission

D. Stage 4: Full thickness tissue loss with exposed bone, tendon or muscle. Slough or eschar may be present on some parts of the wound bed. Often includes undermining and tunneling

Enter Number ☐
1. Number of Stage 4 pressure ulcers - If 0 → Skip to M0300E, Unstageable: Non-removable dressing

Enter Number ☐
2. Number of these Stage 4 pressure ulcers that were present upon admission/reentry - enter how many were noted at the time of admission

M0300 continued on next page

Resident _____   Identifier _____   Date _____

Section M   Skin Conditions

M0300. Current Number of Unhealed (non-epithelialized) Pressure Ulcers at Each Stage - Continued

E. Unstageable - Non-removable dressing: Known but not stageable due to non-removable dressing/device

Enter Number ☐
1. **Number of unstageable pressure ulcers due to non-removable dressing/device** - If 0 → Skip to M0300F, Unstageable: Slough and/or eschar

Enter Number ☐
2. **Number of these unstageable pressure ulcers that were present upon admission/reentry** - enter how many were noted at the time of admission

F. Unstageable - Slough and/or eschar: Known but not stageable due to coverage of wound bed by slough and/or eschar

Enter Number ☐
1. **Number of unstageable pressure ulcers due to coverage of wound bed by slough and/or eschar** - If 0 → Skip to M0300G, Unstageable: Deep tissue

Enter Number ☐
2. **Number of these unstageable pressure ulcers that were present upon admission/reentry** - enter how many were noted at the time of admission

G. Unstageable - Deep tissue: Suspected deep tissue injury in evolution

Enter Number ☐
1. **Number of unstageable pressure ulcers with suspected deep tissue injury in evolution** - If 0 → Skip to M0610, Dimension of Unhealed Stage 3 or 4 Pressure Ulcers or Eschar

Enter Number ☐
2. **Number of these unstageable pressure ulcers that were present upon admission/reentry** - enter how many were noted at the time of admission

M0610. Dimensions of Unhealed Stage 3 or 4 Pressure Ulcers or Eschar
Complete only if M0300C1, M0300D1 or M0300F1 is greater than 0

If the resident has one or more unhealed (non-epithelialized) Stage 3 or 4 pressure ulcers or an unstageable pressure ulcer due to slough or eschar, identify the pressure ulcer with the largest surface area (length x width) and record in centimeters:

☐☐.☐ cm   **A. Pressure ulcer length:** Longest length from head to toe

☐☐.☐ cm   **B. Pressure ulcer width:** Widest width of the same pressure ulcer, side-to-side perpendicular (90-degree angle) to length

☐☐.☐ cm   **C. Pressure ulcer depth:** Depth of the same pressure ulcer from the visible surface to the deepest area (if depth is unknown, enter a dash in each box)

M0700. Most Severe Tissue Type for Any Pressure Ulcer

Enter Code ☐
Select the best description of the most severe type of tissue present in any pressure ulcer bed
1. **Epithelial tissue** - new skin growing in superficial ulcer. It can be light pink and shiny, even in persons with darkly pigmented skin
2. **Granulation tissue** - pink or red tissue with shiny, moist, granular appearance
3. **Slough** - yellow or white tissue that adheres to the ulcer bed in strings or thick clumps, or is mucinous
4. **Necrotic tissue (Eschar)** - black, brown, or tan tissue that adheres firmly to the wound bed or ulcer edges, may be softer or harder than surrounding skin

M0800. Worsening in Pressure Ulcer Status Since Prior Assessment (OBRA, PPS, or Discharge)
Complete only if A0310E = 0

Indicate the number of current pressure ulcers that were **not present or were at a lesser stage** on prior assessment (OBRA, PPS, or Discharge). If no current pressure ulcer at a given stage, enter 0

Enter Number ☐   **A. Stage 2**

Enter Number ☐   **B. Stage 3**

Enter Number ☐   **C. Stage 4**

MDS 3.0 Item Listing-Version 1.00.2 10/01/2010

Resident _____   Identifier _____   Date _____

Section M   Skin Conditions

M0900. Healed Pressure Ulcers
Complete only if A0310E = 0

Enter Code	A. Were pressure ulcers present on the prior assessment (OBRA, PPS, or Discharge)?
☐	0. No → Skip to M1030, Number of Venous and Arterial Ulcers 1. Yes → Continue to M0900B, Stage 2

Indicate the number of pressure ulcers that were noted on the prior assessment (OBRA, PPS, or Discharge) that have completely closed (resurfaced with epithelium). If no healed pressure ulcer at a given stage since the prior assessment (OBRA, PPS, or Discharge), enter 0

Enter Number	
☐	B. Stage 2

Enter Number	
☐	C. Stage 3

Enter Number	
☐	D. Stage 4

M1030. Number of Venous and Arterial Ulcers

Enter Number	
☐	Enter the total number of venous and arterial ulcers present

M1040. Other Ulcers, Wounds and Skin Problems

↓ Check all that apply

Foot Problems

- ☐ A. Infection of the foot (e.g., cellulitis, purulent drainage)
- ☐ B. Diabetic foot ulcer(s)
- ☐ C. Other open lesion(s) on the foot

Other Problems

- ☐ D. Open lesion(s) other than ulcers, rashes, cuts (e.g., cancer lesion)
- ☐ E. Surgical wound(s)
- ☐ F. Burn(s) (second or third degree)

None of the Above

- ☐ Z. None of the above were present

M1200. Skin and Ulcer Treatments

↓ Check all that apply

- ☐ A. Pressure reducing device for chair
- ☐ B. Pressure reducing device for bed
- ☐ C. Turning/repositioning program
- ☐ D. Nutrition or hydration intervention to manage skin problems
- ☐ E. Ulcer care
- ☐ F. Surgical wound care
- ☐ G. Application of nonsurgical dressings (with or without topical medications) other than to feet
- ☐ H. Applications of ointments/medications other than to feet
- ☐ I. Application of dressings to feet (with or without topical medications)
- ☐ Z. None of the above were provided

Resident _____   Identifier _____   Date _____

Section N	Medications

N0300. Injections

Enter Days	
☐	**Record the number of days that injections of any type** were received during the last 7 days or since admission/reentry if less than 7 days. If 0 → Skip to N0400, Medications Received

N0350. Insulin

Enter Days	
☐	**A. Insulin injections - Record the number of days that insulin injections** were received during the last 7 days or since admission/reentry if less than 7 days
Enter Days	
☐	**B. Orders for insulin - Record the number of days the physician (or authorized assistant or practitioner) changed the resident's insulin orders** during the last 7 days or since admission/reentry if less than 7 days

N0400. Medications Received

↓ Check all medications the resident received at any time during the last 7 days or since admission/reentry if less than 7 days

☐	**A. Antipsychotic**
☐	**B. Antianxiety**
☐	**C. Antidepressant**
☐	**D. Hypnotic**
☐	**E. Anticoagulant** (warfarin, heparin, or low-molecular weight heparin)
☐	**F. Antibiotic**
☐	**G. Diuretic**
☐	**Z. None of the above were received**

Resident _____   Identifier _____   Date _____

Section O — Special Treatments, Procedures, and Programs

O0100. Special Treatments, Procedures, and Programs

Check all of the following treatments, procedures, and programs that were performed during the last **14 days**

	1. While NOT a Resident	2. While a Resident
1. While NOT a Resident Performed *while NOT a resident* of this facility and within the *last 14 days*. Only check column 1 If resident entered (admission or reentry) IN THE LAST 14 DAYS. If resident last entered 14 or more days ago, leave column 1 blank **2. While a Resident** Performed *while a resident* of this facility and within the *last 14 days*	↓ Check all that apply ↓	
Cancer Treatments		
A. Chemotherapy	☐	☐
B. Radiation	☐	☐
Respiratory Treatments		
C. Oxygen therapy	☐	☐
D. Suctioning	☐	☐
E. Tracheostomy care	☐	☐
F. Ventilator or respirator	☐	☐
G. BiPAP/CPAP	☐	☐
Other		
H. IV medications	☐	☐
I. Transfusions	☐	☐
J. Dialysis	☐	☐
K. Hospice care	☐	☐
L. Respite care	▉	☐
M. Isolation or quarantine for active infectious disease (does not include standard body/fluid precautions)	☐	☐
None of the Above		
Z. None of the above	☐	☐

O0250. Influenza Vaccine - Refer to current version of RAI manual for current flu season and reporting period

Enter Code ☐   **A.** Did the **resident receive the Influenza vaccine in this facility** for this year's Influenza season?
  0. **No** → Skip to O0250C, If Influenza vaccine not received, state reason
  1. **Yes** → Continue to O0250B, Date vaccine received

B. Date vaccine received → Complete date and skip to O0300A, Is the resident's Pneumococcal vaccination up to date?

☐☐ – ☐☐ – ☐☐☐☐
Month   Day   Year

Enter Code ☐   **C.** If Influenza vaccine not received, state reason:
  1. **Resident not in facility** during this year's flu season
  2. **Received outside of this facility**
  3. **Not eligible** - medical contraindication
  4. **Offered and declined**
  5. **Not offered**
  6. **Inability to obtain vaccine** due to a declared shortage
  9. **None of the above**

O0300. Pneumococcal Vaccine

Enter Code ☐   **A.** Is the resident's Pneumococcal vaccination up to date?
  0. **No** → Continue to O0300B, If Pneumococcal vaccine not received, state reason
  1. **Yes** → Skip to O0400, Therapies

Enter Code ☐   **B.** If Pneumococcal vaccine not received, state reason:
  1. **Not eligible** - medical contraindication
  2. **Offered and declined**
  3. **Not offered**

MDS 3.0 Item Listing-Version 1.00.2 10/01/2010

Resident _____   Identifier _____   Date _____

Section O	**Special Treatments, Procedures, and Programs**

O0400. Therapies

A. Speech-Language Pathology and Audiology Services

Enter Number of Minutes [ ][ ][ ][ ]

1. **Individual minutes** - record the total number of minutes this therapy was administered to the resident **individually** in the last 7 days

Enter Number of Minutes [ ][ ][ ][ ]

2. **Concurrent minutes** - record the total number of minutes this therapy was administered to the resident **concurrently with one other resident** in the last 7 days

Enter Number of Minutes [ ][ ][ ][ ]

3. **Group minutes** - record the total number of minutes this therapy was administered to the resident as **part of a group of residents** in the last 7 days

If the sum of individual, concurrent, and group minutes is zero, ➞ skip to O0400B, Occupational Therapy

Enter Number of Days [ ]

4. **Days** - record the **number of days** this therapy was administered for **at least 15 minutes** a day in the last 7 days

5. **Therapy start date** - record the date the most recent therapy regimen (since the most recent entry) started

[ ][ ] – [ ][ ] – [ ][ ][ ][ ]
Month   Day   Year

6. **Therapy end date** - record the date the most recent therapy regimen (since the most recent entry) ended - enter dashes if therapy is ongoing

[ ][ ] – [ ][ ] – [ ][ ][ ][ ]
Month   Day   Year

B. Occupational Therapy

Enter Number of Minutes [ ][ ][ ][ ]

1. **Individual minutes** - record the total number of minutes this therapy was administered to the resident **individually** in the last 7 days

Enter Number of Minutes [ ][ ][ ][ ]

2. **Concurrent minutes** - record the total number of minutes this therapy was administered to the resident **concurrently with one other resident** in the last 7 days

Enter Number of Minutes [ ][ ][ ][ ]

3. **Group minutes** - record the total number of minutes this therapy was administered to the resident as **part of a group of residents** in the last 7 days

If the sum of individual, concurrent, and group minutes is zero, ➞ skip to O0400C, Physical Therapy

Enter Number of Days [ ]

4. **Days** - record the **number of days** this therapy was administered for **at least 15 minutes** a day in the last 7 days

5. **Therapy start date** - record the date the most recent therapy regimen (since the most recent entry) started

[ ][ ] – [ ][ ] – [ ][ ][ ][ ]
Month   Day   Year

6. **Therapy end date** - record the date the most recent therapy regimen (since the most recent entry) ended - enter dashes if therapy is ongoing

[ ][ ] – [ ][ ] – [ ][ ][ ][ ]
Month   Day   Year

C. Physical Therapy

Enter Number of Minutes [ ][ ][ ][ ]

1. **Individual minutes** - record the total number of minutes this therapy was administered to the resident **individually** in the last 7 days

Enter Number of Minutes [ ][ ][ ][ ]

2. **Concurrent minutes** - record the total number of minutes this therapy was administered to the resident **concurrently with one other resident** in the last 7 days

Enter Number of Minutes [ ][ ][ ][ ]

3. **Group minutes** - record the total number of minutes this therapy was administered to the resident as **part of a group of residents** in the last 7 days

If the sum of individual, concurrent, and group minutes is zero, ➞ skip to O0400D, Respiratory Therapy

Enter Number of Days [ ]

4. **Days** - record the **number of days** this therapy was administered for **at least 15 minutes** a day in the last 7 days

5. **Therapy start date** - record the date the most recent therapy regimen (since the most recent entry) started

[ ][ ] – [ ][ ] – [ ][ ][ ][ ]
Month   Day   Year

6. **Therapy end date** - record the date the most recent therapy regimen (since the most recent entry) ended - enter dashes if therapy is ongoing

[ ][ ] – [ ][ ] – [ ][ ][ ][ ]
Month   Day   Year

O0400 continued on next page

Resident _____ Identifier _____ Date _____

Section O	Special Treatments, Procedures, and Programs

O0400. Therapies - Continued

D. Respiratory Therapy

Enter Number of Minutes

1. **Total minutes** - record the total number of minutes this therapy was administered to the resident in the last 7 days
   If zero, → skip to O0400E, Psychological Therapy

Enter Number of Days

2. **Days** - record the **number of days** this therapy was administered for **at least 15 minutes** a day in the last 7 days

E. Psychological Therapy (by any licensed mental health professional)

Enter Number of Minutes

1. **Total minutes** - record the total number of minutes this therapy was administered to the resident in the last 7 days
   If zero, → skip to O0400F, Recreational Therapy

Enter Number of Days

2. **Days** - record the **number of days** this therapy was administered for **at least 15 minutes** a day in the last 7 days

F. Recreational Therapy (includes recreational and music therapy)

Enter Number of Minutes

1. **Total minutes** - record the total number of minutes this therapy was administered to the resident in the last 7 days
   If zero, → skip to O0500, Restorative Nursing Programs

Enter Number of Days

2. **Days** - record the **number of days** this therapy was administered for **at least 15 minutes** a day in the last 7 days

O0500. Restorative Nursing Programs

Record the **number of days** each of the following restorative programs was performed (for at least 15 minutes a day) in the last 7 calendar days (enter 0 if none or less than 15 minutes daily)

Number of Days	Technique
	A. Range of motion (passive)
	B. Range of motion (active)
	C. Splint or brace assistance

Number of Days	Training and Skill Practice In:
	D. Bed mobility
	E. Transfer
	F. Walking
	G. Dressing and/or grooming
	H. Eating and/or swallowing
	I. Amputation/prostheses care
	J. Communication

O0600. Physician Examinations

Enter Days

Over the last 14 days, **on how many days did the physician (or authorized assistant or practitioner) examine the resident?**

O0700. Physician Orders

Enter Days

Over the last 14 days, **on how many days did the physician (or authorized assistant or practitioner) change the resident's orders?**

MDS 3.0 Item Listing-Version 1.00.2 10/01/2010

Resident _____   Identifier _____   Date _____

Section P	**Restraints**

P0100. Physical Restraints

Physical restraints are any manual method or physical or mechanical device, material or equipment attached or adjacent to the resident's body that the individual cannot remove easily which restricts freedom of movement or normal access to one's body

	↓ **Enter Codes in Boxes**
	Used in Bed
	☐ A. Bed rail
	☐ B. Trunk restraint
	☐ C. Limb restraint
Coding: 0. **Not used** 1. **Used less than daily** 2. **Used daily**	☐ D. Other
	Used in Chair or Out of Bed
	☐ E. Trunk restraint
	☐ F. Limb restraint
	☐ G. Chair prevents rising
	☐ H. Other

Resident _____   Identifier _____   Date _____

Section Q — Participation in Assessment and Goal Setting

Q0100. Participation in Assessment

Enter Code	**A. Resident participated in assessment** 0. **No** 1. **Yes**
Enter Code	**B. Family or significant other participated in assessment** 0. **No** 1. **Yes** 9. **No family or significant other**
Enter Code	**C. Guardian or legally authorized representative participated in assessment** 0. **No** 1. **Yes** 9. **No guardian or legally authorized representative**

Q0300. Resident's Overall Expectation

Complete only if A0310E = 1

Enter Code	**A. Resident's overall goal established during assessment process** 1. Expects to be **discharged to the community** 2. Expects to **remain in this facility** 3. Expects to be **discharged to another facility/institution** 9. **Unknown or uncertain**
Enter Code	**B. Indicate information source for Q0300A** 1. **Resident** 2. If not resident, then **family or significant other** 3. If not resident, family, or significant other, then **guardian or legally authorized representative** 9. **None of the above**

Q0400. Discharge Plan

Enter Code	**A. Is there an active discharge plan in place for the resident to return to the community?** 0. **No** 1. **Yes** → Skip to Q0600, Referral
Enter Code	**B. What determination was made by the resident and the care planning team regarding discharge to the community?** 0. **Determination not made** 1. **Discharge to community determined to be feasible** → Skip to Q0600, Referral 2. **Discharge to community determined to be not feasible** → Skip to next active section (V or X)

Q0500. Return to Community

Enter Code	**A. Has the resident been asked about returning to the community?** 0. **No** 1. **Yes** - previous response was **"no"** 2. **Yes** - previous response was **"yes"** → Skip to Q0600, Referral 3. **Yes** - previous response was **"unknown"**
Enter Code	**B. Ask the resident** (or family or significant other if resident is unable to respond): **"Do you want to talk to someone about the possibility of returning to the community?"** 0. **No** 1. **Yes** 9. **Unknown or uncertain**

Q0600. Referral

Enter Code	**Has a referral been made to the local contact agency?** 0. **No** - determination has been made by the resident and the care planning team that contact is not required 1. **No** - referral not made 2. **Yes**

Resident _____   Identifier _____   Date _____

| **Section V** | **Care Area Assessment (CAA) Summary** |

V0100. Items From the Most Recent Prior OBRA or Scheduled PPS Assessment

Complete only if A0310E = 0 and if the following is true for the **prior assessment**: A0310A = 01- 06 or A0310B = 01- 06

<table>
<tr>
<td>Enter Code
☐☐</td>
<td>
A. Prior Assessment Federal OBRA Reason for Assessment (A0310A value from prior assessment)
   01. Admission assessment (required by day 14)
   02. Quarterly review assessment
   03. Annual assessment
   04. Significant change in status assessment
   05. Significant correction to prior comprehensive assessment
   06. Significant correction to prior quarterly assessment
   99. Not OBRA required assessment
</td>
</tr>
<tr>
<td>Enter Code
☐☐</td>
<td>
B. Prior Assessment PPS Reason for Assessment (A0310B value from prior assessment)
   01. 5-day scheduled assessment
   02. 14-day scheduled assessment
   03. 30-day scheduled assessment
   04. 60-day scheduled assessment
   05. 90-day scheduled assessment
   06. Readmission/return assessment
   07. Unscheduled assessment used for PPS (OMRA, significant or clinical change, or significant correction assessment)
   99. Not PPS assessment
</td>
</tr>
<tr>
<td></td>
<td>
C. Prior Assessment Reference Date (A2300 value from prior assessment)
  ☐☐ – ☐☐ – ☐☐☐☐
  Month   Day   Year
</td>
</tr>
<tr>
<td>Enter Score
☐☐</td>
<td>D. Prior Assessment Brief Interview for Mental Status (BIMS) Summary Score (C0500 value from prior assessment)</td>
</tr>
<tr>
<td>Enter Score
☐☐</td>
<td>E. Prior Assessment Resident Mood Interview (PHQ-9©) Total Severity Score (D0300 value from prior assessment)</td>
</tr>
<tr>
<td>Enter Score
☐☐</td>
<td>F. Prior Assessment Staff Assessment of Resident Mood (PHQ-9-OV) Total Severity Score (D0600 value from prior assessment)</td>
</tr>
</table>

Resident _____ Identifier _____ Date _____

Section V Care Area Assessment (CAA) Summary

V0200. CAAs and Care Planning

1. Check column A if Care Area is triggered.
2. For each triggered Care Area, indicate whether a new care plan, care plan revision, or continuation of current care plan is necessary to address the problem(s) identified in your assessment of the care area. The <u>Addressed in Care Plan</u> column must be completed within 7 days of completing the RAI (MDS and CAA(s)). Check column B if the triggered care area is addressed in the care plan.
3. Indicate in the <u>Location and Date of CAA Information</u> column where information related to the CAA can be found. CAA documentation should include information on the complicating factors, risks, and any referrals for this resident for this care area.

A. CAA Results

Care Area	A. Care Area Triggered	B. Addressed in Care Plan	Location and Date of CAA Information
	↓ Check all that apply ↓		
01. Delirium	☐	☐	
02. Cognitive Loss/Dementia	☐	☐	
03. Visual Function	☐	☐	
04. Communication	☐	☐	
05. ADL Functional/Rehabilitation Potential	☐	☐	
06. Urinary Incontinence and Indwelling Catheter	☐	☐	
07. Psychosocial Well-Being	☐	☐	
08. Mood State	☐	☐	
09. Behavioral Symptoms	☐	☐	
10. Activities	☐	☐	
11. Falls	☐	☐	
12. Nutritional Status	☐	☐	
13. Feeding Tube	☐	☐	
14. Dehydration/Fluid Maintenance	☐	☐	
15. Dental Care	☐	☐	
16. Pressure Ulcer	☐	☐	
17. Psychotropic Drug Use	☐	☐	
18. Physical Restraints	☐	☐	
19. Pain	☐	☐	
20. Return to Community Referral	☐	☐	

B. Signature of RN Coordinator for CAA Process and Date Signed

1. Signature

2. Date ☐☐ - ☐☐ - ☐☐☐☐
   Month   Day   Year

C. Signature of Person Completing Care Plan and Date Signed

1. Signature

2. Date ☐☐ - ☐☐ - ☐☐☐☐
   Month   Day   Year

MDS 3.0 Item Listing-Version 1.00.2 10/01/2010

APPENDIX C

USEFUL SPANISH VOCABULARY AND PHRASES*

ENGLISH	SPANISH	ENGLISH	SPANISH
A bowel movement.	Hacer del baño. (Ah-sehr dehl bah-nyoh) evacuación (eh-bah-coo-ah-see-ohn)	Are you sleepy?	¿Tiene sueño? (Tee-eh-neh soo-eh-nyoh)
A glass of juice?	¿Un vaso de jugo? (oon bah-soh deh hoo-goh)	Are you thirsty?	¿Tiene sed? (Tee-eh-neh sehd)
A glass of water?	¿Un vaso de agua? (oon bah-soh deh ah-goo-ah)	asthma	asma (ahs-mah)
A nurse will see you.	Una enfermera la atenderá. (Ooh-nah ehn-fehr-meh-rah lah ah-tehn-deh-rah)	at eleven thirty.	a las once y media. (ah lahs ohn-seh ee meh-dee-ah)
A virus known as HIV . . .	El virus causal del SIDA se conoce como VIH . . . (Ehl bee-roos kah-oo-sahl dehl see-dah seh koh-noh- seh koh-moh beh-ee-ah- cheh [VIH])	at five PM.	a las cinco de la tarde. (ah lahs seen-koh deh lah tahr-deh)
abdomen	abdomen (ahb-doh-mehn)	at seven am.	a las siete de la mañana. (ah lahs see-eh-teh deh lah mah-nyah-nah)
Activities are part of the plan.	Las actividades son parte del plan. (Lahs ahk-tee-bee-dah-dehs sohn pahr-teh dehl plahn)	At what time do you get up?	¿A qué hora se levanta? (Ah keh oh-rah seh leh-bahn-tah)
After meals.	Después de las comidas. (Dehs-poo-ehs deh lahs koh-mee-dahs)	At what time do you go to bed?	¿A qué hora se acuesta? (Ah keh oh-rah seh ah-koo-ehs-tah)
Among the vegetables that we serve are:	Entre los vegetales que servimos hay: (Ehn-treh lohs beh-heh-tah-lehs keh sehr-bee-mohs ah-ee)	At what time do you go to sleep?	¿A qué hora se acuesta a dormir? (Ah keh oh-rah seh ah-koo-ehs-tah ah dohr-meer)
anesthesia	anestesia (ah-nehs-teh-see-ah)	aunt	tía (tee-ah)
apple	manzana (mahn-sah-nah)	backward	Atrás. (Ah-trahs)
Are you cold?	¿Tiene frío? (Tee-eh-neh free-oh)	bacteria	bacteria (bahk-teh-ree-ah)
Are you comfortable?	¿Está cómoda? (Ehs tah koh-moh-dah)	baked chicken	pollo asado (poh-yoh ah-sah-doh)
Are you constipated?	¿Está estreñida? (Ehs-tah ehs-treh-nyee-dah)	baked potatoes	papas asadas (pah-pahs ah-sah-dahs)
Are you dizzy?	¿Tiene mareos? (Tee-eh-neh mah-reh-ohs)	beans	frijoles/habas (free-hoh-lehs/ah-bahs)
Are you having problems breathing?	¿Tiene problemas al respirar? (Tee-eh-neh proh-bleh-mahs ahl rehs-pee-rahr)	beef	res (rehs)
Are you hot?	¿Tiene calor? (tee-eh-neh kah-lohr)	Bend it.	Dóblala. (Doh-blah-lah)
Are you hungry?	¿Tiene hambre? (Tee-eh-neh ahm-breh)	Bend the wrist.	Dobla la muñeca. (Doh-blah lah moo-nyeh-kah)
Are you hurting?	¿Tiene dolor? (Tee-eh-neh doh-lohr)	Bend your elbow.	Dobla el codo. (doh-blah ehl koh-doh)
Are you nauseated?	¿Está nauseada?/¿Tiene náuseas? (Ehs-tah nah-oo-seh-ah-dah/Tee-eh-neh nah-oo-seh-ahs)	Bend your hip.	Dobla la cadera. (Doh-blah lah kah-deh-rah)
		Bend your toes.	Dobla los dedos (del pie). (Doh-blah lohs deh-dohs [dehl pee-eh]
Are you okay?	¿Está bien?/¿Se siente bien? (Ehs-tah bee-ehn/ Seh see-ehn-teh bee-ehn)	black	negro (neh-groh)
		blue	azul (ah-sool)
		bradycardia	bradicardia (brah-dee-kahr-dee-ah)
		breaded	empanizado (ehm-pah-nee-sah-doh)

*This appendix is presented for your convenience. Please note: This listing does not include all terms or address all chapters.
Translations taken from Joyce EV, Villanueva ME: *Say it in Spanish: a guide for health care professionals,* ed 3, St Louis, 2004, Saunders.

ENGLISH	SPANISH
breast	pechuga (peh-choo-gah)
breast-feeding?	¿tomando pecho? (toh-mahn-doh peh-choh)
Breathe in.	Respire. (Rehs-pee-reh)
Breathe out.	Saque el aire. (Sah-keh ehl ah-ee-reh)
broiled fish	pescado al horno (pehs-kah-doh ahl ohr-noh)
brother	hermano (ehr-mah-noh)
brother-in-law	cuñado (koo-nyah-doh)
Call if you need help.	Llame si necesita ayuda. (Yah-meh see neh-seh-see-tah ah-yoo-dah)
cancer	cáncer (kahn-sehr)
candy	dulces (dool-sehs)
cardiac	cardíaco (kahr-dee-ah-koh)
Change into the gown.	Póngase esta bata. (Phn-gah-seh ehs-tah bah-tah)
chemotherapy	quimioterapia (kee-mee-oh-teh-rah-pee-ah)
chicken	pollo (poh-yoh)
children	hijos (eeh-hohs)
chocolate	chocolate (choh-koh-lah-teh)
chops	chuletas (choo-leh-tahs)
claustrophobia	claustrofobia (klah-oos-troh-foh-bee-ah)
clear	claro (klah-roh)
Close it.	Ciérrala. (See-eh-rah-lah)
coffee	café (kah-feh)
coma	coma (koh-mah)
comatose	comatoso (koh-mah-toh-soh)
communication	comunicación (koh-moo-nee-kah-see-ohn)
cookies	galletas (gah-yeh-tahs)
corn	maíz/elote (mah-ees/eh-loh-teh)
corn flakes	hojitas de maíz/corn flakes (oh-hee-tahs de mah-ees/hohrn fleh-ee-ks)
Cough!	¡Tosa! (Toh-sah)
Cough deeply.	Tosa más fuerte. (Toh-sah mahs foo-ehr-teh)
Cough harder!	¡Tosa más fuerte! (Toh-sah mahs foo-ehr-teh)
cousin (female)	prima (pree-mah)

ENGLISH	SPANISH
cousin (male)	primo (pree-moh)
cousins	primos (pree-mohs)
cream of wheat	crema de trigo (kreh-mah deh tree-goh)
dad	papá (pah-pah)
daughter	hija (ee-hah)
decaffeinated	descafeinado (dehs-kah-feh-ee-nah-doh)
dehydration	deshidratación (deh-see-drah-tah-see-ohn)
delirious	delirio (deh-lee-ree-oh)
Dial 9, wait for the tone, then dial the number you want to call.	Marque el nueve, espere el tono, luego marque el número que quiera llamar. (mahr-keh ehl noo-eh-beh, ehs-peh-reh ehl toh-noh, loo-eh-doh mahr-key ehl noo-meh roh keh kee-eh-rah yah-mahr)
Did you bring a hearing aid?	¿Trajo un aparato para oír? (Trah-hoh oon ah-pah-rah-toh pah-rah oo-eer)
Did you bring an artificial eye?	¿Trajo un ojo artificial? (Trah-hoh oon prohs-teh tee-koh)
Did you bring an artificial limb?	¿Trajo un prostético? (Trah-hoh oon oh-hoh ahr-tee-fee-see-ahl)
Did you bring contact lenses?	¿Trajo lentes de contacto? (Trah-hoh lehn-tehs deh kohn-tahk-toh)
Did you bring dentures?	¿Trajo una dentadura postiza? (Trah-hoh oon-ah dehn-tah-doo-rah pohs-tee-sah)
Did you bring glasses?	¿Trajo anteojos/lentes? (Trah-hoh ahn-teh-oh-hohs/lehn-tehs)
Did you bring jewelry?/cash?	¿Trajo joyas?/dinero? (Trah-hoh hoh-yahs/dee-neh-roh)
Did you fall?	¿Se cayó? (Seh kah-yoh)
Difficulty in swallowing . . .	Dificultad al tragar . . . (Dee-fee-kool-tahd ahl-trah-gahr)
Do not drive!	¡No maneje/conduzca! (Noh mah-neh-heh/ kohn-doos-kah)
Do not operate machinery!	¡No maneje/opere una máquina/maquinaria! (Noh mah-neh-heh/oh-peh- reh oo-nah mah-kee-nah/ah-kee-nah-ree-ah)
Do not put on plastic pants!	¡No le ponga calzones de plástico! (Noh lch pohn-gah kahl-sohn-ehs deh plahs-tee-koh)
Do you feel dizzy?	¿Se siente mareada? (Seh see-ehn-tch mah-rch-ah-dah)
Do you feel nauseated?	¿Se siente nauseada? (Seh see-ehn-teh nah-oo- seh-ah-dah)
Do you feel weak?	¿Se siente débil? (Seh see-ehn-teh deh-beel)

ENGLISH	SPANISH	ENGLISH	SPANISH
Do you have any symptoms: nausea, dizziness, other unusual feelings?	¿Tiene algún síntoma como náuseas, vértigo, otra sensación rara? (Tee-eh-neh ahl-goon seen-toh-mah koh-moh nah-oo-seh-ahs, behr-tee-goh, oh-trah sehn-sah-see-ohn rah-rah)	Do you want a glass of water?	¿Quiere un vaso con agua? (Kee-eh-reh oon bah-soh kohn ah-goo ah)
Do you have chest pain?	¿Tiene dolor en el pecho? (Tee-eh-neh doh-lohr ehn ehl peh-choh)	Do you want something to drink?	¿Quiere algo de tomar/beber? (Kee-eh-reh ahl-goh deh toh-mahr/beh-behr)
Do you have diarrhea?	¿Tiene diarrea? (Tee-eh-neh dee-ah-reh-ah)	Do you want the bedpan?	¿Quiere el pato/el bacín? (Kee-eh-reh ehl pah-toh/ehl bah-seen)
Do you have dizzy spells?	¿Tiene mareos? (Tee-eh-neh mah-reh-ohs)	Do you want to have a bowel movement?	¿Quiere evacuar?¿Quiere obrar? (Kee-eh-reh eh-bah-koo-ahr/Kee-eh-reh oh-brahr)
Do you have pain?	¿Tiene dolor? (Tee-eh-neh doh-lohr)	Do you want to pass urine?	¿Quiere orinar? (Kee-eh-reh oh-ree-nahr)
Do you have problems with starting to urinate?	¿Tiene dificultad para empezar a orinar? (Tee-eh-neh dee-fee-kool-tahd pah-rah ehm-peh-sahr ah oh-ree-nahr)	Do you want water?	¿Quiere agua? (Kee-eh-reh ah-goo-ah)
		Do you want:	¿Quiere: (Kee-eh-reh)
Do you have problems with your teeth?	¿Tiene problemas con los dientes? (Tee-eh-nehs proh-bleh-mahs kohn lohs dee-ehn-tehs)	Do you wear glasses?	¿Usa anteojos/lentes? (Oo-sahs ahn-teh-ohhohs/ lehn-tehs)
Do you have vision problems?	¿Tiene problemas con la visión? (Tee-eh-nehs proh-bleh-mahs kohn lah bee-see-ohn)	Do you wish to have a bowel movement?	¿Quiere evacuar/hacer del baño? (Kee-eh-reh eh-bah-koo-ahr/ ah-sehr dehl bah-nyoh)
Do you know the day?	¿Qué día es hoy? (Keh dee-ah ehs oh-ee)	Does he cry a lot?	¿Llora mucho? (Yoh-rah moo-choh)
Do you know where we are?	¿Sabe dónde está? (Sah-beh dohn-deh ehs-tah)	Does he/she have: fever/ diarrhea/colic?	¿Tiene: fiebre/diarrea/cólico? (Tee-eh-neh: fee-eh-breh/dee-ah-rreh-ah/ koh-lee-koh)
Do you like them hot/ cold?	¿Le gustan calientes/fríos? (Leh goos-tahn kah-lee-ehn-tehs/ free-ohs)	Does it have undigested food?	¿Tiene restos de comida? (Tee-eh-neh rehs-tohs deh koh-mee-dah)
Do you need ice?	¿Necesita hielo? (Neh-seh-see-tah ee-eh-loh)	Does it hurt to breathe?	¿Le duele al respirar? (Leh doo-eh-leh ahl toh-sehr)
Do you need more pillows?	¿Necesita más almohadas? (Neh-seh-see-tah mahs ahl-moh-ah-dahs)	Does it hurt to cough?	¿Le duele al toser? (Leh doo-eh-leh ahl toh-sehr)
Do you need the headboard up?	¿Necesita levantar más la cabecera? (Neh-seh-see-tah leh-bahn-tahr mahs lah kah-beh-seh-rah)	Does it smell bad?	¿Huele mal? (Oo-eh-leh mahl)
		Does it still hurt?	¿Todavía le duele? (Toh-dah-bee-ah leh doo-eh-leh)
Do you sleep during the day?	¿Duerme durante el día? (Doo-ehr-meh doo-rahn-teh ehl dee-ah)	Does the pain get better if you stop and rest?	¿Se mejora el dolor si se detiene y descansa? (Seh meh-hoh-rah ehl doh-lohr see seh deh-tee-eh-neh ee dehs-kahn-sah)
Do you speak English?	¿Habla inglés? (Ah-blah een-glehs)	Does the pain move from one place to another?	¿El dolor se mueve de un lugar a otro? (Ehl doh-lohr seh moo-eh-beh deh oon loo-gahr ah oh-trah)
Do you take a special diet?	¿Toma dieta especial? (Toh-mah dee-eh-tah ehs-peh-see-ah-lehs)	Does the vomit have blood?	¿Tiene sangre el vómito? (Tee-eh-neh sahn-greh ehl boh-mee-toh)
Do you understand?	¿Comprende?/¿Entiende? (Kohm-prehn-deh/ Ehn-tee-ehn-deh)	eggs	huevos (oo-eh-bohs)
Do you wake up at night?	¿Se despierta en la noche? (Seh dehs-pee-ehr-tah ehn lah noh-chen)	embolism	embolismo (ehm-boh-lees-moh)
Do you want a cup of coffee?	¿Quiere una taza de café? (Kee-eh-reh oo-nah tah-sah deh-kah-feh)	employ	emplear (ehm-pleh-ahr)
Do you want a glass of juice?	¿Quiere un vaso con jugo? (Kee-eh-reh oon bah-soh kohn hoo-goh)	epilepsy	epilepsia (eh-peel-ehp-see-ah)

ENGLISH	SPANISH	ENGLISH	SPANISH
Every time you urinate, put it in the container.	Cada vez que orine, póngala en el frasco. (Kah-dah behs keh oh-ree-neh, pohn-gah-lah ehn ehl frahs-koh)	fruit	fruta (froo-tah)
		glaucoma	glaucoma (glah-oo-koh-mah)
Every two hours.	Cada dos horas. (Kah-dah dohs oh-rahs)	godfather	padrino (pah-dree-noh)
Every time you go to the bathroom to void, you must place the urine in the container.	Cada vez que vaya al baño a orinar, debe poner la orina en el recipiente. (Kah-dah behs keh bah-yah ahl bah-nyoh ah oh-ree-nahr, deh-beh poh-nehr lah oh-ree-nah ehn ehl reh-see-pee-ehn-teh)	godmother	madrina (mah-dree-nah)
		godparents	padrinos (pah-dree-nohs)
		Good afternoon.	Buenas tardes. (Boo-eh-nahs tahr-dehs)
Excuse me.	Con permiso. (kohn pehr-mee-soh)	Good afternoon, Miss González.	Buenas tardes, señorita González. (Boo-eh-nahs tahr-dehs, seh-nyoh-ree-tah Gohn-sah-lehs)
exercise	ejercicio (eh-hehr-see-see-oh)	Good evening.	Buenas noches. (Boo-eh-nahs noh-chehs)
Extend it.	Extiéndelia. (Ehx-tee-ehn-deh-lah)	Good luck!	¡Buena suerte! (Boo-eh-nah soo-ehr-teh)
Extend your arm.	Extiende el brazo. (Ehx-tee-ehn-deh ehl brah-soh)	Good morning.	Buenos días. (Boo-eh-nohs dee-ahs)
Extend your leg and foot.	Extiende la pierna y el pie. (Ehx-tee-ehn-deh lah pee-ehr-nah ee ehl pee-eh)	Good morning, doctor!	!Buenos días, doctor! (Boo-eh-nohs dee-ahs, dohk-tohr)
Extend your wrist.	Extiende la muñeca. (Ehx-tee-ehn-deh lah moo-nyeh-kay)	Good morning, Mrs. Ortiz!	!Buenos días, señora Ortiz! (Boo-eh-nohs dee-ahs, seh-nyo-rah ohr-tees)
father	padre (pah-dreh)	Good morning, sir.	Buenos días, señor. (Boo-eh-nohs dee-ahs, seh-nyohr)
father-in-law	suegro (soo-eh-grah)	Good!	¡Bueno! (Boo-eh-noh)
fever	fiebre (fee-eh-bray)	Good-bye!	¡Hasta luego! (Ahs-tah loo-eh-goh)
fish	pescado (pehs-kah-doh)	grandchildren	nietos (nee-eh-tohs)
Flex it.	Dóblala. (Doh-blah-lah)	grandfather	abuelo (ah-boo-eh-loh)
Flex the foot upward.	Dobla el pie hacia arriba. (Doh-blah ehl pee-eh ah-see-ah ah-ree-bah)	grandmother	abuela (ah-boo-eh-lah)
Flex your arm.	Dobla el brazo. (Doh-blah ehl brah-soh)	grandparents	abuelos (ah-boo-eh-lohs)
Flex your foot upward.	Dobla el pie para arriba. (Doh-blah ehl pee-eh pah-rah ah-ree-bah)	grape	uva (oo-bah)
For breakfast:	Para el desayuno: (Pah-rah ehl deh-sah-yoo-noh)	grapefruit	toronja (toh-rohn-hah)
for what?	¿para qué? (pah-rah keh)	great-grandparents	bisabuelos (bee-sah-boo-eh-lohs)
for whom?	¿para quién? (pah-rah kee-ehn)	green	verde (behr-deh)
Forward.	Adelante. (Ah-deh-lahn-teh)	green beans	ejotes/habichuelas (eh-hoh-tehs/ah-bee-choo-eh-lahs)
french fries	papas fritas (pah-pahs free-tahs)	hamburger	hamburguesa (ahm-boor-geh-sah)
Friday	viernes (bee-ehr-nehs)	hard-boiled	duros (doo-rohs)
fried	fritos (free-tohs)	Has the pain gotten worse or gotten better?	¿Se ha puesto el dolor peor o mejor? (Seh ah poo-ehs-toh ehl doh-lohr peh-ohr oh meh-hohr)
fried chicken	pollo frito (poh-yoh free-toh)	Have a good day!	¡Pase un buen día! (Pah-seh oon boo-ehn dee-ah)
		Have you eaten?	¿Ha comido? (Ah koh-mee-doh)

ENGLISH	SPANISH	ENGLISH	SPANISH
Have you had headaches?	¿Ha tenido dolor de cabeza? (Ah teh-nee-doh doh-lohr deh kah-beh-sah)	How often do you have the pain?	¿Con qué frecuencia tiene el dolor? (Kohn keh freh kwen see ah tee-eh-neh ehl doh-lohr)
Have you seen blood in the urine?	¿Ha visto sangre en la orina? (Ah bees-toh sahn-greh ehn lah oh-ree-nah)	How often do you urinate?	¿Con qué frecuencia orina? (Kohn keh freh kwen see ah oh-ree-nah)
Hello.	Hola (Oh-lah)	How severe is the pain?	¿Qué tan severo es el dolor? (Keh tahn seh-beh-roh ehs ehl doh-lohr)
Hello!	¡Hola! (Oh-lah)		
Hello, I'm John Goodguy.	Hola, soy John Goodguy. (Oh-lah, soh-ee John Goodguy)	husband	esposo (ehs-poh-soh)
Hello, Mrs. Mora.	Hola, señora Mora. (Oh-lah, seh-nyoh-rah Moh-rah)	I also need a urine sample.	También necesito una muestra de orina. (Tahm-bee-ehn neh-seh-see-toh oo-nah moo-ehs-trah deh oh-ree-nah)
hematoma	hematoma (eh-mah-toh-mah)		
Here is a glass of water to rinse with.	Aquí está un vaso de agua para que se enjuague. (Ah-kee-ehs-tah oon bah-soh deh ah-goo-ah pah-rah keh seh ehn-hoo-ah-geh)	I am going to ask many questions!	¡Voy a hacerle muchas preguntas! (Boy ah ah-sehr-leh moo-chahs preh-goon-tahs)
		I am going to clean your teeth.	Voy a limpiarle los dientes. (Boy ah leem-pee-ahr-leh lohs dee-ehn-tehs)
Hi!	¡Hola! (Oh-lah)	I am going to cover you.	La voy a cubrir. (Lah boy ah-koo-breer)
How are you?	¿Cómo está? (Koh-moh ehs-tah)	I am going to explain how to collect the urine.	Le voy a explicar cómo juntar la orina. (Leh boy ah ehx-plee-kahr koh-moh hoon-tahr lah oh-ree-nah)
How do you feel?	¿Cómo se siente? (Koh-moh seh see-ehn-teh)		
How do you feel now?	¿Cómo se siente ahora? (Koh-moh seh see-ehn-teh ah-oh-rah)	I am going to explain the collection of the urine.	Le voy a explicar la colección de orina. (Leh boy ah ehx-plee-kahr lah koh-lehk-see-ohn de oh-ree-nah)
How do you like the eggs fixed?	¿Cómo le gustan los huevos? (Koh-moh leh goos-tahn lohs oo-eh-bohs)		
How do you like your coffee?	¿Comó le gusta el café? (Koh-moh leh goos-tah ehl kah-feh)	I am going to give you a list.	Voy a darle una lista. (Boy ah dahr-leh oo-nah lees-tah)
		I am going to give you a tour of the floor.	Voy a darle un recorrido por el piso. (Boy ah dahr-leh oon reh-koh-ree-doh pohr ehl pee-soh)
How long?	¿Cuánto tiempo? (Koo-ahn-toh tee-ehm-poh)		
How many glasses of water do you drink?	¿Cuántos vasos de agua toma? (Koo-ahn-tohs bah-sohs de ah-goo-ah toh-mah)	I am going to help you lie down.	Voy a ayudarla a acostarse. (Boy ah ah-yoo-dahr-lah ah ah-kohs-tahr-seh)
How many hours do you sleep?	¿Cuántas horas duerme? (Koo-ahn-tahs oh Drahs doo-ehr-meh)	I am going to help you lie on the stretcher.	Voy a ayudarla a acostarse en la camilla. (Boy ah ah-yoo-dahr-lah ah ah-kohs-tahr-seh ehn lah kah-mee-yah)
How many ounces does he take?	¿Cuántas onzas toma? (Koo-ahn-tahs ohn sahs-toh-mah)		
How many times do you eat per day?	¿Cuántas veces come por día? (Koo-ahn-tahs beh-sehs koh- meh pohr dee-ah)	I am going to let you rest.	Voy a dejarla descansar. (Boy ah deh-hahr-lah dehs-kahn-sahr)
How many times does he wake up?	¿Cuántas veces se despierta? (Koo-ahn-tahs beh-sehs seh dehs-pee-ehr-tah)	I am through.	Ya terminé. (Yah tehr-mee-neh)
How many times has he vomited?	¿Cuántas veces ha vomitado? (Koo-ahn-tahs beh-sehs ah boh-mee-tah-doh)	I need to ask you some questions.	Necesito hacerle unas preguntas. (Nch-seh-see-toh ah-sehr-leh oo-nahs preh-goon-tahs)
how many?	¿cuántos? (koo-ahn-tohs)	I will ask you to void.	Le diré que orine. (Leh dee-reh keh oh-ree-neh)
How may I help you?	¿En qué puedo servirle? (Ehn keh poo-eh-doh sehr-beer-leh)	I will collect a sample of feces.	Voy a recoger una muestra de excremento. (Boy ah reh-koh-hehr oo-nah moo-ehs-trah deh ehx-kreh-mehn-toh)
how much?	¿cuánto? (koo-ahn-toh)		

ENGLISH	SPANISH
I will help you sit.	Le ayudaré a sentarse. (Leh ah-yoo-dah-reh ah sehn-tahr-seh)
I will put you on the stretcher.	Voy a ponerla en la camilla. (Boy ah poh-nher-lah ehn lah kah-mee-yah)
I will return shortly.	Regresaré en seguida. (Reh-greh-sah-reh ehn seh-ghee-dah)
I will see you tomorrow.	La veré mañana. (Lah beh-reh mah-nyah-nah)
I will show you your room.	Le mostraré su cuarto. (Leh mohs-trah-reh soo koo-ahr-tah)
I will start by taking vital signs.	Voy a empezar por tomar los signos vitales. (Boy ah ehm-peh-sahr pohr toh-mahr lohs seeg-nohs bee-tah-lehs)
I will take the radial pulse.	Voy a tomar su pulso radial. (Boy ah toh-mahr soo pool-soh rah-dee-ahl)
I will take your blood pressure.	Voy a tomar su presión de sangre. (Boy ah toh-mahr soo preh-see-ohn deh sahn-greh)
ice cream	nieve/helado (nee-eh-beh/eh-lah-doh)
If it hurts, tell me.	Si duele, avísame. (See doo-eh-leh, ah-bee-sah-meh)
If there is no ice in the bucket, call me.	Si no hay hielo en la tina, llámeme. (See noh ah-ee ee-eh-loh ehn lah tee-nah, yah-meh-meh)
If you don't understand, please let me know.	Si no entiende, dígame por favor. (See noh ehn-tee-ehn-deh, dee-gah-meh pohr fah-bohr)
In case of fire, take the stairs.	En caso de fuego, use la escalera. (Ehn kah-soh deh foo-eh-goh, oo-seh lah ehs-kah-leh-rah)
independence	independencia (een-deh-pehn-dehn-see-ah)
infancy	infancia (een-fahn-see-ah)
inflammation	inflamación (een-flah-mah-see-ohn)
instant	instantáneo (eens-tahn-tah-neh-oh)
insulin	insulina (een-soo-lee-nah)
intravenous drug abusers	los que abusan de las drogas intravenosas (lohs keh ah-boo-sah deh lahs droh-gahs een-trah-beh-noh-sahs)
Is he coughing?	¿Está tosiendo? (Ehs-tah toh-see-ehn-doh)
Is he urinating well?	¿Orina bien? (Oh-ree-nah bee-ehn)
Is he/she . . .	¿Está . . . (Ehs-tah)
Is it/that a lot?	¿Es mucho? (Ehs moo-choh)

ENGLISH	SPANISH
Is that enough?	¿Es suficiente? (Ehs soo-fee-see-ehn-teh)
Is that too much?	¿Es demasiado? (Ehs deh-mah-see-ah-doh)
Is the pain there all the time, or does it come and go?	¿Está el dolor allí todo el tiempo, o va y viene? (Ehs-tah ehl doh-lohr ah-yee toh-doh ehl tee-ehm-poh, oh bah ee bee-eh-neh?)
Is there a danger from donated blood?	¿Qué peligro hay por sangre donada? (Keh peh-lee-groh ah-ee pohr sahn-greh doh-nah-dah)
Is there any pain?	¿Tiene algún dolor? (Tee-eh-neh ahl-goon doh-lohr)
Is there anything else bothering you?	¿Hay otra cosa que le moleste? (Ah-ee oh-trah koh-sah keh-leh moh-lehs-teh)
Is there anything that worries you?	¿Hay algo que le preocupa? (Ah-ee ahl-goh keh leh preh-oh-koo-pah)
Is there numbness/a tingling sensation/ burning in your leg/ arm/foot/hand?	¿Está entumecido/adormecido/ tiene ardor en su pierna/ brazo/pie/mano? (Ehs-tah ehn-too-meh-see-doh/ ah-dohr-meh-see-do/ tee-eh-neh ahr-dohr ehn soo pee-ehr-nah/brah-soh/ pee-eh/mah-noh)
It can cause drowsiness.	Le puede causar sueño. (Leh poo-eh-deh kah-oo-sahr soo-eh-nyoh)
It keeps the food warm.	Guarda la comida tibia. (Goo-ahr-dah lah koh-mee-dah tee-bee-ah)
juice	jugo (joo-goh)
leg	pierna (pee-ehr-nah)
Let it out.	Exhala. (Ehx-ah-lah)
Let me know how you feel.	Dígame cómo se siente. (Dee-gah-meh koh-moh seh see-ehn-teh)
lettuce	lechuga (leh-choo-gah)
Lift your arm.	Levanta el brazo. (leh-bahn-tah ehl brah-soh)
Lift your foot.	Levanta el pie. (Leh-bahn-tah ehl pee-eh)
Lift your leg.	Levanta la pierna. (Leh-bahn-tah lah pee-ehr-nah)
linen	lino (lee-noh)
Lower your foot.	Baja el pie. (Bah-hah ehl pee-eh)
mashed potatoes	puré de papas (poo-reh deh pah-pahs)
medication	medicamento (meh-dee-kah-mehn-toh)
medicine	medicina (meh-dee-see-nah)

ENGLISH	SPANISH	ENGLISH	SPANISH
milk	leche (leh-cheh)	On a scale from 1 [insignificant] to 10 [unbearable]	En una escala del uno [insignificante] al diez [intolerable] (Ehn oo-nah ehs-kah-lah dehl oo-noh [een-seeg-nee-fee-kahn-teh] ahl deeehs [een- toh-leh-rah-bleh])
Miss	señorita (seh-nyoh-ree-tah)		
Monday	lunes (loo-nehs)		
mother	madre (mah-dreh)	Open the fingers wide.	Separa bien los dedos. (Seh-pah-rah bee-ehn lohs deh-dohs)
mother-in-law	suegra (soo-eh-grah)	Open your hand.	Abre la mano. (Ah-breh lah mah-noh)
Move your leg.	Mueve la pierna. (Moo-eh-beh lah pee-ehr-nah)	Open your mouth, please.	Abra la boca, por favor. (Ah-brah lah boh-kah, pohr fah-bohr)
Mr.	señor (seh-nyohr)		
Mrs.	señora (seh-nyoh-rah)	orange	naranja (nah-rah-hah)
Mrs. . . . , I need to help you change clothes.	Señora . . . , necesito ayudarle a cambiar la ropa. (Señora . . . , neh-seh-see-toh ah-yoo-dahr-leh ah kahm-bee-ahr lah roh-pah)	organ	órgano (ohr-gah-noh)
		over-easy	volteados (bohl-teh-ah-dohs)
		oxygen	oxígeno (ohx-ee-heh-noh)
My name is . . .	Mi nombre es . . . / Me llamo . . . (Mee nohm-breh ehs/Meh yah-moh)	Pain?	¿Dolor? (Doh-lohr)
		pancreas	páncreas (pahn-kreh-ahs)
nausea	náusea (nah-oo-seh-ah)	panic	pánico (pah-nee-koh)
neither	tampoco (tahm-poh-koh)	Pat his back gently.	Dé palmaditas en la espalda. (Deh pahl-mah-dee-tahs ehn lah ehs-pahl-dah)
neither . . . nor	ni . . . ni (nee . . . nee)		
nephew	sobrino (soh-bree-noh)	pathogen	patogénico (pah-toh-heh-nee-koh)
never, not ever	nunca, jamás (noon-kah, hah-mahs)	peas	chícharos (chee-chah-rohs)
niece	sobrina (soh-bree-nah)	pecan	nuez (noo-ehs)
no one, nobody	nadie (nah-dee-eh)	Phone for local calls.	Teléfono para llamadas locales. (Teh-leh-foh-noh pah-rah yah-mah-dahs loh-kah-lehs)
No smoking.	No se permite fumar. (Noh seh pehr-mee-teh foo-mahr)		
no, not	no (noh)	pies	pasteles (pahs-teh-lehs)
normal	normal (nohr-mahl)	pinto beans	frijol pinto (free-hohl peen-toh)
not one, not any	ninguno (neen-goo-noh)	Please stay/remain in bed.	Por favor, quédese en la cama. (Pohr fah-bohr, keh-deh-seh ehn lah kan-mah)
nothing	nada (nah-dah)		
Now raise the left arm.	Ahora levante el brazo izquierdo. (Ah-oh-rah leh-bahn-teh ehl brah-soh ees-kee-ehr-doh)	Please!	¡Por favor! (Pohr fah-bohr)
		Please walk.	Camina, por favor. (Kah-mee-nah, pohr fah-bohr)
Now, take a deep breath.	Ahora, respira hondo. (Ah-oh-rah, rehs-pee-rah ohn-doh)	Point.	Apunte./Señale. (Ah-poon-teh/Seh-nyah-leh)
nutrition	nutrición (noo-tree-see-ohn)	Point where it hurts.	Señale donde duela. (Seh-nyah-leh koo-ahn-doh doo-eh-lah)
oatmeal	harina de avena (ah-ree-nah-day ah-beh-nah)	pork	puerco (poo-ehr-koh)
obsession	obsesión (ohb-seh-see-ohn)	potatoes	papas (pah-pahs)
		prune	ciruela (see-roo-eh-lah)

ENGLISH	SPANISH	ENGLISH	SPANISH
Pull the cord in the bathroom.	Jale el cordón en el baño. (Hah-leh ehl kohr-dohn ehn ehl bah-nyoh)	something to eat?	¿algo de comer? (ahl-goh deh koh-mehr)
pulse	pulso (pool-soh)	something to read?	¿algo de leer? (ahl-goh deh leh-ehr)
rectal	rectal (rehk-tahl)	son	hijo (ee-hoh)
red	rojo (roh-hoh)	spinal	espinal (ehs-pee-nahl)
refried	refritos (reh-free-tohs)	steak	bistec (bees-tehk)
regular	regular (reh-goo-lahr)	stepdaughter	hijastra (ee-hahs-trah)
Remember that you will do this for 24 hours.	Recuerde que hará esto por veinticuatro horas. (Reh-koo-ehr-deh keh ah-rah ehs-toh pohr beh-een-tee-koo-ah-troh oh-rahs)	stepfather	padrastro (pah-drahs-troh)
		stepmother	madrastra (mah-drahs-trah)
		stepson	hijastro (ee-hahs-troh)
respect	respeto (rehs-peh-toh)	stethoscope	estetoscopio (ehs-teh-tohs-koh-pee-oh)
Rest.	Descanse. (Des-kahn-seh)	Straighten your knee.	Endereza la rodilla. (Ehn-deh-reh-sah lah roh-dee-yah)
Rest now.	Descanse ahora. (Dehs-kahn-seh ah-oh-rah)	Straighten your leg.	Endereza la pierna. (Ehn-deh-reh-sah lah pee-ehr-nah)
ribs	costillas (kohs-tee-yahs)	strawberry	fresa (freh-sah)
Rinse your mouth.	Enjuague la boca. (Ehn-hoo ah-geh lah boh-kah)	Sunday	domingo (doh-meen-goh)
roast	rostizado (rohs-tee-sah-doh)	Swelling of the ankles?	¿Hinchazón en los tobillos? (Een-chah-sohn ehn lohs toh-bee-yohs)
Rotate it.	Gíralo./Dale vuelta. (Hee-rah-loh/Dah-leh boo-ehl-tah)	syncope	síncope (seen-koh-peh)
salad	ensalada (ehn-sah-lah-dah)	systole	sístole (sees-toh-leh)
saliva	saliva (sah-lee-bah)	Take it with a full glass of water.	Tómela con un vaso lleno de agua. (Toh-meh-lah kohn oon bah-soh yeh-noh deh ah-goo-a)
salt	sal (sahl)	Take on an empty stomach.	Tómela con el estómago vacío. (Toh-meh-lah kohn ehl ehs-toh-mah-goh bah-see-oh)
sanitary	sanitario (sah-nee-tah-ree-oh)		
Saturday	sábado (sah-bah-doh)	Take one hour before eating.	Tómela una hora antes de comer. (Toh-meh-lah oo-nah oh-rah ahn-tehs de koh-mehr)
scrambled	revueltos (reh-boo-ehl-tohs)		
Select your foods from the menu after breakfast.	Seleccione las comidas del menú después del desayuno. (Seh-lehk-see-oh-neh lahs koh-mee-dahs dehl meh-noo dehs-poo-ehs dehl deh-sah-yoo-noh)	Take the medicine with food.	Tome la medicina con comida. (Toh-meh lah mehdee-see-nah kohn koh-mee-dah)
		Take the medicine with juice.	Tome la medicina con jugo. (Toh-meh lah meh-dee-see-nah kohn joo-goh)
sex	sexo (sehx-oh)	Take the temperature rectally.	Tome la temperatura por el recto. (Toh-meh lah tehm-peh-rah-too-rah pohr ehl rehk-toh)
sexual	sexual (sehx-oo-ahl)		
sister	hermana (ehr-mah-nah)	taking formula?	¿tomando fórmula? (toh-mahn-doh fohr-moo-lah)
sister-in-law	cuñada (koo-nyah-dah)	Tell me if it hurts.	Dime si esto le duele. (Dee-meh see ehs-toh leh doo-eh-leh)
Sit in the chair.	Siéntese en la silla. (See-ehn-teh-seh ehn lah see-yah)		
something to drink?	¿algo de tomar/beber? (ahl-goh deh toh-mahr/beh-behr)	Tell me if there is pain.	Dime si duele. (Dee-meh see doo-eh-leh)

ENGLISH	SPANISH	ENGLISH	SPANISH
Thank you for talking to me!	¡Gracias por hablar conmigo! (Grah-see-ahs pohr ah-blahr kohn-mee-goh)	There are bathrooms for guests in the corner.	Hay baños para las visitas en el rincón. (Hay bah-nyohs pah-rah lahs bee-see-tahs ehn ehl rehn kohn)
Thank you very much!	¡Muchas gracias! (Moo-chahs grah-see-ahs)	There is a shower.	Hay una ducha/regadera. (Ah-ee oo-nah doo-chah/ reh-gah-deh-rah)
Thank you!	¡Gracias! (Grah-see-ahs)	There is a straw.	Hay un popote. (Ah-ee oon poh-poh-teh)
The bell will sound.	La campana sonará. (Lah kahm-pah-nah soh-nah-rah)	There is also a bathtub/tub.	También hay una bañera/tina. (Tahm-bee-ehn ah-ee oo-nah bah-nyeh-rah/tee-nah)
The chair turns into a bed.	Esta silla se hace cama. (Ehs-tah see-yah seh ah-seh kah-mah)	There is an emergency light.	Hay una luz para emergencias.
The container will be kept in the bucket with ice.	El frasco se mantendrá en una tina con hielo. (Ehl frahs-koh seh mahn-tehn-drah ehn oo-nah tee-nah kohn ee-eh-loh)		(Ah-ee oo-nah loos pah-rah eh-mehr-hehn-see-ahs)
		thermometer	termómetro (tehr-moh-meh-troh)
The cover is hot.	La cubierta está caliente. (Lah koo-bee-ehr-tah ehs-tah kah-lee-ehn-teh)	These buttons move the bed up/down.	Estos botones mueven la cama arriba/abajo. (Ehs-tohs boh-tah-nehs moo-eh-behn lah kay-mah ah-ree-bah/ah-bah-hoh)
The elevators work twenty-four hours.	Los elevadores funcionan las veinticuatro horas. (Lohs eh-leh-bah-dohrehs foon-see-oh-nahn lahs beh-een-tee-koo-ah-troh oh-rahs)	This button lowers (raises) the headboard.	Este botón baja (sube) la cabecera de la cama. (Ehs-teh boh-tohn bah-hah (soo-beh) lah kah-beh-seh-rah deh lah kah-mah)
the family	la familia (lah fah-mee-lee-ah)	This is the call bell.	Este es el timbre. (Ehs-teh ehs ehl teem-breh)
The fork, spoon, and knife are wrapped in the napkin.	El tenedor, la cuchara, y el cuchillo están envueltos en la servilleta. (Ehl teh-neh-dohr, lah koo-chah-rah ee ehl koo-chee-yoh ehs-tahn ehn-boo-ehl-tohs ehn lah sehr-bee-yeh-tah)	This is the call bell/buzzer.	Este es la campana/el timbre. (Ehs-teh ehs lah kahm-pah-nah/ehl teem-breh)
		This is the lobby.	Esta es la sala de espera. (Ehs-tah ehs lah sah-lah deh ehs-peh-rah)
The meals are served	Los alimentos se sirven (Lohs ah-lee-mehn-tohs seh seer-behn)	This is the radio.	Este es el radio. (Ehs-teh ehs ehl rah-dee-oh)
The meals are served at . . .	Los alimentos se sirven a . . . (Lohs ah-lee-mehn-tohs seh seer-behn ah)	This is your room.	Este es su cuarto. (Ehs-teh ehs soo koo-ahr-toh)
The pain is in one place?	¿El dolor está fijo? (Ehl doh-lohr ehs-tah fee-hoh)	Thursday	jueves (hoo-eh-behs)
The pain is localized, sharp.	El dolor está fijo, agudo. (Ehl doh-lohr ehs-tah ehn ehl lah-dohl kohs-tah-doh)	toast	pan tostado (pahn tohs-tah-doh)
The pain is on the side.	El dolor está en el lado/costado. (Ehl doh-lohr ehs-tah ehn ehl lah-dohl kohs-tah-doh)	tomato	tomate (toh-mah-teh)
		Tuesday	martes (mahr-tehs)
The pain is sharp?	¿El dolor es agudo? (Ehl doh-lohr ehs ah-goo-doh)	Turn it to the left.	Voltéalo hacia la izquierda. (Bohl-teh-ah-loh ah-see-ah lah ees-kee-ehr-dah)
The rails lower down.	El barandal se baja. (Ehl bah-rahn-dahl seh bah-hah)	Turn it to the right.	Voltéalo hacia la derecha. (Bohl-teh-ah-loh ah-see-ah lah deh-reh-chah)
The salt and pepper are in these packets.	La sal y pimienta están en estos paquetes. (Lah sahl ee pee-mee-ehn-tah ehs-tahn ehn ehs-tohn pah-keh-tehs)	Turn on your side.	Voltéese de lado. (Bhol-teh-eh-seh deh lah-doh)
		Turn the forearm.	Voltea el antebrazo. (Bhol-teh-ah ehl ahn-teh-brah-soh)
The television has four channels.	El televisor tiene cuatro canales. (Ehl teh-leh-bee-sohr tee-eh-neh koo-ah-troh kay-nah-lehs)	Turn to your side.	Voltéate de lado. (Bhol-teh-ah-teh deh lah-doh)
The water is in the glass/pitcher.	El agua está en el vaso/la jarra. (Ehl ah-goo-ah ehs-tah ehn ehl bah-soh/lah hah-rah)	Turn your forearm.	Voltea el antebrazo. (Bohl-teh-ah ehl ahn-teh brah-soh)

ENGLISH	SPANISH	ENGLISH	SPANISH
ulcer	úlcera (ool-seh-rah)	What did you do that caused the pain?	¿Qué hacía cuando apareció el dolor? (Keh ah-see-ah koo-ahn-doh ah-pah-reh-see-oh ehl doh-lohr)
uncle	tío (tee-oh)	What did you eat for breakfast?	¿Qué comió en el desayuno? (Keh koh-mee-oh ehn ehl deh-sah-yoo-noh)
Use dental floss.	Use hilo dental. (Oo-seh ee-loh dehn-tahl)	What did you eat?	¿Qué comió? (Keh koh-mee-oh)
vanilla	vainilla (bah-ee-nee-yah)	What foods do you dislike?	¿Qué alimentos le disgustan? (Keh ah-lee-mehn-tohs leh dees-goos-tahn)
venereal	venéreo (beh-neh-reh-oh)	What foods do you like?	¿Qué alimentos le gustan? (Keh ah-lee-mehn-tohs leh goos-tahn)
vertigo	vértigo (behr-tee-goh)	What formula does he take?	¿Qué fórmula toma? (Keh fohr-moo-lah toh-mah)
vision	visión (bee-see-ohn)	What is hurting you?	¿Qué le duele? (Keh leh doo-eh-leh)
Visiting hours are from nine in the morning to nine at night.	Las horas de visita son de las nueve de la mañana a las nueve de la noche. (Lahs oh-rahs deh bee-see-tah shon deh lahs noo-eh-beh deh lah mah-nyah-nah ah lahs noo-eh-beh deh lah noh-cheh)	What is the matter?	¿Qué le pasa/sucede? (Keh leh pah-sah/soo-seh-deh)
		What is the pain like?	¿Qué tipo de dolor tiene? (Keh tee-oh deh doh-lohr tee-eh-neh)
Visiting hours are from two to eight PM.	Las horas de visita son de las dos a las ocho de la noche. (Lahs oh-rahs deh bee-see- tah sohn deh lahs dohs ah loahs oh-choh deh lah noh-cheh)	What is wrong?	¿Qué pasa? (Keh pah-sah)
		What kind of coffee?	¿Qué clase de café? (Keh klah-seh deh kah-feh)
vomit	vómito (boh-mee-toh)	What kind of juices?	¿Qué clase de jugos? (Keh klah-seh deh joo-gohs)
Wash hands before eating.	Lávese las manos antes de comer. (Lah-beh-seh lahs mah-nohs ahn-tehs deh koh-mehr)	What makes the pain better?	¿Qué hace mejorar el dolor? (Keh ah-seh meh-hoh-rahr ehl doh-lohr)
Wash well all fruits and vegetables.	Lave bien frutas y verduras. (Lah-beh bee-ehn froo-tahs ee behr-doo-rahs)	What other discomfort do you have?	¿Qué otra molestia tiene? (Keh oh-trah moh-lehs-tee-ah tee-eh-neh)
We also have desserts.	También tenemos postres: (Tahm-bee-ehn teh-neh-mohs pohs-trehs)	What symptoms do you have?	¿Qué síntomas tiene? (Keh seen-toh-mahs tee-eh-neh)
We are going in the ambulance.	Vamos en la ambulancia. (Bah-mohs ehn lah ahm-boo-lahn-see-ah)	what?	¿qué?/¿qué tal? (keh/keh tahl)
We are going to the hospital.	Vamos al hospital. (Bah-mohs ahl ohs-pee-tahl)	When did you notice the skin rash?	¿Cuándo se dio cuenta de la piel rosada? (Koo-ahn-doh seh dee-oh koo-ehn-tah deh lah pee-ehl roh-sah-dah)
We have cereals.	Tenemos cereales. (Teh-neh-mohs seh-reh-ah-lehs)		
We have meats.	Tenemos carnes. (Teh-nehmohs kahr-nehs)	When was the last time he had a bowel movement?	¿Cuándo fue la última vez que evacuó/hizo del baño? (Koo-ahn-doh foo-eh lah ool-tee-mah behs keh eh-bah-koo-oh/ ee-soh dehl bah-nyoh)
Wear this bracelet all the time.	Use esta pulsera todo el tiempo. (Oo-seh ehs-tah pool-seh-rah toh-doh ehl tee-ehm-poh)		
Wednesday	miércoles (mee-ehr-koh-lehs)	When was the last time you ate?	¿Cuándo fue la última vez que comió? (Koo-ahn-doh foo-eh lah ool-tee-mah behs keh koh-mee-oh)
What brought you to the hospital?	¿Qué la trajo al hospital? (Keh lah trah-hoh ahl ohs-pee-tahl)		
What can I help you with?	¿En qué puedo ayudarla? (Ehn keh poo-eh-doh ah-yoo-dahr-lah)	When was the last time you used the toilet?	¿Cuándo fue la última vez que hizo del baño/que obró? (Koo-ahn doh foo-eh lah ool-tee-mah behs keh ee-soh dehl bah-nyoh/keh oh-broh)
What caused the pain?	¿Qué causó el dolor? (Keh kah-oo-soh ehl doh-lohr)		
What color?	¿De qué color? (Deh keh koh-lohr)	When you have pain, do you get nauseated?	¿Cuando tiene dolor, ¿le dan náuseas? (Koo-ahn-doh tee-eh-neh doh-lohr, leh dahn nah-oo-seh-ahs)

ENGLISH	SPANISH	ENGLISH	SPANISH
when?	¿cuándo? (koo-ahn-doh)	You have to choose three meals a day.	Tiene que escoger tres comidas diarias. (Tee-eh-neh keh ehs-koh-hehr trehs koh-mee-dahs dee-ah-ree-ahs)
Where does it hurt?	¿Dónde le duele? (Don-deh leh doo-eh-leh)		
where?	¿dónde? (dohn-deh)	Your clothes go in the closet.	La ropa va en el closet/ropero. (Lah roh-pah bah ehn ehl kloh-seht/roh-peh-roh)
which?	¿cuál? (koo-ahl)		
white	blanco (blahn-koh)	Your towels are in the bathroom.	Sus toallas están en el baño. (Soos too-ahyahs ehs-tahn ehn ehl bah-nyoh)
who?	¿quién? (kee-ehn)		
why?	¿por qué? (pohr keh)	**Numbers**	
wife	esposa (ehs-poh-sah)	one (1)	uno (oo-noh)
wings	alas (ah-lahs)	two (2)	dos (dohs)
with cream	con crema (kohn kreh-mah)	three (3)	tres (trehs)
with ham	con jamón (kohn hah-mahn)	four (4)	cuatro (koo-ah-troh)
with sugar	con azúcar (kohn ah-soo-kahr)	five (5)	cinco (seen-koh)
without	sin (seen)	six (6)	seis (seh-ees)
yellow	amarillo (ah-mah-ree-yoh)	seven (7)	siete (see-eh-teh)
Yes, sir.	Sí, señor. (See, seh-nyohr)	eight (8)	ocho (oh-choh)
You are welcome.	De nada. (Deh nah-dah)	nine (9)	nueve (noo-eh-beh)
You can call collect.	Puede llamar por cobrar. (poo-eh-deh yah-mahr pohr koh-brahr)	ten (10)	diez (dee-ehs)
You can have flowers.	Puede tener flores. (Poo-eh-deh teh-nehr floh-rehs)	eleven (11)	once (ohn-seh)
You can make local phone calls.	Puede hacer llamadas locales. (Poo-eh-deh ah sehr-yah-mah-dahs loh-kah-lehs)	twelve (12)	doce (doh-seh)
		thirteen (13)	trece (treh-seh)
You can put cards on the shelf.	Puede poner tarjetas en el estante. (Poo-eh-deh poh-nehr tahr-hehtahs ehn ehl ehs- tahn-teh)	fourteen (14)	catorce (kah-tohr-seh)
		fifteen (15)	quince (keen-seh)
You can raise the feet.	Puede levantar los pies. (Poo-eh-deh leh-bahn-tahr lohs pee-ehs)	sixteen (16)	dieciséis (dee-ehs-ee-seh-ees)
		seventeen (17)	diecisiete (dee-ehs-ee-see-eh-teh)
You can raise the head.	Puede levantar la cabeza. (Poo-eh-deh leh-bahn-tahr lah kah-beh-sah)	eighteen (18)	dieciocho (dee-ehs-ee-oh-choh)
		nineteen (19)	diecinueve (dee-ehs-ee-noo-eh-beh)
You can tape pictures to the wall.	Puede pegar retratos en la pared. (Poo-eh-deh peh-gahr reh-trah-tohs ehn lah pah-rehd)	twenty (20)	veinte (beh-een-teh)
		thirty (30)	treinta (treh-een-tah)
You cannot smoke here.	No puede fumar aquí. (Noh poo-eh-deh foo-mahr ah-kee)	forty (40)	cuarenta (koo-ah-rehn-tah)
		fifty (50)	cincuenta (seen-koo-ehn-tah)
You cannot smoke in your room.	No puede fumar en el cuarto. (Noh poo-eh-deh foo-mahr ehn ehl koo-ahr-toh)	sixty (60)	sesenta (seh-sehn-tah)
You have a private bathroom.	Tiene un baño/inodoro privado. (Tee-eh-neh oon bah-nyoh/ ee-noh-doh-roh pree-bah-doh)	seventy (70)	setenta (seh-tehn-tah)

ENGLISH	SPANISH
eighty (80)	ochenta (oh-chehn-tah)
ninety (90)	noventa (noh-behn-tah)
one hundred (100)	cien (see-ehn)

Time	Standard	Military (hours PM)
one o'clock	la una (la oo-nah)	las trece horas (lahs treh-seh oh-rahs)
two o'clock	las dos (lahs dohs)	las catorce horas (lahs kah-tohr-seh oh-rahs)
three o'clock	las tres (lahs trehs)	las quince horas (lahs keen-seh oh-rahs)
four o'clock	las cuatro (lahs koo-ah-troh)	las dieciséis horas (lahs dee-ehs-ee-seh-ees oh-rahs)
five o'clock	las cinco (lahs seen-koh)	las diecisiete horas (lahs dee-ehs-ee-see-eh-teh oh-rahs)
six o'clock	las seis (lahs seh-ees)	las dieciocho horas (lahs dee-ehs-ee-oh-choh oh-rahs)
seven o'clock	las siete (lahs see-eh-teh)	las diecinueve horas (lahs dee-ehs-ee-noo-eh-beh oh-rahs)
eight o'clock	las ocho (lahs oh-choh)	las veinte horas (lahs beh-een-teh oh-rahs)
nine o'clock	las nueve (lahs noo-eh-beh)	las veintiuna horas (lahs beh-een-tee-oo-nah oh-rahs)
ten o'clock	las diez (lahs dee-ehs)	las veintidós horas (lahs beh-een-tee-dohs oh-rahs)
eleven o'clock	las once (lahs ohn-seh)	las veintitrés horas (lahs beh-een-tee-trehs oh-rahs)
twelve o'clock/ midnight	las doce/la media noche (lahs doh-seh/lah meh-dee-ah non-cheh)	las cero horas (lahs seh-roh-oh-rahs) las veinticuatro horas (lahs beh-een-tee-koo-ah-troh oh-rahs)

GLOSSARY

abbreviation A shortened form of a word or phrase

abduction Moving a body part away from the midline of the body

abrasion A partial-thickness wound caused by the scraping away or rubbing of the skin

abuse The willful infliction of injury, unreasonable confinement, intimidation, or punishment that results in physical harm, pain, or mental anguish; depriving the person (or the person's caretaker) of the goods or services needed to attain or maintain well-being

accountable Being responsible for one's actions and the actions of others who performed delegated tasks; answering questions about and explaining one's actions and the actions of others

acetone See "ketone"

activities of daily living (ADL) The activities usually done during a normal day in a person's life

acute illness A sudden illness from which a person is expected to recover

acute pain Pain that is felt suddenly from injury, disease, trauma, or surgery

adduction Moving a body part toward the midline of the body

admission Official entry of a person into a nursing center

advance directive A document stating a person's wishes about health care when that person cannot make his or her own decisions

affect Feelings and emotions

allergy A sensitivity to a substance that causes the body to react with signs and symptoms

alopecia Hair loss

Alzheimer's disease (AD) A disease that affects brain tissue; memory loss and confusion increase until the person cannot tend to simple personal needs

ambulation The act of walking

AM care See "early morning care"

amputation The removal of all or part of an extremity

anaphylaxis A life-threatening sensitivity to an antigen

anorexia The loss of appetite

anticoagulant A drug that prevents or slows down (*anti*) blood clotting (*coagulate*)

anxiety A vague, uneasy feeling in response to stress

aphasia The total or partial loss (*a*) of the ability to use or understand language (*phasia*); a language disorder resulting from damage to parts of the brain responsible for language

apical-radial pulse Taking the apical and radial pulses at the same time

apnea The lack or absence (*a*) of breathing (*pnea*)

arterial ulcer An open wound on the lower legs or feet caused by poor arterial blood flow

artery A blood vessel that carries blood away from the heart

arthritis Joint (*arthr*) inflammation (*itis*)

arthroplasty The surgical replacement (*plasty*) of a joint (*arthr*)

asepsis Being free of disease-producing microbes

aspiration Breathing fluid, food, vomitus, or an object into the lungs

assault Intentionally attempting or threatening to touch a person's body without the person's consent

assessment Collecting information about the person; a step in the nursing process

assisted living A housing option for older persons who need help with activities of daily living yet wish to remain independent as long as possible

assisted living residence Provides housing, personal care, support services, health care, and activities in a home-like setting

atrophy The decrease in size or the wasting away of tissue

autopsy The examination of the body after death

avoidable pressure ulcer A pressure ulcer that develops from the improper use of the nursing process

base of support The area on which an object rests

battery Touching a person's body without his or her consent

bedfast Confined to bed

bed rail A device that serves as a guard or barrier along the side of the bed; side rail

benign tumor A tumor that does not spread to other body parts; it can grow to a large size

biohazardous waste Items contaminated with blood, body fluids, secretions, or excretions; *bio* means life, and *hazardous* means dangerous or harmful

Biot's respirations Rapid and deep respirations followed by 10 to 30 seconds of apnea

birth defect An abnormality present at birth that can involve a body structure or function

bisexual A person who is attracted to both sexes

blindness The absence of sight

blood pressure (BP) The amount of force exerted against the walls of an artery by the blood

board and care home Provides rooms, meals, laundry, and supervision to independent residents in a home-like setting; group home

body alignment The way the head, trunk, arms, and legs are aligned with one another; posture

body language Messages sent through facial expressions, gestures, posture, hand and body movements, gait, eye contact, and appearance

body mechanics Using the body in an efficient and careful way

body temperature The amount of heat in the body that is a balance between the amount of heat produced and the amount lost by the body

bony prominence An area where the bone sticks out or projects from the flat surface of the body

boundary crossing A brief act or behavior outside of the helpful zone

boundary sign An act, behavior, or thought that warns of a boundary crossing or violation

boundary violation An act or behavior that meets your needs, not the person's

bradycardia A slow (*brady*) heart rate (*cardia*); less than 60 beats per minute

bradypnea Slow (*brady*) breathing (*pnea*); respirations are fewer than 12 per minute

braille A touch reading and writing system that uses raised dots for each letter of the alphabet; the first 10 letters also represent the numbers 0 through 9

Broca's aphasia See "expressive aphasia"

calorie The fuel or energy value of food

cancer See "malignant tumor"

capillary A tiny blood vessel; food, oxygen, and other substances pass from the capillaries into the cells

cardiac arrest See "sudden cardiac arrest"

carrier A human or animal that is a reservoir for microbes but does not have the signs and symptoms of infection

case management A nursing care pattern; a case manager (an RN) coordinates a person's care from admission through discharge and into the home setting

catheter A tube used to drain or inject fluid through a body opening

catheterization The process of inserting a catheter

cell The basic unit of body structure

cerumen Earwax

chairfast Confined to a chair

chart See "medical record"

chemical restraint Any drug that is used for discipline or convenience and not required to treat medical symptoms

Cheyne-Stokes respirations Respirations gradually increase in rate and depth and then become shallow and slow; breathing may stop (*apnea*) for 10 to 20 seconds

chronic illness An ongoing illness, slow or gradual in onset; it has no cure; the illness can be controlled and complications prevented with proper treatment

chronic pain Pain that continues for a long time (months or years) or occurs off and on; persistent pain

chronic wound A wound that does not heal easily

circadian rhythm Daily rhythm based on a 24-hour cycle; the day-night cycle or body rhythm

circulatory ulcer An open sore on the lower legs or feet caused by decreased blood flow through the arteries or veins; vascular ulcer

civil law Laws concerned with relationships between people

clean-contaminated wound Occurs from the surgical entry of the reproductive, urinary, respiratory, or gastro-intestinal system

clean technique See "medical asepsis"

clean wound A wound that is not infected

closed fracture The bone is broken but the skin is intact; simple fracture

closed wound Tissues are injured but the skin is not broken

cognitive function Involves memory, thinking, reasoning, ability to understand, judgment, and behavior

colonized The presence of bacteria on the wound surface or in wound tissue; the person does not have signs and symptoms of an infection

colostomy A surgically created opening (*stomy*) between the colon (*colo*) and abdominal wall

coma A state of being unaware of one's surroundings and being unable to react or respond to people, places, or things

comatose Being unable to respond to verbal stimuli

comfort A state of well-being; the person has no physical or emotional pain and is calm and at peace

communicable disease A disease caused by pathogens that spread easily; a contagious disease

communication The exchange of information—a message sent is received and correctly interpreted by the intended person

compound fracture See "open fracture"

comprehensive care plan A written guide about the care a person should receive; developed by the health team; care plan

compress A soft pad applied over a body area

compulsion Repeating an act over and over again

confidentiality Trusting others with personal and private information

conflict A clash between opposing interests or ideas

constipation The passage of a hard, dry stool

constrict To narrow

contagious disease See "communicable disease"

contaminated wound A wound with a high risk of infection

contamination The process of becoming unclean

contracture The lack of joint mobility caused by abnormal shortening of a muscle

contusion A closed wound caused by a blow to the body; a bruise

convulsion See "seizure"

cotton drawsheet A drawsheet made of cotton; it helps keep the mattress and bottom linens clean

courtesy A polite, considerate, or helpful comment or act

crime An act that violates a criminal law

criminal law Laws concerned with offenses against the public and society in general

culture The characteristics of a group of people—language, values, beliefs, habits, likes, dislikes, customs—passed from one generation to the next

cyanosis Bluish color to the skin, lips, mucous membranes, and nail beds

Daily Value (DV) How a serving fits into the daily diet; expressed in a percent (%) based on a daily diet of 2000 calories

dandruff Excessive amounts of dry, white flakes from the scalp

deafness Hearing loss in which it is impossible for the person to understand speech through hearing alone

deconditioning The loss of muscle strength from inactivity

defamation Injuring a person's name and reputation by making false statements to a third person

defecation The process of excreting feces from the rectum through the anus; a bowel movement

defense mechanism An unconscious reaction that blocks unpleasant or threatening feelings

dehiscence The separation of wound layers

dehydration The excessive loss of water from tissues; a decrease in the amount of water in body tissues

delegate To authorize another person to perform a nursing task in a certain situation

delirium A state of sudden, severe confusion and rapid brain changes

delusion A false belief

delusion of grandeur An exaggerated belief about one's importance, wealth, power, or talents

delusion of persecution A false belief that one is being mistreated, abused, or harassed

dementia The loss of cognitive and social function caused by changes in the brain; the loss of cognitive function that interferes with routine personal, social, and occupational activities

denture An artificial tooth or a set of artificial teeth

development Changes in mental, emotional, and social function

developmental disability (DD) A disability occurring before 22 years of age

developmental task A skill that must be completed during a stage of development

diabetic foot ulcer An open wound on the foot caused by complications from diabetes

dialysis The process of removing waste products from the blood

diarrhea The frequent passage of liquid stools

diastole The period of heart muscle relaxation; the heart is at rest

diastolic pressure The pressure in the arteries when the heart is at rest

digestion The process of physically and chemically breaking down food so that it can be absorbed for use by the cells

dilate To expand or open wider

diplegia Similar body parts are affected on both sides of the body

dirty wound See "infected wound"

disability Any lost, absent, or impaired physical or mental function

disaster A sudden catastrophic event in which people are injured and killed and property is destroyed

discharge Official departure of a person from a nursing center

discomfort See "pain"

disinfection The process of destroying pathogens

distraction To change the person's center of attention

diuresis The process *(esis)* of passing *(di)* urine *(ur)*; large amounts of urine are produced—1000 to 5000 mL (milliliters) a day

dorsal recumbent position The back-lying or supine position; the supine position with the legs together; horizontal recumbent position

dorsiflexion Bending the toes and foot up at the ankle

drawsheet A small sheet placed over the middle of the bottom sheet

dysphagia Difficulty *(dys)* swallowing *(phagia)*

dyspnea Difficult, labored, or painful *(dys)* breathing *(pnea)*

dysuria Painful or difficult *(dys)* urination *(uria)*

early morning care Care given before breakfast; AM care

edema Swelling caused by fluid collecting in tissues; the swelling of body tissues with water

electrical shock When electrical current passes through the body

elopement When a person leaves the center without staff knowledge

embolus A blood clot that travels through the vascular system until it lodges in a vessel

emesis See "vomitus"

emotional illness See "mental disorder"

end-of-life care The support and care given during the time surrounding death

enema The introduction of fluid into the rectum and lower colon

enteral nutrition Giving nutrients into the gastro-intestinal (GI) tract *(enteral)* through a feeding tube

enuresis Urinary incontinence in bed at night

erectile dysfunction (ED) See "impotence"

ergonomics The science of designing a job to fit the worker

eschar Thick, leathery dead tissue that may be loose or adhered to the skin; it is often black or brown

esteem The worth, value, or opinion one has of a person

ethics Knowledge of what is right conduct and wrong conduct

evaluation To measure if goals in the planning step were met; a step in the nursing process

evening care Care given in the evening at bedtime; PM care

evisceration The separation of the wound along with the protrusion of abdominal organs

expressive aphasia Difficulty expressing or sending out thoughts; motor aphasia, Broca's aphasia

expressive-receptive aphasia Difficulty expressing or sending out thoughts and difficulty understanding language; global aphasia, mixed aphasia

extension Straightening a body part

external rotation Turning the joint outward

fainting The sudden loss of consciousness from an inadequate blood supply to the brain

false imprisonment Unlawful restraint or restriction of a person's freedom of movement

fecal impaction The prolonged retention and buildup of feces in the rectum

fecal incontinence The inability to control the passage of feces and gas through the anus

feces The semi-solid mass of waste products in the colon that is expelled through the anus

fever Elevated body temperature

first aid Emergency care given to an ill or injured person before medical help arrives

flashback Reliving the trauma in thoughts during the day and in nightmares during sleep

flatulence The excessive formation of gas or air in the stomach and intestines

flatus Gas or air passed through the anus

flexion Bending a body part

flow rate The number of drops per minute *(gtt/min)*

Foley catheter See "indwelling catheter"

footdrop The foot falls down at the ankle; permanent plantar flexion

Fowler's position A semi-sitting position; the head of the bed is raised between 45 and 60 degrees

fracture A broken bone

fraud Saying or doing something to trick, fool, or deceive a person

freedom of movement Any change in place or position of the body or any part of the body that the person is physically able to control

friction The rubbing of one surface against another

full-thickness wound The dermis, epidermis, and subcutaneous tissue are penetrated; muscle and bone may be involved

full visual privacy Having the means to be completely free from public view while in bed

functional incontinence The person has bladder control but cannot use the toilet in time

functional nursing A nursing care pattern focusing on tasks and jobs; each nursing team member has certain tasks and jobs to do

gait belt See "transfer belt"

gangrene A condition in which there is death of tissue

gastrostomy tube A tube inserted through a surgically created opening (stomy) in the stomach (gastro); stomach tube

gavage The process of giving a tube feeding

genupectoral position See "knee-chest position"

geriatrics The care of aging people

germicide A disinfectant applied to the skin, tissues, or non-living objects

gerontology The study of the aging process

global aphasia See "expressive-receptive aphasia"

glucosuria Sugar (glucos) in the urine (uria); glycosuria

glycosuria Sugar (glycos) in the urine (uria); glucosuria

goal That which is desired for or by a person as a result of nursing care

gossip To spread rumors or talk about the private matters of others

graduate A measuring container for fluid

ground That which carries leaking electricity to the earth and away from an electrical item

group home See "board and care home"

growth The physical changes that are measured and that occur in a steady, orderly manner

guided imagery Creating and focusing on an image

hallucination Seeing, hearing, smelling, or feeling something that is not real

harassment To trouble, torment, offend, or worry a person by one's behavior or comments

hazard Any thing in the person's setting that may cause injury or illness

hazardous substance Any chemical in the workplace that can cause harm

healthcare-associated infection (HAI) An infection that develops in a person cared for in any setting where health care is given; the infection is related to receiving health care

hearing loss Not being able to hear the normal range of sounds associated with normal hearing

heartburn A burning sensation in the chest and sometimes the throat

hematoma A swelling (oma) that contains blood (hemat)

hematuria Blood (hemat) in the urine (uria)

hemiplegia Paralysis (plegia) on one side (hemi) of the body

hemoglobin The substance in red blood cells that carries oxygen and gives blood its color

hemoptysis Bloody (hemo) sputum (ptysis means to spit)

hemorrhage The excessive loss of blood in a short time

hemothorax Blood (hemo) in the pleural space (thorax)

heterosexual A person who is attracted to members of the other sex

high blood pressure See "hypertension"

high-Fowler's position A semi-sitting position; the head of the bed is raised 60 to 90 degrees

hirsutism Excessive body hair

holism A concept that considers the whole person; the whole person has physical, social, psychological, and spiritual parts that are woven together and cannot be separated

homosexual A person who is attracted to members of the same sex

horizontal recumbent position See "dorsal recumbent position"

hormone A chemical substance secreted by the endocrine glands into the bloodstream

hospice A health care agency or program for persons who are dying

hyperextension Excessive straightening of a body part

hyperglycemia High (hyper) sugar (glyc) in the blood (emia)

hypertension Blood pressure measurements remaining above (hyper) a systolic pressure of 140 mm Hg or a diastolic pressure of 90 mm Hg; high blood pressure

hyperthermia A body temperature (thermia) that is much higher (hyper) than the person's normal range

hyperventilation Respirations (ventilation) are rapid (hyper) and deeper than normal

hypoglycemia Low (hypo) sugar (glyc) in the blood (emia)

hypotension When the systolic blood pressure is below (hypo) 90 mm Hg and the diastolic pressure is below 60 mm Hg

hypothermia A very low (hypo) body temperature (thermia)

hypoventilation Respirations (ventilation) are slow (hypo), shallow, and sometimes irregular

hypoxemia A reduced amount (hypo) of oxygen (ox) in the blood (emia)

hypoxia Cells do not have enough (hypo) oxygen (oxia)

ileostomy A surgically created opening (stomy) between the ileum (small intestine [ileo]) and the abdominal wall

immunity Protection against a certain disease or condition; the person will not get or be affected by the disease

implementation To perform or carry out nursing measures in the care plan; a step in the nursing process

impotence The inability of the male to have an erection; erectile dysfunction

incident Any event that has harmed or could harm a resident, visitor, or staff member

incision A cut produced surgically by a sharp instrument; it creates an opening into an organ or body space

independence Not relying on or requiring care from others

indwelling catheter A catheter left in the bladder so urine drains constantly into a drainage bag; retention or Foley catheter

infected wound A wound containing large amounts of microbes that shows signs of infection; a dirty wound

infection A disease state resulting from the invasion and growth of microbes in the body

infection control Practices and procedures that prevent the spread of infection inherited That which is passed down from parents to children

insomnia A chronic condition in which the person cannot sleep or stay asleep all night

intake The amount of fluid taken in

intellectual disability Involves severe limits in intellectual function and adaptive behavior occurring before age 18

intentional wound A wound created for therapy

interdisciplinary health care team The many health care workers whose skills and knowledge focus on the person's total care; health team

internal rotation Turning the joint inward

intravenous (IV) therapy Giving fluids through a needle or catheter inserted into a vein; IV and IV infusion

intubation Inserting an artificial airway

invasion of privacy Violating a person's right not to have his or her name, photo, or private affairs exposed or made public without giving consent

involuntary seclusion Separating a person from others against his or her will, keeping the person to a certain area, or keeping the person away from his or her room without consent

jaundice Yellowish color of the skin or whites of the eyes

jejunostomy tube A feeding tube inserted into a surgically created opening (stomy) in the jejunum of the small intestine

job description A document that describes what the center expects you to do

Kardex A type of card file that summarizes information found in the medical record—drugs, treatments, diagnoses, routine care measures, equipment, and special needs

ketone A substance that appears in urine from the rapid breakdown of fat for energy; acetone, ketone body

ketone body See "ketone"

knee-chest position The person kneels and rests the body on the knees and chest; the head is turned to one side, the arms are above the head or flexed at the elbows, the back is straight, and the body is flexed about 90 degrees at the hips; genupectoral position

Kussmaul respirations Very deep and rapid respirations

laceration An open wound with torn tissues and jagged edges

laryngeal mirror An instrument used to examine the mouth, teeth, and throat

lateral position The person lies on one side or the other; side-lying position

law A rule of conduct made by a government body

libel Making false statements in print, writing, or through pictures or drawings

lice See "pediculosis"

licensed practical nurse (LPN) A nurse who has completed a 1-year nursing program and has passed a licensing test; called licensed vocational nurse (LVN) in some states

licensed vocational nurse (LVN) See "licensed practical nurse"

lithotomy position The woman lies on her back with her hips at the edge of the exam table, her knees are flexed, her hips are externally rotated, and her feet are in stirrups

logrolling Turning the person as a unit, in alignment, with one motion

low vision Eyesight that cannot be corrected with eyeglasses, contact lenses, drugs, or surgery

malignant tumor A tumor that invades and destroys nearby tissue and can spread to other body parts; cancer

malpractice Negligence by a professional person

mechanical ventilation Using a machine to move air into and out of the lungs

Medicaid A health care payment program sponsored by the federal government and operated by the states

medical asepsis Practices used to remove or destroy pathogens and to prevent their spread from one person or place to another person or place; clean technique

medical diagnosis The identification of a disease or condition by a doctor

medical record A written account of a person's condition and response to treatment and care; chart or clinical record

medical symptom An indication or characteristic of a physical or psychological condition

Medicare A federal health insurance program for persons 65 years of age or older and younger people with certain disabilities

medication reminder Reminding the person to take drugs, observing them being taken as prescribed, and charting that they were taken

melena A black, tarry stool

menopause When menstruation stops and there has been at least 1 year without a menstrual period

menstruation The process in which the lining of the uterus breaks up and is discharged from the body through the vagina

mental Relating to the mind; something that exists in the mind or is done by the mind

mental disorder A disturbance in the ability to cope with or adjust to stress; behavior and function are impaired; mental illness, emotional illness, psychiatric disorder

mental health The person copes with and adjusts to everyday stresses in ways accepted by society

mental illness See "mental disorder"

metabolism The burning of food for heat and energy by the cells

metastasis The spread of cancer to other body parts

microbe See "microorganism"

microorganism A small (micro) living plant or animal (organism) seen only with a microscope; a microbe

micturition See "urination"

mite A very small spider-like organism

mixed aphasia See "expressive-receptive aphasia"

mixed incontinence The combination of stress incontinence and urge incontinence

morning care Care given after breakfast; hygiene measures are more thorough at this time

motor aphasia See "expressive aphasia"

nasal speculum An instrument used to examine the inside of the nose

naso-enteral tube A feeding tube inserted through the nose (*naso*) into the small bowel (*enteral*)

naso-gastric (NG) tube A feeding tube inserted through the nose (*naso*) into the stomach (*gastro*)

need Something necessary or desired for maintaining life and mental well-being

neglect Failure to provide the person with the goods or services needed to avoid physical harm, mental anguish, or mental illness

negligence An unintentional wrong in which a person did not act in a reasonable and careful manner and a person or the person's property was harmed

nocturia Frequent urination (*uria*) at night (*noct*)

non-pathogen A microbe that does not usually cause an infection

nonverbal communication Communication that does not use words

normal flora Microbes that live and grow in a certain area

NREM sleep The phase of sleep when there is *no rapid eye movement*; non-REM sleep

nursing assistant A person who gives basic nursing care under the supervision of a licensed nurse; nurse aide, nursing attendant, and health care assistant are some other titles

nursing center Provides health care and nursing care to persons who need regular or continuous care; licensed nurses are required; nursing facility or nursing home

nursing diagnosis Describes a health problem that can be treated by nursing measures; a step in the nursing process

nursing facility (NF) See "nursing center"

nursing home See "nursing center"

nursing intervention An action or measure taken by the nursing team to help the person reach a goal

nursing process The method nurses use to plan and deliver nursing care; its five steps are assessment, nursing diagnosis, planning, implementation, and evaluation

nursing task Nursing care or a nursing function, procedure, activity, or work that can be delegated to nursing assistants when it does not require an RN's professional knowledge or judgment

nursing team Those who provide nursing care—RNs, LPNs/LVNs, and nursing assistants

nutrient A substance that is ingested, digested, absorbed, and used by the body

nutrition The processes involved in the ingestion, digestion, absorption, and use of foods and fluids by the body

objective data Information that is seen, heard, felt, or smelled by an observer; signs

observation Using the senses of sight, hearing, touch, and smell to collect information

obsession A recurrent, unwanted thought, idea, or image

oliguria Scant amount (*olig*) of urine (*uria*); less than 500 mL in 24 hours

ombudsman Someone who supports or promotes the needs and interests of another person

open fracture The broken bone has come through the skin; compound fracture

open wound The skin or mucous membrane is broken

ophthalmoscope A lighted instrument used to examine the internal eye structures

optimal level of function A person's highest potential for mental and physical performance

oral hygiene Mouth care

organ Groups of tissues with the same function

orthopnea Breathing (*pnea*) deeply and comfortably only when sitting (*ortho*)

orthopneic position Sitting up (*ortho*) and leaning over a table to breathe (*pneic*)

orthostatic hypotension Abnormally low (*hypo*) blood pressure when the person suddenly stands up (*ortho* and *static*); postural hypotension

ostomy A surgically created opening for the elimination of body wastes; see "colostomy" and "ileostomy"

otoscope A lighted instrument used to examine the external ear and the eardrum (tympanic membrane)

output The amount of fluid lost

overflow incontinence Small amounts of urine leak from a full bladder

oxygen concentration The amount (percent) of hemoglobin containing oxygen

pack Wrapping a body part with a wet or dry application

pain To ache, hurt, or be sore; discomfort

palliative care Care that involves relieving or reducing the intensity of uncomfortable symptoms without producing a cure

panic An intense and sudden feeling of fear, anxiety, terror, or dread

paralysis Loss of muscle function, loss of sensation, or loss of both muscle function and sensation

paranoia A disorder (*para*) of the mind (*noia*); the person has false beliefs (delusions) and suspicion about a person or situation

paraphrasing Restating the person's message in your own words

paraplegia Paralysis in the legs and lower trunk

parenteral nutrition Giving nutrients through a catheter inserted into a vein; *para* means beyond; *enteral* relates to the bowel

partial-thickness wound The dermis and epidermis of the skin are broken

patent Open and unblocked

pathogen A microbe that is harmful and can cause an infection

pediculosis Infestation with wingless insects; lice

pediculosis capitis Infestation of the scalp (*capitis*) with lice; head lice

pediculosis corporis Infestation of the body (*corporis*) with lice

pediculosis pubis Infestation of the pubic (*pubis*) hair with lice

penetrating wound An open wound that breaks the skin and enters a body area, organ, or cavity

percussion hammer An instrument used to tap body parts to test reflexes; reflex hammer

percutaneous endoscopic gastrostomy (PEG) tube A feeding tube inserted into the stomach (*gastro*) through a small incision (*stomy*) made through (*per*) the skin (*cutaneous*); a lighted instrument (*scope*) is used to see inside a body cavity or organ (*endo*)

pericare See "perineal care"

perineal care Cleaning the genital and anal areas; pericare

peristalsis Involuntary muscle contractions in the digestive system that move food down the esophagus through the alimentary canal; the alternating contraction and relaxation of intestinal muscles

persistent pain See "chronic pain"

phantom pain Pain felt in a body part that is no longer there

phlebitis Inflammation (*itis*) of a vein (*phleb*)

phobia An intense fear

physical restraint Any manual method or physical or mechanical device, material, or equipment attached to or near the person's body that he or she cannot remove easily and that restricts freedom of movement or normal access to one's body

planning Setting priorities and goals; a step in the nursing process

plantar flexion The foot (*plantar*) is bent (*flexion*); bending the foot down at the ankle

plaque A thin film that sticks to the teeth; it contains saliva, microbes, and other substances

pleural effusion The escape and collection of fluid (*effusion*) in the pleural space

PM care See "evening care"

pneumothorax Air (*pneumo*) in the pleural space (*thorax*)

pollutant A harmful chemical or substance in the air or water

polyuria Abnormally large amounts (*poly*) of urine (*uria*)

post-mortem care Care of the body after (*post*) death (*mortem*)

postural hypotension See "orthostatic hypotension"

posture See "body alignment"

preceptor A staff member who guides another staff member

prefix A word element placed before a root; it changes the meaning of the word

pre-hypertension When the systolic pressure is between 120 and 139 mm Hg or the diastolic pressure is between 80 and 89 mm Hg

presbyopia Age-related (*presby*) farsightedness (*opia* means eye)

pressure ulcer A localized injury to the skin and/or underlying tissue

usually over a bony prominence resulting from pressure or pressure in combination with shear; any lesion caused by unrelieved pressure that results in damage to underlying tissues

primary nursing A nursing care pattern; an RN is responsible for the person's total care

priority The most important thing at the time

professional boundary That which separates helpful behaviors from behaviors that are not helpful

professionalism Following laws, being ethical, having good work ethics, and having the skills to do your work

professional sexual misconduct An act, behavior, or comment that is sexual in nature

progress note A written description of the care given and the person's response and progress

pronation Turning the joint downward

prone position Lying on the abdomen with the head turned to one side

prosthesis An artificial replacement for a missing body part

protected health information Identifying information and information about the person's health care that is maintained or sent in any form (paper, electronic, oral)

pseudodementia False (*pseudo*) dementia

psychiatric disorder See "mental disorder"

psychosis A state of severe mental impairment

pulse The beat of the heart felt at an artery as a wave of blood passes through the artery

pulse deficit The difference between the apical and radial pulse rates

pulse rate The number of heartbeats or pulses felt in 1 minute

puncture wound An open wound made by a sharp object

purulent drainage Thick green, yellow, or brown drainage

pyuria Pus (*py*) in the urine (*uria*)

quadriplegia Paralysis in the arms, legs, and trunk; tetraplegia

radiating pain Pain felt at the site of tissue damage and in nearby areas

range of motion (ROM) The movement of a joint to the extent possible without causing pain

receptive aphasia Difficulty understanding language; Wernicke's aphasia

recording The written account of care and observations; charting

reflex incontinence Urine is lost at predictable intervals when the bladder is full

registered nurse (RN) A nurse who has completed a 2-, 3-, or 4-year nursing program and has passed a licensing test

regurgitation The backward flow of stomach contents into the mouth

rehabilitation The process of restoring the person to his or her highest possible level of physical, psychological, social, and economic function

reincarnation The belief that the spirit or soul is reborn in another human body or in another form of life

relaxation To be free from mental and physical stress

religion Spiritual beliefs, needs, and practices

remove easily The manual method, device, material, or equipment used to restrain the person that can be removed intentionally by the person in the same manner it was applied by the staff

REM sleep The phase of sleep when there is *rapid eye movement*

reporting The oral account of care and observations

representative Any person who has the legal right to act on the resident's behalf when he or she cannot do so for himself or herself

reservoir The environment in which a microbe lives and grows; host

resident unit The personal space, furniture, and equipment provided for the person by the nursing center

respiration Breathing air into (*inhalation*) and out of (*exhalation*) the lungs; the process of supplying the cells with oxygen and removing carbon dioxide from them

respiratory arrest When breathing stops; breathing stops but heart action continues for several minutes

respiratory depression Slow, weak respirations at a rate of fewer than 12 per minute

responsibility The duty or obligation to perform some act or function

rest To be calm, at ease, and relaxed; no anxiety or stress

restorative aide A nursing assistant with special training in restorative nursing and rehabilitation skills

restorative nursing care Care that helps persons regain health, strength, and independence

retention catheter See "indwelling catheter"

reverse Trendelenburg's position The head of the bed is raised and the foot of the bed is lowered

rigor mortis The stiffness or rigidity (*rigor*) of skeletal muscles that occurs after death (*mortis*)

root A word element containing the basic meaning of the word

rotation Turning the joint

sanguineous drainage Bloody (*sanguis*) drainage

seizure Violent and sudden contractions or tremors of muscle groups; convulsion

self-actualization Experiencing one's potential

self-esteem Thinking well of oneself and seeing oneself as useful and having value

self-neglect A person's behaviors that threaten his or her health and safety

semi-Fowler's position The head of the bed is raised 30 degrees; or the head of the bed is raised 30 degrees and the knee portion is raised 15 degrees

semi-prone side position See "Sims' position"

serosanguineous drainage Thin, watery drainage (*sero*) that is blood-tinged (*sanguineous*)

serous drainage Clear, watery fluid (*serum*)

service plan A written plan listing the services needed by the person, how much help is needed, and who provides the services

sex Physical activities involving the reproductive organs; done for pleasure or to have children

sexuality The physical, emotional, social, cultural, and spiritual factors that affect a person's feelings and attitudes about his or her sex

shear See "shearing"

shearing When layers of the skin rub against each other; when the skin remains in place and underlying tissues move and stretch and tear underlying capillaries and blood vessels, causing tissue damage; when skin sticks to a surface while muscles slide in the direction the body is moving

shock Results when organs and tissues do not get enough blood

side-lying position See "lateral position"

signs See "objective data"

simple fracture See "closed fracture"

Sims' position A left side-lying position in which the upper leg (right leg) is sharply flexed so it is not on the lower leg (left leg) and the lower arm (left arm) is behind the person; semi-prone side position

skilled nursing facility (SNF) Provides health care and nursing care for residents who have many or severe health problems or who need rehabilitation; may be part of a nursing center or a hospital

skin tear A break or rip in the outer layers of the skin; the epidermis (top skin layer) separates from the underlying tissues

slander Making false statements orally

sleep A state of unconsciousness, reduced voluntary muscle activity, and lowered metabolism

slough Dead tissue that is shed from the skin; it is usually light colored, soft, and moist; it may be stringy at times

spastic Uncontrolled contractions of skeletal muscles

sphygmomanometer A cuff and measuring device used to measure blood pressure

spore A bacterium protected by a hard shell

sputum Mucus from the respiratory system that is expectorated (*expelled*) through the mouth

standard of care The skills, care, and judgments required by a health team member under similar conditions

stasis ulcer See "venous ulcer"

sterile The absence of *all* microbes

sterile field A work area free of *all* pathogens and non-pathogens (including spores)

sterile technique See "surgical asepsis"

sterilization The process of destroying *all* microbes

stethoscope An instrument used to listen to sounds produced by the heart, lungs, and other body organs

stoma An opening that can be seen through the abdominal wall; see "colostomy" and "ileostomy"

stomatitis Inflammation (*itis*) of the mouth (*stomat*)

stool Excreted feces

straight catheter A catheter that drains the bladder and then is removed

stress The response or change in the body caused by any emotional, physical, social, or economic factor

stress incontinence When urine leaks during exercise and certain movements that cause pressure on the bladder

stressor The event or factor that causes stress

subjective data Things a person tells you about that you cannot observe through your senses; symptoms

suction The process of withdrawing or sucking up fluid (secretions)

sudden cardiac arrest (SCA) The heart stops suddenly and without warning; cardiac arrest

suffix A word element placed after a root; it changes the meaning of the word

suffocation When breathing stops from the lack of oxygen

suicide To kill oneself

suicide contagion Exposure to suicide or suicidal behaviors within one's family, one's peer group, or media reports of suicide

sundowning Signs, symptoms, and behaviors of AD increase during hours of darkness

supination Turning the joint upward

supine position The back-lying or dorsal recumbent position

suppository A cone-shaped, solid drug that is inserted into a body opening; it melts at body temperature

surgical asepsis The practices that keep items free of *all* microbes; sterile technique

symptoms See "subjective data"

syncope A brief loss of consciousness; fainting

system Organs that work together to perform special functions

systole The period of heart muscle contraction; the heart is pumping blood

systolic pressure The pressure in the arteries when the heart contracts

tachycardia A rapid (*tachy*) heart rate (*cardia*); more than 100 beats per minute

tachypnea Rapid (*tachy*) breathing (*pnea*); respirations are more than 20 per minute

tartar Hardened plaque

team nursing A nursing care pattern; a team of nursing staff is led by an RN who delegates care to other nurses; some nursing tasks and procedures are delegated to nursing assistants

terminal illness An illness or injury from which the person will not likely recover

tetraplegia See "quadriplegia"

thrombus A blood clot

tinnitus A ringing, roaring, hissing, or buzzing sound in the ears or head

tissue A group of cells with similar functions

tort A wrong committed against a person or the person's property

tracheostomy A surgically created opening (*stomy*) into the trachea (*tracheo*)

transfer Moving the person from one place to another; moving the person to another health care setting; moving the person to a new room within the center

transfer belt A device used to support a person who is unsteady or disabled; gait belt

transgender A broad term used to describe people who express their sexuality or gender in other than the expected ways; persons who are undergoing hormone therapy or surgery for sexual reassignment (female to male; male to female)

transient incontinence Temporary or occasional incontinence that is reversed when the cause is treated

transsexual A person who believes that he or she is a member of the other sex

transvestite A person who dresses and behaves like the other sex for emotional and sexual relief; cross-dresser

trauma An accident or violent act that injures the skin, mucous membranes, bones, and organs

treatment The care provided to maintain or restore health, improve function, or relieve symptoms

Trendelenburg's position The head of the bed is lowered and the foot of the bed is raised

triggers Clues for the Care Area Assessments (CAAs)

tumor A new growth of abnormal cells; tumors are benign or malignant

tuning fork An instrument vibrated to test hearing

ulcer A shallow or deep crater-like sore of the skin or a mucous membrane

unavoidable pressure ulcer A pressure ulcer that occurs despite efforts to prevent one through proper use of the nursing process

unintentional wound A wound resulting from trauma

urge incontinence The loss of urine in response to a sudden, urgent need to void; the person cannot get to a toilet in time

urinary diversion A new pathway for urine to exit the body

urinary frequency Voiding at frequent intervals

urinary incontinence The involuntary loss or leakage of urine

urinary urgency The need to void at once

urination The process of emptying urine from the bladder; micturition or voiding

urostomy A surgically created opening (*stomy*) between a ureter (*uro*) and the abdomen

vaccination Giving a vaccine to produce immunity against an infectious disease

vaccine A preparation containing dead or weakened microbes

vaginal speculum An instrument used to open the vagina for examining it and the cervix

vascular ulcer See "circulatory ulcer"

vein A blood vessel that returns blood to the heart

venous ulcer An open sore on the lower legs or feet caused by poor venous blood flow; stasis ulcer

verbal communication Communication that uses written or spoken words

vertigo Dizziness

vital signs Temperature, pulse, respirations, and blood pressure

voiding See "urination"

vomitus Food and fluids expelled from the stomach through the mouth; emesis

vulnerable adult A person 18 years old or older who has a disability or condition that makes him or her at risk to be wounded, attacked, or damaged

waterproof drawsheet A drawsheet made of plastic, rubber, or absorbent material used to protect the mattress and bottom linens from dampness and soiling

Wernicke's aphasia See "receptive aphasia"

will A legal document of how a person wants property distributed after death

withdrawal syndrome The person's physical and mental response after stopping or severely reducing the use of a substance that was used regularly

word element A part of a word

work ethics Behavior in the workplace

workplace violence Violent acts (including assault and threat of assault) directed toward persons at work or while on duty

wound A break in the skin or mucous membrane

AD	Alzheimer's disease
ADA	Americans With Disabilities Act of 1990
ADL	Activities of daily living
AED	Automated external defibrillator
AFB	American Foundation for the Blind
AHA	American Heart Association
AIDS	Acquired immunodeficiency syndrome
AIIR	Airborne infection isolation room
ALR	Assisted living residence
ALS	Amyotrophic lateral sclerosis
AMD	Age-related macular degeneration
ASL	American Sign Language
BLS	Basic Life Support
BM	Bowel movement
BP	Blood pressure
BPD	Borderline personality disorder
BPH	Benign prostatic hyperplasia
C	Centigrade
CAA	Care Area Assessments
CAD	Coronary artery disease
CCRC	Continuing care retirement community
CDC	Centers for Disease Control and Prevention
cm	Centimeter
CMS	Centers for Medicare & Medicaid Services
CNA	Certified nursing assistant, certified nurse aide
CO_2	Carbon dioxide
COPD	Chronic obstructive pulmonary disease
CP	Cerebral palsy
CPR	Cardiopulmonary resuscitation
CVA	Cerebrovascular accident
DD	Developmental disability
DNR	Do not resuscitate
DON	Director of nursing
DS	Down syndrome
DV	Daily Value
ED	Erectile dysfunction
EMS	Emergency Medical Services
ET	Endotracheal
F	Fahrenheit
FBAO	Foreign-body airway obstruction
FDA	Food and Drug Administration
FXS	Fragile X syndrome
GERD	Gastro-esophageal reflux disease
GI	Gastro-intestinal
gtt	Drops
gtt/min	Drops per minute

HAI	Healthcare-associated infection
HBV	Hepatitis B virus
Hg	Mercury
HIPAA	Health Insurance Portability and Accountability Act of 1996
HIV	Human immunodeficiency virus
HMO	Health maintenance organization
ID	Identification
I&O	Intake and output
IQ	Intelligence quotient
IV	Intravenous
L/min	Liters per minute
LNA	Licensed nursing assistant
LPN	Licensed practical nurse
LVN	Licensed vocational nurse
MDRO	Multidrug-resistant organism
MDS	Minimum Data Set
mg	Milligram
MI	Myocardial infarction
mL	Milliliter
mm	Millimeter
mm Hg	Millimeters of mercury
MRSA	Methicillin-resistant *Staphylococcus aureus*
MS	Multiple sclerosis
MSD	Musculo-skeletal disorder
MSDS	Material safety data sheet
NANDA-I	North American Nursing Diagnosis Association International
NATCEP	Nursing assistant training and competency evaluation program
NCSBN	National Council of State Boards of Nursing
NG	Naso-gastric
NIA	National Institute on Aging
NIAAA	National Institute on Alcohol Abuse and Alcoholism
NIMH	National Institute of Mental Health
NPO	Non per os; nothing by mouth
NREM	No rapid eye movement
O2	Oxygen
OBRA	Omnibus Budget Reconciliation Act of 1987
OCD	Obsessive-compulsive disorder
OPIM	Other potentially infectious materials
OSHA	Occupational Safety and Health Administration
oz	Ounce

PASS	*Pull* the safety pin, *aim* low, *squeeze* the lever, *sweep* back and forth
PEG	Percutaneous endoscopic gastrostomy
PHI	Protected health information
PPE	Personal protective equipment
PPO	Preferred provider organization
PT	Physical therapist
PTSD	Post-traumatic stress disorder
RA	Rheumatoid arthritis
RBC	Red blood cell
REM	Rapid eye movement
RN	Registered nurse
RNA	Registered nurse aide
ROM	Range of motion; range-of-motion
SB	Spina bifida
SCA	Sudden cardiac arrest
SNF	Skilled nursing facility

SpO$_2$	Oxygen saturation (S = saturation; p = pressure; O$_2$ = oxygen)
SSE	Soapsuds enema
STD	Sexually transmitted disease
TB	Tuberculosis
TBI	Traumatic brain injury
TIA	Transient ischemic attack
TJC	The Joint Commission
TPN	Total parenteral nutrition
USDA	United States Department of Agriculture
UTI	Urinary tract infection
VF	Ventricular fibrillation
V-fib	Ventricular fibrillation
VRE	Vancomycin-resistant *Enterococcus*
WBC	White blood cell

A

Abandonment, 39, 41
Abbreviations, 59, 67-69
Abdominal binder, 554, 554f
Abdominal regions, 67, 67f
Abdominal thrusts, 139, 140f
Abduction, 414, 419
Abrasion, 535, 537
Abuse
   child, 40-41, 42b
   definition of, 15, 32, 38
   domestic, 41-42
   economic, 41
   elder, 38-40, 39b, 40b
   emotional, 39, 41, 42b
   mental, 39
   in nursing centers, 40
   physical, 41, 42b
   reporting of, 15, 38-42
   resident's right to freedom from, 15, 467, 717
   sexual, 39, 41, 42b
   social, 41
   substance, 41
   verbal, 39, 41
   vulnerable adults, 38, 38b
Accessory dwelling unit, 123
Accidents
   burns, 136, 137b, 137t, 706-707, 706f
   in dementia patients, 135b
   equipment-related, 141, 141f, 142b, 142f
   falls. See Fall(s)
   poisoning, 137, 137b
   prevention of, 154
   risk factors for, 135
Accountable, 19, 28
Acetone, 502, 508
Acquired immunodeficiency syndrome, 598-599, 599b, 639-640t
Active range-of-motion exercises, 419
Active-assistive range-of-motion exercises, 419
Activities director, 6-7t
Activities of daily living
   assessment of, 76b
   assisted living residents, 466
   definition of, 70b, 682, 684
   flow sheet for, 62, 62f
Activity. See also Exercise
   Dietary Guidelines for Americans recommendations, 373
   groups involved in, 16
   importance of, 415
   MyPyramid guidelines, 375, 377b
   recreational, 429
   resident's right to, 16, 16f
Acute confusion, 656
Acute illness, 1, 3
Acute kidney failure, 637
Acute pain, 431, 433
Addiction
   alcoholism, 648
   drug, 648-649, 649-651t
Adduction, 414, 419
Admission, 522-527
   definition of, 521-522
   first impressions at, 526
   form used in, 524f
   height measurements at, 527, 528b, 529b, 530f, 531b, 531f
   identifying information necessary for, 522-523
   new room

Admission (Continued)
   moving of person to, 531, 532b
   preparation of, 523, 523b, 523f
   of dementia persons, 523
   procedure for, 526, 526-527b
   quality of life considerations, 534b
   safety issues, 522b, 526
   security issues, 526
   weight measurements at, 527, 528b, 528f, 529b, 530f
Admission sheet, 61
Adolescence, 116b
Adrenal cortex, 112
Adrenal glands, 112
Adrenocorticotropic hormone, 111
Adult day-care centers, 123
Adult foster care, 124
Advance directives, 12, 709, 714
Affect, 642, 646
Afternoon care, 282
Age-related macular degeneration, 585-586, 586f
Aggressive behavior
   in Alzheimer's disease, 664
   description of, 87
   sexually, 131-132, 131b
   in workplace, 150b
Aging
   Alzheimer's disease vs., 659b
   digestion affected by, 405
   myths and facts about, 116b
   oxygen needs affected by, 443
   pain and, 434, 434b
   physical changes associated with, 118-122, 119b, 656b
Agitation, 150b, 171, 172b, 663-664
Agonal gasps, 693-694
Agonal respirations, 693
Air flotation bed, 573, 575f
Airborne precautions, 194b
Airway
   artificial. See Artificial airways
   cardiopulmonary resuscitation considerations for, 694, 694f
   head tilt-chin lift method, 140f
   obstruction of, 138
   suctioning of, 459-460, 460b, 460f
Alcohol
   cancer risks, 596
   description of, 45
   Dietary Guidelines for Americans, 374
   oxygen needs affected by, 443
Alcohol abuse, 648
Alcohol-based hand rub, 187
Alcoholism, 648
Alert and oriented residents, 86
Alimentary canal, 107, 108f
Allergy, 442-443
Alopecia, 311, 313
Alveoli, 107
Alzheimer's disease, 658-666. See also Dementia
   age-related changes vs., 659b
   basic needs for, 668
   behaviors and problems associated with, 661-666
      aggression, 664
      agitation, 663-664
      catastrophic reactions, 663
      combativeness, 664
      communication-related, 665, 665b
      delusions, 663, 668
      elopement, 655, 662
      hallucinations, 663, 668
      hiding things, 666
      intimacy, 664
      paranoia, 663, 663b
      repetitive behaviors, 664

Alzheimer's disease (Continued)
      restlessness, 663-664
      rummaging, 666
      screaming, 666
      sexuality, 664
      sundowning, 655, 662, 667
      wandering, 662, 662f, 667
   brain effects, 658, 658f
   caring for, 666-670, 667-668b, 667b, 668f, 669f, 670b
   definition of, 1
   family caregivers, 669-670, 670b
   mild, 660, 661f
   moderate, 660, 661f
   quality of life considerations, 671b
   rights of persons with, 671
   safety considerations, 667, 668f, 669f
   severe, 660, 661f
   signs of, 658, 659b
   sleep promotion in, 668
   special care units for, 669
   stages of, 660, 660b
   validation therapy for, 670
Alzheimer's Disease Education and Referral Center, 343
Alzheimer's units, 4
AM care, 280, 282
Ambu bag, 460, 460f
Ambulation, 424-429
   aids for, 426-429, 426f, 427f, 428f, 429f
   benefits of, 424
   braces for, 429, 429f
   cane for, 428, 428f
   charting of, 425f
   crutches for, 426, 426f, 427f
   definition of, 414, 424
   delegation of, 424b
   guidelines for, 425b
   safety in, 424b
   walkers for, 429, 429f
American Nurses Association code of ethics, 33
American Sign Language, 580, 581f
Amphetamine, 649-651t
Amputation, 601, 615, 615f
Amyotrophic lateral sclerosis, 605
Anabolic steroids, 649-651t
Anaphylactic shock, 704
Anaphylaxis, 691, 704
Anger, 85, 87-88, 91
Angina, 619-620, 620f
Ankle exercises, 423f
Ankle-foot orthosis, 429f
Anorexia, 371, 382
Anterior, 67, 67f, 211f
Antibiotics, 184
Antibodies, 112
Anticoagulant, 311, 319
Antidiuretic hormone, 111
Anti-embolism stockings, 541. See also Elastic stockings
Antigens, 112, 704
Antiperspirants, 291t
Antisocial personality disorder, 647
Anus, 108
Anxiety, 433, 642-643, 643b
Anxiety disorders, 643-645
   nonverbal communication, 653
   obsessive-compulsive disorder, 645
   panic disorder, 644
   phobias, 642, 644
   post-traumatic stress disorder, 645, 645b
Aorta, 106
Apartments, 123
Aphasia, 578, 583-584, 687
Apical pulse, 483, 487, 487b, 487f

Page numbers followed by "*f*" indicate figure(s); "*t*" indicate table(s); "*b*" indicate box(es)

Apical-radial pulse, 473, 488, 488b, 488f
Apnea, 442, 444
Appearance, personal, 45, 46b, 54
Appetite, 76b, 382
Apraxia, 583
Aquathermia pad, 556, 558
Aqueous chamber, 104
Arachnoid space, 103
Armrest, 217f
Arterial blood gases, 445
Arterial ulcers, 535, 545, 545f
Arteries, 97, 106, 106f
Arterioles, 106
Arthritis
    definition of, 601, 607
    osteoarthritis, 607, 607f
    osteoporosis caused by, 610
    rheumatoid, 607-608, 607f
    total joint replacement surgery for, 608, 608f, 609b, 609f
Arthroplasty, 601, 608
Artificial airways, 458-459
    endotracheal tube, 458, 458f
    nasopharyngeal, 459
    oropharyngeal, 458-459, 458f
    tracheostomy, 458, 458f, 459b
Artificial eye. See Ocular prosthesis
Ascending colostomy, 367f
Ascites, 630f
Ascorbic acid, 379t
Asepsis
    definition of, 182, 186
    medical. See Medical asepsis
    surgical, 183, 186
Aspiration
    definition of, 280, 286, 371, 386, 401
    enteral nutrition, 405
    precautions for, 387b
    prevention of, 405
    in unconscious patients, 286
Assault, 32, 37, 149
Assessment
    definition of, 74
    in nursing process, 75, 76b, 77b
Assignment sheets, 80, 80f, 81b
Assist devices, for moving persons up in bed, 229, 229b, 229f
Assisted living
    definition of, 464-465
    purpose of, 466
    safety in, 466b
    service plan for, 468-471, 469b
Assisted living residences, 2-3, 124
    activities in, 471
    definition of, 1
    discharge from, 467, 471
    environment requirements of, 466b
    eviction from, 471
    food safety in, 469, 469f
    laundry services in, 469, 469b
    living areas of, 465, 465f
    medication assistance in, 470-471, 470b, 470f
    nursing services in, 470
        privacy rights, 467
    purpose of, 2
    recreation in, 471
    residents of, 466, 467b, 471b
    safety needs in, 471
    service plan for, 468-471, 469b
    services offered, 465
    special services in, 471
    staff requirements, 468
    transfer from, 467, 471, 532-533
Assisted living units, 465b
Assistive device, 70b
Asthma, 622
Atelectasis, 448
Atherosclerosis, 618, 618f
Athetoid, 677

Athlete's foot, 545, 546f
Atria, 106, 106f
Atrophy, 70b, 414-415, 416f
Attendance, 53, 53b
Attitude, 53
Audiologist, 6-7t
Autism, 678, 678b
Autoclave, 190, 190f
Autoimmune disorders, 597-598
Automated external defibrillators, 698, 699f, 702b, 702f
Autonomic dysreflexia, 606, 606b, 607b
Autonomic nervous system, 103-104
Autopsy, 709, 715
Avoidable pressure ulcer, 564, 566
Axillary measurement, of body temperature, 475, 475t, 477, 480f

B
B lymphocytes, 112
Back injuries, 213-214, 214b
Back massage, 302, 303-304b, 303b, 304f
Bacteria, 183
Bag baths, 297
Bag valve mask, 695, 696f
Ball-and-socket joint, 100, 100f
Barbiturates, 649-651t
Barrel chest, 622, 622f
Barrier device breathing, 695, 695f, 696f
Base of support, 210-211
Basic Life Support, 693-703
    cardiopulmonary resuscitation. See Cardiopulmonary resuscitation
    Chain of Survival, 693
    respiratory arrest, 694
    sudden cardiac arrest, 620, 691, 693
Bath oils, 291t
Bathing, 290-299
    bag baths, 297
    comfort in, 293b
    complete bed bath, 293, 294-295b, 295f, 296f, 297f
    delegation of, 292b
    in dementia persons, 292b
    frequency of, 290
    partial bath, 297, 297-298b, 298f
    safety in, 293b
    showers, 299, 299b, 300f, 301-302b, 301b
    towel baths, 297
    tub baths, 299, 299b, 300f, 301-302b, 301b
Battery, 32, 37
Beans, 378
Beards, 322
Bed, 254-257
    air flotation, 573, 575f
    closed. See Closed bed
    controls for, 254, 255f
    dangling on side of, 236, 236b, 237b, 237f, 238f
    eggcrate-type pads on, 573, 575f
    electrical, 255
    entrapment zones in, 256-257, 257f, 258f
    height measurements of persons in, 531b, 531f
    manually operated, 255, 255f
    moving persons in, 225-231
    occupied. See Occupied bed
    open, 266, 266f, 274, 274b
    positions of, 256, 256f, 257f
    quality of life issues, 279b
    safety issues for, 255b, 256-257, 257f, 258f
    shampooing of hair in, 317, 317f
    sitting on the side of, 236, 236b, 237b, 237f, 238f
    surgical, 266, 266f, 278, 278b, 278f
    types of, 266, 266f
    wheel locks for, 162
Bed cradle, 417, 418f, 573
Bed rails, 156, 160, 160f, 161b, 175f
Bed transfers, 242, 243b
Bed-boards, 417, 417f

Bedfast, 564, 567
Bedmaking, 268-278
    closed bed, 269, 270-271b, 271f, 272f, 273f
    delegation of, 268b
    linens. See Linens
    rules for, 269b
    safety in, 269b
Bedpans, 335, 335f, 336b, 336f, 337b, 338f, 513f
Bedrest, 415-418
    complications of, 415-416, 416b
    exercise during, 418
    positioning support during, 417, 417f, 418f
    types of, 415
Bedside table, 259, 259f
Behavior
    disability-related, 87, 87b, 88b
    illness-related, 87, 87b, 88b
Belonging, 84, 437
Belt restraints, 176, 177f
Benign prostatic hyperplasia, 635-636, 635f
Benign tumor, 594-595, 595f
Benzodiazepines, 649-651t
Between-meal snacks, 396
Bias, 33
Bile, 108, 627
Binders, 554, 554f, 555b
BIOHAZARD symbol, 201f
Biohazardous waste
    definition of, 182, 201
    double-bagging of, 201, 201f
Biological therapy, 597
Biot's respiration, 442, 444
Bipolar disorder, 646, 646b
Birth defect, 673-674
Bisexual, 128-129
Bladder
    anatomy of, 109
    assessment of, 76b
Bladder training, 353, 684
Bland diet, 384-385t
Bleeding. See Hemorrhage
Blindness, 578, 584, 587-590, 588-589b, 589b, 589f
Blisters, 545, 546f
Bloating, 359
Blood
    capillary, 516
    description of, 105, 203b
    glucose levels, testing of, 516-517, 517b, 517f, 518-519b, 518b, 519f
    occult, 513, 514f
    in stool, 513, 513b, 514b
    in urine, 508
Blood pressure, 490-492
    abnormal, 490
    definition of, 473, 490
    factors that affect, 490b
    measurement of
        charting, 494f
        delegation of, 492b
        equipment for, 491, 491b, 491f
        guidelines for, 492b
        sphygmomanometer, 473, 491, 491f
        technique for, 492, 493b, 494f
    normal, 490
Blood vessels
    constriction of, 535, 555, 556f
    description of, 106-107, 106f
    dilation of, 535, 555, 556f
Bloodborne pathogen standard, 203-205
    exposure control plan, 204
    preventive measures, 204-205
    terminology associated with, 203b
Board and care homes, 1-2, 124
Body alignment, 210-211
Body language
    communication through, 91, 91b
    definition of, 82
    in job interview, 51

Body mechanics, 45
    definition of, 210-211
    principles of, 211f, 213
    rules for, 212b
Body temperature, 475-482
    definition of, 473, 475
    normal, 475t
Body temperature measurement
    axillary, 475, 475t, 477, 480f
    oral, 475, 475t, 477, 479f, 482f
    rectal, 475, 475t, 477, 479f
    sites for, 475, 475b
    temporal artery, 475, 475t, 480, 480f, 482
    thermometers
        digital, 482
        disposable oral, 482, 482f
        electronic, 480, 480f, 481b, 482b
        glass, 476-477, 476b, 476f, 477f, 478-479b, 478b
        temperature-sensitive tape, 482, 483f
        tympanic membrane, 475, 475t, 480, 480f, 482, 482f
Body weight, 527, 528b, 528f, 529b, 530f
Bomb threats, 149
Bone marrow, 100
Bones
    age-related changes in, 120
    anatomy of, 100, 100f
Bony prominence, 564-565
Borderline personality disorder, 647
Boundaries, 33-34
Boundary crossing, 32, 34
Boundary signs, 32, 34, 35b
Boundary violation, 32, 34
Bowel elimination
    constipation, 121-122, 355, 357-358, 607
    diarrhea, 355, 358, 359b
    dietary factors, 357
    factors that affect, 356-357
    flatulence, 355, 359
    normal, 356, 356b
    privacy issues, 357
    problems involving, 357-359
    quality of life issues, 370b
Bowel movement, 356-357, 359, 360f
Bowel training, 359, 360f
Bowman's capsule, 109
Braces, 429, 429f
Braden Scale for Predicting Pressure Sore Risk, 570, 571f
Bradycardia, 473, 484
Bradypnea, 442, 444
Braille, 578, 589, 590f
Brain
    age-related changes in, 120
    Alzheimer's disease effects, 658, 658f
    anatomy of, 103, 103f, 658f
    stroke effects on, 602f
    traumatic injury to, 605
Brainstem, 103
Breaks, 55
Breast binder, 554, 554f
Breasts, 110, 111f
Breathing. See also Respiration(s)
    cardiopulmonary resuscitation, 694-696, 695f
    during death and dying, 713
Broca's aphasia, 578, 583
Bronchioles, 107
Bronchitis, chronic, 621-622
Bronchoscopy, 445
Bronchus, 107
Brushing
    of hair, 314, 314b, 315-316b
    of teeth, 283, 284b, 284f
Bunions, 545, 546f
Burns, 136, 137b, 137t, 706-707, 706f

C
Caffeine, 439
Calcium, 380t

Calculi
    renal. See Kidney stones
    urinary, 510
Call system, for resident unit, 260-261, 260f, 261b, 261f
Callus, 517, 545
Calorie, 371-372
Calorie counts, 396
Calorie-controlled diet, 384-385t
Cancer, 595-597, 595f, 596b
    definition of, 594
Cane, 428, 428f, 590
Cannabinoids, 649-651t
Cannula
    nasal, 452, 453f
    tracheostomy, 458f
Capillaries, 97, 106
Capillary blood, 516
Car safety, 151b, 152f
Carbohydrates, 374, 379
Cardiac arrest
    description of, 138
    sudden. See Sudden cardiac arrest
Cardiac muscle, 101
Cardiopulmonary resuscitation, 694-700
    adult, 699-700, 699b, 700b, 701b, 702b
    airway, 694, 694f
    breathing, 694-696, 695f
    circulation, 697, 697f, 698f
    defibrillation, 698, 699f, 702b, 702f
    hands-only, 700
    one-rescuer, 700b
    recovery position after, 703, 703f
    safety in, 694b
    technique for, 699-700, 699b, 700b, 701b, 702b
    two-rescuer, 701b, 701f, 702b
Cardiovascular disorders, 618-621
    angina, 619-620, 620f
    coronary artery disease, 618-619, 618f, 619b, 619f
    heart failure, 621
    myocardial infarction, 620, 620f, 621b
    risk factors for, 618b
Care plan, 70b
Caregivers
    Alzheimer's disease, 669-670, 670b
    children as, 118
Carotid pulse, 697f
Carpooling, 52
Carrier, 182, 185
Cartilage, 100
Case management, 1, 6
Case manager, 6
Case mix groups, 9
Casts, 611, 611f, 612b, 612f
Cataracts, 585, 585f
Catastrophic reactions, 663
Catheter, 344-351
    care of, 346b, 347f
    clamped, 348f, 353
    condom, 351, 351b, 351f, 352b, 353f
    definition of, 333, 344
    delegation of, 345b
    drainage systems for, 347-348, 348b, 349b, 350b, 350f
    indwelling, 333, 344, 344f, 345b
    intravenous, 409, 409f
    securing of, 344f
    straight, 333, 344
Catheter plug, 348f
Catheterization, 333, 344
Catholicism, 381
Cell, 98-99
    definition of, 97
    division of, 98f
    parts of, 98f
Cell membrane, 98, 98f
Centers for Medicare & Medicaid Services
    comfort requirements, 432
    description of, 126, 126b
    incontinence, 342
    nutritional assessment requirements, 372

Centers for Medicare & Medicaid Services (Continued)
    pressure ulcers, 566
    range-of-motion exercises, 419
    resident unit requirements, 263b
    restraint rules, 167
Central nervous system, 102-103, 102f, 103f
Cerebellum, 103
Cerebral cortex, 103
Cerebral hemispheres, 103
Cerebral palsy, 677-678
Cerebrospinal fluid, 103
Cerebrovascular accident. See Stroke
Cerebrum, 103
Certification, 21, 22-23
Cerumen, 104, 121, 578, 580
Cervical traction, 605-606
Cervix, 110
Chair
    repositioning in, 250
    in resident unit, 259
    transfer of persons, 239, 239b, 240-241b, 241f, 242, 242f
Chair position, 217, 217f
Chairfast, 564, 567
Charge nurse, 4-5
Chart, 59
Charting
    ambulation, 425f
    blood pressure measurement, 494f
    choking, 139f
    cold applications, 561f
    computer, 71f
    dangling on side of bed, 237f
    enema, 363f
    falls, 161f
    grooming, 332f
    heat applications, 561f
    pressure ulcer, 576f
    restraints, 169f, 176f
    sample of, 65, 66f
Chemical disinfectants, 189
Chemical restraint, 166-167, 170
Chemotherapy, 597
Chest compressions, 697, 697f, 698f
Chest pain, 619, 620f
Chest tubes, 462, 462f, 463b
Chest x-ray, 445
Chewing, 382
Cheyne-Stokes respirations, 442, 444
Child abuse, 40-41, 42b
Child pornography, 41
Child prostitution, 41
Childcare, 52
Chlamydia, 639-640t
Choking, 138-139, 138f, 139-140b, 139f
Choroid, 104
Chromosomes, 98
Chronic bronchitis, 621-622
Chronic illness, 1, 3, 115
Chronic kidney failure, 638, 639b
Chronic obstructive pulmonary disease, 621-622
Chronic pain, 431, 433
Chronic wound, 535, 537
Church of Jesus Christ of Latter-day Saints, 381
Chyme, 108, 356
Circadian rhythm, 431, 437
Circulatory system, 105-107
    age-related changes in, 119b, 121
    blood, 105
    blood vessels. See Blood vessels
    cardiopulmonary resuscitation of, 697, 697f, 698f. See also Cardiopulmonary resuscitation
    functions of, 105
    heart. See Heart
    oxygen needs affected by, 443
Circulatory ulcers, 539-545
    arterial ulcers, 535, 545, 545f
    definition of, 535, 539
    diabetic foot ulcer, 535, 545, 545b
    venous. See Venous ulcers

Circumcision, 305, 347f
Cirrhosis, 629-630, 630b, 630f
Civil laws, 32, 34
Clamped catheter, 348f, 353
Clean technique, 182, 186
Clean wound, 535, 537
Clean-catch urine specimen. See Midstream urine
    specimen
Clean-contaminated wound, 535, 537
Cleansing enema, 361, 362-363b
Clean-voided urine specimen. See Midstream urine
    specimen
Clear-liquid diet, 384-385t
Cleric, 6-7t
Clinical nurse specialist, 6-7t
Clitoris, 110, 110f
Closed bed
    definition of, 266
    illustration of, 266f
    making of, 269, 270-271b, 271f, 272f, 273f
Closed fracture, 601, 610
Closed wound, 535, 537
Closet space, 262, 262b, 262f
CMS. See Centers for Medicare & Medicaid
    Services
Cocaine, 649-651t
Cochlea, 104-105
Code of conduct, 34b
Codeine, 649-651t
Codes of ethics, 33
Cognitive function, 70b, 655-656
Cold, common, 623t
Cold applications, for wound healing, 555-561,
    557b, 557t, 558b, 559-560b, 560f, 561f
Cold compress, 557
Cold packs, 557-558
Collecting specimens. See Specimen collection
Colonized, 564, 575
Color-coded wristbands, 152, 152f
Colostomy, 355, 366, 367f
Coma, 133, 135
Comatose, 82, 87, 94
Combativeness, 664
Combing of hair, 314, 314b, 315-316b
Comfort, 432
    bowel elimination, 357b
    brushing and combing of hair, 315b
    during death and dying, 712-714
    definition of, 431-432
    enemas, 360b, 361b
    hand hygiene, 188b
    isolation precautions, 192
    mechanical lift, 244
    nail care, 322b
    nursing measures for, 436, 436b
    Omnibus Budget Reconciliation Act
        requirements, 432
    perineal care, 306b
    in positioning the person, 215, 215b
    promotion of, 136b
    pulse oximetry, 446b
    shampooing of hair, 318b
    shaving, 320b
    stethoscope, 484, 484f
    transfer of persons, 238b
Commodes, 340, 340b, 340f, 341b
Communicable diseases
    definition of, 182, 191
    prevention of, 3
Communication, 60
    aids for, 89-90f, 90f
    with Alzheimer's disease persons, 665, 665b
    barriers to, 93, 93b
    blind persons, 582
    clarifying, 93
    cultural barriers to, 93, 93b
    definition of, 59-60
    in delegation, 28-29
    direct questions for, 92
    eye contact during, 92b, 92f

Communication (Continued)
    focusing, 93
    health team members, 73b
    hearing loss persons, 580, 581f
    listening, 92
    methods of, 92-93
    nonverbal. See Nonverbal communication
    open-ended questions for, 92
    paraphrasing, 92
    rehabilitation of, 687, 687b
    with residents, 88-91, 89-90f, 90f, 92-93
    silence, 93, 93b
    speech-impaired person, 583b
    verbal, 88-89, 89-90f, 90f
    visually impaired persons, 582
Compensation, 644
Competency evaluation, 21-22, 47
Complete bed bath, 293, 294-295b, 295f, 296f, 297f
Complete care residents, 86
Compound fracture, 601
Comprehensive care plan, 74, 77, 79
Compress
    cold, 557
    definition of, 535
    hot, 555, 556f
Compulsion, 642, 645
Computers, 70, 71b
Condom catheters, 351, 351b, 351f, 352b, 353f
Confidentiality
    definition of, 44, 53-54
    exposure incidents, 205
    resident information, 73
    resident's right to, 12-14, 717
    at work, 53-54, 54b
Conflict
    dealing with, 72, 72b
    definition of, 59, 72
Confused residents, 86
Confusion
    description of, 656, 656b, 656f
    restraints as cause of, 171, 172b
Congregate housing, 123
Connective tissue, 98
Consent, informed, 37, 37b
Constipation, 121-122, 355, 357-358, 607
Constrict, 535, 555, 556f
Contact lenses, 592, 592b
Contact precautions, 194b
Contagious disease, 182, 191
Contaminated laundry, 203b
Contaminated sharps, 203b
Contaminated wound, 535, 537
Contamination, 182, 186, 203b
Continuing care retirement communities, 124
Contracture, 70b, 414-415, 416f
Controlled substance, 41
Contusion, 535, 537, 537f
Conversion, 644
Convulsion, 691
Cooling blanket, 561
Cornea, 104
Corns, 545, 546f
Coronary artery disease, 618-619, 618f, 619b, 619f
Corporal punishment, 38
Corrective lenses, 590, 591b, 591f
Cotton drawsheet, 265, 268
Cough, 192-193b
Coughing
    oxygen promotion through, 448, 448b,
        449b, 450f
    postural drainage for, 515, 515f
    sputum specimen collection, 515, 515f
Courtesy, 44, 54
Cranial nerves, 103
Creams, 291t
Crime, 21, 32, 34
Criminal background check, 23
Criminal laws, 32, 34
Crutches, 426, 426f, 427f

Culture, 84-85
    communication affected by, 93, 93b
    death rites and, 711, 711b
    definition of, 82, 84
    food practices affected by, 381, 381b
    health care beliefs, 84b
    hygiene practices affected by, 281, 281b
    meal time practices affected by, 372b
    pain reactions affected by, 434, 434b
    sick care practices affected by, 85b
Cyanosis, 442
Cystitis, 635
Cytoplasm, 98, 98f

D
Daily care, 282
Daily Value, 371, 380
Dandruff, 311, 313
Dangling, 236, 236b, 237b, 237f, 238f
Day-care centers, for older persons, 123
Day-night cycle, 437
Deafness, 578-579
Death and dying
    age-related understanding of, 711-712
    attitudes about, 710-712
    breathing problems during, 713
    care of body after, 715, 715b, 716b, 717f
    children's understanding of, 711-712
    comfort needs during, 712-714
    cultural considerations, 711, 711b
    elimination during, 714
    family care during, 714
    hearing during, 713
    incontinence during, 714
    legal issues during, 714-715
    mental and emotional needs during, 714
    mouth care during, 713
    nutrition during, 714
    of partner, 118
    older person's view of, 712
    pain during, 713
    physical needs during, 713-714
    resident's rights, 717, 718b
    shroud, 717f
    signs of, 715
    skin care during, 713
    spiritual needs, 711-712
    stages of, 712
    vision changes during, 713
Death rattle, 713, 715
Deconditioning, 3, 414-415
Decontamination, 203b
Deep breathing, 448, 448b, 449b
Defamation, 32, 36
Defecation, 355-356
Defense mechanisms, 642, 644, 644b
Defibrillation, 698, 699f, 702b, 702f
Defibrillator, 698, 699f
Degenerative joint disease, 607
Dehiscence, of wound, 535, 548, 549f
Dehydration
    causes of, 388b
    definition of, 355, 371, 388
    description of, 358
Delayed wound healing, 561
Delegate
    definition of, 19, 25
    persons eligible to, 28
Delegation, 25-30
    ambulation, 424b
    bathing, 292b
    bedmaking, 268b
    blood glucose testing, 517b
    blood pressure measurement, 492b
    body temperature measurement, 478b
    brushing and combing of hair, 315b
    cold applications, 558b
    counting respirations, 489b
    deep breathing, 448b
    elastic bandages, 543b

Delegation *(Continued)*
  elastic stockings, 541b
  enema, 361b
  heat applications, 558b
  intravenous therapy, 412b
  isolation precautions, 191b
  meal preparation, 392b
  moving of residents, 225b
  perineal care, 305b
  physical examination preparations, 498b
  post-mortem care, 715b
  process of, 28-29
  pulse oximetry, 447b
  pulse taking, 485b
  restraints, 178b
  rights of, 29, 30b
  role in, 29-30
  shampooing of hair, 317b
  sputum specimen collection, 515b
  steps involved in, 28-29
  stool specimen collection, 511b, 513b
  transfer of persons, 238b
  tube feedings, 406b
  turning persons, 233b
  urine specimen collection, 503b
  wound dressings, 552b
Delirium, 655, 657, 657b
Delusion(s)
  in Alzheimer's disease, 663, 668
  characteristics of, 645-646
  definition of, 642, 655
  of grandeur, 642, 645
  of persecution, 642, 645
Demanding behavior, 87
Dementia, 657-658. *See also* Alzheimer's disease
  accident risk factors, 135b
  admission considerations, 523
  aseptic practices in, 186b
  basic needs in, 202b, 713b
  bathing procedures in, 292b
  caring for, 666-670, 667-668b, 667b, 668f, 669f, 670b
  causes of, 657, 657b
  definition of, 70b, 133, 655, 657
  delirium, 655, 657, 657b
  falls and, 164b
  fecal incontinence in, 359b
  feeding considerations, 396b
  otitis media in, 579b
  pain in, 434b
  permanent, 657, 657b
  physical examination in, 500b
  quality of life considerations, 671b
  restraints, 178b
  shaving in, 320b
  sleep promotion in, 440b
  treatable causes of, 657
  urinary incontinence in, 343b
  vital signs measurements and reporting in, 474b, 475b
  warning signs of, 657
  work-related injuries, 224b
Denial, 644
Dental hygienist, 6-7t
Dentist, 6-7t
Denture
  care of, 288, 288b, 288f, 289-290b
  cleaning of, 288, 290f
  definition of, 280, 288
  full, 288f
  partial, 288f
  removal of, 290f
Deodorants, 291t
Dependability, 47
Depressants, 649-651t
Depression, 647, 647b, 658
Dermis, 99, 99f
Development, 114. *See also* Growth and
  development

Developmental disabilities. *See also* Intellectual
  disabilities
  autism, 678, 678b
  cerebral palsy, 677-678
  definition of, 86, 673-674
  Down syndrome, 676-677, 676f
  family effects, 674
  fragile X syndrome, 677
  hydrocephalus, 680, 680f
  limited function areas associated with, 86
  quality of life considerations, 681b
  special services for, 674
  spina bifida, 679, 679f, 680f
Developmental task, 114-115
Diabetes meal plan, 384-385t, 386
Diabetes mellitus, 631
  complications of, 631
  definition of, 386
  description of, 112
  gestational, 631
  signs and symptoms of, 631
  stroke risks, 603
  treatment of, 631
  types of, 627, 631
Diabetic foot ulcer, 535, 545, 545b
Diabetic retinopathy, 586-587, 586f
Diagnosis. *See* Medical diagnosis; Nursing
  diagnosis
Dialysis, 634, 638, 638f
Diarrhea, 355, 358, 359b
Diastole, 106, 473
Diastolic pressure, 473, 490
Diet. *See also* Nutrition
  bowel elimination affected by, 357
  cultural influences on, 381, 381b
  diabetes meal plan, 384-385t, 386
  dysphagia, 386, 386b
  Omnibus Budget Reconciliation Act require-
    ments, 382, 383f
  poor, 372
  religious influences on, 381, 381b
  sodium-controlled, 383, 384-385t, 385b
  special types of, 383-386, 384-385t, 385b, 388-390
Dietary Guidelines for Americans, 373, 373-374b
Diethylstilbestrol, 596
Dietitian, 6-7t
Digestion, 97, 107, 405
Digestive disorders, 626-630
  cirrhosis, 629-630, 630b, 630f
  diverticular disease, 626-627, 626f
  gallstones, 627, 627f, 628b
  gastro-esophageal reflux disease, 626
  hepatitis, 628-629, 628b, 629b
  vomiting, 625-626
Digestive system
  age-related changes in, 119b, 121-122
  anatomy of, 107-108, 108f
Digital rectal examination, for fecal impaction, 358, 358f
Dignity, 15, 15-16b
Dilate, 535, 555, 556f
Dining programs, 391, 392f
Diplegia, 673, 677
Direct questions, 92
Director of nursing, 4
Dirty wound, 535
Disability
  age-related, 115
  anger responses to, 85, 87-88
  behavior issues associated with, 87, 87b, 88b
  causes of, 683
  criteria for, 674
  definition of, 82, 85, 673-674, 682-683
  developmental. *See* Developmental disabilities
  effects of, 85
  etiquette for, 94b
  intellectual. *See* Intellectual disabilities
  residents with, 94
Disasters, 133, 149

Discharge, 532-533, 533b
  from assisted living residence, 467, 471
  definition of, 521-522
  from nursing center, 532-533, 533b
  safety issues, 522b
Discipline, 169
Discomfort, 431
Disinfection, 182, 189
Disoriented residents, 86
Displacement, 644
Dissociative anesthetics, 649-651t
Distal, 67, 67f
Distraction, 431, 436, 436f
Diuresis, 634, 637
Diverticular disease, 626-627, 626f
Diverticulitis, 626
Diverticulosis, 626, 626f
Diverticulum, 626
"Do Not Resuscitate" orders, 715
Domestic abuse, 41-42
Donning
  of mask, 200b, 200f
  of personal protective equipment, 195, 196f
Dorsal recumbent position, 496, 499, 499f
Dorsiflexion, 414, 419
Double-bagging, of biohazardous waste, 201, 201f
Double-barrel colostomy, 367f
Down syndrome, 676-677, 676f
Drainage systems
  chest tubes, 462, 462f
  urinary, 347-348, 348b, 349b, 350b, 350f
  wound, 548, 550f
Draping, for perineal care, 306f
Drawsheets, 230f, 265, 268, 268f
Dressing (attire)
  for job interview, 51b
  of person, 325, 325b, 328-329b, 329f
Dressings (wound), 550-551
  application of, 551, 552b, 553b
  dry, 551
  functions of, 550
  gauze, 550
  pressure ulcer prevention, 575
  securing of, 551, 551b, 551f
  transparent adhesive film, 550
  types of, 550-551, 550f
  wet-to-dry, 551
  wet-to-wet, 551
Drinking water, 397, 397b, 398b, 399f
Droplet precautions, 194b
Drug(s)
  accidents caused by side effects of, 135
  administration of, 470
  bowel elimination affected by, 357
  effects of, 45
  medication record about, 471
  oxygen needs affected by, 443
  sleep affected by, 439
  storage of, 471
Drug abuse and addiction, 648-649, 649-651t
Drug errors, 471
Drug testing, 57
Dry cold applications, 557, 560f
Dry dressings, 551
Dry heat application, 556
Dura mater, 103
Durable power of attorney for health care, 714
Dust mite, 314f
Dying. *See* Death and dying
Dysarthria, 583
Dysphagia, 70b, 114, 121, 371, 386, 386b
Dysphagia diet, 386, 386b
Dyspnea, 70b, 114, 121, 442, 444
Dysuria, 333, 335t, 634-635

E
Ear(s)
  age-related changes in, 121
  anatomy of, 104-105, 105f
  assessment of, 76b
  pressure ulcers on, 570

Ear disorders, 579-582
  hearing loss. *See* Hearing loss
  Meniere's disease, 579
  otitis media, 579, 579b
Early morning care, 200, 202
Earwax. *See* Cerumen
Eating devices, 684, 684f
Eating utensils, 383f
Edema
  definition of, 371, 535, 539
  pulmonary, 621
Education
  licensed practical nurse, 5, 6-7t
  licensed vocational nurse, 6-7t
  nursing center programs, 22-23
  registered nurse, 5, 6-7t
Eggcrate-type pads, 573, 575f
Elastic bandages, 543, 543b, 544b, 544f
Elastic stockings, 541, 541b, 542b, 542f
Elbow exercises, 420f
Elbow protectors, 573, 574f
Elder abuse, 38-40, 39b, 40b
Elder Cottage Housing Opportunity, 123
Electrical injuries, 141, 141f, 142b, 142f, 706f
Electrical shock, 133, 141
Electrocardiogram, 485f
Electronic devices, 70, 71b
Electronic thermometers, 480, 480f, 481b, 482b
Elimination
  bowel. *See* Bowel elimination
  during death and dying, 714
  rehabilitation of, 684
  urinary. *See* Urinary elimination
Elopement, 655, 662
Embarrassment, 91
Embolus, 535, 541
Emergency care, 692
  Basic Life Support. *See* Basic Life Support
  burns, 706-707, 706f
  cardiopulmonary resuscitation. *See* Cardiopulmo-
    nary resuscitation
  fainting, 691, 704
  hemorrhage, 703, 703f, 704b
  privacy protection during, 707
  rules of, 692b
  safety in, 693b
  seizures, 705-706, 706f
  shock, 691, 704
  stroke, 602-603, 602b, 602f, 603b, 705
Emergency medical services, 692
Emesis, 625-626
Emotional abuse, 39, 41, 42b
Emotional illness, 642-643
Empathy, 47
Emphysema, 622, 622f
Employers, 46-47
Endocardium, 105
Endocrine system, 111-112, 111f, 631
End-of-life care, 709. *See also* Death and dying
End-of-shift report, 64, 64b
Endometrium, 110
Endoscope, 402
Endotracheal tube, 458, 458f
Enema, 360-365
  charting of, 363f
  cleansing, 361, 362-363b
  definition of, 355, 360
  delegation of, 361b
  oil-retention, 360, 365, 365b, 366b
  safety and comfort measures, 360b, 361b
  small-volume, 360, 364, 364-365b, 365f
  solutions, 360
  technique for, 363f
Enema tubing, 363f
Engineering controls, 203b, 204
Enteral nutrition, 402-406
  aspiration prevention, 405
  comfort measures, 405
  definition of, 401-402
  feeding times, 404, 404f, 405f

Enteral nutrition *(Continued)*
  feeding tubes, 402, 403f, 405-406, 406b, 406f, 407b
  formulas, 404, 404b
  observations during, 404
Entrapment zones, in bed, 256-257, 257f, 258f
Enuresis, 431
Environment
  for blind persons, 582
  resident's right to, 17
  for visually impaired persons, 582
Epidermis, 99, 99f
Epididymis, 109
Epiglottis, 107
Epilepsy, 705
Epinephrine, 112
Epithelial tissue, 98
Equipment accidents, 141, 141f, 142b, 142f
Erectile dysfunction, 128, 130
Ergonomics, 210, 213-214
Erythrocytes, 105
Eschar, 564, 567
Escherichia coli, 186
Esophagitis, 626
Esteem, 82, 84, 437
Estrogen, 110
Ethics
  codes of, 33
  definition of, 32-33
Eustachian tube, 104
Evaluation
  definition of, 74
  in nursing process, 29, 81
Evening care, 280, 282
Eviction, from assisted living residence, 471
Evisceration, of wound, 535, 548, 549f
Exercise. *See also* Activity
  during bedrest, 418
  Dietary Guidelines for Americans recommendations,
    373
  importance of, 45
  MyPyramid guidelines, 375, 377b
  oxygen needs affected by, 443
  range-of-motion, 419, 419b, 420b, 420f, 421-422b,
    422f, 423f
  sleep affected by, 439
  walking. *See* Ambulation
Expiration, 107
Exposure incidents, 203b, 205
Expressive aphasia, 578, 583-584
Expressive-receptive aphasia, 578, 584
Extension, 414, 419
External female genitalia, 110, 110f
External rotation, 414, 419
Extubation, 459
Eye(s)
  age-related changes in, 121
  anatomy of, 104, 104f
  artificial. *See* Ocular prosthesis
  assessment of, 76b
Eye contact, during communication, 92b, 92f
Eye disorders, 584-592
  age-related macular degeneration, 585-586,
    586f
  blindness, 578, 584, 587-590, 588-589b, 589b,
    589f
  cataracts, 585, 585f
  contact lenses for, 592, 592b
  corrective lenses for, 590, 591b, 591f
  diabetic retinopathy, 586-587, 586f
  glaucoma, 584, 584f
  low vision, 578, 587
  ocular prosthesis, 592, 592b, 592f
  signs and symptoms of, 587b
Eyeglasses, 590, 590b

F
Face shields, 200f, 201, 201b
Facial expressions, 91b
Fainting, 691, 704
Fall(s)

  in bathrooms, 158-159b
  bed rails to prevent, 156, 160, 160f, 161b, 175f
  causes of, 157, 157b
  charting of, 161f
  color-coded wristbands to indicate risk for, 152,
    158-159b
  in dementia patients, 164b
  dizziness as cause of, 120
  fracture risks, 164
  grab bars to prevent, 161, 162f
  hand rails to prevent, 161, 161f
  prevention of, 158-159b, 158-162, 159b
  restraints as cause of, 167
  risk factors for, 157, 157b
  statistics regarding, 157
  time of occurrence, 157
Falling, 163, 164b, 164f
Fallopian tubes, 110
False imprisonment, 32, 36, 171, 171b
Family
  of Alzheimer's disease person, 669-670, 670b
  of resident, 94-95, 95f
  older person living with, 122-123
Fat-controlled diet, 384-385t
Fats, 373, 379
Faxes, 71b
Fear, 91
Fecal impaction, 355, 358, 358f, 607
Fecal incontinence, 355, 358-359, 359b, 567
Feces, 70b, 108, 355-356, 357, 627
Federal laws, 20-25
Feedback, 29
Feeding, 395, 396b, 397b
Feeding tubes, 402, 403f, 405-406, 406b, 406f, 407b
Female perineal care, 306f, 307-308b
Female reproductive system
  age-related changes in, 119b, 122
  anatomy of, 110, 110f
Fentanyl, 649-651t
Fertilization, 111
Fever, 70b, 473, 475
Fiber-restricted diet, 384-385t
Financial exploitation, 39
Finger exercises, 422f
Fingernail trimming, 322, 324f
Fire
  elements necessary for, 145
  evacuation techniques, 148, 148f
  oxygen and, 145, 145b
  prevention of, 145, 146b
  safety considerations, 145-148, 146b, 146f, 147b
  what to do during, 146
Fire extinguisher, 146-148, 147b, 147f
First aid, 691-692
First degree burn, 136
First intention wound healing, 546, 547f
Flashback, 642, 645
Flat bones, 100
Flatulence, 355, 359
Flatus, 355
Flexion, 414, 419
Flossing, 283, 284b, 286f
Flow rate
  intravenous therapy, 401, 410, 410b, 410f
  oxygen therapy, 453, 453f
Flow sheets, 62, 62f, 63f
Flowmeter, 453f
Flu. *See* Influenza
Fluid balance, 388-390
  fluid requirements for, 388
  intake and output records, 388-390, 389f,
    390-391b, 390b, 390f
  need for, 388
Fluid orders, 388
Flunitrazepam, 649-651t
Foam cushions, 573, 574f
Focusing, 93
Folate, 379t
Folic acid, 379t

Food. *See also* Nutrition
    cultural influences on, 381, 381b
    dining programs, 391, 392f
    high-sodium types of, 385b
    meals, 392-393, 392b, 393b, 394-395b, 394b
    needs for, 391-397, 391b, 398b
Food groups, 374
Food labels, 380, 380f
Food safety, 374, 469, 469f
Food temperature guide, 375f
Foodborne illnesses, 399, 399b
Foot care, 322, 322b, 323-324b, 323b, 323f, 324f, 327f
Foot elevator, 573
Foot exercises, 423f
Foot-boards, 417, 417f
Footdrop, 414, 417
Forceps, 206f
Forearm crutches, 426f
Forearm exercises, 420f
Foreign body airway obstruction, 138
Foreign-born persons, 117b
Four-point gait, 427f
Fowler's position, 70b, 210, 215, 215f, 252, 256, 256f
    high-, 252, 256, 256f
    semi-, 70b, 252, 256, 256f
Fracture(s), 610-614
    casts for, 611, 611f, 612b, 612f
    closed, 601, 610
    definition of, 601, 610
    fixation of, 610, 611f
    hip, 614, 614b
    open, 601, 610, 610f
    reduction of, 610, 611f
    signs and symptoms of, 610
    traction for, 613, 613b, 613f
Fracture pans, 335, 335f, 336b, 336f
Fragile X syndrome, 677
Fraud, 32, 37
Freedom of movement, 166-167
Friction, 219, 225, 564, 566
Friends, of resident, 94-95, 95f
Full denture, 288f
Full visual privacy, 252
Full-liquid diet, 384-385t
Full-thickness burns, 706f, 707
Full-thickness wound, 535, 537
Functional incontinence, 333, 342
Functional nursing, 1, 5
Fungi, 183

G
Gait belt, 156, 162, 162f, 163b, 222
Gait patterns, for crutches, 426, 427f
Gallbladder, 108
Gallstones, 627, 627f, 628b
Gangrene, 535, 539, 601, 615, 615f
Gastro-esophageal reflux disease, 626
Gastrointestinal tract
    aging effects on, 357, 382
    anatomy of, 107, 108f
Gastrostomy tube, 401-402, 403f
Gauze dressings, 550
Gavage, 401-402
Gay, 129
Gel cushions, 573, 574f
Generalized absence seizure, 705
Generalized tonic-clonic seizure, 705
Genital warts, 639-640t
Geriatrics, 114-115
Germicides, 182, 189
Gerontology, 114-115
Gestational diabetes mellitus, 631
GHB, 649-651t
Glass thermometers, 476-477, 476b, 476f, 477f, 478-479b, 478b
Glasses. *See* Eyeglasses
Glaucoma, 584, 584f
Global aphasia, 578, 584
Glomerulus, 109
Gloves, 192-193b, 194b, 197, 197b, 197f, 198b, 198f

Gloving, sterile, 207, 207b, 208f
Glucocorticoids, 112
Glucose
    blood, testing of, 516-517, 517b, 517f, 518-519b, 518b, 519f
    in urine, 508
Glucose meter, 517, 518f
Glucosuria, 502, 508
Glycosuria, 502, 508
Goal, 74, 77
Goggles, 201, 201b
Gonads, 112
Gonorrhea, 639-640t
Gossip, 44, 53
Gowns
    changing of, 325-330, 325b, 326b, 330b, 330f, 331b
    description of, 192-193b, 194b, 198, 199b
Grab bars, 161, 162f, 261
Graduate, 371, 389, 390f
Grains, 377
Grandchildren, 118
Graves' disease, 597, 598f
Greek Orthodox, 381
Grievances, 14
Grooming
    charting of, 332f
    clothing changes, 325-330, 325b, 326b
    dressing, 325, 325b, 328-329b, 329f
    equipment for, 312b, 313f
    foot care, 322, 322b, 323-324b, 323b, 323f, 324f, 327f
    gown changing, 325-330, 325b, 326b, 330b, 330f, 331b
    hair care, 312-314, 313b, 315-316b, 315b, 316f
    for job interview, 51b
    nail care, 322, 322b, 323-324b, 323b, 323f, 324f, 327f
    quality of life considerations, 331b
    shampooing, 317, 317b, 317f, 318-319b, 318b
    shaving, 319-322, 319b, 320b, 320f, 321b
    undressing, 325, 325b, 326b, 327f, 328f
Ground, 133
Group insurance, 8
Growth and development, 115
    definition of, 114
    late adulthood, 115, 116b
    measurement of, 115
    stages of, 116b
Growth hormone, 111
Guided imagery, 431, 436

H
Hair
    brushing and combing of, 312-314, 313b, 315-316b, 315b, 316f
    care of, 312-314, 313b, 315-316b, 315b, 316f
    description of, 99, 120
    shampooing of, 317, 317b, 317f, 318-319b, 318b
Hallucinations
    in Alzheimer's disease, 663, 668
    definition of, 642, 655
    description of, 645
Hallucinogens, 649-651t
Hammer toes, 545, 546f
Hand grips, 417, 418f
Hand hygiene, 186, 187b, 187f, 188b, 188f, 189b, 192-193b
Hand rails, 161, 161f
Hand rolls, 417
Hand washing facilities, 203b
Harassment, 44, 56-57, 56b
Hashish, 649-651t
Hazard
    definition of, 133-134
    types of, 143
Hazardous substances. *See also* Biohazardous waste
    definition of, 133, 143
    employee training about, 145
    handling of, 143-145
    labeling of, 144, 144f
    material safety data sheets, 144, 144f
    safety measures for, 145b

Head tilt-chin lift method, 140f, 694, 694f
Health, 45
Health care
    cost reductions, 20
    goals for, 8
    paying for, 8-9
    pre-approval process for, 9
Health care beliefs, 84b
Health care proxy, 714
Health care systems, 20
Health Insurance Portability and Accountability Act, 37
Health maintenance organization, 9
Health team, 6, 6-7t
Healthcare-associated infection, 182, 185-186
Hearing
    during death and dying, 713
    devices for, 582, 582f
Hearing aids, 582, 582f
Hearing assistance dogs, 580
Hearing loss, 579-582
    causes of, 580
    communication methods, 580, 581f
    definition of, 578-579
    description of, 135
    prevalence of, 579
    signs and symptoms of, 580
    speech affected by, 580
    terminology for, 580b
Hearing promotion, 582b
Heart
    anatomy of, 105-106, 106f
    chest compressions of, 697, 697f, 698f
Heart disease, 603
Heart failure, 621
Heartburn, 625-626
Heat applications, for wound healing, 555-561, 556f, 557b, 557t, 558b, 559-560b
Heat stroke, 561
Heberden nodes, 607f
Heel elevator, 573, 574f
Heel protectors, 573, 574f
Height measurements, 527, 528b, 529b, 530f, 531b, 531f
Hematoma, 502, 517
Hematuria, 333, 335f, 502, 508, 634-635
Hemiplegia, 133, 135, 601, 603, 677
Hemodialysis, 638
Hemoglobin, 97, 105, 446
Hemoptysis, 442, 502, 515
Hemorrhage, 691, 703, 703f, 704b
Hemothorax, 457, 462
Hemovac, 548, 550f
Hepatitis, 203-204, 628-629, 628b, 629b
Heroin, 649-651t
Herpes, 639-640t, 640f
Herpes zoster, 599, 600f
Heterosexual, 128-129
High-calorie diet, 384-385t
High-fiber diet, 384-385t
High-Fowler's position, 252, 256, 256f
High-iron diet, 384-385t
High-protein diet, 384-385t
Hinduism, 381
Hinge joint, 100, 100f
Hip
    fractures of, 614, 614b
    range-of-motion exercises for, 423f
Hip abduction wedges, 417, 417f
Hip protector, 169f
Hip replacement surgery, 608, 608f, 609b, 609f
Hirsutism, 311, 313
Holism, 82-83
Home care, 20
Home-sharing, 123
Homosexual, 128-129
Horizontal recumbent position, 496, 499
Hormone(s). *See also specific hormone*
    definition of, 97, 111
    pituitary, 111

Hormone replacement therapy, 596
Hormone therapy, 597
Hospice, 1, 3, 710
Hospital(s)
    closings of, 20
    mergers of, 20
Hot compress, 555, 556f
Hot packs, 555-556, 556f, 558
Hot soaks, 555, 556f
Hot-cold balance, 84
Housekeeping, 205
Housing, for older persons, 122-126. *See also specific*
        housing
Human immunodeficiency virus, 203, 598, 639-640t
Humidifier, 454f
Hydrocephalus, 680, 680f
Hydrocodone bitartrate, 649-651t
Hygiene
    adaptive devices for, 281f
    back massage, 302, 303-304b, 303b, 304f
    bathing. *See* Bathing
    cultural influences on, 281, 281b
    daily care, 282
    factors that affect, 281
    oral. *See* Oral hygiene
    perineal care. *See* Perineal care
    personal, 45, 46f, 54
    purposes of, 281
    rehabilitation considerations, 281b
    reporting and reporting of, 309, 309f
    self-esteem affected by, 437
Hymen, 110
Hyperextension, 414, 419
Hyperglycemia, 625, 631, 632t
Hypersexuality, 664
Hypertension
    definition of, 473, 617
    description of, 490, 603
Hyperthermia, 535, 561
Hyperventilation, 442, 444
Hypoglycemia, 625, 631, 632t
Hypotension
    definition of, 473, 490
    orthostatic, 414, 415-416, 416b
    postural, 414, 415-416
Hypothermia, 536, 561
Hypoventilation, 442, 444
Hypoxemia, 442
Hypoxia, 442, 444, 444b, 459

I
Identification bracelet, 135-136, 135f, 136f
Identification (defense mechanism), 644
Identification (of person), 135-136, 135f, 136b
Ileostomy, 355, 366-367, 367f
Illness
    acute, 1, 3
    anger responses to, 85, 87-88
    appetite affected by, 382
    behavior issues associated with, 87, 87b, 88b
    chronic, 1, 3
    effects of, 85
    pain reactions affected by, 434
    sleep affected by, 439
Immune system
    description of, 112, 112f
    disorders of, 597-599, 598f, 599b
Immunity
    definition of, 182, 204
    description of, 97, 112
Immunotherapy, 597
Implementation, 74, 80, 80f, 81b
Impotence, 128, 130
Incentive spirometry, 450, 451b, 451f
Incest, 41
Incident
    definition of, 133, 153
    reporting of, 153-154
    types of, 154b

Incident report, 154
Incision, 536-537, 538f
Incontinence
    definition of, 70b
    fecal, 355, 358-359, 359b, 567
    urinary. *See* Urinary incontinence
Incus, 104
Independence, 1
Indwelling catheter, 333, 344, 344f, 345b
Infancy, 116b
Infected wound, 536-537
Infection
    chain of, 184-185, 185f
    definition of, 182-183, 184-186
    healthcare-associated, 185-186
    nosocomial, 185
    in older persons, 184
    prevention of, 141
    signs and symptoms of, 184b
    urinary tract, 635
    wound, 536, 548, 561, 575
Infection control, 182
Inferior vena cava, 106-107, 106f
Influenza, 622, 623t
Information, resident's right to, 12, 61, 467
Informed consent, 37, 37b, 171
In-grown toenails, 545, 546f
Inhalants, 649-651t
Inherited, 673, 677
Insomnia, 431, 439
Inspiration, 107
Insulin, 112
Intake, 371, 388
Intake and output records, 388-390, 389f, 390-391b,
        390b, 390f
Integumentary system
    age-related changes in, 119b, 120
    anatomy of, 99, 99f
Intellectual disabilities, 674-676
    causes of, 675b
    criteria for, 675
    definition of, 673-674
    life-long residents, 86
    sexuality issues, 676
    types of, 674b
Intentional torts, 36-37
Intentional wound, 536-537
Interdisciplinary care planning conference, 62,
        77-79, 80b
Interdisciplinary health care team, 1
Internal jugular vein, 409, 409f
Internal rotation, 414, 419
Interview, for job, 47-49, 50b, 51-52, 51b, 51f
Intimacy, 664
Intravenous therapy, 408-411
    assisting with, 411, 412b
    catheter, 409, 409f
    central venous sites for, 408-409, 409f
    complications of, 412b
    definition of, 401, 408
    equipment for, 408f, 409, 409f
    flow rate, 401, 410, 410b, 410f
    peripheral sites for, 408, 408f
    pump used in, 410f
    safety considerations for, 411b, 411f
    sites for, 408, 408f, 409f
Intubation, 457-458
Invasion of privacy, 32, 36, 36b
Involuntary seclusion, 11, 15, 38
Iodine, 380t
Ionizing radiation, 596
Iris, 104
Iron, 380t
Irregular bones, 100
Islam, 381
Isolation precautions, 191-202, 191b
    guidelines for, 195b
    protective measures, 195-202
    standard precautions, 192, 192-193b
    transmission-based precautions, 192, 192b

J
Jacket restraints, 177, 178f
Jackson-Pratt drain, 548, 550f
Jaundice, 625, 628f
Jejunostomy tube, 401-402, 403f
Job, 45-52
    acceptance of, 52
    attendance at, 53, 53b
    drug testing for, 57
    losing of, 52, 57, 57b
    new employee orientation, 52
    preparations for, 52-53
    resigning from, 57
    sources for finding, 45
Job applications, 47, 48f, 50b
Job description, 25
    definition of, 19
    example of, 26f
    written, 25
Job interview, 47-49, 50b, 51-52, 51b, 51f
Job safety, 55
Job skills and training, 47
Joints
    anatomy of, 100, 100f, 101f
    degenerative disease of, 607
    movements of, 419b
Judaism, 381

K
Kardex, 59, 62, 63f
Ketamine, 649-651t
Ketone body, 502
Ketones, 502, 508
Kidney(s)
    anatomy of, 108, 108f, 109f
    failure of, 637-638, 638b, 638f, 639b
Kidney stones, 637, 637f
Knee exercises, 423f
Knee replacement surgery, 608, 608f, 609b
Knee-chest position, 496, 499, 499f
Kübler-Ross, Elisabeth, 712
Kussmaul respirations, 442, 444

L
Labeling of hazardous substances, 144, 144f
Labia majora, 110, 110f
Labia minora, 110, 110f
Laceration, 536-537, 538f
Lancet, 517, 517f
Language, 54
Large intestine, 108
Laryngeal mirror, 496-497
Larynx, 107
Late adulthood, 115, 116b
Lateral (direction), 67, 67f, 211f
Lateral position, 210, 215, 216f
Lateral transfers, 221-222
Latex allergies, 197
Laundry, 205, 469, 469b
Law(s)
    civil, 34
    criminal, 34
    definition of, 32, 34
    federal, 20-25
    state, 20-25
Left lower quadrant, 67f
Left upper quadrant, 67f
Leg prostheses, 615, 615f
Leg shaving, 322
Lesbian, 129
Leukemia, 676
Leukocytes, 105
Liability, 36
Libel, 32, 36
Lice, 311. *See also* Pediculosis; Pubic lice
Licensed practical nurse, 5
    as charge nurse, 4-5
    definition of, 1
    delegation by, 28

Licensed practical nurse (Continued)
  education of, 5, 6-7t
  supervision of, 5
Licensed vocational nurse
  as charge nurse, 4-5
  definition of, 1
  delegation by, 28
  education of, 6-7t
  supervision of, 5
Life support, 693-703
  cardiopulmonary resuscitation. See Cardiopulmonary resuscitation
  Chain of Survival, 693
  respiratory arrest, 694
  sudden cardiac arrest, 620, 691, 693
Life-long residents, 86
"Lift teams," 224
Ligaments, 100
Lighting, in resident unit, 254
Linens, 267-268
  drawsheets, 265, 268, 268f
  handling of, 267, 267f
Liquid oxygen, 452
Lithotomy position, 496, 499, 499f
Liver, 108
Liver spots, 120
Living will, 714
Logrolling, 219, 233, 235, 235b, 236f
Loneliness, 118, 126, 647
Long bones, 100
Long-term care centers, 2-5
  board and care homes, 1-2
  function of, 2
  goals of, 3
  nursing centers. See Nursing centers
  nursing service, 4-5
  purposes of, 3
  residents of, 2
  skilled nursing facilities, 2-3
Loss of limb, 615, 615f
Lotions, 291t
Lou Gehrig's disease. See Amyotrophic lateral sclerosis
Love, 84
Low vision, 578, 587
LPN. See Licensed practical nurse
LSD, 649-651t
Lung(s), 107
Lung cancer, 595f
Lung scan, 445
Lupus, 597, 598f
LVN. See Licensed vocational nurse
Lymphocytes, 112

M
Macular degeneration, age-related, 585-586, 586f
Mail, 14
Major depression, 647, 647b, 658
Male perineal care, 308b, 309f
Male reproductive system
  age-related changes in, 119b, 122
  anatomy of, 109, 109f
Malignant tumor, 594-595, 595f
Malleus, 104
Malpractice, 32, 36
Mammary glands, 110
Managed care, 9, 9b
Manual lifting, 221
Marijuana, 649-651t
Masks, 199, 199f, 200b, 200f
Maslow's theory of basic needs, 77, 83, 83f
Masturbation, 130-131
Material safety data sheets, 144, 144f
MDMA, 649-651t
Meal(s)
  preparation of, 392, 392b, 393b
  serving of, 393, 394-395b, 394b
Meal breaks, 55
Meal time practices, 372b
Meal trays, 394-395b

Meats, 378
Mechanical lifts, 223f, 244, 244b, 245b, 246f
Mechanical soft diet, 384-385t
Mechanical ventilation, 457, 461, 461b, 461f, 687
Medial, 67, 67f
Medicaid, 8. See also Centers for Medicare & Medicaid Services
  definition of, 1
  nursing center funding by, 126
Medical asepsis, 186-190
  cleaning, 189
  definition of, 182, 186
  hand hygiene, 186, 187b, 187f, 188b, 188f, 189b, 192-193b
  measures of, 190, 190-191b
  practices of, 186, 186b
  supplies and equipment for, 189-190, 190-191b
Medical diagnosis, 74, 77
Medical director, 4
Medical laboratory technician, 6-7t
Medical record, 60-62
  activities of daily living flow sheet, 62, 62f
  admission sheet, 61
  components of, 60
  definition of, 59-60
  flow sheets, 62, 62f, 63f
  illustration of, 61f
  progress notes, 61-62, 61f
  recording of. See Recording
Medical records and health information technician, 6-7t
Medical symptom, 166, 169
Medical technologist, 6-7t
Medical terms, 67-69, 67f, 68b, 70b
MedicAlert + Safe Return, 662
Medicare. See also Centers for Medicare & Medicaid Services
  definition of, 1, 8
  nursing center funding by, 126
Medication assistant-certified, 6-7t, 30
Medication record, 471
Medication reminder, 464, 470
Medulla, 103
Melena, 502, 513
Meniere's disease, 579
Meninges, 103
Meningocele, 679, 679f
Meningomyelocele, 679, 679f
Menopause, 114, 122
Menstrual cycle, 110
Menstruation, 97, 110
Mental, 642-643
Mental abuse, 39
Mental disorder, 642-643
Mental health, 642
Mental health problems
  anxiety disorders. See Anxiety disorders
  mood disorders, 646-647, 646b, 647b
  personality disorders, 647
  quality of life considerations, 653b
  schizophrenia, 645-646, 646b
  sleep affected by, 439
  suicide, 642, 652-653, 652b, 653b
Mental illness, 642-643
Mental retardation. See Intellectual disabilities
Mentally ill residents, 87
Mescaline, 649-651t
Metabolism, 97, 111, 437
Metastasis, 594
Methamphetamine, 649-651t
Methaqualone, 649-651t
Methicillin-resistant Staphylococcus aureus, 184
Methylphenidate, 649-651t
Mexican Americans, 84
Microbes, 182-183, 185f
Microorganisms, 182-184
Micturition, 333-334
Midbrain, 103
Middle adulthood, 116b
Midstream urine specimen, 505, 505-506b, 505b, 505f

Mild cognitive impairment, 658
Military time, 66, 66b, 66f
Milk, 378
Mineralocorticoids, 112
Minerals, 379, 380t
Minimum data set, 75, 77-79
Misappropriation, 39
Mistreatment, 15, 717
Mite, 311
Mitered corner, 272f
Mitosis, 98
Mitral valve, 106, 106f
Mitt restraints, 176, 177f
Mixed aphasia, 578, 584
Mixed incontinence, 333, 342
mm Hg, 490
Mobility
  rehabilitation of, 684, 685f, 686f
  vision loss effects on, 590
Moist heat application, 555-556, 556f
Molestation, 41
Mons pubis, 110
Montgomery ties, 551, 551f
Mood disorders, 646-647, 646b, 647b
Mormons, 381
Morning care, 280, 282
Morphine, 649-651t
Motor aphasia, 578, 583
Mouth, 76b
Mouth-to-mouth breathing, 695, 695f
Mouth-to-nose breathing, 696, 696f
Mouth-to-stoma breathing, 696, 697f
Moving, of persons
  in bed, 225-231
  delegation for, 225b
  dependence level considerations, 221, 222-223b
  head and shoulders, 225, 226b, 226f, 227f
  lateral transfers, 221-222
  manual lifting in, 221
  mechanical lift for, 223f
  safety and comfort in, 220b
  to side of bed, 231, 231b, 231f, 232b
  up in bed, 227, 227b, 227f, 228b, 229, 229b, 229f
  work-related injuries in, 221, 221-222b, 224b
Multidrug-resistant organisms, 184
Multiple sclerosis, 604
Muscle tissue, 98
Muscles, 101-102, 101f
Musculo-skeletal disorders, 607-615
  arthritis. See Arthritis
  definition of, 213
  description of, 213
  fractures. See Fracture(s)
  loss of limb, 615, 615f
  osteoporosis, 610
  risk factors for, 213
  work-related, 213
Musculo-skeletal system, 100-102
  age-related changes in, 119b, 120
  bones, 100, 100f
  joints. See Joints
  muscles, 101-102, 101f
Mustaches, 322
Myelin sheath, 102
Myocardial infarction, 620, 620f, 621b
Myocardium, 105
MyPyramid, 375-379, 376f, 377b, 377t
Myths, 115, 116b

N
Nails
  care of, 322, 322b, 323-324b, 323b, 323f, 324f, 327f
  description of, 99, 120
  in-grown toenails, 545, 546f
NANDA-I nursing diagnoses, 78-79b
Narcotics, 443
Nasal cannula, 452, 453f
Nasal speculum, 496-497
Naso-enteral tube, 401-402, 403f
Naso-gastric tube, 401-402, 403f

Nasopharyngeal airway, 459
National Council of State Boards of Nursing
    delegation steps, 28-29
    description of, 21
    nursing assistant standards, 25, 25b
    range of functions, 23-24
National Federation of Licensed Practical Nurses,
        33, 34b
National Nurse Aide Assessment Program, 722
Neck exercises, 420f
Need(s)
    in Alzheimer's disease persons, 668
    basic, 83-84, 202, 202b, 561-562
    belonging, 84
    definition of, 82-83
    in dementia persons, 202b, 713b
    love, 84
    Maslow's theory of, 77, 83, 83f
    physical, 84
    safety, 84
    security, 84
    self-actualization, 82, 84
    self-esteem, 84
    sexual, 130-131
    wound effects on, 561-562
Neglect
    child, 40-41, 42b
    definition of, 32
    elder, 39
    resident's right to freedom from, 15, 717
Negligence, 55
    definition of, 32, 34
    malpractice, 36
Nephron, 109, 109f
Nerve tissue, 98
Nervous system, 102-105
    age-related changes in, 119b, 120-121, 656b
    central, 102-103, 102f, 103f
    functions of, 102
    oxygen needs affected by, 443
    peripheral, 102, 103-104, 103f
Nervous system disorders, 602-606
    amyotrophic lateral sclerosis, 605
    multiple sclerosis, 604
    Parkinson's disease, 604, 604f
    spinal cord injury, 605-606, 606b, 606f
    stroke, 602-603, 602b, 602f, 603b
    traumatic brain injury, 605
New employee orientation, 52
Niacin, 379t
Nicotine, 649-651t
Nipple, 110, 111f
Nitroglycerin, 619
Nocturia, 333, 335t
Noise, in resident unit, 254, 254b
Non-pathogens, 182-183
Non-rebreather mask, 452, 453f
Nonspecific immunity, 112
Nonverbal communication, 89-91, 653
    body language, 91, 91b
    definition of, 82, 89
    sign language, 90f
    touch, 91, 91b
Norepinephrine, 112
Normal flora, 182, 184
Nose
    assessment of, 76b
    mouth-to-nose breathing, 696, 696f
Nosocomial infections, 185
Nothing by mouth, 388
NREM sleep, 431, 438
Nucleus, of cell, 98, 98f
Nurse managers, 4
Nurse practice acts, 20-21, 25
Nurse practitioner, 6-7t
Nursing assistant(s), 5
    credentials of, 6-7t
    definition of, 1
    history of, 20
    nurse practice acts, 21
    trends in, 20

Nursing assistant registry, 22
Nursing assistant standard, 25, 25b
Nursing care patterns, 5, 6b
Nursing centers, 3-4
    abuse in, 40
    accreditation of, 9
    certification of, 9
    deficiencies in, 9, 10b
    definition of, 2
    dining programs in, 391, 392f
    discharge from, 532-533, 533b
    educational programs, 22-23
    environment requirements, 126b
    features of, 125b
    illustration of, 124f
    licensure of, 9
    married couples in, 131
    Medicare/Medicaid funding of, 126
    Omnibus Budget Reconciliation Act requirements
        for, 17, 126, 134
    organization of, 4, 4f
    quality of life considerations, 126b, 218b
    relationships in, 131f
    resident unit in. See Resident unit
    residents of, 3, 86-87, 124
    rooms in, 125b
    safety of, 134
    services offered by, 3-4
    settings in, 124, 124f, 125b
    staff of, 125b
    standards for, 9
    transfer from, 532-533, 533b
Nursing diagnosis, 77
    definition of, 74, 77
    NANDA-I, 78-79b
Nursing education, 5
Nursing intervention, 74, 77
Nursing process
    assessment, 74-75, 76b, 77b
    definition of, 74-75
    evaluation, 29, 81
    implementation, 74, 80, 80f, 81b
    nursing diagnosis, 74, 77, 78-79b
    planning, 74, 77-79
    steps of, 75
Nursing services
    in assisted living residences, 470
    definition of, 4-5
Nursing task
    acceptance of, 30
    definition of, 19, 24
    delegated, 29
    refusing of, 30, 30b
Nursing team, 5
    definition of, 2
    licensed practical nurse. See Licensed practical
        nurse
    licensed vocational nurse. See Licensed vocational
        nurse
    registered nurses. See Registered nurse
Nursing-assistant training and competency
        evaluation program, 21-22
Nutrients, 371-372, 379
Nutrition, 372-380. See also Diet; Food; Nutritional
        support
    beans, 378
    definition of, 371-372
    Dietary Guidelines for Americans, 373, 373-374b
    drinking water, 397, 397b, 398b, 399f
    enteral. See Enteral nutrition
    factors that affect, 381-382
    feeding, 395, 396b, 397b
    fruits, 378
    grains, 377
    meats, 378
    milk, 378
    MyPyramid, 375-379, 376f, 377b
    oils, 378-379
    rehabilitation of, 687
    sleep affected by, 439

Nutrition (Continued)
    vegetables, 378
    wound healing, 561
Nutritional support
    cessation of, 412
    enteral nutrition. See Enteral nutrition
    intravenous therapy. See Intravenous therapy
    parenteral nutrition, 401, 407, 407f

O
Obesity, 603
Objective data, 74-75
OBRA. See Omnibus Budget Reconciliation Act
Observation, 74-75, 76b, 77b
Obsession, 642, 645
Obsessive-compulsive disorder, 645
Occult blood, 513, 514f
Occupational exposure, 203b
Occupational Safety and Health Association
    personal protective equipment, 204
    violence prevention program, 149
    work practice controls, 204
Occupational therapist, 6-7t
Occupational therapist assistant, 6-7t
Occupied bed
    definition of, 266
    illustration of, 266f
    making of, 274, 274b, 275-276b, 276f, 277f
Ocular prosthesis, 592, 592b, 592f
Odors, in resident unit, 253
Oil glands, 99
Oil-retention enema, 360, 365, 365b, 366b
Oils, 378-379
Old, 114-115
Older Americans Act, 17
Older person
    alcohol use in, 648
    children as caregivers of, 118
    circulatory system in, 119b, 121
    death of partner, 118
    depression in, 647
    digestive system in, 119b, 121-122
    housing options for, 122-126
    income reductions in, 117
    integumentary system in, 119b, 120
    musculo-skeletal system in, 119b, 120
    physical changes in, 118-122, 119b
    psychological changes, 117-118
    reproductive system in, 119b, 122
    respiratory system in, 119b, 121
    retirement, 117
    sexuality in, 130, 130f
    social changes, 117-118, 118b
    social relationships of, 117-118
    suicide in, 652
    urinary system in, 119b, 122
Old-old, 114-115
Oliguria, 333, 335t, 634-635
Ombudsman, 11, 17
Omnibus Budget Reconciliation Act, 21-22
    activity programs, 429
    comfort requirements, 432
    competency evaluation, 21-22, 47
    description of, 17
    developmental disability protections, 674
    dietary requirements, 382, 383f
    discharge requirements, 532
    food preparation requirements, 399
    minimum data set, 75, 77-79
    nursing center requirements, 17, 126
    passage of, 12
    purpose of, 21
    quality of life, 42b
    range-of-motion exercises, 419
    rehabilitation requirements, 689
    requirements, 22, 23b
    resident unit requirements, 263b
    training program, 21, 22f
    transfer requirements, 532
Open bed, 266, 266f, 274, 274b

Open fracture, 601, 610, 610f
Open wound, 536-537
Open-ended questions, 92
Ophthalmoscope, 496-497
Opioids, 649-651t
Opium, 649-651t
Optic nerve, 104
Optimal level of function, 82, 85
Oral hygiene, 282-288
    benefits of, 282
    brushing of teeth, 283, 284b, 284f
    definition of, 280
    dentures. *See* Denture
    flossing, 283, 284b, 286f
    safety considerations, 283, 287b
    in unconscious persons, 286-287, 286f, 287-288b,
        287b
Oral measurement, of body temperature, 475, 475t,
    477, 479f, 482f
Organs, 97, 99
Oropharyngeal airway, 458-459, 458f
Orthopnea, 442, 444
Orthopneic position, 442, 448
Orthostatic hypotension, 414, 415-416, 416b
Ossicles, 104
Osteoarthritis, 607, 607f
Osteomyelitis, 575
Osteoporosis, 610
Ostomy, 366-368
    colostomy, 355, 366, 367f
    definition of, 355
    ileostomy, 355, 366-367, 367f
Ostomy pouch, 367-368, 368b, 369b
Other potentially infectious materials, 203b
Otitis media, 579, 579b
Otoscope, 496-497
Output, 371, 388
Ovaries, 110
Overbed table, 253f, 259
Overflow incontinence, 333, 342
Ovulation, 110
Oxycodone, 649-651t
Oxygen concentration, 442, 446
Oxygen needs, 443
    factors that affect, 443
    promotion of, 448-450
        coughing, 448, 448b, 449b, 450f
        deep breathing, 448, 448b, 449b
        incentive spirometry, 450, 451b, 451f
        positioning for, 448, 448f
    respiratory function alterations, 444, 444f, 445b
Oxygen tank, 451, 451f
Oxygen therapy, 451-454
    administration set-up, 454, 454b, 454f, 455b
    devices used in, 452, 453f
    flow rates, 453, 453f
    quality of life issues, 456b
    safety concerns, 454, 455b
    sources for, 451, 451f, 452b, 452f
Oxytocin, 111

P
Pack, 536, 555, 556f
Padded tongue blade, 286, 286f
Pain, 432-436
    acute, 431, 433
    aging and, 434, 434b
    anxiety and, 433
    attention to, 433
    chronic, 431, 433
    communication about, 432b
    cultural influences, 434, 434b
    during death and dying, 713
    definition of, 431-432
    in dementia persons, 434b
    differences in, 432
    factors that affect, 433-434
    illness effects, 434
    intensity of, 434, 435f
    localizing of, 434, 435f

Pain (*Continued*)
    meaning of, 433
    nursing measures to relieve, 436, 436b
    oxygen needs affected by, 443
    past experiences with, 433
    persistent, 431, 433
    phantom, 431, 433, 615
    precipitating factors, 434
    pressure ulcer, 575
    radiating, 431, 433, 433f
    signs and symptoms of, 434, 435b
    support for, 433
    types of, 433
    words used to describe, 435b
Pain rating scales, 434, 435f
Palliative care, 709-710
Pancreas, 112
Panic, 642
Panic disorder, 644
Paralysis, 133, 135
Paranoia, 642, 645, 655, 663, 663b
Paraphrasing, 82, 92
Paraplegia, 133, 135, 601, 605, 606b, 606f
Parasympathetic nervous system, 104
Parathormone, 112
Parathyroid glands, 112
Parenteral, 203b, 205
Parenteral nutrition, 401, 407, 407f
Parkinson's disease, 604, 604f
Partial bath, 297, 297-298b, 298f
Partial denture, 288f
Partial seizure, 705
Partial-rebreather mask, 452, 453f
Partial-thickness burns, 707
Partial-thickness wound, 536-537
Passive range-of-motion exercises, 419
Patent, 457-458
Pathogens
    definition of, 182-183
    foodborne, 399
Patient Self-Determination Act, 714
PCP, 649-651t
Pediculosis, 311, 313
Pediculosis capitis, 311, 313
Pediculosis corporis, 311, 313
Pediculosis pubis, 311, 313
Penetrating wound, 536-537, 538f
Penis
    anatomy of, 109
    hygiene of, 308b, 309f
Penrose drain, 548, 550f
Percussion hammer, 496-497
Percutaneous endoscopic gastrostomy tube,
    401-402, 403f
Pericardium, 105
Pericare, 280, 305
Perineal care, 305
    comfort in, 306b
    definition of, 280, 305
    delegation of, 305b
    draping for, 306f
    female, 306f, 307-308b
    male, 308b, 309f
    safety in, 306b
Periodontal disease, 282
Peripheral nervous system, 102, 103-104, 103f
Peripherally inserted central catheters, 409
Peristalsis, 97, 108, 355-356
Peritoneal dialysis, 638, 638f
Persistent pain, 431, 433
Personal appearance, 45, 46b, 54
Personal belongings, 152-153, 153f
Personal care items, 259, 259f
Personal choice, resident's right to, 14, 717
Personal digital assistants, 71b
Personal matters, 55
Personal protective equipment, 204
    definition of, 203b
    description of, 189, 191-192, 192-193b
    donning of, 195, 196f

Personal protective equipment (*Continued*)
    face shields, 200f, 201, 201b
    gloves, 192-193b, 194b, 197, 197b, 197f, 198b, 198f
    goggles, 201, 201b
    masks, 199, 199f, 200b, 200f
    Occupational Safety and Health Association
        guidelines for, 204
    types of, 204
Personal safety, 151b
Personality disorders, 647
Phagocytes, 112, 112f
Phantom pain, 431, 433, 615
Pharmacist, 6-7t
Pharynx, 108
Phencyclidine, 649-651t
Phlebitis, 536, 540
Phobia, 642, 644
Phone communications, 70, 72b
Phosphorus, 380t
Photo identification systems, 136, 136f
Physical abuse, 41, 42b
Physical activity. *See* Activity
Physical examination
    assisting with, 500, 500b
    in dementia persons, 500b
    equipment used in, 497, 497f
    nursing assistant's role in, 497
    positioning for, 499, 499f
    preparing the person for, 497, 498b
    privacy during, 497
    quality of life considerations, 501b
Physical needs, 84
Physical restraint, 166-167, 170
Physical therapist, 6-7t
Physical therapy assistant, 6-7t
Physician's assistant, 6-7t
Picking up objects, 212f
Picture board, 90f
Pill organizers, 470, 470f
Pillowcases, 273f
Pituitary gland, 111
Pivot joint, 100, 100f
Planning, 74, 77-79
Plantar flexion, 414, 417, 419
Plantar warts, 545, 546f
Plaque, 280, 282, 618, 618f
Plasma, 105
Platelets, 105
Pleura, 107
Pleural effusion, 457, 462
PM care, 280, 282
Pneumonia, 623, 623b
Pneumothorax, 457, 462
Podiatrist, 6-7t
Poisoning, 137, 137b
Pollutant, 442-443
Polyuria, 333
Pons, 103
Portal of entry, 185, 190-191b
Posey quick-release tie, 174f
Positioning, 214-217, 214b
    bedrest, 417, 417f, 418f
    chair position, 217, 217f
    dorsal recumbent, 496, 499, 499f
    Fowler's position, 70b, 210, 215, 215f, 252, 256,
        256f
    horizontal recumbent, 496, 499
    knee-chest, 496, 499, 499f
    lateral, 210, 215, 216f
    lithotomy, 496, 499, 499f
    oxygenation promotion, 448, 448f
    physical examination, 499, 499f
    pressure ulcer prevention, 572, 573f
    prone, 215, 216f
    safety in, 215b
    Sims' position, 210, 215, 216f, 499, 499f
    supine position, 210, 215, 216f
Posterior, 67, 67f
Post-mortem care, 709, 715, 716b
Post-traumatic stress disorder, 645, 645b

Postural drainage, 515, 515f
Postural hypotension, 414, 415-416
Postural supports, 217, 217f
Posture, 210-211
Potassium, 374, 380t
Powders, 291t
Preceptor, 44
Preferred provider organizations, 9
Prefixes, 59, 67, 68b
Pre-hypertension, 617-618
Prejudice, 33
Presbyopia, 114, 121
Preschool, 116b
Pressure points, 565f, 703f
Pressure ulcers
    at-risk persons for, 567, 570, 571f
    Braden Scale for Predicting Pressure Sore Risk, 570, 571f
    causes of, 566, 566f
    charting of, 576f
    costs of, 570
    definition of, 70b, 564-565, 566
    dressing considerations, 575
    illustration of, 565f
    onset of, 566
    pain caused by, 575
    positioning to prevent, 572, 573f
    prevention of, 570-575, 571f, 572b, 573f, 574f, 575f
    quality of life considerations, 576b
    reporting and recording of, 575, 576b, 576f
    risk factors for, 566
    sites of, 570
    skin care for, 572
    stages of, 567, 567b, 568f, 569f
    treatment of, 570-575
    unstageable, 568f, 570f
Primary nursing, 2, 5
Primary-progressive multiple sclerosis, 604
Priority, 44, 55
Privacy
    assisted living residences, 467
    bowel elimination, 357
    emergency care, 707
    Health Insurance Portability and Accountability Act protection of, 37
    invasion of, 32, 36, 36b
    protection of, 13, 37f
    resident unit, 263
    resident's right to, 12-14, 15, 15-16b, 717
    sexuality-related, 130
    transfer of persons, 250
    urinary elimination, 353
    vital signs, 494
Privacy curtains, 259
Private insurance, 8
Problem solving, 72
Problem-focused conference, 62
Professional boundaries, 33-34, 34f, 35b
Professional sexual misconduct, 33-34
Professionalism, 44-45
Progesterone, 110, 112
Progress notes, 59, 61-62, 61f
Progressive-relapsing multiple sclerosis, 604
Projection, 644
Pronation, 414, 419
Prone position, 70b, 210, 215, 216f
Prospective payment systems, 9
Prostate gland, 109
Prosthesis
    definition of, 682, 684
    leg, 615, 615f
    ocular, 592, 592b, 592f
Protected health information, 33, 37, 70
Protein, 379
Protoplasm, 98
Protozoa, 183
Proximal, 67, 67f
Pseudodementia, 655, 657
Psilocybin, 649-651t
Psychiatric disorder, 642-643

Psychosis, 642, 645-646
Pubic lice, 639-640t
Pulmonary edema, 621
Pulmonary embolism, 541
Pulmonary function tests, 445, 446f
Pulse, 483-488
    apical, 483, 487, 487b, 487f
    apical-radial, 473, 488, 488b, 488f
    carotid, 697f
    definition of, 473, 483
    electrocardiographic recording of, 485f
    force of, 485
    radial, 483, 486, 486b, 486f
    ranges for, 484t
    rhythm of, 485
    taking of
        delegation of, 485b
        safety during, 485b
        sites for, 483, 483f
        stethoscope for, 473, 483, 483f, 484b, 484f
        techniques for, 486-487, 486b, 486f, 487b, 487f, 488, 488b, 488f
Pulse deficit, 473, 488
Pulse oximetry, 446, 446b, 446f, 447b
Pulse rate, 473, 484
Puncture wound, 536-537, 538f
Pupil, 104
Purulent drainage, 536, 548, 549f
Pyelonephritis, 635
Pyuria, 634-635

Q
Quadriplegia, 133, 135, 601, 606f, 677
Quality of life
    admission, 534b
    Alzheimer's disease, 671b
    bed, 279b
    bowel elimination, 370b
    dementia, 671b
    developmental disabilities, 681b
    grooming, 331b
    mental health problems, 653b
    nursing centers, 126b
    Omnibus Budget Reconciliation Act provisions, 42b
    oxygen therapy, 456b
    physical examination, 501b
    pressure ulcers, 576b
    rehabilitation, 689-690b
    reproductive disorders, 641
    resident's right to, 15, 15-16b
    respiratory support, 463b
    restraints, 180-181b
    urinary system disorders, 641
    wound, 562b
Questions, 92

R
Radial pulse, 483, 486, 486b, 486f
Radiating pain, 431, 433, 433f
Radiation therapy, 596
Radioactive, 445
Radiographer, 6-7t
Radioisotope, 445
Radiologic technologist, 6-7t
Random urine specimen, 503, 504b, 504f
Range of functions, 23-24
Range of motion, 414
Range-of-motion exercises, 419, 419b, 420b, 420f, 421-422b, 422f, 423f
Rape, 41
Rationalization, 644
Reaction formation, 644
Reagent strips
    for blood glucose testing, 518f, 519f
    for urine testing, 508, 509b, 509f
Receptive aphasia, 578, 583
Recording, 65-66
    definition of, 59, 62
    rules for, 65b
    time used in, 66, 66b, 66f

Recreational activities, 429
Rectal measurement, of body temperature, 475, 475t, 477, 479f
Rectum, 108
Red blood cell count, 443
Red blood cells, 105, 443
Reflex incontinence, 333, 342
Registered nurse, 5
    definition of, 2
    delegation by, 28
    education of, 5, 6-7t
    responsibilities of, 5
    in team nursing, 20
Regression, 644
Regulated waste, 203b
Regurgitation, 401, 405
Rehabilitation
    communication, 687, 687b
    definition of, 682-683
    economic aspects of, 687
    elimination, 684
    equipment for, 263
    health problems that require, 683b
    hygiene, 281b
    mobility, 684, 685f, 686f
    in nursing centers, 4
    nutrition, 687
    Omnibus Budget Reconciliation Act requirements, 689
    physical aspects of, 684-687
    programs for, 689
    psychological aspects of, 687, 687b
    purpose of, 3
    quality of life considerations, 689-690b
    self-care, 684
    self-help devices, 684, 685f
    services for, 689
    social aspects of, 687, 687b
    speech, 583b
    spinal cord injury, 606b
    vision loss, 589b
    whole-person approach to, 683-687
Rehabilitation team, 688, 688b
Reincarnation, 709, 711
Relapsing-remitting multiple sclerosis, 604
Relaxation, 431, 436
Religion, 84-85
    definition of, 82, 85
    dietary practices affected by, 381, 381b
REM sleep, 431, 438
Remove easily, 166-167
Repetitive behaviors, 664
Reporting, 64b
    definition of, 59, 62
    end-of-shift report, 64, 64b
    rules for, 65b
Repositioning of person, 250, 250f
Representative, 11-12
Repression, 644
Reproduction, 109
Reproductive disorders, 639, 639-640t, 640f, 641, 641b
Reproductive system, 109-111
    age-related changes in, 119b, 122
    female, 110, 110f, 119b, 122
    male, 109, 109f, 119b, 122
Reservoir, 182-183, 185, 190-191b
Resident(s)
    alert and oriented, 86
    assisted living residences, 466, 467b
    caring for, 83
    communication with, 88-91, 89-90f, 90f, 92-93
    complete care, 86
    confused, 86
    disability, 94
    disoriented, 86
    family and friends of, 94-95, 95f
    life-long, 86
    mentally ill, 87
    of board and care homes, 2

Resident(s) (Continued)
of nursing centers, 3, 86-87
short-term, 86
terminally ill, 87
Resident assessment protocols, 77-79
Resident care conferences, 62
Resident groups, 14
Resident handling
comfort in, 220b
communication in, 220b
lateral transfers, 221-222
manual lifting, 221
safety during, 220b
work-related injuries in, 221, 221-222b, 224b
Resident rights, 12-17
activities, 16, 16f
Alzheimer's disease residents, 671
assisted living residences, 466, 467b, 471b
care planning, 81
confidentiality, 12-14, 717
during death and dying, 717, 718b
dignity, 15, 15-16b
environment, 17
freedom from abuse, mistreatment, neglect, 15,
467, 717
grievances, 14
information, 12, 61, 467
personal choice, 14, 717
personal items, 14-15, 717
posting of, 12f, 13b
privacy, 15, 15-16b, 717
quality of life, 15, 15-16b
refusing treatment, 12, 567
restraint, freedom from, 15, 467, 717
work, 14
Resident unit
bathroom, 261, 262f
bed in. See Bed
bedside table, 259, 259f
call system, 260-261, 260f, 261b, 261f
Centers for Medicare & Medicaid Services
requirements, 263b
chairs, 259
closet space in, 262, 262b, 262f
comfort features, 253-254
definition of, 252-253
drawer space in, 262, 262b
equipment in, 254-257, 259, 260-261, 262
furniture in, 254-257, 259, 260-261, 262
illustration of, 253f
lighting in, 254
maintenance of, 263b
noise in, 254, 254b
odors in, 253
Omnibus Budget Reconciliation Act requirements, 263b
overbed table, 253f, 259
personal care items in, 259, 259f
privacy curtains, 259
privacy issues, 263
rules for, 262
temperature in, 253
ventilation in, 253
Residential hotels, 123
Residual urine, 344
Residue-restricted diet, 384-385t
Resource utilization groups, 9
Respect, 47
Respiration(s), 489. See also Breathing
abnormal, 444, 444f
assessment of, 76b
Biot's, 442, 444
Cheyne-Stokes, 442, 444
counting of, 489, 489b
definition of, 97, 107, 473
Kussmaul, 442, 444
Respiratory arrest, 442-443, 691, 694
Respiratory depression, 442-443

Respiratory disorders, 621-624
asthma, 622
chronic obstructive pulmonary disease, 621-622
emphysema, 622, 622f
influenza, 622, 623t
pneumonia, 623, 623t
tuberculosis, 623-624
Respiratory function alterations, 444
assessment of, 445-448
hypoxia, 442, 444, 444b
pulse oximetry evaluations, 446, 446b, 446f, 447b
respiration abnormalities, 444, 444f
signs and symptoms of, 445b
sputum specimens, 448
Respiratory hygiene, 192-193b
Respiratory protection, 199
Respiratory support
artificial airways. See Artificial airways
chest tubes, 462, 462f, 463b
mechanical ventilation, 457, 461, 461b, 461f, 687
quality of life issues, 463b
Respiratory system
age-related changes in, 119b, 121
anatomy of, 107, 107f
oxygen needs affected by, 443
Respiratory therapist, 6-7t
Respite care, 122
Responsibility, 19, 25
Rest, 431, 437
Restlessness, 663-664
Restorative aide, 682-683
Restorative care, 3
Restorative nursing care, 682-683
Restraint(s)
agitation caused by, 171, 172b
alternatives to, 168, 168b, 170f
applying of, 172-173b, 173f, 174f, 175f, 176-177,
177f, 178b, 179-180b
belt, 176, 177f
Centers for Medicare & Medicaid Services rules
for, 167
charting of, 169f, 176f
chemical, 166-167, 170
complications of, 170
confusion caused by, 171, 172b
delegation of, 178b
in dementia patients, 178b
doctor's order for, 170
falls caused by, 167
guidelines for, 171, 172-173b, 178b
history of, 167
informed consent for, 171
injuries caused by, 167b
jacket, 177, 178f
legal aspects of, 170-171, 171b
mitt, 176, 177f
physical, 166-167, 170
Posey quick-release tie, 174f
protection uses of, 170
quality of life issues, 180-181b
reporting and recording of, 176, 176f
resident's right to freedom from, 15, 467, 717
safe use of, 169-171, 172-173b, 176-177, 178b
strangulation caused by, 175f
vest, 173f, 177
wrist, 176, 177f
Restraint straps, 174f
Retina, 104
Retirement, 117
Reverse Trendelenburg's position, 252, 256, 257f
Rheumatoid arthritis, 607-608, 607f
Riboflavin, 379t
Rickettsiae, 183
Right lower quadrant, 67f
Right upper quadrant, 67f
Rights
delegation, 29, 30b
resident. See Resident rights
Rigor mortis, 709, 715
Risk management, 152-154, 152f, 153f, 154b

Roles and responsibilities, 23-25, 24b
Roll guard, 169f
Roman Catholic, 381
Root, 59, 67, 68b
Rotation, 414, 419

S
Safe Medical Device Act, 170
Safe setting, 134, 134b
Safety
accident risk factors, 135, 135b
admission, 522b
airway suctioning, 460b
Alzheimer's disease persons, 667, 668f, 669f
ambulation, 424b
assisted living, 466b
assisted living residences, 471
bathing, 293b
bed, 255b, 256-257, 257f, 258f
bedmaking, 269b
blood glucose testing, 518b
bowel elimination, 357b
brushing and combing of hair, 315b
building, 150b
burn prevention, 136, 137b, 137t
cardiopulmonary resuscitation, 694b
catheters, 345b
cold applications, 558b
discharge, 522b
elastic bandages, 543b
elastic stockings, 541b
electrical, 141, 141f, 142b, 142f
emergency care, 693b
end-of-shift report, 64b
enemas, 360b, 361b
fire. See Fire
glass thermometers, 476b
hand hygiene, 188b
hazardous substances. See Hazardous substances
heat applications, 558b
identification of person, 135-136, 135f, 136b
infection prevention, 141
intravenous flow rate, 410b
intravenous therapy, 411b, 411f
isolation precautions, 192
mechanical lift, 244
nail care, 322b
need for, 84
oral hygiene, 283, 287b
oxygen therapy, 454, 455b
paranoia, 663b
perineal care, 306b
personal, 151b
personal protective equipment, 195
poisoning prevention, 137, 137b
positioning the person, 215b
promotion of, 136b
pulse oximetry, 446b
pulse taking, 485b
range-of-motion exercises, 420, 420b
restraints, 171, 172-173b
shampooing of hair, 318b
shaving, 320b
showers, 301b
smoking, 137
sphygmomanometer, 491
sputum specimen collection, 515b
sterile procedures, 205b
stethoscope, 484
stool specimen collection, 511b
stretcher, 142, 143b, 143f
thermometers, 476b, 478b
transfer of persons, 238b
tub baths, 301b
tube feedings, 407b
24-hour urine specimen, 506b
urinary diversions, 636b
urine testing, 508, 509b
wheelchair, 142, 142f, 143b, 239

Safety *(Continued)*
  worker, 192-193b
  wound dressings, 552b
Safety belt, 175f
Safety razors, 319, 321b
Saline enema, 360-361
Salivary glands, 108
Sandwich generation, 669
Sanguineous drainage, 536, 548, 549f
Scabies, 313-314, 314f
Scales, 527, 528f, 530f
Schizophrenia, 645-646, 646b
School age, 116b
Sclera, 104
Scope of practice, 23
Scrotum, 109
Second degree burn, 136
Second intention wound healing, 546, 547f
Secondary-progressive multiple sclerosis, 604
Security needs, 84
Seizures, 691, 705-706, 706f
Self-actualization, 82, 84
Self-care, 684
Self-centered behavior, 87
Self-determination rights, 467
Self-directed medication management, 470
Self-esteem, 82, 84, 437
Self-help devices, 684, 685f
Self-neglect
  definition of, 33
  signs of, 38
Semen, 109
Semicircular canals, 104-105
Semi-Fowler's position, 70b, 252, 256, 256f, 713
Senior citizen housing, 123
Sense organs. *See* Ear(s); Eye(s)
Serosanguineous drainage, 536, 548, 549f
Serous drainage, 536, 548, 549f
Service plan, 464, 468-471, 469b
Seventh-Day Adventists, 381
Sex, 128-129
Sexual abuse, 39, 41, 42b
Sexual harassment, 56-57
Sexual needs, 130-131
Sexual relationships, 129
Sexuality
  in Alzheimer's disease persons, 664
  definition of, 128-129
  description of, 132
  intellectual disability persons, 676
  in older persons, 130
  promotion of, 130b
Sexually aggressive person, 131-132, 131b
Sexually transmitted diseases, 639, 639-640t, 640f, 641
Shampooing, 317, 317b, 317f, 318-319b, 318b
Shaving, 319-322, 319b, 320b, 320f, 321b
Shear, 564, 566
Shearing, 219, 225, 225f
Shingles, 599, 600f
Shock, 691, 704
Short bones, 100
Short-term residents, 86
Shoulder exercises, 420f
Showers, 299, 299b, 300f, 301-302b, 301b
Shroud, 717f
Sick care
  cultural influences on, 85b
  family roles in, 95b
Sick role, 85
Sigmoid colostomy, 367f
Sign language, 90f, 580, 581f
Signal light, 70b
Signs, 74-75
Silence, 93, 93b
Simple face mask, 452, 453f
Simple fracture, 601
Sims' position, 210, 215, 216f, 499, 499f
Sitting on the side of the bed, 236, 236b, 237b, 237f, 238f

Sitz baths, 555, 556f, 558
Skeletal muscle, 101
Skeletal traction, 613, 613f
Skilled nursing facilities, 2-3
Skin
  age-related changes in, 120
  anatomy of, 99
  assessment of, 76b
  breakdown of, 566b. *See also* Pressure ulcers
  cracked, 545, 546f
  disorders of, 599, 600f
  dry, 290, 291t, 545, 546f
  functions of, 99
  malignant tumor on, 595f
  nerve endings in, 99
  thermoregulatory functions of, 99
Skin appendages, 99
Skin care
  during death and dying, 713
  pressure ulcer prevention, 572
  products for, 291t
Skin conditions, 313-314
  alopecia, 313
  dandruff, 313
  hirsutism, 313
  lice. *See* Pediculosis
  scabies, 313-314, 314f
Skin puncture, 516, 517f
Skin tears, 536, 538-539, 538f, 539b
Skin traction, 613, 613f
Slander, 33, 36
Sleep
  in Alzheimer's disease persons, 668
  circadian rhythm, 431, 437
  definition of, 431, 437
  in dementia persons, 440b
  factors that affect, 439
  importance of, 45
  NREM, 431, 438
  in older persons, 120
  promotion of, 440, 440b
  REM, 431, 438
  requirements for, 438, 438t
  restorative effects of, 433
  routines for, 440
Sleep cycle, 438, 438b, 438f
Sleep deprivation, 440
Sleep disorders, 439-440, 439b
Sleepwalking, 440, 440b
Slide board, 223f
Slide sheet, 229f
Slings, 244
Slough, 564, 567
Small intestine, 108
Small-volume enema, 360, 364, 364-365b, 365f
Smell, 121
Smoker's cough, 622
Smoking
  cancer risks, 443, 596
  chronic obstructive pulmonary disease risks, 621
  effects of, 45
  odors caused by, 253
  safety measures for, 137
  stroke risks, 603
Smooth muscle, 101
Soap, 291t
Soapsuds enema, 360-361
Social abuse, 41
Social relationships, 117-118
Social worker, 6-7t
Sodium, 374, 380t
Sodium-controlled diet, 383, 384-385t, 385b
Source individual, 203b
Spastic, 673, 677
Specific immunity, 112
Specimen collection, 202
  blood glucose testing, 516-517, 517b, 517f, 518-519b, 518b, 519f
  reasons for, 503
  rules for, 503b

Specimen collection *(Continued)*
  sputum, 448, 515, 515b, 515f, 516b, 516f, 520
  stool. *See* Stool specimens
  urine. *See* Urine specimens
Speech
  description of, 54
  functions of, 583
  hearing loss effects on, 580
Speech disorders, 583-584
  aphasia, 583-584
  communication methods, 583b
  rehabilitation for, 583b
Speech-language pathologist, 6-7t
Sperm, 111
Sphygmomanometer, 473, 491, 491f
Spina bifida, 679, 679f, 680f
Spinal cord
  anatomy of, 103
  injury to, 605-606, 606b, 606f
Spinal nerves, 103
Splints, 417, 418f
Spores, 183, 189
Sputum
  definition of, 442, 502, 515
  specimen of, 448, 515, 515b, 515f, 516b, 516f, 520
Staff/staffing, 20
  assisted living residence, 468
  nursing center, 125b
  safety for, 150b
Standard of care
  definition of, 33, 36
  sources of, 36
Standard precautions, 192, 192-193b
Stand-assist lift, 223f
Stand-pivot transfers, 222
Stapes, 104
Stasis ulcers, 536, 539
State, working in another, 23
State laws, 20-25
Sterile, 183
Sterile cap, 348f
Sterile field, 183, 205
Sterile gloving, 207, 207b, 208f
Sterile procedures, 205b
Sterilization, 183, 186, 190, 190f, 676
Sterilize, 203b
Stethoscope, 473, 483, 483f, 484b, 484f
Stimulants, 649-651t
Stoma
  definition of, 355
  mouth-to-stoma breathing, 696, 697f
Stomach, 108
Stomatitis, 594, 597
Stool
  blood in, testing for, 513, 513b, 514b
  definition of, 355
  description of, 356
Stool specimens, 511-513
  collection of, 512b, 513f
  delegation of, 511b, 513b
  safety concerns, 511b
Straight catheter, 333, 344
Straining of urine, 510, 510b, 511f
Strangulation, 175f
Stress
  definition of, 44, 55, 642-643
  health effects of, 56
  management of, 55-56
Stress incontinence, 333, 342
Stressor, 44, 55, 642-643
Stretcher
  safety considerations, 142, 143b, 143f
  shampooing of hair on, 317, 317f
  transfer of persons to, 248, 248b, 249b, 249f
Striated muscle, 101
Stroke, 602-603, 602b, 602f, 603b, 705
Subacute care, 4
Subclavian vein, 409, 409f
Subcutaneous tissue, 99, 99f
Subjective data, 74-75

Substance abuse and addiction, 648-649
    alcohol abuse, 648
    alcoholism, 648
    description of, 41
    drug abuse and addiction, 648-649, 649-651t
Suction/suctioning, 457, 459-460, 460b, 460f
Sudden cardiac arrest, 620, 691, 693
Suffix, 59, 67, 68b
Suffocation
    choking, 138-139, 138f, 139-140b, 139f
    definition of, 133, 138
    prevention of, 138-139, 138b
Suicide, 642, 652-653, 652b, 653b
Suicide contagion, 643, 652
Sundowning, 655, 662, 667
Superior vena cava, 106-107, 106f, 409, 409f
Supervision, 29
Supination, 414, 419
Supine position, 70b, 210, 215, 216f
Suppository, 355, 359, 360f
Surgical asepsis, 183, 186, 205-207, 206b
Surgical bed, 266, 266f, 278, 278b, 278f
Surveillance, 29
Surveys, 9
Sustained maximal inspiration, 450
Swallowing, 382, 387f. See also Dysphagia
Sweat glands, 99
Swing-through gait, 427f
Swing-to gait, 427f
Sympathetic nervous system, 104
Symptoms, 74-75
Syncope, 414
Synkoptein, 415-416
Synovial fluid, 100
Synovial membrane, 100
Syphilis, 639-640t
System, 97
Systole, 106, 473, 490
Systolic pressure, 473, 490

T
T lymphocytes, 112
Tachycardia, 473, 484
Tachypnea, 442, 444
Tap water enema, 360-361
Tape, for wound dressings, 551, 551b, 551f
Tartar, 280, 282
Taste, 121
Team nursing, 5
    definition of, 2
    history of, 20
Teamwork, 53-55
Temperature
    body. See Body temperature
    hot and cold, 557t
Temperature-sensitive tape, for body temperature
    measurement, 482, 483f
Temporal artery measurement, of body tempera-
    ture, 475, 475t, 480, 480f, 482
Tendons, 102
Terminal illness, 87, 709-710
Testes, 109
Testosterone, 109, 112, 122
Tetany, 112
Tetraplegia, 601
Thank-you note, 52, 52f
Thermometers
    digital, 482
    disposable oral, 482, 482f
    electronic, 480, 480f, 481b, 482b
    glass, 476-477, 476b, 476f, 477f, 478-479b, 478b
    temperature-sensitive tape, 482, 483f
Thiamine, 379t
Third degree burn, 136, 137t
Third intention wound healing, 546, 547f
Thoracentesis, 445, 446f
Thrombocytes, 105
Thrombo-embolic hose. See Elastic stockings
Thrombus, 536, 541, 541f

Thumb exercises, 420f
Thyroid gland, 111
Thyroid hormone, 111
Thyroid-stimulating hormone, 111
Thyroxine, 111
Time, 66, 66b, 66f
Tinnitus, 578-579
Tissue
    connective, 98
    definition of, 97
    epithelial, 98
    muscle, 98
    nerve, 98
Toddlerhood, 116b
Toe exercises, 423f
Toilet, transfer of persons to and from, 246, 246b,
    247b, 248f
Tongs, 613f
Torts, 34-37
    defamation, 36
    definition of, 33-34
    intentional, 36-37
    negligence. See Negligence
    unintentional, 34-36
Total joint replacement surgery, 608, 608f, 609b, 609f
Total parenteral nutrition. See Parenteral nutrition
Touch, 91, 91b, 120-121, 131, 669f, 712
Towel baths, 297
Trachea, 107
Tracheostomy, 457-459, 458f, 459b
Traction, 613, 613b, 613f
Training
    job, 47
    Omnibus Budget Reconciliation Act require-
        ments, 21, 22f
Transfer, from assisted living residence, 467, 471
Transfer belt, 156, 162, 162f, 163b, 222, 239
Transfer board, 685f
Transfer of persons, 238-248, 532-533
    bed to chair or wheelchair, 239, 239b, 240-241b,
        241f, 242f
    chair or wheelchair to bed transfers, 242, 243b,
        685f, 686f
    comfort in, 238b
    definition of, 219, 521-522
    delegation of, 238b
    mechanical lift for, 244, 244b, 245b, 246f
    from nursing center, 532-533, 533b
    privacy protections in, 250
    safety in, 238b, 522b
    to stretcher, 248, 248b, 249b, 249f
    toilet, 246, 246b, 247b, 248f
    wheelchair, 239, 239b, 240-241b, 241f, 242, 242f,
        243b, 685f, 686f
Transgender, 128-129
Transient incontinence, 333, 342
Transient ischemic attack, 602
Transmission-based precautions, 192, 192b
Transparent adhesive film, 550
Transportation
    considerations for, 202
    to job, 52-53
Transsexual, 128-129
Transurethral resection of the prostate, 636
Transverse colostomy, 367f
Transvestite, 128-129
Trapeze, 418, 418f
Trauma, 536
Traumatic brain injury, 605
Treatment
    confidentiality, 12-14
    definition of, 11
    privacy, 12-14
    resident's right to refuse, 12, 567
Tremors, 604
Trendelenburg's position, 252, 256, 256f
Trichomoniasis, 639-640t
Tricuspid valve, 106, 106f
Triggers, 74
Trochanter rolls, 417, 417f

Trustworthiness, 47
Tryptophan, 439
Tub baths, 299, 299b, 300f, 301-302b, 301b
Tube feedings, 402, 403f, 405-406, 406b, 406f, 407b
Tuberculosis, 623-624
Tuberculosis respirators, 199, 199f
Tumor
    benign, 594-595, 595f
    definition of, 594-595
    malignant, 594-595, 595f
Tuning fork, 496-497
Turning pad, 229f
Turning persons, 233-235
    delegation of, 233b
    guidelines for, 233-234b
    logrolling, 219, 233, 235, 235b, 236f
    safety in, 233b
    technique for, 233-234b, 234f
24-hour urine specimen, 506, 506b, 507b
Two-point gait, 427f
Tympanic membrane
    anatomy of, 104
    body temperature measurements, 475, 475t, 480,
        480f, 482, 482f

U
Ulcer
    arterial, 535, 545, 545f
    definition of, 536-537
    diabetic foot, 535, 545, 545b
    pressure. See Pressure ulcers
    venous. See Venous ulcers
Unavoidable pressure ulcer, 564, 566
Unconscious persons
    mouth care for, 286-287, 286f, 287-288b, 287b
    oral hygiene in, 286-287, 286f, 287-288b, 287b
Underarm crutches, 426f
Underarm shaving, 322
Undressing, 325, 325b, 326b, 327f, 328f
Unintentional torts, 34-36
Unintentional wound, 536-537
Ureter, 109
Urethra, 109
Urge incontinence, 333, 342
Urinals, 338, 338b, 338f, 339b
Urinary diversions, 634, 636, 636b, 636f
Urinary elimination
    bedpans, 335, 335f, 336b, 336f, 337b, 338f
    bladder training, 353
    catheters for. See Catheter
    commodes, 340, 340b, 340f, 341b
    drainage systems, 347-348, 348b, 349b, 350b,
        350f
    privacy during, 353
Urinary frequency, 333, 335t
Urinary incontinence, 342
    definition of, 333, 342
    in dementia patients, 343b
    mixed, 342
    nursing measures for, 343b
    pressure ulcer risks, 567
    reflex, 333, 342
    stress, 333, 342
    transient, 333, 342
    types of, 335t, 342
Urinary system
    age-related changes in, 119b, 122
    anatomy of, 108-109, 108f, 109f
    disorders of, 635-638
        benign prostatic hyperplasia, 635-636, 635f
        cystitis, 635
        kidney failure, 637-638, 638b, 638f, 639b
        kidney stones, 637, 637f
        pyelonephritis, 635
        quality of life considerations, 641
        urinary diversions, 634, 636, 636b, 636f
        urinary tract infections. See Urinary tract
            infections
Urinary tract infections, 345, 635
Urinary urgency, 333, 335t

Urination, 333
  bedpans, 335, 335f, 336b, 336f, 337b, 338f
  commodes, 340, 340b, 340f, 341b
  normal, 334-340, 334b
Urine
  blood testing, 508
  color of, 335f
  flow of, 635f
  glucose testing of, 508
  observations of, 335
  pH testing of, 508
  residual, 344
  storage of, 109
  straining of, 510, 510b, 511f
  testing of, 508-510, 508b, 511f
Urine specimens, 503-510
  delegation of, 503b
  midstream, 505, 505-506b, 505b, 505f
  random, 503, 504b, 504f
  self-collection of, 520
  24-hour, 506, 506b, 507b
Urostomy, 634, 636
Utensils, 383f
Uterus, 110

V
Vaccination
  definition of, 183, 204
  hepatitis B, 204
Vaccine, 183, 204
Vagina, 110
Vaginal speculum, 496-497
Validation therapy, 670
Vancomycin-resistant Enterococcus, 184
Varicose veins, 540f
Vas deferens, 109
Vascular ulcers, 536, 539
Vegetables, 378
Veins, 97, 106-107, 106f
Venous ulcers, 539-543
  definition of, 536, 539
  elastic bandages for, 543, 543b, 544b, 544f
  elastic stockings for, 541, 541b, 542b, 542f
  pathophysiology of, 539
  prevention of, 540-543, 540b
  risk factors for, 540
Ventricles, of heart, 106, 106f
Ventricular fibrillation, 693, 698
Venturi mask, 452, 453f
Verbal abuse, 39, 41
Verbal communication, 82, 88-89, 89-90f, 90f
Vertigo, 578-579
Vest restraint, 173f, 177
Vietnamese Americans, 84
Viruses, 183
Vision impairments, 587-590, 587b
Vision loss
  braille for communication, 578, 589, 590f
  cataracts as cause of, 585, 585f
  description of, 135
  glaucoma as cause of, 584, 584f
  mobility issues, 590
  signs and symptoms of, 587b

Visually impaired persons
  communication with, 582
  environment considerations for, 582
  feeding of, 395
Vital signs, 70b
  blood pressure. See Blood pressure
  body temperature. See Body temperature
  definition of, 473
  in dementia persons, 474b
  measuring of, 474, 474b, 475b
  privacy rights, 494
  pulse. See Pulse
  reporting of, 474, 474b, 475b
  respirations, 489, 489b
  types of, 474
Vitamin(s), 379, 379t
Vitamin A, 379t
Vitamin B₁, 379t
Vitamin B₂, 379t
Vitamin B₃, 379t
Vitamin B₁₂, 379t
Vitamin C, 379t
Vitamin D, 379t
Vitamin E, 379t
Vitamin K, 379t
Vitreous humor, 104
Voiding, 70b, 333-334
Vomiting, 625-626
Vomitus, 625
Vulnerable adults, 38
  definition of, 33, 38
  dementia, 38b

W
Walker, 429, 429f
Walking aids, 426-429, 426f, 427f, 428f, 429f. See also
    Ambulation
Wandering, by Alzheimer's disease persons, 662,
    662f, 667
Warming blanket, 561
Waste
  biohazardous. See Biohazardous waste
  regulated, 205
Water, drinking, 397, 397b, 398b, 399f
Waterproof drawsheet, 265, 268
Weapons, 150b, 152f
Weight measurements, at admission, 527, 528b, 528f,
    529b, 530f
Wernicke's aphasia, 578, 583
Wet-to-dry dressings, 551
Wet-to-wet wound dressings, 551
Wheel locks, 162
Wheelchair
  repositioning in, 250, 250f
  safety for, 142, 142f, 143b, 239
  transfer of persons, 239, 239b, 240-241b, 241f, 242,
      242f, 685f, 686f
White blood cells, 105
Will, 33, 38
Withdrawal, 87, 649
Withdrawal syndrome, 643, 649
Wong-Baker FACES Pain Rating Scale, 435f
Word elements, 59, 67

Work
  attendance at, 53, 53b
  drug testing at, 57
  planning your, 55, 56b
  preparations for, 52-53
  resident's right to, 14
Work ethics
  definition of, 44-45
  qualities and traits associated with, 46, 47b
Work practice controls, 203b, 204
Workplace violence, 133, 149, 150b
Wound. See also specific wound
  appearance of, 548, 549b
  basic needs affected by, 561-562
  definition of, 536
  dehiscence of, 548, 549f
  drainage from, 548, 549f, 550f
  evisceration of, 535, 548, 549f
  intentional, 537
  measurement of, 549f
  quality of life considerations, 562b
  resident's reaction to, 562
  skin tears, 536, 538-539, 538f, 539b
  types of, 537, 537b, 537f, 538f
  unintentional, 537
Wound care
  binders, 554, 554f, 555b
  circulatory ulcers. See Circulatory ulcers
  delegation of, 552b
  infection risks, 536, 548, 561, 575
Wound dressings, 550-551
  application of, 551, 552b, 553b
  complications of, 575
  dry, 551
  functions of, 550
  gauze, 550
  pressure ulcer prevention, 575
  securing of, 551, 551b, 551f
  transparent adhesive film, 550
  types of, 550-551, 550f
  wet-to-dry, 551
  wet-to-wet, 551
Wound healing, 546-548
  cold applications for, 555-561, 557b, 557t, 558b,
      559-560b, 560f, 561f
  complications of, 548, 548b
  delayed, 561
  heat applications for, 555-561, 556f, 557b, 557t,
      558b, 559-560b
  nutrition for, 561
  phases of, 546
  types of, 546, 547f
Wrist exercises, 420f
Wrist restraints, 176, 177f

Y
Yankauer suction catheter, 459, 460f
Young adulthood, 116b
Young-old, 114-115